THIRD EDITION

FUNDAMENTALS OF SLEEP TECHNOLOGY

THIRD EDITION

FUNDAMENTALS OF SLEEP TECHNOLOGY

Cynthia D. Mattice, MS, RPSGT, RST
Sleep Center Manager
Oklahoma Heart Hospital
Oklahoma City, Oklahoma

Rita Brooks, MEd, R. EEG/EP T., RPSGT
Director of Diagnostic Services
Capital Health System
Trenton, New Jersey

Teofilo L. Lee-Chiong, MD
Professor of Medicine
National Jewish Health
Denver, Colorado
Professor of Medicine
University of Colorado Denver
Aurora, Colorado
Chief Medical Liaison
Philips SRC
Murrysville, Pennsylvania

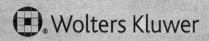

Philadelphia · Baltimore · New York · London
Buenos Aires · Hong Kong · Sydney · Tokyo

Acquisitions Editor: Chris Teja
Development Editor: Carole Wonsiewicz
Editorial Coordinator: Lauren Pecarich/Julie Kostelnik
Marketing Manager: Rachel Mante Leung
Production Project Manager: Marian Bellus
Design Coordinator: Holly McLaughlin
Artist/Illustrator: Holly R. Fischer
Manufacturing Coordinator: Beth Welsh
Prepress Vendor: S4Carlisle Publishing Services

Third edition

9 8 7

Printed in the United States of America

Library of Congress Cataloging-in-Publication Data

Names: Mattice, Cynthia, editor. | Brooks, Rita, editor. | Lee-Chiong,
    Teofilo L., 1960- editor. | American Association of Sleep Technologists,
    issuing body.
Title: Fundamentals of sleep technology / [edited by] Cynthia D. Mattice,
    Rita Brooks, Teofilo L. Lee-Chiong.
Description: Third edition. | Philadelphia: Wolters Kluwer Health, [2020] |
    Includes bibliographical references and index.
Identifiers: LCCN 2018059468 | ISBN 9781975111625 (pbk.)
Subjects: | MESH: Sleep Wake Disorders—diagnosis | Polysomnography—methods
    | Sleep—physiology
Classification: LCC RC547 | NLM WL 108 | DDC 616.8/498075—dc23
LC record available at https://lccn.loc.gov/2018059468

shop.lww.com

Preface

During the 8 years since the previous edition of *Fundamentals of Sleep Technology*, there have been not only remarkable advances in the science and profession of sleep technology—automation, portable testing, advanced positive airway pressure technologies, and telemedicine, to name a few, but also many vexing challenges. In many areas, sleep testing and treatments are still unavailable or unaffordable, adequate numbers of sleep health professionals lacking, and patients with sleep-related illnesses remain undiagnosed or untreated. Although opportunities for sleep technologists are expanding in education, research, industry, business, and government, many practitioners are increasingly anxious about their career longevity and professional advancement. In some countries, sleep technology has established curricula, certification, professional societies, and educational conferences; yet in others, none of these exist. Regardless of location around the globe, the sleep technologist has a profound responsibility to serve as an example of a healthy lifestyle, use health resources responsibly, reduce health inequalities, increase access to and support sustainable health programs, and promote cultural sensitivity in our health systems. Let us continue to work toward these positive changes.

Sleep technology needs to be reimagined—from sleep disorders to sleep wellness, one-size fits-all approach to patient-oriented choices, and fragmented to integrated treatment. It is during these crossroads of our journey that the best insights might come not from the skillful experience of years but from the unbiased clarity of youth; not from successful sleep centers, but from start-ups trying to compete by offering novel programs.

Last, with a global collaborative perspective, important lessons can be learned not only from nations with established sleep medicine systems but also from those working to address the needs of their vulnerable populations with limited resources. Let us change the conversation and start listening to their narratives.

This textbook is written by and for sleep technologists who are eyewitnesses and participants in this ongoing transformation. In this new edition, we have expanded and updated content to reflect the latest advancements in sleep technology and the broader responsibilities of the technologist, adding several key chapters on advanced technologies, new treatments for sleep disorders, sleep health and the technologist's role in education, and other new roles that sleep technologists are embracing. Additional topics on sleep center management are also available as part of your complementary expanded eBook (see the inside front cover for instructions). This textbook is a comprehensive, practical resource for educators, students, and practitioners of sleep technology, but should not be used as a static reference for this rapidly evolving discipline. The inter- and cross-disciplinary nature of medicine is nowhere more evident than in the sleep sciences. Let us continue our efforts to build communities of learning, collaboration, and dialogue and, in so doing, empower them to change our world.

It is time we imagined what the profession of sleep technology *could* be.

Cynthia D. Mattice
Rita Brooks
Teofilo L. Lee-Chiong

Acknowledgements and Dedication

The editors extend appreciation and thanks to all the authors who contributed chapters to this edition and the associate editors who dedicated significant time to review and edit many of the chapters, namely, Debbie Guerrero, Daniel Lane, Tripat Deep Singh, and Chad Whittlef.

We also thank Chris Teja, acquisitions editor at Wolters Kluwer and the AAST Board of Directors for their untiring assistance and counsel throughout the process.

Finally, this textbook would not have been possible without the support of the following individuals—it is to them that we dedicate this third edition of *Fundamentals of Sleep Technology*:

Keely Mattice, Lucy Gordon and Elly Gordon, Richard Brooks, Dolores Grace Zamudio, and Zoe Lee-Chiong.

Cynthia D. Mattice
Rita Brooks
Teofilo L. Lee-Chiong

Contributors

Fayçal Abdenbi, PhD
Clinical Manager
Philips Sleep & Respiratory Care
Goussainville, France

Sonya Abercrombie, BS, RPSGT
Sleep Technologist
St. Mary's Sleep Disorders Center
Enid, Oklahoma

Saad S. Ahmad, MD
Medical Director
Huron Medical Sleep Center
McLaren Thumb Region
Bad Axe, Michigan

Debbie Akers, RRT, RPSGT
Account Relations Manager
Medical Equipment Distributors
Virginia Beach, Virginia

Matthew W. Anastasi, BS, RST, RPSGT
Principal Sleep Consultant
Limina Sleep Consulting, LLC
Pittsburgh, Pennsylvania
Committee Member
American Association of Sleep Technologists
Chicago, Illinois

Joseph W. Anderson, RPSGT, CCSH, RPFT, CRT-NPS
Sleep Center Coordinator
SOVAH Sleep Center
Martinsville, Virginia

Jon W. Atkinson, BA, RPSGT, CCSH, FAAST
President
Ohio Sleep Consulting and Recording Services, LLC
Lancaster, Ohio

Matthew J. Balog, MPH, CCSH, RPSGT
Pediatric Clinical Sleep Educator
Department of Pediatric Sleep Medicine
Advocate Aurora Health
Park Ridge, Illinois
Adjunct Faculty
Health Sciences
Moraine Valley Community College
Palos Hills, Illinois

Richard B. Berry, MD
Professor of Medicine
Division of Pulmonary, Critical Care and Sleep Medicine
University of Florida
Medical Director
UF Health Sleep Center
Gainesville, Florida

Joyce M. Black, BS, CRT, RPSGT
Retired—Guest Faculty
School of Sleep Medicine
Palo Alto, California
Retired—Senior Clinical Sales Trainer
Philips Respironics
Murrysville, Pennsylvania

Lisa M. Bond, RST, RPSGT
Director
Clinical Services/Scoring
Advanced Sleep Management, LLC
Richardson, Texas

Allen Boone, AS, CCRA, CCRC, RPSGT, RST
Director, Clinical Research
Forefront Management, LLC
Principal CRA, Clinical Research
Louisville, Kentucky

Nicole Brecht, CRT
Rocky Mountain Medical Equipment
Loveland, Colorado

Lee J. Brooks, MD
Pediatric Pulmonology and Sleep Medicine
Children's Hospital of Philadelphia
Philadelphia, Pennsylvania

Rita Brooks, MEd, RPSGT, R. EEG/EP T.
Director of Diagnostic Services
Capital Health System
Trenton, New Jersey

Paul R. Carney, MD
Professor
Neurology and Pediatrics
University of North Carolina at Chapel Hill
Chapel Hill, North Carolina

David A. Davis, MD, (Retired)
Neurology and Sleep Medicine
Fayetteville, Arkansas

Reana Davis, RPSGT
Director of Sleep Disorders Center and Neurodiagnostic
    Center Opelika
East Alabama Medical Center
Opelika, AL

Julie DeWitte, RPSGT, RST, RCP
Assistant Department Administrator
Fontana Sleep Center
Kaiser Permanente
Fontana, California

Aleshia L. Dorst, RPSGT
Sleep Lab Supervisor
Department of Sleep
National Jewish Health Hospital
Denver, Colorado

Todd Eiken, RPSGT, FAAST
Vice President
Product Development
Dymedix Diagnostics
Shoreview, Minnesota

Lawrence J. Epstein, MD
Instructor
Department of Medicine
Harvard Medical School
Sleep Medicine Fellowship Program Director
Division of Sleep and Circadian Disorders
Brigham and Women's Hospital
Boston, Massachusetts

Carla A. Evans, BSc (Hons), PhD
Chief Senior Sleep Technologist
Adult Paediatric Sleep Service
Woolcock Institute of Medical Research
Sydney, Australia

Laree J. Fordyce, BTech, RPSGT, RST, CCSH
Director of Sleep Services
Maple Respiratory Group
Calgary, Alberta, Canada

Robin E. Foster, RPSGT
Sleep/Wake Healthcare Solutions
La Conner, Washington

Zack Freeman, RPGST, CCSH
Sleep Care Manager
Huron Medical Sleep Center
McLaren Thumb Region
Bad Axe, Michigan

Michael R. Furgason, RPSGT, RST, CCSH
Supervisor
Sleep Disorders Center
Martin Health System
Palm City, Florida

Sonia Garcia, RRT
Rocky Mountain Medical Equipment
Loveland, Colorado

James D. Geyer, MD, FAASM, FAES
Director of Sleep Medicine
Alabama Neurology and Sleep Medicine
Medical Director
Clinical Neurophysiology and Sleep Medicine
DCH Health System
Tuscaloosa, Alabama

Debra A. Guerrero, MS, RPSGT, CCSH, RRT
Sleep Technology Program Coordinator
    and Professor
Department of Health Sciences
Moraine Valley Community College
Palos Hills, Illinois

Kathryn Hansen, BS, CPC, CPMA, REEGT
Executive Director
Kentucky Sleep Society
Lexington, Kentucky

Susan Harpham, BS
Sleep Program Manager
Major Medical
Rocky Mountain Medical Equipment Company
Fort Collins, Colorado

Monica M. Henderson, RN, RPSGT
Sleep Education Coordinator
Sleep Medicine
Alabama Neurology and Sleep Medicine
Tuscaloosa, Alabama

Robert Hendrickson, RPSGT
Retired
Jacksonville, Florida

Mary Kay Hobby, RRT, RPSGT, CCSH, BAS
President
Sleep Health Management Resources, Inc
Stillman Valley, Illinois

Henry L. Johns, BS, RPSGT, CRT, CPFT
Sleep Lab Supervisor
VHA
Lawrence, Kansas

Danieliza Juniis-Johnson, MSE, LPN, RPSGT, RST
Sleep Technologist and Clinical Coordinator
Sleep Center
Sleep Services of America—MedBridge Healthcare
    Company
Valhalla, New York

Sharon A. Keenan, PhD, R. EEG. T, RPSGT, D-ABSM
Founder and Director
The School of Sleep Medicine
La Honda, California
Adjunct Lecturer
Department of Psychiatry and Behavioral Sciences
Division of Interdisciplinary Brain Sciences
Stanford University, School of Medicine
Stanford, California

Shawn Kimbro, RST, RPSGT
Sleep Program Manager
Department of Pulmonary, Critical Care, and
    Sleep Disorders
The George Washington University Medical
    Faculty Associates
Washington, District of Columbia

Amy Korn-Reavis, MBA, RRT, RPSGT, CCHS
Clinical Manager
Total Sleep Management
Orlando, Florida

Theresa A. Krupski, BS, RRT, RPSGT
Polysomnographic Technologist
Sleep Disorder Center
Rose Medical Center
Denver, Colorado

Eileen B. Leary, MS, RPSGT, RST
Senior Manager of Clinical Research
Center for Sleep Sciences and Medicine
Stanford University
Palo Alto, California

Teofilo L. Lee-Chiong, MD
Professor of Medicine
National Jewish Health
Denver, Colorado
Professor of Medicine
University of Colorado Denver
Aurora, Colorado
Chief Medical Liaison
Philips SRC
Murrysville, Pennsylvania

Laura S. Lehnert, RPSGT, RRT, BA
Sleep Technologist
Sleep Center
Kaiser Permanente
Bellevue Medical Center
Bellevue, Washington

Laura A. Linley, CRT, RPSGT
VP of Clinical Operations
Advanced Sleep Management, LLC
Fargo, North Dakota

Su Jeong Linstrom, BS, RPSGT
Clinical Program Coordinator
The Breathing Institute
Children's Hospital Colorado
Aurora, Colorado

Darius Loghmanee, RPSGT
Sleep Technologist
Sleep Center
Advocate Children's Hospital
Park Ridge, Illinois

Elise A. Maher, MA, RPSGT
Manager
Sleep and Neurodiagnostic Services
North Shore Medical Center
Salem, Massachusetts

Raman K. Malhotra, MD
Associate Professor
Department of Neurology, Sleep Medicine Center
Washington University in St. Louis School of Medicine
St. Louis, Missouri

Jayme R. Matchinski, JD
Greensfelder, Hemker & Gale, PC
Chicago, Illinois

Cynthia D. Mattice, MS, RPSGT, RST
Sleep Center Manager
Oklahoma Heart Hospital
Oklahoma City, Oklahoma

Lisa J. Meltzer, PhD
Associate Professor
Department of Pediatrics
National Jewish Health
Denver, Colorado

David Moore, RPSGT
Chief Polysomnographic Technologist
Sleep Center
University of Alabama at Birmingham
Birmingham, Alabama

Jennifer Parr-Christmas, CRT, RPSGT
Chief Sleep Technologist
Sleep Center
Northport Medical Center
Northport, Alabama

Regina Patrick, BA, RPSGT, RST
Medical Writer/Editor
Patrick Writing Service
Toledo, OH

Emmanuel (Joel) Porquez, BS, CCSH, RPSGT, RST
Clinical Manager of Sleep Lab
Sleep Medicine
Mercy Medical Center
Canton, Ohio

Janet Pruett, RRT
Clinical Director
Medical Equipment Distributors
Virginia Beach, VA

Susan Purdy, AA, RPSGT, RST
Sleep Tech II, Research Coordinator
Sleep Disorder Center
UF Health
Gainesville, Florida

Richard S. Rosenberg, PhD
Adjunct Faculty
Psychology and Human Development
California State University
Long Beach, California

Thomas Russell, RRT (Adv.)
Retired
Victoria, British Columbia Canada

Brian J. Schultz, RPSGT
Clinical Supervisor
Sleep Lab
Children's Hospital of Philadelphia
Philadelphia, Pennsylvania

Tamara Kaye Sellman, BA (Journ), RPSGT, CCSH
Principal and Curator
SleepyHeadCENTRAL.com
Bainbridge Island, Washington

Kristine Bresnehan Servidio, BBS, RCP, CRTT, RPSGT
Consulting Education Coordinator
Sleep Disorders and Pulmonary Labs
Complete Sleep Solutions
Murrieta, California

John Seymour, RRT
Retired
New Kensington, Pennsylvania

Katherine M. Sharkey, MD, PhD, FAASM
Assistant Professor of Medicine
Warren Alpert Medical School of Brown University
Physician
Rhode Island Hospital
Providence, Rhode Island

Stephen H. Sheldon, DO, FAAP
Professor of Pediatrics
Northwestern University Feinberg School of Medicine
Director, Sleep Medicine Center
Ann & Robert H. Lurie Children's Hospital of Chicago
Chicago, Illinois

Tripat Deep Singh, MBBS, MD, RPSGT, RST
International Sleep Specialist
World Sleep Federation Program
Clinical Manager, Sleep Medicine
Philips Respironics
Singapore, Singapore

Connstance Shivers Smith, BA, RPSGT
Polysomnographer
Shawnee Mission Health
Sleep Disorder Center
Shawnee Mission, Kansas

Patrick Sorenson, MA, RPSGT
Manager, Sleep Laboratory
Department of Sleep Medicine
Children's National Medical Center
Washington, District of Columbia
Polysomnography Program
Montgomery County Community College
Takoma Park, Maryland

Rui M. de Sousa, BSc, RPSGT, RST
Polysomnographic Technologist
Department of Neurophysiology
Sunnybrook Health Sciences Centre
Toronto, Ontario, Canada

Tim A. Statza, BA, CRT, RPSGT, RST
Director
Neurophysiology and Pulmonary Sleep
DCH Health System
Northport, Alabama

Stephen Tarnoczy, BS, RRT/SDS, RPSGT, CCSH
Sleep Technologist
Sleep Center
Oklahoma Heart Hospital
Oklahoma City, Oklahoma

S. Justin Thomas, PhD
Assistant Professor
Psychiatry and Behavioral Neurobiology
University of Alabama at Birmingham
Birmingham, Alabama

Cheryl Thomas-Yvanauskas, RRT RPSGT
Polysomnographic Technologist
Sleep Center
Advocate Sherman Hospital
Elgin, Illinois

Lauren Tribou, BS, RPSGT
Registered Sleep Technologist
Department of Sleep
National Jewish Health
Denver, Colorado

Melinda O. Trimble, RPSGT, RST, LCRP
Clinical Specialist
Philips Respironics
Springdale, Arkansas

Kimberly A. Trotter, MA, RPSGT
Administrative Director
Sleep Disorders Center
University of California, San Francisco
San Francisco, California

Robert N. Turner, MS, RPSGT, LPC
Clinical Supervisor
Rose Medical Center
Sleep Center
Denver, Colorado

Matthew Lee Uhles, MS, RPSGT, RST
Adjunct Instructor, Department of Sleep
St. Louis University
St. Louis, Missouri
Chief Operating Officer, Department of Sleep
Clayton Sleep Institute
Maplewood, Missouri

Carla Uy, BMedSc
Scientific Officer
Department of Sleep Medicine
The Children's Hospital at Westmead
Westmead, Australia

Edwin M. Valladares, MS, RPSGT
Manager
USC Sleep Disorder Center
Keck Hospital of USC
ACGME Lecturer
LAC+USC Sleep Medicine Fellowship
Keck School of Medicine of USC
University of Southern California
Los Angeles, California

Robert D. Vorona, MD
Associate Professor of Sleep Medicine
Eastern Virginia Medical School
Sleep Center
Norfolk, Virginia

Frank Walther, RPSGT, RST, BSChE
Consultant
Natus Medical Incorporated
Pleasanton, California

J. Catesby Ware, PhD, ABSM
Professor and Chief of Sleep Medicine
Eastern Virginia Medical School
Sleep Center
Norfolk, Virginia

Karen Waters, MBBS, FRACP, PhD
Conjoint Professor, Discipline of Child and Adolescent Health
The University of Sydney
Camperdown, Australia
Head, Sleep Medicine/Long Term Ventilation Unit
The Children's Hospital at Westmead, Sydney Children's
    Hospital Network
Westmead, Australia

Michael R. Watson, BS, CRT
Rocky Mountain Medical Equipment
Loveland, Colorado

Kristina Weaver, EMPT-P, RPSGT
Director of Care Navigation
Parrish Medical Center
Sleep Disorders Center
Titusville, Florida

Harry Whitmore, RPSGT
Clinical Sleep Coordinator
Sleep Disorders Center, Department of Pulmonary and
    Critical Care
University of Chicago Medicine
Chicago, Illinois

Chad Whittlef, BS, RPSGT
Sleep Technologist
Royal Papworth Hospital
Cambridge, England

Robyn V. Woidtke, MSN, RN, RPSGT, CCSH
Principal
RVW Clinical and Sleep Consulting
Castro Valley, California

David F. Wolfe, MSEd, RRT-SDS, RST, RPSGT
Adjunct Assistant Professor
Respiratory Therapy Education
State University of New York Upstate
    Medical University
Educational Coordinator
Educational and Professional Development
Crouse Health
Syracuse, New York

Carol Wood, RSCN, BSc (Hons)
Specialist
Nursing Practice (Paediatrics)
Clinical Nurse Consultant
Department of Sleep Medicine
The Children's Hospital at Westmead
Westmead, Australia

Rochelle Zozula, PhD, D-ABSM
Clinical Associate Professor
Department of Neuroscience
Seton Hall University, School of Health and
    Medical Sciences
South Orange, New Jersey

Associate Editors

Debra A. Guerrero, MS, RPSGT, CCSH, RRT
Sleep Technology Program Coordinator and Professor
Department of Health Sciences
Moraine Valley Community College
Palos Hills, Illinois

Daniel D. Lane, BS, RPSGT, CCSH
Senior Sleep Technologist
Apnea Solutions
Yorba Linda, California

Tripat Deep Singh, MBBS, MD, RPSGT, RST
International Sleep Specialist
World Sleep Federation Program
Clinical Manager, Sleep Medicine
Philips Respironics
Singapore, Singapore

Chad Whittlef, BS, RPSGT
Sleep Technologist
Royal Papworth Hospital
Cambridge, England

Contents

SECTION X Appendix 877

Appendices and Glossary are available online as a supplement.

SECTION 1
Overview of Sleep Medicine

chapter 1

Sleep Technology: Past, Present, and Future

JON W. ATKINSON

LEARNING OBJECTIVES

On completion of this chapter, the reader should be able to:

1. Outline an overview of the key people involved in the development of sleep medicine and technology.
2. Describe some of the hallmark publications related to sleep medicine and technology.
3. Describe the technologic advances in recording and treating sleep disorders.
4. Describe the history of the sleep technology professional organizations (American Association of Sleep Technologists [AAST] and Board of Registered Polysomnographic Technologists [BRPT]).
5. Outline an overview of legislative and licensure status.
6. Define the evolving role of the sleep technologist.

KEY TERMS

Analog (paper) polysomnography
Association of Polysomnographic Technologists (APT)
American Association of Sleep Technologists (AAST)
Board of Registered Polysomnographic Technologists (BRPT)
Continuous positive airway pressure (CPAP)
Digital polysomnography
Hallmark publications
Technologic advances

HISTORY

The seed of polysomnographic technology was sown during the late 1920s and 1930s with research studies in physiology and psychology/psychiatry. William Dement's chronicle of the history of sleep physiology and medicine provides an insight from the perspective of one of the pioneers of sleep medicine (1). Since the first recording of the electroencephalogram (EEG) in

humans by Hans Berger (2) in the late 1920s, the following five decades provided the substrate upon which the current level of sleep medicine and polysomnographic technology was built. Much of the information came out of efforts to determine the state of sleep in which dreaming was most likely to occur (3–6). It was not until the 1950s when papers by Eugene Aserinsky and Nathaniel Kleitman (7, 8) describing the electrographic characteristics of rapid eye movement (REM) sleep and the association of REM sleep and dream report, as well as the work by Dement and Kleitman (9) describing the cyclic variation of sleep depth in normal subjects, that the science of sleep technology began to be established.

One of the events that shaped the evolution of sleep medicine and technology was the development of a standardized manual for terminology and scoring by Alan Rechtschaffen and Anthony Kales in 1968 (10). This hallmark publication, likely the most quoted and referenced source in sleep medicine, provided a nomenclature, technical methodology recommendations, and sleep scoring method needed to provide a common reference point for future development of the science. This reference has been replaced by a comprehensive guide for scoring sleep stages and related events initially published in 2007 by the American Academy of Sleep Medicine (AASM) (11). This manual also outlines technical specifications for performance of polysomnography. AASM sleep center accreditation standards require that accredited sleep facilities follow these standards (12). This manual has undergone multiple revisions and modifications since the original publication. The current version, 4.5, was published in 2018 (13). It is expected that the manual will continue to undergo annual updates.

In the early to mid-1960s, the electrographic description of sleep-onset REM periods was established (14–16), interest in sleep problems from a clinical perspective developed in Europe (17), and the discovery of sleep apnea (18, 19) entrenched sleep as a clinical, medical entity. In 1974, the term "polysomnography" was coined by Jerome Holland at Stanford University following the routine employment of multiple physiologic parameters, adding respiratory and cardiac sensors to the routine EEG, electrooculography, and chin electromyography sensors to sleep studies. The addition of these derivations was instituted following the arrival of Christian Guilleminault at Stanford, based on his experience with sleep apnea in Europe (1, 20).

The body of knowledge of sleep disorders and sleep medicine advanced, and several key resources were published, including the Peter Hauri and William C. Orr's classic monograph, *The Sleep Disorders* (21); the Guilleminault-edited *Sleeping and Waking Disorders: Indications and Techniques* (22); the first edition of *Principles and Practice of Sleep Medicine* (23), edited by Meir Kryger, Thomas Roth, and William Dement; and the *Atlas of Clinical Polysomnography* (24) by Nic Butkov.

TECHNOLOGIC ADVANCES

The development of sleep science, sleep medicine, and sleep technology has been codependent on advances in both recording and treatment technology.

It is fascinating to read some of the early information on methodology for recording sleep studies. These recordings were performed on analog equipment, using paper and ink EEG machines with direct current capabilities and limited channel availability. Because of the limitations in the number of recording channels, montages had to be well devised to provide adequate information for proper diagnosis, often sacrificing a recording derivation for one that may be more important, based on the presentation of a particular patient. Recording devices with 8, 10, or 12 channels were commonplace; 16, 18, or 21 channels were a luxury. Sleep technologists had to possess a good understanding of amplifiers and filters as well as expected frequency ranges of the physiologic parameters recorded. Improper use of filters or sensitivity controls could make stage N3 sleep look like wakefulness or make normal breathing appear to be apnea . . . and there was no return. Once on paper, it was there for good. Sleep technologists had to unclog polygraph pens, change broken galvanometers, fill inkwells, and carefully align and tape together boxes of folded paper to ensure that a single overnight recording was properly acquired. It was extremely awkward to go back and review previous portions of the recording. Scoring was performed manually and data tabulation was done with pencil and paper, sometimes with the assistance of a calculator. It often took longer to generate the requisite sleep report statistics than to identify sleep stages and abnormal events. The recording technologist could hear the sound of sleep spindles, REM sleep, slow-wave sleep, arousals, cardiac dysrhythmias, and periodic limb movements. Each had its own distinct sound generated by the scratching of the pens on the moving paper chart. This was actually quite helpful because it drew the attention of the attending technologist to a particular patient, when concentration may have been focused elsewhere.

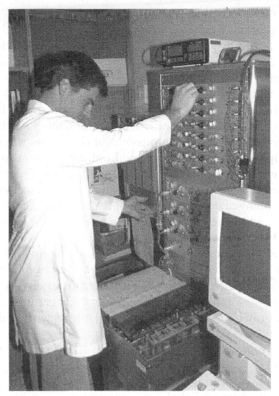

Figure 1-1 Grass Model 78 polygraph for analog (paper) polysomnography.

The polygraphs were massive, veritable monoliths, with approximate dimensions of 5 to 6 ft height, 4 ft width, and 2.5 to 3 ft depth, each weighing several hundred pounds (see Fig. 1-1). Storage and archival of recorded data was an enormous and expensive problem. The cost of the paper alone for four recordings was over $200 and required about 2.3 ft^3 of storage space for a minimum of 7 years (see Fig. 1-2). This is not to say that these behemoths were not wonderful, highly reliable workhorses. They seldom failed in such a way that a recording needed to be rescheduled. Fairly simple

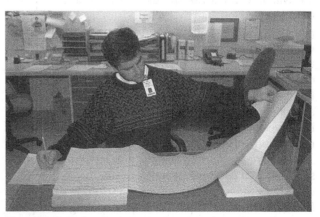

Figure 1-2 Technologist reviewing a single-night analog (paper) recording.

pen or galvanometer replacement, or occasional swapping of an amplifier board "on the fly," that is, while the recording was still being performed, put you back in business. There are times when many of "the old guard" sleep technologists long for the days of analog recorders with stable amplifiers and filters, in place of nebulous software glitches and corruptions, or the whims and fancies of computer hardware, networks, and interfaces that can put one out of commission for days. Days when a couple of more beds added did not mean several days or weeks of troubleshooting, as often seen today, even when using the same brand of equipment and software.

Many of the sensors for peripheral devices were constructed in the laboratory. Snore sensors, flow sensors, and mercury strain gauges were often homemade, and chasing down spilled mercury balls with a syringe or pipette was a challenge. Burns and blisters from dropped or mishandled soldering irons were painful. Ear oximeters were bulky and cumbersome, even painful, and performed poorly or not at all on patients with highly pigmented skin.

Huge technologic strides have been made in the past 25 to 30 years. In the late 1980s and early 1990s, computer technology had advanced sufficiently for the introduction of digital polysomnography. As with any new technology, digital recordings were not without problems. Hard drive capacities were insufficient to run the acquisition program and store the raw data. Thirty to 50 MB hard drives were the standard. Raw data had to be stored on optical media at a cost of about $100 per optical disk. Processor speeds were slow (<100 MHz per second), and frequent computer crashes because of data overload were a common occurrence. Waveform definition on the computer screen was mediocre at best. Automated sleep staging and scoring algorithms were very inaccurate. However, by the late 1990s, computer technology had advanced far enough to make digital polysomnography the rule rather than the exception. With current technology, massive terabyte hard drives are available, processor speeds have increased to several GHz per second, archival media storage is very inexpensive (<$1 per patient), and several years of recording data can be stored in the space required for one or two nights of paper studies. Resolution of the monitors can produce paper-like, crisp-appearing records (see Fig. 1-3). Although automated sleep staging is still not accurate, computer recognition of abnormal events has improved dramatically but still requires technologists' review and editing.

Despite all these advances, the technologist must still possess a good working understanding of the basics of polysomnographic technology, including amplifiers, filters, sensitivities, expected frequency ranges of physiologic parameters, and troubleshooting. In addition, the technologist must understand the Nyquist theorem,

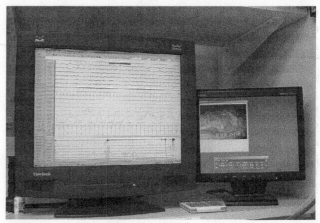

Figure 1-3 Contemporary workstation with dual high-resolution monitors.

sampling rates, signal resolution, hardware versus software filters, common referencing, basic networking, and data file management. Indeed, there are more potential recording and troubleshooting issues now than ever before.

There are currently more than 20 manufacturers and suppliers of digital polysomnography systems. Today's recording technologist has high-quality snore sensors, pressure transducers, thermocouples and thermistors, respiratory effort sensors, and so on, available from multiple commercial companies. There are also multiple vendors supplying a variety of preparation materials and supplies needed for polysomnographic recordings. Pulse oximetry devices placed on the finger have replaced the ear oximeter.

In the past, patients with obstructive sleep apnea that could not be ameliorated significantly by weight loss, by maintaining a side sleeping position, or by changing bed elevation were often subjected to a tracheotomy. It was not uncommon, even in a modest-sized laboratory, to encounter one or two such cases per week. This provided the impetus for the massive growth in sleep medicine and technology, such as the demonstration of treating obstructive sleep apnea through nasal continuous positive airway pressure (CPAP) by Colin Sullivan and colleagues in 1981 (25). An effective, nonsurgical treatment for a debilitating, potentially life-threatening disorder had been discovered.

In the early years, CPAP masks were individually molded to the patient, and adhesive was used to apply the mask. The flow generators were noisy and cumbersome, weighing close to 16 lb (7.25 kg). Early commercial CPAP devices became available in the mid-1980s (Fig. 1-4). Competition among manufacturers continues to lead to increasingly smaller and less noisy flow generators and more comfortable interfaces. Some of the newer flow generators are less than a tenth the size and weight of the early models and are very quiet during operation.

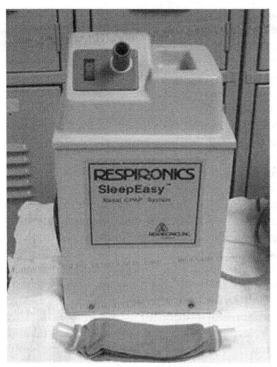

Figure 1-4 Respironics SleepEasy, circa 1985.

Advances in positive airway pressure device technology led to the availability of flow generators that can provide pressure reduction on exhalation (C-Flex and C-Flex+, EPR), auto-adjusting CPAP, and BiLevel positive airway pressure devices, which are in common usage. Other advances include auto servo ventilation and respiratory assist devices such as average volume assured pressure support (AVAPS) produced by several manufacturers.

ASSOCIATION OF POLYSOMNOGRAPHIC TECHNOLOGISTS/AMERICAN ASSOCIATION OF SLEEP TECHNOLOGISTS

The Association of Polysomnographic Technologists (APT) was formed in 1978, spurred by the vision of Peter McGregor, the organization's first president and the first registered polysomnographic technologist (RPSGT).

The early years were those of a closely knit group of individuals gathering for the purpose of promoting the field, sharing ideas about a burgeoning technology, and administering the registration examination. To encompass the expansion of the sleep technologist's role in the growing field of sleep medicine, in 2007, the APT changed its name as the American Association of Sleep Technologists (AAST). The following individuals served as presidents of the APT/AAST: Peter McGregor, 1978

to 1983; Sharon Keenan, 1983 to 1991; Cameron Harris, 1991 to 1993; Todd Eiken, 1993 to 1996; Pamela Minkley, 1996 to 1998; Robert Turner, 1998 to 2000; Kelly Million, 2000 to 2002; Rose Ann Zumstein, 2002 to 2005; Cynthia Mattice, 2005 to 2007; Jon Atkinson, 2007 to 2009; Cindy Kistner, 2009 to 2011; Melinda Trimble, 2011 to 2013; Rita Brooks, 2013 to 2015 and 2017 to 2019; and Laura Linley, 2015 to 2017.

Working through the years, the APT leadership successfully advanced the profession, culminating in April 2003 when the profession of polysomnographic technology was recognized by the Commission on Accreditation of Allied Health Education Programs (CAAHEP) and the Committee on Accreditation for Polysomnographic Technologist Education (CoA PSG) was formed. The CoA PSG is currently sponsored by two organizations: the AAST and the Board of Registered Polysomnographic Technologists (BRPT). The CoA PSG established standards and guidelines for the accreditation of educational programs in sleep technology and recommended the first community college educational programs in polysomnographic technology to CAAHEP for accreditation in 2006.

Within the last few years, the AAST has experienced tremendous growth, leading to the development of numerous educational programs and continuing education credits for members of the association and those credentialed in sleep technology. The AAST offers comprehensive review courses to technicians preparing for certification examinations, scientific sessions, courses, and workshops at its annual meetings; position papers; career opportunities listed on the association's website; and other valuable resources. The association's goal is to prepare individuals for a rewarding career in the field of sleep technology and to enhance their skills and knowledge as the profession continues to expand. The AAST continues to engage new initiatives that promote sleep technology as a separate and distinct profession and that direct the advancement of the profession by increasing recognition in many venues including the medical community, educational institutions, and the public. New technologies are continually being developed that provide state-of-the-art methods that are used in the evaluation and diagnosis of sleep disorders. The future is certainly difficult to predict, but given the recent developments on multiple fronts, the field will provide sleep technologists with opportunities for continued career growth and development for years to come.

BRPT, THE RPSGT, AND OTHER CREDENTIALS

Initially a standing committee of the APT, the BRPT is an independent nonprofit corporation established in the year 2000. Although a standing committee of the APT, chairpersons included Moshe Reitman, Cynthia Mattice, David Franklin, Jan McAninch, Robin Foster, Andrea Patterson, Gregory Landholt, Gary Hansen, Dan Herold, Bonnie Robertson, and Cameron Harris. The following people have served as president of the BRPT board of directors: Cameron Harris, Marietta Bellamy-Bibbs, Mark DiPhillipo, Bonnie Robertson, Becky Appenzeller, Janice East, Cindy Altman, Theresa Krupski, Daniel Lane, and Jessica Schmidt.

The early examinations consisted of four stations, each 2 hours in duration, which were modeled after the EEG credentialing examinations of the period. The stations were as follows: written examination, scoring, record review with a physician or PhD, and practical examination adjudicated by a technologist. Beginning in 1990, a professional examination company, Applied Measurement Professionals, was hired to professionally construct and administer the examination. It was during this period that the examination changed to a two-part written and third part practical construct. Around 1996, the test transitioned to a single-hurdle written examination with no practical portion. Several factors led to the elimination of the practical portion of the examination, which are as follows:

1. The increasing use of digital polysomnographs and the infeasibility of providing the same or similar equipment at examination sites;
2. The volume of candidates waiting to take the practical portion of the examination;
3. The expense of travel and housing for the examiners and site supervisors; and
4. The potential liability for injury to subject volunteers during the examination process.

The following is paraphrased from former BRPT President Mark DiPhillipo's "President's Perspective" column in 2004 and provides some insight into the very first BRPT examination (26, 27):

> The initially certified individuals were Peter Mc-Gregor, Sharon Keenan, Norman Shubert, Jane Skinner, Moshe Reitman, Gerald McCoy, and Deborah Starr. Moshe Reitman was appointed as the first chairperson. Examiners for this first examination administration included doctors Helmut Schmidt, Merrill Mitler, Peter Hauri, and William Orr; technologists Linda Fortin, Deborah Starr, Jane Skinner, Cleo Hanlon; and graduate student Mark Pressman. A technologist was paired with a polysomnographer for an intimidating two-on-one examination experience.

The first administration of the RPSGT examination involved both practical and written components. During the practical phase, the Grass polygraph was purposely sabotaged to test the applicant's ability to troubleshoot the recording. There was also a record review session with the clinical polysomnographer and an oral review with an examining technologist. The examination also included equipment review and a brief written test. Certainly, by today's standards, this would not constitute a valid, reliable examination format. Nevertheless, passing was no small task.

This labor-intensive examination format continued for many years with sections being added and formalized over the years. Each subsequent board of directors contributed to the improved reliability and validity while meeting the growing demand for the examination. Owing to the growing interest in the RPSGT credential, candidates had to wait increasingly longer to get tested, and examiners found themselves picking up frequent flyer miles while losing touch with their families to meet the demand. To resolve this problem, the examination was streamlined by instituting a process whereby candidates had to pass the written and scoring sections before taking the practical portion of the examination. This helped for several years, but the forces of demand and modern test theory necessitated the creation of a more valid and reliable measurement tool.

The massive growth in the number of certified individuals can be seen in Figure 1-5. As of June 2011, there were nearly 17,000 technologists registered by the BRPT. Current statistics reveal that there have been 24,220 RPSGT credentials issued (28).

Over the years, there has been a gradual evolution of the examination process from the original four-component (written, scoring, recorded review, and practical) examination lasting 8 hours to the current 4-hour, 200-question single-hurdle examination. Since June 2010, the examination has been available "on demand" instead of only during discrete 2-week periods. In addition, the candidate receives immediate notification of the examination results. Previously, it was customary to receive the examination results in 6 to 8 weeks. As of

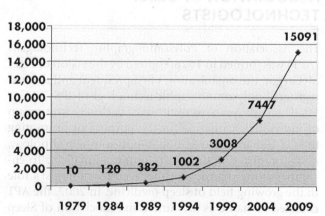

Figure 1-5 Growth of Board of Registered Polysomnographic Technologists membership, 1979 to 2009.

September 2017, the RPSGT examination is 3 hours and has 175 questions instead of the previous 4 hours and 200 questions (28). Since the first edition of this book, several other credentials have been introduced for sleep technologists. In late 2009, the BRPT developed a new certificate for sleep technicians, the certified polysomnographic technician (CPSGT). The purpose was to provide an early, entry-level time-limited credential for persons new to the sleep technology field. Over 1,500 technicians have been certified since the first examination in early 2010 (28).

In December 2008, the National Board of Respiratory Care (NBRC) introduced the sleep disorders specialist (SDS) credential for registered respiratory therapists (RRT) and certified respiratory therapists (CRT). As of the date of this writing (March 2018), 687 RRTs or CRTs have been credentialed by the NBRC (29).

Early in 2011, the American Board of Sleep Medicine (ABSM) announced its intent to provide another pathway for sleep technologist credentialing; the initial examination was in November 2011. The current number of registered sleep technologist (RST) credential holders listed on the ABSM website as of March 2018 is 6,907; however, many of these credential holders were issued the RST credential based on their current holding of the RPSGT credential.

The ABSM developed the examination to cover the educational components of standardized sleep education programs and the day-to-day responsibilities of the sleep technologist in a clinical setting. It is specifically designed to be reflective of the education and training pathways currently available for the sleep technology profession. The ABSM sleep technologist examination requires candidates to have completed either a CAAHEP-accredited educational program in sleep technology or the full ASTEP program. Successful candidates will earn the RST credential. At this time, the ABSM's RST credential is not National Commission on Certifying Agencies (NCCA) accredited nor is ABSM seeking NCCA accreditation (30).

In 2014 and 2015, the BRPT developed a new, advanced credential, the Certificate in Clinical Sleep Health (CCSH). The CCSH examination is an advanced-level examination for health care providers and educators who work directly with sleep medicine patients, families, and practitioners to coordinate and manage patient care, improve outcomes, educate patients and the community, and advocate for the importance of good sleep. Since the first examinations in late 2014 and early 2015, 962 CCSH credentials have been issued (28).

Legislation/Licensure

Since the late 1990s, the sleep technology profession has seen challenges in the regulation of scope of practice in many states. Threats to the ability of the sleep technologists to practice their profession were real and largely related to overlapping scopes of practice between the respiratory care and sleep technology professions. Sleep technologists must be responsible for monitoring potential legislative activity in their individual states and, where possible, be proactive rather than reactive to the environment.

There are basically five different categories under which sleep technology is regulated (31).

The first category is *Licensure*. Licensure provides sleep technologists a specific education, training, and examination pathway to obtain licensure/certification. As of April 2018, 13 states and the District of Columbia required licensure: California, Delaware, Idaho, Louisiana, Maryland, New Jersey, New Mexico, North Carolina, North Dakota, Oregon, Tennessee, Virginia, New York, and Washington, DC.

The second category is *Exemption*. General exemption language allows sleep technologists to work within their scope of practice while under the direction of a licensed physician. Twenty-nine states contain general exemption language in their respective Respiratory Care Acts (state names abbreviated): AL, AZ, AR, CO, GA, HI, IL, IN, IA, KS, ME, MA, MI, MN, MS, MO, NE, NV, OH, OK, PA, SC, SD, TX, UT, VT, WA, WV, and WY.

The third category consists of *Respiratory Care Acts that specifically define the education and training for sleep technologists*. Currently, New Hampshire is the only state that specifically defines sleep technology and its scope of practice in the state's respective Respiratory Care Acts.

The fourth category consists of *Respiratory Care Practice Acts that do not address sleep technology*. This includes six states that have a Respiratory Practice Care Act that does not address the practice of sleep technology. These states include CT, FL, KY, MT, RI, and WI.

Finally, one state, Alaska, has *no Polysomnography or Respiratory Care Practice Act*.

FUTURE AND EVOLVING ROLES OF SLEEP TECHNOLOGISTS

The tide of sleep medicine and technology and, for that matter, medicine in general is in a constant state of flux; the future is certainly difficult to predict. Given the past and recent developments on multiple fronts, the following will likely occur.

A formal educational requirement for sleep technologists sitting for credentialing examinations may become mandatory in the next 5 to 10 years. As of January 2009, the AASM has mandated 80 hours of didactic education before becoming a trainee, with additional successful completion of competency tests in various educational modules required during the training period, or enrollment in a CAAHEP-accredited program with a sleep component for personnel in accredited sleep centers (12). With the establishment of accreditation of educational programs, it becomes a matter of sufficient availability of these programs for the credentialing body to mandate formal education.

Technology will continue to improve. Industry is in constant search of the "ultimate" PAP interface, with smaller and quieter flow generators and more potential "bells and whistles" to establish a better control of the marketplace. Computer equipment will improve with higher quality amplifiers, higher resolution monitors, faster processors to handle more information, and larger, cheaper storage devices. Software will become increasingly user-friendly. We can expect to see more manufacturers of software and recording devices in the next few years and then perhaps a decline in those numbers when the market consolidates.

Opportunities for technologists to specialize will become more abundant. In the early days, most technologists were appliers of electrodes and sensors, maintainers of recordings, and observers. When the growth of sleep medicine and technology progressed, particularly after the advent of nasal CPAP, technologists became therapeutic interventionists. Sleep center growth in size and numbers of personnel has led to the need for lead technologists, supervisors, and managers.

Many larger facilities are employing sleep technologists who function specifically in the role of patient educator for PAP and sleep apnea as well as other sleep disorders. They also monitor PAP patients for adherence to therapeutic regimes, increasingly mandated by the Centers for Medicare and Medicaid Services (CMS) and other third-party payers. In other centers, this task falls to the multitasking day shift technologist who is constantly "changing hats" from scoring, to acquisition, to scheduling secretary, and so on. These sleep technologists work closely with the sleep physicians when patient volumes increase.

Industry growth will provide opportunities for sales, marketing, and installation and training positions. Industry will continue to expand, and new technology will continue to develop with a continuing need for sleep technology professionals to fill multiple roles.

As the growth in facilities continues, opportunities for traveling technologists and training consultants will be created. Soon, positions for sleep technologist educators will become prevalent at community colleges and in stand-alone training programs. We are indeed no longer merely denizens of the night. We have become a diverse group of individuals with varying interests who have one thing in common: a passion for sleep. It is that passion that keeps sleep technologists involved in sleep medicine and technology whatever the capacity,

for without it, they do not survive in this profession. It is just too arduous to pursue for any length of time without the love of sleep medicine instilled in our beings.

In the past few years, the CMS has begun reimbursement for some technologies (procedures) that have been available for many years, namely portable, unattended polysomnography and actigraphy. With reimbursement for these procedures, one would expect to see increased use of these diagnostic tools. At the time of this writing, the use of portable in-home unattended polysomnography is expanding, particularly in the self-insured arena. The usage has been fairly limited in the private sector because reimbursement does not cover or barely covers the costs involved. Actigraphy is a very useful tool particularly for diagnosis and treatment of insomnia and circadian rhythm disorders. Reimbursement for actigraphy is often tied to precertification or is not available because some payers still consider the procedure as investigational at this time.

REFERENCES

1. Dement, W. (2005). History of sleep physiology and medicine. In M. Kryger, T. Roth, & W. Dement (Eds.), *Principles and practice of sleep medicine* (4th ed.). Philadelphia, PA: Elsevier.
2. Berger, H. (1929). Hans Berger on the electroencephalogramm of man: the fourteen original reports on the human electroencephalogram. *NervKrankh, 87*, 527.
3. Kiloh, L., McComas, A., & Osselton, J. (1972). *Clinical electroencephalography* (3rd ed., p. 210). London, UK: Butterworths.
4. Loomis, A., Harvey, E., & Hobart, G. (1937). Cerebral states during sleep, as studied by human brain potentials. *Journal of Experimental Psychology, 21*, 127.
5. Blake, H., Girard, R., & Kleitman, N. (1929). Factors influencing brain potentials during sleep. *Journal of Neurophysiology, 25*, 48.
6. Knott, J., Henry, C., & Hadley, J. (1939). Brain potentials during sleep: A comparative study of dominant and non-dominant alpha groups. *Journal of Experimental Psychology, 24*, 157.
7. Aserinsky, E., & Kleitman, N. (1953). Regularly occurring periods of eye motility, and concomitant phenomena, during sleep. *Science, 118*, 273–274.
8. Aserinsky, E., & Kleitman, N. (1955). Two types of ocular motility occurring in sleep. *Journal of Applied Physiology, 8*, 1.
9. Dement, W., & Kleitman, N. (1957). Cyclic variations in EEG during sleep and their relation to eye movements, body motility, and dreaming. *Electroencephalography and Clinical Neurophysiology, 9*, 673–690.
10. Rechtschaffen, A., & Kales, A. (Eds.). (1968). *A manual of standardized terminology: Techniques and scoring*

system for sleep stages of human subjects. Los Angeles, CA: UCLA Brain Information Service/Brain Research Institute.

11. Iber, C., Ancoli-Israel, S., Chesson, A., et al. (Eds.). (2007). *The AASM manual for the scoring of sleep and associated events: Rules, terminology and technical specifications* (1st ed.). Westchester, IL: American Academy of Sleep Medicine.

12. American Academy of Sleep Medicine. (2011). *Center accreditation standards.* Darien, IL: Author.

13. Berry, R. B., Albertario, C. L., Harding, S. M., et al. for the American Academy of Sleep Medicine. (2018). *The AASM Manual for the scoring of sleep and associated events: Rules, terminology and technical specifications* [Version 2.5]. Darien, IL: Author.

14. Vogel, G. (1960). Studies in the psychophysiology of dreams, III: The dream of narcolepsy. *Archives of General Psychiatry, 3,* 421–428.

15. Rechtschaffen, A., Wolpert, E., Dement, W., et al. (1963). Nocturnal sleep of narcoleptics. *Electroencephalography and Clinical Neurophysiology, 15,* 599–609.

16. Dement, W., Rechtschaffen, A., & Gulevich, G. (1966). The nature of the narcoleptic sleep attack. *Neurology, 16,* 18–33.

17. Fischgold, H. (Ed.). (1965). *La sommeil de nuit normal et pathologique: Etudes electroencephalographiques* [Normal and pathological sleep at night: Electroencephalographic studies]. Paris, France: Masson et Cie.

18. Gastaut, H., Tassinari, C., & Duron, B. (1965). Polysomnographic study of manifestations of episodes (of sleep and respirations) of Pickwickian Syndrome. *Revista de Neurologia, 112,* 568–579.

19. Jung, R., & Kuhlo, W. (1965). Neurophysiological studies of abnormal night sleep and the Pickwickian syndrome. *Progressive Brain Research, 18,* 140–159.

20. Butkov, N. (2002). Polysomnography. In T. Lee-Chiong, M. Sateia, & M. Carskadon (Eds.), *Sleep medicine.* Philadelphia, PA: Hanley and Belfus.

21. Hauri, P., & Orr, W. (1982). *The sleep disorders.* Kalamazoo, MI: Upjohn.

22. Guilleminault, C. (Ed.). (1982). *Sleeping and waking disorders: Indications and techniques.* Menlo Park, CA: Addison-Wesley.

23. Kryger, M., Roth, T., & Dement, W. (Eds.). (1989). *Principles and practice of sleep medicine.* Philadelphia, PA: Elsevier.

24. Butkov, N. (1996). *Atlas of clinical polysomnography.* Medford, OR: Synapse Media.

25. Sullivan, C., Issa, F., Berthon-Jones, M., et al. (1981). Reversal of obstructive sleep apnea by continuous positive airway pressure applied through the nares. *Lancet, 1,* 862–865.

26. DiPhillipo, M. (2004). *President's perspective.* Board of Registered Polysomnographic Technologists. McLean, VA. Retrieved from http://www.brpt.org/Newsletter/2004/spring04.htm

27. Board of Registered Polysomnographic Technologists. (2004). *BRPT 2004 annual report.* McLean, VA. Retrieved from http://www.brpt.org/aboutbrpt.htm

28. Board of Registered Polysomnographic Technologists. Retrieved March 21, 2018, from https://www.brpt.org

29. National Board of Respiratory Care. Retrieved March 21, 2018, from https://practitionerportal.nbrc.org/directory/all

30. American Board of Sleep Medicine. *American Board of Sleep Medicine sleep technologist registry examination.* Retrieved March 21, 2018, from http://absm.org/techcertification.aspx

31. American Association of Sleep Technologists. *Government affairs.* Retrieved March 21, 2018, from https://www.aastweb.org/governmentaffairs

chapter 2

Sleep Technology: A Global Perspective

TRIPAT DEEP SINGH

LEARNING OBJECTIVES

On completion of this chapter, the reader should be able to:

1. Discuss new developments in sleep technology and sleep diagnostics.
2. Describe the role of computer-assisted scoring and interscorer reliability (ISR).
3. Discuss the role of consumer sleep technologies (CSTs).
4. Describe the role of home sleep apnea testing (HSAT).
5. Describe the development of the global sleep medicine and technology field.

KEY TERMS

Chemogenetics
CRISPR-Cas system
Gene therapy
Home sleep apnea testing (HSAT)
Optogenetics

INTRODUCTION

Sleep technology has evolved rapidly in the last 50 years. Polysomnography (PSG) has transitioned from analog to digital machines, positive airway pressure (PAP) therapy was identified as a treatment for obstructive sleep apnea (OSA), and various advanced forms of PAP therapy and interfaces were introduced to treat sleep-disordered breathing (SDB). In the last decade with advancements in mobile phone technology, mobile apps and wearables have been marketed to monitor health including sleep.

The first professional bodies involved in the development of sleep medicine and sleep technology were established in the United States and Europe. In the past 20 years, additional professional bodies have formed including in many countries that are performing important work in the development of sleep medicine and technology.

MECHANISMS OF SLEEP AND WAKEFULNESS

Hans Berger, a German psychiatrist, discovered electroencephalography (EEG) in 1929 (1), which later led to the study of sleep states in humans and the discovery of rapid eye movement (REM) sleep (2). Jouvet, Bremer, and Moruzzi used brain cuttings to study sleep and wakefulness in animals (3, 4). To study the role of specific cell groups and neurochemicals, researchers used various techniques like cell-specific lesions (5, 6), cellular electrophysiology (7), and measurement of neurotransmitters (8–10). With c-Fos technique, it became clear that these neurons were embedded in groups of neurons controlling other behaviors, but how they also controlled specific sleep behaviors was unclear (11, 12). Newer techniques like genetic approaches, gene therapy, optogenetics, and chemogenetics and clustered regularly interspaced short palindromic repeats (CRISPR)-Cas now allow researchers to understand the finer details of sleep–wake regulation and are also assisting to better understand the causes and treatments of sleep disorders.

The genetic approach has improved understanding of two sleep disorders: narcolepsy and advanced sleep phase syndrome. Emmanuel Mignot found mutation in hypocretin receptor 2 in canine narcolepsy using forward genetics, and Masashi Yanagisawa's group found narcoleptic symptoms in orexin knockout mouse (13). In advanced sleep phase syndrome, forward genetics revealed that individuals with this disorder have a mutation in the *hPer2* gene (14), and reverse genetics established that mice with this mutation also demonstrated a shorter period of sleep–activity cycle (15).

Optogenetics

Optogenetics ("opto" for optical stimulation and "genetics" for genetically targeted cell types) uses light-sensitive proteins channelrhodopsin-2 (ChR2) and halorhodopsin (NpHR) to either activate or inhibit, respectively, the activity of neurons in which they are targeted (16). The ChR2-expressing cells depolarize when exposed to blue light, and NpHR-expressing cells hyperpolarize when exposed to yellow light. These two proteins can be inserted into specific cells, which allow to control the activity of a particular cell in neural network with millisecond precision.

Optogenetics has helped resolve the mystery of which neurons, cholinergic or γ-aminobutyric acid (GABA), in the basal forebrain produce wakefulness. GABA neurons in the basal forebrain are active during wakefulness (17) and hypocretin cells function to promote arousal (18, 19). Optogenetic stimulation helped to identify specific cell groups in the basal forebrain that promote nonrapid eye movement (NREM) sleep; optogenetic stimulation of GABA+ somatostatin neurons in the basal forebrain produced transition from wakefulness to NREM sleep and also increased the amount of NREM sleep (17).

Melanin-concentrating hormone (MCH) neurons fire during NREM sleep and become most active during REM sleep (20). Optogenetic technique provided new evidence about the role of MCH neurons in sleep; MCH neurons increased both NREM and REM sleep and delta power. They also increased sleep at night, suggesting that MCH neurons inhibit arousal-promoting circuits and drive sleep in mammals (21, 22). Activation of MCH neurons during NREM sleep produces transition to REM sleep (23).

Optogenetics has highlighted the role of the ventral medulla in the control of REM sleep. Optogenetically activating GABA cells in the ventral medulla increase the probability of REM sleep episodes, and chemogenetic inactivation of these same cells reduced REM sleep (24). For the first time with optogenetic stimulation of non-neural structure, glial cells in the hypothalamus show that glial cell activation increases both NREM and REM sleep (25). It is thought that it is glial rather than neuronal adenosine that may regulate the homeostatic sleep drive response before waking (26).

Astrocytes are a key component of a glymphatic system in the central nervous system that is responsible for waste disposal and distribution of lipids, glucose, and other nutrients (27). The glymphatic system is active during natural sleep and anesthesia but not during wakefulness (28). The glymphatic system also clears brain lactate that accumulates during wakefulness (29). These studies provide the first direct evidence of the role of sleep in clearing brain waste accumulated during wakefulness. One of the drawbacks of optogenetics is that this technique generates heat, and this may be problematic if cells under study are heat sensitive. Also, if cells under study are scattered, the light may not be able to reach all the opsin-containing cells.

Chemogenetics

Also called pharmacogenetics, a drug-based approach is used to control cell activity. Chemogenetics differs from optogenetics in that it can activate or suppress the activity of broadly scattered neuron populations, which makes it a more useful approach than optogenetics for manipulating distributed cell groups. This technique has contributed to the understanding of sleep–wake mechanisms including the following:
- Activation of hypocretin neurons increasing wakefulness (30)
- Role of GABA neurons in lateral hypothalamus in regulating waking (31, 32)
- Activation of GABAergic neurons in the medullary parafacial zone rapidly inducing NREM sleep regardless of circadian time (33)
- Inactivation of GABA cells in the ventral medulla increasing wakefulness and decreasing NREM and REM sleep (24)
- Activation of MCH neurons leading to increase in slow-wave sleep (SWS) depth and acceleration in the extinction of SWS episodes. These two processes facilitate the transition from SWS to REM sleep and assist in REM sleep onset (34).

Gene Therapy

Gene therapy may be attempted as a treatment strategy for treating narcolepsy. Several animal studies have shown that restoring hypocretin gene expression in different neuronal groups improves symptoms of cataplexy and consolidates wakefulness (35–38).

CRISPR-Cas System

The CRISPR-Cas system is a new gene-editing tool that allows researchers to delete, silence, enhance, or insert genes at a precise location in the genome (39–41). CRISPR is a segment of DNA containing short repetitions of base sequences, with each repeat sequence followed by pieces of *spacer DNA*. This technique has been used to show the role of the entire N-methyl-D-aspartate receptor family in sleep regulation in mice (42). This technique can be applied across all eukaryotes including humans and reduces the time, cost, and effort compared with conventional genetic strategies of gene manipulation.

TECHNOLOGY AND SLEEP DIAGNOSTICS

Computer-Assisted Sleep Scoring and Interscorer Reliability

Manual scoring of sleep and associated events has been the standard worldwide, and interscorer reliability (ISR) is an important issue in quality control. The American Academy of Sleep Medicine (AASM) frequently revises the scoring manual, the latest manual being released in April 2018, to refine the scoring rules and improve ISR.

Younes et al. have highlighted that inattention errors and bias contribute little to interscorer variability (43); rather, the difference is due to equivocal epochs that can be assigned one or two sleep stages by trained technologists (43). They indicate digital information regarding key sleep staging variables (spindles, delta wave duration, and objective sleep depth) is needed to reduce scoring variability and that better training or refining the scoring rules is not going to improve ISR (43). As a continuation to this study, Younes et al. showed that providing digital information regarding key sleep staging variables (spindles, delta wave duration, and objective sleep depth) improved ISR (44). Younes et al. also showed that manual scoring of NREM sleep stages is highly variable and unreliable among experienced sleep technologists (45). Technologists varied widely in scoring N1 and N3 sleep stages (45). The AASM also reported the lowest agreement in scoring of N1 and N3 sleep among different scorers globally in their ISR program (46). They also identified that scoring the first epoch of N3 after N2 sleep has low agreement among scorers and suggested the use of automated analysis of slow-wave activity as a potential solution (46). Several computer-assisted sleep scoring systems have been validated against human scoring, which has not only improved interscorer variability but also shortened the time required to score one sleep study considerably (43, 44, 47, 48). Recently, researchers in Singapore developed a real-time automatic sleep staging system that can be cloud based, allowing multiple users to perform real-time sleep staging at the same time (49). This system can score an entire night's sleep recording with an accuracy on par with expert human scorers but much faster (5 seconds compared with 30 to 60 minutes). This system also facilitates the automatic delivery of acoustic stimuli at the targeted phase of slow-sleep oscillations to enhance SWS (49).

It requires considerable practice and knowledge to learn manual sleep staging. There are very few technologists trained in manual scoring of sleep stages in developing countries, which is a limiting factor in starting more sleep labs in these countries. Computer-assisted sleep scoring systems make scoring simple and may be very useful in extending the reach of sleep facilities to patients in developing countries.

Automated scoring of respiratory events faces several impediments: determining the baseline to compute a 30% or 90% reduction in flow amplitude to score hypopneas or apneas, measuring airflow with nasal pressure and not with a pneumotachograph, and therefore overestimating the flow signal at small amplitudes with oronasal interfaces and difficulty automating methods (flow morphology, paradox between thorax and abdominal belts) on which manual scoring of obstructive versus central hypopnea depends (50).

Two methods have been described to automate the scoring of EEG arousals based on absolute power of EEG (51, 52). Both methods are limited because the absolute power of EEG may be affected by scalp properties and impedance values (43, 44, 47, 48). These computer-assisted scoring systems should not be a threat to sleep technologists. The sleep technologist can focus more on patient-centric activities like educating the patients about disease, explaining PAP therapy, proper mask fit, and troubleshooting their issues with PAP therapy. The role of experienced technologists is indispensable even if these new technologies are adopted in the day-to-day practice of sleep labs.

Consumer Sleep Technologies

Consumer sleep technologies (CSTs) have become very popular within our society for self-monitoring sleep. They are primarily used for sleep induction, wake induction, self-guided sleep assessment, entertainment, social connection, information sharing, and sleep education (53). A recent review classified the primary delivery platforms for CSTs into five categories:

- Mobile device platforms,
- Wearable platforms,
- Embedded platforms,
- Desktop or website platforms, and
- Accessory appliance platforms (53).

The manufacturers of these technologies update them at a rapid pace and the medical community cannot keep up. By the time any study is published validating the technology, a new version of the technology has already been released.

A recent study reported that only 32.9% of sleep apps contained information supporting their claims, 15.8% included clinical input, and 13.2% contained links to sleep literature. Also, apps contained information on how sleep is affected by alcohol or drugs (23.7%), food, daily activities, and stress (13.2%). Users gave a high rating to apps that contained a sleep tip function (54). However, no guidelines or validation of data generated by CSTs shows how sleep is affected by different disease states and how to use the data to manage different disease states long term.

Recently, a study protocol published studying the clinical applicability of a wearable device (Fitbit Charge HR or Fitbit Charge 2) generated data on the management of thyrotoxicosis by analyzing continuously monitored data for heart rate, physical activity, and sleep in patients with thyrotoxicosis during their clinical course after treatment (55). In patients with major depressive disorders, Fitbit Flex (FBF) in a normal setting significantly overestimated sleep time and efficiency and displayed poor ability to correctly identify wake epochs.

In the sensitive setting, the FBF significantly underestimated sleep time and efficiency relative to PSG (56).

Validation of data across different age groups is not available, and scant available data show different results across age groups. In healthy adults, Fitbit Charge 2 when compared with gold standard PSG overestimated total sleep time (TST) and time spent in N1 + N2 sleep stage and underestimated sleep onset latency and stage N3 but did not differ in estimation of wake time after sleep onset and time spent in REM sleep. Fitbit Charge 2 correctly identified 82% of PSG-defined NREM–REM sleep cycles across the night in healthy adults and also in subjects with periodic leg movements during sleep (57). In the pediatric population (3 to 17 years), Fitbit Ultra significantly overestimated TST (41 minutes) and sleep efficiency (SE) (8%) in normal mode and underestimated TST (105 minutes) and SE (21%) in sensitive mode (58). In adolescents, Fitbit Charge HR significantly but negligibly overestimated TST by 8 minutes and sleep efficiency by 1.8% and underestimated wake time after sleep onset by 5.6 minutes ($p < 0.05$) (59, 60).

Some studies have tested the proof of concept that these technologies can be used as diagnostic tools. A recent study compared data from PSG with snore data recorded from a smartphone taped to the patient's chest and found good agreement between the respiratory disturbance index (RDI) obtained from the smartphone and the apnea–hypopnea index (AHI) from PSG (61). However, in real-life settings, the recordings may be affected by the presence of a bed partner and other sounds in the sleeping environment including bed partner snoring (61).

Sonomat, a contactless sleep monitoring system embedded into a foam mattress which detects apneas and hypopneas, was found to have good correlation for AHI, apnea index, and hypopnea index for AHI less than 50 events per hour when compared with PSG (62). Sonomat has recently been validated for detecting SDB in children as well (63).

Another contact-free monitoring system (EarlySense, Ltd., Israel) was compared with PSG (64). It comprises an under-the-mattress piezoelectric sensor and a smartphone application to collect vital signs and analyze sleep. TST estimates with the EarlySense were closely correlated with the PSG. This system also showed good sleep staging capability with improved performance over accelerometer-based apps (64). It can also collect additional physiologic information on heart rate and respiratory rate (64).

Sleep on Cue, an iPhone-based app, was compared with PSG to detect sleep onset (65). The Sleep on Cue app uses behavioral responses to auditory stimuli to detect sleep onset and it overestimates sleep onset latency by 3.17 minutes (65). TST and sleep latency estimated by another iPhone app, Sleep Cycle, in children (2 to 14 years) did not correlate with PSG (66).

Technology is becoming an integral part of human lives. Whether we like it or not, patients will come to the clinic asking us to interpret the data from these devices. Instead of throwing the data away in light of no evidence, we should take a look at the data to see whether it makes any sense clinically. These technologies are at least engaging consumers and making them self-aware and interested in their own health. There is a danger that these CSTs may prevent few patients from seeking professional evaluation and treatment, however, or even destroy the physician–patient relationship by providing conflicting advice.

Home Sleep Apnea Testing

Prevalence of OSA has increased in the US population over the past two decades (67). In a population-based Spanish study (Hypnolaus study), the prevalence of moderate-to-severe SDB (≥ 15 events per hour) was 23.4% in women and 49.7% in men (68). In recent years, there is a trend toward increased Home Sleep Apnea Testing (HSAT) use because the number of patients has increased and PSG being an expensive test is a big burden on public health systems. In Western societies where PSG and PAP treatments are reimbursed, economic analysis has found HSAT to be a more cost-effective test compared to PSG for payers but not for service providers (69).

OSA in the Asian population is not different from that in Western societies. A recent study found the prevalence of moderate-to-severe SDB of 30.5% in the Singapore population (70). The authors also reported that 91% of subjects with moderate-to-severe SDB were previously undiagnosed (70). The authors used HSAT for their study citing limited availability of PSG in Singapore (70). In a population-based study in Vietnam, prevalence of OSA with AHI greater than 5 per hour was 8.5% and of OSA with AHI greater than 15 per hour was 5.2% (71).

However, in most Asian countries (except Japan) where PSG and PAP treatments are not reimbursed by the public health system or private insurance companies, the high costs of PSG and PAP treatments impede the diagnostic and treatment process. The number of trained professionals in the field of sleep medicine and sleep technology is few in developing countries. Given the high burden of SDB in the Asian population, the high cost of PSG which is not reimbursed by public health systems or private insurance companies, and few trained professionals, there is a need for a simple, low-cost, and reliable test to diagnose patients with SDB in developing countries. HSAT and computer-assisted sleep scoring may play an important role in developing countries to extend services of sleep diagnostics to patients with SDB.

The AASM updated guidelines for diagnostic testing of OSA in adult patients (72) recommend HSAT for diagnosing uncomplicated adult OSA patients with increased risk of moderate-to-severe OSA. If a single HSAT is negative, inconclusive, or technically inadequate, a PSG can be performed for the diagnosis of OSA. HSAT should not be used for the diagnosis of OSA in patients with significant cardiorespiratory disease, potential respiratory muscle weakness because of neuromuscular condition, awake hypoventilation or suspicion of sleep-related hypoventilation, chronic opioid medication use, and history of stroke or severe insomnia (72).

A study in stroke patients reported that unattended HSAT can be easily implemented after stroke or transient ischemic attack, which facilitates early diagnosis and start of treatment in both inpatient and outpatient settings (73). Another study in diabetic patients reported that screening for OSA using questionnaires is suboptimal, and the authors suggested that OSA screening should be performed using HSAT in diabetic patients (74).

Another study reported that comorbidities were associated in 56.2% of patients diagnosed with mild OSA, in 67.6% with moderate OSA, and in 70% with severe OSA. Therefore, 30% to 40% of moderate-to-severe OSA patients do not have any major comorbidity (obesity, hypertension, depression, gastroesophageal reflux disease, diabetes, hypercholesterolemia, and asthma) (75). In yet another study, 38% patients were eligible for HSAT (76). These figures highlight the fact that a large proportion of patients may be eligible for HSAT in developing countries where PSG and PAP therapies are not reimbursed. Several studies have shown that in selected OSA patients without comorbidities, HSAT followed by auto-PAP (APAP) treatment is as effective as a PSG–CPAP titration strategy (77, 78). HSAT–APAP strategy in selected patients with OSA may be beneficial to many patients in developing countries.

With increased adoption of HSAT, there is a need for uniform standards. The AASM has included detailed guidelines for HSAT in the scoring manual, highlighting technical requirements and reporting parameters including scoring rules for respiratory events (79).

However, HSAT is not free of limitations. Some HSAT devices do not record body position, which makes it difficult to study positional OSA and recommend positional therapy. Choosing a device that records body position may overcome this limitation. Most HSAT devices do not record sleep, but only total recording time (TRT). As a result, AHI may be underestimated with HSAT.

The AASM scoring manual has proposed a new parameter to determine the severity of OSA assessed by HSAT. The respiratory event index (79) is defined as the number of apneas plus the number of hypopneas divided by monitoring time (not TST). Monitoring time is defined as TRT minus time patient was awake as assessed by asking the patient, upright body position, regularity of respiration, or actigraphy minus the time of artifact (79). This gives a close approximation to TST and a more reliable estimation of AHI. A recent study showed that manual editing of TRT improves sensitivity of HSAT studies to detect SDB (80).

Because HSAT does not record sleep and hence arousals cannot be scored, it may lead to underscoring of hypopneas that are not associated with desaturation but are associated with arousal. This limitation can be overcome by choosing an HSAT device that records sleep.

Several studies have shown that snoring characteristics provide very useful information about OSA severity (81–85). A recent study compared data from PSG with snore data recorded from a smartphone taped to a patient's chest and found good agreement between an RDI estimated from the smartphone snoring data and AHI from PSG (61). The study was performed in a sleep lab. At home, the recordings may be affected by the presence of a bed partner and other sounds in the sleeping environment including bed partner snoring (61). Central apneas are another challenge for this technology because snoring generally does not occur in patients with central apnea.

Global Sleep Medicine and Technology

In Europe, the European Sleep Research Society (ESRS) and other local sleep societies are leading the way in the development of sleep medicine and technology; however, very little has been published regarding the state of sleep medicine and technology in South Asia, Asia-Pacific, and other global organizations.

World Sleep Society

This society was formed in 2016 with the merger of the World Association of Sleep Medicine (WASM) and the World Sleep Federation (WSF). The official society website is www.worldsleepsociety.org. There are currently 28 members associated with this society from across the globe. The society has four different types of individual membership options including full, regular, student, and technician memberships.

A primary focus of the association is education and curriculum development. This program is focused on developing a sleep medicine curriculum and materials that associated societies offer in their respective countries including study materials, study questions, and self-assessment tools.

The journal *Sleep Medicine* is the official society journal. The society conducts World Sleep Day in the month of March every year. Recognition for those performing research and working in sleep medicine includes awards in different areas of sleep medicine and sleep research.

- The Christian Guilleminault WASM Award for sleep research
- The Elio Lugaresi Award for sleep medicine
- IRLSSG Wayne Hening Young Investigator Award
- Annual Young Investigator Award

The World Sleep Congress is held every 2 years in one of the member countries across the globe. The association also conducts the Sleep Medicine Specialist examination to certify sleep specialists. Information about the examination is available at http://worldsleepsociety.org/about/committees/sleep-specialist-certification/.

Sleep Medicine and Sleep Technology in Asia

In a survey conducted in Asia-Pacific countries, authors reported very limited coverage of sleep and sleep disorders in medical school curriculum (86). Countries like Malaysia, Indonesia, and Vietnam reported no coverage at all (86). Some countries like India did not respond to the survey (86). This study highlights the poor state of affairs in Asia; the overall response rate to the survey was only 25%.

There are two organizations in Asia involved in the development of sleep medicine and sleep technology:

- Asian Sleep Research Society (ASRS)
- Asian Society of Sleep Medicine (ASSM)

Sleep societies in different Asian countries are members of one of these two sleep societies. Each society conducts an annual 2- to 3-day conference in one of the Asian countries. The conferences include various activities such as symposiums, keynote lectures, workshops, and special lectures.

The official journal of ASRS is *Sleep and Biological Rhythms* and of ASSM is *Sleep Medicine Research*. Both ASRS and ASSM are associate society members of the World Sleep Society (WSS).

Different Asian countries are at different levels of development in sleep medicine and technology. Some specific developments in the field in specific Asian countries are discussed below.

Sleep Medicine and Sleep Technology in India

The population of India is 1.3 billion. There are strong epidemiologic data on the burden of OSA in the Indian population. The prevalence of OSA and obstructive sleep apnea syndrome (OSAS) in India is 9.3% and 2.8%, respectively (87). There is a huge burden of OSA

in the Indian population. However, there are less than 300 sleep labs in all of India (88).

Sleep medicine and sleep technology are developing fields in India. Currently, different specialties including pulmonary medicine, ENT, psychiatry, neurology, and physiology practice sleep medicine. Because there is no separate job title for sleep technologists, EEG technologists, pulmonary function technologists, and nurses work as sleep technologists in various sleep centers across India. There is no professional body regulating the profession of sleep technologists. There are no courses in medical school curriculum teaching sleep medicine or sleep technology, and training is on the job and by attending various conferences and courses. There is no reimbursement for PSG or PAP devices in India except for central government employees. The patient has to pay out of his pocket for diagnosis and treatment.

There are four societies in India promoting the fields of sleep medicine and sleep technology.

- Indian Society for Sleep Research (ISSR)— www.issr.in
- Indian Sleep Disorder Association (ISDA)— www.isda.co.in
- Indian Association of Surgeons for Sleep Apnoea (IASSA)—www.iassa.in
- South East Asian Academy of Sleep Medicine (SEAASM)—www.seaasm.org

Indian Society of Sleep Research

The ISSR was founded in 1992 (88). It is an associate society member of the WSS and ASRS. The society conducts educational activities to develop the fields of sleep technology and sleep medicine in India.

The National Sleep Medicine Course (NSMC), founded in 2006, is held annually and covers different aspects of sleep medicine in a comprehensive manner. Faculties from the United States, Japan, India, and Singapore attend and conduct the course (88). The National Sleep Technology Course (NSTC) was founded in 2014 and holds an annual 1-day meeting covering different aspects of sleep technology in a comprehensive manner with faculties from the United States, India, and Singapore attending and conducting the course. This course is designed for beginners and is also used as refresher by trained technologists (88). In 2018, the society initiated an Advanced Sleep Technology Course to discuss advanced topics in the field of sleep technology that is held in New Delhi.

Certification Examination for Sleep Specialists

An Indian Board of Sleep Medicine was constituted by the ISSR in 2010. This board, in collaboration with the WSF, conducts the Transitional Board Certification Examination for Indian sleep specialists. The examination is conducted annually in July (88). The first examination was conducted in 2012, and at the time of this writing, six examinations have been conducted and 25 physicians have earned certification in sleep medicine.

Certification Examination for Sleep Technologists

The ISSR conducts a certification examination to certify sleep technologists once every year (88). The examination was initiated in 2015, and at the time of this writing, examinations have been conducted three times, with 18 sleep technologists earning certification.

Sleep Lab Accreditation Program

This program was instituted to bring uniformity to sleep laboratory standards across the country and improve patient care (88).

Publications

The society launched their journal in 2016. *Sleep and Vigilance* is published two times a year. The ISSR also publishes a newsletter titled *SleepWatching India* highlighting various activities in India, including educational topics, sleep laboratory details, sleep technologist interviews, and other news related to sleep from India and across the world. It is also published twice annually. All the issues of the newsletter are available on the website at www.issr.in. The ISSR also publishes a summary of important studies in the field of sleep medicine and sleep technology from January to June and July to December every year. These publications are also available on the website at www.issr.in.

Indian Sleep Disorder Association

The ISDA was established in 1995 as an associate society member of the ASSM. ISDA's activities are focused on the development of the fields of sleep medicine and sleep technology in India as highlighted on their website at www.isda.co.in.

The society conducts a certification examination for sleep specialists; at this time, 23 physicians have been awarded fellowship status for passing this examination. The ISDA also plans to begin a 1-year diploma program for sleep technologists. The society publishes their own journal titled *Indian Journal of Sleep Medicine* four times a year. The ISDA conducts an annual conference "SleepCon" as well.

Indian Association of Surgeons for Sleep Apnoea

This society was established in 2012 and comprises mostly surgeons. The focus of this association is promoting and developing the role of surgery for the management of sleep apnea. The IASSA is an associate society member of the WSS. Experts in the field of sleep apnea surgery from across the globe are invited to their annual conference "IASSACON." The society conducts training programs in surgery for sleep apnea in different parts of India.

South East Asian Academy of Sleep Medicine

Established in 2013, the SEAASM is an associate society member of the WSS. They hold an annual conference called the "International Conference on Sleep Disorders (ICSD)." The society's goal is to develop training pathways and credentials for physicians and technologists.

Additional Sleep Medicine Organizations in India

There are other private organizations assisting to develop the field of sleep medicine in India. Two of these organizations are the Nithra Institute of Sleep Medicine established in 2004 and the ACE School of Sleep Medicine. The Nithra Institute of Sleep Medicine is a comprehensive center for diagnosing and treating sleep disorders in Chennai that has established a 1-year fellowship in sleep medicine, which is accredited by The Tamil Nadu Dr. M. G. R. Medical University. The university also conducts short-term courses of 1- to 2-week duration and a certified PSG Technician Program of 6 months duration.

The ACE School of Sleep Medicine conducts 1- to 2-day training courses in sleep medicine and sleep technology two to three times each year in different parts of the country. In 2017, they conducted 19 training programs. Every 2 years, they also conduct a regular event titled "Sleep Update." Their official website is located at www.assm.in.

Sleep Medicine and Sleep Technology in Singapore

The prevalence of moderate-to-severe SDB and sleep apnea in Singapore's population of five million is 30.5% and 18.1%, respectively (70). It is also reported that 91% of patients with moderate-to-severe SDB in Singapore were previously undiagnosed (70).

Most physicians practicing sleep medicine in Singapore have completed a 1-year fellowship in sleep medicine after their specialization; some are American Board certified in sleep medicine, and a few have taken the WASM examination.

Most of the sleep technologists working in the sleep laboratories have attained the Registered Polysomnographic Technologist (RPSGT) credential. There is no formal certification program in medical school curriculum for physicians in sleep medicine or for technologists in sleep technology. Different specialties including ENT, pulmonary medicine, neurology, psychiatry, and cardiology practice sleep medicine in Singapore. There are at least three government multispecialty multibed sleep centers along with few private hospital sleep labs and independent facilities in Singapore.

Singapore Sleep Society

The Singapore Sleep Society (SSS) is the professional body working to develop the fields of sleep research, sleep medicine, and sleep technology. The SSS was established in 2002 and is an associate society member of the ASSM. SSS members are actively involved in the following research areas:

- Functional imaging of sleep deprivation,
- Behavioral studies of sleep deprivation,
- Sleep and aging,
- Adolescent sleep,
- Markers of vulnerability to sleep deprivation,
- Circadian variation in physiology,
- School sleep habits, and
- Pediatric sleep patterns.

The SSS also participates in the annual conference organized by the Singapore General Hospital. This conference is 2 days in duration and is attended by physicians and sleep techs from across the Association of Southeast Asian Nations (ASEAN) region. As part of this conference, a 1-day sleep tech forum was begun in 2016 where sleep technologists from different hospitals in Singapore share knowledge with their colleagues and overseas participants. The sleep technologist forum is a first of its kind event in the ASEAN region and entirely focuses on sleep technology topics.

There is no reimbursement for PSG or PAP devices in Singapore. HSAT is well accepted, and efforts are being made to empower general practitioners to begin ordering HSAT to screen their patients for OSA.

Sleep Medicine and Sleep Technology in the Philippines

There are no prevalence studies on the burden of sleep disorders in the Philippines. Many Philippine specialists go to the United States for fellowship training in sleep medicine and some have American Board of Sleep Medicine certification. There are 20 sleep laboratories in the Philippines—which is an archipelago of 7,107 islands—most in Manila city.

The Philippine Society of Sleep Medicine (PSSM) is the professional body involved in developing the fields of sleep medicine and sleep technology. The PSSM was established in 2002 and is an associate society member of the ASSM. One of the major achievements of PSSM includes formulation of a sleep fellowship program. Currently, 42 physicians have become fellows of PSSM

after completing this program. The PSSM has also created the Philippine Board of Sleep Medicine and a sleep laboratory accreditation committee, and they host an annual 3-day conference.

Currently, there is no separate certification program for sleep technologists. Most are trained on the job or through an apprenticeship. Many sleep technologists are respiratory therapists. There is no reimbursement for PSG or PAP devices in the Philippines.

Sleep Medicine and Sleep Technology in Indonesia

There are no published data on the prevalence of sleep disorders in Indonesia where the population is 245 million. There are only six to eight level 1 sleep laboratories in Indonesia where specialties including neurology, pulmonary medicine, and ENT practice sleep medicine, and training is on the job or through attending conferences, short-duration courses, or an apprenticeship. There are no certification programs in sleep medicine or sleep technology.

The Indonesian Society of Sleep Medicine is the professional body and is an associate society member of ASSM. Sleep technologists are nurses or medical assistants who have no formal training or certification in sleep technology. There are two RPSGT-credentialed technologists in Indonesia. There is no reimbursement for PSG or PAP devices in Indonesia.

Sleep Medicine and Sleep Technology in Thailand

The prevalence of OSA and OSAS in Thai men is 15.4% and 4.8% and in Thai women is 6.3% and 1.9%, respectively (89). In Thai children who underwent PSG at a single sleep center in Thailand, OSA was the most common diagnosis with a prevalence of 92.7%; 40.4% of these patients were diagnosed with severe OSA (90).

In 1974, PSG was used for the first time to evaluate treatment of a patient with snoring and sleep apnea. In 1984, the first sleep laboratory was established at Mahidol University to study the sudden unexplained deaths of Thai construction workers. In 1991, Thai Sleep Research and Sleep Medicine Society was established, and it conducted an International Sleep Conference in Bangkok in 2000 and hosted the WASM Conference in 2007. In 2009, the Sleep Society of Thailand was established as an associate society member of the ASSM (91). Specialties including neurology, pulmonary medicine, ENT, psychiatry, and pediatric pulmonology practice sleep medicine. Most have gone to the United States or Canada for fellowship training in sleep medicine. Some are American Board of Sleep Medicine–certified sleep specialists. The AASM certified 10 Thai sleep specialists in 2010 (91).

There is a certification program in sleep medicine and master of science in sleep medicine program in some universities in Thailand. Some sleep centers also take foreign students for training in sleep medicine for a period of 6 months to 1 year. Sleep medicine has been included in the undergraduate medical curriculum since 2010 (91).

Since 2010, training courses have been organized for sleep technologists. There are two levels of training: a 5-day basic-level course and a 4-day advanced-level course. Thailand Sleep Society has two certification examinations for sleep technologists: basic and advanced. Some sleep technologists have gone to the United States for training. Thailand Sleep Society has started a 4-month training program for technologists as well. The training program involves five sleep centers in Thailand, and trainees will rotate through all five sleep centers over the 4-month period (91).

There are a total of 48 sleep laboratories in Thailand, mostly in Bangkok. The PSG is free in public hospitals for civil servants and their families, referred under the civil service welfare system, social security for private employees, and a universal coverage scheme. No private insurance covers the sleep study in Thailand (91).

In 2015, the Thailand Sleep Society started a sleep laboratory accreditation program to provide uniform standards for sleep laboratories across the country (91).

Sleep Medicine and Sleep Technology in Korea

In a questionnaire-based study in Korean population, prevalence of high-risk factors for OSA was 15.8% (92). The prevalence of OSAS was 4.5% in men and 3.2% in women (93).

Specialties including ENT, neurology, psychiatry, pediatrics, and pulmonary medicine practice sleep medicine in Korea (94). There is no formal certification program for sleep medicine in Korea. Thirteen Korean medical schools reported that psychiatry/psychology and respiratory departments teach sleep medicine in their curriculum (86). Insomnia, pediatric parasomnias, and adult sleep apnea were the most frequently covered topics (86). Many physicians have gone to the United States for sleep medicine fellowship training, some are American Board of Sleep Medicine–certified sleep specialists, and some have taken the WASM examination.

Several sleep societies are involved in the development of the fields of sleep medicine and sleep technology in Korea (94). These include the Korean Sleep Research Society, an associate society member of the Asian Society for Sleep Research; the Korean Society of Sleep Medicine, an associate society member of the Asian Society for Sleep Medicine; and the Korean Academy of Sleep Medicine, also an associate society member of the Asian Society for Sleep Research.

There are no formal training or certification programs for sleep technologists. Most are trained on the job or by attending conferences or short-duration workshops conducted by the Korean Sleep Societies (94). Recently, the Korean government has begun to reimburse PSG for diagnosis and PAP therapy on a monthly rental basis. At the time of this writing, reimbursement has been approved but not implemented.

Sleep Medicine and Sleep Technology in Malaysia

In a published study on 289 Malaysian express bus drivers, 128 (44.3%) subjects were diagnosed as having OSA, with 83 (28.7%), 26 (9.0%), and 26 (6.6%) classified as mild, moderate, and severe OSA, respectively (95). There are no published prevalence data for the general population of 30 million Malaysians.

Sleep medicine is practiced by pulmonary medicine, ENT, neurology, psychiatry, and pediatrics specialists in Malaysia. There is no formal certification program in sleep medicine. Some physicians have traveled to the United States and some have gone to Thailand for 6 months to 1-year training programs, and some are WASM-certified sleep specialists.

The Sleep Disorder Society of Malaysia (SDSM) holds an annual conference and sometimes conducts a road show on sleep medicine in different parts of Malaysia. There is also a 1-day program for sleep technologists held during the conference. There are no training or certification programs for sleep technologists. Most are trained on the job and by attending the conferences or short-duration training courses. Most sleep technologists are medical assistants, nurses, or pulmonary function technologists who do sleep studies at night and work in the ward or clinic during the daytime.

No private insurance companies reimburse for PSG or PAP devices in Malaysia. There are some government agencies who pay for PAP devices for government employees, but reimbursement is a lengthy process. Patients often have to pay out of pocket for PSG and PAP devices.

SUMMARY

There have been many new developments in sleep diagnostics and technology, and new ways of doing things are emerging rapidly. Computer technology is rapidly becoming integrated with medicine, including in the practices of sleep medicine and technology. Telemedicine, HSAT, and computer-assisted technologies along with consumer devices that track sleep are mainstream practices today. Technology is likely to continue to make sleep medicine more accessible across the world and to assist physicians and sleep technologists to improve the sleep of our patients. These practices are growing rapidly, and many are being developed and utilized successfully across the globe where the cost of care for patients with sleep disorders has been prohibitive in the past. As the sleep medicine and technology fields continue to grow globally, we can anticipate better diagnostics and treatments for our patients throughout the world.

REFERENCES

1. Tudor, M., Tudor, L., & Tudor, K. I. (2005). Hans Berger (1873-1941)—The history of electroencephalography. *Acta Medica Croatica, 59*(4), 307–313.

2. Aserinsky, E., & Kleitman, N. (1953). Regularly occurring periods of eye motility, and concomitant phenomena, during sleep. *Science, 118*(3062), 273–274.

3. Jouvet, M. (1972). The role of monoamines and acetylcholine-containing neurons in the regulation of the sleep-waking cycle. *Ergebnisse der Physiologie, 64,* 166–307.

4. Moruzzi, G. (1972). The sleep-waking cycle. *Ergebnisse der Physiologie, 64,* 1–165.

5. Gerashchenko, D., Kohls, M. D., Greco, M., et al. (2001). Hypocretin-2-saporin lesions of the lateral hypothalamus produce narcoleptic-like sleep behavior in the rat. *Journal of Neuroscience, 21*(18), 7273–7283.

6. Blanco-Centurion, C., Gerashchenko, D., & Shiromani, P. J. (2007). Effects of saporin-induced lesions of three arousal populations on daily levels of sleep and wake. *Journal of Neuroscience, 27*(51), 14041–14048

7. Siegel, J. M. (1979). Behavioral functions of the reticular formation. *Brain Research, 180*(1), 69–105.

8. Nitz, D., & Siegel, J. M. (1996). GABA release in posterior hypothalamus across sleep–wake cycle. *American Journal of Physiology, 271*(6, Pt. 2), R1707–R1712.

9. Lydic, R., Baghdoyan, H. A., & Lorinc, Z. (1991). Microdialysis of cat pons reveals enhanced acetylcholine release during state-dependent respiratory depression. *American Journal of Physiology, 261*(3, Pt. 2), R766–R770.

10. George, R., Haslett, W. L., & Jenden, D. J. (1964). A cholinergic mechanism in the brainstem reticular formation: Induction of paradoxical sleep. *International Journal of Neuropharmacology, 3,* 541–552.

11. Shiromani, P. J., Kilduff, T. S., Bloom, F. E., et al. (1992). Cholinergically induced REM sleep triggers Fos-like immunoreactivity in dorsolateral pontine regions associated with REM sleep. *Brain Research, 580*(1/2), 351–357.

12. Sherin, J. E., Shiromani, P. J., McCarley, R. W., et al. (1996). Activation of ventrolateral preoptic neurons during sleep. *Science, 271*(5246), 216–219.

13. Willie, J. T., Chemelli, R. M., Sinton, C. M., et al. (2003). Distinct narcolepsy syndromes in Orexin receptor-2 and Orexin null mice: Molecular genetic dissection of non-REM and REM sleep regulatory processes. *Neuron, 38*(5), 715–730.

14. Toh, K. L., Jones, C. R., He, Y., et al. (2001). An hPer2 phosphorylation site mutation in familial advanced sleep phase syndrome. *Science, 291*(5506), 1040–1043.

15. Xu, Y., Padiath, Q. S., Shapiro, R. E., et al. (2005). Functional consequences of a CKIdelta mutation causing familial advanced sleep phase syndrome. *Nature, 434*(7033), 640–644.

16. Yizhar, O., Fenno, L. E., Davidson, T. J., et al. (2011). Optogenetics in neural systems. *Neuron, 71*(1), 9–34.

17. Xu, M., Chung, S., Zhang, S., et al. (2015). Basal forebrain circuit for sleep–wake control. *Nature Neuroscience, 18*(11), 1641–1647.

18. Adamantidis, A. R., Zhang, F., Aravanis, A. M., et al. (2007). Neural substrates of awakening probed with optogenetic control of hypocretin neurons. *Nature, 450*(7168), 420–424.

19. Carter, M. E., Yizhar, O., Chikahisa, S., et al. (2010). Tuning arousal with optogenetic modulation of locus coeruleus neurons. *Nature Neuroscience, 13*(12), 1526–1533.

20. Hassani, O. K., Lee, M. G., & Jones, B. E. (2009). Melanin-concentrating hormone neurons discharge in a reciprocal manner to orexin neurons across the sleep–wake cycle. *Proceedings of the National Academy of Sciences of the United States of America, 106*(7), 2418–2422.

21. Konadhode, R. R., Pelluru, D., Blanco-Centurion, C., et al. (2013). Optogenetic stimulation of MCH neurons increases sleep. *Journal of Neuroscience, 33*(25), 10257–10263.

22. Blanco-Centurion, C., Liu, M., Konadhode, R. P., et al. (2016). Optogenetic activation of melanin-concentrating hormone neurons increases non-rapid eye movement and rapid eye movement sleep during the night in rats. *European Journal of Neuroscience, 44*(10), 2846–2857.

23. Jego, S., Glasgow, S. D., Herrera, C. G., et al. (2013). Optogenetic identification of a rapid eye movement sleep modulatory circuit in the hypothalamus. *Nature Neuroscience, 16*(11), 1637–1643.

24. Weber, F., Chung, S., Beier, K. T., et al. (2015). Control of REM sleep by ventral medulla GABAergic neurons. *Nature, 526*(7573), 435–438.

25. Pelluru, D., Konadhode, R. R., Bhat, N. R., et al. (2016). Optogenetic stimulation of astrocytes in the posterior hypothalamus increases sleep at night in C57BL/6J mice. *European Journal of Neuroscience, 43*(10), 1298–1306.

26. Bjorness, T. E., Dale, N., Mettlach, G., et al. (2016). An adenosine-mediated glial-neuronal circuit for homeostatic sleep. *Journal of Neuroscience, 36*(13), 3709–3721.

27. Jessen, N. A., Munk, A. S., Lundgaard, I., et al. (2015). The glymphatic system: A beginner's guide. *Neurochemical Research, 40*(12), 2583–2599.

28. Xie, L., Kang, H., Xu, Q., et al. (2013). Sleep drives metabolite clearance from the adult brain. *Science, 342*(6156), 373–377.

29. Lundgaard, I., Lu, M. L., Yang, E., et al. (2017). Glymphatic clearance controls state-dependent changes in brain lactate concentration. *Journal of Cerebral Blood Flow and Metabolism, 37*(6), 2112–2124.

30. Sasaki, K., Suzuki, M., Mieda, M., et al. (2011). Pharmacogenetic modulation of orexin neurons alters sleep/wakefulness states in mice. *PLoS One, 6*(5), e8760.

31. Herrera, C. G., Cadavieco, M. C., Jego, S., et al. (2016). Hypothalamic feedforward inhibition of thalamocortical network controls arousal and consciousness. *Nature Neuroscience, 19*(2), 290–298.

32. Venner, A., Anaclet, C., Broadhurst, R. Y., et al. (2016). A novel population of wake-promoting GABAergic neurons in the ventral lateral hypothalamus. *Current Biology, 26*(16), 2137–2143.

33. Anaclet, C., Ferrari, L., Arrigoni, E., et al. (2014). The GABAergic parafacial zone is a medullary slow wave sleep-promoting center. *Nature Neuroscience, 17*(9), 1217–1224.

34. Varin, C., Luppi, P. H., & Fort, P. (2018). Melanin-concentrating hormone-expressing neurons adjust slow-wave sleep dynamics to catalyze paradoxical (REM) sleep. *Sleep, 41*(6), zsy068.

35. Brooks, P. L., & Peever, J. H. (2012). Identification of the transmitter and receptor mechanisms responsible for REM sleep paralysis. *Journal of Neuroscience, 32*(29), 9785–9795.

36. Blanco-Centurion, C., Liu, M., Konadhode, R., et al. (2013). Effects of orexin gene transfer in the dorsolateral pons in orexin knockout mice. *Sleep, 36*(1), 31–40.

37. Liu, M., Thankachan, S., Kaur, S., et al. (2008). Orexin (hypocretin) gene transfer diminishes narcoleptic sleep behavior in mice. *European Journal of Neuroscience, 28*(7), 1382–1393.

38. Kantor, S., Mochizuki, T., Lops, S. N., et al. (2013). Orexin gene therapy restores the timing and maintenance of wakefulness in narcoleptic mice. *Sleep, 36*(8), 1129–1138.

39. Ran, F. A., Hsu, P. D., Lin, C. Y., et al. (2013). Double nicking by RNA-guided CRISPR Cas9 for enhanced genome editing specificity. *Cell, 154*(6), 1380–1389.

40. de la Fuente-Nunez, C., & Lu, T. K. (2017). CRISPR-Cas9 technology: Applications in genome engineering, development of sequence-specific antimicrobials, and future prospects. *Integrative Biology, 9*(2), 109–122.

41. Hsu, P. D., Lander, E. S., & Zhang, F. (2014). Development and applications of CRISPR-Cas9 for genome engineering. *Cell, 157*(6), 1262–1278.

42. Sunagawa, G. A., Sumiyama, K., Ukai-Tadenuma, M., et al. (2016). Mammalian reverse genetics without crossing reveals Nr3a as a short-sleeper gene. *Cell Reports, 14*(3), 662–677.

43. Younes, M., Raneri, J., & Hanly, P. (2016). Staging sleep in polysomnograms: Analysis of inter-scorer variability. *Journal of Clinical Sleep Medicine, 12*(6), 885–894.

44. Younes, M., & Hanly, P. J. (2016). Minimizing interrater variability in staging sleep by use of computer-derived features. *Journal of Clinical Sleep Medicine, 12*(10), 1347–1356.

45. Younes, M., Kuna, S. T., Pack, A. I., et al. (2018). Reliability of the American Academy of Sleep Medicine rules for assessing sleep depth in clinical practice. *Journal of Clinical Sleep Medicine, 14*(2), 205–213.

46. Rosenberg, R. S., & Van Hout, S. (2013). The American Academy of Sleep Medicine inter-scorer reliability program: Sleep stage scoring. *Journal of Clinical Sleep Medicine, 9*(1), 81–87.

47. Younes, M., Younes, M., & Giannouli, E. (2016). Accuracy of automatic polysomnography scoring using frontal electrodes. *Journal of Clinical Sleep Medicine, 12*(5), 735–746.

48. Punjabi, N. M., Shifa, N., Dorffner, G., et al. (2015). Computer-assisted automated scoring of polysomnograms using the somnolyzer system. *Sleep, 38*(10), 1555–1566.

49. Patanaik, A., Ong, J. L., Gooley, J. J., et al. (2018). An end-to-end framework for real-time automatic sleep stage classification. *Sleep, 41*(5), zsy041.

50. Sands, S. A., Owens, R. L., & Malhotra, A. (2016). New approaches to diagnosing sleep-disordered breathing. *Sleep Medicine Clinics, 11*(2), 143–152.

51. Asyali, M. H., Berry, R. B., Khoo, M. C., et al. (2007). Determining a continuous marker for sleep depth. *Computers in Biology and Medicine, 37*(11), 1600–1609.

52. Younes, M., Ostrowski, M., Soiferman, M., et al. (2015). Odds ratio product of sleep EEG as a continuous measure of sleep state. *Sleep, 38*(4), 641–654.

53. Ko, P. R., Kientz, J. A., Choe, E. K., et al. (2015). Consumer sleep technologies: A review of the landscape. *Journal of Clinical Sleep Medicine, 11*(12), 1455–1461.

54. Lee-Tobin, P. A., Ogeil, R. P., Savic, M., et al. (2017). Rate my sleep: Examining the information, function, and basis in empirical evidence within sleep applications for mobile devices. *Journal of Clinical Sleep Medicine, 13*(11), 1349–1354.

55. Lee, J. E., Lee, D. H., Oh, T. J., et al. (2018). Clinical feasibility of continuously monitored data for heart rate, physical activity, and sleeping by wearable activity trackers in patients with thyrotoxicosis: Protocol for a prospective longitudinal observational study. *JMIR Research Protocols, 7*(2), e49.

56. Cook, J. D., Prairie, M. L., & Plante, D. T. (2017). Utility of the Fitbit Flex to evaluate sleep in major depressive disorder: A comparison against polysomnography and wrist-worn actigraphy. *Journal of Affective Disorders, 217*, 299–305.

57. de Zambotti, M., Goldstone, A., Claudatos, S., et al. (2018). A validation study of Fitbit Charge 2 compared with polysomnography in adults. *Chronobiology International, 35*(4), 465–476.

58. Meltzer, L. J., Hiruma, L. S., Avis, K., et al. (2015). Comparison of a commercial accelerometer with polysomnography and actigraphy in children and adolescents. *Sleep, 38*(8), 1323–1330.

59. de Zambotti, M., Baker, F. C., Willoughby, A. R., et al. (2016). Measures of sleep and cardiac functioning during sleep using a multi-sensory commercially-available wristband in adolescents. *Physiology and Behavior, 158*, 143–149.

60. Bauer, J. S., Consolvo, S., Greenstein, B., et al. (2012). ShutEye: Encouraging awareness of healthy sleep recommendations with a mobile, peripheral display. In *Proceedings of the SIGCHI Conference on Human Factors in Computing Systems* (pp. 1401–1410). CHI '12, Austin, TX, May 5–10, 2012. New York, NY: ACM.

61. Nakano, H., Hirayama, K., Sadamitsu, Y., et al. (2014). Monitoring sound to quantify snoring and sleep apnea severity using a smartphone: Proof of concept. *Journal of Clinical Sleep Medicine, 10*(1), 73–78.

62. Norman, M. B., Middleton, S., Erskine, O., et al. (2014). Validation of the Sonomat: A contactless monitoring system used for the diagnosis of sleep disordered breathing. *Sleep, 37*(9), 1477–1487.

63. Norman, M. B., Pithers, S. M., Teng, A. Y., et al. (2017). Validation of the Sonomat against PSG and quantitative measurement of partial upper airway obstruction in children with sleep-disordered breathing. *Sleep, 40*(3), zsx017.

64. Tal, A., Shinar, Z., Shaki, D., et al. (2017). Validation of contact-free sleep monitoring device with comparison to polysomnography. *Journal of Clinical Sleep Medicine, 13*(3), 517–522.

65. Scott, H., Lack, L., & Lovato, N. (2018). A pilot study of a novel smartphone application for the estimation of sleep onset. *Journal of Sleep Research, 27*(1), 90–97.

66. Patel, P., Kim, J. Y., & Brooks, L. J. (2017). Accuracy of a smartphone application in estimating sleep in children. *Sleep Breath, 21*(2), 505–511.

67. Peppard, P. E., Young, T., Barnet, J. H., et al. (2013). Increased prevalence of sleep-disordered breathing in adults. *American Journal of Epidemiology, 177*(9), 1006–1014.

68. Heinzer, R., Vat, S., Marques-Vidal, P., et al. (2015). Prevalence of sleep-disordered breathing in the general population: The HypnoLaus study. *Lancet Respiratory Medicine, 3*(4), 310–318.

69. Kim, R. D., Kapur, V. K., Redline Bruch, J., et al. (2015). An economic evaluation of home versus laboratory-based diagnosis of obstructive sleep apnea. *Sleep, 38*(7), 1027–1037.

70. Tan, A., Cheung, Y. Y., Yin, J., et al. (2016). Prevalence of sleep-disordered breathing in a multiethnic Asian population in Singapore: A community-based study. *Respirology, 21*(5), 943–950.

71. Duong-Quy, S., Dang Thi Mai, K., Tran Van, N., et al. (2018). Étude de la prévalence du syndrome d'apnées obstructives du sommeil au Vietnam [Study of the prevalence of obstructive sleep apnea syndrome]. *Revue des maladies respiratoires, 35*(1), 14–24.

72. Kapur, V. K., Auckley, D. H., Chowdhuri, S., et al. (2017). Clinical practice guideline for diagnostic testing for adult obstructive sleep apnea: An American Academy of Sleep Medicine Clinical Practice Guideline. *Journal of Clinical Sleep Medicine, 13*(3), 479–504.

73. Boulos, M. I., Elias, S., Wan, A., et al. (2017). Unattended hospital and home sleep apnea testing following cerebrovascular events. *Journal of Stroke and Cerebrovascular Diseases, 26*(1), 143–149.

74. Westlake, K., Plihalova, A., Pretl, M., et al. (2016). Screening for obstructive sleep apnea syndrome in patients with type 2 diabetes mellitus: A prospective study on sensitivity of Berlin and STOP-Bang questionnaires. *Sleep Medicine, 26*, 71–76.

75. Pinto, J. A., Ribeiro, D. K., Cavallini, A. F., et al. (2016). Comorbidities associated with obstructive sleep apnea: A retrospective study. *International Archives of Otorhinolaryngology, 20*(2), 145–150.

76. Skomro, R. P., Gjevre, J., Reid, J., et al. (2010). Outcomes of home-based diagnosis and treatment of obstructive sleep apnea. *Chest, 138*(2), 257–263.

77. Berry, R. B., & Sriram, P. (2014). Auto-adjusting positive airway pressure treatment for sleep apnea diagnosed by home sleep testing. *Journal of Clinical Sleep Medicine, 10*(12), 1269–1275.

78. Rosen, C. L., Auckley, D., Benca, R., et al. (2012). A multisite randomized trial of portable sleep studies and positive airway pressure autotitration versus laboratory-based polysomnography for the diagnosis and treatment of obstructive sleep apnea: The HomePAP study. *Sleep, 35*(6), 757–767.

79. Berry, R. B., Brooks, R., Gamaldo, C., et al. (2017). AASM Scoring Manual Updates for 2017 (Version 2.4). *Journal of Clinical Sleep Medicine, 13*(5), 665–666.

80. Zhao, Y. Y., Weng, J., Mobley, D. R., et al. (2017). Effect of manual editing of total recording time: Implications for home sleep apnea testing. *Journal of Clinical Sleep Medicine, 13*(1), 121–126.

81. Maimon, N., & Hanly, P. J. (2010). Does snoring intensity correlate with the severity of obstructive sleep apnea? *Journal of Clinical Sleep Medicine, 6*(5), 475–478.

82. Fiz, J. A., Jane, R., Sola-Soler, J., et al. (2010). Continuous analysis and monitoring of snores and their relationship to the apnea–hypopnea index. *Laryngoscope, 120*(4), 854–862.

83. Karci, E., Dogrusoz, Y. S., & Ciloglu, T. (2011). Detection of post apnea sounds and apnea periods from sleep sounds. *Conference Proceedings: Annual International Conference of the IEEE Engineering in Medicine and Biology Society, 2011*, 6075–6078.

84. Sola-Soler, J., Fiz, J. A., Morera, J., et al. (2011). Bayes classification of snoring subjects with and without sleep apnea–hypopnea syndrome, using a Kernel method. *Conference Proceedings: Annual International Conference of the IEEE Engineering in Medicine and Biology Society, 2011*, 6071–6074.

85. Lee, L. A., Yu, J. F., Lo, Y. L., et al. (2012). Energy types of snoring sounds in patients with obstructive sleep apnea syndrome: A preliminary observation. *PLoS One, 7*(12), e53481.

86. Mindell, J. A., Bartle, A., Wahab, N. A., et al. (2011). Sleep education in medical school curriculum: A glimpse across countries. *Sleep Medicine, 12*(9), 928–931.

87. Reddy, E. V., Kadhiravan, T., Mishra, H. K., et al. (2009). Prevalence and risk factors of obstructive sleep apnea among middle-aged urban Indians: A community-based study. *Sleep Medicine, 10*(8), 913–918.

88. Mallick, H. N., & Kumar, V. M. (2016). Sleep medicine education in India. *Sleep and Biological Rhythms, 14*(1), 37–44.

89. Neruntarat, C., & Chantapant, S. (2011). Prevalence of sleep apnea in HRH Princess Maha Chakri Srinthorn Medical Center, Thailand. *Sleep Breath, 15*(4), 641–648.

90. Veeravigrom, M., & Desudchit, T. (2016). Prevalence of sleep disorders in Thai children. *Indian Journal of Pediatrics, 83*(11), 1237–1241.

91. Tantrakul, V., Preutthipan, A., & Maranetra, N. (2016). Sleep medicine in Thailand. *Sleep and Biological Rhythms, 14*(1), 31–35.

92. Sunwoo, J. S., Hwangbo, Y., Kim, W. J., et al. (2018). Prevalence, sleep characteristics, and comorbidities in a population at high risk for obstructive sleep apnea: A nationwide questionnaire study in South Korea. *PLoS One, 13*(2), e0193549.

93. Kim, J., In, K., Kim, J., et al. (2004). Prevalence of sleep-disordered breathing in middle-aged Korean men and women. *American Journal of Respiratory and Critical Care Medicine, 170*(10), 1108–1113.

94. Shin, C. (2016). Sleep education in Korea. *Sleep and Biological Rhythms, 14*(1), 27–29.

95. Yusoff, M. F., Baki, M. M., Mohamed, N., et al. (2010). Obstructive sleep apnea among express bus drivers in Malaysia: Important indicators for screening. *Traffic Injury Prevention, 11*(6), 594–599.

chapter 3
Modern Sleep Medicine

SHARON A. KEENAN   ROBIN E. FOSTER

LEARNING OBJECTIVES

On completion of this chapter, the reader should be able to:

1. Outline the fundamental development of modern sleep medicine.
2. Describe modern sleep medicine and current scope of practice.
3. Define the impact of undiagnosed sleep problems.
4. Appreciate the role of the polysomnographic technologist in modern sleep medicine.
5. Describe the potential scope of sleep health care, education, and the urgency for social change.

KEY TERMS

Sleep medicine
History
Polysomnography
Clinic model
Public health/consequences/education

There is agreement on a number of important conclusions (1) regarding sleep. These include the following:

- Sleep is a process necessary to ensure normal physiologic, mental, and emotional functions during waking hours.
- In the development of the central nervous system (CNS), sleep provides a foundation for the development of normal alertness, attention, and productive wakefulness.
- Perturbations in the development of sleep mechanisms in early childhood pose a higher risk of problems with attention, alertness, and emotional well-being later in life.
- Sleep is a necessary healing and recovery state.
- Abnormal sleep can cause psychological or physical illness or death.
- Treatment of sleep disorders improves physical well-being and quality of life and can be instrumental in the treatment of medical and psychiatric disease.

The history of sleep medicine is relatively brief but extremely rich. It includes brilliant basic science developed around the world throughout the 20th century until now. Dr. Nathaniel Kleitman, who is regarded as the father of American sleep research, began his work in the 1920s examining sleep and wakefulness and the nature of circadian rhythms (2). In 1953 Kleitman and one of his students, Dr. Eugene Aserinsky, made the landmark discovery of rapid eye movement (REM) during sleep. Another of Kleitman's students, Dr. William C. Dement, extended Dr. Kleitman's path of research. Dement described the "cyclical" nature of nocturnal sleep in 1955, and in 1957 and 1958 established the relationship between REM sleep and dreaming (3).

The Sleep Research Society (SRS) was established in 1961 when a small group of sleep researchers met at the University of Chicago to share ideas and data. The host scientists that year were Drs. Nathaniel Kleitman, Allan Rechtschaffen, and William Dement (4). The SRS fosters research from basic sleep research to clinical sleep medicine practice research across the different disciplines in sleep medicine.

Subsequent rapid development of clinical practice in sleep medicine has occurred over the past 40 years. The clinical specialty began in 1970 when Dr. William C. Dement established the world's first sleep disorders clinic at Stanford University. It was Dr. Jerome Holland, a member of the Stanford group, who first coined the term *polysomnography* (2). Sleep medicine has expanded to include sleep centers throughout the world.

According to the National Sleep Foundation, a lack of sleep health education and consequent undiagnosed sleep disorders represents a major public health problem. There are a limited number of sleep medicine specialists who provide health care to individuals with difficulties sleeping or staying awake. The integration of information about physiology and pathophysiology during sleep into the overall evaluation of patient health is a cornerstone of modern sleep medicine and should be a part of every routine physical examination. This critical integration of information about sleep does not happen on a broad-enough scale—partly because of a lack of systematic education about sleep in medical school.

The challenge for clinicians and researchers alike is to understand sleep-related changes in physiology and their impact on the quality and quantity of sleep and consequent impact on waking function. Only recently has there been recognition of the role of healthy sleep for optimal physical and emotional well-being and performance.

The Association of Sleep Disorders Centers (ASDC) was founded in 1976. In 1987, the ASDC changed its name to the American Sleep Disorders Association (ASDA), and in 1999, the ASDA was renamed the American Academy of Sleep Medicine (AASM) (5).

The Association of Polysomnographic Technologists (APT) was established in 1978. It was renamed the American Association of Sleep Technologists (AAST) in 2007. The Board of Registered Polysomnographic Technologists (BRPT) was established as a committee of the APT. In 2000, the BRPT became a separate organization with a primary focus on technologist credentialing. In 2005, the AASM commissioned a Polysomnographic Technologist Issues Committee consisting of educators, clinicians, and technologists. Their goal was to meet the educational needs of sleep technologists. They developed the Accredited Sleep Technologist Education Program (ASTEP) to promote the standardization of sleep technologist education and training and to equip students with the knowledge and skills they need to excel in the profession of sleep technology (6). These programs are AASM accredited and are provided by AASM-accredited sleep centers.

The ASTEP consists of an 80-hour didactic introductory course provided in an AASM-accredited sleep center or affiliated academic institution and an e-learning program consisting of AASM-developed ASTEP online self-study modules completed while the technician completes 18 months of on-the-job training provided by their employer (7). The standards for accreditation of educational programs in sleep technology are available on the AASM website. The AASM began accepting applications for accreditation of ASTEPs in January 2006.

The ultimate educational goal for sleep technologists is formal college-based education in sleep technology. Accredited college programs in sleep technology have been developed across the country. These programs are accredited through the Commission on Accreditation of Allied Health Education Programs (CAAHEP). The Committee on Accreditation for Polysomnographic Technologist Education (CoA PSG) is sponsored by the AAST and the BRPT and comprises nine members (3). The committee's purpose is to facilitate the accreditation of allied health programs through CAAHEP by establishing standards and guidelines for college programs in polysomnographic technology and reviewing applications for accreditation of such programs.

At the time of this writing, CAAHEP has accredited 45 programs in polysomnography. Some programs offer both a certificate and an associate degree. Currently, there are 25 certificate programs, 17 associate degree programs, 2 bachelor's degree programs, and 7 accredited online/distance education programs (8). At the time of this publication, there is one master's degree program in the process of achieving accreditation. This programmatic accreditation process continues to grow until there are enough college programs accredited to meet the educational needs of this field that has grown so rapidly. There is also a distance education program offering an MSc in sleep medicine through Nuffield Department of Clinical Neurosciences at the University of Oxford, UK (9).

Although sleep medicine has its roots in psychiatry and neurology, specialists from many areas of medicine provide sleep health care. Pulmonologists became active in clinical practice of sleep medicine after the initial description of obstructive sleep apnea (OSA) in the mid-1970s. Pediatricians, pediatric neurologists, pediatric pulmonologists, and pediatric psychiatrists also recognize that sleep disorders are common in children. Psychologists play an important role in the care and treatment of sleep disorder patients.

In 2003, the first behavioral sleep medicine board examination was administered to approximately 30 individuals by the AASM's Behavioral Sleep Medicine Committee. "Following the completion of the 2008 examination cycle, the administration of the certification examination in behavioral sleep medicine was transferred to the American Board of Sleep Medicine." As of this writing, there were 214 individuals certified in behavioral sleep medicine (10). Sleep medicine is an interdisciplinary field that includes practitioners from internal medicine and its relevant subspecialties including otolaryngology, neuroscience, dentistry, pharmacology, gerontology, and nursing.

There are more nurses serving as health care providers than any other professional group in the United States. Nurses are a valuable resource for advocating healthy sleep as well as promoting the diagnosis and treatment of sleep disorders. They are in a unique position in all areas of medicine to contribute to diagnosis and treatment of sleep disorders because of the amount of contact they have with patients and their ability to educate them. Nurses, nurse practitioners, and physician assistants make excellent case managers for patients suffering from sleep disorders. They have the same problem as all health care professionals: a limited availability of education in the interdisciplinary field of sleep medicine. Courses in sleep medicine are being added to nursing educational programs for both undergraduate and graduate degrees. Unfortunately, this is only occurring on a limited basis.

Education in sleep medicine will expand in time. The traditional order of implementation of a new medical science is that research informs and guides clinical practice. Institutions are slow to incorporate newly acquired knowledge into curricula. Sleep professionals and the AASM provide critical input into curriculum development and have been instrumental in providing education for the public and the professional sectors as well as supporting legislation for licensure of practitioners.

In June 1996, the AASM was granted a seat in the House of Delegates of the American Medical Association (AMA). In December 2003, the AMA awarded the Resident Recognition of Excellence distinction to the AASM for their efforts with the "Sleep, Fatigue, and Medical Training" conference in October 2001, and the Sleep, Alertness, and Fatigue Education in Residency (SAFER) educational module (11).

The American Board of Medical Specialties (ABMS) has recognized the ABSM certification examination for sleep medicine. This was an important milestone in the further recognition of sleep medicine as a medical specialty. Four ABMS boards have developed a sleep medicine certification program and as of 2007 administer the examination for certification in the subspecialty of sleep medicine. They include the American Board of Pulmonology, the American Board of Psychiatry and Neurology, the American Board of Otolaryngology, and the American Board of Pediatrics. The member boards of the American Osteopathic Association have also approved a subspecialty examination in sleep medicine. The American Osteopathic Board of Internal Medicine administered the first certification examination in sleep medicine in 2009.

MEDICAL–TECHNICAL INTERFACE

Sleep medicine is unique in the level of cooperation, support, and information exchange required between medical and technical teams in the diagnosis and treatment of sleep disorders. Technologists enter the field from a variety of allied health professions including neurodiagnostics, respiratory therapy, biomedical engineering, and nursing. Many receive technical and clinical training without medical background, and many technologists spend time in the rich clinical and technical environment of the sleep laboratory while continuing on their path to graduate or medical school. Other seasoned, highly esteemed technologists have spent over a quarter of a century dedicated to clinical polysomnography and patient care.

The technical advances in sleep medicine and technology have been very exciting. A recent report describes the use of a wireless wide area network to conduct polysomnography on hospitalized patients (12). It is likely that in the next couple of decades we will see the systematic integration of the collection of numerous physiologic parameters during sleep in all hospitalized patients.

SCOPE OF PRACTICE

Who has sleep disorders? Infants, children, adolescents, adults, and seniors of either sex experience problems with sleep. First published in 1979 (13), the 2014 revised edition of the *International Classification of Sleep Disorders*, or *ICSD-3*, describes multiple diagnoses for symptoms related to insufficient sleep, excessive sleepiness, or a mismatch of sleep and circadian or environmental factors (14).

Currently insomnia, the most common sleep disorder, is often left untreated. Estimates from the National Sleep Foundation (NSF) Sleep in America poll show that approximately one-third of the US population suffers from insomnia, and as many as 47 million adults may be at risk for injury and/or death and behavior problems because they do not get as much sleep as they need. The 2018 poll demonstrated that people understand the link between sleep and effectiveness but only a few prioritize sleep and plan for adequate sleep at the right time (15). And, "people have inherently different threshold susceptibility to fatigue and comorbidities induced by sleep deprivation" (16). Individuals with insomnia report difficulty initiating or maintaining sleep, waking too early in the morning, or having sleep that is not refreshing. Effective cognitive, behavioral, and pharmacologic treatments are available for patients who suffer from insomnia.

There are a limited number of sleep centers that offer specialized services for the treatment of insomnia. The polysomnogram (PSG), a sleep study and standard diagnostic tool, is not required according to the AASM guidelines set forth in the practice parameters for the treatment of insomnia. *However*, if there is a suspected comorbid physiologic sleep-related problem *or* if the patient is not responding to behavioral and/or pharmacologic therapy after a reasonable period of time, a PSG may be indicated. It is important to obtain objective data during sleep for these patients to rule out an underlying physiologic etiology for their insomnia complaint. Sadly, at the time of this writing, sleep studies for patients with the complaint of insomnia are not reimbursed by third-party payers. Consequently, insomniacs are often referred to psychiatrists or psychologists (also often not supported by insurance) (16). Clearly, this is yet another example of the multidisciplinary nature of sleep disturbance and the need for a collaborative approach in supporting our patients in the goal of optimal sleep health.

Many patients who suffer from OSA syndrome and other sleep-related breathing problems often report snoring. They suffer from the inability to sleep and breathe effectively at the same time. Often they report difficulty with staying awake and alert. Most commonly, they come to the clinic because of complaints of the bed partner or family member (17 to 22).

Narcolepsy, another disorder of the sleep–wake system, is characterized by difficulty maintaining wakefulness. Patients with narcolepsy suffer lack of CNS organization of wakefulness, non-REM sleep, and REM sleep. These patients are effectively treated with stimulant medication and medication that reduces REM sleep. Narcolepsy is a brilliant example of a disorder that allows opportunity to gain insight into the function of the brain. Some of the most exciting basic science in the last decade has been in the study of narcolepsy and the identification of a novel neurotransmitter system (23) and the elucidation of genetics specific to the disorder (24).

Other common sleep disorders such as restless legs syndrome and periodic limb movements during sleep are less well understood but under intense investigation (25). Restless legs syndrome is a disorder characterized by painful or uncomfortable sensations in the legs and an urge to move in order to relieve the discomfort. Basic science research has resulted in the development of numerous medications and techniques for the treatment of these disorders.

LACK OF RECOGNITION

Patients often suffer for many years before finding appropriate diagnosis and treatment for their sleep disorders. There are two important reasons. The first is that, as mentioned previously, sleep medicine is not systematically taught in medical schools. A survey of US medical schools conducted under the auspices of the National Commission of Sleep Disorders Research found that most medical schools do not teach normal sleep or fundamentals of sleep disorders. This survey also reported that medical students receive an average of 20 minutes to 2 hours of sleep education during their entire time in medical school (26). The AASM and others are working aggressively to change this. Second, the general population does not recognize disordered sleep as a legitimate medical complaint. Sleep complaints are normalized or expected as a consequence of aging or a stressful lifestyle.

Sound argument can be made that every *health care practitioner*, and every *mental health care practitioner*, *should ask their patients about sleep*. Pediatricians need to recognize the impact of lack of sleep or poor quality of sleep on a child's behavior and his or her ability to perform in an academic setting (27). Failure to thrive is seen in neonates, and growth retardation is seen in children with sleep-related breathing problems (28, 29). In April of 2003, the American Academy of Pediatrics released a position paper stating that snoring is not normal for a child and that if a child snores on a regular basis there is a need for evaluation (30). Recent literature points to the importance of recognizing the

association between OSA and preeclampsia in pregnant women (31). Use of continuous positive airway pressure has been demonstrated to improve clinical outcomes for patients with preeclampsia (32). Indeed, any patient with any medical disorder may suffer poor sleep secondary to medication, other treatments, or simply suffering from the disease.

The National Institute of Aging has reported that the second most common reason for institutionalization of the elderly is the family's inability to manage sleep-related problems, such as nocturnal wandering. Often the sleep-related problems of elderly family members have a negative impact on the sleep of family wage earners and their performance at work. The list goes on to describe negative consequences with the lack of recognition and education on the importance of healthy sleep.

MODELS OF CLINICAL PRACTICE

Historically, health care for sleep disorders has been delivered in a clinic model. In the ideal circumstance, the patient is seen in a sleep center for consultation, physical examination, and polysomnographic evaluation and is treated and followed to evaluate the effectiveness of treatment.

Highly trained sleep technologists collect objective data for various physiologic parameters, including brain and muscular activity, eye movement, heart rate, breathing patterns, level of blood oxygen saturation and carbon dioxide levels, movement, temperature, body position, and a host of other parameters that may be important for the individual patient. The clinic model is still the gold standard of sleep medicine practice. However, it is well recognized that in order to meet the needs of the millions of undiagnosed patients, alternatives to this model must be considered. This is especially true in light of limitations of critical resources such as trained professionals and clinical services. Currently, there is a lack of well-trained sleep technologists and clinicians. Satellite centers exist where data are collected in remote centers and sent to a central location for analysis and interpretation. Diagnostic testing also occurs within patients' homes. Some devices focus exclusively on cardiopulmonary aspects and have been used for screening and follow-up for patients with sleep-related breathing disorders.

We can accomplish a great deal simply by asking questions. A brief sleep questionnaire must be administered as part of the annual examination or when patients present for medical problems. As children enter the school system, they typically are required to have a physical examination. This is an opportunity to systematically evaluate for sleep disorders with simple questionnaires and triage children who are at high risk for sleep disorders. This interface would also provide a chance to educate parents, teachers, and children about healthy sleep.

General practitioners, family practitioners, internists, and nurses should ask every patient about the quality and quantity of his or her sleep. It must become the standard of practice for patients to be asked about their sleep upon admission to a hospital, when checking into the emergency department, and before having surgery. All clinicians should help identify patients who are at risk for sleep disorders and refer them for more comprehensive evaluation, diagnosis, and treatment.

SUMMARY

It is clear that the scope of sleep medicine is broad. Every physician, health care worker, and mental health care worker should have knowledge of the essentials of optimal sleep health and awareness of sleep disorders and complications when they are left untreated. Engel (33) argued for the understanding of every patient from a biologic, psychological, and social perspective. Sleep is an essential physiologic process, and it is well recognized that perturbations of this process have consequences on biologic, physiologic, psychological, and societal levels. From a psychological perspective, individuals who suffer sleep deprivation often report irritability and anxiety as well as poor performance, health, and quality of life. The social consequences of untreated sleep disorders are profound. If the biologic and psychological consequences of individual patients are ignored, we as a society share the consequences in terms of increased risk of accidents and a decrease in public health and safety. Some examples of these consequences include the following (34):

- The annual direct cost of sleep-related problems in the United States is in the billions.
- Over 100,000 motor vehicle accidents that occur annually are sleep related.
- Disasters such as Chernobyl, Three Mile Island, Challenger, Bhopal, and Exxon Valdez were officially attributed to errors in judgment induced by sleepiness or fatigue.

Data have demonstrated that patients undiagnosed for sleep disorders use health care resources at a higher rate. Also, recent findings regarding cardiovascular morbidity and undiagnosed sleep disordered breathing (SDB), as well as the findings linking SDB and menopause, point to the possibility for early intervention and prevention. Not only do millions of patients suffer needlessly, but it is also possible to save millions of dollars in health care costs with early diagnosis and treatment of sleep disorders and foster improved quality of life for millions of people.

Sleep affects and is affected by every system of the body in ways that we have yet to understand completely. Sleep medicine is still an emerging field that offers a unique opportunity to positively impact the lives of millions of patients and improve quality of life. The backgrounds and expertise of those who practice sleep medicine and sleep technology are wide ranging and varied. This heterogeneity lends strength to the discipline and speaks to the broad scope of our field. The challenge we face as clinicians, scientists, and technologists is to remain open minded and committed to the cause. It is an exciting adventure and provides great opportunity to increase our appreciation and understanding of the wonders of sleep and decrease suffering for some of our fellow humans.

REFERENCES

1. Golbin, A., Kravitz, H., & Keith, L. G. (2004). *Sleep psychiatry*. London, UK: Taylor & Francis Publishing/CRC Group.
2. Todman, D. (2008). A history of sleep medicine. *The Internet Journal of Neurology, 9*(2). Retrieved from www.ispub.com
3. Stanford University. (1999). *A brief history of sleep research*. Retrieved from www.stanford.edu/~dement/history.html
4. Shepard, J. W., Jr., Buysse, D. J., Chesson, A. L., Jr., et al. (2005). History of the development of sleep medicine in the United States. *Journal of Clinical Sleep Medicine, 1*(1), 61–82.
5. Talk About Sleep. (2011). *A brief history of sleep medicine*. Retrieved from www.talkaboutsleep.com/sleep-disorders/archives/history.htm
6. Epstein, L. J. (2006). The profession of sleep technology. *Sleep Review: The Journal for Sleep Specialists*. Retrieved from www.sleepreviewmag.com/issues/articles/2006-0-07.asp
7. American Academy of Sleep Medicine. (2009). *Accredited sleep technology education program*. Retrieved from www.aasmnet.org/astep
8. Commission on Accreditation of Allied Health Education Programs. (2011). *Accredited program search—CAAHEP*. Retrieved from https://www.caahep.org/Students/Find-a-Program.aspx
9. University of Oxford. (2018). *MSc in sleep medicine*. Retrieved from https://www.ox.ac.uk/admissions/graduate/courses/msc-sleep-medicine?wssl=1
10. American Board of Sleep Medicine. (2011). *Certification—Behavioral sleep medicine*. Retrieved from www.absm.org/BSMCertification.aspx
11. Owens, J. A. (2001). Sleep loss and fatigue in medical training: Sleep, alertness and fatigue education in residency (SAFER). *Current Opinions in Pulmonary Medicine, 7*(6), 411–418.

12. Farney, R. J., Walker, J. M., Cloward, T. V., et al. (2006). Polysomnography in hospitalized patients using a wireless wide area network. *Journal of Clinical Sleep Medicine, 2*(1), 28–34.

13. Association of Sleep Disorders Centers and the Association for the Psychophysiological Study of Sleep. (1979). Diagnostic classification of sleep and arousal disorders. *Sleep, 2*(1), 1–154.

14. American Academy of Sleep Medicine. (2014). *The international classification of sleep disorders: Diagnostic and coding manual* (3rd ed.). Darien, IL: Author.

15. Sleep.org. (1999–2018). *NSF sleep in America poll.* Retrieved from www.sleep.org

16. Candaras, M. M. (2011). *Current understanding of sleep, its disorders and treatment trends.* Retrieved from www.sleepreviewmag.com

17. Apnex Medical. (2011). *Obstructive sleep apnea FAQs.* Retrieved from www.apnexmedical.com

18. Young, T., Palta, M., Dempsey, J., et al. (1993). The occurrence of sleep-disordered breathing among middle-aged adults. *New England Journal of Medicine, 328*(17), 1230–1235.

19. Lee, K. A. (1998). Alterations in sleep during pregnancy and post-partum: A review of 30 years of research. *Sleep Medicine Review, 2*(4), 231–242.

20. Edwards, N., Middleton, P. G., Blyton, D. M., et al. (2002). Sleep-disordered breathing and pregnancy. *Thorax, 57*(6), 555–558.

21. Young, T., Blustein, J., Finn, L., et al. (1997). Sleep-disordered breathing and motor vehicle accidents in a population-based sample of employed adults. *Sleep, 20*(8), 608–613.

22. Quan, S. F., Howard, B. V., Iber, C., et al. (1997). The Sleep Heart Health Study: Design, rationale, and methods. *Sleep, 20*(12), 1077–1085.

23. Mignot, E., Lammers, G. J., Ripley, B., et al. (2002). The role of cerebrospinal fluid hypocretin measurement in the diagnosis of narcolepsy and other hypersomnias. *Archives of Neurology, 59,* 1553–1562.

24. Lin, L., Faraco, J., Li, R., et al. (1999). Sleep disorder canine narcolepsy is caused by a mutation in the hypocretin (orexin) receptor 2 gene. *Cell, 98,* 365–376.

25. Chokroverty, S., Hening, W., & Walters, A. (Eds.). (2002). *Sleep and movement disorders.* Boston, MA: Butterworth-Heinemann.

26. Rosen, R. C., Rosekind, M., Rosevear, C., et al. (1993). Physician education in sleep and sleep disorders: A national survey of U.S. medical schools. *Sleep, 16*(3), 249–254.

27. Owens, J. A., & Mindell, J. A. (2006). Pediatric sleep medicine: Priorities for research, patient care, policy and education. (A report from the conference held February 19–20, 2005, Amelia Island, Florida.) *Journal of Clinical Sleep Medicine, 2*(1), 77–88.

28. Everett, A. D., Koch, W. C., & Saulsbury, F. T. (1987). Failure to thrive due to obstructive sleep apnea. *Clinical Pediatrics, 26,* 90–92.

29. Freezer, N. F., Bucins, L. K., & Robertson, C. F. (1995). Obstructive sleep apnea presenting as failure to thrive in infancy. *Journal of Pediatric Child Health, 31,* 172–175.

30. American Academy of Pediatrics. (2016). Policy statement, clinical practice guideline: Diagnosis and management of childhood obstructive sleep apnea syndrome. *Pediatrics, 190*(4), 704–712.

31. Edwards, N., Blyton, C. M., Kesby, G. J., et al. (2000). Pre-eclampsia is associated with marked alterations in sleep architecture. *Sleep, 23*(5), 609–625.

32. Blyton, D. M., Sullivan, C. E., & Edwards, N. (2004). Reduced nocturnal cardiac output associated with preeclampsia is minimized with the use of nocturnal nasal CPAP. *Sleep, 27*(1), 79–84.

33. Engel, G. L. (1997). The need for a new medical model: A challenge for biomedicine. *Science, 196,* 129–136.

34. University of Maryland Medical Center. (2010). *Sleep disorders center.* Retrieved from www.umm.edu/sleep/sleep_dis_main.htm

SECTION 2
Anatomy and Physiology

chapter 4

The Biologic, Anatomic, and Physiologic Aspects of the Biopotentials of Sleep

REGINA PATRICK

LEARNING OBJECTIVES

On completion of this chapter, the reader should be able to:

1. Describe how individual cells generate electrical potentials.
2. Appreciate that surface electrodes attached to the skin record the electrical potentials associated with many cells and not individual cells.
3. Describe skin anatomy and the principles of recording biopotentials using surface electrodes.
4. Describe the biopotentials of the heart, muscles, skin, and eyes.
5. Describe the basic anatomy of the eye, brain, heart, and respiratory system.

KEY TERMS

Biopotential
Electroencephalogram
Electromyogram
Electrooculogram
Neuron
Neurotransmitter
Reticular formation
Suprachiasmatic nucleus

A polysomnograph (PSG) is a device that measures the electrical activity generated by the brain, heart, skeletal muscles, and eyes. The activity is extremely small, but a PSG is able to record this activity through sensors placed on the scalp, chest, chin, legs, and outer canthus of the eyes. The sensors relay the electrical activity to amplifiers that increase the signal. The electrical activity can then be viewed in a visual form on a polysomnogram (i.e., the recording produced by a PSG). On a polysomnogram, the recording of the electrical activity of the brain is called an electroencephalogram (EEG); the electrical activity of the heart, an electrocardiogram (ECG); the

electrical activity of the muscles, an electromyogram (EMG); and the electrical activity of the eyes, an electrooculogram (EOG). A polysomnogram also presents information on respiratory activity, which is transmitted by respiratory sensors that detect airflow and air pressure changes through the nose and mouth and by sensors that detect mechanical activity created by respiratory movements of the chest and the abdomen. The signals from these sensors are transformed into an electrical signal, amplified, and viewed on the respiratory channels of a polysomnogram.

The first portion of this chapter describes how biopotentials are generated and briefly describes the biopotentials of the heart, brain, muscle, integumentary (i.e., skin) cells, and eye. The second portion of this chapter gives a basic description of the anatomy of the brain, heart, and respiratory system with an emphasis on their physiologic relation to sleep.

BIOPOTENTIALS

In living organisms, a biopotential is electrical activity that results from chemical processes (i.e., biochemical processes). In living cells, biopotentials result from the movement of ions (i.e., electrically charged atoms or molecules) across a cell's membrane. The fluid within a cell (i.e., intracellular fluid or cytoplasm) contains ions such as sodium (Na^+), potassium (K^+), chloride (Cl^-), and calcium (Ca^{2+}). The fluid that surrounds a cell is called "extracellular fluid"; it contains these same ions but at a different concentration.

The relative difference in the net charge between the intracellular and extracellular fluid of a cell creates an electrical potential across the cell's membrane. Potential (from Latin *potentia*, meaning "power") refers to the work needed to move ions across a cell's membrane. A cell's baseline electrical potential—that is, when it is not transmitting a signal—is called its "resting potential" or "membrane polarization." A decrease in a cell's electrical potential (i.e., a decrease in the electrical difference across the cell membrane) is called "depolarization." An increase in a cell's electrical potential (i.e., an increase in the electrical difference across the cell membrane) is called "hyperpolarization."

Depolarization and hyperpolarization come about through the movement of ions across a cell's membrane. Depolarization can occur if an excess of positively charged ions enters from the extracellular fluid into the intracellular fluid or an excess of negatively charged ions exits from the intracellular fluid and enters the extracellular fluid. Hyperpolarization can occur if an excess of negatively charged ions enters from the extracellular fluid into the intracellular fluid or an excess of positively charged ions exits from the intracellular fluid and enters the extracellular fluid.

A cell's potential is usually expressed by the electrical charge, usually in millivolts (mV), of its intracellular fluid with respect to the fluid outside the cell. A cell's potential is expressed as a positive value (e.g., +55 mV) when the electrical charge of the intracellular fluid is more positive than that of the extracellular fluid, and a cell's potential is expressed as a negative value (e.g., −55 mV) when the electrical charge of the intracellular fluid is more negative than that of the extracellular fluid.

Ions move across a cell's membrane through ion channels, which are proteins interspersed on the surface of a cell's membrane. The molecular structure of the proteins that make up an ion channel is arranged in a way that gives the ion channel a unique "shape." This shape allows only certain ions to flow into or out of a cell. A change in the shape of an ion channel changes how it functions. For example, a small change in an ion channel's shape may allow a sudden increase or decrease in the rate at which certain ions flow through the ion channel. In the process, the electrical potential between intracellular and extracellular fluids changes and a cell may become depolarized or hyperpolarized.

After the process of depolarization or hyperpolarization begins, ion channels quickly work to restore the resting potential. Restoration of the resting potential is called "repolarization." However, as one area of a cell's membrane undergoes repolarization, the process of depolarization (or hyperpolarization) continues along the length of the cell's membrane like a wave. Newly depolarized (or hyperpolarized) areas quickly undergo repolarization as the wave of depolarization (or hyperpolarization) continues along the cell's membrane. Depolarization typically enhances the propagation of a signal from cell to cell, and hyperpolarization typically inhibits the transmission of signals from cell to cell (Fig. 4-1).

Nerve cells (i.e., neurons), muscle cells, and heart cells are unable to transmit an impulse until the electrical potential decreases (i.e., depolarizes) to a certain level. The point at which an impulse becomes possible is called the "threshold potential." The electrical potential that exists when a cell is transmitting an impulse is called its "action potential."

Biopotentials measured on the surface of the body are extremely small—one-millionth or one-thousandth of a volt (microvolts [μV] or mV, respectively). The following sections briefly describe the biopotentials that occur in the heart, brain, muscles, and skin.

Cardiac Biopotentials

Biopotential changes in the heart are involved in the rhythmicity of heart contractions. The sinoatrial (SA) node is the pacemaker of the heart. It is in the right atrium, which is one of two upper chambers of the heart. (The plural of atrium is "atria.") The resting potential of the SA node cells is −90 mV. Certain ion channels in the cells of the SA node allow a continuous outflow of K^+ and inflow of Na^+ ions, which causes the cell's intracellular environment to become more positive (i.e., the cells depolarize). When the cells depolarize to their threshold potential at approximately −60 mV, calcium ion channels suddenly open, which allows the sudden influx of Ca^{2+} ions into the cells, further enhancing the depolarization process. An impulse results and spreads quickly throughout the heart's left and right atria. The impulse spreads so quickly that the atrial myocytes (i.e., heart muscle cells) contract in synchrony. After the atrial contraction, the atria repolarize. Meanwhile, the wave of depolarization spreads downward toward the atrioventricular (AV) node, which is another set of pacemaker cells. The AV node is at the bottom of the right atrium and just above the right ventricle. The AV node acts as a relay point between the atria and ventricles. The resting potential of the AV node cells is −60 mV. Once these cells become depolarized, they relay the signal to the bundle of His (also called the AV bundle; this bundle travels down the ventricular septum and then spreads over both ventricles). Depolarization of the bundle of

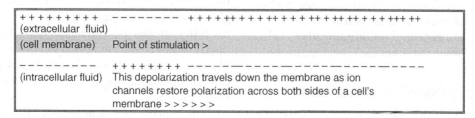

Figure 4-1 Net electrical charges across a cell membrane during depolarization.

His causes the ventricles to contract in synchrony. One heart contraction takes approximately 0.8 seconds.

Brain Biopotentials

The brain is made up of billions of neurons. A brain wave represents the collective activity of biopotential changes occurring among the neurons. A neuron has a central portion (i.e., the cell body) and extensions branching from the cell body. A neuron may have one or more short extensions (i.e., dendrites) and a single long extension (i.e., axon) branching from the cell body. Dendrites receive impulses and transmit them through the cell body; an axon carries the impulse away from the cell body. A neuron's resting potential ranges between −60 and −70 mV; its threshold potential is approximately −55 mV. When a neuron reaches its action potential, an impulse travels down the neuron's axon to the axon's terminal. At the terminal, the axon releases neurotransmitters such as serotonin, acetylcholine, and glutamic acid. On exiting the axonal terminal, a neurotransmitter enters a small space between the neuron's axonal terminal and the dendrite of an adjacent neuron. This space is called the "synaptic cleft." The average distance between cells in the synaptic cleft is approximately 20 to 30 nm. (A nanometer is one-billionth of a meter.) The neurotransmitter travels across the synaptic cleft and attaches to a receptor on the surface of an adjacent neuron's dendrites or cell body. Once the neurotransmitter is attached to the receptor, it can depolarize the neuron and cause the neuron to reach its action potential. In this way, electrical impulses are transmitted from neuron to neuron.

Muscle Biopotentials

A muscle contraction begins when a stimulus triggers an action potential within a neuron that innervates the muscle. The action potential travels down the neuron's axon toward the axonal terminal. At the terminal, neurotransmitters are released into the neuromuscular junction (i.e., the synapse between the axon of a neuron and a muscle fiber). The neurotransmitter travels across the neuromuscular junction to attach to receptors on the muscle fiber. The resting potential of skeletal muscle is −95 mV, and the threshold potential is −50 mV. Once the neurotransmitter attaches to the receptors on the muscle fiber, Na$^+$ ions flood into the muscle fiber. The muscle fiber depolarizes until it reaches its action potential. The action potential quickly spreads to other muscle fibers and results in a muscle contraction.

Integumentary (Skin) Biopotentials

The outermost layer of the skin (i.e., epidermis) consists of dead cells, which do not have electrical activity.

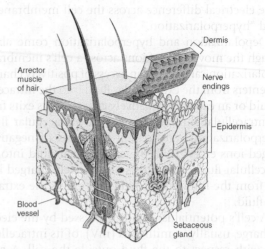

Figure 4-2 Basic overview of the skin. (Adapted from Neil O. Hardy, Neil Hardy Art Collection, Westport, Connecticut.)

However, two layers beneath the epidermis—the dermis and, below it, the hypodermis—have electrical activity (Fig. 4-2). In polysomnography, the biopotentials of the skin (i.e., dermis and hypodermis) are not measured. However, oil, sweat, and dead skin cells on the surface of the skin can create a barrier between the skin's surface and an electrode. This electrical barrier is called "resistance." Resistance can interfere with the recording of EEG, EMG, and ECG signals.

The metal of the electrode and the conductive electrode paste used in electrodes can retain some of the electrical charge recorded from the body. This storage is called "capacitance." The combination of capacitance and resistance is called "impedance." Excessive impedance can hinder the recording of a signal received by an electrode and affect the quality of a recording. An impedance meter is an instrument used to measure the impedance formed between an electrode and the surface of the skin. In polysomnography, impedance is measured in kilo-ohms. Properly cleaned skin should ideally have a reading of 5.0 kΩ or less.

Eye Biopotentials

The eye is a fluid-filled, globe-shaped organ. A round, clear, convex membrane—the cornea—extends slightly outward from the front of the eye. A circular-colored membrane—the iris—is visible though the cornea and gives a person's eye its color. The iris opens and contracts in response to light. Light enters the eye though an open circular center (the pupil) in the iris. A transparent biconvex lens situated behind the iris focuses the light onto a membrane, the retina, which lines much of the eye globe (Fig. 4-3).

The process of vision begins in the retina, following the refraction of light through the cornea and lens.

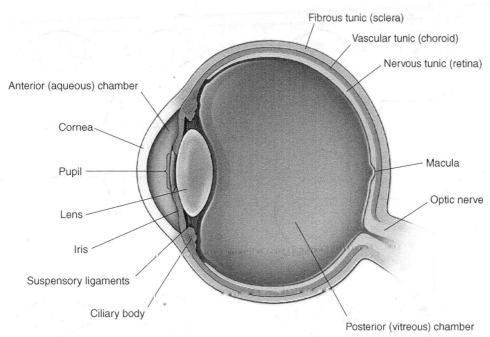

Figure 4-3 Basic eye anatomy. (Reprinted with permission from Detton AJ. *Grant's dissector, 16th ed.* [Figure 7-57]. Philadelphia, PA: ©Lippincott Williams & Wilkins/Wolters Kluwer, 2016.)

Through chemical reactions triggered by light (i.e., photochemical reaction), visual cells in the retina (e.g., cones, rods) transform light energy into a neurologic impulse that is transmitted from the retina, through the optic nerve, to the visual center of the brain where it is interpreted.

The electrical potential of the retina's visual cells before undergoing a photochemical reaction (i.e., the retina's resting potential) is approximately −30 to −40 mV. When a particle of light (i.e., a photon) strikes the rods and cones, ion channels on the surface of these cells change their shape. The shape change prevents positively charged sodium and potassium ions from entering the cells while allowing positively charged calcium ions to exit the cells. These two actions cause the intracellular environment of the rods and cones to become more negatively charged (i.e., hyperpolarized). Hyperpolarization of the rods and cones can approach −80 mV.

Epithelial cells that line the outer surface of the cornea secrete positively charged ions such as sodium (Na^+) and potassium (K^+) into the cornea and excrete negatively charged ions out of the cornea. This process creates a potential of approximately +30 to +40 mV across the membrane of the cornea. Because of the positive charge of the cornea and the negative charge of the retina, an electrical potential exists between the front and the back of the eye. This potential is called the "corneoretinal potential."

An EOG records changes that occur in the corneoretinal potential with eye movement. In polysomnography, two electrodes are used to record an EOG. Both electrodes are placed on the outer canthus (i.e., eye socket ridge), with one electrode placed above the midline of the outer canthus and the other placed below the midline of the outer canthus. (The right electrode is typically placed above the midline and the left electrode is placed below the midline [Fig. 4-4].)

As eyes move in tandem (i.e., conjugate eye movements), one electrode will be closer to the cornea, whereas the other will be closer to the retina. Hence, one electrode will record a positive impulse (recorded as a downward deflection), whereas the other electrode will record a negative impulse (recorded as an upward deflection) as the eyes move around (Fig. 4-5).

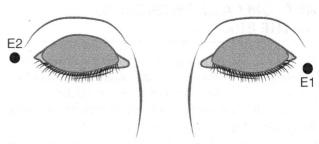

Figure 4-4 Electrode placement on the outer canthus.

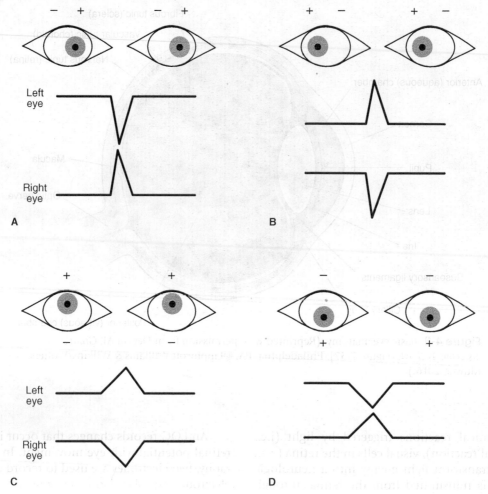

Figure 4-5 Positive and negative changes of the eyes and the left eye and right eye signals on the electrooculogram with eye movements. **A:** Eyes looking left. **B:** Eyes looking right. **C:** Eyes looking up. **D:** Eyes looking down.

Therefore, it is important that one electrode is placed above the midline and the other below the midline on the outer canthus. If both electrodes are placed in the same horizontal plane, vertical eye movements would be recorded as moving conjunctively (i.e., both EOG channels deflect in the same direction, or "in phase") rather than disjunctively (i.e., both EOG channels deflect in opposite directions, or "out of phase").

ANATOMY AND PHYSIOLOGY OF THE BRAIN

The brain consists of the cerebrum (which has two hemispheres), the midbrain, the brainstem (the stalk-like portion of the brain that connects the cerebral hemispheres with the spinal cord; the brainstem contains the midbrain, pons, and medulla), and the cerebellum (which has two hemispheres and extends from the back

of the brainstem). Several brain structures involved in sleep and wakefulness are in the brainstem (e.g., locus ceruleus, reticular formation, raphe nuclei) or near the base of the brain (e.g., thalamus, suprachiasmatic nucleus, hypothalamus, and the pineal gland). These structures have the following roles in sleep.

Locus Ceruleus

The locus ceruleus (pronounced "LOH-kus suh-ROO-lee-us"), a small blue-tinged area in the back of the brainstem, is involved in rapid eye movement (REM) sleep and in wakefulness (Fig. 4-6). The locus ceruleus contains neurons that release or are activated by norepinephrine, serotonin, and choline (i.e., norepinephrinergic, serotoninergic, and cholinergic neurons, respectively). These neurons fire quickly during wake, begin slow firing with the onset of sleep, continue to slow as sleep deepens, and then nearly stop firing during REM sleep. The locus ceruleus contains

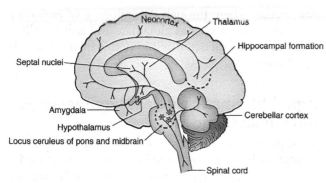

Figure 4-6 Locus ceruleus. (Reprinted with permission from Gould DJ, Brueckner-Collings JK, and Fix JD. *High-yield neuroanatomy, 5th ed*. Philadelphia, PA: ©Wolters Kluwer, 2015.)

a group of neurons, "REM-off" cells, that inhibit REM sleep (i.e., the action of these cells ends a REM period). The REM-off cells become increasingly active as REM sleep progresses and ultimately hinder the activity of the "REM-on" cells (i.e., these cells induce the onset of a REM period), which are in the pons and basal forebrain.

Reticular Formation

The reticular formation consists of diffuse groups of nerve cells that are embedded within a wealth of nerve fibers (Fig. 4-7), which gives it a mesh-like appearance when examined using a microscope. (In Latin, *reticulo* means "net.") The reticular formation runs throughout the inner core of the midbrain, pons, and medulla and fills the spaces between major nuclei and nerve tracts in the brainstem.

The alternation between sleep and wake cycles results from the neural interplay between the reticular formation and the cerebral cortex. The thalamus, a structure located just above the brainstem, relays signals between the cerebral cortex and the reticular formation. Increased cerebral activation results in activation of the reticular formation and consequently wakefulness. During sleep, fewer impulses arise from the cerebral cortex; therefore, there is decreased activation of the reticular formation.

The reticular formation has two components: the ascending reticular formation and the descending reticular formation. Of these two components, the ascending reticular formation (also called the "reticular activating system") is most directly involved in sleep and wake cycles and has a role in the overall degree of central nervous system activity. The ascending reticular formation receives sensory signals traveling from the periphery toward the brain; the signals are first relayed to the thalamus. From there, the signals are relayed to the cerebral cortex of the brain. The pathway from the thalamus to the cortex is called the "thalamocortical pathway." Neurons of the thalamocortical pathway release excitatory neurotransmitters such as glutamate, dopamine, noradrenaline, serotonin, and histamine to the cerebral cortex. These neurotransmitters are involved in wakefulness.

The descending reticular formation receives information from the hypothalamus and is involved in the degree of activity in the autonomic nervous system (i.e., the sympathetic and parasympathetic nervous systems collectively). Activation of the descending reticular formation allows the body to withstand the increase in autonomic nervous activity that occurs with wakefulness. An increase in the heart rate, respiratory rate, and muscle tone activates the descending reticular formation and thereby forms a positive feedback loop (i.e., as one factor increases, another factor also increases). The positive feedback loop is controlled by various dampening neural systems in the brain. If it were not dampened, the result would be an extreme arousal state and consequently a seizure.

Another arousal pathway in the brain extends from the reticular formation to the hypothalamus and, finally, to the cerebral cortex. This pathway is called the "reticulo-hypothalamo-cortical pathway." In the hypothalamus, a group of cells, called the "tuberomammillary nucleus," releases histamine to the cerebral cortex. The greatest amount of histamine in the cerebral cortex is synthesized during wake. A second group of cells in the hypothalamus produces the wake-promoting excitatory neurotransmitter orexin, which is also called "hypocretin."

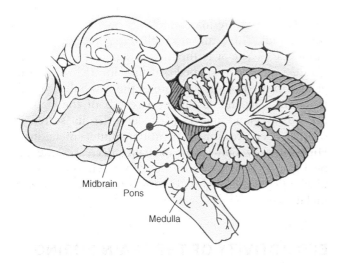

Figure 4-7 Ascending and descending axons in the reticular formation. (Reprinted with permission from Siegel A and Sapru HN. *Essential neuroscience 4th ed.*, [Figure 22.6]. Philadelphia, PA. ©Lippincott Williams & Wilkins/Wolters Kluwer, 2018.)

The basal forebrain (i.e., the base of the frontal lobe) has pathways that are involved in arousal and in REM sleep. Acetylcholine-synthesizing neurons in the basal forebrain project to the cerebral cortex. The neurotransmitter acetylcholine is involved in wakefulness and facilitates REM sleep, and the highest brain level of acetylcholine is synthesized during wake and REM sleep. The pons also contains a group of cholinergic neurons (i.e., REM-on cells) that facilitate REM sleep.

Reticular deactivation leads to sleep. This deactivation results from neuronal activity in the forebrain, pons, medulla, and cerebellum. For example, the basal forebrain contains neurons that synthesize the inhibitory neurotransmitter γ-amino butyric acid (GABA). These neurons project to the cerebral cortex, to the histamine-producing neurons of the tuberomammillary nucleus in the hypothalamus, and to the reticular formation. In these regions, GABA inhibits the activation of the reticular activating system through a negative feedback system (i.e., as one factor increases, another factor decreases) and thereby induces sleep.

Raphe Nuclei

The reticular formation contains several groups of cells, collectively called the "raphe nuclei," which consist of the caudal linear nucleus, dorsal raphe nucleus, median raphe nucleus, raphe magnus nucleus, raphe obscurus nucleus, and raphe pallidus nucleus. The raphe nuclei are clustered near the junction that separates the left and right sides of the brainstem. This junction is called the "raphe" (in Greek, *raphe* means "seam"). Nerve fibers that project from the raphe nuclei release the excitatory neurotransmitter serotonin to all parts of the brain, which contributes to wakefulness. During wake, the raphe nuclei neurons fire rapidly. They reduce their firing rate with sleep onset and increasingly reduce firing until nearly becoming quiescent in REM sleep. Exactly what triggers the cells to reduce their firing rate with sleep onset is unknown. A possibility is that other neurons (e.g., GABAergic neurons) indirectly or directly regulate the activity of other neurotransmitters involved in sleep.

Thalamus

The thalamic reticular nuclei are embedded within a thin layer of myelinated fibers, called the "internal medullary lamina," in the thalamus. The thalamic reticular nuclei neurons are GABAergic (i.e., they are activated by or synthesize GABA) and project from the thalamus to the reticular formation. During slow-wave sleep, the thalamic reticular nuclei neurons rhythmically shift between depolarization and hyperpolarization and result in the rhythmic bursting pattern of slow waves that occur during slow-wave sleep. The transition from sleep to wake occurs when, through the influence of excitatory neurotransmitters such as glutamate and acetylcholine, the thalamocortical neurons inhibit this rhythmic bursting pattern.

Suprachiasmatic Nuclei, Hypothalamus, and Pineal Gland

The suprachiasmatic nuclei (SCN) are important in the alternation between sleep and wake cycles. These nuclei are in the anterior hypothalamus. They receive signals by way of the retinohypothalamic tract, the geniculohypothalamic tract (i.e., the pathway between the geniculate bodies [i.e., four small round masses just beneath the thalamus] in the upper brainstem and the nearby hypothalamus), and the raphe nuclei.

The retinohypothalamic tract lies between the retina of each eye and the hypothalamus and is important in establishing the circadian rhythmicity of the sleep–wake cycle. The retina, a thin multilayered lining inside the eye, contains two types of light-sensitive visual cells: rods and cones. Rods make it possible for a person to see in dim light settings and to detect motion; cones make it possible for a person to perceive color.

When light strikes the rods and cones, photopigments (e.g., the protein rhodopsin) in these cells chemically transform the light energy into an action potential. The signal is relayed from the rods and cones to bipolar cells and finally to the ganglion cell layer in the retina. Fibers extending from the ganglion cells exit from the back of the eye as the optic nerve and project into the lateral geniculate bodies, which are involved in vision. From there, the signals are relayed to the visual center in the occipital lobe.

Some fibers from the retinal ganglion cells relay signals from the retina to the SCN in the anterior hypothalamus. This pathway is called the "retinohypothalamic tract." The SCN then relays signals to the pineal gland, a pine cone–shaped structure, located within the groove formed by the juncture of the two halves of the thalamus. Depending on the strength of the signals, the pineal gland increases or decreases its secretion of the sleep-promoting neurotransmitter melatonin. High-intensity light (e.g., daylight) decreases the pineal gland's production of melatonin, whereas low-intensity light (e.g., nightfall) increases its production of melatonin.

EEG ACTIVITY OF THE BRAIN DURING SLEEP

Electrodes used for recording EEG signals in polysomnography are too large to detect the activity of a single neuron. The signal recorded from an EEG electrode

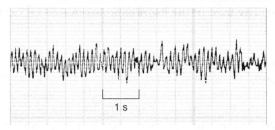

Figure 4-8 Alpha waves in stage N1 sleep.

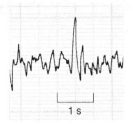

Figure 4-10 Sharp vertex wave in stage N2 sleep.

actually reflects the change in the collective electrical activity of numerous neurons on the surface of the brain beneath the site of the electrode. The change in the collective neuronal activity is called a "brainwave." On the EEG channels of a PSG, brainwaves fluctuate in characteristic ways for each stage of sleep and for wake. Brain waves of interest in polysomnography are alpha waves, theta waves, beta waves, spindles, K-complex waveforms, sharp vertex waves, delta waves (i.e., slow waves), and sawtooth waves. These waveforms are identified by frequency (i.e., the number of waves [cycles] per second, usually expressed in Hertz [Hz]); by peak-to-peak amplitude (representing the signal voltage); and by morphology (i.e., shape). Each stage of sleep has unique EEG waveforms.

Wake

During wake, the EEG shows low-amplitude, high-frequency activity. With the eyes closed during relaxed wakefulness, alpha waves (so named because they were the first brain waves discovered) initially appear intermittently among low-amplitude, high-frequency waves and ultimately become the dominant wave. (On opening the eyes, the waves drop out.) Alpha waves have a frequency of 8 to 13 Hz and are most prominent in the occipital region (Fig. 4-8).

Stage N1 Sleep

Alpha waves drop out and theta waves appear with the onset of sleep (i.e., stage N1). Theta waves have a frequency of 4 to 7 Hz (Fig. 4-9) and are the predominant waves of stage N1 sleep.

Stage N2 Sleep

A sharp vertex wave is a transient wave that commonly appears during the transition from stage N1 to stage N2 sleep. These waves have a negative (i.e., upward) deflection and last less than 0.5 seconds. The amplitude of these waves is maximal in the central channels; however, there is no amplitude criterion for a sharp vertex wave (Fig. 4-10).

As sleep progresses from stage N1 sleep to stage N2 sleep, the EEG amplitude remains somewhat low, but short bursts of fast, short-lasting activity begin to appear. These bursts are called "spindles" and are one indicator of the onset of stage N2 sleep. Spindles have a frequency of 11 to 16 Hz (more commonly 12 to 14 Hz) and typically last approximately 0.5 seconds or longer. Their maximal amplitude occurs in the central channels.

A second waveform that can indicate the onset of stage N2 sleep is the K-complex. A K-complex is a short lasting wave that begins with a sharp negative (i.e., upward) deflection, followed by a slower positive (i.e., downward) component. The duration of a K-complex is 0.5 seconds or longer. The maximal amplitude is usually in the frontal channels (Fig. 4-11).

Stage N3 Sleep (Slow-Wave Sleep)

As sleep progresses from stage N2 to slow-wave (i.e., stage N3) sleep, high-amplitude waves—slow waves (also called "delta waves")—begin to appear. Slow waves have a frequency of 0.5 to 2 Hz and a voltage of 75 μV or greater (Fig. 4-12). As N3 sleep progresses, the

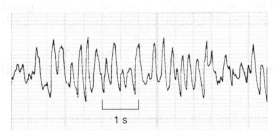

Figure 4-9 Theta waves in stage N1 sleep.

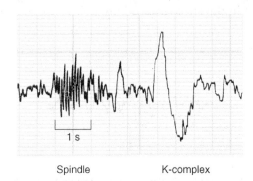

Spindle   K-complex

Figure 4-11 K-complex and spindle in stage N2 sleep.

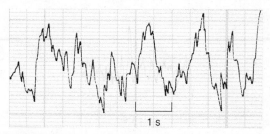

Figure 4-12 Slow waves in slow-wave sleep.

slow waves become increasingly dominant. They are most readily detected in the frontal channels.

Stage R Sleep (REM Sleep)

As sleep progresses from N3 sleep to REM sleep (i.e., stage R sleep), the voltage of the EEG waves dramatically decreases and the EEG appears very similar to stage N1. However, other channels on the PSG reveal features in this sleep stage that do not occur in N1 sleep. Just before stage R sleep, the electromyography channel (i.e., chin channel) shows the sudden loss of muscle tone, as reflected by a thick line suddenly becoming a thin line on the chin EMG channel. Bursts of waves, called "sawtooth waves," which resemble jagged theta waves, intermittently appear. The frequency of sawtooth waves (2 to 6 Hz) is within the theta frequency range of 4 to 7 Hz (Fig. 4-13). The amplitude of sawtooth waves is highest in the central channels. Sawtooth waves often appear just before the onset of conjunctive eye movements (i.e., the eyes move in unison; however, signals of the left and right eye movements are recorded in opposite directions on the EOG). Because the EEG of REM sleep is very similar to stage N1 sleep, REM sleep is distinguished from stage N1 sleep by non-EEG features (i.e., lack of muscle tone and REMs).

ANATOMY AND PHYSIOLOGY OF THE HEART

The heart is a cone-shaped, four-chambered muscular organ. Its apex points downward and slightly to the left in the chest and its base points upward in the

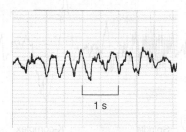

Figure 4-13 Sawtooth waves in rapid eye movement sleep.

chest. The base of the heart contains two atria and the apex of the heart contains two ventricles. The atria and ventricles make up the four chambers of the heart. The cardiac septum is a muscular wall that splits the heart longitudinally into left and right halves. The atrial septum forms a border between the left and right atria and the ventricular septum forms a border between the left and right ventricles. Valves separate each atrium from its corresponding ventricle. The tricuspid valve separates the right atrium from the right ventricle, and the mitral valve separates the left atrium from the left ventricle.

A heartbeat begins with the simultaneous contraction of the atria. When they contract, the tricuspid and mitral valves open to allow blood to flow from each atrium into its corresponding ventricle. After the ventricles are filled, the tricuspid and mitral valves close as the ventricles contract. Ventricular contraction expels the blood into the pulmonary trunk (right ventricle) and into the aorta (left ventricle). The pulmonary trunk takes the blood to the lungs for oxygenation while blood from the aorta travels throughout the body to oxygenate the body's tissues. Blood that is oxygenated in the lungs is returned to the left atrium by the pulmonary vein. Blood that has gone through the body tissues ultimately loses oxygenation and is returned to the right atrium by the inferior and superior venae cavae (singular, vena cava; these veins are the largest in the body). Once the atria are filled, this process begins again.

A heart muscle cell is called a "cardiomyocyte." Cardiomyocytes are short, flat, branching quadrangular cells shaped somewhat like a thick X. The branches of a cardiomyocyte are joined with the branches of another myocyte by dense fibrous bands called "intercalated discs." Gap junctions and desmosomes of one myocyte are juxtaposed with those of another myocyte through the intercalated discs.

A gap junction is a channel that is formed by a hexagon-shaped protein on a cell's membrane. Within the center of the hexagonal protein is a pore (i.e., channel) through which ions and proteins and other small molecules can pass from one cell into the next. The distance between the gap junctions of adjacent cells is extremely small, approximately 2 to 3 nm. Such a short distance allows electrical energy to be transmitted quickly from cell to cell, so that an impulse originating in one part of the heart can spread quickly enough to cause the myocytes to beat in synchrony.

Desmosomes are dense circular bodies scattered just beneath and attached to the cell membrane. Thin fibers extend from each desmosome and insert into the desmosome of adjacent myocytes. The thin fibers anchor myocytes tightly together so that myocytes do not come apart during contractions.

An impulse for a heartbeat normally begins in the SA node. The SA node is functionally and histologically a specialized group of cells in the upper right atrium. The SA node cells usually act as the heart's pacemaker. However, under certain conditions, other cells can take over as the heart's pacemaker, which will be discussed later in this section. Pacemaker cells are modified myocytes that do not contract. They instead transmit rhythmic impulses by undergoing a continual process of depolarization and repolarization.

The rhythmic impulses from the SA pacemaker cells induce rhythmic depolarization of the myocytes of the atria (i.e., atrial contraction). The signal is relayed to the AV node, a group of pacemaker cells that lie at the bottom of the right atrium. The AV node depolarizes and relays the signal to the bundle of His, which is a group of specialized pacemaker fibers. The bundle of His fibers exit from the AV node and travel downward through the septum (i.e., the muscular portion of the ventricular septum). In the upper region of the interventricular septum, the bundle of His breaks into left and right branches. These branches travel down the interventricular septum toward the heart's apex. At the apex, the left bundle branch breaks into many fibers as it spreads itself throughout the muscular wall of the left ventricle, and the right bundle branch similarly spreads itself throughout the muscular wall of the right ventricle. When an impulse passes through the bundle of His, the ventricular myocytes depolarize, which causes the ventricles to contract. A heartbeat (i.e., atrial contraction followed by ventricular contraction) normally takes approximately 0.8 seconds.

The AV node cells or the bundle of His fibers can set the heart's rhythm in case disease or injury to the SA node prevents it from transmitting a signal. The AV node or bundle of His fibers can take over as pacemaker because each has its own intrinsic rhythm: The AV node can generate 40 to 60 impulses per minute and the bundle of His fibers can generate 30 to 40 impulses per minute. The SA node normally sets the heart's rhythm because it can generate impulses at a rate of 60 to 100 impulses per minute and therefore can override the impulses of the AV node or the bundle of His fibers. If an injury occurs at or near the SA node, the AV node takes over as the heart's pacemaker because it can generate signals more quickly than the bundle of His fibers. If injury affects the SA node and AV node, the His fibers may then take over as the heart's pacemaker (Fig. 4-14).

Pulmonary and Systemic Circulation

Two separate cardiovascular circuits exist for blood flowing into and out of the heart. The first circuit is the pulmonary circuit. In this circuit, blood flows from the heart to the lungs and back to the heart. The second

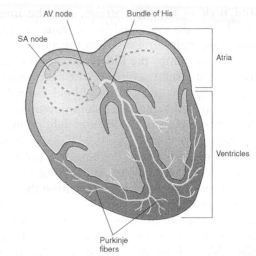

Figure 4-14 The conducting system of the heart. Impulses originating in the sinoatrial (SA) node are transmitted through the atria, into the atrioventricular (AV) node to the bundle of His, and by way of Purkinje fibers through the ventricles. (Reprinted with permission from Frandsen G and Pennington SS. *Abrams' clinical drug therapy*, 10th ed. [Figure 25.1]. Philadelphia, PA: ©Lippincott Williams & Wilkins/Wolters Kluwer, 2013.)

circuit is the systemic circuit. In this circuit, blood flows from the heart, throughout the body to oxygenate all of the body's cells, and then returns to the heart (Fig. 4-15).

The pulmonary circuit begins at the right atrium. Deoxygenated blood from the body's tissues is returned to the right atrium by way of the venae cavae. The superior vena cava brings deoxygenated blood from the

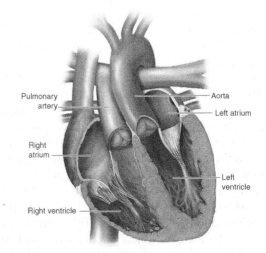

Figure 4-15 Pulmonary blood flow. (Reprinted with permission from Lee EY, Laya BF, Liszewski MC, et al. *Pediatric thoracic imaging*. [Figure 4.27] Philadelphia, PA: ©Wolters Kluwer, 2018.)

head and neck to the right atrium, and the inferior vena cava brings deoxygenated blood from the rest of the body to the right atrium. When the atria contract, the right atrium pumps the blood through the tricuspid valve into the right ventricle. When the ventricles contract, the right ventricle pumps blood through the pulmonary valve and into the pulmonary trunk. This vessel branches to become the left and right pulmonary arteries, which carry the deoxygenated blood away from the heart and to the lungs. In the lungs, the pulmonary arteries branch and become increasingly smaller as they travel to the alveoli, where the blood within the vessels undergoes gas exchange.

The lungs contain millions of alveoli, saclike outpouchings that contain air that flows into and out of the lungs with each breath. The outer surface of each alveolus is surrounded by a mass of capillaries consisting of a network of microscopic vessels that connect the venous system with the arterial system. Oxygen in the alveolar air diffuses through the alveolar wall and enters the surrounding pulmonary capillaries. Hemoglobin molecules in the red blood cells in the capillaries pick up oxygen—thereby oxygenating the blood—whereas carbon dioxide in the blood diffuses out of the capillaries and through the alveolar wall to be released into the alveolar air. Once the blood is oxygenated, it flows out of the arterial capillaries and enters the venous capillaries. The oxygenated blood flows through venous system and is returned to the heart through the left and right pulmonary veins to the left atrium.

Once in the left atrium, the blood enters the systemic circuit. When the atria contract, the now oxygenated blood is pushed through the mitral valve and enters the left ventricle. On ventricular contraction, the left ventricle pumps the blood through the aortic valve into the aorta, which is the largest artery in the body. The aorta arches over the heart and then descends through the thorax and abdomen to the lower trunk of the body, where it splits into two main branches that carry blood to the legs. Throughout its descent through the trunk, arteries branch off the aorta. Each of these branches becomes increasingly smaller until joining a capillary bed associated with a tissue (e.g., tendons, organs such as the liver). At the capillary bed, the oxygenated arterial blood provides oxygen to the body's tissues. As the blood travels from the arterial capillaries to the venous capillaries, the blood ultimately flows into the inferior and superior vena cava, both of which take the blood to the right atria. On atrial contraction, the right atrium pumps blood into the right ventricle, and blood reenters the pulmonary circuit. Thus, with each heartbeat, some blood is always entering the pulmonary circuit and some blood is entering the systemic circuit.

It is often erroneously believed that all arteries transport red oxygenated blood and all veins transport blue deoxygenated blood. However, an artery carries blood away from the heart and a vein carries blood to the heart. Therefore, in the pulmonary system, arteries are blue because the blood is deoxygenated and veins are red because the blood is oxygenated. In the systemic system, the converse is true.

Cardiac Waveforms

In polysomnography, cardiac waveforms of interest on an ECG channel are the P wave, the QRS complex, and the T wave (Fig. 4-16). The P wave represents the depolarization (i.e., contraction) of the atria. It appears as a small upwardly curved stroke. It is quickly followed by the QRS complex, an angular down–up–down stroke that represents the depolarization of the ventricles. Repolarization of the atria occurs at the same time as the contraction of the ventricles; however, the QRS complex has a larger voltage and therefore is more easily recorded than the waveform for atrial repolarization. The T wave represents the repolarization of the ventricles. Its shape is somewhat similar to the P wave, except that it is a little broader.

ANATOMY AND PHYSIOLOGY OF THE RESPIRATORY SYSTEM

Oxygenating the blood is the function of the respiratory system. The respiratory system consists of the upper airway and the lower airway (Fig. 4-17). The upper airway consists of the nose and nasal passages, the oral cavity (i.e., mouth), and the pharynx (i.e., throat cavity). The nasal passage and oral cavity open into the pharynx.

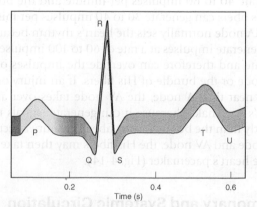

Figure 4-16 The cardiac waveforms: P, QRS, and T waves. (Reprinted with permission from Plowman S & Smith D. *Exercise physiology for health fitness and performance.* Philadelphia, PA. ©Lippincott Williams & Wilkins/Wolters Kluwer, 2017.)

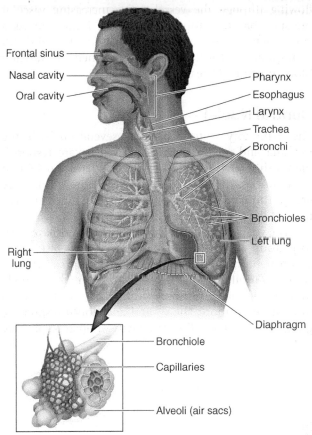

Frontal sinus

Nasal cavity

Oral cavity

Pharynx

Esophagus

Larynx

Trachea

Bronchi

Bronchioles

Left lung

Right lung

Diaphragm

Bronchiole

Capillaries

Alveoli (air sacs)

Figure 4-17 The respiratory system. (Reprinted with permission from McConnell TH and Hull KL. *Human form, human function* (*North American edition.* [Figure 13-2], Philadelphia, PA: ©Lippincott Williams & Wilkins/Wolters Kluwer, 2010.)

The pharynx begins at the back of the nasal cavity and ends at the larynx and is divided into three major regions: the nasopharynx (i.e., the region extending from the back of the nasal cavity to the soft palate), the oropharynx (i.e., the region extending from the soft palate to above the epiglottis [the cartilaginous membrane that covers the larynx when a person swallows]), and the laryngopharynx (i.e., the region extending from below the epiglottis to the larynx). The larynx contains the vocal cords, which expand and contract to control the entrance of air into and out of the lungs when a person is talking or breathing.

The larynx opens into a cartilage-ringed, rigid tube-like structure called the "trachea" (often called the "windpipe"). The trachea branches into two bronchi (singular, bronchus), which are also ringed by cartilage. As the bronchi descend into the lungs, they become smaller and smaller while increasingly losing the protective rings of cartilage. Minute extensions of the bronchi, called "bronchioles," consist of smooth muscle supported by connective tissue. A bronchiole continues

to divide until it forms a terminal bronchiole, which branches into respiratory bronchioles, each of which is capped by an alveolar sac. The surface of an alveolar sac contains grapelike clusters of air sacs (i.e., alveoli). Air enters and exits an alveolar sac through the respiratory bronchiole.

Gas exchange—the movement of oxygen into the blood and carbon dioxide out of the blood—occurs on the surface of each alveolus on an alveolar sac. On inhalation, the oxygen in the alveolar air diffuses through the alveolar wall, passes through the wall of surrounding capillaries, and finally enters the capillary blood. Once in the capillary blood, most of the oxygen is picked up by hemoglobin molecules in red blood cells and is ultimately transported throughout the body tissues. Carbon dioxide in the capillary blood diffuses out of the capillaries, passes through the alveolar wall, and enters the alveolar air. On exhalation, the carbon dioxide is expelled from the lungs.

Breathing Control Mechanisms

The rhythmicity of inhalation and exhalation involves the interplay between several nuclei in the brainstem (collectively called the "respiratory center"), the aorta, and the carotid arteries. Nuclei outside the brain are called "peripheral nuclei" and nuclei within the brain are called "central nuclei." Peripheral nuclei that are involved in respiration are the aortic bodies, the carotid body, and baroreceptors in the aorta and carotid arteries. Some central nuclei that are involved in respiration are the apneustic center, pneumotaxic center, ventral respiratory group, and dorsal respiratory group.

Peripheral Nuclei

Aortic bodies lie along the aorta. These bodies are small groups of cells that are especially sensitive to changes in the blood level of oxygen (O_2); they also respond to changes in the blood level of carbon dioxide (CO_2) and changes in the blood concentration of hydrogen ions (i.e., pH, a measure of acidity or alkalinity). The aortic bodies increase their firing rate in response to a low blood O_2 level (i.e., hypoxemia); high CO_2 blood level (i.e., hypercapnia); or a pH level less than or equal to 7.35, which represents increased blood acidity (i.e., acidemia). The increased firing rate of the aortic bodies induced by hypoxemia, hypercapnia, or acidemia results in a person taking deep, fast breaths.

The aortic bodies decrease their firing rate in response to a high blood O_2 level (i.e., hyperoxemia), low CO_2 blood level (i.e., hypocapnia), or a pH level greater than or equal to 7.45 (i.e., alkalemia [increased blood alkalinity]). The decreased firing rate of the aortic bodies induced by hyperoxemia, hypocapnia, or alkalemia results in a person breathing in shallow, slow breaths.

The carotid body is a mass of cells lodged within the carotid bifurcation of each carotid artery (Fig. 4-18). The left and right carotid artery each extend from the top of the aorta, pass through the neck, and supply oxygenated blood to the neck, face, skull, and brain. At the level of the neck, each carotid artery splits into two branches. The point where a carotid artery splits is called the "carotid bifurcation."

The carotid bodies are sensitive to changes in blood levels of O_2, blood pH, and CO_2. The aortic bodies increase their firing rate in response to hypoxemia, hypercapnia, or acidemia and decrease their firing rate in response to hyperoxemia, hypocapnia, or alkalemia. The carotid and aortic bodies relay signals to the respiratory center. The respiratory center neurons increase or decrease their firing rate in correlation with the frequency of signals received from the carotid bodies and aortic bodies. The depth and rate of respiration correspondingly increases or decreases.

Baroreceptors (in Greek, *baros* means "pressure") are embedded within the wall of a blood vessel and respond to changes in the pressure exerted by blood flowing through the vessel. With increasing vascular pressure, baroreceptors increase their firing rate. As a consequence, a person has an increased rate and depth of respiration. The converse occurs when the vascular blood pressure decreases.

Central Nuclei

The respiratory center consists of several nuclei in the medulla and pons. These central nuclei are responsible for different aspects of respiration. Four nuclei that are important in respiration are the ventral respiratory group, the dorsal respiratory group, the apneustic center, and the pneumotaxic center (Fig. 4-19).

The ventral respiratory group and the dorsal respiratory group are in the medulla. The ventral respiratory group neurons become stimulated during strong, active respiration; they are involved in respiratory muscle movement when a person voluntarily controls inspiration and expiration. The ventral and dorsal respiratory group nuclei can modify the activity of other respiratory

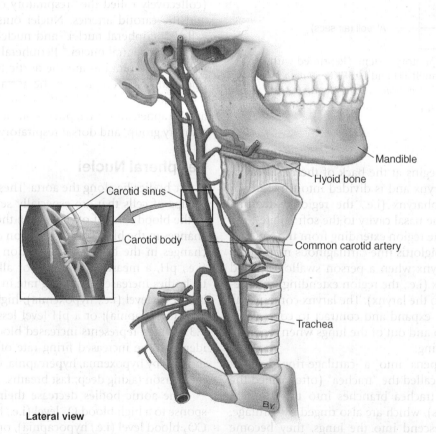

Lateral view

Figure 4-18 The carotid body is an ovoid mass of tissue that lies at the bifurcation of the common carotid artery. It is a chemoreceptor that monitors the level of oxygen in the blood. (Modified with permission from Agur AMR and Dalley AF. *Grant's atlas of anatomy* 14 ed., [Figure 8.15 C]. Philadelphia, PA: ©Lippincott Williams & Wilkins/Wolters Kluwer, 2016.)

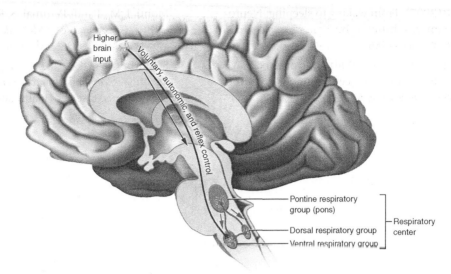

Figure 4-19 Respiratory control centers. The pontine and dorsal respiratory groups send information to the ventral respiratory group, which sets the basic respiratory rhythm by altering motor nerve activity supplying inspiratory muscles. The respiratory center, in turn, receives inputs from peripheral and central chemoreceptors and higher brain regions. (Reprinted with permission from McConnell TH and Hull KL. *Human form, human function* (*North American edition.* [Figure 13-15], Philadelphia, PA: ©Lippincott Williams & Wilkins/ Wolters Kluwer, 2010.)

motor neurons. The dorsal respiratory group neurons control the basic rhythm of respiration.

The pontine nuclei consist of the apneustic center and the pneumotaxic center. The apneustic center promotes the inspiratory phase of a breath. The pneumotaxic center rhythmically inhibits the inspirations induced by the apneustic center and thereby sets the stage for the expiratory phase of a breath. The interplay between these four nuclei within the respiratory center makes respiration possible, whether breaths are occurring automatically (i.e., involuntary) or a person is voluntarily changing the breathing rate and frequency.

SUMMARY

It is important for sleep technologists to understand how the brain, heart, skeletal muscles, and eyes generate electrical activity. Without understanding why certain settings are used on a channel, a technologist will be unable to recognize artifacts and quickly make corrections when an artifact occurs in a channel. Without understanding how normal physiologic signals are produced, a technologist will be unable to determine when an abnormal physiologic signal is occurring (i.e., normal EEG waves vs. abnormal EEG waves during a seizure; a normal heart rhythm on an ECG vs. heart arrhythmias such as premature ventricular contractions), which can potentially put a patient's life at risk. Without an understanding of how certain factors such as blindness or

a skin problem can alter the biochemical generation of signals, a technologist will not adjust electrode placement on a patient or adjust the PSG recording settings to produce a desired signal on the sleep record. Most importantly, by having a clear understanding of the anatomy and the physiology of biopotentials, a technologist will be capable of producing a sleep record with signals that are accurately recorded (e.g., with the correct polarity) and channels that are artifact-free.

SUGGESTED READINGS

Alcamo, I. E., & Krumhardt, B. (2004). *Anatomy and physiology the easy way: Barron's E-Z series.* Hauppauge, NY: Barron's Educational Series, Inc.

Brown, R. E., Basheer, R., McKenna, J. T., et al. (2012). Control of sleep and wakefulness. *Physiological Reviews, 92*(3), 1087–1187.

Chu, N.-S., & Bloom, F. E. (1973). Norepinephrine-containing neurons: Changes in spontaneous discharge patterns during sleeping and waking. *Science, 179*(4076), 908–910.

Fuller, P. M., Saper, C. B., & Lu, J. (2007). The pontine REM switch: Past and present. *Journal of Physiology, 584*(Pt. 3), 735–741.

Hobson, J. A., McCarley, R. W., & Wyzinski, P. W. (1973). Sleep cycle oscillation: Reciprocal discharge by two brainstem neuronal groups. *Science, 189*(4196), 55–58.

Jones, B. E. (2005). From waking to sleeping: Neuronal and chemical substrates. *Trends in Pharmacological Sciences, 26*(11), 578–586.

Monti, J. M., & Monti, D. (2000). Role of dorsal raphe nucleus serotonin 5-HT1A receptor in the regulation of REM sleep. *Life Science, 66*(21), 1999–2012.

Monti, J. M., Pandi-Perumal, S. R., & Möhler, H. (Eds.). (2010). *GABA and sleep: Molecular, functional and clinical aspects.* Basel, Switzerland: Springer Basel AG.

Standring, S. (Ed.). (2015). *Gray's anatomy: The anatomical basis of clinical practice ebook.* Amsterdam, the Netherlands: Elsevier Health Sciences.

chapter 5

Regulating Sleep and Waking— Circadian and Homeostasis

DAVID F. WOLFE

LEARNING OBJECTIVES

On completion of this chapter, the reader should be able to:

1. Describe the ascending reticular activating system's role in maintaining wakefulness.
2. Describe the brain structures and processes for activating rapid eye movement (REM) and non-REM sleep.
3. Describe the circadian and homeostatic influences on the regulation of sleep.

KEY TERMS

Circadian rhythm
Homeostatic drive
Suprachiasmatic nucleus
Hypothalamus
Ventrolateral preoptic area
Raphe nuclei
Reticular formation
Thalamus
Pons
Locus ceruleus
Basal forebrain
Ascending reticular activating system
Pineal gland
Zeitgebers
Aminergic
Cholinergic
γ-Aminobutyric acid
Melatonin
Galanin
Adenosine
Serotonin
Acetylcholine
Norepinephrine
Glutamate

INTRODUCTION

Various areas of the brain are responsible for allowing the body to enter different sleep stages, as well as regulate sleep and wake. Two of the most important processes in regulating sleep and wake are the circadian rhythm and homeostatic sleep drive. The balance of each of these processes helps individuals sleep well, whereas disturbances of each of these systems may cause difficulty sleeping.

CIRCADIAN AND HOMEOSTATIC PROCESSES

The homeostatic drive for sleep decreases during sleep and increases during wakefulness, whereas the circadian process diminishes its alerting signal during the night to help promote sleep and increases during the day to promote alertness (1).

Homeostatic Drive

The homeostatic sleep drive increases with sleep debt—the more hours awake, the higher the drive to sleep. Although processes exist that cause continued alertness within an individual with excessive sleep debt, the only way to satisfy the homeostatic drive to sleep is by sleeping. High cognitive workload promotes sleep homeostatic responses by increasing subjective sleepiness and fatigue, but it also delays sleep onset, producing a global sleep homeostatic response by reducing wake after sleep onset (2).

Circadian Rhythm

With its alerting effects, the circadian rhythm opposes the homeostatic drive to sleep. Through specialized retinal photoreceptors containing melanopsin, the suprachiasmatic nucleus (SCN), located in the anterior hypothalamus, receives input from light. The input of light to the SCN inhibits melatonin secretion by the pineal gland

(1), producing alertness. When the SCN receives input from low levels of light (dark), melatonin is secreted from the pineal gland, causing a decrease in alertness.

The pineal gland produces melatonin from the amino acid tryptophan. Melatonin is secreted not only into the blood but also into the cerebrospinal fluid. Daytime plasma melatonin concentrations are at least 10-fold lower than nocturnal concentrations (3, 4). The secretion of melatonin begins at 3 or 4 months of age, concurrent with sleep consolidation at night. Nighttime melatonin levels then increase rapidly, peaking at 1 to 3 years of age, at which point it begins to decline (5): melatonin nocturnal serum concentrations decline across puberty (6). Peak nocturnal melatonin concentrations in 70-year-olds decrease to only a quarter or less of what they are in young adults (7).

Ocular light exposure induces a range of neurobehavioral, neuroendocrine, and circadian responses, including melatonin suppression, circadian phase resetting, and enhancement of alertness and performance. These responses are most sensitive to blue (short-wavelength, 450 to 480 nm) visible light (8). Before bedtime, sleep improves when subjects looked through amber lenses (blocking blue wavelength light) instead of clear lenses (9). Nighttime light exposure acutely suppresses melatonin and increases alertness in a dose-dependent manner. Independent of melatonin suppression, daytime white light exposure has also been shown to increase alertness (8).

Although inherent and set genetically, the circadian system is modifiable. Zeitgebers, meaning "time givers" in German, entrain or align the internal clock, which cycles with a period slightly longer than 24 hours: about 24.2 hours in adults (10) and 24.3 hours in adolescents (11). Although zeitgebers include meals, exercise, and social contact, the most potent stimuli to entrain the circadian phase is bright light (12).

VENTROLATERAL PREOPTIC AREA

In addition to the SCN, the hypothalamus contains another important system for sleep: the ventrolateral preoptic (VLPO) area. The VLPO and the median preoptic nuclei contain sleep-active neurons. Insomnia and sleep fragmentation are produced by a loss of VLPO neurons (13). Neurons in the VLPO contain γ-aminobutyric acid (GABA) and galanin—they are relatively inactive during wake. Most sleep-active neurons in the VLPO are active during nonrapid eye movement (NREM) and REM sleep and are activated by sleep-inducing factors including prostaglandin D2 and adenosine (14). Caffeine is an adenosine antagonist, causing arousal (15).

LOCUS CERULEUS

Located in the brainstem (pons), the locus ceruleus inhibits the VLPO, leading to wakefulness. In addition, norepinephrine-, choline-, and serotonin-containing neurons, within the locus ceruleus, fire quickly during wake. With the onset of sleep, the neurons fire slower and continue to slow as sleep deepens. During REM sleep, the neurons cease firing (16). The locus ceruleus is involved in inhibiting REM sleep with REM sleep-off neurons. As REM sleep progresses, these cells become increasingly active, eventually obstructing the activity of REM sleep-on neurons, found in the pons and basal forebrain (17, 18).

BASAL FOREBRAIN

Activation of the basal forebrain leads to acetylcholine release, resulting in wakefulness or REM sleep. Inhibition of acetylcholine release in the basal forebrain, by adenosine, leads to slow-wave sleep (16). Major cholinergic output of the central nervous system occurs in the basal forebrain (19).

RAPHE NUCLEI

The raphe nuclei are located in the reticular formation of the brainstem. By way of the thalamus, serotonin-containing neurons of the raphe nuclei promote the emergence of slow-wave cortical activity (20). Similar to the locus ceruleus, raphe nuclei cells are most active and variable during waking, particularly in response to novel stimuli. Also similar to the locus ceruleus, these cells do not fire in REM sleep (16) because of the decrease in aminergic system activity (serotonin-containing raphe neurons and norepinephrine-containing locus ceruleus) (18) and fire relatively slowly during slow-wave sleep (16).

ASCENDING RETICULAR ACTIVATING SYSTEM

The ascending reticular activating system (ARAS) comprises several neuronal circuits, traveling through the thalamus, connecting the brainstem (reticular formation) to the cerebral cortex. The ARAS also includes the hypothalamus and basal forebrain (21) and consists of dorsal and ventral pathways. Both pathways are involved in cortical activation (22), causing neurons in the ARAS to fire at a higher rate during wakefulness. Because of external stimuli, the ARAS provides an inhibitory influence by reducing afferent (sensory neurons) activity during sleep. In other words, during sleep, fewer impulses arise from the cerebral cortex and decrease ARAS activation.

The ARAS is also involved in REM sleep. Interaction of brainstem aminergic, cholinergic, and GABAergic neurons controls the activity of glutamatergic reticular formation neurons. This leads to REM sleep, resulting in rapid eye movements, muscle atonia, cortical activation, and dreaming (19).

THALAMUS

Located just above the brainstem is the thalamus. Within the thalamus is the thalamic reticular nuclei, which contain GABAergic neurons that project from the thalamus to the reticular formation. The rhythmic bursting pattern of slow waves seen during slow-wave sleep is caused by the thalamic reticular nuclei neurons rhythmically shifting between depolarization and hyperpolarization (23). The thalamocortical neurons inhibit this rhythmic bursting pattern through the influence of excitatory neurotransmitters, such as acetylcholine and glutamate, causing the transition from sleep to wake (23, 24).

CONCLUSION

The reticular formation is the primary generator of wakefulness. As the circadian rhythm and homeostatic sleep drive balance to achieve sleep and wakefulness, the hypothalamus, brainstem, basal forebrain, and thalamus assist in sleep–wake balance and maintaining REM and NREM sleep.

REFERENCES

1. Malkani, R., & Zee, P. C. (2014). Basic circadian rhythms and circadian sleep disorders. In S. Chokroverty, & R. J. Thomas (Eds.), *Atlas of sleep medicine* (2nd ed., p. 119). Philadelphia, PA: Elsevier.

2. Goel, N., Abe, T., Braun, M. E., et al. (2014). Cognitive workload and sleep restriction interact to influence sleep homeostatic responses. *Sleep, 37*(11), 1745.

3. Lynch, H. J., Wurtman, R. J., Moskowitz, M. A., et al. (1975). Daily rhythm in human urinary melatonin. *Science, 187*(4172), 169.

4. Lynch, H. J., Jimerson, D. C., Ozaki, Y., et al. (1978). Entrainment of rhythmic melatonin secretion in man to a 12-hour phase shift in the light/dark cycle. *Life Sciences, 23*(15), 1557.

5. Kennaway, D. J., Stamp, G. E., & Goble, F. C. (1992). Development of melatonin production in infants and the impact of prematurity. *Journal of Clinical Endocrinology and Metabolism, 75*, 367.

6. Waldhauser, F., Weiszenbacher, G., Frisch, H., et al. (1984). Fall in nocturnal serum melatonin during prepuberty and pubescence. *Lancet, 1*, 362.

7. Waldhauser, F., Lynch, H. J., & Wurtman, R. J. (1984). Melatonin in human body fluids: Clinical significance. In R. J. Reiter (Ed.), *The pineal gland (comprehensive endocrinology)* (p. 345). New York, NY: Raven Press.

8. Rahman, S. A., Flynn-Evans, E. E., Aeschbach, D., et al. (2014). Diurnal spectral sensitivity of the acute alerting effects of light. *Sleep, 37*(2), 271–281.

9. Shechter, A., Kim, E. W., St-Onge, M. P., et al. (2018). Blocking nocturnal blue light for insomnia: A randomized controlled trial. *Journal of Psychiatric Research, 96*, 196.

10. Czeisler, C. A., Duffy, J. F., Shanahan, T. L., et al. (1999). Stability, precision, and near-24-hour period of the human circadian pacemaker. *Science, 284*, 2177.

11. Carskadon, M. A., Labyak, S. E., Acebo, C., et al. (1999). Intrinsic circadian period of adolescent humans measured in conditions of forced desynchrony. *Neuroscience Letters, 260*, 129.

12. Dunlap, J. C., Loros, J. L., & DeCoursey, P. J. (2004). *Chronobiology: Biological timekeeping.* Sunderland, MA: Oxford University Press.

13. Fuller, P. M., Zee, P. C., & Buxton, O. M. (2014). Sleep mechanisms. In M. Kryger, A. Avidan, & R. Berry (Eds.), *Atlas of clinical sleep medicine* (2nd ed.). Philadelphia, PA: Elsevier.

14. Berry, R. B. (2012). Neurobiology of sleep. In R. B. Berry (Ed.), *Fundamentals of sleep medicine* (pp. 91–100). Philadelphia, PA: Elsevier.

15. McGinty, D., & Szymusiak, R. (2005). Sleep-promoting mechanisms in mammals. In M. H. Kryger, T. Roth, & W. C. Dement (Eds.), *Principles and practice of sleep medicine* (4th ed., p. 179). Philadelphia, PA: Elsevier.

16. Garcia-Rill, E. (2002). Mechanisms of sleep and wakefulness. In T. L. Lee-Chiong Jr., M. J. Sateia, & M. A. Carskadon (Eds.), *Sleep medicine* (p. 33). Philadelphia, PA: Hanley & Belfus.

17. Patrick, R. (2012). Anatomy and physiology of the biopotentials of sleep. In C. Mattice, R. Brooks, & T. Lee-Chiong (Eds.), *Fundamentals of sleep technology* (2nd ed., pp. 39–40). Philadelphia, PA: Lippincott Williams & Wilkins.

18. Reinoso-Suarez, F., de Andres, I., Rodrigo-Angulo, M., et al. (2001). Brain structures and mechanisms involved in the generation of REM sleep. *Sleep Medicine Reviews, 5*(1), 68.

19. Brown, R. E., Basheer, R., McKenna, J. T., et al. (2012). Control of sleep and wakefulness. *Physiological Reviews, 92*(3), 1087.

20. Culebras, A. (2002). Normal sleep. In T. L. Lee-Chiong Jr., M. J. Sateia, & M. A. Carskadon (Eds.), *Sleep medicine* (p. 2). Philadelphia, PA: Hanley & Belfus.

21. Brown, R. E., Basheer, R., McKenna, J. T., et al. (2012). Control of sleep and wakefulness. *Physiological Reviews, 92*(3), 1094.

22. Brown, R. E., Basheer, R., McKenna, J. T., et al. (2012). Control of sleep and wakefulness. *Physiological Reviews, 92*(3), 1094–1095.

23. Patrick, R. (2012). Anatomy and physiology of the biopotentials of sleep. In C. Mattice, R. Brooks, & T. Lee-Chiong (Eds.), *Fundamentals of sleep technology* (2nd ed., p. 41). Philadelphia, PA: Lippincott Williams & Wilkins.

24. Reinoso-Suarez, F., de Andres, I., Rodrigo-Angulo, M., et al. (2001). Brain structures and mechanisms involved in the generation of REM sleep. *Sleep Medicine Reviews, 5*(1), 65.

chapter 6
Sleep Deprivation

LISA M. BOND

LEARNING OBJECTIVES

On completion of this chapter, the reader should be able to:

1. State the recommended sleep requirements for all age groups.
2. Describe the adverse effects of sleep deprivation.
3. Differentiate acute total sleep deprivation from chronic partial sleep deprivation.
4. Explain the methods employed in the diagnosis of sleep deprivation.
5. Describe the clinical features of insufficient sleep syndrome.
6. Outline the countermeasures available to combat sleep deprivation associated with shift work.

KEY TERMS

Sleep duration
Sleep deprivation
Sleep fragmentation
Shift work
Strategic napping
Bright light
Caffeine
Modafinil
Armodafinil
Melatonin

Sleep technologists are in a unique position both to evaluate and to experience the consequences of sleep deprivation. Because most sleep disorders evaluated by polysomnography (PSG) are the result of qualitative or quantitative disturbances in sleep, the technologist is at the front line of the evaluation. In addition, most sleep recordings are made during the patient's usual sleep hours, requiring sleep technologists to work during the evening and night. Often, the shift is 10 to 12 hours in length and the workweek is sometimes limited to three nights per week. As shift workers, technologists are likely to experience sleep deprivation and will need to have a working knowledge of the consequences and countermeasures available. A recent ad representing a training program for sleep technologists indicated that candidates would need to "remain awake, alert and maintain good interpersonal skills throughout the night as well as demonstrate the ability to get proper sleep during the day." The challenges for the sleep technologist are significant.

NORMAL SLEEP REQUIREMENTS

Sleep requirements differ among individuals and within different age groups. In recognition of this, in 2015, the National Sleep Foundation (NSF) updated what is considered normal sleep requirements for various age groups (1). The NSF also broke down recommendations for sleep for adults into three categories rather than just one for all adult ages and created new age grouping for younger adults ages 18 to 25, adults ages 26 to 64, and adults ages 65 or older. The scientifically grounded guidelines were developed on the basis of a rigorous, systematic review of scientific literature on sleep duration, health, performance, and safety. The different age categories now have recommended sleep amounts, what may be appropriate, and what is not recommended.

It is no longer sufficient to simply say an adult should get 8 hours of sleep each night. Sleep technologists need to be aware of how much sleep is recommended for each age group. Even with sufficient sleep time, sleep quality is still important to enable best function. The best indicator of sufficient good-quality sleep is waking up feeling refreshed, alert, and performing at a peak level during wake time.

DEFINITION OF SLEEP DEPRIVATION

Sleep deprivation in an individual can be caused by insufficient duration of sleep (quantitative sleep deprivation), a fragmented or interrupted sleep period (qualitative sleep deprivation), or a combination of both factors. Sleep deprivation can be either chronic or acute. The subjective assessment of the quality of sleep is based on the amount of sleep, continuity of sleep, and depth of the sleep. See Table 6-1 for the NSF's sleep duration recommendations (2).

Table 6-1 National Sleep Foundation's Sleep Duration Recommendations

Age	Recommended (hours)	May Be Appropriate (hours)	Not Recommended (hours)
Newborns 0–3 mo	14–17	11–13 18–19	<11 >19
Infants 4–11 mo	12–15	10–11 16–18	<10 >18
Toddlers 1–2 y	11–14	9–10 15–16	<9 >16
Preschoolers 3–5 y	10–13	8–9 14	<8 >14
School-aged children 6–13 y	9–11	7–8 12	<7 >12
Teenagers 14–17 y	8–10	7 11	<7 >11
Young adults 18–25 y	7–9	6 10–11	<6 >11
Adults 26–64 y	7–9	6 10	<6 >10
Older adults ≥65 y	7–8	5–6 9	<5 >9

From: Hirshkowitz, M., Whiton, K., Albert, S. M., et al. (2015). National Sleep Foundation's sleep time duration recommendations: Methodology and results summary. *Sleep Health, 1*(1), 40–43.

Acute sleep deprivation refers to no sleep or a reduction in the usual total sleep time, usually lasting 1 or 2 days (3). Chronic sleep insufficiency (also called sleep restriction) exists when an individual routinely sleeps less than the amount required for optimal functioning.

PREVALENCE OF SLEEP DEPRIVATION

The prevalence of sleep deprivation in the industrialized world appears to be on the rise. In February of 2017, the Centers for Disease Control and Prevention's (CDC) Morbidity and Mortality weekly report estimated that more than a third of Americans were not getting enough sleep on a regular basis. The major consequences of chronic sleep deprivation are fatigue, excessive daytime sleepiness, clumsiness, weight changes, and adversely affected cognitive function. Consequences can also include motor vehicle or industrial accidents, negative socioeconomic and public health outcomes, reduced academic and job performance, and a reduced sense of well-being. According to Johns Hopkins sleep researcher Patrick Finan, sleep deprivation can affect your judgment in such a way that you don't notice its effects (4). In a world that is increasingly changing into a "global community," the encroaching demands on the sleep–wake cycle of an individual pose a significant dilemma.

Major industrial disasters, such as those at Chernobyl, Three Mile Island, and Bhopal, and serious accidents, such as those involving the Exxon Valdez and the Space Shuttle Challenger, have been officially attributed to errors in judgment caused at least in part by sleepiness in the workplace (5). One in 25 adults in the United States report falling asleep at the wheel at least once in a month. There are nearly 6,000 fatal car crashes caused by drowsy driving each year. People who are sleep deprived have nearly three times the risk for type 2 diabetes than nonsleep-deprived individuals and have an increased risk for high blood pressure, and a 48% increased chance of developing heart disease. Getting less than 5 hours of sleep nightly puts an individual at a 50% higher risk of obesity as there is an increase in the hunger hormone ghrelin and a decrease in the appetite-control hormone leptin.

The 2014 NSF Health Index revealed that as many as 35% of Americans reported that their sleep quality was "poor" or "only fair" and that Americans slept 40 minutes longer on nonwork days. Nearly 40% indicated that they snored more than a few nights per week, with 17% of respondents being told by their physician that they have a sleep disorder; 24% of women reported they woke up feeling well-rested 0 days out of 4 as against 16% of men. Adding up, nearly 15% of the US workforce works for hours outside of the traditional 9-a.m.-to-5-p.m. workday. Most sleep technologists are part of that workforce. Even if shift workers technically get sufficient sleep during the day, they may still experience some symptoms of shift work disorder.

Approximately 10% of shift workers are believed to be suffering from shift work disorder. Roughly between 25% and 30% of shift workers experience symptoms of excessive sleepiness or insomnia. This is especially problematic when most shift workers, such as those in the medical field or transportation industry, are required to be alert and able to make quick and important decisions (6).

TYPES OF SLEEP DEPRIVATION

Acute, Chronic, and Total Sleep Deprivation

Acute sleep deprivation refers to no sleep or a reduction in the usual total sleep time, usually lasting 1 or 2 days. Chronic sleep insufficiency or deprivation (also called sleep restriction) exists when an individual routinely sleeps less than the amount required for optimal functioning. Chronic sleep restriction has been shown to cause similar deficient cognitive performance as two nights of total sleep deprivation (TSD), meaning that even moderate sleep restriction can seriously impair the functioning of healthy adults (7).

A study published in 2001 examined the effect of TSD on the brain. TSD was noted to be associated with increased activation in the bilateral prefrontal cortex and parietal lobes. It appears that at least with short-term TSD, various brain regions show increased response in an attempt to compensate (8). However, we know from studies done in 1894 on puppies, 1898 on dogs (9), different rat studies, and in 1896 on humans (10), as well as from individuals who have prion disease referred to as fatal familial insomnia, that prolonged sleep loss leads to a range of psychological problems and death.

Accumulating research in both animals and humans has demonstrated profound behavioral and physiologic consequences from sleep deprivation. Animal sleep deprivation studies have suggested that sleep is critically important for survival and is probably vitally important in thermoregulation, energy balance, and immune function. Totally sleep-deprived rats show a characteristic picture of weight loss, skin lesions, and ultimately death after 11 to 22 days of TSD (5, 11). As they deteriorate, the animals exhibit marked increases in energy expenditure, an increase in heart rate, large increases in food intake, rises in plasma norepinephrine, and declines in plasma thyroxine. It is theorized that the increased energy expenditure is an attempt to maintain body temperature despite excessive heat loss during sleep deprivation. Available studies in humans suggest a far less profound physiologic response to sleep deprivation over periods of up to 11 days (12).

The studies of sleep deprivation in humans suffer from certain methodologic limitations. It is unethical to deprive human subjects of sleep to the point of producing medical consequences. Motivations of both experimenter and subject can have a large impact on results, particularly on data related to behavior and mood (12).

Despite these methodologic limitations, numerous studies of human sleep deprivation have been published. The most obvious consequence of acute sleep loss is excessive sleepiness. Even one night of TSD can reduce the latency of sleep onset on the Multiple Sleep Latency Test (MSLT) by 60% (13). Various studies have addressed the impact of sleep deprivation on subjective and objective measures of sleepiness, as well as psychomotor vigilance, performance, memory tasks, and mood. This will be described later in this chapter. Technologists should keep in mind that the characteristics of each individual, such as age, may affect the severity of sleep loss consequence and ability to recover (12).

Recovery from TSD

The sleep technologist will be asked, and will need to know, if sleep loss can be recovered. Early studies suggested that only a small fraction (10% to 20%) of the total sleep time lost during deprivation is recoverable (14, 15). However, those studies allowed ad-lib time in bed, and an individual's motivation to get out of bed resulted in an underestimation of the true recovery. In a study that enforced a 24-hour time in bed following sleep deprivation, subjects recovered 72% and 42% of the total sleep lost during the 24- and 48-hour periods, respectively, of deprivation (16).

For recovery sleep, both the hours slept and the intensity of the sleep are important. Some of the most refreshing sleep occurs during deep sleep. Although such sleep's true effects are still being studied, it is generally considered a restorative period for the brain. Sleeping more hours allows the brain more time in this rejuvenating period (17).

Chronic and Partial Sleep Deprivation

More common than acute TSD is chronic partial sleep deprivation, which may accumulate over several days. This type of sleep restriction occurs in everyday life in those who voluntarily restrict their sleep time or during travel across time zones. For example, when a person with a usual nocturnal sleep need of 8 hours gets only 7, a 1-hour "sleep deficit" or "sleep debt" is created. If this pattern is sustained over 1 week, the "sleep debt" is roughly equivalent to a full night of total sleep loss. Despite the frequent occurrence of this type of chronic partial sleep deprivation in the population, it is not readily recognizable.

Several experimental studies have looked closely at this issue. In a study evaluating partial sleep restriction over a 2-week period, Van Dongen et al. (7) showed that chronic restriction of sleep to 6 hours or less per night produced cognitive performance deficits equivalent to up to two nights of TSD. Equally important, subjects in the study were largely unaware of the increasing cognitive deficits. In a related study from the same group (18), impairment from sleep loss was significantly different among individuals and stable within individuals, suggesting that an individual's vulnerability to sleep loss was an inherent trait.

Dinges et al. (19) evaluated the impact of a 33% reduction in sleep duration for seven consecutive nights in 16 healthy young adults. The average sleep time was 4.98 hours per night. A cumulative and escalating adverse effect on measures of daytime sleepiness, fatigue, mood disturbance, stress, and psychomotor vigilance testing was demonstrated. The worst deficits were seen on the final day of sleep restriction. Recovery from deficits created by sleep restriction required two full nights of sleep.

Chronic sleep restriction is also associated with a higher overall mortality rate. In fact, both short and long sleep durations are associated with an increase in mortality from cardiovascular disease as well as total mortality (20, 21). A large-scale prospective study of Japanese men and women aged 40 to 79 years confirmed that, compared with 7 hours of sleep, short sleep duration of 4 hours or less was associated with a 2-fold increase in mortality from coronary heart disease for women and a 1.5-fold increase in mortality from noncardiovascular disease/noncancer and a 1.3-fold increase in total mortality for both men and women. Clearly, optimal sleep duration is a key factor in overall health (22).

DIAGNOSING QUANTITATIVE SLEEP DEPRIVATION

The *International Classification of Sleep Disorders*, 3rd edition, lists insufficient sleep syndrome (ISS) also known as behaviorally induced ISS, insufficient nocturnal sleep, chronic sleep deprivation, and sleep restriction, under Central Disorders of Hypersomnolence (23). This sleep disorder is extrinsic—it originates from causes outside of the body. Diagnostic criteria consist of daily need to sleep, or lapses into sleep, during the day (for children there is a complaint of behavior abnormalities attributed to sleepiness).

The sleep time, obtained via personal history, sleep logs, or actigraphy, is shorter than expected for the age group. The patient curtails sleep by an alarm clock or wakening by others and generally sleeps longer on weekends and vacations. The curtailing of sleep is present most days for at least 3 months. Extending the total sleep time resolves symptoms of sleepiness. The symptoms are also not better explained by another untreated sleep disorder, medication effects, or a medical, neurologic, or mental disorder. Actigraphy is commonly used

with sleep diaries for 2 to 3 weeks to help document the patient's time in bed, sleep latency, total sleep time, and sleep efficiency. PSG and MSLT are not required to establish this diagnosis. Rather, a therapeutic trial of longer sleep episodes is used and if the longer sleep durations lead to resolution of the symptoms this is sufficient to diagnose ISS.

If PSG is performed, it would reveal reduced sleep latency and a greater-than-90% sleep efficiency, reflecting the need for more sleep. It is also common to see slow-wave sleep (SWS) rebound (23–25) at the expense of other nonrapid eye movement (NREM) stages (7). An MSLT would show excessive sleepiness with N1 in most naps and a short sleep onset. It is often common to see N2 in 80% of the MSLT NAPS, and sleep-onset rapid eye movement periods (SOREMPs) can occur. As the MSLT can have two SOREMPs and a short sleep latency, ISS can be confused with narcolepsy along with other disorders of hypersomnolence. This confusion can be heightened with the epidemic we see of adolescents and young adults that frequently suffer from ISS. It is therefore important that a clear and accurate sleep history of normal sleep amounts be obtained.

SELECTIVE SLEEP DEPRIVATION AND RECOVERY

REM Sleep Deprivation

Animal experiments have shown that selective rapid eye movement (REM) sleep deprivation leads to increased motor activity (26) and aggression (27) as well as reduced pain thresholds (28), memory impairment for recently acquired tasks (29), and a decrease in the seizure threshold (30). Selective deprivation studies in humans suggest that this leads to increasingly shorter REM sleep latencies (31). A REM rebound, or temporary increases in REM sleep activity, may also be observed. Short REM sleep latencies and REM rebound suggest that REM pressure exists; if so, it is postulated to be related to the composition of prior sleep rather than prior wakefulness. Through unknown mechanisms, selective REM deprivation actually enhances alertness in experimental human subjects (32).

SWS Deprivation

In human experimental studies, it was found to be more difficult to deprive a person of stage N3, or SWS, than REM sleep (33). Subjects required five to seven times as many arousals to deprive them of stage N3 sleep than to deprive them of REM sleep during each night of selective sleep deprivation. Daytime performance after selective stage N3 and REM sleep deprivation conditions in humans has also been tested, yet decrements were not found after as many as seven nights of either stage N3 or REM sleep deprivation (34, 35). It is clear from the available research that the major predictor of performance during these sleep loss paradigms was the total amount of time spent asleep, regardless of sleep stage parameters.

However, even though the deprivation of SWS may not objectively affect daytime performance, SWS deprivation appears to result in meaningful changes in daytime pain levels and the sensation of fatigue. In a study of healthy subjects, both REM sleep and SWS interruption decreased mechanical pain thresholds (36). An increase in pain thresholds followed recovery sleep. Similar studies in middle-aged women without musculoskeletal complaints showed that three nights of selective SWS deprivation decreased pain thresholds (37). The subjects also reported generalized discomfort, fatigue, and reduced vigor. The qualitative changes of alpha wave intrusion into SWS have been associated with chronic syndromes (e.g., fibromyalgia), but critical reviews by numerous investigators have failed to show a direct connection between the alpha–delta electroencephalography (EEG) sleep pattern and pain complaints among patients with chronic pain (38–40).

SLEEP FRAGMENTATION

Sleep fragmentation is best described as the interruption of sleep with frequent, brief arousals characterized by increases in EEG frequency or bursts of alpha activity and, occasionally, transient increases in skeletal muscle tone (41). These arousals generally last 3 to 15 seconds, usually do not result in prolonged wakefulness, and may not alter the sleep stage scoring of a standard 30-second epoch on a polysomnogram. Many times, the sleep technologist will be able to identify the arousing condition or stimulus (apneas, leg movements, and pain), and other times, no arousing stimulus will be identifiable.

Several studies have shown that sleep fragmentation without overall sleep loss per se is associated with reduced daytime function similar to that seen from acute sleep deprivation and TSD (42–44). Bonnet (42) evaluated this phenomenon by simulating the sleep-disrupting effects of apnea. This study involved performing a standardized awakening after each minute of sleep for two consecutive nights in normal adults. Following this experimental sleep disruption, subjects were significantly sleepier than they were at their baseline. The level of impairment was similar to that seen after periods of total sleep loss of 40 to 64 hours. In a similar study, Roehrs et al. (44) confirmed these effects. The latter study showed that brief EEG arousals on average of once every 4 to 5 minutes led to a 30% reduction

in sleep latency, as measured by the MSLT during the following day. In addition, it was noted that as sleepiness increases, the threshold for arousal during subsequent nights rises as well.

ADVERSE EFFECTS OF SLEEP DEPRIVATION

The adverse effects of sleep deprivation on human function are wide ranging and include excessive sleepiness; alterations in immune, cardiovascular, and hemodynamic changes; and alterations in hormone production. Not getting enough sleep, and enough good-quality sleep, has been shown to increase the risk of or exacerbate high blood pressure, heart disease, obesity, diabetes, anxiety, depression, and irritability (that can damage relationships) and profoundly affect the ability to think clearly, react quickly as well as form memories. Being sleep deprived can be very dangerous. Testing done in 2000 showed that the hand–eye coordination of individuals driving while sleep deprived was just as bad as, if not worse than, that of drunk drivers (45). Being sleep deprived magnifies the effect of alcohol on the sleep-deprived body beyond what is seen in a normal rested individual (46). Most of these issues are beyond the scope and purpose of this review, but some of the behavioral changes described earlier in this chapter deserve elaboration.

Every sleep technologist should know and recognize the basic signs of sleep deprivation, which include irritability and moodiness, reduced ability to cope and deal with stress, lack of motivation, difficulty concentrating, memory problems, impaired motor skills, drowsiness when driving, feeling sluggish in the afternoon, needing a nap to get through the day, difficulty getting out of bed in the morning, relying on the snooze button, weight gain, frequent colds, and infections.

Daytime Sleepiness

Daytime sleepiness is the feeling of being drowsy and sluggish most days to the extent that it can interfere with work, school, or relationships. It is not the same as fatigue, which is characterized as low energy. It is also not depression, where there is a reduced desire to perform normal activities, even those that are enjoyable. Though this is not a disorder, it is a serious symptom and the one most people list as a chief complaint for why they are seeking help in a sleep clinic. Daytime sleepiness can be measured subjectively by use of the Stanford Sleepiness Scale (SSS) or the more commonly used Epworth Sleepiness Scale (ESS). However, for an objective measurement one would need to perform the MSLT after an adequate overnight PSG test.

The SSS was developed in 1972 by William Dement and colleagues as a means of measuring sleepiness throughout the day and is generally used to track overall alertness each hour of the day. The ESS was developed by Dr. Murray Johns in 1990 and was slightly modified in 1997 to include the instruction that it is important to answer the questions as best as you can. That one sentence change decreased the frequency of questions being skipped down to less than 1%. The questionnaire is named after the Epworth Hospital in Melbourne, where Dr. Johns established his sleep center in 1988. A result of greater than 10 is considered significant and requires further medical assessment (47). Sleep questionnaires have also been developed for both pediatrics and adolescents with variations on the questions above. For example, "sitting and watching TV" would be changed to "sitting, watching TV or a video." "Sitting in a classroom at school during the morning" may be substituted for "sitting inactive in a public place (theater, movie, meeting, etc.)."

The two-process model described by Borbely (48) best answers the question: Why do we feel sleepy? The homeostatic sleep drive is driven by the amount of prior wakefulness. It is physiologic, linear, and cumulative. The "sleep load" or sleep need increases as an individual becomes progressively sleepier with each passing hour. Superimposed is a second process, the circadian rhythm, driven by the "biologic clock" and influenced by the time of the day. A reduction in circadian alertness leads to increased sleepiness that occurs roughly at the same time each day. These two processes interact with each other—the circadian rhythm influences how sleepy a sleep-deprived individual feels. After a night without sleep, one may be fairly alert at 10 a.m. because the circadian increase in alertness counteracts the accumulated physiologic sleep need, but in the afternoon, the biologic and physiologic influences may combine to create an intense need for sleep. The most vulnerable times to feel sleepy appear to be between 5 and 8 a.m. and 2 and 4 p.m. (independent of a lunch-time meal), and the most likely times to feel alert seem to be between 10 a.m. and 12 noon and also again in the evening. Carskadon (49) has summarized the concept nicely: "Regardless of how many hours you've been awake, the most sleepy time occurs as the circadian 'night' is ending; the least sleepy time occurs at the end of the circadian day."

Cognitive Functioning, Memory, and Mood Disturbance

Various studies have addressed the impact of sleep deprivation on subjective and objective measures of sleepiness, as well as psychomotor vigilance, performance, memory tasks, and mood. Impairment of immediate recall for elements placed in short-term memory is a classic finding in sleep deprivation experiments. The pattern of memory deficits shows some functional similarities to adult aging and alcohol intoxication (50).

Degradation of nonexecutive components of cognition, such as information intake, that accounted for the overall impairment in subjects' performance on cognitive tasks also occurs. A study on the effects of sleep deprivation published in the journal *Sleep* in 2010 appeared to show that the sleep-deprived brain is capable of processing information, but this information may be distorted before it can be processed. Sleep deprivation in individuals such as emergency responders, police officers, military personnel, and medical personnel, who often have little opportunity for adequate sleep, risk their ability to make sound decisions in safety critical environments (51).

A meta-analysis of available data suggested that mood is more affected by sleep deprivation than either cognitive or motor performance. Despite the possibility of self-reporting errors, it is likely that sleep deprivation has a negative effect on mood (52). For example, the therapeutic effects of sleep deprivation on endogenous depression have long been recognized. Because depression can be associated with a decrease of functional serotoninergic neurotransmission, afflicted patients may exhibit significant mood improvement after one night of sleep deprivation even though they may complain of sleep loss. This antidepressant effect is likely related to the enhancement of central serotoninergic neurotransmission, similar to that described for antidepressants such as selective serotonin reuptake inhibitors (53). When selective REM sleep deprivation was employed in patients with endogenous depression, mood improved and was associated with improvement in the abnormal temporal distribution of REM sleep (54).

Dietary Changes and Increases in Obesity

The CDC reports 70.7% of the US adult population age 20 and up are overweight or obese. There are several factors including sleep deprivation that influence this growing problem of obesity. Studies have demonstrated an association between insufficient sleep and an increased appetite (55). Individuals with adequate amount of sleep are more likely to make healthy food choices. Conversely, sleep deprivation promotes overeating and inactivity, with the increase in caloric consumption derived from less healthy choices such as snack foods (56). Several studies have demonstrated that sleep curtailment leads to decreased leptin and elevated ghrelin, agents that provide feedback to hypothalamic regulatory centers that control food intake (57, 58). The changes reported would likely lead to increased food consumption and weight gain. Chronic or partial sleep loss may increase the risk of obesity and diabetes by affecting glucose regulation and increasing insulin resistance (59). During experimentally induced sleep loss, healthy individuals showed decreased insulin sensitivity without adequate compensation in beta-cell function, resulting in an impaired glucose tolerance and increased diabetes risk (60). Another report demonstrated that school-age children (4 to 10 years of age) with more variable sleep schedules and shorter sleep durations were at higher health risk for altered insulin levels and adverse metabolic outcomes leading to obesity (61). Weight gain from sleep deprivation has also been shown to result from a dysregulation of the neuroendocrine control of appetite, leading to excessive food intake and decreased energy expenditure (59).

Effects on Pain Thresholds and Increases in Spontaneous Pain

Improving sleep quantity and quality is important in the treatment of patients with chronic pain disorders. Studies performed on female patients at Johns Hopkins University School of Medicine have shown that sleep-deprived individuals have a decrease or absence of SWS, which can be a risk factor for the exacerbation of chronic pain ranging from tension headaches to fibromyalgia (62). These findings support the need for aggressive treatment of insomnia and other sleep quality issues as an adjunct to other modalities directed at treating chronic pain.

Motor Vehicle Accidents

Excessive sleepiness is the second leading cause of automobile crashes and a major cause of truck accidents in the United States (63, 64). In a recent study done by AAA, drowsiness was assessed using a validated measure of the percentage of time that an individual's eyes are closed. Using this measure, drowsiness was identified in 8.8% to 9.5% of all crashes reviewed and 10.6% to 10.8% of crashes that resulted in significant property damage, airbag deployment, or injury (65). This is significantly more than previous reports by the National Highway Traffic Safety Administration (NHTSA), which showed that of an estimated 1.4% of all police-reported crashes between 2011 and 2015 nationwide, 2.0% of crashes that resulted in injuries and 2.4% of crashes that resulted in a death were related to driver drowsiness. These differences may be related to how the observations of the police at the time of a vehicular accident are reported. Regardless of how the data are gathered and analyzed, sleep-related accidents are estimated to cost billions of dollars each year (66). Studies have shown that fatigue-related crashes are more common for truck drivers with irregular schedules (67%) than

those with regular schedules (38%). The challenges that face us are predicting performance and vehicular safety on the basis of driver fatigue. Previous studies have shown that the most important crash predictor is the duration of the driver's most recent sleep period (67). In the future, artificial intelligence will be used to develop an analytic approach to predict fatigue and drowsiness and the effect on reducing vigilance and the impact on reaction time.

In a review of vehicle accidents specifically attributed to driver "fatigue," a prominent 24-hour pattern was identified, showing a major peak at 3 a.m. and a minor peak at 3 p.m. (68). This bimodal pattern closely mirrors the known circadian propensity to sleep (2 to 7 a.m. and 2 to 5 p.m.) seen in human studies of healthy, noncomplaining individuals (69).

Studies have also affirmed that sleep-deprived drivers are just as dangerous as drunk drivers. Subjects who drove after being awake for 17 to 19 hours performed worse than those with a blood alcohol level of 0.05% (45). Twenty to 25 hours of wakefulness produced performance decrements equivalent to those observed at a blood alcohol concentration of 0.10%, a level deemed unsafe and unacceptable when working or driving (70, 71).

Driver risk factors for sleep-related crashes were identified in a population-based case–control study (72). Police reports identified 312 drivers who were asleep or fatigued at the time of a motor vehicle accident. Drivers in sleep-related crashes were more likely to work multiple jobs or night shifts, or opt for other unusual work schedules. They averaged fewer hours of sleep per night, reported poorer quality sleep, were less likely to feel that they received enough sleep, were sleepier during the day, drove more often late at night, and had more prior instances of drowsy driving. Compared with drivers in nonsleep-related crashes, they had been driving for longer times, had been awake more hours, had slept fewer hours the night before, and were more likely to have used sleep-promoting medications.

INTERVENTIONS TO COMBAT SLEEP DEPRIVATION IN SHIFT WORKERS

Sleep technologists may suffer from shift work disorder because of the nature of the field. Most people sleep at night, and most technologists work at night, monitoring, recording, and intervening with treatment for many sleep disorders. Sleep technologists are intimately familiar with shift work and are in a unique position to help others that need to deal with a 24-hour society. The traditional 9-a.m.-to-5-p.m. day shift has been replaced in many industries with evening shifts, night shifts, and rotating shifts.

According to the NSF, roughly 15% of our full-time labor force is working shift work. In the 2008 NSF poll, 63% of shift workers (vs. 89% of nonshift workers) reported that their jobs allowed them to get enough sleep. Though not all shift workers suffer from shift work disorder, about 10% of those working rotating shifts are believed to have a shift disorder of some type, and roughly 25% to 30% of any type of shift worker do suffer from symptoms such as excessive sleepiness and insomnia regularly (73).

The diagnostic criteria for shift work disorder in the *International Classification of Sleep Disorders*, 3rd edition, list the following requirements to diagnose shift work disorder:

1. Insomnia or excessive sleepiness paired with a reduction of total sleep time that is associated with a recurring work schedule that overlaps the usual sleep times.
2. The symptoms must have been present for, and the patient must have been working shift work for, at least 3 months.
3. A disrupted sleep-and-wake pattern demonstrated by a sleep log or actigraphy monitoring over a minimum of 14 days that includes both work and free days.
4. There is no other current sleep disorder, medical, neurologic, or mental disorder present, medication use, or poor sleep hygiene or substance use that can explain the symptoms.

Several strategies have been developed to address the impairments associated with shift work.

Education

In 1999, the US Department of Transportation targeted shift workers and teens in a new program implemented to combat the problem that fatigue and sleepiness present for highway safety. A National Highway Traffic Safety Administration (NHTSA) program provided materials and guidance for employers, shift workers, and shift workers' families. NHTSA administrator Ricardo Martinez stated, "Shift workers cannot be expected to adapt to society's schedules. Society must adapt to these workers' schedules." The NHTSA's program to combat drowsy driving is available at the NHTSA's web site at https://www.nhtsa.gov/risky-driving/drowsy-driving.

Several preventive strategies have been suggested to minimize the effect of sleep deprivation on shift workers. The effective use of days off to catch up on sleep is critical. However, studies of medical residents working the night float shift (rotating night shift) revealed that they slept less even though they had ample opportunity to sleep during the day after each night shift. Furthermore, they had decreased vigor and increased fatigue during the night float shift, and their fatigue scores correlated significantly with omission errors during the night float rotations but not during daytime rotations (74).

Sleep loss is cumulative; it is important to begin a new work schedule without an existing sleep debt. This generally requires two nights of unrestricted sleep, as it is not possible to stock up in anticipation of sleep debt in the future. Exercise also has a role in helping to cope with shift work. Moderate exercise is preferred to intensive training. For day shifts, exercise is best timed after the shift. For night shifts, exercise should be timed before an evening nap (75). Detailed recommendations designed to achieve chronobiologically sound shift schedule systems have been provided by Knauth (76).

The following recommendations may help individuals (including sleep technologists) who are coping with shift work remember that there is no substitute for sleep:

1. Limit continuous performance schedules to 12 to 16 hours.
2. Schedule adequate time off duty to protect sleep and sanity.
3. Know the times of greatest impairment and maximum alertness.
4. Avoid driving between 2 and 9 a.m.
5. Recognize behavioral changes as an indication of dangerous levels of fatigue.
6. Provide performance backups during times of impairment.
7. Avoid alcohol.
8. Realize that there is no substitute for sleep.

Work Environment

It is important when working evening or night shifts that the workplace be bright and cool to support alertness and productivity on the job. Bright light doesn't need to be constant, even 20 to 30 minutes can help shift workers to be more alert. If possible, schedule the work that requires the most concentration and skill when workers are in their most alert state. The drowsiest time for night shift workers is roughly 3 to 5 a.m. Workers should avoid working more than a few consecutive nights and if possible schedule at least 2 days off after working a night shift rotation (73).

Dealing with Rotating Shifts

Some jobs require working rotating shifts, which is possibly the most physically demanding adjustment for shift workers. Still there are things that can be done to make even rotating shifts easier to handle. A clockwise rotation is much easier to adapt to than a counterclockwise rotation. This is a more natural change for the body. A pattern of day shift to evening shift to night shift to day shift would be the preferred pattern to follow. Rotating every 2 to 3 days is also easier on you physically than rotating every 5 to 7 days or randomly rotating even when following the clockwise pattern. Rotating-shift workers should also begin to adjust before their shift change if possible. Delaying sleep by an hour or two before the day of the change can also make the change a bit easier (73).

Sleep Schedule

Shift workers should maintain consistent bed times and rise times, including nights off work. Delaying sleep by an hour or two to allow some daytime activities that cannot be avoided can be appropriate. However, flipping completely back to days and then back to nights is not healthy or advised. Doing so can make it more difficult to return to work and function optimally and to sleep again during the daytime when needed.

Bright Light

Evidence supports a role for appropriately timed bright-light exposure. Yoon and colleagues (77) demonstrated improvement in nocturnal alertness and daytime sleep in night shift workers who were exposed to bright light in their workplace followed by attenuating morning light (using dark sunglasses) on the way home from work. Light boxes, which produce 10,000 lux, once large and cumbersome, now can be easily purchased and are small and more compact. Working with a sleep specialist can help determine the best time and the appropriate amount of time for bright-light sessions for maximum effectiveness. Sessions are normally between 15 and 30 minutes in length. Light boxes are familiar devices to most sleep technologists in that they are aware of light therapy for treating circadian rhythm disorders and seasonal affective disorder. However, light therapy can also be used to help with managing working the night shift.

Blue Light

More recent findings (78) have shown that low-intensity blue light exposure can promote alertness during prolonged nighttime performance testing. Low-intensity blue light exposure may be a valuable option to be applied in situations where bright-light therapy may not be appropriate, such as in certain occupational settings. Testing on daytime workers has demonstrated subjective improvement in alertness, performance, and even fatigue when working under blue-enriched white lights instead of standard white lighting (79). However, it should also be noted that the blue light emitted by electronic devices can also affect individuals and delay sleep onset. Shift workers, like all workers, should be attentive to turning off and discontinuing the use of such devices before sleep.

Eating Habits

Eating healthy is important for shift workers, regardless of shift, though it may be difficult. The best practices for night shift workers include having a lunch like meal upon awakening to energize for your "day." Early in the shift, a small dinner meal or snack is appropriate. Later in the shift small healthy snacks every couple of hours can help to maintain alertness and energy. At the end of the shift, a small breakfast is best to improve daytime sleep.

Meals should be balanced between proteins, low glycemic index foods, fruits and vegetables, and carbohydrates (80). Eat for energy and avoid junk foods that cause sluggishness. Preplanning meals and snacks ahead of time is also a best practice and assists with wiser choices. To achieve better eating habits, bring your own food to work. Most to-go foods and vending machine foods are high in salt, fat, and sugars, and the temptation to upsize is high. Drink plenty of water and stay away from soft drinks because even the diet versions are unhealthy.

Napping

Napping is an effective strategy for those who suffer sleep deprivation as the result of shift work or prolonged work schedules. It is important to take advantage of the circadian rhythm and normal periods of sleepiness. Night shift workers who took a 90-minute-to-2-hour nap before their shift were able to prevent sleepiness. Later naps produced deeper sleep, but workers awakened with grogginess because of sleep inertia (81). When time will not allow a 90-minute-to-2-hour nap, the nap timing should be limited to 45 minutes to avoid entering SWS. Even a 20-minute nap at work on the night shift between 1 and 3 a.m. can improve performance on the first night shift but not the second (82). In a study of emergency physicians working a 24-hour shift, a 1-hour afternoon nap had a vigilance-promoting effect (83). The same study showed that performance in brief psychometric tests was unchanged (83). The beneficial effect of a nap seems to be delayed several hours among individuals subjected to acute sleep loss (84).

Exercise

Exercise triggers an increase in body temperature and improves alertness. Shift workers that engage in brief bouts of aerobic exercise experience less sleepiness and more alertness during their shift.

Sleep Aids

The temptation to use a sleeping pill to fall asleep during the day is high and many over-the-counter sleep aids are available. However, they cannot reset the circadian clock; not even the prescription sleep aids can do that. Many sleep aids also become less and less effective over time. Antihistamines are a common ingredient in over-the-counter items that people use as sleep aids, but the side effect of drowsiness when awake can be severe. This could lead to drowsy driving or difficulty being alert while working.

Sleep Hygiene

The practice of following basic sleep hygiene is important. Black out curtains to darken rooms, and the use of "white noise" to help block daytime sounds is even more important for shift workers. Schedule repairs and deliveries outside of scheduled sleep hours as much as possible. Silence phones and consider setting up an alternate contact for an emergency during sleep hours. Protect sleep time and maintain good sleep habits to improve functioning during a night shift.

Stimulants
Caffeine

The alerting effect of caffeine has been recognized for centuries. Caffeine-containing beverages and over-the-counter tablets help individuals ameliorate the impact of both voluntary and involuntary sleep deprivation. In general, its effects last 3 to 5 hours yet may last for 10 or more hours in caffeine-sensitive individuals. The alerting effect is dependent on habitual use, body mass index, and previous food intake. Strategies for caffeine use have been developed for workers and call for avoidance when already alert (e.g., the beginning of a daytime shift or just after a nap). Caffeine is best ingested 1 hour before the expected time of decreased alertness, which on the night shift would probably be between 3 and 5 a.m. Consumption should be stopped at least 3 hours ahead of the planned bedtime. Users of caffeine need to be aware of the potential side effects, such as diuresis (dehydration), anxiety, irritability, tremulousness, and insomnia. One team of investigators (85) suggested the combined use of caffeine and a nap to counteract sleepiness in drivers. Knowing that the effect of caffeine is usually delayed by 30 minutes after ingestion, drivers who employed the use of caffeine followed by a short nap incurred the benefits of both.

Studies have also examined the use of caffeine to counteract the fatigue and sleepiness of shift work. Muehlbach and Walsh (86) demonstrated a decreased physiologic tendency to sleep on the night shift compared with placebo; however, both the placebo and caffeine group performed assembly-line tasks equally. A recent study suggests that caffeine improves vigilance and athletic performance for special forces personnel who were subjected to 27 hours of sustained wakefulness during field operations (87).

Modafinil

Medications should not be the first line of treatment for shift workers. Modafinil, a unique wake-promoting agent, is approved for use in treating sleepiness associated with shift work. This drug was originally developed for the treatment of narcolepsy. Generally well tolerated and associated with few side effects, it is relatively long acting and does not usually cause peripheral sympathetic stimulation. Studies have suggested a lower abuse and dependency potential when compared with older stimulant drugs. Modafinil has been shown to attenuate physiologic sleepiness and neurobehavioral deficits that occur during the hours of a typical night shift (88–90). In a study exploring the efficacy of modafinil prophylactically given for maintaining the performance of aviators in simulators despite 40 hours (2 days and 1 night) of continued wakefulness, the drug showed some promise, but nausea, vertigo, and dizziness were common (91). When compared with D-amphetamine, modafinil had comparable beneficial effects on mood, fatigue, and cognitive performance with fewer side effects (92). When compared with 600 mg of caffeine in normal adults following 40 continuous hours of wakefulness, both drugs improved performance and vigilance equally (93). In a randomized, placebo-controlled study (94), improvements in alertness and performance were found with 200 mg of modafinil in measures of sleep latency, clinical impression rating, sustained-attention performance, and patient-estimated sleepiness. However, the benefits were small, and in those treated, high levels of sleepiness and impaired performance persisted at night.

Many sleep technologists, like other night workers, suffer from shift work sleep disorder (SWSD), which is caused by an inability of some shift workers to adapt to the major misalignment between their work and rest schedules. The US Modafinil Study Group reported that the effect of modafinil taken 30 minutes before the night shift in patients with excessive sleepiness was the result of SWSD. Modafinil significantly improved functioning and quality of life and at the same time did not show adverse effects on intended sleep. The drug was well tolerated and did not lead to meaningful changes in safety parameters when compared with placebo (95).

Armodafinil

Armodafinil is another oral wakefulness-promoting agent used in the treatment of narcolepsy, SWSD, and residual daytime sleepiness complaints in obstructive sleep apnea patients treated with continuous positive airway pressure. The Food and Drug Administration–approved dose of armodafinil is 150 to 250 mg taken as a single dose in the morning or 150 mg taken 1 hour before the start of the night shift in patients with SWSD. Armodafinil dose reductions should be considered for patients with severe hepatic impairment or for elderly patients in whom elimination may be slowed. Unlike modafinil, there is a lower risk of serious rash or hypersensitivity reaction with the use of armodafinil. The incidence and type of psychiatric symptoms associated with armodafinil are expected to be similar to those of modafinil (96).

Melatonin

Melatonin, a secretory product of the pineal gland, is known to be important in synchronization of circadian rhythms. Exogenous melatonin has been used to treat the symptoms of circadian maladaptation associated with night shift work and jet lag (97–99). By taking melatonin before the start of the first four of eight afternoon/evening sleep episodes before night shift (a 7-hour advance of the sleep schedule), subjects were found to have larger phase advances than those who took placebo (100). However, only a few studies have addressed the impact of melatonin in practical, real-life situations. Cavallo et al. (101) gave melatonin or placebo to physicians training in pediatrics during the morning after night shift work and found no improvement in measures of sleep, mood, and five of six measures of attention in the melatonin group when compared with the placebo group. It is safe to say that there is insufficient evidence to recommend melatonin as part of the strategy to combat sleep loss in night shift workers.

SUMMARY

Quantitative and qualitative sleep deprivation is a widespread problem with serious health consequences both for the individual and for society. Sleep technologists are in a unique position to understand sleep deprivation from a "personal" perspective and to employ their knowledge of sleep physiology to advise their patients and improve their own performance.

REFERENCES

1. Malik, S. W., & Kaplan, J. (2005). Sleep deprivation. *Primary Care: Clinics in Office Practice, 32*, 475–490.
2. Hirshkowitz, M., Whiton, K., Albert, S. M., et al. (2015). National Sleep Foundation's sleep time duration recommendations: Methodology and results summary. *Sleep Health, 1*(1), 40–43.
3. Cirelli, C. (2018). *Insufficient sleep: Definition, epidemiology, and adverse outcomes.* UpToDate. Retrieved June 23, 2018, from https://www.uptodate.com/contents/insufficient-sleep-definition-epidemiology-and-adverse-outcomes
4. Finan, P. *The effects of sleep deprivation.* Johns Hopkins Medicine. Retrieved June 23, 2018, from https://www.hopkinsmedicine.org/health/healthy-sleep/health-risks/the-effects-of-sleep-deprivation
5. Mitler, M. M., Carskadon, M. A., Czeisler, C. A., et al. (1988). Catastrophes, sleep, and public policy: Consensus report. *Sleep, 11*, 100–109.
6. National Sleep Foundation. (2014). *2014 Sleep Health Index.* Retrieved June 23, 2018, from https://sleepfoundation.org/sites/default/files/2014%20Sleep%20Health%20Index-FINAL_0.PDF
7. Van Dongen, H., Maislin, G., Mullington, J. M., et al. (2003). The cumulative cost of additional wakefulness: Dose-response effects on neurobehavioral functions and sleep physiology from chronic sleep restriction and total sleep deprivation. *Sleep, 26*(2), 117–126. doi:10.1093/sleep/26.2.117
8. Drummond, S. P. A., & Brown, G. G. (2001). The effects of total sleep deprivation on cerebral responses to cognitive performance. *Neuropsychopharmacology, 25*, S68–S73. doi:10.1016/S0893-133X(01)00325-6
9. Bentivoglio, M., & Grassi-Zucconi, G. (1997). The pioneering experimental studies on sleep deprivation. *Sleep, 20*(7), 570–576.
10. Patrick, G. T. W., & Gilbert, J. A. (1896). On the effect of loss of sleep. *Psychological Review, 3*, 469–483.
11. Rechtschaffen, A., Bergmann, B. M., Everson, C. A., et al. (1989). Sleep deprivation in the rat: Integration and discussion of the findings. *Sleep, 25*, 68–87.
12. Bonnet, M. H. (2005). Acute sleep deprivation. In M. H. Kryger, T. Roth, & W. C. Dement (Eds.), *Principles and practice of sleep medicine* (4th ed., pp. 51–57). Philadelphia, PA: WB Saunders.
13. Bonnet, M. H. (1986). Performance and sleepiness as a function of frequency and placement of sleep disruption. *Psychophysiology, 23*, 263–271.
14. Webb, W. B., & Agnew, H. W. (1975). The effects on subsequent sleep of an acute restriction of sleep length. *Psychophysiology, 12*, 367–370.
15. Benoit, O., Foret, J., Bouard, G., et al. (1980). Habitual sleep length and patterns of recovery sleep after 14 hour and 36 hour sleep deprivation. *Electroencephalography and Clinical Neurophysiology, 50*, 477–485.
16. Rosenthal, L., Merlotti, L., Roehrs, T. A., et al. (1991). Enforced 24-hour recovery following sleep deprivation. *Sleep, 14*, 448–453.
17. Dispersyn, G., Sauvet, F., Gomez-Merino, D., et al. (2017). The homeostatic and circadian sleep recovery

responses after total sleep deprivation in mice. *Journal of Sleep Research, 26,* 531–538. doi:10.1111/jsr.12541

18. Van Dongen, H. P. A., Baynard, M. D., & Maislin, G. (2004). Systematic interindividual differences in neurobehavioral impairment from sleep loss: Evidence of trait-like differential vulnerability. *Sleep, 27,* 423–433.

19. Dinges, D. F., Pack, F., Williams, K., et al. (1997). Cumulative sleepiness, mood disturbance, and psychomotor vigilance performance decrements during a week of sleep restricted to 4–5 hours per night. *Sleep, 20,* 267–277.

20. Qureshi, A. I., Giles, W. H., Croft, J. B., et al. (1997). Habitual sleep patterns and risk for stroke and coronary heart disease: A 10-year follow-up from NHANES I. *Neurology, 48,* 904–911.

21. Ferrie, J. E., Shipley, M. J., Cappuccio, F. P., et al. (2007). A prospective study of change in sleep duration: Associations with mortality in the Whitehall II cohort. *Sleep, 30,* 1659–1666.

22. Satoyo, I., Hiroyasu, I., & Chigusa, D. (2009). Association of sleep duration with mortality from cardiovascular disease and other causes for Japanese men and women: The JACC study. *Sleep, 32*(3), 259–301.

23. American Academy of Sleep Medicine. (2014). *International classification of sleep disorders* (3rd ed.). Darien, IL: Author.

24. Carskadon, M. A., & Dement, W. C. (1981). Cumulative effects of sleep restriction on daytime sleepiness. *Psychophysiology, 18,* 107–113.

25. Dement, W., & Greenberg, S. (1966). Changes in total amount of stage four sleep as a function of partial sleep deprivation. *Electroencephalography and Clinical Neurophysiology, 20,* 523–526.

26. Albert, I., Cicala, G. A., & Siegel, J. (1970). The behavioral effects of REM sleep deprivation in rats. *Psychophysiology, 6,* 550–560.

27. Peder, M., Elomaa, E., & Johansson, G. (1986). Increased aggression after rapid eye movement sleep deprivation in Wistar rats is not influenced by reduction of dimensions of enclosure. *Behavioral Neural Biology, 45,* 287–291.

28. Hicks, R. A., Moore, J. D., Findley, P., et al. (1978). REM sleep deprivation and pain thresholds in rats. *Perception and Motor Skills, 47,* 848–850.

29. Smith, C. (1996). Sleep states, memory processes, and synaptic plasticity. *Behavioral Brain Research, 78,* 49–56.

30. Cohen, H. B., & Dement, W. C. (1965). Sleep: Changes in threshold to electroconvulsive shock in rats after deprivation of "paradoxical" phase. *Science, 150,* 1318–1319.

31. Dement, W., Greenberg, S., & Klein, R. (1966). The effect of partial REM sleep deprivation and delayed recovery. *Journal of Psychiatric Research, 4,* 141–152.

32. Nykamp, K., Rosenthal, L., Folkerts, M., et al. (1988). The effects of REM sleep deprivation on the level of sleepiness/alertness. *Sleep, 21,* 609–614.

33. Agnew, H. W., Jr., Webb, W. B., & Williams, R. L. (1964). The effects of stage four sleep deprivation. *Electroencephalography and Clinical Neurophysiology, 17,* 68–70.

34. Johnson, L. C., Naitoh, P., Moses, J. M., et al. (1974). Interaction of REM deprivation and stage 4 deprivation with total sleep loss: Experiment 2. *Psychophysiology, 11,* 147–159.

35. Devoto, A., Lucidi, F., Violani, C., et al. (1999). Effects of different sleep reductions on daytime sleepiness. *Sleep, 22,* 336–343.

36. Onen, S. H., Alloui, A., Gross, A., et al. (2001). The effects of total sleep deprivation, selective sleep interruption and sleep recovery on pain tolerance thresholds in healthy subjects. *Journal of Sleep Research, 10,* 35–42.

37. Lentz, M. J., Landis, C. A., Rothermel, J., et al. (1999). Effects of selective slow wave sleep disruption on musculoskeletal pain and fatigue in middle-aged women. *The Journal of Rheumatology, 26,* 1586–1592.

38. Carette, S., Oakson, G., Guimont, C., et al. (1995). Sleep electroencephalography and the clinical response to amitriptyline in patients with fibromyalgia. *Arthritis and Rheumatology, 38,* 1211–1217.

39. Mahowald, M. L., & Mahowald, M. W. (2000). Nighttime sleep and daytime functioning (sleepiness and fatigue) in less well-defined chronic rheumatic diseases with particular reference to the "alpha delta NREM sleep anomaly" *Sleep Medicine, 1,* 195–207.

40. Rains, J. C., & Penzien, D. B. (2003). Sleep and chronic pain challenges to the α-EEG sleep pattern as a pain specific sleep anomaly. *Journal of Psychosomatic Research, 54,* 77–83.

41. Roth, T., Hartse, K. M., Zorick, F., et al. (1980). Multiple naps and the evaluation of daytime sleepiness in patients with upper airway sleep apnea. *Sleep, 3,* 425–439.

42. Bonnet, M. H. (1985). Effect of sleep disruption on sleep, performance, and mood. *Sleep, 8,* 11–19.

43. Levine, B., Roehrs, T., Stepanski, E., et al. (1987). Fragmenting sleep diminishes its recuperative value. *Sleep, 10,* 590–599.

44. Roehrs, T., Merlotti, L., Petrucelli, N., et al. (1994). Experimental sleep fragmentation. *Sleep, 17,* 438–443.

45. Williamson, A. M., & Feyer, A. M. (2000). Moderate sleep deprivation produces impairments in cognitive and motor performance equivalent to legally prescribed levels of alcohol intoxication. *Occupational and Environmental Medicine, 57*(10), 649–655.

46. National Institute of Neurological Disorders and Stroke. (2007). *Brain basics: Understanding sleep: How much sleep do we need?* Retrieved June 23, 2018, from

http://www.ninds.nih.gov/disorders/brain_basics/understanding_sleep.htm#how_much

47. Johns, M. *About the ESS*. Retrieved June 23, 2018, from http://epworthsleepinessscale.com/about-the-ess/

48. Borbely, A. A. (1982). A two process model of sleep regulation. *Human Neurobiology, 1*, 195–204.

49. Carskadon, M. A., & Roth, T. (1991). Sleep restriction. In T. Monk (Ed.), *Sleep, sleepiness and performance* (pp. 151–167). Chichester, UK: John Wiley & Sons.

50. Nilsson, L. G., Backman, L., & Karlsson, T. (1989). Priming and cued recall in elderly, alcohol intoxicated and sleep deprived subjects: A case of functionally similar memory deficits. *Psychology in Medicine, 19*, 423–433.

51. Tucker, A. M., Whitney, P., Belenky, G., et al. (2010). Effects of sleep deprivation on dissociated components of executive functioning. *Sleep, 33*(1), 47–57.

52. Pilcher, J. J., & Huffcutt, A. I. (1996). Effects of sleep deprivation on performance: A meta-analysis. *Sleep, 19*, 318–326.

53. Adrien, J. (2002). Neurobiological bases for the relation between sleep and depression. *Sleep Medicine Review, 6*, 341–351.

54. Vogel, G. W., Vogel, F., McAbee, R. S., et al. (1980). Improvement of depression by REM sleep deprivation: New findings and a theory. *Archives of General Psychiatry, 37*, 247–253.

55. Buxton, O. M., Quintiliani, L. M., Yang, M. H., et al. (2009). Association of sleep adequacy with more healthful food choices and positive workplace experiences among motor freight workers. *American Journal of Public Health, 3*, S636–S643.

56. Nedeltcheva, A., Kilkus, J., Imperial, J., et al. (2009). Sleep curtailment is accompanied by increased intake of calories from snacks. *American Journal of Clinical Nutrition, 89*, 126–133.

57. Spiegel, K., Tasali, E., Penev, P., et al. (2004). Sleep curtailment in healthy young men is associated with decreased leptin levels, elevated ghrelin levels, and increased hunger and appetite. *Annals of Internal Medicine, 141*, 846–851.

58. Taheri, S., Lin, L., Austin, D., et al. (2004). Short sleep duration is associated with reduced leptin, elevated ghrelin, and increased body mass index. *PLoS Medicine, 1*, e62.

59. Knutson, K., Spiegel, K., Penev, P., et al. (2007). The metabolic consequences of sleep deprivation. *Sleep Medicine Review, 11*, 163–178.

60. Morselli, L., Leproult, R., Balbo, M., et al. (2010). Role of sleep duration in the regulation of glucose metabolism and appetite. *Best Practice and Research: Clinical Endocrinology and Metabolism, 24*, 687–702.

61. Sprunyt, K., Molfese, D., & Gozal, D. (2011). Sleep duration, sleep regularity, body weight and metabolic homeostasis in school aged children. *Pediatrics, 127*, e345–e352.

62. Smith, M., Edwards, R., McCann, U., et al. (2007). The effects of sleep deprivation on pain inhibition and spontaneous pain in women. *Sleep, 30*, 494–505.

63. Mitler, M. M., Dinges, D. F., & Dement, W. C. (1994). Sleep medicine, public policy, and public health. In M. H. Kryger, T. Roth, & W. C. Dement (Eds.), *Principles and practice of sleep medicine* (2nd ed., pp. 453–462). Philadelphia, PA: WB Saunders.

64. Summala, H., & Mikkola, T. (1994). Fatal accidents among car and truck drivers: Effects of fatigue, age and alcohol consumption. *Human Factors, 36*, 315–326.

65. Owens, J. M., Dingus, T. A., Guo, F., et al. (2018). Prevalence of drowsy driving crashes: Estimates from a large-scale naturalistic driving study. *AAA Foundation for Traffic Safety*.

66. Leger, D. (1994). The cost of sleep related accidents: A report for the National Commission on Sleep Disorders Research. *Sleep, 17*, 84–93.

67. Safety Study NTSB/SS-95/01. (1995). *Factors that affect fatigue in heavy truck accidents* (Vol. 1). Washington, DC: National Transportation Safety Board.

68. Langlois, P. H., Smolensky, M. H., His, B. P., et al. (1985). Temporal patterns of reported single-vessel car and truck accidents in Texas, U.S.A. *Chronobiology International, 2*, 131–140.

69. Richardson, G. S., Carskadon, M. A., Orav, E. J., et al. (1982). Circadian variation of sleep tendency in elderly and young subjects. *Sleep, 5*, S82–S92.

70. Lamond, N., & Dawson, D. (1999). Quantifying the performance impairment associated with fatigue. *Journal of Sleep Research, 8*, 255–262.

71. Dawson, D., & Reid, K. (1997). Fatigue, alcohol and performance impairment. *Nature, 388*, 235.

72. Stutts, J. C., Wilkins, J. W., Scott Osberg, J., et al. (2003). Driver risk factors for sleep-related crashes. *Accident Analysis and Prevention, 35*, 321–331.

73. National Sleep Foundation. (2008). 2008 *Sleep in America Poll*. Retrieved June 23, 2018, from https://sleepfoundation.org/sites/default/files/2008%20POLL%20SOF.PDF

74. Cavallo, A., Ris, M. D., & Succop, P. (2003). The night float paradigm to decrease sleep deprivation: Good solution or new problem? *Ergonomics, 46*, 653–663.

75. Harma, M. I., Ilmarinen, J., Knauth, P., et al. (1988). Physical training intervention in female shift workers: II. The effects of intervention on the circadian rhythms of alertness, short-term memory, and body temperature. Aging, physical fitness and shiftwork tolerance. *Ergonomics, 31*, 51–63.

76. Knauth, P. (1987). Changing schedules: Shiftwork. *Chronobiology International, 14*, 159–171.

77. Yoon, I., Jeong, D., Kwon, K., et al. (2002). Bright light exposure at night and light attenuation in the morning improve adaptation of night shift workers. *Sleep, 25,* 351–356.

78. Phipps-Nelson, J., Redman, J., Schlangen, L., et al. (2009). Blue light exposure reduces objective measures of sleepiness during prolonged nighttime performance testing. *Chronobiology International, 26,* 891–912.

79. Viola, A. U., James, L. M., Schlangen, L. J. M., et al. (2008). Blue-enriched white light in the workplace improves self-reported alertness, performance and sleep quality. *Scandinavian Journal of Work Environment Health, 34,* 297–306.

80. A Shift Workers' Guide to Nutrition. *Shifting nutrition: A shift workers guide to nutrition.* Retrieved June 23, 2018, from https://www.worksafe.qld.gov.au/__data/assets/pdf_file/0009/109773/shifting-nutrition.pdf

81. Dinges, D. F., Orne, M. T., Whitehouse, W. G., et al. (1987). Temporal placement of a nap for alertness: Contribution of circadian phase and prior wakefulness. *Sleep, 10,* 313–329.

82. Purnell, M. T., Feyer, A. M., & Herbison, G. P. (2002). The impact of a nap opportunity during the night shift on the performance and alertness of 12-hour shift workers. *Journal of Sleep Research, 11,* 219–227.

83. Frey, R., Decker, M. A., Lutz, R., et al. (2002). Effect of rest on physicians' performance in an emergency department, objectified by electroencephalographic analyses and psychometric tests. *Critical Care Medicine, 30,* 2322–2329.

84. Lumley, M., Roehrs, T., Zorick, F., et al. (1986). The alerting effects of naps in sleep-deprived subjects. *Psychophysiology, 23,* 403–408.

85. Reyner, L. A., & Horne, J. A. (1997). Suppression of sleepiness in drivers: Combination of caffeine with a short nap. *Psychophysiology, 34,* 721–725.

86. Muehlbach, M. J., & Walsh, J. K. (1995). The effects of caffeine on simulated night-shift work and subsequent daytime sleep. *Sleep, 18,* 22–29.

87. McLellan, T. M., Kamimori, G. H., Voss, D. M., et al. (2005). Caffeine maintains vigilance and improves run times during night operations for Special Forces. *Aviation and Space Environment Medicine, 76,* 647–654.

88. Walsh, J. K., Randazzo, A. C., Stone, K. L., et al. (2004). Modafinil improves alertness, vigilance, and executive function during simulated night shifts. *Sleep, 27,* 434–439.

89. Dinges, D. F., Wright, K. P., Walsh, J. K., et al. (2003). Modafinil improves psychomotor vigilance performance in shift work sleep disorder. *Sleep, 26,* A87.

90. Czeisler, C. A., Dinges, D. F., Walsh, J. K., et al. (2003). Modafinil for the treatment of excessive sleepiness in chronic shift work sleep disorder. *Sleep, 26,* A114.

91. Caldwell, J. A., Jr., Caldwell, J. L., Smythe, N. K., III, et al. (2000). A double-blind, placebo-controlled investigation of the efficacy of modafinil for sustaining the alertness and performance of aviators: A helicopter simulator study. *Psychopharmacology (Berlin), 150,* 272–282.

92. Pigeau, R., Naitoh, P., Buguet, A., et al. (1995). Modafinil, d-amphetamine and placebo during 64 hours of sustained mental work: Effects on mood, fatigue, cognitive performance and body temperature. *Journal of Sleep Research, 4,* 212–228.

93. Wesenstein, N. J., Belenky, G., Kautz, M. A., et al. (2002). Maintaining alertness and performance during sleep deprivation. Modafinil versus caffeine. *Psychopharmacology (Berlin), 159,* 238–247.

94. Czeisler, C. A., Walsh, J. K., Roth, T., et al. (2005). Modafinil for excessive sleepiness associated with shift-work sleep disorder. *New England Journal of Medicine, 353,* 476–486.

95. Erman, F., & Rosenburg, R. (2007). Modafinil for excessive sleepiness associated with chronic shift work sleep disorder: Effects on patient functioning and health related quality of life. *Primary Care Companion to the Journal of Clinical Psychiatry, 9,* 188–194.

96. Schwartz, J., Roth, T., & Drake, C. (2010). Armodafinil in the treatment of sleep/wake disorders. *Neuropsychiatric Disease and Treatment, 6,* 417–427.

97. Folkard, S., Arendt, J., & Clark, M. (1993). Can melatonin improve shift workers' tolerance of the night shift? Some preliminary findings. *Chronobiology International, 10,* 315–320.

98. James, M., Tremea, M. O., Jones, J. S., et al. (1998). Can melatonin improve adaptation to night shift? *American Journal of Emergency Medicine, 16,* 367–370.

99. Jorgensen, K. M., & Witting, M. D. (1998). Does exogenous melatonin improve day sleep or night alertness in emergency physicians working night shifts? *American Journal of Emergency Medicine, 31,* 699–704.

100. Sharkey, K. M., & Eastman, C. I. (2002). Melatonin phase shifts human circadian rhythms in a placebo-controlled simulated night-work study. *American Journal of Physiology and Regular Integrated Comprehensive Physiology, 282,* R454–R463.

101. Cavallo, A., Ris, D., Succop, P., et al. (2005). Melatonin treatment of pediatric residents for adaptation to night shift work. *Ambulatory Pediatrics, 5,* 172–177.

chapter 7
Respiratory Anatomy and Physiology

DAVID F. WOLFE

LEARNING OBJECTIVES

On completion of this chapter, the reader should be able to:

1. Identify the anatomic name and location of each portion of the respiratory system from the mouth to the blood flowing through the lungs including the relevant respiratory muscles and their control.
2. Discuss the physics of respiratory gas exchange, the role of oxygen and carbon dioxide concentration gradients, and the thin membranes involved in gas exchange.
3. Describe several aspects of the relationship between ventilation and perfusion of the lungs, including anatomy, gas exchange, and neural/chemical control of ventilation.
4. Describe the general effects of sleep on respiratory and cardiovascular control of ventilation.
5. Describe the differential effects of waking, nonrapid eye movement sleep, and rapid eye movement sleep on ventilation and heart rate.
6. Identify and describe the more common pathologic states associated with breathing control mechanisms including central apnea/hypopnea, obstructive apnea/hypopnea, treatment-emergent central sleep apnea, Cheyne–Stokes respiration, and periodic breathing.

KEY TERMS

Alveoli
Aortic bodies
Apnea
Atrium
Bicarbonate
Carbon dioxide (CO_2)
Carbonic acid
Carbonic anhydrase
Carotid bodies
C-fiber receptors
Chemoreceptors
Cheyne-Stokes respiration
Concentration gradients
Cranial nerves
Dead space
Diaphragm
Diffusion
Expiratory reserve volume
Functional residual capacity
Hypercapnia
Hypopnea
Hypoxia
Inspiratory capacity
Inspiratory reserve volume
Intercostals
Intrapleural space
Larynx
Mediastinum
Medulla
Obstructive sleep apnea (OSA)
Oxygen (O_2)
Oxyhemoglobin dissociation curve
Parietal pleura
Pharynx
Phrenic nerve
Pneumocytes
Pneumothorax
Pons
Pulmonary capillaries
Rapidly adapting receptors
Residual volume
Respiration
Shunt
Slowly adapting receptors
Surfactant
Tidal volume
Total lung capacity
Trachea
Tricuspid valve
Vena cava
Ventricle
Visceral pleura
Vital capacity

Respiration is, in all animals, a vital process responsible for the delivery of oxygen (O_2) to the tissues to support metabolism and the removal of the metabolic waste gas, carbon dioxide (CO_2). The major mechanisms of this exchange of gases between the external and internal environments are (1) simple passive diffusion along concentration gradients and (2) transport of these gases by the circulatory system. Concentration gradients refer to the difference in the concentration of a gas or liquid across a semipermeable barrier. In very small animals, such as single-celled organisms, gaseous diffusion occurs across their cell membranes, but larger organisms have distances that are too great for passive diffusion. Animals evolved a small number of very effective solutions, for example, a closed circulatory system and highly vascularized lungs or gills. Lungs (or gills) provide a specialized structure for placing a large amount of circulating body fluid (e.g., blood) very close (<1 mm) to a large amount of environmental media (e.g., air). Proximity across a permeable membrane that separates different concentrations of O_2 and CO_2 allows rapid movements of both gases down their concentration gradients, normally in opposite directions.

In higher chordate animals, respiratory transfer of CO_2 and O_2 is a two-step, cyclic process. The first step is at the interface between the body tissues (e.g., muscle cells, liver cells) and the circulating lung capillary blood. This step is characterized by O_2 movement from blood plasma across the thin separating membrane that makes up the capillary wall and into a metabolizing tissue (e.g., muscle or brain). Concurrently, the CO_2 liberated by tissue metabolism diffuses from the metabolizing cells across the tissue capillary membrane and into the circulating blood.

The second step occurs in the lungs between the lungs' airspaces and the circulating blood in very small capillaries within the lungs. Opposite from the tissue part of the cycle, gas movements in the lung are characterized by O_2 movement from the air within the lung into the pulmonary capillary blood, whereas CO_2 moves from the capillary blood into the minute air spaces called "alveoli" within the lung. The next expiration then expels most of the CO_2, and the next inspiration replenishes the O_2 supply. This two-part process is termed "gas exchange." The transfers of metabolic gases are passive processes because both gases are simply moving down their concentration gradients at both the pulmonary and the tissue locations.

Necessary and complementary components of this process are the circulation of blood and ventilation of the lungs. Therefore, the heart and blood vessels are essential components of respiration and are intimately involved in blood gas homeostasis. Breathing control mechanisms exist to control the concentrations of O_2 and CO_2 in the lung air and, subsequently, blood within the lung, which is carried to the tissues to support normal metabolism. In other words, the controls of respiratory movements are mostly based on sensory signals from the brain and body chemoreceptors, sensing O_2 levels, and CO_2/pH levels. These sensory signals mostly come from chemosensitive neurons in the brainstem, especially the medulla, the carotid bodies in the neck, and the aortic bodies on the aortic arch. The carotid and aortic bodies are chemosensitive to O_2 and CO_2/pH. These signals then "feed back" to the brainstem controllers, which then reduce hypercapnia (an excess of CO_2) or hypoxia (a deficiency of O_2 in the airways) by increasing ventilation and cardiac output. This is a classic example of a negative feedback loop used to control some critical physiologic variable. These respiratory actions are well coordinated with the cardiovascular system to achieve effective blood gas homeostasis.

In humans and other mammals, the respiratory drive to ventilate the lungs is mostly performed by neural networks in the brain. In fact, much of the brainstem and significant portions of certain "higher" areas of the brain are devoted to respiratory and cardiovascular control, especially cardiopulmonary coordination. Although purely physical and biochemical factors can and do affect respiration, by far, most mechanisms for maintaining and adjusting pulmonary ventilation are found in the brainstem and spinal cord. As a first step into the mechanisms used to control gas exchange, we review the structural components of the system, because a basic biologic principle is the intricate interdependence between form (anatomy) and function (physiology).

A REVIEW OF RESPIRATORY-RELATED ANATOMY AND PHYSIOLOGY

Any comprehensive discussion of respiratory function requires a review of thoracic, circulatory, and central nervous system (CNS) structure. Respiration and respiratory control encompass many anatomic and physiologic features that interact to meet very specific goals of homeostasis. One excellent example of this interaction is that of the circulatory and respiratory systems. The O_2 content and the CO_2 content within the circulatory system are the focus of the homeostatic controllers of ventilation.

Upper Respiratory Tract

Air drawn into the nasal passages and oral cavity is humidified, filtered, and warmed (in cooler climates) at the beginning of the pathway (see Fig. 7-1). Humidification of the incoming air is complete, resulting in pulmonary airspaces with 100% water saturation. The inside surfaces of the oral cavity and tongue contribute to water saturation of the incoming breath and

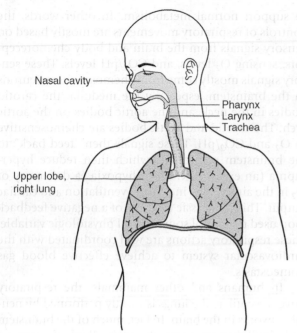

Figure 7-1 A schematic of the respiratory system with the most important anatomic features emphasized. Note the narrowing of the airspace around the pharynx and larynx.

also collect particulates from the incoming air, using surface water and turbulent airflow. In addition to humidification, the mucus membranes of the irregularly shaped turbinates within the nasal passages promote turbulence in the airflow, which assists the filtering of particulates. Air turbulence serves to increase filtering efficiency because small particles in the inhaled, turbulent air are more likely to eventually contact a mucus membrane than would particles within a straight streamlined airflow. Nasal hairs also serve to create turbulence in the nasal airflow to maximize the filtering and humidification of the inspired air. These hairs also screen out large particles in the air stream. The captured particles (dust, ash, pollen, skin flakes, etc.) are then swallowed, coughed out, or blown out of the nose by a sneeze. The main utility of this physical process is that the amount of particulate matter going into the lung is minimized.

Just behind the nasal passages and the oral cavity is the pharynx, essentially the upper part of the throat. As suggested by Figure 7-1, nasal and oral air mix here before passing into the larynx; this portion of the upper airway is located between the pharynx and the trachea and contains the vocal cords. The pharynx is a common site for airway collapse or partial obstruction, especially during supine sleep. The collapse may lead to a complete occlusion, called an apnea, or a partial collapse allowing some airflow, called a hypopnea. Muscles of the larynx and pharynx respond to sleep like most other skeletal muscles, with a significant decrease in muscle tone and reactivity (1). Most of the upper airway is surrounded by

pharyngeal and laryngeal muscles that are important in airway rigidity, airway size, coughing, and speech. A bolus of food or water activates complex laryngeal motor reflexes, which guide the bolus into the esophagus, away from the vocal cords and trachea.

The pharynx and the larynx are the usual sites for obstructive ventilatory events; that is, both structures tend to collapse and occlude the airway. One common scenario is when the back of the tongue relapses onto the posterior walls of the pharynx. The relapse is often caused by insufficient tongue muscle activation during sleep, especially in supine sleep and obesity. This is the classic description of obstructive sleep apnea (OSA), or obstructive hypopnea. The insufficiency is partly related not only to the normal decrease in motor tone during sleep, but also to anatomic features, such as the tongue's size and mass and/or micrognathia (small, recessed chin). The most important aspect of obesity in relation to obstructive apnea is when the area under the chin is obese and flaccid, allowing the tissue to sag into the mouth cavity leading to obstructions (2). Obviously, supine sleep significantly exacerbates the obstruction. In that position, the tissue sags toward the back of the throat, increasing the effect of an obstruction in the airway.

Other airway obstructions often occur because of sleep-related relaxation of the pharyngeal and/or laryngeal muscles, allowing negative airway pressure to pull the posterior wall of the airway forward toward the tongue and the front side of the airway. This obstruction usually creates either an apnea or a hypopnea. Airflow through the vocal cords and trachea is low resistance and generally unremarkable. This continuum from the mouth and nares to the superior end of the trachea represents the upper respiratory tract.

Lower Respiratory Tract

The lower respiratory tract begins at the upper end of the trachea (Fig. 7-1); this then connects to the pulmonary trunk that soon branches into the right and left bronchi (Fig. 7-2). At the first branching level, the trachea splits into right and left bronchi. The left bronchus branches into two smaller sections, whereas the right bronchus branches into three. The lung tissue supplied by these five bronchi corresponds to the five lobes of the lung: three lobes of the right lung and two lobes of the left lung. Branching continues, ending with the alveoli and the alveolar ducts. These levels are where gas exchange takes place.

The walls of the alveoli are composed of pulmonary epithelial cells and pulmonary capillaries carrying deoxygenated venous blood. There are two important cell types lining the alveolus: type I pneumocytes and type II pneumocytes. Type I cells make up the cell membrane or walls. The less numerous type II cells are the source of a substance called "surfactant," which reduces surface tension on the inner alveolar walls. The reduced (and

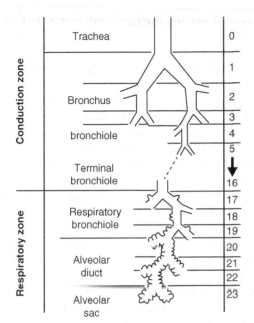

Figure 7-2 This diagram represents the branching of the respiratory conduction system of the lung. There is no real "airflow" after the terminal bronchioles; the distances are so short that diffusion moves the gases. Note that from the trachea to the later branches and terminal bronchioles total airway volume is increasing as the individual airway size decreases.

variable) surface tension stabilizes the alveolus, making collapse less likely (3). The narrow divide (0.5 μm) between air in the alveoli and venous blood in the capillaries greatly facilitates gas exchange across the alveolar membrane with the nearby red blood cells (RBCs).

When a reduced RBC (depleted of O_2) reaches the alveolar membrane, the venous O_2 pressure is approximately 40 mm Hg and the alveolar air, half a micron away, is about 100 mm Hg. This concentration gradient moves alveolar O_2 easily across the membrane into the blood plasma and then into the RBC. The PO_2 value for the exiting capillary blood, on its way to the left atrium of the heart, is approximately 150 mm Hg. In contrast, the CO_2 pressure is about 45 mm Hg in venous blood and about 40 mm Hg in oxygenated alveoli, a relatively small concentration gradient. In healthy people, the transfer of that 5 mm Hg of CO_2 takes about one-fourth second (similar to the time for RBC oxygenation), well before the RBC exits the pulmonary capillary (~0.75 seconds).

Vascular Anatomy of the Lungs and Heart

It should be clear that the cardiovascular system is intimately involved in breathing control mechanisms. The flow of blood generated by the heart is how O_2 reaches the tissues and how CO_2 gets to the alveoli to be expired. There is a considerable symmetry between the vascular structure and the airway structure in the lower reaches of the lungs. This is necessary to bring the smallest airways and the very small pulmonary capillaries into close contact while maintaining sufficient blood pressure to keep the small vessels open and sufficient airway pressure to keep the most vulnerable airways open.

Venous blood from the body reaches the heart through two large veins: the superior vena cava and the inferior vena cava. The superior vena cava carries blood from the head, arms, and upper torso; the inferior vena cava carries blood from the legs and lower torso. These two large veins converge on the right atrium. During the part of the cycle when the cardiac muscle is relaxed, blood flows through the right atrium via the tricuspid valve and pools in the right ventricle (see Fig. 7-3). When the ventricle is full, systole (cardiac muscle contraction) begins with contraction of the right atrium, forcing atrial venous blood into the already-full ventricle. This stretches the ventricular muscle, raising the ventricular blood volume and pressure. The tricuspid valve between the right atrium and the right ventricle closes just as the right ventricle contracts. Contraction of the right ventricle expels the venous blood, forcing it through the pulmonary valve of the heart into the pulmonary artery and, eventually, the pulmonary capillaries of the alveoli within the lung. For the now-oxygenated blood exiting the alveoli, it is the same process back to the heart. The pulmonary capillaries come together to form very small veins, which merge with others to form a somewhat larger vein and so on. Finally, this O_2-saturated blood travels the pulmonary vein back to the left atrium of the heart. As with the right side, the left atrium is essentially a primer pump to create sufficient intraventricular pressure to stretch the cardiac muscle and maximize the efficiency of the ventricular contraction. The left ventricle then expels its volume of oxygenated, low CO_2 content blood into the arterial circulation (see Fig. 7-3).

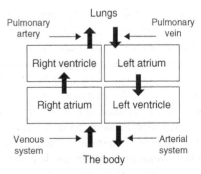

Figure 7-3 A simple schematic of the circulatory cycle within the heart, lungs, and body. Large arrows demonstrate the direction of blood flow in and out of the lungs and heart. Small arrows indicate body anatomy involved: right heart (pulmonary artery and venous system) and left heart (pulmonary vein and arterial system).

The circulatory structure of the cardiopulmonary system is the one place in the body where venous blood is carried in an "artery," because it is exiting the right ventricle but is still deoxygenated and hypercapnic (an excess of CO_2). Similar to the airway conduction system, the large pulmonary artery coming from the right ventricle enters the lung and branches down to the level of the alveolar ducts and alveoli. Once the venous blood is into the pulmonary capillaries surrounding an alveolus, the CO_2 within that blood flows down its concentration gradient, across the pulmonary membrane, into the alveolar air. At the same time, inspired O_2 moves down its concentration gradient, across the alveolar membrane into the "venous" blood in the pulmonary capillaries, changing it to oxygenated arterial blood.

Thoracic Anatomy and Function

The main muscles of inspiration are the diaphragm and the external intercostals. Both are common skeletal muscles controlled by spinal motor nerves. The diaphragm and the external intercostals act in concert to create negative intrapulmonary pressure, resulting in airflow into the trachea, or inspiration. During an inspiration, ambient air enters the body through the nares, mouth, or both. Then, the air stream passes through the many branches of the airways, eventually reaching the vicinity of many alveoli. Diffusion moves the O_2 the rest of the way into the alveoli and their capillaries.

The air within the pathways from the mouth and nares down to the terminal airways constitutes a significant volume that is not involved in an exchange of O_2 and CO_2. This is because air is in the passageways of the lung, not in the portions involved in gas exchange. This is the "conduction" portion of the respiratory system. The "respiratory" portion of the lungs is composed of the alveoli, alveolar ducts, and respiratory bronchioles. These are the levels at which gas exchange occurs. The airway conduction system is graphically demonstrated in Figure 7-2.

One of the two respiratory "pump" muscles is the diaphragm, necessary for normal ventilation, although many other muscles assist the diaphragm in producing ventilation. Ventilation is the physical consequence of normal cyclic respiratory muscle activity. Diaphragmatic contraction, due to CNS activation, causes the thoracic cavity floor to descend, making the thoracic cavity larger and creating negative pressure to draw in air from the environment, that is, inspiration. The diaphragm has almost no involvement in expiring air from the lungs. The other major inspiratory pump muscles are the external intercostals, which connect adjacent ribs. During inspiration, the external intercostals contract to pull the chest wall outward and upward to increase thoracic cavity size, contributing to the decrease of intrapulmonary

pressure and making the chest wall stiffer (less compliant). There are also several sets of secondary, or accessory, inspiratory muscles. Accessory respiratory muscles include those in the abdomen, neck, pharynx, larynx, nose, tongue, and upper chest.

In polysomnography, changes in abdominal and thoracic circumference are usually recorded to assess ventilatory effort. This technique is actually measuring the displacement because of the external intercostals—diaphragmatic contraction does not increase chest circumference. This is still useful because it provides a relatively easy index of respiration, without complicated and invasive procedures or imaging.

In normal "at-rest" ventilation, expiration is entirely passive. Because during normal breathing no expiratory muscle activity is required, cyclic inspiration is the emphasis of the control system at rest. Of course, active expiration by expiratory muscles is often necessary, such as in exercise, to more quickly expel the breath and allow for appropriately rapid ventilation. The main expiratory muscles are the internal intercostals and abdominal muscles, but others also assist. Expiratory pump muscles act to increase intrathoracic pressure in order to increase intrapulmonary pressure and push air out of the lungs more quickly.

The conducting airways, from the mouth and nose to the lungs, are not involved in gas exchange, but are surrounded by both skeletal and smooth muscles that act to control the flow of air to and from the lungs (Fig. 7-2). Muscles of the upper respiratory tract are especially relevant in sleep medicine because of their involvement in OSA. The usual site of an obstruction is an area of the upper airway where muscles are relatively flaccid, or abnormally large. Muscles of the pharynx, larynx, and tongue make up this group. These too are skeletal muscles and, like the other accessory respiratory muscles, have functions other than ventilation—for example, swallowing, speech, and movement of the head, neck, or shoulders. Airway muscles are activated in a specific phase of respiration (inspiration or expiration), but they are not responsible for controlling intrathoracic pressures and, therefore, are not respiratory pump muscles.

OSA/hypopnea arises from insufficient compensation by muscular control systems for certain anatomic and postural features or deficiencies, such as the chin and neck obesity described earlier. This insufficiency is often not due to any change in the CNS controllers or blood gas reflexes, but simply due to the weight of the tongue (or tonsils) and the lack of physical support while sleeping supine. Sleep is a critical factor in apneas/hypopneas because neural output to all skeletal muscles, except the diaphragm, is reduced during sleep (4). OSA is an excellent illustration of the interaction between structure and function and of the impact of the neurophysiologic state, sleep, on those interactions.

The lungs themselves have no muscles for movement and are not physically attached to the chest wall; instead, an alternate mechanism evolved to couple the lungs to the thoracic wall. The outer surface of the lungs is called the "visceral pleura." The visceral pleura also covers the mediastinum, a midline "structure" between the lungs that includes the trachea, heart, great vessels, thymus, and esophagus. The inside surface of the thoracic cavity is lined by a layer of epithelium called the "parietal pleura." The visceral pleura is held to the parietal pleura by negative intrapleural pressure. It is important to realize that there are no anatomic features that hold the lungs against the inner thoracic walls. This physical coupling of the two pleura, resulting from the negative intrapleural pressure, ensures that the volume of the lungs varies directly with the size of the thoracic cavity. The pleura are mostly impervious to gases, helping maintain the negative pressure. Because there is normally almost no "space" in the "intrapleural space" (2 to 5 mL), it is often referred to as a "potential space." Negative intrapleural pressure results from elastic recoil of the respiratory muscles and lungs and the surface tension of the aqueous film lining the inner alveolar surface. Elasticity is a structural property of lung tissue. Emphysema reduces elastic recoil through the destruction of alveolar walls and their pulmonary capillaries (5). The resulting enlargement of that airspace represents a greatly reduced surface area for gas exchange.

The term "pneumothorax" is used to convey a loss of negative pressure in the intrapleural space because of an opening to the atmosphere or into the lung. When the negative pressure is lost, the two pleura separate and air flows into the newly enlarged space. This effectively uncouples the close adhesion between inspiratory chest wall movement and lung expansion, that is, the lung collapses. A pneumothorax may occur spontaneously or as a result of trauma involving an opening in either of the pleura. For example, a stab or gunshot wound that penetrates both pleura can allow air from the atmosphere into the intrapleural space and the lung, removing the negative pressure gradient. This is a medical emergency requiring immediate assistance.

In patients without penetrating trauma of the chest wall, the diagnosis is usually based on the presence of chest pain, increased heart rate, tachypnea, hypoxemia, and shortness of breath. X-rays are also helpful in diagnosing a pneumothorax. Acute pneumothorax is usually treated with a needle aspiration of the intrapleural space and/or a chest tube. Both procedures require hospitalization. Other treatments include supplemental O_2 and positive pressure ventilation. A chronic spontaneous pneumothorax can occur in the lung, often near the apex, and creates a hole in the visceral pleura, allowing lung air to flow into the negative pressure of the intrapleural space.

Innervation of the Respiratory Muscles and Blood Vessels

The diaphragm and external intercostals are driven by specific motor nerves from the spinal cord. The diaphragm is the main controller of ventilatory movements and is driven by the phrenic nerves. The external intercostals are the most relevant to respiratory control mechanisms. The output carried by the phrenic nerve is from the bilateral phrenic areas of the spinal cord gray matter. The spinal phrenic area is, in turn, controlled from specific areas in the brainstem. Neural control is addressed later in this chapter.

In addition to the inspiratory muscles, there are important expiratory muscles as well. The most important expiratory muscles are the internal intercostals and the abdominal muscles. Like the external intercostals, the internal intercostals are driven by nerves that emanate from the full length of the thoracic segment of the spinal cord. Motor nerves to the abdominal muscles derive from the lumbar portion of the spinal cord.

Blood vessel diameter, and subsequently pressure, is actively controlled by the sympathetic nervous system. The main output nuclei controlling cardiovascular sympathetic neurons are located in the brainstem and hypothalamus; these areas are driven by many inputs from several brain areas. The parasympathetic system has no known significant impact on the control of blood pressure. The other major controlling variable is the heart rate. The intrinsic heart rate is derived from the sinoatrial (SA) node, located in the right atrium. This "baseline" rate is normally modulated by many factors but mostly by the sympathetic system and the parasympathetic system. Usually, sympathetic excitation is associated with increased heart rate, enhanced cardiac muscle contractility (force of contraction), increased motor tone throughout the body, and often an increase in blood pressure. The parasympathetic effects are mostly the opposite of the sympathetic effects.

RESPIRATORY PHYSIOLOGY

Respiratory function is based on the need to acquire O_2 for normal metabolism and to remove the metabolic waste gas, CO_2. A paradox of this physiologic mechanism is that the respiratory system does not try to eliminate *all* of the CO_2 in the lungs. Instead, the neurally mediated respiratory control system actively maintains CO_2 at approximately 40 mm Hg. The respiratory system is an important component of acid–base (pH) balance within the body. Within RBCs, the combination of CO_2 and water (H_2O) into carbonic acid (H_2CO_3) is catalyzed by carbonic anhydrase. Blood plasma does not have this important enzyme. Carbonic acid dissociates

Controller effects on the oxyhemoglobin dissociation curve

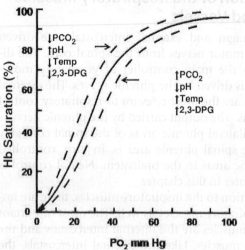

Figure 7-4 The oxyhemoglobin dissociation curve. This graph illustrates that the basic function for hemoglobin (Hb) is the uptake of, or dissociation from, oxygen (O_2) molecules. The broken lines describe the effect of four variables on O_2 release from Hb. These effects are much greater when the patient is on the steep part of the curve. 2,3-DPG, 2,3-diphosphoglycerate.

to hydrogen (H^+) and bicarbonate ions (HCO_3^-). Maintaining CO_2 at approximately 40 mm Hg results in an O_2 pressure lower than it would be without the high level of CO_2, illustrating the importance of the role played by the respiratory system in acid–base balance. Figure 7-4 shows the effects of various agents on the oxyhemoglobin dissociation curve, including acidity and PCO_2: decreased PCO_2 or increased pH shifts the curve to the left, decreasing PO_2 for a given hemoglobin (Hb) saturation (increasing the Hb's affinity for O_2). Most relevant to the patient is where he or she is on the x-axis when the controlling factors are expressed ($\uparrow PCO_2$, $\downarrow pH$).

In what follows, there are many descriptions of gradients and concentration differences. Often, it is important to know the quantity of some gas, mixed with other gases and contained within some space (like a lung, or the earth's atmosphere). The quantitative measure of that specific gas is the partial pressure (Table 7-1), conventionally in millimeters of mercury (mm Hg). The total of all partial pressures in the earth's atmosphere is the barometric pressure, approximately 760 mm Hg. The partial pressure of O_2 in our atmosphere is 158 mm Hg. Because 158 divided by 760 equals 0.208, the O_2 in our atmosphere is approximately 21%. Almost all the rest is nitrogen, with a partial pressure of 596 mm Hg (78.4% of barometric pressure). Also, there is usually water in the atmosphere, with some obvious exceptions. A generalized value for the partial pressure of water in the atmosphere is 5.7 mm Hg or 0.008%. Therefore,

$$P_{baro} = PO_2 + PN_2 + PH_2O = 759.7.$$

Table 7-1 Partial Pressures (mm Hg)

Compartment	O_2	CO_2
Atmosphere	158	0.3
Alveolar air	97–100	~40
Pulmonary capillary	100–45	~46
Arterial blood	~100	36–44
Arterial capillary	60–65	~40
Tissues	~40	45–48
Venous blood	40–50	46.0

There is a very small amount of other gases in the atmosphere, such as argon (0.93%) and CO_2 (0.03%). Still more gases are also present in air, but at very low concentrations.

The following is an illustrative example of a gradient: if the partial pressure of O_2 in arterial capillary blood is 62 mm Hg and the partial pressure of O_2 in an adjacent metabolizing cell is 35 mm Hg, then the O_2 gradient is 27 mm Hg, from blood to tissue cells. The steeper the gradient, the greater is the force or speed of gas movement.

Respiratory Volumes and Capacities

There are several "compartments" within the respiratory system: first, the body trunk cavity lined with parietal pleura, then the thoracic cavity, then the lungs themselves within the visceral pleura, the upper airway, the trachea, the conducting portion of the bronchial tree, and, finally, the cavities within alveoli and alveolar ducts. These compartments comprise the pulmonary structure.

It is necessary to know the various volumes and capacities to understand the usual clinical pulmonary function testing (PFT) (Table 7-2). The first example is tidal volume (V^T), the volume of air moved in a single breath, usually in milliliters (mL) or liters (L). V^T multiplied by the respiratory rate (breaths per minute) gives the minute ventilation (liters per minute), an important clinical parameter describing the amount of air moved in 1 minute. Low levels of minute ventilation are a common accessory to apnea of any type. The maximum volume that one can inspire beginning at the end of a normal inspiration is the inspiratory reserve volume (IRV). Similarly, the expiratory reserve volume (ERV) is the volume that can be expired from the end of a normal expiration. This information from the reserve volumes can indicate deficiencies that do not become evident until the patient tries to exercise.

Table 7-2 Respiratory Volumes and Capacities[a]

Space/Structure	Volumes (mL)	Capacities (mL)
Tidal volume (V^T)	500	
Inspiratory reserve volume (IRV)	3,000	
Expiratory reserve volume (ERV)	1,100	
Residual volume (RV)	1,300	
Total lung capacity	IRV + V^T + ERV + RV	5,900
Vital capacity	IRV + V^T + ERV	4,600
Function residual capacity	ERV + RV	2,400
Inspiratory capacity	V^T + IRV	3,500
Physiologic dead space	155	
Anatomic dead space	150	
Intrapleural space	2–5	

[a]All values approximate.

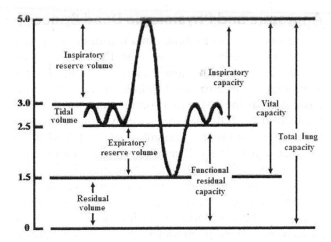

Figure 7-5 The various lung volumes and capacities as defined by a spirometry trace. These volumes are measured using specific breathing maneuvers while attached to a spirometer. y-axis is in liters (L).

Exertion requires extra energy and O_2, and the removal of excess CO_2 created by the increase in metabolism with exertion. This need to restore normal or optimal concentrations requires ventilation to increase and move into the IRV and likely the ERV as well. Different pathologies affect different volumes in different ways and can be quite valuable in diagnosis.

Measures of various volumes within the respiratory system are very important in diagnosing disease or injury in the lungs (see Fig. 7-5 and Table 7-2); examples include pulmonary fibrosis, asthma, and chronic obstructive pulmonary disease (COPD). Knowledge of these pressures, volumes, and capacities is essential in PFT.

Almost all the lung volumes can be measured by a device called a "spirometer," a clinical instrument for measuring ventilatory movements in terms of relative volume changes. The spirometer measures and records the changes in the volume of inhaled or exhaled air continuously across ongoing respiratory cycles. A change in spirometer volume is equal to the amount of air expired (or inspired) by the patient. Performing several ventilatory maneuvers allows assessment of specific volumes using spirometry, which is very useful in the diagnosis of several obstructive diseases, for example, asthma and COPD.

The volume in the lung remaining at the end of a normal expiration is the functional residual capacity (FRC). The FRC is composed of the ERV and the residual volume (RV): FRC = ERV + RV. RV is the volume of air remaining after a maximum expiration. RV cannot be quantified by spirometry, but it can be estimated or quantified by other more extensive, and sometimes invasive, tests.

In another spirometric test, the patient is asked for a maximal inspiration followed by a maximal expiration; the difference (range) between the peak and trough volumes defines vital capacity (VC). VC is the combination of V^T, ERV, and IRV: VC = V^T + ERV + IRV. In many texts, the VC is referred to as the forced vital capacity, which refers to the use of maximum force on both inspiration and expiration. As may be clear by now, a capacity is the sum of two or more volumes. Total lung capacity (TLC) is the sum of VC (V^T + IRV + ERV) and RV.

RV is the only volume that cannot be measured by spirometry. This derivation is problematic because one of the limits of the RV range is zero (0). FRC also cannot be derived by spirometry because FRC contains RV, along with ERV. Spirometry measures volumes as differences between two definable limits or landmarks, such as ERV derived from the volume at the end of a maximal expiration *relative to* the lung volume at the end of a normal expiration. RV cannot be measured by spirometry because absolute values are needed, not relative values. Therefore, other procedures must be used to measure an absolute value such as RV. Because RV cannot be directly measured (quantitatively), TLC cannot be derived from spirometry as that would require absolute values for RV.

RV is one portion of the lung that does not directly participate in normal gas exchange. In this area, lacking sufficient ventilation, diffusion distances are large and inefficient. This volume is not adequately replenished with atmospheric air, and removal of CO_2 is slow. Therefore, in RV, O_2 levels are low (hypoxia) and CO_2 accumulates (hypercapnia).

Anatomic and Physiologic Dead Space

"Dead space" refers to those areas within the lung that are not participating in gas exchange. These are volumes of great importance because they represent the useless ventilation of an area that has little or no blood flow. Dead space is inevitable in a complex structure like the lung, but changes in dead space usually indicate a pathologic process or event. Essentially, increased dead space represents inefficiency in ventilation. There are two important types of dead space: anatomic and physiologic.

Most of the anatomic dead space is represented by the volume of the conducting airways: nares, pharynx, larynx, trachea, bronchi, bronchioles, and terminal bronchioles. Their membranes are thick and fibrous, resulting in rigidity; effective gas exchange is practically impossible in those tissues. Anatomic dead space (in milliliters) is roughly equal to a person's weight in pounds (6, 7).

Another type of dead space is physiologic dead space. This represents areas that could engage in gas exchange but do not for some reason, for example, insufficient pulmonary blood flow (Q) to some portion of the lung to maintain normal gas exchange. Dead space reduces gas exchange and can lower O_2 levels in the arterial system.

Circulatory abnormalities can also create shunting. This refers to the absence of ventilation through some area in the lung while perfusion of that area continues. Ventilation of the area affected by shunt does not include gas exchange between atmospheric air in the lung and circulating blood because there is no, or very little, blood flow. One hallmark of shunt is an increase in the difference between the PO_2 in the alveolus (PAO_2) and PaO_2 (partial pressure of O_2 in the arterial blood); normally, this difference is due to a drop in PaO_2 rather than an increase in PAO_2. The normal difference is small (<5 mm Hg). A larger difference normally results from a reduced PaO_2 and indicates incomplete oxygenation of the arterial blood.

The magnitude of the shunt can be expressed by the shunt fraction, which expresses the percentage of blood in the cardiac output that is not ventilated. Intrapulmonary shunting (low ventilation with normal right heart output) can be a major cause of hypoxemia in pulmonary edema and pneumonia.

The application of supplemental O_2 to a patient will either increase the PaO_2 or have no significant effect. If the patient shows an increased level of arterial O_2 in response to supplemental O_2, he or she probably has a ventilation/perfusion mismatch; if the patient has nearly the same PaO_2 with supplemental O_2, the problem is likely a shunt.

Measuring the PAO_2 for comparison with the PaO_2 is problematic regarding access to small groups of alveoli, which are microscopic blind sacs. A good estimate for the partial pressure of alveolar O_2 can be derived with the alveolar gas equation:

$$P_AO_2 = FIO_2 \left(P_{atm} - PH_2O\right) - PaCO_2/R$$

The uppercase P represents partial pressure, "A" denotes alveolar, "a" denotes arterial, FI is fraction inspired (normally 0.21), P_{atm} indicates atmospheric (barometric) pressure (usually near 760 mm Hg), and R signifies the respiratory quotient, which is the ratio between the O_2 consumed and the CO_2 produced. The normal value for R is 0.8 but varies from approximately 0.6 to 1.1, usually because of dietary differences. For example, a diet high in carbohydrates may result in a higher respiratory quotient.

Lastly, a blood clot (embolus) in a pulmonary arteriole in the wall of ventilated alveoli creates physiologic dead space because perfusion is reduced in that area. The RV also contributes to physiologic dead space. However, most physiologic dead space results from low blood flow creating an inequality between ventilation and perfusion. A rough average for normal anatomic dead space is 150 mL, and physiologic dead space is about 155 mL, for a total of approximately 305 mL in a normally functioning respiratory system. Refer to Table 7-3 for normal values for several of the most relevant respiratory variables.

Gas Exchange and Transport

Gas exchange refers to the movements of O_2 and CO_2 between the atmosphere and the metabolizing cells of the body. Respiratory gas exchange occurs in two different areas of the body. One is the membrane between alveolar air spaces and the deoxygenated, CO_2-laden blood entering the pulmonary capillaries, that is, alveolar capillaries. This particular exchange includes the movement of CO_2 from the blood into the alveolar air spaces and O_2 moving from the air spaces into the pulmonary/alveolar capillary blood. Although it takes a RBC about 0.75 seconds, to traverse a typical pulmonary capillary, it takes only 0.25 seconds for about 95% of the blood to be oxygenated (6). Note that the equilibration point is only one-third of the way through the capillary. This is another example of "built-in" extra capacity to increase the rate of blood flow and ventilation. The second area for gas exchange is between the arterial capillaries and the metabolizing tissues, for example, muscle cells, liver cells, or neurons. In this exchange, the gas movements are reversed. Here, O_2 in the blood diffuses into the tissues to support metabolism, whereas CO_2 moves from the tissue into the local venous capillaries. In both locations, the movements of both respiratory gases are driven by their respective concentration (or partial pressure) gradients.

There is another important factor at work that greatly increases the O_2-carrying capacity of the blood,

Table 7-3 Normative Values

Term	Parameter	Value	Other
Partial pressure O_2	PO_2	100 mm Hg	Value—lung, arterial blood
Tidal volume	V^T	400 mL	Normal value
Minute ventilation	Vdot	6 L/min	Normal value
Breath frequency	f	10 breaths/min	Normal value
Minute circulation	Qdot	100 mL/min	Value—bronchial circ./flow
Barometric pressure	B	760 mm Hg	Atmospheric press, sea level
Dead space	D	~150 mL	
Arterial O_2	PO_{2a}	95 mm Hg	
Venous O_2	PO_{2v}	40 mm Hg	Also for "mixed" venous
O_2 conc. in air/inhaled	FIO_2	0.2094	Inhaled air is 21% O_2
CO_2 conc./exhaled	$FECO_2$	0.045	Exhaled air is 4.5% CO_2

but at the same time has little effect on the PO_2 gradient between the blood and the tissues. That factor is Hb, a complex molecule with a proteinaceous part (a globin molecule) and an iron-dependent pigment molecule with four heme groups attached (heme is an organic molecule containing nitrogen). Each heme group contains an atom of ferrous iron (Fe^{2+}) and each Fe^{2+} atom can carry one molecule of O_2. Hence, one Hb molecule can carry up to four O_2 molecules. The globin molecule actively controls the affinity of the iron atoms for O_2 and plays a major role in gas exchange between Hb and the tissues and efficient oxidation in the lungs.

The O_2–Hb Dissociation Curve

The complex relationship between HbO_2 (percent saturation) and plasma PO_2 (mm Hg) is commonly illustrated with the O_2–Hb dissociation curve (Fig. 7-4). The most obvious feature of this curve is the sigmoid (S-shaped) nature of the relationship. This shape is a direct result of particular properties of the Hb molecule, especially that once the first heme is oxidized, there is an increase in O_2 affinity of the three remaining hemes. Stated differently, the shape of the curve represents a facilitation of the *release* of O_2 when exposed to the low O_2 levels characteristic of metabolizing tissues ($\downarrow PO_2$, <60 mm Hg) and, conversely, the quick, efficient capture of O_2 when exposed to ventilated alveolar air ($\uparrow PO_2$, >60 to 70 mm Hg). The flat portion of the curve at the top of the graph represents a weak effect of PO_2 on percent Hb saturation in that area of the curve when both PO_2 and HbO_2 are high. In that upper area, Hb-bound O_2 is relatively unaffected by modest falls in PO_2, which can happen when there are lung regions that are underventilated or underperfused. In spite of the fall in PO_2, the blood maintains a lower, but still adequate, O_2 storage. While sitting (or during mild exercise in fit people), most of the O_2 needs of the body are supplied by dissolved O_2 and a small amount of Hb-bound O_2. Dissolved O_2 must fall approximately 40 mm Hg (40%) for a fall in Hb saturation of only 7% to 10%. Because most O_2 is carried by Hb, not dissolved, O_2 content (= HbO_2 + PO_2) is mostly preserved. However, once the inflection of the curve is reached, a much smaller further drop in PO_2 is accompanied by a rapid, large drop in saturation (and O_2 content), that is, the steep portion of the curve. These unique properties of Hb provide considerable extra capacity for effective gas exchange. The sheer volume of HbO_2 in the blood provides a ready source of O_2 to maintain metabolism and appropriate gas concentration gradients, even during intense exercise.

One example of biophysical factors modulating the O_2 affinity of Hb, the Bohr effect, describes the effects of local acidity (H^+) on affinity between heme and O_2 (Fig. 7-4). As PCO_2 rises (e.g., during exercise), the amount of coupling of CO_2 with water (H_2O + CO_2) also rises, creating more of the intermediate form H_2CO_3 (carbonic acid). Carbonic acid quickly dissociates into hydrogen ions (H^+) and bicarbonate ions (HCO_3^-). Bicarbonate ions are essential in acid–base homeostasis, in that bicarbonate ions are the main base (opposite of acid) within that regulatory system. The release of hydrogen ions lowers the pH, which reduces the affinity of heme for O_2. In other words, if during exercise the H^+ concentration goes up (lower pH), the heme groups tend to release their O_2 molecules to maintain the exercise. This is referred to as the Bohr effect, which occurs in the metabolizing tissues ($\uparrow PCO_2$, $\downarrow pH$, $\downarrow PO_2$)

and increases O_2 availability to counteract the acidosis. Other factors modulating heme affinity for O_2 include temperature and concentrations of CO_2, adenosine triphosphate, and phosphate. Increases in muscle temperature, for example, tend to release O_2 from Hb.

It is noteworthy that much of the mechanism for the fine control of O_2 delivery to the tissues is accounted for by the interaction between many metabolic factors (PO_2, temperature, pH, PCO_2, etc.), all shifting the basic controller, the slope, and/or shape of the oxyhemoglobin dissociation curve, to the left or right (Fig. 7-4). Using the single factor of acidity may illustrate the impact of moderate changes in pH on Hb saturation and O_2 content. With PO_2 at 45 mm Hg and a normal pH of 7.4, the Hb saturation is approximately 80%; however, at the same PO_2, but with a more acidic pH of 7.2, Hb saturation is approximately 70%. Therefore, an acidosis of 7.2 leads to a considerable loss of Hb saturation and O_2 content of the blood. Under the same conditions, but with an alkalosis (pH 7.6), the percentage of Hb that is saturated is 85% to 90%, a 5- to 10-point increase from the normal condition. The degree of change is smaller in alkalosis than in acidosis because of the very small slope of the upper part of the dissociation curve. Other important variables such as increased temperature and increased levels of inorganic phosphate in the body shift the oxyhemoglobin dissociation curve to the right, as with acidosis. Generally, an increase in metabolism is associated with a shift of the curve to the right, favoring O_2 release to maintain activity and oxygenation.

CO_2 Storage and Transfer

Practically all of the CO_2 in the body is generated by tissue metabolism. About 10% of the CO_2 is in the plasma and 90% within the RBC. However, only about 5% of total CO_2 in the blood is dissolved and another 5% reacts within the plasma, which alters the form of the CO_2. For example, a noncatalyzed reaction with water incorporates the CO_2 into a bicarbonate ion, but very slowly (3). The presence of carbonic anhydrase within the RBC catalyzes the reaction, creating large amounts of bicarbonate ions; this is the reason for the large difference in the percentage of CO_2 between plasma and within the RBC. In fact, the majority of the CO_2 in the body is held in bicarbonate ions—HCO_3—not as CO_2. Some of the hydrogen ions liberated by the carbonic acid bind to Hb, triggering O_2 release from the Hb molecule into the RBC plasma and, then, into the blood.

Ventilation–Perfusion Ratios (V_A/Q)

A common occurrence in the normal lung is the temporary partial collapse of small areas of alveoli and alveolar ducts, which reduces the effectiveness of gas exchange. Most of these underventilated alveoli are still perfused with deoxygenated pulmonary capillary blood. This condition significantly reduces gas exchange in that area, whereas in other areas of the lung, gas exchange is normal or even elevated. The ventilation–perfusion ratio (V_A/Q) of this local area of partly or completely collapsed alveoli will fall substantially because the local alveolar collapse represents a decrease in the numerator, V_A, whereas Q is relatively unchanged. The O_2 content of the arterial blood, as it leaves the lung, is diluted by the low or absent contribution from the fully or partially collapsed areas. Normal healthy people at rest have some small amount of collapsed alveoli and dilution ($\leq$4%) but can still be fully functional, that is, these small few collapsed areas have little impact on the normal values of PO_2, O_2 content, or PCO_2. The unchanged pulmonary arterial blood (still hypoxic and hypercapnic) then mixes with and dilutes the plasma gas concentrations, altering the O_2 and CO_2 stores. The result is a small decrease in the whole-body average arterial O_2 level (6).

When an abnormally low amount of ventilation occurs (hypopnea or apnea), V_A is reduced. This is commonly because of increased amounts of alveolar collapse, while Q remains normal, and the V_A/Q falls. The airway blockage also leads to changes in the gas concentrations of the unventilated alveoli; there, gas concentrations become equal to those of venous blood. Alveolar O_2 falls from a PO_2 of 100 to 40 mm Hg, and alveolar PCO_2 increases from 40 to 45 mm Hg (7).

A somewhat different result is seen when the lungs are ventilated normally but underperfused in some area, again effectively reducing or preventing gas exchange within that area. In this case, alveolar O_2 levels can go up as the blood flow drops, increasing the V_A/Q above 1. This is because O_2 is not being absorbed from the alveoli because of the underperfusion. However, the increase in PO_2 has little effect on total body O_2 content. PCO_2 is essentially zero when V_A/Q is high.

Another way of describing this two-way V_A/Q pathology is that a low (<1) V_A/Q is associated with a respiratory pathology (collapsed alveoli), whereas a high V_A/Q is normally associated with a cardiovascular problem. Usually, the problem is a full or partial blockage of pulmonary capillaries or of the upstream arteries that feed the pulmonary capillaries. Deficiencies in either V_A or pulmonary blood flow are referred to as a "V_A/Q mismatch."

Disease or injury may adversely affect cardiac output or lung surface area and consequently decrease blood flow through the lung. Moderately low blood flow does not usually result in significant hypoxia because of the extra unused capacity for gas exchange. If it takes 0.6 seconds (more than twice the normal 0.25 seconds) to accomplish adequate gas exchange, it is still accomplished. This rapid equilibration is mostly due to the thinness of the alveolar membrane (<0.5 μm), but the substantial concentration gradient for O_2 (95% arterial to 40% venous) also contributes to rapid O_2 movement.

Because the normal V_A in humans is approximately 5,250 mL per minute and the normal cardiac output (Q) is 5,000 to 6,000 mL per minute, the normal V_A/Q ratio is approximately 1. If an obstructive problem arises upstream from the pulmonary capillaries, effectively occluding blood flow into the alveoli, then the alveolar gases soon become equal to inspired gas (PO_2 = 150 mm Hg; PCO_2 = 0 mm Hg) but are not absorbed into the blood. In this case, supplemental O_2 can help increase mean arterial O_2. However, if a total blockage occurs in the airways, then the alveolar gas concentrations mimic those of the "venous" blood arriving through the pulmonary arteries. With the airway blockage, supplemental O_2 has little effect on arterial saturation mainly because a greater supply of O_2 does not matter if the O_2 is not absorbed. In a situation where blood flow is compromised and V_A is normal or higher, the V_A/Q is large (>1) because Q is low. Similarly, when blood flow is normal but ventilation is significantly reduced, the V_A/Q is small in magnitude (<1). Hypoxia is one of several factors that causes pulmonary arterial vasoconstriction in the lungs. In patients with cardiopulmonary disease, hypoxemia is usually caused by V_A/Q mismatch.

From the clinical perspective, an important distinction must be made for the effects of gravity on blood and lung tissue. The effect of gravity varies somewhat between upright and reclining; upright posture results in a greater effect on the blood, which is massive compared with the nearly weightless air. When upright, gas and blood stratify between the base of the lung and the apex but in different directions. In that posture, blood pressure is higher in the base of the lung than in the apex while air stratifies in the opposite direction. Volume is one parameter affected by gravity, such that the base of the lung contains more volume than the apex. Also, at the base of the lung, PCO_2 and O_2 content is higher than at the apex. Nearer to the apex, V_A/Q and PO_2 are larger than values at the base. It is important to acknowledge that the posture of a patient under examination has an impact on several aspects of cardiopulmonary function and must be taken into account during a clinical measurement. Likewise, it is clear that alveolar function in one region of the lung is not equal to the function in another area.

Work of Breathing

The work of breathing is a relevant topic owing to the high levels of exertion and muscle activity that accompany many respiratory pathologies, such as emphysema and OSA. Of course, normal respiration also incurs work. The "work" is muscular work used in inspiration and often in expiration too. Most of the muscular work is overcoming elasticity of the lungs and thorax, and part of that elasticity results from the natural tendency of alveoli to collapse from surface tension, even with

surfactant. Another important component of the work of breathing is overcoming airway resistance, especially during high airflow rates, as with exercise. The type of airflow is an important factor in airway resistance. A laminar flow incurs less airway (or vascular) resistance than a turbulent flow. A third source of work of breathing is related to moving inelastic structures such as the liver and stomach, particularly an issue in obese patients. The proportions of the overall work of breathing are overcoming elasticity—65%, airway resistance—28%, and displacement of organs and tissues—7% (3).

NEURAL CONTROL OF VENTILATION

The nervous system is essential for the act of breathing and is responsible for the signals transmitted by nerves to the respiratory muscles. The neural signals also modulate respiratory sensitivity to CO_2 and O_2, which is especially relevant during sleep when the incoming neural signals are reduced in strength. Many neural structures participate in the control of respiration; a few have already been mentioned. Most of the areas responsible for the control of normal breathing are in the medulla, pons, and cerebellum.

Respiratory Rhythm Generation

The basic respiratory rhythm is created and controlled by the CNS. The phrenic nerve output to the diaphragm comes from cervical spinal nuclei called the "phrenic nucleus" (C3 to C5). The medulla is that portion of the brain just "above" (rostral to) the spinal cord. The basic, at-rest, respiratory rhythm is created by a network of neurons in the medulla that fire mostly together, resulting in sustained (~1 to 3 seconds) muscle contractions of the diaphragm and external intercostals, followed by the loss of inspiratory muscle activity, and relaxation of the respiratory muscles. Expiration occurs passively when at rest, as stretched muscles and lungs shorten (elastic recoil), pushing out the breath (8).

Central sleep apnea is caused by a lack of respiratory drive from the brainstem and phrenic nucleus. Most likely, this event is caused by insufficient neural activity in the respiratory rhythm generator within the medulla. This lack of respiratory drive occurs only in sleep, suggesting that the central pattern generator, in some relatively rare individuals, requires greater brainstem arousal to allow normal function. Common treatments for central sleep apnea are respiratory stimulants such as theophylline and related compounds; caffeine is used in some central apnea cases.

Many influences converge in the nucleus of the tractus solitarius (NTS), also known as the solitary tract, and nearby structures that not only control respiration but also affect the autonomic system (heart rate, arterial pressure, cardiac force, etc.). In fact, there is quite a bit of spatial and physiologic overlap between the respiratory and autonomic controllers. These other autonomic influences modulating respiration come from all levels of the nervous system, but most importantly, from the pons (just above the medulla), hypothalamus, and cerebellum (3).

Neurally mediated coordination between the cardiovascular and respiratory control systems serves to appropriately match respiratory airflow and blood flow through the lungs. The main controlling influences on the phrenic nucleus are the respiratory pattern generator (in the brainstem), PCO_2/pH, and PO_2. The brain's response to increased CO_2 is more robust than the response to hypoxia. The neural control system uses these many incoming sensory signals concerning PCO_2/pH, hypoxia, stretch, blood pressure, temperature, and so on to determine how *much* gas exchange is needed. The required change in ventilation requires alterations in the activity of the muscles controlling ventilation and, thus, of those controlling the respiratory gas pressure gradients. These mechanisms of blood gas maintenance are extremely rapid and efficient in healthy people.

NERVOUS SYSTEM ANATOMY AND FUNCTION

The two most relevant CNS areas for respiration are the medulla and the pons (see Fig. 7-6). There are two main areas within the medulla that drive respiratory muscles: the dorsal respiratory group, which is mostly inspiratory, and the ventral respiratory group (VRG), which is related to both inspiration and expiration. Many other brainstem and higher CNS areas modulate those two outputs to "fine-tune" respiration. The pons is also an important source of the effects of rapid eye movement

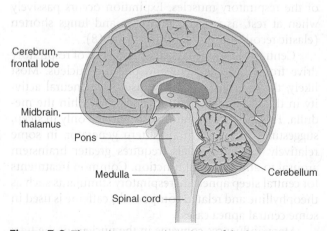

Cerebrum, frontal lobe

Midbrain, thalamus

Pons

Medulla

Cerebellum

Spinal cord

Figure 7-6 The major anatomic regions of the brain. Respiratory and most cardiovascular control is centered in the medulla and pons and assisted by the fastigial nucleus of the cerebellum and the hypothalamus.

(REM) sleep on respiration in which respiratory variability increases in both amplitude and frequency.

There are an unknown number of chemosensory areas that monitor the amount of O_2, CO_2, and acidity in the blood, but the most well-known group of brain chemoreceptors lies on the ventral surface of the medulla. This group of medullary neurons makes up the classical central chemoreceptors. Central chemoreceptors seem to provide the major drive to the basic respiratory rhythm; that is, without some CO_2 sensory stimulation in this area, respiration tends to slow or stop. This is an important reason why the respiratory control system does not completely eliminate CO_2, because CO_2 is essential to the acid–base balance of the body and, likely, the centrally mediated drive to breathe. Central chemoreceptors are the main sensors for CO_2, but they also respond to acidic pH and low PO_2.

There are two sets of peripheral chemoreceptors, that are similar to the central chemoreceptors but not identical. These sensors are called "peripheral" because they reside outside the CNS. One set of peripheral chemoreceptors is in the carotid bodies, which are located at the bifurcation of the common carotid arteries in the neck. The other set is located in the aortic arch of the upper chest. Most of the monitoring of O_2 in the blood is performed by the peripheral chemoreceptors. It is now known that several other brain sites are also chemoreceptive to CO_2 (9), but their relative contribution to respiration is largely unknown.

The carotid bodies' sensory nerve fibers make up a part of the carotid sinus nerve and also carry information on arterial blood pressure. Those arterial pressure sensors, called "baroreceptors," are in the carotid sinus, adjacent to the carotid bodies. Chemoreceptor information from the aortic arch conducts baroreceptor information. Both sets of peripheral chemoreceptors (and their associated baroreceptors) send their sensory information back to the NTS. The NTS is the first target for many important peripheral sensory inputs from the respiratory and cardiovascular systems, such as oxygenation, CO_2, arterial blood pressure, lung stretch, pulmonary irritant receptors, and others.

Practically all of the secondary respiratory muscles, for example, shoulder muscles, chest muscles, and abdominals, are also controlled by brainstem cell groups, especially the VRG, but these muscles are also controlled by more conventional motor systems located outside of the brainstem. An important point concerning neuromuscular control of ventilation is that many of those muscle actions must also accommodate the other nonventilatory functions of the respiratory system, such as swallowing, talking, postural control, defecation, vomiting, and locomotion.

One of the more important brainstem controllers is the NTS, which processes sensory signals from both respiratory and cardiovascular systems, although mostly in different subregions (10). The medulla is also the major source of sympathetic (autonomic) drive to constrict the blood vessels of skeletal muscles, the kidneys, and other viscera and to participate in the control of the heart rate. In fact, it is possible that the chemoreceptors and the sympathetic neurons of the ventral medulla are one and the same. The extensive anatomic overlap between respiratory and cardiovascular control is just one reflection of the complex functional coupling of the two systems. For example, increased blood flow through exercising muscles, mediated in part by the medulla, is necessary to carry the additional CO_2 away from the tissues, modulating the CO_2 concentration gradient between the intracellular environment and the blood plasma. Respiratory insufficiency, leading to low oxygenation (hypoxia), causes increased sympathetic activity that leads to higher heart rate and blood pressure. These changes in sympathetic activity compensate for the low O_2 levels by increasing the delivery rate of blood. Therefore, respiration and cardiovascular control are fundamentally linked by common goals of cardiopulmonary homeostasis.

Innervation of the Respiratory Muscles

The intercostal muscles (both external and internal) and other thoracic and abdominal muscles also receive innervation from spinal motor neurons in the ventral parts of the lower cervical and thoracic spinal cord. These spinal motor neurons receive input from many of the same medullary cell groups that project to the phrenic nucleus (10, 11). Other accessory respiratory muscles, such as those in the upper airway (pharynx, larynx, and tongue), are innervated by cranial motor nerves such as the facial (VII), the glossopharyngeal (IX), and the hypoglossal (XII) nerves. Although the primary function of the upper airway muscles is to maintain an open airway during inspiration, a secondary function is the regulation of the rate of expiratory airflow using constriction and relaxation of the airway. The change from nasal breathing to mouth breathing (and vice versa) is also controlled by upper airway muscles (pharyngeal). Although many of these ventilatory muscles are driven by the same medullary cell groups, they often have maximal activity during a selective portion of the inspiratory (or expiratory) phase, such as late inspiration or early expiration. Different timing of accessory muscle activations in both inspiration and expiration are important control features that serve to reduce the work of breathing and maximize gas exchange. In addition, as respiratory activation is intensified by large blood gas disturbances, the degree of accessory muscle participation increases.

Although skeletal muscles make up the main functional component of ventilation, smooth muscle is used in the tracheal and bronchial airways for constriction or relaxation. The parasympathetic branch of the autonomic nervous system innervates these muscles. Although this aspect of respiratory control is mediated by autonomic (parasympathetic) structures, it is incorrect to refer to respiratory control as an "autonomic" system; it is a somatomotor system (albeit a very specialized one) in a similar way as the control of chewing or walking is a somatomotor system. The parasympathetic innervation of the airways is mainly from the vagus nerve and uses acetylcholine to constrict the airways; therefore, anticholinergic drugs can be used for airway muscle relaxation, for example, in asthma (12).

Basic Respiratory Pattern Generation

The source of the cyclical alternation of inspiration and expiration is a long-running controversy in various branches of the biomedical community. The arguments fall into two major groups: the pacemaker hypothesis and the network hypothesis (10). However, there is little controversy that the basic respiratory rhythm is generated in the medulla, regardless of how it is generated. The basic respiratory rhythm produced by either scenario is then modified and controlled by reflexes and other influences to match ventilation to changing physiologic needs, such as exercise and sleep.

The pacemaker hypothesis states that there exists a group (or groups) of medullary neurons that independently create the basic respiratory rhythm, similar to the pacemaker cells in the SA node of the heart. A group of pacemaker neurons does seem to exist in the ventrolateral part of the medulla, very near to a major output path to the phrenic nucleus (in the VRG), but it is doubtful that these neurons are solely responsible for normal respiration (10).

The network hypothesis states that the basic respiratory rhythm arises from a complex interplay between various types of inspiratory and expiratory neurons. These cell types are, once again, localized to the medulla but are distributed over several nuclei (5, 10, 13). In rather simplistic terms, neurons that depolarize preferentially in the early part of the inspiratory phase inhibit all other cell types but have decreasing influence over the course of the inspiration. This network concept has somewhat greater acceptance than the pure pacemaker hypothesis, although there are medullary neurons (surgically isolated) that cyclically activate inspiratory or expiratory muscles, constituting a pacemaker. However, it is unclear whether this greatly reduced ventilation can be sustained for long periods and increased metabolism. The basic oscillation between inspiratory and postinspiratory cells likely requires stimulation from outside the respiratory pattern–generating network; that external stimulation may come from central chemoreceptors (10).

Because this chapter addresses the control of breathing, this brief introduction to rhythm generation is useful in spite of the fact that rhythm generation is not well understood; it provides some physiologic separation between the centralized, respiratory pattern generator and the multitude of respiratory-related reflexes that adjust that basic respiratory rhythm. This diversity of controlling influences is a reflection of the necessity to coordinate many different physiologic and behavioral demands on the respiratory system. Although most of the reflexes act on various brainstem respiratory neuronal groups, some act more directly on the phrenic nucleus and the other spinal areas controlling the intercostals and other accessory respiratory muscles (14).

Chemical (Blood Gas) Control of Ventilation

The primary function of the respiratory control system is regulation of the partial pressures of CO_2 and O_2 in arterial blood and plasma. This is accomplished by sensory signals from the various chemoreceptors and is the main driver of respiration. This sensory information is used by the brain to adjust ventilation to bring the gas concentrations back to their respective "set points." In most scenarios, the peripheral chemoreceptors respond to blood gas disturbances more quickly than the central chemoreceptors, allowing very rapid responses to transient changes. Those set points for CO_2 and O_2 vary with sleep and disease states and are reflected in their arterial concentrations. For example, part of the reason that respiration during non-REM sleep is slower and deeper is a reduced sensitivity of chemoreceptors to CO_2.

It is important to remember that pH is also a variable controlled by the respiratory system, especially CO_2 control. The level of CO_2 has a direct effect on pH because CO_2 and H_2O naturally combine to form carbonic acid, which dissociates into H^+ and bicarbonate (HCO_3^-). Carbonic anhydrase is an important catalyst (enzyme) in the reactions of CO_2 and water but only within RBCs (not plasma). Bicarbonate and certain proteins are important buffers for acidity in the plasma and cerebrospinal fluid (CSF). The main problem with high CO_2 levels in the blood is its influence on the production of H^+ ions in the body. Acidity must be tightly controlled because small deviations ($\sim$0.2 pH units) can adversely affect many different biochemical and physiologic processes, and extremes of pH can be toxic.

Increases in PCO_2 (or decreases in PO_2) activate the chemoreceptors, which then directly influence the medullary respiratory networks to increase V^T (the volume of a single breath) and, likely, respiratory frequency as well. There are varying degrees of relative change in the two parameters depending on the particular disturbance and physiologic context. In mild exertion, it is common to have the augmentation of V^T but not frequency. The increase in ventilation leads to an enhanced excretion of CO_2, which leads to a decreased stimulation of the chemoreceptors—another classic example of a negative feedback loop. The changes in blood gases that elicit alterations in respiration are so small, and the effectiveness of the chemical control of respiration is so great, that during mild-to-moderate exercise almost no differences can be detected in arterial PCO_2.

Because the classical chemoreceptors lie on or just beneath the surface of the medulla, they respond to pH/PCO_2 disturbances in CSF, not the blood. However, CSF levels of respiratory gases depend on the arterial plasma levels. Therefore, CSF is an important intermediary between the blood and the central chemoreceptors. The normal value of arterial pH is approximately 7.4, whereas the usual pH of CSF is about 7.32.

These blood gas sensory stimuli also influence cardiovascular reflexes, with hypoxia, hypercapnia (high PCO_2), or acidity being generally sympathetically activating. Hypoxia, hypercapnia, and/or a pH of less than 7.3 initiate sympathetic reflexes to increase heart rate, cardiac output, and often blood pressure. The dual action of chemoreceptors in blood gas homeostasis is another reflection of the coupling between respiratory and cardiovascular control systems and the requirements of efficient gas exchange. An increase in ventilation would be ineffective without a corresponding increase in blood perfusion of the lungs and tissues.

Imagine a possible real-life occurrence—you are about to miss your bus to campus. You cognitively recognize the need to hurry, so you begin to run. Muscles throughout your body increase activity for locomotion and balance. The increased muscular activity requires greater metabolism, which consumes more O_2 and produces more CO_2. These changes are reflected by your falling concentrations of O_2 and rising concentration of CO_2, altering the concentration gradients that existed before you began to run. That is, more O_2 diffuses from the blood to the tissues because tissue O_2 levels are lowered (because of increased consumption), which then increases the concentration gradient from arterial blood to the tissue. CO_2 diffuses from the working tissues into the blood, raising your PCO_2 and lowering pH.

These changes in blood gases are sensed by the various chemoreceptors in contact with the arterial blood and CSF that then activate respiration through neuronal networks. Just as importantly, this sudden bout of exercise requires that blood flow through the lungs be increased to make best use of the increased ventilation and exchange of gases; therefore, cardiac output must be increased. This is accomplished by increasing your heart rate and making adjustments to the strength of each beat, which are, in part, mediated by neural systems. Blood pressure may or may not change depending on the type of exercise and other factors. In addition to increased activation of the phrenic nucleus, the expiratory muscles are activated by medullary respiratory networks (recall that during rest, expiration is passive, i.e., not driven by muscular contraction) and the participation of accessory inspiratory muscles is increased, as is necessary for rapid respiratory rates. This increase in ventilation then enhances the expiration of CO_2 and the delivery of O_2, which offsets the changes caused by the dash for the bus. Homeostasis is maintained and you just make the bus—a little acidic maybe, but your knowledge of respiratory control assures you that as soon as your chemoreceptors detect the correction, your breathlessness will subside.

Other Respiratory Reflexes

Several respiratory reflexes act to protect the respiratory system (e.g., cough, antioverinflation). At least three broad classes of sensory receptors are involved in these protective reflexes: slowly adapting receptors, rapidly adapting receptors, and C-fiber nerve endings. There is some degree of overlap in the function of the reflexes mediated by these three classes of receptors, all of which reside in the lungs and airways and practically all of which use the vagus nerve to transmit their information back to the brainstem.

Slowly adapting receptors are mainly stretch receptors residing in the smooth muscle of the conducting airways, which mediate the Hering–Breuer inflation reflex. This most well-known of the respiratory protective reflexes acts to restrict overinflation of the lung. An important role for this reflex in neonates and infants is widely accepted; however, another role for the reflex in adults during exercise seems likely. Bronchoconstriction and, possibly, lung deflation below normal expiratory volume also activate these receptors.

The second major type of pulmonary receptor is the rapidly adapting type, which is also referred to as irritant receptors and which can initiate many different responses, such as cough, rapid breathing (tachypnea), breath holding, and/or airway constriction. Several activators for the rapidly adapting receptors exist, including hyperinflation and deflation, but unlike the slowly adapting receptors, which are mechanoreceptors, the rapidly adapting type is also quite sensitive to several different noxious chemicals—hence the name "irritant receptors." Examples of chemical stimulants of these receptors are ammonia, cigarette smoke, edema, distilled water, and sulfur dioxide, but other stimulants also exist. In addition, irritant receptors may be involved in asthma "attacks" in which certain asthma mediators stimulate airway irritant receptors that are pathologically hypersensitive, initiating a strong airway constrictor reflex involving increased vagal parasympathetic activity (12). Other factors, both neural and nonneural, are also involved in asthma.

C-fiber endings are the most numerous of the pulmonary receptors and are stimulated by both mechanical and chemical stimuli. The activating stimuli and the resulting respiratory reflexes of these receptors are very similar to those for rapidly adapting irritant receptors. There are two classes of C-fiber receptors based mainly on where they are found: pulmonary and bronchial. Activation of pulmonary C-fiber receptors usually evokes apnea, bradycardia, hypotension, and bronchoconstriction. Activation of the bronchial receptors elicits rapid shallow breathing, bronchoconstriction, and increased secretion of mucus onto the surface of the airways. Both classes of C-fiber receptors (and rapidly adapting receptors) can cause cough.

Cardiovascular reflexes also affect respiration. One example is the effect of changes in blood pressure on respiration. Increases in blood pressure are sensed by the baroreceptors in the carotid sinus and the aortic arch, which then increase their firing rates. These sensory signals are passed to the NTS, which distributes the information to various brain sites, where the signal causes a reduction in sympathetic drive to the blood vessels and returns blood pressure to "normal" levels. The respiratory component of the baroreflex involves a reduction in ventilation during hypertension and a small increase during low blood pressure (hypotension) (8). This is the classic baroreceptor reflex (or baroreflex).

SLEEP AND RESPIRATION

Sleep is a very important modulator of respiration and cardiovascular function. Part of that effect is caused by the general reduction in muscle tone characteristic of sleep. Another effect on breathing is that during sleep, energy needs are considerably lower than during waking and especially so for active waking. A reduced need for energy and O_2 is representative of the behavioral aspect of sleep, that is, reduced metabolism.

Effects of Normal Sleep on Respiratory Control

Sleep affects respiration in several ways. Most notable is the reduction in respiratory rate during non-REM sleep compared with waking. In addition, respiratory variability is lowest in non-REM sleep. Generally, the deeper stages of non-REM sleep (i.e., N3, slow-wave sleep) are associated with slower, deeper, and less variable breathing than non-REM sleep stages N1 and N2. Heart rate and heart rate variability are also lowest in non-REM sleep. Respiration during REM sleep is more like waking than during non-REM sleep in terms of rate, depth, and variability.

The sensitivity of the respiratory system to CO_2 is affected by the sleep–wake state. CO_2 sensitivity is highest during waking and lowest during quiet, non-REM sleep, with REM sleep having intermediate sensitivity (9). A difference in sensitivity means that for a given increase in PCO_2, the respiratory response is greater in waking than in non-REM sleep. This is a large part of the reason respiration is slower during non-REM sleep (especially N3, slow-wave sleep) than waking or REM sleep. Concentrations of CO_2 in the blood are slightly higher during non-REM sleep. The abrupt decrease in PCO_2 sensitivity at sleep onset while the "waking" PCO_2 level persists (for a few dozen seconds) may be a mechanism of sleep-onset central apneas (15, 16).

Compared with non-REM sleep, REM sleep is associated with respiratory frequency increases, smaller V^T, and greater variability. A significant portion of that greater variability is caused by changes in respiratory pattern (e.g., tachypnea) associated with periods of REMs. In addition, the reduction in muscle tone during non-REM sleep and the loss of accessory respiratory muscle activity in REM sleep are factors in sleep-related respiratory patterns and variability.

Arousal as a Respiratory Drive

Waking respiratory frequencies are higher and more variable than either type of sleep. These state-related differences are a result of the higher metabolic needs during waking and activity and of the neural-stimulating action of arousal or wakefulness (13) on respiratory control systems, cardiovascular systems, and other brain networks. In other words, the major effect of sleep on respiration may be the removal of the stimulating effect of waking.

Respiration is affected by sleep and arousal in another way that has even more clinical significance—that of a sleep-related decrease in the basal level of skeletal muscular activity. Compared with waking, non-REM sleep is characterized by a reduction in muscle tone throughout the body; in REM sleep, muscle activity is at its lowest. In fact, a scoring criterion for REM sleep is muscular paralysis, as reflected by a nearly flat electromyographic signal during polysomnography (17). The diaphragm is the only skeletal muscle not inhibited by sleep (or at least not *as* inhibited). The large decline in tonic muscle activation includes the accessory respiratory muscles; consequently, the rhythmic drive to assist in ventilation is reduced during non-REM sleep and practically disappears in REM sleep.

Sleep-Disordered Breathing

There are many kinds of sleep-disordered breathing, including not only the common obstructive and central apnea/hypopnea but also Cheyne–Stokes respiration/periodic breathing and treatment-emergent central sleep apnea. Loss of muscular tone in the upper airways during supine sleep is the major factor in OSA. OSA is easily the most common type of apnea, partly because of the increase in the incidence of obesity. During an obstruction, the airway muscles are unable to maintain an open airway because of the loss of the wakefulness stimulus, usually in conjunction with supine sleeping,

obesity, airway narrowing, muscular disease, and/or abnormal craniofacial structure. The reduction in muscle tone during non-REM sleep can lead to airway turbulence, airway narrowing, or complete occlusion.

Central apnea is the lack of respiratory drive to the diaphragm and the subsequent lack of airflow. The mechanisms for this are uncertain, but in healthy adults, many central apneas are likely because of a short-lasting drop in PCO_2 during sleep that can happen after a sigh or hyperventilation (18). The occasional central apnea is not pathologic. On the contrary, those patients with clinically significant central apnea or hypopnea are more difficult to treat compared with those with obstructive symptoms. A relative lack of arousal stimuli to the central pattern generator is the usual way a central apnea is initiated.

Cheyne–Stokes respiration is characterized by a period of central apnea followed by gradually increasing ventilation, usually to hyperventilation, then gradually decreasing back to apnea. The entire cycle takes 30 to 90 seconds and can reflect slow chemoreceptor responses or impaired circulatory function associated with heart failure. These symptoms are suggestive of a neurologic problem, usually in association with congestive heart failure (CHF).

Treatment-emergent central sleep apnea is seen in a relatively small subset of OSA patients when positive airway pressure is applied. Central apneas emerge during the titration portion of a polysomnographic recording. In these patients, the resolution of their obstructive and mixed events seems to lead to a greater propensity for central apneas. Continuous positive airway pressure may be contraindicated for these patients. The common therapy for treatment-emergent central sleep apnea is the use of adaptive servo-ventilation (ASV). Note that recent warnings have been posted by equipment manufacturers and the American Academy of Sleep Medicine suggesting that ASV should not be used in patients with CHF with an ejection fraction of less than 45% because of the risk of mortality. ASV devices respond to arrhythmic ventilatory movement, usually central and obstructive apneas, with appropriate pressure support and disengage when the respiratory pattern stabilizes. Much research is directed at processes of treatment-emergent central sleep apnea and, subsequently, more effective treatments.

SUMMARY

The primary function of the respiratory system is to maintain blood gases (O_2 and CO_2) and pH at optimal levels. O_2 and CO_2 move down their respective concentration gradients between the blood and the cells and then again between the blood and air within the alveoli of the lungs. Rhythmic ventilation by respiratory muscles exchanges the air in the lungs with fresh air to remove the CO_2 and replenish O_2. These blood gases must be tightly controlled to allow sufficient metabolism and vigorous activity.

CNS networks not only are centered in the medulla and spinal cord but are also affected by neural systems in other brain areas. The respiratory rhythm of inspiration and expiration is generated in the medulla, most likely by several different neuronal types, although a single type may form the basis of the inspiratory phase. This basic rhythm is powerfully affected by sensory signals concerning the level of CO_2 and O_2 in the blood and the CSF. There are two categories of chemoreceptors: the central chemoreceptors, mainly near the surface of the rostral part of the ventrolateral medulla; and peripheral chemoreceptors, which are in the carotid bodies and aortic arch. These sensory signals are used to adjust ventilation to compensate for a change in blood gases, returning them to their optimal levels.

The diaphragm is the main respiratory muscle, and therefore output from the medulla is mainly directed at the phrenic nucleus of the spinal cord that innervates the diaphragm. However, accessory respiratory muscles play an essential role in ventilation, especially during physical activity. These accessory muscles are powerfully affected by sleep and the sleeping body position (reclining), which can contribute to pathologic processes and conditions. Sleep and arousal are powerful modulators of respiratory and cardiovascular function to the extent that arousal and wakefulness are significant activating factors for both systems and are notably absent during sleep.

REFERENCES

1. Ayappa, I., & Rapoport, D. M. (2003). The upper airway in sleep: Physiology of the pharynx. *Sleep Medicine Review, 7*(1), 9–33.

2. Victor, L. (n.d.). *Obstructive sleep apnea.* Retrieved from www.aafp.org/afp/991115ap/2279.html

3. Lambertson, C. (1980). Respiration. In V. B. Mountcastle (Ed.), *Medical physiology* (14th ed., pp. 1677–1842). St. Louis, MO: Mosby.

4. Horner, R. L., Liu, X., Gill, H., et al. (2002). Selected contribution: Effects of sleep-wake state on the genioglossus vs. diaphragm muscle responses to CO_2 in rats. *Journal of Applied Physiology, 92*(2), 878–887.

5. West, J. B. (1982). *Pulmonary pathophysiology: The essentials* (2nd ed., pp. 61–64). Baltimore, MD: Williams & Wilkins.

6. West, J. B. (1979). Pulmonary gas exchange. In J. Brobeck (Ed.), *Best and Taylor's physiological basis of medical practice* (10th ed.). Baltimore, MD: Williams & Wilkins.

7. Schwartzstein, R. M., & Parker, M. J. (2006). The gas exchanger: Matching ventilation and perfusion. In *Respiratory physiology: A clinical approach.* Baltimore, MD: Lippincott, Williams & Wilkins.

8. West, J. B. (1985). *Respiratory physiology: The essentials* (3rd ed.). Baltimore, MD: Williams & Wilkins.

9. Nattie, E. E. (2001). Central chemosensitivity, sleep, and wakefulness. *Respiration Physiology, 129*(1–2), 257–268.

10. Feldman, J. L., & McCrimmon, D. R. (2003). Neural control of breathing. In L. E. Squire, F. E. Bloom, S. K. McConnell, et al. (Eds.), *Fundamental neuroscience* (2nd ed., pp. 967–990). San Diego, CA: Academic Press.

11. West, J. B. (1979). Control of breathing. In J. Brobeck (Ed.), *Best & Taylor's physiological basis of medical practice* (10th ed.). Baltimore, MD: Williams & Wilkins.

12. de Jongste, J. C., Longejan, R. C., & Kerrebijn, K. F. (1991). Control of airway caliber by autonomic nerves in asthma and in chronic obstructive pulmonary disease. *American Review of Respiratory Disease, 143*(6), 1421–1426.

13. Richter, D. W. (1982). Generation and maintenance of the respiratory rhythm. *Journal of Experimental Biology, 100,* 93–107.

14. Mack, S. O., Kc, P., Wu, M., et al. (2002). Paraventricular oxytocin neurons are involved in neural control of breathing. *Journal of Applied Physiology, 92*(2), 826–834.

15. Horner, R. L., Rivera, M. P., Kozar, L. F., et al. (2001). The ventilatory response to arousal from sleep is not fully explained by differences in CO_2 levels between sleep and wakefulness. *Journal of Physiology, 534*(Pt. 3), 881–890.

16. Nakayama, H., Smith, C. A., Rodman, J. R., et al. (2002). Effect of ventilatory drive on carbon dioxide sensitivity below eupnea during sleep. *American Journal of Respiratory and Critical Care Medicine, 165,* 1251–1260.

17. Rechtschaffen, A., & Kales, A. (Eds.). (1968). *A manual of standardized terminology, techniques and scoring system for sleep stages of human subjects.* Los Angeles, CA: UCLA Brain Information Service/Brain Research Institute.

18. Dempsey, J. A., Smith, C. A., Harms, C. A., et al. (1996). Sleep-induced breathing instability. *Sleep, 19*(3), 236–247.

chapter 8

Oxygen and Gas Exchange in the Body

STEPHEN TARNOCZY

LEARNING OBJECTIVES

On completion of this chapter, the reader should be able to:

1. Describe the basic exchange of gases within the body as well as the outside environment.
2. Discuss the methods for oxygen delivery to the tissues throughout the body.
3. Define the relationship between oxygen and hemoglobin and factors that alter their relationship.
4. Describe how disease may impact oxygen diffusion, transport, and/or delivery.
5. Define the different types of hypoxia, hypoxemia, and ischemia.
6. Describe how supplemental oxygen affects the healthy and compromised patient.

KEY TERMS

Ventilation
External respiration
Internal respiration
Room air
Alveoli
Hypoxia
Anemic hypoxia
Circulatory hypoxia
Hypoxemia
Ischemia
Anemia
Hemoglobin

The human organism is a magnificent yet complex machine that operates with the precision of a fine Swiss watch. Like any mechanical device, the human organism is the sum of all its parts. Rather than analyzing gears, springs, and pendulums as the primary makeup of our machine, we will be referring to organs, tissues, and cells to describe the processes of the body and the wonderment of respiration.

RESPIRATION VERSUS VENTILATION

A very important concept surrounding this topic of discussion is the distinction between respiration and ventilation, which are two very different processes. Ventilation is defined as "the process of moving gas (usually air) in and out of the lungs" (1). This is completely independent of respiration, where the exchange of gas actually occurs either in the lungs (external respiration) or at the level of the tissues inside the body (internal respiration). These two very important areas will be addressed, but only respiration will be covered in this chapter. The mechanism of ventilation (moving air in and out of the lungs) will be covered in another forum. It is important to realize that ventilating a patient does not ensure that respiration is actually taking place and vice versa. Rather than dwelling on these two distinctions, let us examine the forces and laws that govern the miracle of respiration.

External Respiration

The exchange of gas between the body and the outside environment is referred to as "external respiration." The process of external respiration takes place between the lungs and the atmospheric air we breathe. This takes place in the tiny spherical sacs of the lungs called "alveoli" and the blood supply carried in by very tiny blood vessels in the lungs called the "pulmonary capillaries." Collectively, we refer to the conjoining of these two systems as the "alveolar–capillary membrane" (ACM). The process of gas exchange at this level is one of physics and pure diffusion, the movement of gas from an area of high concentration to an area of low concentration, until the two areas are equilibrated or equal. As we take air in or inhale air (inhalation), we are bringing in a gas (air) that comprises primarily nitrogen (N_2) and 20.9% oxygen (O_2). The amount of oxygen in the inspired air, or the fraction of inspired oxygen (FiO_2), is greater inside the alveoli than the amount of oxygen contained in the pulmonary capillaries. Utilizing the gradient of diffusion and movement of gas from a high to a low concentration, oxygen leaves the alveoli, crosses the ACM, and enters the red blood cell (RBC). As oxygen moves in, carbon dioxide (CO_2) is simultaneously moving out. Again, under the laws of diffusion, the amount of CO_2

inside the RBC is significantly higher than the amount of CO_2 inside the alveoli, and CO_2 diffuses from the RBC into the alveoli to be excreted or expired during exhalation. Under normal conditions, this takes place very quickly at the level of the ACM, usually in about 0.25 seconds. The amount of contact time that the average RBC has with the ACM is about 0.75 seconds.

Internal Respiration

After the exchange of gas in the lungs, oxygenated blood returns to the heart to be distributed throughout the body through the left ventricle, arteries, and the body's systemic circulation. The blood travels the arterial circulation to be distributed throughout the body and to its many organ systems. As the RBCs make their way through the smaller blood vessels, they eventually reach the arterial capillaries of the body. These capillaries are the end point of a network of blood vessels that feed the entire body with nutrients, electrolytes, and oxygen. At the capillary level, much as in the capillaries of the lungs, the RBC comes into contact with the capillary wall and the adjoining tissues.

Under normal circumstances, internal or cellular respiration utilizes oxygen to create energy, with the waste product primarily being CO_2 through the aerobic pathway of the Krebs cycle. At the tissue level, the amount of oxygen inside the RBC is greater than the amount outside the RBC in the tissues, and O_2 moves out of the RBC and into the tissues. Again, simultaneous exchange of CO_2 is taking place as CO_2 leaves the tissues and moves into the plasma and RBC for return to the lungs and elimination; then the process starts all over again. The concentration of CO_2 is greater in the tissues compared with the RBC, so CO_2 leaves the tissues and diffuses out into the plasma and RBC. The transport of both CO_2 and O_2 within the body is a bit more complex than described here, but it sets the foundation for further discussion.

ATMOSPHERIC GAS AND PARTIAL PRESSURES OF OXYGEN

Depending on where you live, the atmosphere of the air you breathe exerts a pressure that is equal to about 760 mm Hg, 1 atm, or 14.7 pounds per square inch (psi). At higher altitudes above sea level, that pressure gradually begins to decrease. As you go below the sea level, the opposite occurs and the pressure actually increases by 760 mm Hg, 1 atm, or 14.7 psi for every 33 ft you are below the water's surface! The concentration of gas or the amount of oxygen in room air of 21% never changes, but rather the pressure that it is under in the atmosphere changes, causing the gas to behave differently. Take a

balloon and blow it up. You have a balance of air pressures that keep the balloon inflated. You have air inside the balloon exerting a force outward in all directions against the inside wall. You have air in the atmosphere exerting pressure on the balloon at 760 mm Hg. *Keeping all other variables constant*, if you were to take the balloon and submerge it under a pool of water, the balloon would shrink in size. Elevating the same balloon several thousand feet will cause it to expand. The gas in the balloon never went anywhere, but the environmental pressure on the outside of the balloon changed! Now notice the phrase *keeping all other variables constant* because that is very important when you are dealing with any gas and demonstrating its physical properties.

Regardless of the units of measure used, the atmospheric pressure (760 mm Hg) is a combination of all the gases in room air. Because room air is made up primarily of nitrogen and oxygen, these two gases make up the greatest percentage of the atmospheric pressure of 760 mm Hg. For example, room air is 21% oxygen and 79% nitrogen. There are additional "trace" gases or elements also present in extremely small amounts, but the air we breathe is primarily nitrogen and oxygen. Of the 760 mm Hg pressure exerted by the atmosphere, 160 mm Hg pressure is exerted by oxygen and 600 mm Hg pressure is exerted by nitrogen. Because air does not comprise 100% pure gas but rather is a mixture of these two elements, we refer to the pressures exerted by nitrogen and oxygen as *partial pressures*. Adding these two pressures together, we get the 760 mm Hg of total pressure exerted by our atmosphere on an average day. This calculation is known as Dalton's law of partial pressure: *The partial pressure of a gas is equal to the concentration of that gas (expressed as a decimal) × the atmospheric pressure (760 mm Hg in our example).*

Therefore,

The partial pressure of nitrogen (PN_2)
$$= 0.79 \times 760 \text{ mm Hg}$$
$$= 600 \text{ mm Hg}$$

The partial pressure of oxygen (PO_2)
$$= 0.21 \times 760 \text{ mm Hg}$$
$$= 160 \text{ mm Hg}$$

Total atmospheric pressure
$$= PN_2 (600) + PO_2 (160)$$
$$= 760 \text{ mm Hg}$$

The change in atmospheric pressure at higher elevations requires hikers or climbers attempting summit assaults on Everest to bring canisters of oxygen to facilitate their climb. As you reach altitudes of one mile or greater, the air becomes "thinner" or, better phrased, the atmospheric pressure significantly decreases as you rise in altitude.

Let us calculate partial pressures of these gases at 30,000 ft elevation where atmospheric pressure is about 250 mm Hg:

The partial pressure of nitrogen (PN$_2$) $\left.\right\}$ = 0.79 × 250 mm Hg = 197.5 mm Hg

The partial pressure of oxygen (PO$_2$) $\left.\right\}$ = 0.21 × 250 mm Hg = 52.5 mm Hg

Total atmospheric pressure at 30,000 ft $\left.\right\}$ = PN$_2$ 197.5 + PO$_2$ (52.5) = 250 mm Hg

Notice that the concentration of gases or the composition of air did not change, but the partial pressures of both gases dropped markedly compared with a sea-level pressure of 760 mm Hg. The PO$_2$ dropped by more than one-third! This is why there are emergency oxygen masks in airline cabins; if the internal pressure suddenly drops, supplemental oxygen is required because the surrounding air at 30,000 ft contains insufficient oxygen.

This is also why patients with abnormally low levels of oxygen in their blood (hypoxemia) are treated by giving them supplemental oxygen to breathe through a mask or oxygen cannula. Although we are not changing atmospheric pressure by administering oxygen, we are changing the concentration of oxygen that the patient inspires, or more correctly, we are increasing the patient's FiO$_2$.

So, to complete our sample calculations, let us calculate the partial pressure of these gases while climbing our mountain, breathing extra oxygen from a tank, estimating that we have increased the FiO$_2$ from 0.21 of room air to 0.40 by putting our oxygen masks on . . .

The partial pressure of nitrogen (PN$_2$) $\left.\right\}$ = 0.60 × 250 mm Hg = 150 mm Hg

The partial pressure of oxygen (PO$_2$) $\left.\right\}$ = 0.40 × 250 mm Hg = 100 mm Hg

Total atmospheric pressure at 30,000 on O$_2$ $\left.\right\}$ = PN$_2$ (150) + PO$_2$ (100) =250 mm Hg

Using a higher FiO$_2$ with supplemental oxygen, we were able to correct for the lower partial pressure of oxygen at the higher altitude. We will utilize similar strategies to treat patients with lower than normal blood oxygen levels (hypoxemia).

DIFFUSION OF RESPIRATORY GASES ACROSS THE ACM

When gas (room air) enters the body through inhalation, it makes its way through the conducting airways of the respiratory system and eventually to the level of the alveolus. Only gas that comes into contact with the alveolus has the potential to participate in gas exchange. The word potential is used because there are a variety of factors that must exist in order for the transfer of gases

or external respiration to occur. The presence of disease, as well as the equally important role of pulmonary capillary perfusion, determines how well gases diffuse or exchange across the alveolar–capillary junction.

There are multiple factors associated with the diffusion process, any one of which can fail or become impaired, leading to impaired gas exchange and resulting in harm to the patient. We will analyze the anatomy first and then specifically talk about CO$_2$ and O$_2$ exchange in the alveoli.

The alveoli are small saclike structures attached to the terminal bronchioles that are recognized as the last branching or division of the tracheobronchial tree. Starting with the trachea, the airways branch off into 23 divisions until they split into the terminal bronchioles. Air is brought in and out of the chest as a result of changing pressures in the thorax, but gas movement at this level is through Brownian movement of pure diffusion from an area of high concentration to an area of low concentration. This pressure gradient or drive can be altered or accelerated depending on the general health of the structural system and the presence of either pulmonary or cardiovascular disease (2).

Each alveolus is wrapped in a net of capillaries that surround the spherical lung unit to provide blood supply and enable gas exchange. As oxygen moves out of the alveolus, it crosses a series of thin yet significant layers of tissue on its journey out of the alveolus, moves across the alveolar cell wall, through the capillary membrane wall, into the blood plasma, across the membrane wall of the RBC, and finally adheres to the hemoglobin (HBG) molecule in the RBC. Depending on the overall health of the individual, this process may occur unhindered, or there may be significant barriers at the tissue level that impede the diffusion of oxygen. All these structures and tissues can be diseased, scarred, or underperfused, which will make gas exchange significantly less efficient. The end result is lower oxygen content in the arterial circulation and potentially a simultaneous increase in carbon dioxide in the bloodstream when damage becomes severe.

A similar process of diffusion occurs at the tissue level of the arterial capillaries. When an RBC comes into contact with tissue that is in need of O$_2$, the drive or diffusion gradient causes the relatively higher concentration of O$_2$ to move out of the RBC and across the barriers and diffuse into the cellular tissue that is in need of oxygen. However, if not enough oxygen was efficiently exchanged at the alveoli, there will be insufficient oxygen available when the RBC arrives at the tissue level, resulting in hypoxemia.

Patients with a history of pulmonary disease such as emphysema or fibrosis can suffer from a variety of conditions that alter the normal diffusion process. Changes in the alveoli and eventual destruction of lung function because of smoking or by scar tissue formed as the lungs tried to repair themselves from previous disease resulting in fibrosis produces varying degrees of damage from unnoticeable to extremely debilitating. It is sometimes very difficult for the clinician to determine through physical examination and history the extent of damage and the potential challenges the patient may present in the sleep center. Key indicators for potential ACM damage are a history of smoking, occupational health exposure, or any type of pulmonary fibrosis, to name a few. The definitive test to evaluate ACM function is pulmonary function testing with arterial blood gases. Pulmonary function testing is used to determine a patient's baseline status and level of damage. The results of this testing in the patient record are an invaluable tool in assessing patients with significant pulmonary disease that we sometimes see in the sleep center.

Gas exchange, as previously stated, is just as much a function of ventilation as of perfusion. The circulatory system is the delivery pathway back and forth to where respiration can occur. The first component of gas exchange is getting the RBC to the lungs and exchanging gases across a healthy ACM. The second component is the delivery system and getting the RBC to the tissue level where it is needed and perfusing the areas where gas exchange needs to occur. When these two systems become unbalanced, significant impairment of gas exchange and/or delivery of oxygen or elimination of CO_2 can result. The body has a unique system that accommodates these potential challenges that lead us to discuss the relationship between hemoglobin (Hgb) and oxygen.

OXYGEN–HEMOGLOBIN DISSOCIATION CURVE

The relationship between oxygen and Hgb of the RBC is a complex one; however, it is quite simple to understand. Oxygen and Hgb, just like two magnets, have an attraction to each other. The closer the magnets, the stronger the attraction, and the opposite is true as you spread the magnets further away. There are a few conditions that can make oxygen more or less attractive to Hgb. Temperature, blood pH, and CO_2 levels of the blood can all affect the attraction or *affinity* of oxygen and Hgb. Factors that make oxygen more attractive to Hgb are decreased CO_2, decreased temperature, and increased pH. These factors result in oxygen binding more readily at the lungs and staying bound to the RBC more strongly at the tissue level. Factors that make oxygen less attractive to Hgb include increased CO_2, increased temperature, and decreased pH. With these factors in place, oxygen binds at the alveolar level less readily and is freed up at the tissue level much more easily. So, what does this mean?

Under normal circumstances in healthy individuals, there is really no significant alteration in gas exchange related to these differences in affinity. There is a problem, however, in individuals who do not have normal oxygen levels. The oxygen–Hgb relationship curve is not linear but rather is S-shaped with a rapid downward slope in the middle of the curve. In patients who have less than normal blood oxygen levels because of cardiopulmonary disease, these shifts in affinity can be most detrimental. In the real world of health care, a majority of patients who are sick will have an increased temperature and an increased CO_2 level, which often results in a decreased pH. As you recall, these factors make oxygen slightly less attractive to Hgb, and the uptake at the ACM level may not be ideal, resulting in a less than normal oxygen level in the blood. This is our patient with chronic obstructive pulmonary disease, emphysema, and cardiopulmonary disease who has such significant impairment of gas exchange that they fall in the middle of the S-shaped oxyhemoglobin dissociation curve, and any slight shift or movement on that curve (affinity) can have huge consequences on the amount of oxygen available at the tissue level. So, how do we compensate?

Fortunately, the body's rate of oxygen consumption is not all or nothing, and there is a great deal of oxygen in reserve. As each Hgb molecule can hold up to four oxygen molecules, there is a tremendous carrying capacity evident. If we assume that the arterial Hgb sites are all bound with oxygen, yielding a 100% oxygen saturation, at the tissue level when oxygen is released, generally only one oxygen molecule unbinds from Hgb, leaving the other three oxygen molecules intact. The remaining three of the four Hgb molecules with bound oxygen yield an oxygen saturation equal to 75% as the RBC returns in the venous circulation back to the heart. This also clearly demonstrates that the body consumes only about 25% of the oxygen available under normal conditions. This leaves a tremendous amount of oxygen available in reserves if needed. As an individual increases his or her demand for oxygen, the body is normally able to accommodate without issue. Again, the difficulty arises for those individuals who have less than normal arterial Hgb saturation to start with, leaving their oxygen reserves severely compromised to the point where the slightest increase in demand for oxygen can tax them to the point of respiratory insufficiency.

HYPOXEMIA/HYPOXIA/ISCHEMIA

These two terms, unfortunately, are interchangeably used quite often, yet they mean very distinctly different things. Although both of these terms relate to lower than normal oxygen levels, hypoxemia is specifically a lower than normal oxygen level in the blood, whereas hypoxia is lower than normal oxygen level in the tissues, which leads to ischemia. Theoretically, it is possible to have one without the other, and their clinical significance varies and therefore warrants discussion.

Hypoxemia is usually related to the integrity and efficiency of gas exchange at the ACM. If not enough oxygen diffuses across in the lungs, then the RBC will not pick up sufficient oxygen to saturate the Hgb in the arterial circulation (generally 97% or greater). Hypoxia occurs when there is not enough oxygen present at the level of the tissues resulting in ischemia; there are several different causes and types of hypoxia.

This is where the nomenclature starts to get a bit tricky. Review the definition of hypoxemia; if there are low oxygen levels to start with at the level of gas exchange in the lungs, then it makes sense that there will be lower than normal oxygen available to the tissues. Therefore, hypoxia, caused by hypoxemia, is referred to as *hypoxic hypoxia*. Another type of hypoxia is caused by insufficient RBCs in the blood (anemia). When there are an insufficient number of Hgb molecules to accept oxygen, there will not be enough oxygen delivered to the tissues. This is referred to as *anemic hypoxia*.

Remember that oxygen delivery is reliant just as much on the circulatory system to transport the RBC as it is on the gas exchange that occurs in the lungs; if the body has vascular damage or underperfusion of the tissues, it is called *circulatory hypoxia*. In circulatory hypoxia, the arterial oxygen content may be completely normal, but there is a problem with the delivery system, and the oxygen-rich blood cannot reach the site where gas exchange occurs because of a fault in the circulatory system.

The last and rarer form of hypoxia is caused by any condition that interferes with or impedes the body's ability to use oxygen normally. The example often used is cyanide poisoning resulting in *histotoxic hypoxia*.

Correcting Hypoxemia

In the sleep center environment, frequent desaturation events related to sleep-disordered breathing (SDB) are a nightly occurrence. Pressurization of the upper airway using continuous positive airway pressure (CPAP), bilevel, or adaptive servoventilation can benefit the alveolar exchange mechanism by enabling the alveoli to remain distended and participate in gas exchange. Many times, pressurization alone can maintain a patient's oxygen level within a normal range. Occasionally, in the presence of severe SDB or in concert with pulmonary disease, the need to increase FiO_2 may arise and necessitate the adjunct of supplemental oxygen.

Assuming that the patient has no preexisting cardiopulmonary conditions, the primary cause of hypoxemia is the interruption of gas exchange in the lung and does not usually involve damage to the airway control mechanism. Logically, this should be corrected by resolving the upper airway obstruction, and normal oxygen levels in the blood should resume. These otherwise healthy patients may suffer from normal alveolar hypoventilation changes associated with the resumption of restored physiologic sleep. This can sometimes result in borderline hypoxemia that responds in the sleep lab with an additional 1- to 2-cm H_2O increase in baseline CPAP. Occasionally, increasing the FiO_2 may be necessary to address persistent hypoxemia in the absence of breathing-related events. Implementation of supplemental oxygen should be initiated following department protocols and parameters as established by the center medical director.

SUMMARY

The exchange of gases with the atmosphere as well as within the body occurs utilizing well-defined processes in the field of biochemistry and within the laws of physics. If these normal processes are disturbed or interrupted, then the consequence of altered gas exchange mechanisms may occur. By understanding the laws that govern these processes, it is possible to apply concepts that we use in the sleep center to create mechanisms to correct this disturbance. The challenge is that sometimes we get only a few brief hours of diagnostic and therapeutic time to evaluate and treat individuals in a single night. A good understanding of the normal gas exchange process allows the technologist to apply that knowledge to understanding how the body responds to an alteration in that normal mechanism and take corrective action in an effort to restore normal physiologic function.

REFERENCES

1. Wilkins, R. L., Stoller, J. K., & Kacmarek, R. M. (2009). *Egan's fundamentals of respiratory care* (9th ed.). St. Louis, MO: Mosby.
2. West, J. B. (2008). *Pulmonary pathophysiology* (7th ed.). Baltimore, MD: Lippincott Williams & Wilkins.

SUGGESTED READINGS

Des Jardins, T. (2008). *Cardiopulmonary anatomy & physiology* (4th ed.). Champagne, IL: Delmar.

Des Jardins, T., & Burton, G. G. (2011). *Clinical manifestations and assessment of respiratory disease* (6th ed.). Maryland Heights, MO: Mosby.

chapter 9
Cardiac Anatomy and Physiology

MICHAEL R. FURGASON

LEARNING OBJECTIVES

On completion of this chapter, the reader should be able to:

1. Describe normal cardiac anatomy and explain the functions of the conduction system.
2. Demonstrate basic knowledge of the cardiac cycle, cardiac circulation, and systemic vascular system.
3. Understand the basic concepts of cardiac electrophysiology.
4. Identify the main components of the electrocardiogram (ECG).
5. Understand the importance of basic ECG recognition for the sleep technologist.

KEY TERMS

Endocardium
Action potential
Transmission of impulses
Cardiac cycle
Systole
Diastole
Preload
Afterload
Depolarization
Repolarization
Conduction system

FUNCTIONAL ANATOMY OF THE CARDIOVASCULAR SYSTEM

An essential part of a full-night polysomnogram is the electrocardiogram (ECG). The ECG is a graphic illustration of the electrical activity of the heart and is crucial to monitoring a patient's cardiovascular status. A knowledge of basic cardiac anatomy and electrophysiology will assist the reader to achieve a better understanding of the ECG and its components.

Heart Anatomy

The heart is a four-chambered muscular organ that lies in the thorax, posterior to the sternum and intercostal cartilages. It sits on the superior surface of the diaphragm and is the largest organ in the mediastinum, weighing approximately 2 g per lb of ideal body weight. The wall of the heart is composed of three layers. The most superficial of these layers is the epicardium. The epicardium contains an outer fibrous connective tissue and an inner serous pericardium. The space between these layers, the pericardial sac, contains about 25 mL of fluid that acts to reduce friction of the beating heart. Just underneath the pericardium is the muscular middle layer of the heart, the myocardium, which in addition to its contractile properties has the capacity to conduct electrical impulses to its cells. The endocardium, a sheet of endothelium resting on a thin layer of connective tissue, is the innermost layer of the heart and extends outward to include the valves of the heart.

The four chambers of the heart are the right and left atria, superiorly, and the right and left ventricles, inferiorly. The two sides of the heart are divided internally by the interventricular septum. Atrioventricular (AV) valves are made up of leaflets of connective tissue connected to fibrous cords called chordae tendineae. They connect to muscular projections (papillary muscles) from the inner surface of the heart wall. The AV valves sit between the atria and the ventricles and function to prevent backward blood flow. Specifically, the tricuspid valve contains three leaflets and lies between the right atrium and the right ventricle. The mitral or bicuspid valve contains two leaflets and sits between the left atrium and the left ventricle. The two semilunar valves are made up of leaflets attached to a fibrous ring of endothelium: The pulmonic semilunar valve lies between the right ventricle and the pulmonary trunk, whereas the aortic semilunar valve sits between the left ventricle and the aorta (see Fig. 9-1).

The right atrium is the receiving chamber for deoxygenated blood returning from systemic circulation and is fed by the superior vena cava, inferior vena cava, and coronary sinus. Deoxygenated blood enters the right atrium and flows through the tricuspid valve into the right ventricle. The right ventricle pumps the blood through the pulmonic semilunar valve and into the lungs for oxygenation. Once oxygenated, the blood then returns to the left atrium of the heart. Here, it

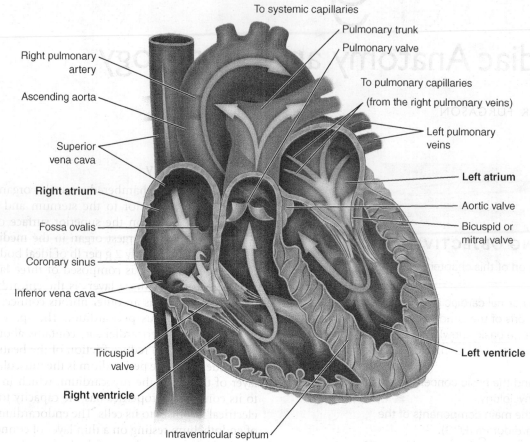

Figure 9-1 Anatomic view of cardiac blood flow. (Reprinted with permission from Archer P and Nelson LA. *Applied anatomy & physiology for manual therapists.* [Figure 10.8A]. Baltimore, MD: ©Lippincott Williams & Wilkins/Wolters Kluwer, 2012.)

passes through the mitral valve into the left ventricle. With each beat of the heart, the left ventricle pumps this oxygen-rich blood through the aortic valve into the aorta and out to the body, where it delivers a fresh supply of oxygen to the tissues.

Coronary Circulation

The heart itself is nourished with a rich blood supply by coronary arteries extending over the surface of the epicardium. The right and left coronary arteries arise from the base of the aorta and surround the heart like a crown. The left coronary artery passes posterior to the pulmonary trunk and then divides into two. The left anterior descending (LAD) artery runs anterior and downward toward the apex of the heart. In its path, the LAD artery branches to supply the free wall of the right and left ventricles, anterior papillary muscle, anterior two-thirds of the septum, and much of the conduction tissue, namely, the bundle of His and right and left bundle branches. The circumflex artery follows the coronary sulcus, the groove between the left atrium and ventricle, and runs posteriorly to supply the left atrium and the posterior and lateral portions of the left ventricle. In approximately 45% of people, the circumflex branch also supplies blood to the sinoatrial (SA) node. The right coronary artery (RCA)

travels in the coronary sulcus between the right atrium and right ventricle on the anterior surface of the heart. At the top of the ventricular septum posteriorly, the RCA becomes the posterior descending branch and runs parallel to the ventricular septum, supplying most of the right atrium and right ventricle. At the inferior border of the heart, the RCA branches off to become the marginal artery. It then sends a penetrating branch to the AV node and part of the bundle of His (see Fig. 9-2).

The coronary veins return deoxygenated blood from the heart wall into the right atrium. Specifically, the great (anterior), middle (posterior), and small (inferior) cardiac veins drain into the coronary sinus, located in the posterior coronary sulcus. Coronary artery anatomy can vary significantly among people. The anatomic distribution has no physiologic implications in the normal healthy heart. However, in those people with disease of the coronary arteries, a blockage in an artery that supplies a great deal of cardiac tissue can be fatal.

Conduction System

The conducting system of the heart includes the SA node, the AV node, the bundle of His, right and left bundle branches, and the Purkinje fibers. This specialized network of cells making up the conduction system

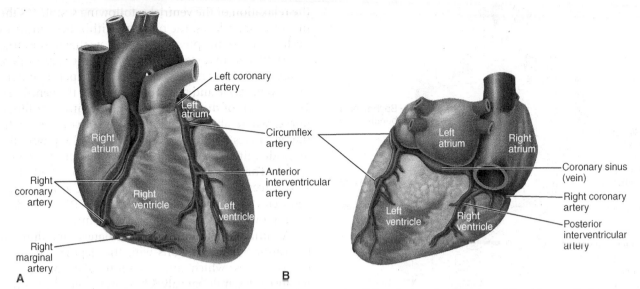

Figure 9-2 Coronary circulation. The coronary circulation, anterior (**A**) and posterior (**B**) views. Blood is supplied to the heart muscle via the coronary vessels. The major vessels of the coronary circulatory loop are shown here. (Reprinted with permission from Nath J. *Stedman's medical terminology, 2nd ed.* [Figure 10.5]. Baltimore, MD: ©Lippincott Williams & Wilkins/Wolters Kluwer, 2016.)

is the cardiac muscle cells modified for spontaneous excitation and rapid conduction of an action potential. The primary pacemaker of the heart, the SA node, is located in the posterior wall of the right atrium near the opening to the superior vena cava. All of the cells in the conducting system have automaticity, that is, the ability of self-excitation. However, those in the SA node fire spontaneously at a faster rate than the others, at a frequency between 60 and 80 bpm.

Once an impulse is generated at the SA node, the action potential spreads quickly through the cardiac muscle cells and internodal pathways of the right atrium and left atria, causing simultaneous depolarization and contraction. At the same time, the impulse is conducted through the conduction pathway to the AV node located in the interatrial septum. Because the AV node is the only connection of impulse between the atria and the ventricles, the action potential slows here, causing a slight delay and allowing time for atrial kick and ventricular filling. This delay in conduction at the AV node also has the protective function of preventing excessive impulse rates from entering the ventricles. Consequently, the AV node also can serve as a backup pacemaker should the SA node fail to initiate an impulse. Thus, the AV node has a significant role in preserving cardiac function.

The action potential continues from the point of origin to the bundle of His, a fibrous projection of cells, which enters the interventricular septum and divides into right and left bundle branches. About 1 cm down the septum, the bundle branches become bundles of Purkinje fibers. These fibers approach the apex of the heart and turn superiorly into the ventricular walls, extending into the myocardium on the inner surfaces of the ventricles. Once an electrical impulse enters the bundle of His, the conduction through the bundle branches and Purkinje fibers is extremely fast, about 1 to 4 ms. This rapid conduction of the impulse to the apex of the heart allows simultaneous depolarization of both ventricles, with a wave of contraction traveling superiorly, effectively pumping blood up and out through the great vessels (see Fig. 9-3).

Innervation

Cardiac muscle fibers generate spontaneous contractions that are coordinated into a functional heartbeat by the electrical conduction mechanisms inherent in the heart itself. However, the activity of the heart is also influenced by inputs from the nervous system.

The heart receives two opposing neural inputs belonging to the autonomic nervous system. Both send motor neurons to certain cardiac muscle cells. One input comes from the cells of the parasympathetic nervous system, whose synaptic terminals in the heart release the neurotransmitter acetylcholine. The effect of acetylcholine is to decrease the rate of depolarization during the pacemaker potential of the SA node. This has the effect of increasing the interval between successive action potentials, thereby decreasing the rate at which the pacemaker drives the rate of the heartbeat.

The second neural input to the heart comes from cells of the sympathetic nervous system, whose synaptic terminals release the neurotransmitter norepinephrine. Activation of this input increases the heart rate. This effect is also mediated through the pacemaker potential, which depolarizes more rapidly after the activation of the sympathetic input. Both factors accentuate the depolarizing trend during the pacemaker potential.

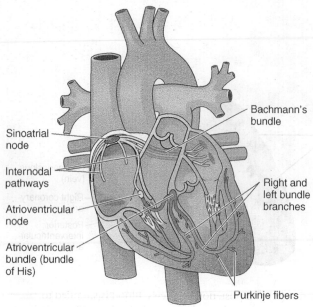

Figure 9-3 Conduction pathway of the heart. (Reprinted with permission from Plowman S and Smith D. *Exercise physiology for health fitness and performance, 5th ed.,* [Figure 11.4] Philadelphia, PA: ©Wolters Kluwer, 2017.)

Cardiac Muscle

A cardiac muscle cell is made up of contractile units known as sarcomeres. Within the sarcomere are long thread-like structures called myofibrils. Myofibrils are made up of two types of contractile proteins, or myofilaments, called actin and myosin. Cross-bridges that project from myosin fibers link themselves to the thinner actin filaments, giving the muscle cell a striated appearance. When cardiac muscle cells receive an electrical impulse, the actin filaments slide over myosin filaments, shortening the sarcomere. The shortening of adjacent sarcomeres effectively shortens the entire muscle cell.

The plasma membranes of adjacent myocardial cells form a structure known as intercalated discs. These junctions contain desmosomes, which join adjacent cells, and gap junctions, which allow electrical signals to pass directly from cell to cell. This complex network of electrically linked cells, through which an impulse can travel quickly, sets the environment for the simultaneous contraction of many cells. This is crucial for the heart to pump efficiently.

Cardiac Cycle

The cardiac cycle describes the mechanical events of the heart involving pressure and volume changes and path of blood flow. One cardiac cycle is one beat of the heart and lasts approximately 0.8 seconds in duration during a normal resting heart rate. The cardiac cycle can be divided into two phases: systole, the contractile phase, and diastole, the filling or relaxation phase.

The diastolic phase is normally about 500 ms in duration, or two-thirds of the cardiac cycle. It begins with

the relaxation of the ventricles following systole. As the myocardium relaxes, the pressure within the ventricles declines. When the pressure falls below that of the atria, the AV valves are forced open. When these valves open, venous blood enters the atria from the superior and inferior vena cavae and passively flows into the ventricles. This portion of diastole is called the ventricular filling phase, where about 75% of the blood volume enters the ventricles passively. At the end of this phase, the SA node initiates an impulse and atrial depolarization occurs. The contraction of the atria, also called atrial kick, forces the remaining blood from the atria into the ventricles. Atrial kick contributes about 20% to 30% of the total ventricular end diastolic volume.

Ventricular systole is approximately one-third of the cardiac cycle. It begins with the depolarization of the ventricles, which initiates ventricular contraction. Because the semilunar valves have not opened yet, myocardial contraction causes pressure to rise within the ventricles. When the pressure inside the ventricles exceeds that of the atria, the AV valves close. With both valves closed and blood volume constant, continued contraction of the myocardium causes pressures to rise within the ventricles. This phase is known as *isovolumetric contraction*.

When the pressure in the left ventricle reaches about 80 mm Hg and the right ventricle about 8 mm Hg, the semilunar valves are forced open, because these pressures exceed those of the aorta and pulmonary artery, respectively. At this point, the cardiac cycle enters the rapid ejection phase. With the semilunar valves open, contraction of the myocardium forces blood rapidly out of the ventricles into the great vessels. The aorta receives oxygenated blood from the left ventricle to be circulated throughout the body, whereas the pulmonary artery receives deoxygenated blood from the right ventricle to participate in gas exchange in the lungs.

As the blood flow out of the ventricles slows and the myocardium relaxes, intraventricular pressure declines. When the pressure falls below that of the great vessels, the semilunar valves close. This marks the end of systole. With both valves closed, the ventricles enter a phase of *isovolumetric relaxation;* pressure within the ventricles declines until it falls below that of the atria, the AV valves open, and the cycle repeats.

Regulation of Cardiac Activity

Both intrinsic and extrinsic factors are responsible for the regulation of cardiac activity. Extrinsic regulation of cardiovascular activity involves, most notably, the autonomic nervous system. The role of sympathetic and parasympathetic nerve pathways has been discussed previously. Chemical and pharmacologic influences have also become incredibly specific in the extrinsic regulation of cardiovascular activity; however, they are too numerous and beyond the scope of this text. Our discussion will focus instead on the intrinsic mechanisms involved in the regulation of cardiac activity.

Cardiac output is the amount of blood pumped by one ventricle and is measured in liters per minute. It is a product of heart rate (beats per minute) and stroke volume (liters per beat). Stroke volume, in turn, is dependent on several different factors, including preload, afterload, and contractility. Preload of the heart describes the stretch on the ventricular myocardium prior to contraction. The Frank–Starling model describes the recoil properties of an elastic object. Specifically, the greater the stretch on an elastic object up to the outer limit of normal, the greater the recoil. In this case, a greater stretch on the ventricular myocardium will result in a greater force of contraction. Because the ventricular myocardium is stretched by the amount of blood that exists in the ventricle prior to contraction, an increased venous return will produce greater tension on the myocardial wall, resulting in a greater force of contraction and stroke volume.

Afterload describes the resistance against which the heart must pump blood, or the systemic vascular resistance. Thus, changes in vascular tone will affect stroke volume and, ultimately, cardiac output. For example, increased systemic vascular resistance, or arterial vasoconstriction, results in a greater afterload and will cause a decrease in the strength, velocity, and/or duration of ventricular contraction.

Normal cardiac output is approximately 5 to 6 L per minute. By increasing stroke volume and/or heart rate, the heart can increase its cardiac output up to 25 L per minute. This portrays the heart's ability to intrinsically adjust its pumping capacity to alterations in venous return. In addition, the heart matches the outputs of the two ventricles to keep a balance of the systemic and pulmonary circuits.

THE SYSTEMIC VASCULAR SYSTEM

The vascular system is an intricate network of passages that delivers oxygen-rich blood to needy cells of the body. Oxygenated blood, originating in the heart, is pumped out of the aorta and channeled into arteries, arterioles, and capillaries, where major organ systems such as the heart, brain, skeletal muscle, liver, gastrointestinal tract, glands, skin, and reproductive organs are nourished. Veins carry deoxygenated blood containing metabolic by-products from the tissues back to the heart. Here, it is channeled into the pulmonary vascular system to reclaim its oxygen supply and dispose of waste products. Oxygen-rich blood then reenters the heart, and the endless loop of circulating blood continues. Blood flow within the vascular system is maintained by pressure gradients between different blood vessels. Specifically, the aortic blood pressure is normally about 90 mm Hg, whereas the central venous pressure, measured at the

vena cava, is normally close to 0 mm Hg. Changes in vascular resistance, or resistance to flow, within different organ systems or tissues control the distribution of blood according to the need. For example, tissues with increased metabolic demand will signal nervous system inputs to decrease blood vessel tone. This results in vasodilatation, making blood more available to the starved tissue.

Systemic arterial blood pressure is the pressure exerted by blood against the walls of a blood vessel per unit area. It is normally measured at the brachial artery by a sphygmomanometer (blood pressure cuff), which temporarily occludes blood flow and measures the pressure at which blood flow returns to the artery. Arterial blood pressure consists of a higher systolic pressure, which represents the contraction of the ventricles and outflow of blood, and a lower diastolic component, which corresponds to the relaxation of the ventricles. Normal systemic arterial blood pressure is approximately 120/80 mm Hg.

The cardiovascular system is extremely efficient in maintaining an adequate and effective blood pressure to drive blood throughout the entire body despite changes in body position or fluid volume. In addition, it has the intrinsic ability to adjust blood pressure to local tissue oxygen requirements and metabolic demands. Specialized sensory neurons such as baroreceptors and chemoreceptors, found within the walls of the arteries and specific areas of the heart, sense changes in volume and blood chemistry. Feedback loops involving the cardiovascular regulatory center found in the medulla oblongata of the brain respond with appropriate adjustments to variables such as heart rate, vascular tone, and cardiac output.

CARDIAC ELECTROPHYSIOLOGY

Membrane Potentials

The plasma membrane, the outside casing holding the cell intact, possesses selective permeability that is referred to as a potential. The potential directly influences the movement of charged particles (positive and negative ions) across the cell membrane. Electrical energy stored in the membrane potential is tapped to generate signals that can be passed from one cell to another. The common molecules that exist in the body are water and simple inorganic molecules. Fluids in the body can be divided into one of two parts. They can be part of either the extracellular fluid (ECF) or the intracellular fluid (ICF). The barrier between these two compartments is the plasma membrane of the cell. The ECF is high in both sodium, a positively charged ion, and chloride, a negatively charged ion, but low in potassium, whereas the ICF is low in sodium and chloride, but high in potassium. This difference is maintained and regulated by control mechanisms residing in the plasma membrane, which acts as a selective permeable barrier permitting some substances to cross while excluding others. Major organic cellular anions inside the cell, such as protein, are the cell's biochemical machinery, and the plasma membrane is impermeable to this special group of molecules.

Ion Channels and Gates

An electrical voltage difference exists between the inside and the outside of the cell, the inside being more negative than the outside. The difference is measured in millivolts (mV) and is referred to as the membrane potential of the cell. The membrane is permeable only to some ions. Ion channels are the routes that ions travel to gain access into the cell. These channels exhibit ion selectivity, which allows some inorganic ions to pass through but not others. These channels are designed to permit entry only to certain permeating ions of appropriate size and charge. This enables the cell to limit their rate of passage. However, these ion channels are gated and not always open. The gates open only for a brief period and are then closed again. In most cases, the gates open in response to specific stimuli. There are different ways in which these channels are gated and different types of stimulation that cause them to open. One of the main types of stimuli is caused by an intracellular mediator, referred to as an ion-gated channel (see Table 9-1).

Action Potentials

Action potentials are defined as rapid, transient electrical excitations of the cell's membrane. Action potentials are simply impulses that allow for long-distance signaling within the system. Cardiac action potentials can last for several hundred milliseconds. There is a timed sequence of permeability changes underlying the action potentials of cardiac fibers. The sequence consists of a depolarizing phase, a long-lasting plateau phase, and a concluding repolarizing phase. In a cardiac muscle fiber, the duration of the action potential is explained by the maintained calcium influx during the plateau of the action potential. Therefore, the characteristics of the

action potential can have a direct influence on the duration and strength of each cardiac contraction.

The initial rising phase of the cardiac action potential is caused by the sodium channel. This channel drives the rapid depolarization phase and is responsible for the brief initial spike of the cardiac action potential before the plateau phase kicks in. The sodium channel rapidly closes with maintained depolarization. This rapid closing is not complete, as there remains a small constant increase in sodium permeability during the plateau portion (Table 9-1).

There are a few things that are responsible for terminating the cardiac action potential, causing the last phase of the cycle, repolarization, to occur. One implication of the prolonged cardiac action potential is that the duration of the contraction in cardiac muscle is controlled by the duration of the action potential itself. In cardiac muscle fibers, the contraction is maintained by the influx of calcium ions across the plasma membrane during the plateau phase of the cardiac action potential. The change in the duration of the action potential in the cardiac muscle fibers can alter the duration of the contraction of the heart. This provides an important mechanism by which the pumping action of the heart can be regulated.

Transmission of Impulses

For the contraction of a chamber in the heart to be able to perform a pumping action, all of the individual muscle fibers making up the walls of that chamber must contract simultaneously. It is this unified contraction that constricts the cavity of the chamber and drives out the blood to the blood vessels involved in the circulation process.

When an action potential is generated in a cardiac muscle fiber, it causes action potentials in their surrounding neighbors. This type of excitation spreads rapidly through all the muscle fibers of the heart chamber, ensuring that all the muscle fibers within that chamber contract together.

At the ends of each cardiac cell, the plasma membranes of neighboring cells come into close contact at the intercalated discs. The contact at this point is sufficiently close to enable the electrical current flowing inside of

Table $9\text{-}1$ Summary of Ionic Channels of Cardiac Muscle Membrane

Principal Ion	Response to Depolarization	Speed of Response	Inactivation	Function
Na^+	Opens	Fast	Fast, but incomplete	Initial depolarization
K^+	Closes	Fast	None	Maintains plateau
K^+	Opens	Slow	Little	Repolarization
K^+	Opens because of Ca^+ influx	Slow	Closes as internal Ca^+ falls	Repolarization
Ca^+	Opens	Slow	Slow	Maintains plateau and prolongs contraction

one fiber to cross directly into the interior of the next fiber. This electrical current will pass through the point of least resistance. This low-resistance path from one cell to another becomes possible through gap junctions. These structures directly connect the interiors on the joined cells, so ions can pass directly from one cell to another.

When electrical current passes from cell to another, as in cardiac muscle, those cells are considered to be electrically coupled. If two cells are coupled through gap junctions, a response to the injected current occurs in both cells because the ions carrying the current inside of the cell can pass directly through the gap junction. This electrical coupling among cardiac muscle fibers explains how contraction occurs synchronously in all of the fibers of a chamber.

Within the electrical membrane potential of a spontaneously beating cardiac cell lie a series of spontaneous action potentials. After each action potential, the potential falls back to its normal negative resting value and then begins to depolarize slowly. This slow depolarization is called a pacemaker potential and is caused by spontaneous changes in ionic permeability within the membrane.

THE ECG

The ECG records specific waveforms produced by the cells within the atrium and ventricles. Consider the function of the ECG recording as a voltmeter that records the differences in electrical voltages (potentials) generated by depolarization of heart muscle. This electrical activity of the heart is visually recorded through electrodes connected by cables to an ECG machine, one end of the cable being attached to the patient at the electrode site and the other end connected to the machine.

Lead Placement

Electrodes are applied to specific sites on the chest wall and extremities and can range from a simple 2-lead placement to a full-scale 12-lead placement, which provides the ability to view the heart's electrical activity from different angles and planes. A lead is a record of electrical activity between two electrodes. Each lead records the average current flow at a specific time during the cardiac cycle in a particular portion of the heart. There are three types of leads: standard limb, augmented, and precordial (chest) leads. Each lead has both a positive and a negative electrode that senses the magnitude and direction of the electrical forces caused by the spread of waves of both the depolarization and repolarization throughout the myocardium. Any of the electrodes can be made positive or negative simply by changing the lead selector on the ECG machine.

The position of the positive electrode on the body determines the portion of the heart that is seen by each of the leads. If the wave of depolarization (electrical impulse) moves toward the positive electrode, the waveform recorded on the ECG graph paper will appear upright, relaying a positive deflection.[1] If the wave of depolarization moves toward the negative electrode, the waveform recorded will be inverted, appearing downward or as a negative deflection. A biphasic waveform, which is both partly positive and partly negative, is recorded when the wave of depolarization moves perpendicularly to the positive electrode.

A polysomnogram requires a simple two- or three-lead placement, using electrodes aVR and aVL, which are placed midclavicular, under both the right and the left sides in the first intercostal space, and aV6, which is placed midaxillary, in the sixth intercostal space. Although it is only necessary to have two ECG leads to obtain enough diagnostic information, a 3-lead placement may be used in the sleep lab, as it provides a backup channel for re-referencing if one should become displaced during the course of the testing (1).

Normal ECG Rhythm

A normal ECG rhythm includes the appearance of a P, QRS, and T wave during one cardiac cycle. The P wave portion represents atrial depolarization (contraction). This waveform is normally less than 0.08 seconds in duration. The QRS wave represents ventricular depolarization (contraction) and atrial repolarization and should be less than 0.12 seconds in duration. Finally, the ECG resolves with the T wave, where ventricular repolarization occurs (see Fig. 9-4). In the normal heart, all of these waves will be conducted through electrical impulses and seen in precise timing in relation to one another and in correct sequence. The heart rate is determined by the number of QRS complexes per minute. Normal heart rates for adults range from 60 to 100 bpm.

Respiration may alter the rhythm and the rate of cardiac pacing. For example, it is quite common to see sinus arrhythmia in children. This benign condition is caused by the pressure fluctuation within the thorax during normal breathing. Specifically, during inhalation you may see a heart rate deceleration, whereas cardiac acceleration may be noted during exhalation.

ECG Patterns Commonly Seen in Sleep

A typical sleep study includes an ECG channel for the purpose of monitoring a patient's cardiac status throughout the testing. Many of the parameters that define a sleep disorder can cause changes in the cardiac rate and rhythm. Therefore, it is important that the sleep technologist be able to recognize abnormal cardiac rhythms. Apnea and hypopnea episodes, typical of obstructive sleep apnea (OSA), are often followed by arousals and/or hypoxia.

---

[1]This differs from standard EEG and polysomnography polarity convention, whereby a positive voltage produces a *downward* deflection. When recording ECG in polysomnography (using a modified lead II derivation), the electrode connections are arranged to produce an upward deflection of the "R" wave of the ECG.

Frequent arousals and/or hypoxia during sleep commonly result in changes in heart rate. Bradycardia (heart rate < 50 bpm) may be noted during an apneic/hypoxic episode, whereas tachycardia (heart rate > 90 bpm) or rate acceleration may accompany the arousal that follows. If the patient has severe OSA, this pattern may be observed throughout the night. Repeated episodes of apnea and hypopnea with oxygen desaturation may also be associated with premature atrial contractions or other atrial dysrhythmias such as atrial fibrillation or atrial flutter. Supraventricular tachycardia is an example of a supraventricular dysrhythmia that may be noted and is characterized by a fast, narrow complex rhythm that begins and ends very abruptly. Lastly, the sleep technologist may encounter patients who have other comorbidities, such as underlying cardiac disease. In this case, ventricular dysrhythmias, such as premature ventricular contractions and bigeminy, or conduction abnormalities, may be noted. For this reason, it is important that the sleep technologist carefully review the patient's past medical and cardiopulmonary history as well as current medications before beginning the sleep study. This can better prepare the technologist for what to expect while monitoring the patient.

Besides obtaining a quality sleep study, the most important role of the sleep technologist is to maintain patient safety. Sleep technologists should all be certified in basic life support and be familiar with emergency

protocols. By monitoring the cardiac rate and rhythm, they will be prepared to recognize changing and deteriorating rhythms and know when it becomes necessary to call for help. For a more detailed discussion of cardiac arrhythmias, refer Chapter 40.

CONCLUSION

This section has provided a brief overview of the normal anatomy and electrophysiology of the heart, including the specialized functions and mechanics of the cardiac muscle, cardiac cycle, the electrical impulse conduction pathways, and the way in which this relates to the entire cardiovascular system. Patients undergoing sleep studies may exhibit any number of cardiac dysrhythmias. Sleep technologists must be prepared to recognize and identify these rhythms and, when necessary, act appropriately. A strong understanding of the anatomy and electrophysiology of the heart can better prepare them for this task and greatly improve patient safety.

REFERENCES

1. Berry, R. B., Albertario, C. L., Harding, S. M., et al.; for the American Academy of Sleep Medicine. (2018). *The AASM manual for the scoring of sleep and associated events: Rules, terminology and technical specifications* [Version 2.5]. Darien, IL: American Academy of Sleep Medicine.

SUGGESTED READINGS

Aehlert, B. (2006). *ECG's made easy* (3rd ed.). St. Louis, MO: Mosby.

Alberts, B., Bray, D., Lewis, J., et al. (1983). *Molecular biology of the cell* (3rd ed.). New York, NY: Garland Publishing.

Darovic, G. O. (1985). *Hemodynamic monitoring: Invasive and noninvasive clinical application* (2nd ed., pp. 77–116). Philadelphia, PA: W.B. Saunders Company.

Hicks, G. H. (2000). *Cardiopulmonary anatomy and physiology*. Philadelphia, PA: W.B. Saunders Company.

Matthews, G. G. (1991). *Cellular physiology of nerve and muscle* (2nd ed.). Cambridge, MA: Blackwell Scientific Publications.

Smith, J. J., & Kampine, J. P. (1984). *Circulatory physiology: The essentials* (2nd ed.). Baltimore, MD: Williams & Wilkins.

Stalheim-Smith, A., & Fitch, G. K. (1993). *Understanding human anatomy and physiology* (pp. 581–615). St. Paul, MN: West Publishing Company.

Vander, A. J., Sherman, J. H., & Luciano, D. S. (1990). *Human physiology* (5th ed.). New York, NY: McGraw-Hill Publishing Company.

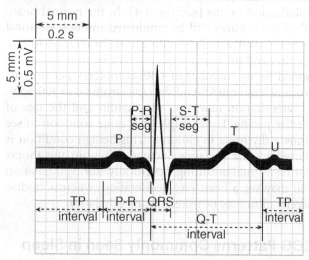

P wave (0.08–0.10 s)   QRS (0.06–0.10 s)
P-R interval (0.12–0.20 s)   Q-T$_C$ interval (≤ 0.44 s)*

$$*QT_C = \frac{QT}{\sqrt{RR}}$$

Figure 9-4 Normal electrocardiography tracing showing a normal sinus rhythm. Shown are the P, QRS, T, and U waves, which represent electrical activity in different parts of the heart. Intervals measure from one wave to the next; segments are smaller components of the tracing. (Reprinted with permission from Smeltzer SC and Brunner, LS. *Brunner and Suddarth's textbook of medical-surgical nursing, 12th ed.* Philadelphia, PA: ©Lippincott Williams & Wilkins/Wolters Kluwer, 2010.)

chapter 10

General Human Physiology for the Sleep Technologist

REGINA PATRICK

LEARNING OBJECTIVES

On completion of this chapter, the reader should be able to:

1. Have a basic understanding of human anatomy and physiology.
2. Understand the unique functions of the endocrine system, the renal system, the digestive system, the immune system, the genitourinary system, the musculoskeletal system, metabolism, and thermoregulation in humans.
3. Understand how dysfunction in these systems can impact sleep.
4. Understand why certain sleep disorders are associated with dysfunction in one or more of these systems.

KEY TERMS

Acid–base balance
Digestive system
Electrolyte
Endocrine system
Genitourinary system
Immune system
Metabolism
Musculoskeletal system
pH
Renal system
Thermoregulation

The brain is the primary organ that controls sleep and wake. However, the function of many other body systems can impact sleep. This chapter will discuss the basic functions of the endocrine system, the renal system, the digestive system, the immune system, the genitourinary system, the musculoskeletal system, metabolism, and thermoregulation. This chapter will also discuss sleep disorders that are associated with dysfunctions in these systems.

THE ENDOCRINE SYSTEM

The endocrine system consists of several glands that secrete hormones that affect a different organ (i.e., target organ). The glands release their hormones directly into the bloodstream or into lymph (i.e., a transparent yellow liquid that flows through lymphatic vessels). Once the hormone travels to a target organ, it may affect the metabolism or function of the target organ. The hypothalamus, pituitary, pineal gland, thyroid, parathyroid glands, adrenal glands, gonads, and pancreas are a few of the organs that make up the endocrine system (Fig. 10-1).

Overview of Endocrine Hormone Classification

Three types of hormones produced in the endocrine system are steroid hormones, protein hormones (also called "peptide hormones"), and amine hormones. Steroid hormones are synthesized from cholesterol and secreted by the adrenal cortex, testes, and ovaries. Examples of steroid hormones are cortisol, aldosterone, testosterone, and estrogen. Protein hormones consist of amino acids that are bound together with peptide bonds. In a peptide bond, the amine group ($-NH_2$) of one amino acid binds with the carboxyl group ($-COOH$) of another amino acid. Most hormones in the body are protein hormones. Insulin and calcitonin are examples of protein hormones. Amine hormones contain amino acids, but the acids do not form peptide bonds. Melatonin, thyroxine, and epinephrine are examples of amine hormones.

The release of many hormones is controlled by a negative feedback system. In such a system, when one substance reaches a certain level, it inhibits the release of another. For example, when the blood glucose level is high, the release of insulin inhibits the release of glucagon; when the blood glucose level is low, the release of glucagon inhibits the release of insulin. A negative feedback loop helps maintain proper levels of other substances (in this case, glucose) and proper functioning of the body. See Table 10-1 for a synopsis of the endocrine hormones and their main functions.

Table 10-1 The Source and Main Action of Various Endocrine Hormones

Source Organ	Endocrine Hormone	Target Organ	Action of the Hormone
Adrenal gland			
Medulla (inner core)	Epinephrine*	Blood vessels, liver, lungs, brain	Involved in the "fight-or-flight" response in times of stress (e.g., increases blood pressure by increasing the strength and rate of heart contractions and vasoconstriction)
			Assists in the breakdown of glycogen to glucose in the liver to provide energy during times of stress
			Bronchodilation
			Acts as a neurotransmitter in the brain (e.g., activates the reticular formation in the brain)
	Norepinephrine*	Blood vessels, heart	Increases heart rate and vasoconstriction in response to hypotension (i.e., low blood pressure)
Cortex (outer portion)			
Inner layer	Sex hormones: testosterone, estrogen	Reproductive organs	Involved in the development of sex characteristics
Middle layer	Glucocorticoids: cortisol	Immune cells, liver, kidney	Involved in the metabolism of carbohydrates, protein, and fat
			Promotes diuresis
			Reduces inflammatory processes
Outer layer	Mineralocorticoids: Aldosterone	Kidney	Promotes water retention
			Regulates the concentration of electrolytes (e.g., sodium, potassium)
Gonads			
Ovaries (women)	Estrogen	Female genitalia (e.g., uterus)	Involved in menstruation, the development of female reproductive organs and secondary sex characteristics (e.g., pubic hair)
Testes (men)	Testosterone	Male reproductive organs	Involved in the development of male reproductive organs and secondary sex characteristics (e.g., pubic hair, facial hair), spermatozoa formation, muscle growth
Heart			
Atrial wall	Atrial natriuretic peptide	Kidney	Stimulates the retention of sodium and water, which increases fluid within blood vessels and body tissues
			Reduces the levels of renin, aldosterone, and antidiuretic hormone
Hypothalamus			
Anterior hypothalamus	Corticotropin-releasing hormone	Anterior pituitary	Stimulates the anterior pituitary to release adrenocorticotropic hormone (ACTH)
	Dopamine	Brain, kidneys, adrenal gland, anterior pituitary	Involved in the transmission of signals from neuron to neuron in the brain; in sleep, mood, and motor function; and in the regulation of blood flow in the kidneys
			It is a precursor to norepinephrine
			It inhibits the anterior pituitary's release of prolactin (a hormone that is involved in lactation)

Table 10-1 The Source and Main Action of Various Endocrine Hormones (continued)

Source Organ	Endocrine Hormone	Target Organ	Action of the Hormone
	Growth hormone-releasing hormone	Anterior pituitary	Stimulates the anterior pituitary to release growth hormone
	Somatostatin	Anterior pituitary	Inhibits the anterior pituitary production of growth hormone
	Thyrotropin-releasing hormone	Anterior pituitary	Stimulates the anterior pituitary to produce thyroid-stimulating hormone
Posterior hypothalamus	Antidiuretic hormone	Posterior pituitary	Antidiuretic hormone is stored in the posterior pituitary
Pancreas			
Islets of Langerhans			
Alpha cells	Glucagon	Liver, fat tissue	Stimulates the conversion of glycogen into glucose, which is then released into the bloodstream, when blood glucose levels are low
Beta cells	Insulin	Liver, muscles, many other body cells	Promotes the removal of glucose from the blood into cells (thereby reducing blood glucose levels) when blood glucose levels are high Involved in protein and glycogen synthesis Involved in the conversion of glucose to glycogen in the liver
Parathyroid gland	Parathyroid hormone (also called parathormone)	Intestine, kidneys, and skeletal system	Involved in the utilization of calcium and phosphate in the body
Pineal gland	Melatonin	Suprachiasmatic nuclei	Promotes sleep and is involved in the circadian rhythm
Pituitary gland			
Anterior pituitary	Adrenocorticotropic hormone (ACTH)	Adrenal cortex	Stimulates the adrenal cortex to increase its secretion of hormones such as cortisol
	Gonadotropic hormones Follicle-stimulating hormone, luteinizing hormone	Ovaries, testes	Promotes estrogen and testosterone production, involved in menstrual cycle, stimulates spermatozoa formation
	Thyroid-stimulating hormone	Thyroid	Stimulates the release of thyroid hormones
Posterior pituitary	Antidiuretic hormone (also called "vasopressin")	Kidney, smooth muscles of arterioles	Stimulates the resorption of water from urine into the blood, which reduces urine output Increases the constriction of blood vessels
Thyroid	Calcitonin	Skeletal bones	Inhibits the breakdown of bone
	Thyroxine (also called T_4) and tri-iodothyronine (also called T_3)	All cells	Stimulate energy metabolism in cells

*Epinephrine and norepinephrine are commonly called adrenaline and noradrenaline, respectively.

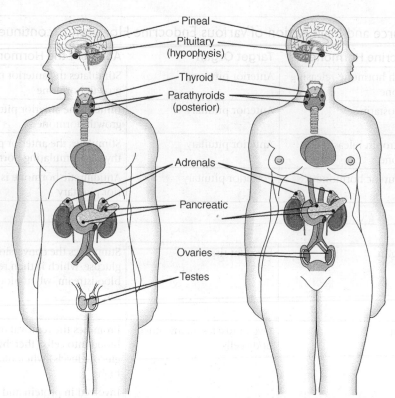

Pineal
Pituitary
(hypophysis)
Thyroid
Parathyroids
(posterior)
Adrenals
Pancreatic
Ovaries
Testes

Figure 10-1 The endocrine system is comprised of glands with a primary function of hormone secretion. (Reprinted with permission from Cohen, B. J. (2012). *Memmler's structure and function of the human body*. Philadelphia, PA: Lippincott Williams & Wilkins/Wolters Kluwer. Copyright © Lippincott Williams & Wilkins/Wolters Kluwer.)

ENDOCRINE ORGANS

Hypothalamus

The hypothalamus is a structure that lies at the base of the brain. The optic tract and optic chiasm (the point at which fibers of the left and right optic nerves cross to the opposite side of the brain) form part of the hypothalamus. The hypothalamus also contains various nuclei (i.e., groups of cells having a specialized function) that are involved in water balance, maintaining body temperature (i.e., thermoregulation), sleep, and food intake. Extending by a stalk from the hypothalamus is the pituitary, a gland that contains an anterior lobe and a posterior lobe. The anterior hypothalamus (i.e., front portion of the hypothalamus) produces various hormones that are transported into the anterior pituitary by way of a special blood capillary network; on arriving to the anterior pituitary, the posterior hypothalamic hormones stimulate the release of or inhibit the production and release of anterior pituitary hormones. In the posterior hypothalamus (i.e., the back portion of the hypothalamus), the axons of neurosecretory cells (i.e., neurons or nerve-like cells that secrete substances

that act on another structure) extend from the posterior hypothalamus into the posterior pituitary. These neurosecretory cells synthesize hormones in the posterior hypothalamus; the hormones are then transported to the terminals of the axons in the posterior pituitary where they are stored and then released when necessary.

Pituitary Gland

The pituitary gland, which is located below the hypothalamus, extends from the hypothalamus by a stalk and consists of two distinct parts: a front portion (i.e., the anterior pituitary) and a rear portion (i.e., the posterior pituitary). The anterior pituitary receives various releasing and inhibiting hormones from the hypothalamus. As their name implies, these hormones cause the anterior pituitary to release hormones (e.g., the growth hormone–releasing hormone stimulates the anterior pituitary to release growth hormone) or inhibit their production and release of hormones (e.g., somatostatin inhibits the anterior pituitary's production of growth hormone). The posterior pituitary gland acts as a reservoir for various hypothalamic hormones such as antidiuretic hormone and releases them into the bloodstream when needed. The anterior pituitary histologically consists of the endocrine tissue, whereas the posterior pituitary histologically has the structure of nerve tissue.

Pineal Gland

The pineal gland is a small, flattened, cone-shaped gland in the upper rear brainstem. It receives sensory information from the optic nerves such as the level of light. It produces several hormones, the most important of which is the sleep-promoting hormone melatonin.

Thyroid

The thyroid is a butterfly shaped gland that lies in front of the lower portion of the throat, just above the trachea. It secretes and stores various thyroid hormones (e.g., thyroxine [T_4], triiodothyronine [T_3], and calcitonin). Thyroxine and triiodothyronine are involved in regulating a person's metabolic rate, and calcitonin is involved in maintaining proper calcium levels in the body.

Parathyroid Glands

The parathyroid glands are four small glands on the posterior surface of the thyroid. The parathyroid glands produce parathyroid hormone (also called "parathormone"), which has a role in the regulation of calcium and phosphate levels in the body.

Adrenal Gland

The adrenal gland is a small organ that lies on the top of the kidney. It consists of an inner core (i.e., the medulla) and an outer portion (i.e., cortex) that covers the medulla. The medulla secretes epinephrine and norepinephrine, which are released to prepare the body for the "flight or fight" response in times of stress. The adrenal cortex has three layers, each of which secretes different hormones. The cortex's outermost layer secretes mineralocorticoids. These chemicals maintain the level of mineral salts (e.g., sodium chloride) in the body. The main mineralocorticoid produced by the adrenal cortex is aldosterone. The middle layer of the cortex produces glucocorticoids. These chemicals are involved in maintaining the blood glucose level and maintaining blood pressure. The main glucocorticoid produced by the adrenal cortex is cortisol. The innermost level of the cortex secretes small amounts of sex hormones (e.g., testosterone and estrogen).

Gonads

The gonads are organs that produce the reproductive cells. The gonads in men are the testes, which produce spermatozoa; the gonads in women are the ovaries, which produce ova (i.e., egg cells). The testes produce the sex hormone testosterone, and the ovaries produce estrogen. These hormones are involved in reproductive behavior, fertility, and the development of secondary sex characteristics (e.g., facial hair in men).

Pancreas

The pancreas is an oblong gland situated behind the stomach. On the surface of the pancreas, microscopic groups of specialized cells are scattered like islands among the pancreatic cells. These cells are called the "islets (or islands) of Langerhans." Two types of cells exist within each islet of Langerhans—alpha and beta cells. The alpha cells secrete the hormone glucagon, which converts the liver starch glycogen into glucose when blood glucose levels are low; the beta cells secrete insulin, which reduces the blood glucose level when glucose levels are too high. Insulin and glucagon are antagonistic in their actions.

Endocrine Function and Sleep Disorders

The secretion of endocrine hormones increases and decreases with circadian rhythmicity. For example, the production of melatonin normally increases in the evening (thereby promoting sleep) and decreases in the morning (thereby promoting wakefulness). Factors such as night shift work, blindness, or dysfunction of certain hypothalamic cells can disrupt the rhythmic production of endocrine hormones. This disruption can lead to sleep and wake cycles that occur at undesired times (e.g., advanced or delayed sleep phase) or lead to the destruction of the cyclicity of a person's sleep and wake cycles (e.g., free-running rhythm). As a result, a person may struggle with sleep problems such as insomnia or excessive daytime sleepiness (EDS).

The production of melatonin is influenced by a person's exposure to light. In the normal eye, light stimulates the retina, which relays signals through the optic nerves. The signals ultimately reach the pineal gland, which produces melatonin. The greater the amount of light, the greater the number of signals reaching the pineal gland and the less the amount of melatonin it produces. As dark progresses through the evening, melatonin production increases and ultimately induces sleep. Night shift work, working frequently changing shifts, and blindness can alter a person's exposure to light and disrupt the production of melatonin and lead to sleep problems.

Night Shift Work/Frequently Changing Shifts

A person who works third shift typically works all night in a lighted setting and drives home in the bright light of morning. Both of these factors reduce the production of melatonin. Once the person arrives home, he or she may have difficulty going to sleep at a desired time because of the reduced melatonin level. Once a person falls asleep, the delayed sleep onset can shorten the person's sleep time and result in struggles with sleepiness when the person is awake during a work shift.

It is possible for a shift worker to shift when the greatest amount of melatonin production occurs. Reducing daytime exposure to light can help shift the greatest melatonin production to daytime hours and thereby promote sleep during the day. For example, after working a shift, the worker could drive home with dark sunglasses on and use room-darkening shades in the bedroom. However, the ability to reset and maintain a consistent rhythm of melatonin production may not be possible if shift changes are frequent (e.g., every week).

Blindness

Some blind people—especially people who have no light perception—have a free-running circadian rhythm. In a free-running rhythm, a person's sleep–wake phases move forward every day, rather than remaining stable at the same time every day. For example, the person may fall asleep at 8:00 p.m. one night, fall asleep the next night at 9:00 p.m., fall asleep the following night at 10:00 p.m., and so forth. When trying to follow a normal sleep–wake schedule, people with a free-running rhythm will experience a period of excessive sleepiness, a period in which they can sleep "normally," and a period of wakefulness (i.e., insomnia) because their sleep–wake phases do not occur at the same time every day, and, therefore, flow into and out of phase with the societal norm.

Dysfunction of Hypothalamic Cells

Scientists have recently discovered that hypothalamic cells that produce the wake-promoting excitatory neuropeptide orexin (also called "hypocretin") are inexplicably and irreversibly destroyed in some patients with narcolepsy. The primary symptom of narcolepsy is EDS. This symptom may be accompanied by cataplexy (i.e., the sudden, temporary loss of skeletal muscle tone), hypnagogic or hypnopompic hallucinations (i.e., realistic dream imagery occurring with sleep onset or on awakening, respectively), and paralysis on awakening from sleep or on going to sleep (i.e., sleep paralysis). The latter three symptoms may be the result of the muscle atonia and dream imagery features of rapid eye movement (REM) sleep intruding into wake. In recent years, scientists have noted another symptom in people with narcolepsy: sleep disrupted by frequent arousals that occur for no apparent reason such as apnea. The arousals may reflect a dysfunction in the neural control of sleep and wake.

Orexin-producing neurons project from the hypothalamus into brainstem areas such as the locus ceruleus, raphe nuclei, and reticular formation. These areas are involved in various aspects of REM sleep and wakefulness. Therefore, the destruction of orexin-producing hypothalamic cells may be involved in the improper manifestation of REM sleep features in wake, sleep disruption, and sleepiness in narcolepsy.

THE RENAL SYSTEM

The renal system consists of the kidneys, ureters, and urinary bladder (Fig. 10-2). The urinary system maintains blood volume, removes waste, regulates blood pressure, and is involved in maintaining pH balance in the blood.

The kidney is a bean-shaped organ that is approximately the size of a fist. The ureter is a fibromuscular tubular structure that descends from the kidney to the urinary bladder. It transports urine (an amber fluid that is a waste product) from the kidney to the urinary bladder. The urinary bladder is a musculomembranous sac in the front portion of the pelvis. It receives urine and voids it to the exterior of the body through the urethra (a membranous canal).

Each kidney contains millions of nephrons (Fig. 10-3), which are the structural component of the kidney. Each nephron contains a glomerulus (a ball-like cluster of capillaries), a proximal convoluted tubule and distal convoluted tubule, and a collecting tubule. Afferent arterioles (i.e., microscopic arteries) bring blood from the renal artery into the glomerulus. A hollow-walled structure, called Bowman's capsule, surrounds each glomerulus. (To use an analogy, imagine a fist that is pushed into a balloon, so that the balloon surrounds the fist; the fist represents the glomerulus and the balloon, Bowman's capsule.) Some amount of

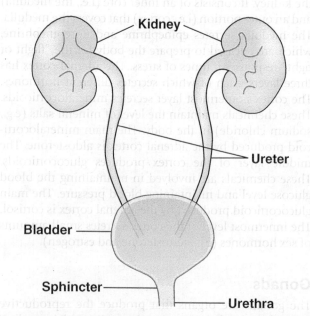

Figure 10-2 The renal system. (National Institute of Diabetes and Digestive and Kidney Diseases, National Institutes of Health, Bethesda, Maryland.)

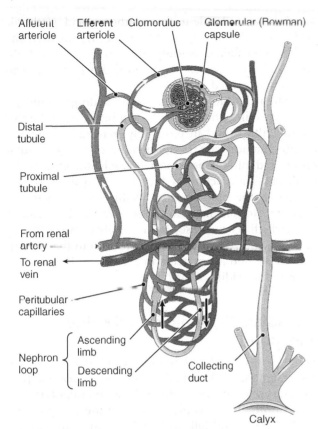

Figure 10-3 A nephron and its blood supply. The nephron regulates the proportion of water, waste, and other materials in urine according to the body's constantly changing needs. A nephron consists of a glomerular capsule, convoluted tubules, the nephron loop (loop of Henle), and a collecting duct. Blood filtration occurs through the glomerulus in the glomerular capsule. Materials that enter the nephron can be returned to the blood through the surrounding peritubular capillaries. (Reprinted with permission from Knight, L. (2013). *Medical terminology: An illustrated guide Canadian edition* (2nd ed., Figure 13.3). Philadelphia, PA: Lippincott Williams & Wilkins/Wolters Kluwer. Copyright © Lippincott Williams & Wilkins/Wolters Kluwer.)

blood plasma exits from the glomerular capillaries and enters the hollow wall of the surrounding Bowman's capsule. The remaining blood flows out of the glomerulus through the efferent arteriole. The efferent arteriole branches to form a capillary network, called the "peritubular capillaries," that surrounds a nephron's tubules. The peritubular capillaries drain blood into veins that ultimately feed into the renal vein. The renal vein takes blood away from the kidney.

The blood plasma in the hollow wall of Bowman's capsule empties into the proximal convoluted tubule. This fluid is called the "glomerular filtrate." Once the glomerular filtrate is in the proximal convoluted tubule, ions such as sodium and chloride, glucose, and amino acids exit from the glomerular filtrate and enter

the surrounding perivascular capillaries, and thereby reenter the bloodstream. This process is called "reabsorption." Through reabsorption, most nutrients and approximately 65% of salt and water in the glomerular filtrate in the proximal tubule are returned to the blood. Electrolytes, which are positively or negatively charged molecules or atoms such as sodium (Na^+), potassium (K^+), bicarbonate (HCO_3^-), and calcium (Ca^{2+}), are also reabsorbed from the glomerular filtrate. Some nitrogen-containing compounds (e.g., urea), ions, salts, and water are not reabsorbed from the glomerular filtrate and are excreted as waste.

The glomerular filtrate next passes through the loop of Henle, which has a descending arm and an ascending arm. The glomerular filtrate becomes increasingly concentrated as it flows down the descending arm and then up the ascending arm of the loop of Henle. The glomerular filtrate then travels to the distal convoluted tubule. In the distal convoluted tubule, salt and water continue to be reabsorbed into the bloodstream. As the filtrate passes through the loop of Henle, chemical compounds such as uric acid, creatinine, ammonia, hydrogen ions, and drugs (e.g., penicillin) exit from the perivascular capillaries and enter the glomerular filtrate. In this way, these compounds are removed from the blood. By the time the glomerular filtrate passes through the distal convoluted tubule, it is urine. The urine drips into the collecting duct and descends through the collecting duct to the renal pelvis, which joins the ureter. The ureter transports the urine into the urinary bladder.

Renal Control of Electrolyte Balance

The kidneys maintain the balance of electrolytes in the body. Electrolytes are ingested with foods and are lost through perspiration and feces. Some important electrolytes are Na^+, K^+, Ca^{2+}, HCO_3^-, phosphate (PO_4^{3-}), and chloride (Cl^-). The amount of electrolytes taken into the body must equal the amount lost by the body. Losing a greater amount of electrolytes than what is consumed can set the stage for heart arrhythmias, muscle cramps, and other problems.

The steroid hormone aldosterone, which is produced and released by the adrenal gland, regulates sodium and potassium levels in the body. Aldosterone is released when the blood sodium level is low. It acts on the tubules to increase sodium reabsorption into the blood. When the blood potassium level is high, aldosterone causes potassium ions to be excreted into the glomerular filtrate and exit the body through urine. Potassium is usually excreted in the form of potassium salts such as potassium chloride (KCl).

Other hormones can impact the kidney's regulation of electrolytes. For example, the distal tubules are sensitive to the actions of parathyroid hormone (i.e., parathormone) and calcitonin. Parathyroid hormone causes calcium to be reabsorbed from the distal tubules into the blood and thereby raises the blood calcium level. Calcitonin decreases the reabsorption of calcium, phosphate, and sodium ions from the distal tubules and thereby allows these electrolytes to be excreted in the urine.

Atrial natriuretic peptide has the opposite action of aldosterone. Atrial natriuretic peptide is secreted from the heart's atrial wall in response to increased intravascular volume or stretching of the atria beyond the normal dimension. It stimulates kidney tubules to excrete sodium into the urine (i.e., natriuresis), which leads to more water entering the urine. Natriuresis reduces fluid volume in body tissues and blood pressure.

Renal Control of Acid–Base Balance

The kidneys also regulate the acid–base balance (i.e., pH, the concentration of hydrogen ions [H^+]) of the body fluids. An improper acid–base balance can result in problems such as sleep-disordered breathing, excessive sleepiness, coma, and death.

In a solution, acids release hydrogen ions (thereby increasing the hydrogen concentration of the solution) and bases remove hydrogen ions (thereby decreasing the hydrogen concentration of the solution). The concentration of hydrogen ions is expressed by pH. A fluid with a pH of 7 is neutral, a fluid with a pH less than 7 is acidic, and a fluid with a pH greater than 7 is basic (i.e., alkaline).

The pH of many body fluids is normally maintained within a narrow range. For example, the normal pH of arterial blood ranges between 7.35 and 7.45. A person experiences acidosis (i.e., too acidic) if the arterial blood pH is less than 7.35 and experiences alkalosis (i.e., too alkaline) if the arterial blood pH is greater than 7.45. The narrow pH range in the blood and the other body fluids is maintained by various buffers.

A buffer is a solution containing two or more chemical compounds that prevent drastic changes in pH when an acid or a base enters a system (e.g., the bloodstream). A buffer usually contains a weak acid and the salt of that acid. In the salt of an acid, some of the hydrogen atoms in the acid have been replaced by other molecules. An example of a buffer is carbonic acid (H_2CO_3) and its salt sodium bicarbonate ($NaHCO_3$).

A buffer helps the kidneys regulate the acid–base balance. For example, lactic acid, a waste product of muscle metabolism, easily dissociates in solution. In a solution such as blood, lactic acid dissociates into lactate ($C_3H_5O_3^-$) and hydrogen (H^+) ions. The negatively charged lactate ions interact with the sodium ions from the sodium bicarbonate molecules to form sodium lactate. The remaining hydrogen ions from the lactic acid bind with the bicarbonate ions from the sodium

bicarbonate molecule to form carbonic acid. Carbonic acid is a weak acid and therefore does not increase the acidity of the fluid drastically. In this way, the pH is buffered against the greater increase in acidity that lactic acid would have caused.

When the blood is too acidic, hydrogen ions are transported into the lumen of the tubules, enter the glomerular filtrate, and are ultimately excreted in urine. The bicarbonate ions are transported out of the glomerular filtrate and into the perivascular vessels surrounding the nephrons. These actions reduce the acidity of the blood.

When the blood is too alkaline, fewer hydrogen ions are excreted into the urine. Because bicarbonate ions (which act as a base) are not easily reabsorbed into the blood from the tubules, they remain in the glomerular filtrate and are excreted in the urine. These actions increase the acidity of the blood.

Circadian Rhythmicity and Kidney Function

Kidney function (e.g., filtration, urine production, salt and water balance) normally varies on a circadian (i.e., 24-hour) rhythm. For example, the glomerular filtration rate is normally at its highest during the day (peaking at ~2–3 p.m.) and falls to its minimum in the middle of the night; sodium excretion and urine production are highest during the day and fall to their minimum at night; and urine is more dilute in the day and more concentrated at night.

It is unclear to what extent circadian rhythmicity in kidney function is influenced by external factors or is intrinsic to kidneys (i.e., internally driven, regardless of external factors such as light or dark). Some research indicates that this fluctuation is driven by light and dark phases. For example, the excretion of urine is increased in the day (i.e., light phase) and decreased at night (i.e., dark phase). However, some research indicates that circadian rhythmicity in kidney function is intrinsic. In animals that are bred to lack certain genes that control the circadian rhythm, the circadian variation in kidney function is abolished, even when the animals are exposed to consistent light/dark cycles.

Circadian Rhythmicity of Normal Kidney Function

The interrelation between renin (a protein and enzyme), angiotensin (a hormone), and aldosterone (a mineralocorticoid) helps maintain proper sodium balance, fluid volume, and blood pressure. When blood flow in the kidneys decreases, the kidneys release renin, which is involved in the production of the powerful vasoconstrictor angiotensin II. Angiotensin II also stimulates the production of aldosterone, which promotes sodium and water retention and thereby raises blood pressure. The production of renin decreases once blood pressure is sufficiently raised. The levels of renin, angiotensin II, and aldosterone are generally higher in the morning and lower in the afternoon and evening. However, the production of these substances—as well as other substances such as cortisol (a glucocorticoid that is involved in diuresis [i.e., increased urine excretion] and natriuresis [i.e., excretion of sodium]) and atrial natriuretic peptide (a small protein that reduces renin, angiotensin II, and aldosterone levels and thereby lowers blood pressure)—varies with sleep stages.

During sleep, the production of hormones involved in kidney function fluctuates with the sleep state. The secretion of renin increases during non-REM sleep and decreases during REM sleep. Aldosterone increases and decreases in correlation with renin production during sleep. However, aldosterone and cortisol quickly increase dramatically when a person awakens from sleep. This sudden rise in aldosterone and cortisol may be related to the activation of the hypothalamus–pituitary–adrenal (HPA) axis with wake. The HPA axis is involved in the interplay between hormones produced by the hypothalamus, pituitary, and adrenal cortex. For example, the hypothalamus produces corticotrophin-releasing hormone, which causes the anterior pituitary to release adrenocorticotropic hormone, which then induces the release of aldosterone from the adrenal glands. Thus, aldosterone production appears to be under the influence of changes in renin production during non-REM and REM sleep but may be under the influence of cortisol during wake. By contrast, cortisol production appears to be weakly linked with REM sleep and non-REM sleep.

Impaired Kidney Function and Sleep Disorders

Kidney failure (i.e., the inability of the kidneys to excrete metabolites or to retain electrolytes at normal physiologic levels in the blood) can occur if there is decreased blood supply to the kidneys, damage to the kidney tissues, or obstruction to the outflow of urine. Kidney failure can be acute (i.e., sudden onset) or chronic. Acute kidney failure, if diagnosed quickly, can often be reversed with medical treatment. Acute kidney failure can progress to end-stage renal disease, uremic syndrome (i.e., kidney failure comprising a group of symptoms such as a metallic taste in the mouth, the formation of a layer of uric acid crystals on the surface of the skin [i.e., uremic frost], muscular twitching, pain, hypertension, mental confusion, and edema), and death. Poorly controlled diabetes, high blood pressure, and chronic glomerulonephritis (i.e., inflammation of the glomeruli) are some common causes of chronic kidney failure. Impaired kidney function or kidney failure can cause the blood to

become too acidic or too alkaline and negatively impact sleep. People with impaired kidney function or kidney failure can experience sleep-disordered breathing, insomnia, alterations in the circadian rhythm, restless legs syndrome (RLS), and EDS.

Sleep-Disordered Breathing
Central Apnea and Cheyne–Stokes Breathing

Neurons in the respiratory center in the brain are sensitive to pH changes in the blood. Therefore, blood pH is involved in the rhythmicity of breathing and in the depth of breathing. Acidosis normally induces increased firing of the respiratory center neurons and causes a person to take deep, fast breaths. Alkalosis normally induces decreased firing of the respiratory center neurons and causes a person to take shallow, slow breaths. However, a chronic state of acidosis or alkalosis, which may occur with impaired kidney function or chronic kidney failure, can alter the respiratory center's response to acidosis and alkalosis.

Improper responses to pH can set the stage for the manifestation of central sleep apnea (i.e., the cessation in the respiratory drive, resulting in a lack of respiratory movements) and Cheyne–Stokes respiration (i.e., a rhythmic breathing pattern in which a person takes increasingly shallow breaths—sometimes to the point of a central apnea—that are followed by increasingly deeper breaths). Frequent arousals resulting from these respiratory events during the night can result in EDS, fatigue, difficulty concentrating, and other symptoms associated with insufficient sleep.

Obstructive Sleep Apnea

Obstructive sleep apnea (OSA) is the cessation in breathing (i.e., apnea; from the Greek *apnoia*, meaning "no breath") caused by upper airway tissues (e.g., fat tissue, tonsils, adenoids) blocking the upper airway during sleep. With airflow impeded, the blood oxygen level falls. However, a person continues to make respiratory movements. Once the blood oxygen falls to a certain level, an arousal occurs and a person awakens briefly (usually a few seconds) to take some deep breaths, which restores the oxygen level. Once the oxygen level is restored, the person promptly resumes sleep. Many episodes of apnea can occur during a sleep period. A person who has five or more episodes of apnea per hour may be diagnosed with OSA. Because of the arousals from sleep, a person may struggle with symptoms such as EDS, impaired cognition, and diminished daytime functioning.

OSA is very common among people with end-stage renal disease. Exactly why OSA is so prevalent in patients with end-stage renal disease is unclear. A possibility may be a phenomenon called "rostral fluid shift." During the day when a person is awake and mobile, fluid volume is greater in the lower extremities because of gravity. However, when a person lies horizontally in bed, fluid shifts from the legs toward the neck (i.e., fluid moves rostrally [toward the oronasal region]). Excess fluid accumulation in the upper airway tissues can swell the tissues and contribute to upper airway narrowing and blockage, and thereby lead to OSA.

Insomnia

Insomnia is difficulty in initiating or maintaining sleep. It is usually secondary to (i.e., the result of) another problem. In people with end-stage renal disease, insomnia may occur because of the physical stress of managing their disease (e.g., the time of the hemodialysis session), whether a person is a long-term dialysis patient, and pain.

For unclear reasons, people whose hemodialysis sessions are scheduled for early morning appear to have a greater problem with insomnia, compared with people whose sessions are scheduled for the afternoon. A possible explanation is that patients with the early morning session may become conditioned to waking up early. By contrast, patients whose sessions are scheduled in the afternoon are often tired and sleepy after hemodialysis, which may enhance their sleep; thus, they report fewer problems with insomnia.

Long-term hemodialysis patients and elderly hemodialysis patients have greater problems with insomnia, compared with younger hemodialysis patients. With aging or long-term dialysis treatment, symptoms associated with chronic dialysis treatment (e.g., itchiness, bone pain) can delay the onset of sleep at a desired time or disrupt sleep. The effect of concurrent diseases such as cardiovascular disease (e.g., heart failure with Cheyne–Stokes breathing) and neurologic disease (e.g., RLS) can also contribute to insomnia in patients on long-term dialysis treatment.

Pain or discomfort due to changes in bone structure, muscle cramps, abdominal pain, etc., can delay the onset of sleep at a desired time. Pain may be so intense that it awakens a person and causes difficulty going back to sleep. High levels of parathyroid hormone can contribute to bone pain. Parathyroid hormone causes the release of calcium from the bone into the blood and other fluids. Excess levels of the hormone weaken the bone structure (i.e., osteoporosis), and thereby result in bone pain, fractures, and tenderness, and affect other organs such as the kidneys (e.g., kidney stones), the muscles (e.g., weakness, tremors, cramps), and the gastrointestinal system (e.g., abdominal pain, nausea, vomiting).

Alteration in the Circadian Rhythm

The level of the sleep-promoting hormone melatonin is normally highest during the night and lowest during the day. People with chronic kidney disease have lower nocturnal production of melatonin, compared with healthy individuals. In addition, the circadian rhythmicity of melatonin production is abolished in some people who are on hemodialysis. This reduced production may contribute to problems with initiating or maintaining sleep. Why the melatonin concentration is lower in hemodialyzed patients is unclear.

Restless Legs Syndrome

Symptoms of RLS begin to manifest in the evening soon before bedtime as a person sits or lies relaxed. Unpleasant sensations in the calves or legs cause a person to irresistibly move the legs to relieve the sensations (e.g., walking, rubbing them against bed sheets). The relief is short-lived and a person has to repeatedly go through efforts to relieve the sensations. These efforts at relief can delay the onset of sleep. The sensations usually drop out just as a person is falling asleep. However, if the person awakens during the night, the symptoms can recur and a person will go through the same efforts to relieve them, thereby delaying sleep. In healthy individuals without kidney disease, RLS has been associated with low levels of iron in the brain. Iron is involved in the production of the hormone dopamine (which has a role in motor function). However, some people with RLS have normal levels of iron. Therefore, the relationship between iron and RLS is unclear. In people undergoing hemodialysis, RLS may be related to increased levels of urea, creatinine, or other nitrogen-containing substances. The excess levels of these substances may contribute to central and peripheral nerve damage and thereby contribute to symptoms of RLS.

Excessive Daytime Sleepiness

As with insomnia, EDS is usually secondary to other problems in people with chronic kidney disease or kidney failure. Uremia (i.e., high blood levels of nitrogen-containing substances such as ammonia), disrupted sleep because of RLS or periodic limb movement disorder (i.e., a disorder in which the foot or leg rhythmically contracts intermittently during sleep and can induce arousals from sleep), or sleep apnea can lead to EDS. Neurologic changes such as uremic encephalopathy (i.e., brain disorder caused by uremia); low levels of the amino acid tyrosine, which is involved in dopamine production; the release of inflammatory cytokines during dialysis; high diurnal levels of melatonin; and a change in the circadian rhythmicity of body temperature may lead to problems with sleepiness at unwanted times. Addressing these factors can help alleviate daytime sleepiness. For example, switching to nocturnal hemodialysis treatment—a slower, longer hemodialysis treatment that takes place at night while a person sleeps—can remove toxic substances from the blood on a more frequent basis, compared with three times weekly hemodialysis treatment, and thereby reduce the impact of toxic substances on the brain and other body tissues.

THE DIGESTIVE SYSTEM

The digestive system begins at the mouth and ends at the anus (Fig. 10-4). The digestive system consists of the gastrointestinal tract and several accessory organs. The mouth, esophagus, stomach, and the small and large intestines make up the gastrointestinal tract. The salivary gland, liver, gallbladder, and pancreas are the accessory organs of the digestive tract. Two major functions of the digestive system are (1) to break down large food molecules into small molecules and (2) to absorb small molecules into the body.

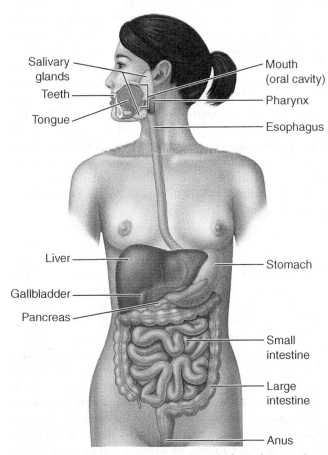

Figure 10-4 The digestive system extends from the mouth to the anus. Accessory organs secrete into the digestive tract. (Reprinted with permission from Cohen, B. J., & Hull, K. (2014). *Memmler's the human body in health and disease* (13th ed., Figure 19.1). Philadelphia, PA: Lippincott Williams & Wilkins/Wolters Kluwer. Copyright © Lippincott Williams & Wilkins/Wolters Kluwer.)

Digestion and Absorption

Digestion is the conversion of food into sugars, carbohydrates, lipids, and other chemical substances that can be absorbed and used by body tissues. Digestion begins when food is taken into the mouth and ground down (i.e., chewed) by the teeth. In the process of chewing, the salivary glands secrete fluids such as mucus that lubricate the food and enzymes such as amylase that break down starches into sugars. Once the food is chewed sufficiently, it is swallowed and the mass of food (i.e., a bolus) begins to travel down the esophagus. Rhythmic muscular contractions (i.e., peristalsis) push the bolus downward toward the stomach. At the lower portion of the esophagus, the bolus passes through the lower esophageal sphincter (LES, which is just above the diaphragm) and the cardiac sphincter (which is below the diaphragm). Once the bolus has passed through the cardiac sphincter, it enters the stomach.

In the stomach, the bolus is subjected to the physical churning actions of the muscular layers of the stomach and to the chemical actions of gastric juice, which is secreted by gastric glands and contains strong protein-digesting enzymes, mucus, and hydrochloric acid. These processes change the bolus into a soup-like liquid called "chyme." The chyme is pushed in spurts from the stomach into the duodenum, the first portion of the small intestine. Most digestion takes place in the duodenum.

Glands within the duodenum release enzymes that further break down chyme. Pancreatic juice and bile are also released into the duodenum from the pancreas and gallbladder, respectively. Pancreatic juice contains bicarbonate ions, protein-digesting enzymes (i.e., peptidases), and other enzymes (e.g., trypsin). Bile is a golden brown to green-yellow alkaline fluid that contains various chemicals such as electrolytes, cholesterol, and bile salts. Bile is synthesized in the liver but is stored in and released by the gallbladder. The pancreas releases pancreatic juice through the pancreatic duct. The gallbladder squeezes bile through the cystic duct. It then flows through the common bile duct, which merges with the pancreatic duct just before inserting into the duodenum. Bile helps break down large fat globules into small globules. The small fat globules are further broken down by enzymes, a process called "emulsification." The duodenum also produces mucus, which helps neutralize the acidity of chyme.

Chyme next passes through the jejunum and finally passes through the last portion of the small intestine, the ileum. The jejunum and ileum contain villi and microvilli. The villi are fingerlike projections that extend from the inner surface of the jejunum and ileum. The microvilli are fingerlike projections that extend from each epithelial (i.e., surface) cell of a villus. Within each villus is a network of capillaries and lymph vessels (called "lacteals"). The products of protein, carbohydrate, and nucleic acid digestion are actively transported or diffused out of the chyme and into the blood vessels within a villus, whereas the products of fat digestion enter the lacteals. The villi also absorb water from chyme as it passes through the jejunum and ileum. As a result, chyme becomes an increasingly concentrated semisolid liquid.

From the ileum, the semisolid liquid (now called "feces" or "stool") enters the first portion of the large intestine, a large saclike structure called the "cecum" (pronounced "SEE-kum"). The large intestines do not have villi or microvilli, and no chemical digestion occurs in these intestines. However, the large intestines reabsorb some water and ions. These intestines contain bacteria that break down the undigested material in the stool. This bacterial action results in the release of nutrients and the synthesis of vitamins (e.g., vitamin K and certain B vitamins) that then enter the bloodstream from the large intestines.

After passing through the cecum, the stool travels up the ascending colon (which is on the right side of the abdomen), then travels horizontally through the transverse colon (which is just beneath the liver, gallbladder, and stomach), and finally travels down the descending colon (which is on the left side of the abdomen). At the level of the pelvis, the colon makes an S-like curve (i.e., the sigmoid colon) and becomes the rectum. The rectum terminates in the anal canal. At the end of the anal canal is a sphincter called the "anal sphincter." By the time the stool has reached the anus, much of its water has been reabsorbed and it has been compacted into a firm mass that primarily contains undigested material (e.g., fiber), bacteria, and other material. The release of stool through the anus is called "defecation."

Neural and Hormonal Mechanisms of Digestion

In recent years, three hormones—leptin, orexin (i.e., hypocretin), and ghrelin (pronounced "GRELL-in")—have been investigated to clarify their roles in digestion and sleep. Each of these hormones has neurotransmitter and hormonal properties. Some of the effects these hormones have on digestion are described in the following paragraphs.

Leptin is produced by many body tissues, but especially by fat tissue. Leptin receptors exist in the brain, in fat, and in other tissues. Insulin regulates leptin production, and cross-talk between insulin and leptin receptors has been observed in the brain.

In the hypothalamus, leptin inhibits the actions of orexin-secreting cells. Hence, there is an antagonistic interplay between orexin (which promotes appetite) and leptin (which reduces appetite). This interplay may be involved in weight control.

Orexin increases appetite and food intake. It is produced within the hypothalamus by a group of specialized neurons (i.e., orexinergic neurons). Orexin stimulates glucose uptake and the formation of fat tissue. Orexin may temporarily regulate energy utilization. The orexin level rises immediately before eating (i.e., when glucose levels are low) and falls immediately after food has been ingested.

Ghrelin increases appetite and promotes food intake. It is produced and secreted primarily by the stomach and, to a lesser extent, by the hypothalamus. The vagus nerve, which contains ghrelin receptors, relays signals from stomach-derived ghrelin to the brain. An increased level of glucose inhibits the production of orexin, whereas prolonged fasting can increase the ghrelin level.

Digestive Function and Sleep Disorders

A digestive disorder that affects sleep is gastroesophageal reflux disorder (GERD). In GERD, gastric juices flow backward (i.e., reflux) from the stomach, through the LES, and into the esophagus during sleep. Gastric juices are very acidic; therefore, if reflux occurs frequently, esophageal tissues can become irritated or destroyed.

GERD occurs when the LES is weak or when there is excessive pressure in the stomach that the LES cannot withstand. In some people, decreased LES pressure and consequently gastric reflux can be promoted by the ingestion of certain foods (e.g., orange juice and chocolate), substances (e.g., alcohol and nicotine), or drugs (e.g., atropine, diazepam, and calcium channel blockers). Any factor that increases the intra-abdominal pressure—including OSA—can also lower the LES pressure and contribute to GERD.

Symptoms of GERD can occur during wake or during sleep. The most common symptom of GERD is heartburn (i.e., a sense of warmth or pain felt behind the breastbone that may travel up toward the neck). The heartburn may be severe enough to mimic angina (i.e., spasmodic thoracic pain that may radiate to the arms and be associated with a sense of suffocation). Other GERD symptoms are pain on swallowing, difficulty swallowing (irritation from gastric juices may induce stricture at the level of the LES because of esophageal spasm or esophagitis, which would then hinder the passage of food through the esophagus), and regurgitation during sleep. When GERD occurs during sleep, a person will complain of having episodes of abrupt awakenings with coughing, choking, or a mouth full of saliva. These actions can interfere with a person's sleep and result in symptoms of insufficient sleep (e.g., EDS).

Leptin is involved in decreasing appetite. In animal studies, the administration of leptin induces weight loss and decreases appetite. However, some people have a higher-than-normal leptin level but are obese.

For example, people with OSA tend to be obese and have higher-than-normal leptin levels. The resistance of leptin receptors to the effects of leptin may explain this finding. However, scientists continue research to clarify the association between leptin resistance and obesity.

THE IMMUNE SYSTEM

The immune system helps the body resist harmful substances and microorganisms through the actions of immune cells or through chemical means. Immunity involving the actions of immune cells is called "cell-mediated immunity." Immunity involving chemical factors is called "antibody-mediated immunity."

The process of immunity begins after a foreign microorganism or substance enters the body. Macrophages, a type of white blood cell, engulf, consume, and digest the offending microorganism. Pieces of the microorganism's proteins (i.e., antigens) are preserved and displayed on the surface of the macrophage. The macrophage moves toward lymph vessels, which convey the cell to lymphoid tissues (e.g., lymph nodes). In a lymph node, the macrophage encounters a helper T-lymphocyte, which is a type of immune cell. The foreign proteins on the surface of the macrophage interact with receptors on the surface of the helper T-lymphocyte. This interaction causes the helper T-lymphocyte to produce various proteins called "lymphokines." Depending on the type of lymphokine produced, one of two types of immune cells becomes stimulated: T-or B-lymphocytes. If T-lymphocytes are stimulated, the immune response is cell-mediated immunity. If B-lymphocytes are stimulated, the immune response is antibody-mediated immunity.

Cell-Mediated Immunity

In cell-mediated immunity, an immune cell directly interacts with a microorganism or a foreign molecule. The T-lymphocytes stimulate the multiplication of cytotoxic T-lymphocytes, which search for cells displaying the foreign antigen. On finding a cell with the antigen, the cytotoxic cell attacks and destroys the foreign cell. To prevent this immune response from destroying normal tissue, another type of lymphocyte, called a "suppressor T-lymphocyte," inhibits the activity of the cytotoxic T-lymphocyte as an increasing number of antigen-containing foreign cells are destroyed.

Antibody-Mediated Immunity

In antibody-mediated immunity, a macrophage (which ingests a foreign cell and displays the foreign cell's antigen on its surface) encounters different types of B-lymphocytes in lymphoid tissue. It ultimately encounters a B-lymphocyte that has the specific antibody to its antigen. An antibody is a large protein that is also called an immunoglobulin (Ig). The presence of an antigen induces the synthesis of an antibody. An antibody is the chemical complement to an antigen, so that only it can chemically react with the antigen. A helper T-lymphocyte binds with a B-lymphocyte and a T-lymphocyte. Only when this complex is formed does the B-lymphocyte begin to multiply and produce sister cells that are programmed to produce the antibody. B-lymphocytes produce antigen-specific antibody molecules at a fast rate. Within hours, many B-lymphocytes are transformed into plasma cells, which only produce the antibody.

Five types of antibodies are immunoglobulin G (IgG), immunoglobulin M (IgM), immunoglobulin A (IgA), immunoglobulin D (IgD), and immunoglobulin E (IgE). IgG is the most common; it confers resistance to disease. IgM is the first antibody to appear when an infection occurs. IgA interacts with microorganisms at the body surface and along other tracts that are open to the environment (e.g., respiratory tract). IgD acts as a receptor site on the B-lymphocyte. IgE is produced during allergic reactions.

Cell-mediated immunity is involved in the delayed allergic response, and antibody-mediated immunity is involved in the immediate allergic response. An immediate allergic response (also called "type I allergic response") manifests minutes after exposure to an allergen (i.e., an antigen). A delayed allergic response, also called "type IV allergic response," manifests 12 to 48 hours after exposure to an antigen. In the immediate allergic response, symptoms can appear within minutes because antibodies produced by B-cells can quickly enter the blood and travel to the site of an antigen. Symptoms of cell-mediated immunity take longer to manifest because it takes longer for T-cells to multiply and then travel to the site of the antigen. Whether a person undergoes an immediate or delayed response is determined by which immune cells—B- or T-cells—are most active.

Immune Function and Sleep Disorders

Neurons that control sleep interact closely with the immune system. This is evidenced, for example, when a person has an infectious disease such as the flu and feels sleepy. During the infection, the production of certain immune factors such as cytokines induces sleep. Two sleep disorders that may involve a dysfunctional immune response are narcolepsy and Kleine–Levin syndrome. Both disorders involve hypersomnia (i.e., the excessive need for sleep or excessive sleepiness when awake).

Narcolepsy

Several factors support the involvement of the immune system in narcolepsy. Some people with narcolepsy report that their symptoms began after an infection. A high percentage of people with narcolepsy have the HLA-DQB1*0602 gene, which belongs to a class of genes (HLA-DQB1) that is associated with other immune disorders. As stated earlier in this chapter, scientists have found that hypocretin-producing hypothalamic cells in people with narcolepsy are inexplicably destroyed, a possible result of autoimmune destruction.

Kleine–Levin Syndrome

Kleine–Levin syndrome consists of several symptoms, the foremost of which is hypersomnia. A person with Kleine–Levin syndrome experiences hypersomnia lasting 16 to 20 hours per day that occurs one or more times per year, with the hypersomnia phase ranging from 2 days to 4 weeks at a time. The hypersomnia is not secondary to another factor such as a mental disorder (e.g., depression), the physiologic effects of a substance (e.g., a drug of abuse or medication), or a medical condition (e.g., a metabolic disorder). In addition to the hypersomnia, one or more of the following symptoms will be present:

- The person is rousable during the episode, but when awake, the person has abnormal cognition or mood (e.g., confusion and lethargy).
- The person has excessive, compulsive eating.
- The person has abnormal behavior (e.g., irritability and aggression).
- The person is hypersexual and exhibits inappropriate sexual behavior (e.g., masturbating in public and making unwanted sexual advances).

After the episode of hypersomnia, the person's alertness, cognition, and behavior return to normal. The person may not remember what occurred during the episode. Nearly one-half of people with Kleine–Levin syndrome report having had an infection days before the onset of symptoms.

THE GENITOURINARY SYSTEM

The genitourinary system consists of the ureters, the urinary bladder, and the urethra (see Fig. 10-2). A ureter is a long tube extending from each kidney that carries urine from the kidney to the urinary bladder. The urinary bladder expels urine through the urethra, a tube that extends from the base of the urinary bladder.

In men and women, the sphincter muscle of the urethra lies slightly below the neck of the bladder (i.e., where the urethra extends from the bladder). It encircles the urethra and compresses it to keep urine in the bladder. Another muscle, called the "sphincter muscle of the urinary bladder," is a circular layer of fibers that surrounds the opening of the urethra at the level of the bladder.

As the bladder fills, stretch receptors in the urinary bladder become stimulated. As a result, the receptors induce a reflexive contraction of the bladder and relaxation of the urethral and urinary bladder sphincter muscles. This action allows urine to be voided from the bladder.

Genitourinary Function and Sleep Disorders

Genitourinary phenomena that may occur during sleep are enuresis, nocturia, and erectile dysfunction. The first two phenomena can disrupt sleep. The third phenomenon does not disrupt sleep, but its manifestation during sleep can be related to other problems.

Enuresis

A person is normally able to sense when the bladder needs voiding. The uncontrolled voiding of urine (i.e., urinary incontinence) can occur for a variety of reasons such as neurologic disorders (e.g., stroke), enlarged prostate (in men), and urinary tract infection. In some people, uncontrolled voiding occurs only during sleep. Urinary incontinence that occurs only during sleep is called "enuresis" (i.e., bed-wetting).

Enuresis typically occurs in children (especially boys) who are past the age that urinary control during the night is normally achieved. However, enuresis can occur in adults. In children, enuresis tends to occur during slow-wave sleep. Scientists are unsure why enuresis tends to occur in this stage.

A factor that may contribute to enuresis in children is OSA. Enuresis may be induced by the excessive intra-abdominal pressures that occur during a child's efforts to breathe. The excessive pressure may be strong enough to induce relaxation of the urethral sphincter muscle, which then results in enuresis. Other factors that can contribute to enuresis are urinary tract infection, urinary tract obstruction, and psychological stress.

Nocturia

A person with nocturia awakens one or more times during the night to urinate. Nocturia can result from a disruption in the normal circadian rhythm in urine concentration. Urine is normally less concentrated in the daytime and more concentrated in the night. The circadian rhythmicity in the production of antidiuretic hormone, which reduces the excretion of urine, contributes to this variation. Antidiuretic hormone levels are higher at night (thereby reducing the urine, which allows a person to sleep through the night) and lower during the day when a person is active and consuming fluids and needs to excrete more urine. Nocturia can result from a medication effect (e.g., diuretics); overactive bladder; kidney or lower urinary tract disorders; or cardiovascular, endocrine, or metabolic disorders.

Erectile Dysfunction (Impotence)

During the night, men normally have an erection during each REM sleep period. (The erection is unrelated to the dream content.) The lack of an erection (i.e., erectile dysfunction) can occur because of psychological factors. People with erectile dysfunction due to psychological factors can have normal REM sleep–related erections. Therefore, the lack of an erection during a REM sleep period indicates that physiologic, rather than psychological, factors are responsible. Some physiologic factors that can contribute to erectile dysfunction are vascular disease, type II diabetes, and spinal cord lesion. Erectile dysfunction can also be the result of an adverse drug effect. For example, some antihypertension drugs block α-adrenergic receptors on nerves that are involved in an erection, and thereby contribute to erectile dysfunction. Newer antihypertension drugs are able to reduce blood pressure by acting on β-adrenergic receptors while allowing the α-adrenergic receptors to remain functional. This action makes it possible for a man to have an erection while allowing the antihypertension drug to exert its blood pressure–lowering effect.

THE MUSCULOSKELETAL SYSTEM

Skeletal muscle is an organ that originates from and inserts into some part of the skeleton. For example, the anterior tibialis muscle, which can be felt on the outer side of the shin bone (i.e., tibia), originates from the upper lateral surface of the tibia and inserts onto the first metatarsal bone (located beneath the base of the big toe) and onto the medial cuneiform bone (located within the instep). The contraction of a skeletal muscle causes the skeleton to move. For example, contraction of the anterior tibialis muscle flexes the foot. Muscle movement induced by contractions can be voluntary (e.g., skeletal muscles) or involuntary (e.g., muscles of the intestines, bladder, and blood vessels).

Skeletal muscle is often called "striated muscle" because of its striped appearance (Fig. 10-5). A muscle is in actuality a bundle of muscle fibers. Each muscle fiber contains 4 to 20 rodlike filaments (i.e., myofibrils). A myofibril is approximately 1 to 2 μm in diameter and 100 μm in length. Each myofibril consists of shorter disk-like units called "sarcomeres." Sarcomeres are stacked end to end (somewhat like a stack of checkers) to create the myofibrils. Sarcomeres give a muscle fiber its striped appearance.

A sarcomere is composed of two types of filaments: thin and thick filaments. A black line (Z line) exists where the thin filaments of one sarcomere interweave with the thin filaments of an adjacent sarcomere. Thick filaments overlap thin filaments in the center of the sarcomere, resulting in another darkened area called the "A

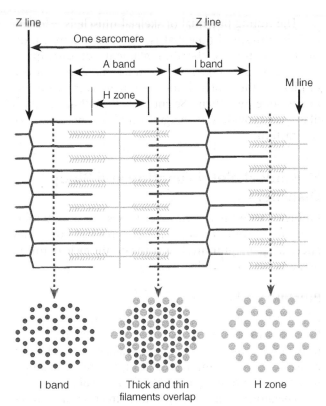

Figure 10-5 Molecular organization of the sarcomere. The arrangement of the elements in a sarcomere viewed longitudinally and as cross sections through selected regions of the sarcomere. Note the overlap of myofilaments at different parts of the sarcomere. (Reprinted with permission from Rhoades, R. A., & Bell, D. R. (2017). *Medical physiology* (5th ed., Figure 8.2). Philadelphia, PA: Lippincott Williams & Wilkins/Wolters Kluwer. Copyright © Lippincott Williams & Wilkins/Wolters Kluwer.)

band." A thin darkened region, the H zone, exists within the very center of the A band. The A band consists of only thick filaments. The lightest portion of the sarcomere is the I band, which exists between the edge of the Z line and the outer edge of the A band.

A muscle contraction begins when a stimulus triggers an action potential within a neuron that innervates a muscle fiber. The action potential travels down the axon of the neuron. When the action potential reaches the axon's terminal, a neurotransmitter is released from the terminal into the neuromuscular junction (NMJ), which is the synapse between the axons of a neuron and a muscle fiber. The neurotransmitter travels across the NMJ to attach to receptors on a muscle fiber.

It is at this point that the process is set in motion for the contraction of a muscle. Once a neurotransmitter is attached to the muscle receptor, sodium ions flood into the muscle fiber and thereby reduce its electrical potential (i.e., depolarizing it). The action potential then travels through the muscle fiber and ultimately spreads to other muscle fibers.

The resting potential of skeletal muscle is −95 mV and the threshold potential is −50 mV. When a muscle fiber contracts, the thin filaments of sarcomeres are drawn close together. The thick filaments remain in place in the center of the sarcomere as the thin filaments slide over them. Scientists believe that the thick filaments provide the energy to the thin filaments for contraction.

Musculoskeletal Function and Sleep Disorders

Problems with the musculoskeletal system can interfere with sleep. Some musculoskeletal problems that may affect sleep are fibromyalgia, arthritis, thoracic deformities, and neuromuscular disorders.

Fibromyalgia

Fibromyalgia is a chronic pain syndrome involving fatigue, morning stiffness, widespread muscle pain, cognitive problems, and poor sleep quality. No pathology exists such as inflammation or degenerative changes that can explain the symptoms of fibromyalgia.

Diagnosing fibromyalgia and treating it can be problematic. It has many symptoms in common with other disorders. For example, hypocalcemia (i.e., low blood calcium level) and low vitamin D level can result in muscle soreness and tenderness, hypothyroidism can result in fatigue, and infections such as Lyme disease and arthritis can result in pain that is similar to fibromyalgia. However, these disorders can be easily diagnosed through testing; there is no definitive test for fibromyalgia. Adding to the difficulty in diagnosing fibromyalgia, people with fibromyalgia may also have nonpain complaints such as gastrointestinal problems (e.g., irritable bowel-like symptoms and nausea), mood disorders (e.g., depression), and sleep disturbances (e.g., insomnia and RLS). People with fibromyalgia tend to have alpha-delta sleep, which manifests on an electroencephalogram (EEG) as alpha waves superimposed on the delta waves of slow-wave sleep. This pattern indicates that the person is awake and asleep at the same time. People with the abnormal EEG pattern of alpha-delta sleep—even those without a diagnosis of fibromyalgia—complain of feeling unrested.

Arthritis

Arthritis is inflammation of the joints. It can occur as a result of an infection (e.g., rheumatic fever), noninfectious degenerative processes (e.g., osteoarthritis), or genetic factors (e.g., ankylosing spondylitis). A person with arthritis has pain, stiffness, and/or swelling of the joints. The pain may be most noticeable in the morning or after sitting or lying in one position for a long time.

Arthritis may affect the small joints of the hands or feet or larger joints such as the hip and spine. People with arthritis may complain of being unable to go to sleep at a desired time because of joint pain or being unable to remain asleep because the pain awakens them.

Thoracic Deformities

A thoracic deformity can result from a deformity in the alignment of the spine, a ribcage deformity, or both. A thoracic deformity can impede normal respiratory movements and consequently impact sleep. Examples of thoracic deformities are kyphosis and scoliosis, and examples of ribcage deformities are pectus excavatum (commonly called "funnel chest") and pectus carinatum (commonly called "pigeon chest").

Kyphosis and Scoliosis

Kyphosis and scoliosis both involve a deformity in the alignment of the spine. In kyphosis, the spine curves in an anteroposterior direction at the level of the thorax or thoracolumbar region or sacrum, giving the back an excessively rounded appearance. Kyphosis is commonly called a "hunchback." In scoliosis, the spine curves at the level of the thorax, lumbar region, or thoracolumbar region in a lateral direction (i.e., to the left or right), giving an S-like curve to the spine. In some people with scoliosis, the spine twists on its axis in addition to having a lateral curvature. Scoliosis often occurs in association with kyphosis and lordosis (i.e., an anterior curvature of the spine in the lumbar region, often called a "swayback").

The spinal curvature in kyphosis and scoliosis can result from collapse of the vertebrae because of disease (e.g., arthritis and osteoporosis), deformity of the vertebrae, genetic factors, compression fractures of the vertebrae, and disk degeneration. Backache or back pain can be associated with kyphosis and scoliosis and may impact the onset of sleep or the maintenance of sleep.

Kyphosis and scoliosis can impede a person's ability to expand the chest wall and thereby reduce lung capacity. Reduced lung capacity may lead to hypoventilation and, consequently, chronic hypoxemia (i.e., low blood oxygen level) and hypercapnia (i.e., excessive blood carbon dioxide). Prolonged hypoventilation can alter the normal physiologic responses to improper levels of oxygen and carbon dioxide. The result can be sleep-related breathing disorders such as hypopnea (i.e., shallow breathing), central sleep apnea (i.e., cessation in breathing due to the lack of the respiratory drive), and OSA (i.e., cessation of breathing due to upper airway blockage).

In some cases of kyphosis and scoliosis, the curvature of the spine may be severe enough to compress and damage the spinal cord, which then may result in spastic paraplegia (i.e., spasticity [stiffness] and paralysis of the lower portion of the body from the point of injury downward). This injury may negatively affect the movement of the respiratory muscles and contribute to hypoventilation or sleep-related breathing disorders.

Ribcage Deformity

Pectus excavatum and pectus carinatum both result from a deformity of the ribcage and sternum (i.e., breastbone). In pectus excavatum (from Latin meaning "excavated chest"), the sternum has the appearance of being sunken. In pectus carinatum (from Latin meaning "keel [as in the keel of a ship] chest"), the chest is narrow but protrudes abnormally in the front. Depending on the severity of the deformity, pectus excavatum and pectus carinatum may restrict lung movement, thereby affecting lung function (e.g., hypoxemia) and may cause pain. These factors may then disrupt sleep.

Neuromuscular Disorders

Neuromuscular disorders such as multiple sclerosis, postpolio syndrome, and quadriplegia (i.e., paralysis affecting all four limbs) affect the transmission of neurologic signals involved in muscular movement. When impaired neurologic signals affect the muscles of respiration (e.g., diaphragm, intercostal muscles), respiratory movements can be altered and make it difficult to ventilate the lungs sufficiently. Chronic insufficient respiratory movements may lead to hypoventilation and improper blood levels of oxygen and carbon dioxide and induce a dysfunction in the sensitivity of receptors that detect oxygen and carbon dioxide levels. People with neuromuscular disorders may consequently develop respiratory failure (i.e., persistent abnormally low level of oxygen or abnormally high level of carbon dioxide) and sleep-related breathing disorders such as hypopnea and OSA. Severe oxygen desaturations and hypercapnia (i.e., excessively high blood levels of carbon dioxide) can occur, especially during REM sleep. In people with neuromuscular disease, low nocturnal levels of oxygen may contribute to nocturnal or morning headache and disrupted sleep may contribute to daytime sleepiness.

METABOLISM

Metabolism is the sum of all physical and chemical processes in a living organism that maintain its various physiologic activities (e.g., respiration) and provide energy. Metabolism can be affected by a person's nutrition: the consumption of foods containing the proper amounts of carbohydrates, fats, proteins, vitamins, and minerals. Improper amounts of these substances can result in malnutrition.

The liver has important roles in metabolism. For example, the liver secretes bile, which breaks fat molecules into smaller molecules; it synthesizes and releases into the bloodstream protein molecules such as albumin; and it stores minerals such as iron and certain vitamins such as vitamins A, D, and K.

The pancreas also has an important role in metabolism. It synthesizes insulin and glucagon. The opposing effects of these hormones normally maintain proper blood glucose levels.

Metabolism consists of two components: catabolism (i.e., the breakdown of large molecules into smaller molecules) and anabolism (i.e., the buildup of large molecules from smaller molecules). Catabolism releases energy, whereas anabolism requires energy. Carbohydrates, fats, proteins, vitamins, and minerals undergo metabolism in the following ways.

Carbohydrate Metabolism

Carbohydrates are molecules that are composed only of carbon, oxygen, and hydrogen atoms. A carbohydrate can be simple sugars such as glucose, fructose, galactose, or a starch (i.e., a complex molecule composed of several sugar molecules). During digestion, simple sugars are absorbed from the small intestines and enter the bloodstream. The bloodstream transports the sugars through the hepatic portal vein into the liver. The sugars are converted into glucose. The glucose is then available for use by other body tissues.

The body's cells take carbohydrates into their cytoplasm (i.e., the fluid surrounding a cell's nucleus). In the cytoplasm, carbohydrate molecules are broken down and release carbon dioxide and water as waste products.

Insulin facilitates the transfer of glucose through a cell's membrane (i.e., it facilitates the uptake of glucose into the cell). This uptake removes glucose from the blood. If insulin is produced in insufficient amounts or if insulin receptors on the surface of a cell cannot respond to the effects of insulin (i.e., insulin resistance), glucose cannot enter the cell. The result is excess amounts of glucose remaining in the blood, a condition called "diabetes mellitus" (i.e., diabetes type II).

In liver cells and in muscle cells, an excess amount of glucose is stored as glycogen, which is a large branched molecule consisting of several glucose molecules joined together. The process of creating glycogen from glucose is called "glycogenesis." When the glucose level is low, liver cells break down glycogen into its glucose components. The breakdown of glycogen into glucose is called "glycolysis." If the available sources of glucose are depleted (e.g., during starvation), glucose can be synthesized from noncarbohydrate sources such as fatty acids, amino acids, and glycerol. Fatty acids are a group of organic (i.e., carbon-containing) molecules that are a constituent of fat. Amino acids are molecules that are the basic components of proteins. Amino acids are joined together in a unique sequence to form a specific protein. Glycerol is a sugar alcohol that is a constituent of many lipids (i.e., fat and fat-like substances).

Fat Metabolism

In the process of digestion, fat molecules are broken down into fatty acids and glycerol. Three fatty acid molecules bind with a glycerol molecule to form a triglyceride molecule. Enzymes in the liver break down a triglyceride molecule into its glycerol and fatty acid components. However, some triglycerides are stored in fat tissue. A fatty acid must be bound with a blood plasma protein such as albumin to allow it to enter a cell.

Before a lipid (e.g., cholesterol) can travel through the blood to a cell, it must be bound with a protein to form a lipoprotein. Lipoproteins are classed by their density (the greater the amount of protein the denser the molecule). Three classes of lipoprotein are very low-density lipoprotein (VLDL), low-density lipoprotein (LDL), and high-density lipoprotein (HDL). Two other classes of lipoproteins are chylomicron (also called "ultra low-density lipoprotein"), which consist of 85% triglyceride, 13% lipid, and 2% protein and are less dense than the VLDL, and intermediate lipoproteins, which consist of approximately 24% to 30% triglyceride, 8% to 10% cholesterol, and 10% to 12% protein and have a density between that of VLDL and LDL.

A VLDL particle consists of approximately 60% triglyceride, 15% cholesterol, and 10% protein; a LDL particle consists of approximately 50% triglyceride, 50% cholesterol, and 25% protein; and an HDL particle consists of approximately 5% triglyceride, 20% cholesterol, and 50% protein. Lipoproteins transport cholesterol to the liver. The liver then breaks down lipoproteins into their lipid and protein constituents. LDL is often called "bad cholesterol" because of its high percentage of cholesterol. HDL is often called "good cholesterol" because of its lower percentage of cholesterol. In addition, LDL carries cholesterol to cells (including the cells of blood vessels), whereas HDL carries cholesterol away from the body's cells to the liver for elimination. These actions contribute to the "bad" and "good" qualities of LDL and HDL, respectively.

The breakdown of fat occurs in the cytoplasm of cells. Once glycerol is separated from fatty acid molecules, glucose may be synthesized from the glycerol, depending on the body's needs. Mitochondria in a cell's cytoplasm break down fatty acids for energy.

A by-product of fat metabolism is the formation of ketone bodies, which comprise three organic molecules: acetone, β-hydroxybutyric acid, and acetoacetic acid. Ketone bodies can be used for energy when glucose levels are depleted. An excessive amount of ketone bodies in body tissues and fluids is a condition called "ketosis." Ketosis causes the body to become acidic. If left untreated, ketosis can lead to coma and death. Ketosis can occur in diabetics because the reduced level of insulin or insulin resistance results in an insufficient amount of glucose molecules entering the body's cells, although an excessive amount of glucose remains in the blood. The body senses a starvation state and begins to form glucose from fat tissue. During the process, ketone bodies are produced as a waste product. As a result of the excessive level of ketone bodies, a person may have a fruity smell to his or her body and breath. Other situations that can set the stage for ketosis is starvation (e.g., anorexia nervosa) and a high-fat, low-protein diet.

The anabolism of fat (i.e., fat storage) normally occurs if there is too much glucose in the blood. In this situation, glucose is converted to fatty acids. In the liver, the fatty acids are used to form triglycerides.

Protein Metabolism

In the gastrointestinal tract, protein molecules are broken down into amino acids. From the intestines, the amino acids are transported to the liver. In the liver, the amino acids may be reassembled into proteins or released into the bloodstream to be transported to other cells. In the cells, the amino acids are linked into specific sequences to form specific proteins. Some amino acids are used for energy. An amino acid may be essential (i.e., it must be obtained from the diet) or nonessential (i.e., it can be synthesized in the body, even if there is no dietary source).

Vitamin Metabolism

Vitamins generally act as coenzymes. They bind with a protein molecule to form an active enzyme. The active enzyme takes part in vital metabolic processes such as fatty acid production and energy expenditure. A vitamin can be fat- or water-soluble. A fat-soluble vitamin is absorbed with dietary fats. Vitamins A, D, E, and K are fat-soluble. They are not normally excreted in the urine, but instead are stored in the fat tissue in the body. Taking fat-soluble vitamins in excess can be toxic. A water-soluble vitamin is absorbed with water from the gastrointestinal tract. All B vitamins and vitamin C are water-soluble. These vitamins are excreted in the urine and must be replaced daily through the diet. The vitamins have the following roles in metabolism.

Fat-Soluble Vitamins

Vitamin A is important for many biologic activities affected by metabolism such as bone growth, reproduction, immune response, and proper functioning of the retina. Vitamin D affects the utilization of calcium, which has a role in enzymatic processes involved in metabolism. Vitamin E is important in the formation of red blood cells, which carry oxygen to the body's tissues. Oxygen is then used in various metabolic processes. Vitamin K is needed for the production of some B vitamins.

Water-Soluble Vitamins

The B vitamins consist of several molecules. Some of the more commonly known B vitamins are vitamin B_1 (i.e., thiamine), B_2 (i.e., riboflavin), B_3 (i.e., niacin), B_5 (i.e., pantothenic acid), B_6 (i.e., pyridoxine), B_{12} (i.e., cyanocobalamin), biotin, and folic acid. Vitamins B_1, B_2, and B_3 are involved in energy expenditure at the cellular level. Vitamin B_5 aids the actions of enzymes that are involved in fat and carbohydrate metabolism. Vitamin B_6 aids the actions of enzymes that break down amino acids (e.g., the degradation of tryptophan), is involved in the conversion of glycogen to glucose, and is involved in fat metabolism. Vitamin B_{12} is required for the synthesis of proteins. Biotin is involved in the degradation of amino acids and in the metabolism of fatty acids. Folic acid is involved in the breakdown of amino acids and energy expenditure in cells.

Vitamin C (also called "ascorbic acid") is needed for certain enzymes to function optimally. It improves the absorption of iron, a metallic element that has a role in energy expenditure in the cells and in the transport of oxygen to cells.

Mineral Metabolism

Inorganic elements (i.e., minerals) are needed for various metabolic processes. Minerals are involved in a variety of physiologic processes such as enhancing the activity of various enzymes and contributing to maintaining osmotic pressure in body fluids. Some minerals that are involved in metabolism are calcium, sodium, potassium, phosphorus, magnesium, iodine, sulfur, copper, cobalt, manganese, and zinc. These minerals have the following effects on metabolic processes.

Calcium and phosphorus have a role in many enzymatic processes involved in metabolism. Sodium and potassium have a role in protein synthesis, maintaining water balance in body tissues, and transporting molecules such as glucose across a cell membrane. Magnesium is a component of many enzymes involved in metabolism and is involved in the creation of energy in cells. Iodine is necessary for the formation of thyroid hormones (e.g., thyroxine and triiodothyronine) that regulate the metabolic rate of all cells. Sulfur is used in the production of several amino acids and is a constituent of some vitamins such as thiamine, which is involved in carbohydrate metabolism. Copper is a constituent of many proteins and enzymes involved in metabolism. Cobalt is a constituent of vitamin B_{12}, which is needed for the synthesis of various proteins. Manganese activates a number of enzymes that are involved in metabolism. Zinc is a constituent of several enzymes involved with metabolism and has a role in protein synthesis.

Metabolism and Sleep Disorders

Faulty metabolism of carbohydrates, fats, proteins, minerals, and vitamins can negatively affect sleep. Two sleep disorders that may result from impaired metabolism are metabolic syndrome and RLS.

Metabolic Syndrome

Metabolic syndrome is a cluster of symptoms that reflect impaired metabolism. A person with metabolic syndrome has the following features: (1) fasting hyperglycemia (i.e., excess blood sugar level) resulting from diabetes mellitus type II or from impaired glucose tolerance and/or insulin resistance; (2) high blood pressure; (3) overweight with abdominal obesity (i.e., fat deposits primarily around the waist); (4) dyslipidemia (i.e., improper levels of fat and fat-like substances in the blood) with a decreased HDL cholesterol level and an elevated triglyceride level. Obesity can increase the amount of fat tissue in the upper airway; therefore, a person with metabolic syndrome may be at greater risk of having sleep-disordered breathing, in particular OSA. Owing to frequent sleep-disordered breathing–related arousals from sleep, people with metabolic syndrome who have OSA may struggle with sleepiness, inattentiveness, and other symptoms of insufficient sleep. In some people with metabolic syndrome, OSA may make it more difficult to control glucose levels and high blood pressure.

Restless Legs Syndrome

In a person with RLS, uncomfortable sensations in the legs begin in the evening soon before bedtime. For some people, the uncomfortable sensations affect the legs and the arms. To relieve such sensations, the person feels compelled to move the legs by walking, by rubbing them against the bedsheet, by stretching, or by other actions. The relief is short-lived, and a person must repeat the actions frequently to obtain relief. These efforts at relief can delay a person going to sleep at the desired time. The sensations drop out soon before or just at the onset of sleep. If a person awakens during the night, the same sensations may recur and thus delay the onset of sleep. A person with RLS may struggle with EDS because of disturbed sleep at night.

Scientists are not sure why RLS occurs. For some people, the cause appears to be related to low levels of iron or improper utilization of iron. However, some people with RLS have normal iron levels. Iron-containing dopamine (D_2) receptors exist on the basal ganglia neurons. The basal ganglia are a collection of nuclei at the base of the brain. Some of the nuclei are involved in movement. Insufficient amounts of iron or the impaired metabolism of iron may, therefore, be involved in the sensations and irresistible urge to move the legs. Scientists continue to investigate the role of iron in RLS.

THERMOREGULATION

Thermoregulation is the maintenance of heat within a certain range. The maintenance of the body temperature between 97° F (36.1° C) and 100° F (37.7° C) is an example of thermoregulation. The maintenance of the body temperature results from the combination of heat production and heat loss. Heat production in the body is primarily a consequence of metabolism—much energy is released as food is broken down into molecules. Other factors such as muscle movement can produce heat in the body.

Four factors that can result in heat loss are radiation, evaporation, conduction, and convection. In radiation, heat is lost from the body in infrared waves to the external environment; in evaporation, heat-retaining water in sweat and exhaled air vaporizes, thereby drawing heat away from the body; in conduction, heat is directly transferred from the body through contact with an external object such as water or air; and in convection, atoms and molecules in contact with the body absorb heat from the body (i.e., through conduction), but move away from the body, only to be replaced by more atoms and molecules that similarly absorb heat from the body. (Wind or water currents can enhance the process of convection.)

The hypothalamus is responsible for thermoregulation in the body. Certain neurons within the hypothalamus function as a thermostat. When the body temperature falls below a certain point (i.e., the set point), blood flow to internal organs increases, whereas blood flow to extremities decreases. These actions conserve heat in the core of the body. When the body temperature rises above the set point, the opposite process occurs.

Temperature-sensing receptors in the skin (i.e., peripheral thermal receptors) relay signals to temperature-sensing receptors in the hypothalamus (i.e., central thermal receptors). Central thermal receptors in the hypothalamus are sensitive to temperature changes in the blood. The peripheral thermal receptors form a negative feedback loop with the central thermal receptors in the hypothalamus to maintain body temperature.

If the central thermal receptors sense that the blood is too hot, blood flow to the extremities increases, whereas blood flow to the internal organs decreases. At the skin, radiation, evaporation, conduction, and convection occur and reduce the temperature of the blood. The cooled blood then travels to the inner organs, thereby cooling them.

Fever-inducing chemicals, called "pyrogens" (from the Greek *pyro-* meaning "fire" and *gen-* meaning "to produce"), induce the hypothalamus to reset the set point to a higher level. As a result, a person with a fever will feel cold and the body will make efforts to conserve or produce body heat (e.g., vasoconstriction of skin vessels and shivering). When the fever is over, other chemicals (e.g., prostaglandins) act on the hypothalamus to reduce the set point. As a consequence, a person will feel hot and the body will make efforts to reduce the body heat (e.g., sweating and vasodilation of skin vessels).

Thermoregulation during Sleep

A person's core body temperature cycles in correlation with the sleep–wake rhythm. Core body temperature decreases during the sleep phase and increases during the wake phase. During sleep, thermoregulatory responses differ, depending on the sleep stage. As a consequence, when a person is exposed to an excessively cold or hot environment during sleep, responses such as shivering to increase body temperature or sweating to decrease body temperature are altered. For example, sensitivity to a hot or cold environment is reduced in REM sleep, compared with non-REM sleep and wakefulness. In a cold environment, shivering occurs during stages 1 and 2 sleep but not during slow-wave sleep or REM sleep; and sweating is increased in slow-wave sleep, compared with other sleep stages, whereas the onset of sweating is delayed in REM sleep.

Such alterations in thermoregulation during sleep can affect sleep architecture when a person is exposed to an excessively hot or cold environmental temperature. For example, the duration of REM sleep and, to a lesser extent, slow-wave sleep decreases because a person awakens more easily when a room is excessively hot or cold.

With sleep onset, the vasodilation of skin vessels occurs, which cools the blood. The cooled blood ultimately travels to the organs in the body, which lowers the core body temperature and further promotes sleep. Some scientists, therefore, believe that skin temperature rather than core body temperature may promote sleep. In addition, research has indicated that brain temperature decreases during slow-wave sleep but increases during REM sleep. To what extent brain temperature contributes to the thermosensitivity of the body during sleep is unclear.

Thermoregulation and Sleep Disorders

Shift Work/Frequently Changing Shifts

A person's core body temperature rises and falls on a circadian rhythm, rising to its highest point during the evening from approximately 4:00 to 6:00 p.m. and falling to its lowest point during the night at approximately 4:00 a.m. Attempting to sleep when the core body temperature is at its highest can lead to difficulty initiating and maintaining sleep (i.e., insomnia), and attempting to remain awake when the body temperature is at its lowest may be difficult. Many physiologic processes such as melatonin secretion easily change their rhythms (i.e., become entrained) to a new schedule somewhat quickly; however, the rhythmicity of core body temperature is not as easily entrained. When shifting to a new schedule, the core body temperature is one of the last biologic rhythms to become entrained. Because it takes a long time for body temperature to become entrained, one-third of shift workers may continue to struggle with sleepiness or insomnia at undesired times—even though the worker is carefully avoiding excessive exposure to daylight and maintaining a regular sleep–wake schedule.

Hot Flash

Some menopausal women experience the consequences of a sudden, temporary fluctuation in temperature control, commonly called a "hot flash." A hot flash is a heat dissipation response that begins with a sudden sense of warmth that is associated with sweating on the face, neck, and chest and peripheral vasodilation (e.g., the face may become suddenly red). The sense of warmth is soon after followed by a sense of extreme cold that may be associated with shivering. A hot flash can occur during wake or during sleep (in which case a woman may awaken with her bedsheets drenched in sweat).

Hot flashes are often reported by menopausal women, leading to the common belief that they are related to low levels of estrogen. However, hot flashes can also occur in other stages of a woman's life (e.g., during breastfeeding) when estrogen levels are still elevated. Some research also indicates that estrogen levels do not differ between symptomatic and asymptomatic menopausal women.

Scientists initially believed that hot flashes were triggered by a sudden downward resetting of the hypothalamic set point because a woman's core body temperature does not increase during the episode. Hence, a woman would feel warm, although the environmental temperature did not change. Evidence obtained using telemetry pills indicates that a small elevation in the core body temperature occurs immediately before a hot flash and that the thermoneutral zone (i.e., the range in which sweating, peripheral vasodilation, and shivering do not occur) is virtually nonexistent in symptomatic women. By contrast, the thermoneutral zone exists in asymptomatic women. It is possible that the small temperature elevation occurring within a reduced thermoneutral zone triggers a hot flash. Animal studies suggest that increased central sympathetic activation reduces the thermoneutral zone. Research has revealed that central sympathetic activation is elevated in women who have hot flashes.

Hot flashes can occur anytime. When experienced at night, they may disrupt sleep. Some women who have hot flashes during sleep awaken cold and with drenched sheets. These consequences can interrupt sleep—especially if she needs to change bedsheets after an episode or if she has several episodes during the night.

SUMMARY

Problems with sleep and wake are not limited to a dysfunction in the brain. As this chapter discussed, many factors in the function of the endocrine system, the renal system, the digestive system, the immune system, the genitourinary system, the musculoskeletal system, metabolism, and thermoregulation can contribute to impaired sleep or wakefulness by impacting brain function or by other means.

SUGGESTED READING

Alcamo, I. E., & Krumhardt, B. (2004). *Anatomy and physiology the easy way: Barron's E-Z series.* Hauppauge, NY: Barron's Educational Series, Inc.

Atrah, H. I., & Davidson, R. J. L. (1988). Mechanism of action of intravenous immunoglobulin in immune-mediated cytopenias. *Journal of Clinical Pathology, 41,* 1249–1255.

Bourgin, P., Huitrón-Reséndiz, S., Spier, A. D., et al. (2000). Hypocretin-1 modulates rapid eye movement sleep through activation of locus coeruleus neurons. *Journal of Neuroscience, 20*(20), 7760–7765.

Buckley, R. H. (1998). Agammaglobulinemia, by Col. Ogden C. Bruton, MC, USA, *Pediatrics,* 1952;9:722–728 [Commentary]. *Pediatrics, 102*(1), 213–215.

Charloux, A., Gronfier, C., Lonsdorfer-Wolf, E., et al. (1999). Aldosterone release during the sleep–wake cycle in humans. *American Journal of Physiology, 276*(1), E43–E49.

Crujeiras, A. B., Carreira, M. C., Cabia, B., et al. (2015). Leptin resistance in obesity: An epigenetic landscape. *Life Sciences, 140,* 57–63.

Dauvilliers, Y., Carlander, B., Rivier, F., et al. (2004). Successful management of cataplexy with intravenous immunoglobulins at narcolepsy onset. *Annals of Neurology, 56*(6), 905–908.

de Lecea, L., Kilduff, T. S., Peyron, C., et al. (1998). The hypocretins: Hypothalamus-specific peptides with neuroexcitatory activity. *Proceedings of the National Academy of Sciences of the USA (PNAS), 95,* 322–327.

Dorland's illustrated medical dictionary (28th ed.). (1996). Philadelphia, PA: W.B. Saunders Company.

Freedman, R. R. (2001). Physiology of hot flashes. *American Journal of Human Biology, 13*(4), 453–464.

Hecht, M., Lin, L., Kushida, C. A., et al. (2003). Report of a case of immunosuppression with prednisone in an 8-year-old boy with an acute onset of hypocretin-deficiency narcolepsy. *Sleep, 26*(7), 809–810.

Johnston, J. G., & Pollock, D. M. (2018). Circadian regulation of renal function. *Free Radical Biology and Medicine, 119,* 93–107. doi:10.1016/j.freeradbiomed.2018.01.018

Karasek, M., Szuflet, A., Chrzanowski, W., et al. (2005). Decreased melatonin nocturnal concentrations in hemodialyzed patients. *Neuro-Endocrinology Letters, 26,* 653–656.

Krahn, L. E., Black, J. L., & Silber, M. H. (2001). Narcolepsy: New understanding of irresistible sleep. *Mayo Clinic Proceedings, 76,* 185–194.

Lecendreux, M., Maret, S., Bassetti, C., et al. (2003). Clinical efficacy of high-dose intravenous immunoglobulins near the onset of narcolepsy in a 10 year old boy. *Journal of Sleep Research, 12,* 347–348.

Leslie, M. (1999/2000, Winter). Dogs and cataplexy. *Stanford Medicine.* Retrieved from http://stanmed.stanford.edu/1999_2000winter/dogs.html

Marcheva, B., Ramsey, K. M., Affinati, A., et al. (2009). Clock genes and metabolic disease. *Journal of Applied Physiology, 107*(5), 1638–1646.

Maret, S., & Tafti, M. (2005). Genetics of narcolepsy and other major sleep disorders. *Swiss Medical Weekly, 135*(45–46), 662–665.

Maung, S. C., El Sara, A., Chapman, C., et al. (2016). Sleep disorders and chronic kidney disease. *World Journal of Nephrology, 5,* 224–232.

National Institutes of Health. (2011). National Institute of Neurological Disorders and Stroke (NINDS).

Narcolepsy Fact Sheet. NIH Publication No. 03-1637. Retrieved from http://www.ninds.nih.gov/disorders/narcolepsy/detail_narcolepsy.htm

Netter, F. H., & Colacino, S. (Eds.). (1989). *Atlas of human anatomy.* Summit, NJ: Ciba-Geigy Corporation.

Norris, J. (Ed.). (1995). *Professional guide to diseases* (5th ed.). Springhouse, PA: Springhouse Corporation.

Okamoto-Mizuno, K., & Mizuno, K. (2012). Effects of thermal environment on sleep and circadian rhythm. *Journal of Physiological Anthropology, 31*(1), 14.

Pan, H., Guo, J., & Su, Z. (2014). Advances in understanding the interrelations between leptin resistance and obesity. *Physiology and Behavior, 130,* 157–169.

Parkes, J. D., Langdon, N., & Lock, C. (1986). Narcolepsy and immunity. *British Medical Journal, 292*(6517), 359–360.

Piper, D. C., Upton, N., Smith, M. I., et al. (2000). The novel brain neuropeptide, orexin-A, modulates the sleep–wake cycle of rats. *European Journal of Neuroscience, 12*(2), 726–730.

Professional guide to signs and symptoms (2nd ed.). (1997). Springhouse, PA: Springhouse Corporation.

Roth, T., Dauvilliers, Y., Mignot, E., et al. (2013). Disrupted nighttime sleep in narcolepsy. *Journal of Clinical Sleep Medicine, 9*(9), 955–965.

Sabbatini, M., Minale, B., Crispo, A., et al. (2002). Insomnia in maintenance haemodialysis patients. *Nephrology, Dialysis, Transplantation, 17,* 852–856.

Sáinz, N., Barrenetxe, J., Moreno-Aliaga, M. J., et al. (2015). Leptin resistance and diet-induced obesity: Central and peripheral actions of leptin. *Metabolism, 64*(1), 35–46.

Sakurai, T., Amemiya, A., Ishii, M., et al. (1998). Orexins and orexin receptors: A family of hypothalamic neuropeptides and G protein-coupled receptors that regulate feeding behavior. *Cell, 92*(4), 573–585.

Siebold, C., Hansen, B. E., Wyer, J. R., et al. (2004). Crystal structure of HLA-DQ0602 that protects against type I diabetes and confers strong susceptibility to narcolepsy. *Proceedings of the National Academy of Sciences of the United States of America (PNAS), 101*(7), 1999–2004.

Stryer, L. (1981). *Biochemistry* (2nd ed.). San Francisco, CA: W.H. Freeman and Company.

Thibodeau, G. A., & Patton, K. T. (2000). *Structure and function of the body* (11th ed.). St. Louis, MO: Mosby.

chapter 11
Sleep Across the Life Cycle

DEBRA A. GUERRERO

LEARNING OBJECTIVES

On completion of this chapter, the reader should be able to:

1. Define sleep.
2. Describe characteristic aspects of normal sleep in different age groups.
3. State the current recommended amount of sleep for people, from birth to old age.

KEY TERMS

Sleep cycle
Sleep architecture
Hypnogram
Sleep consolidation
Sleep regulation
Gestational age
Chronologic age
Conceptional age
Phase delay
Phase advance

Sleep is a vital component of health. Along with proper nutrition and physical activity, good sleep provides a foundation for physical and emotional wellness. For sleep to be "healthy," it needs to be of sufficient duration and timing, and without abnormalities or disturbances (1). Sleep technologists must be well versed in the nature of human sleep across the life span. This knowledge allows technologists to compare the sleep and sleep habits of patients studied to what is expected for their age group. Sleep health education is an important component of the sleep technologist's core job responsibilities. The role of the sleep technologist is expanding with a new focus on patient education and therapy management. Technologists with specific education and a certification in clinical sleep health are assuming a larger role in providing sleep hygiene and disease-specific education for patients with sleep disorders and assisting in the management of their therapies.

Caring for patients at all levels includes a discussion of basic sleep health. Questions relating to sleep needs and basic sleep hygiene practices are routinely discussed in sleep centers, often during polysomnography hookup procedures. Every patient interaction is an opportunity for sleep technologists to enhance patient knowledge regarding the importance of sleep.

SLEEP CHARACTERISTICS

Sleep is a state of being unaware of and unresponsive to the outside world that is immediately reversible (2). Resting with eyes closed in a recumbent position in darkness may look like sleep, but there is no disconnection from the surroundings. Likewise, coma or a state of unconsciousness is not sleep. A person in a coma may be disconnected from the outside world as if asleep, but cannot be immediately awakened. In the sleep center, sleep is identified by observation of a combination of behavioral, physiologic, and electroencephalographic (EEG) features. Sleep in people of all ages is classified into two states: rapid eye movement (REM) and non-REM (NREM) sleep. The rhythmic cycling of REM and NREM patterns, including wake, and the NREM stages of N1, N2, and N3, and REM throughout the course of the sleep period is referred to as sleep architecture. A visual graph of sleep architecture, called a hypnogram, provides an overview of the patient's night of sleep. Figure 11-1 demonstrates the sleep-stage hypnograms of three patients who underwent an in-laboratory polysomnogram. There are physiologic variables and EEG parameters specific to a certain state of sleep and wakefulness. Sleep stages are determined by assessing EEG, electrooculogram and electromyogram activities, and patient observation. The evaluation of these parameters will be discussed in detail in Chapter 38. Sleep is essential for the maintenance of brain and bodily functions in all age groups.

Sleep behaviors demonstrate great variability between individuals, cultures, societies, and geographical regions (3). They are affected by external factors such as parental beliefs, cultural traditions, socioeconomic status, work and school schedules, use of media, and education about sleep hygiene. Nevertheless, extensive sleep research makes it possible to understand and predict

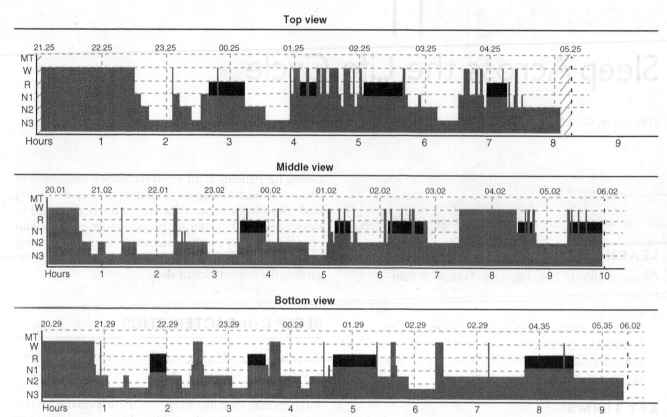

Figure 11-1 Three sleep-stage hypnograms.

sleep–wake patterns in different periods of the life cycle (3). The most noticeable age-related developments in sleep and sleep–wake rhythms take place around birth and during the first year of life. They include consolidation of sleep, reductions in the number and duration of naps, and changes in EEG. In the span of infancy through young childhood, sleep is considered particularly essential to development. By age 2, a child has spent about half of his or her life sleeping (2). Significant changes in sleep occur throughout the life span. See Figure 11-2 for the National Sleep Foundation's (NSF) recommended sleep duration requirements (4).

DEVELOPMENT OF SLEEP–WAKE PATTERNS IN INFANTS AND CHILDREN

Newborns: 0 to 3 Months

Full-term infants are those who are born between 39 and less than 41 weeks of gestation (5). The American Academy of Sleep Medicine (AASM) classifies infants as premature if less than 37 weeks' gestation, full-term if 37 to 42 weeks, and postterm if born after 42 weeks' gestation (6). Sleep technologists need to know and document three "ages" of their newborn patients: gestational,

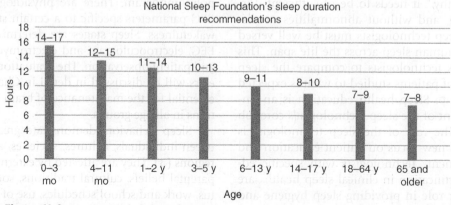

Figure 11-2 Recommended sleep durations.

conceptional, and chronologic. The term "gestational age" (GA) refers to the time from the first day of the mother's last menstrual period to the day of delivery, expressed in weeks. The conceptional age (CA) is the GA plus the number of weeks since birth. The baby's chronologic age is simply the number of weeks since birth. It is necessary to know the CA of newborns and infants in the sleep center in order to accurately interpret the EEG. EEG characteristics of sleep differ based on conceptional, not chronologic age. A baby born 6 weeks ago is considered 6 weeks of chronologic age, but if born 9 weeks before term will have a CA of 37 weeks. That infant's sleep patterns would appear similar to those of a newborn who was born at 37 weeks' gestation. For sleep-stage scoring purposes, the AASM identifies a patient from full-term birth to 2 months' chronologic age as newborn. For sleep study scoring purposes, the AASM uses the term neonate for a baby's first 28 days after birth, and infant at age 1 month to 1 year (6).

Full-term newborns sleep approximately 14 to 17 hours per day. Unfortunately for new parents, that sleep occurs in short bouts distributed throughout the day and night, regardless of light or other environmental cues. Bottle-fed babies tend to sleep for approximately 2 to 5 hours at a time versus breastfed babies who sleep in 1- to 3-hour periods (7). Within the sleep period, sleep cycles occur in which the sleep state alternates between REM and NREM, lasting approximately 50 minutes. Interspersed are periods of wakefulness lasting between less than 1 and 2 hours. Sleep–wake cycles depend not so much on circadian rhythm, which is not fully developed at birth, but on hunger and satiety (7) and comfort. An observer can recognize sleep visually, as the eyes remain closed, with noticeable squirming, sucking motions, and small body movements and twitches upon falling asleep. Newborns enter sleep through REM. At this age, approximately half the baby's sleep is REM, and the other half is NREM. Preterm infants have a higher percentage, as much as 80%, of REM sleep. Undisturbed sleep periods are vital to newborn development, and special care should be taken to preserve the natural sleep periods of the newborn. Particular attention should be paid to preterm babies in the neonatal intensive care area. These patients should have as few disruptions to their REM sleep as possible. Studies have shown that undisturbed sleep periods, when compared to unnaturally disturbed sleep periods, improve cognition in later development (8). There is wisdom in the old saying "never wake a sleeping baby," particularly in the first few months of life.

Issues related to sleep in newborns are often in association with congenital abnormalities or prematurity. Airway compromise with resulting hypoxia and hypercapnia may be seen. Sleep studies on patients in the neonatal intensive care unit are not uncommon.

Sleep-disordered breathing is seen in this and all other age groups. Sudden infant death syndrome is most likely to occur between birth and 4 months postterm. Digestive issues can create sleep–wake problems. Colic and gastroesophageal reflux are seen. Other issues relate to parental expectations of the newborn that are not in concert with their newborn's sleep behaviors. The NSF's expert panel recommends that babies in the 0- to 3-month age group sleep between 14 and 17 hours (4). Babies should sleep in a safe environment, supine, on a firm mattress, and without a pillow (7).

Infants: 4 to 11 Months

As infants develop, their sleep undergoes many changes. The overall sleep needs reduce to approximately 12 to 15 hours, although there is significant variation among infants. Sleep begins to consolidate at night, with longer nighttime sleep periods and shorter day sleeps. Sleep regulation, the infant's ability to self-soothe and fall asleep without assistance, often begins at about 3 months postterm (7). Infants and young children with poor sleep regulation can be a source of great stress for parents. At about 3 to 4 months of age, the sleep cycles begin to increase in length, and the infant enters sleep through NREM, although the transition may not be complete until 8 months of age (9). About this time, EEG develops patterns that will be evident in childhood and beyond. These EEG changes allow for categorizing NREM sleep into three separate stages. Stage N1 is the light stage of sleep that usually occurs at sleep onset. This stage lasts only a few minutes before the infant transitions to stage N2. This stage of sleep is identified by the brain waves named K-complexes and sleep spindles. K-complexes generally appear beginning at 5 months postterm, and sleep spindles become evident between 4 and 6 weeks postterm. The initial cycle of stage N2 generally lasts from 5 to 25 minutes. Stage N3 sleep, also known as slow-wave sleep (SWS) or deep sleep, is identified electrographically by the predominance of high-voltage slow waves, which can first appear anywhere from 2 months postterm to 5 months postterm. Stage N3 usually lasts about 30 minutes. REM sleep appears in the infant EEG as low-voltage high-frequency waves. REMs occur, as do decreased muscle tone and the grimaces, twitches, and sucking motions previously mentioned. Between birth and age 1, there is a reduction in the amount of REM sleep.

By about 6 months of age, infants should be sleeping through the night with longer periods of daytime wakefulness and shorter daytime naps. REM percentage decreases to about 30%. Many healthy infants have given up nighttime feedings at around 6 months of age. Continued nighttime feedings may result more from a learned behavior or parental preference than from hunger. By 1 year of age, overall sleep will likely be reduced by another hour, and naps may decrease from a total of 3 to 4 hours to 1 hour or less. The number of naps needed may be as few as one.

Issues with infants at this age include those associated within the first 3 months postterm, although the likelihood of sudden infant death syndrome is very low at age 1. Nighttime awakenings and sleep-related rhythmic movement are also common around age 1. The NSF recommends that infants between 4 and 11 months of age sleep between 12 and 15 hours, including naps, with normal ranges of as few as 10 and as many as 18 hours of sleep (4). The AASM recommends infants from 4 to 12 months sleep 12 to 16 hours for optimum health (1). Good sleep habits, including consistent bedtimes, bedtime routines, and putting the infant to bed drowsy, are important. Special items such as blankets or stuffed animals can help infants self-soothe and develop the ability to fall asleep on their own.

Toddlers: 1 to 2 Years

At this age, total sleep time averages 11 to 14 hours, including one or two naps of approximately 2 to 3 hours. By age 1, babies generally enter sleep via NREM sleep, which continues throughout the life span. Toddlers begin to develop signs of morningness or eveningness, in terms of their natural propensity for wakefulness, tiredness, and sleep times. The REM–NREM sleep cycle increases to 60 to 70 minutes. The proportion of REM to NREM sleep decreases to 30% between 1 and 2 years (9). Stage N3 sleep occupies much of NREM. During this stage of development, as parents can attest, sleep restriction or deprivation, even of a very short duration (missed afternoon nap) may create an inability to self-regulate, often resulting in a temper tantrum or inconsolable crying spell. Also at this age, sleep issues associated with moving from cosleeping to independent sleeping or moving from crib to bed are common. Bedtime routines are important to develop to help with easy transition to sleep. Other issues can include problems with falling asleep, nighttime awakenings, and head-banging. Both the AASM and the NSF recommend a total sleep time of 11 to 14 hours in this age group, including naps, for optimal health (1, 4). A range of as few as 10 hours and as many as 18 may be within normal.

Preschoolers: 3 to 5 Years

By ages 3 to 5, children sleep about an hour less than toddlers. Naps are reduced to one by age 3 and most likely eliminated by age 5. REM percentage continues to decline closer to the level of adulthood (20% to 25%), and the sleep cycle increases to 90 minutes. A significant

portion of NREM sleep is stage N3 sleep, which is associated with a high arousal threshold. It can be difficult to awaken a child from SWS. Disorders of arousal, usually as a result of waking from SWS, include confusional arousals, sleep walking, and sleep terrors. Other sleep issues that may arise for the first time in this age group are often a result of imagination and inability to distinguish fantasy from reality. Fear of monsters, ghosts, witches, and werewolves can create bedtime resistance and fearful awakenings. Increased language skills allow children to negotiate, stall, and challenge parents regarding bedtime rituals. Other issues at this age include nightmares and bedwetting, in addition to the sleep problems of infants and toddlers. Both the AASM and the NSF expert panels recommend 10 to 13 hours of sleep per 24-hour period, including naps (1, 4).

School Age: 6 to 12 Years

In the period from about 5 years to puberty, nighttime sleep is typically a consistent 10 hours per night. With parental oversight, school routines often require early rise times, which is generally not a problem for grade-school-aged children. They often wake by themselves and rise early even on nonschool days. Sleep propensity during the day is very low (10). Perhaps the term "sleeps like a baby" should be "sleeps like a grade schooler," because children of this age normally have boundless energy during the day and little trouble going to bed, falling asleep, and staying asleep at night. REM approaches adult proportions, and nearing puberty, stage N3 declines in amount and percentage. Throughout the childhood stage, N3 is prominent in the beginning of the night. Disorders common in the younger age groups also appear in school-aged children, although battles over bedtime and requests for nighttime comforting to return to sleep may become less common. Other issues can include insufficient sleep from later bedtimes, sleep disruption from caffeine, and poor sleep hygiene. Restless legs syndrome, periodic limb movement disorder, and narcolepsy can also be seen. The AASM recommends between 9 and 12 hours of sleep, and the NSF recommends 9 to 11 hours for optimal health, with a range as few as 7 to as many as 12 hours per night (1, 4).

Teenagers: 13 to 18 Years

Sleep–wake schedules and total sleep times change dramatically in the teenage years. Around puberty, there is a significant phase delay: a shift in the sleep and wake times caused by circadian rhythm alteration. Where prepubertal children's circadian timing correlate well with early bedtimes and grade school start times, high school students tend to stay up later at night and have difficulty waking for school. This almost 2-hour shift causes a reduction in total sleep time, and increase in sleep debt, which is the difference between what is required to be fully rested and what is achieved. In addition to the biologic propensity to stay up late, many high school students have extracurricular activities, jobs, social lives, virtual lives on social media, and family obligations that make a reasonable bedtime difficult. Most students needing to be at a bus stop at 6 a.m. will accrue a large sleep debt. Children 13 to 18 years old need about 8 to 10 hours of sleep per night. The sleep debt that builds up during the week, along with staying up extra late on Friday and Saturday nights, often creates very late rise times on Saturday and Sunday. Although the sleep debt may be partially repaid on the weekend, there is difficulty falling asleep on Sunday night. Then the weekly cycle begins again. The student is required to rise early, against their natural tendency, until the weekend. As parents can attest, high school students tend to be sleepy, mopey, groggy, and crabby in the morning, yet have a "second wind" in the late evening, making an early bedtime even more difficult.

Sleep-stage changes occur across adolescence. In addition to a decrease in total sleep time by about an hour, there is a significant decrease in SWS. Sleep efficiency may decrease because it can be difficult to fall asleep at bedtime (prolonged sleep latency). Although total sleep time recommended for optimal health by both the AASM and the NSF is 8 to 10 hours, with a normal range of 7 to 11 hours (1, 4), many in this age group get less sleep. A host of issues related to insufficient sleep may occur, including drowsy driving, psychomotor impairment, and behavioral issues such as moodiness, lack of motivation, and poor judgment (7). Sleep disorders that may appear in this age group include delayed sleep–wake phase disorder and insomnia, in addition to the disorders associated with younger children.

SLEEP AND WAKE IN YOUNG AND MIDDLE-AGED ADULTS

Young and middle-aged adults with no sleep problems sleep on average 7 to 9 hours per night. A typical night consists of a fairly short sleep latency, a few minutes of N1, progressing to N2 and N3 sleep, followed by the first REM period about 90 minutes after falling asleep. This ultradian (occurs rhythmically more than once per day) pattern repeats itself every 90 to 110 minutes, with less N3 as the night progresses, but longer REM periods. Healthy sleepers will have a sleep efficiency (the percentage of time in bed asleep) of over 90%. REM occupies 20% to 25% of sleep, occurring in four to six discrete episodes (11). As adults reach middle age, their total sleep time decreases by about an hour. The N3 sleep

percentage continues to decline throughout adulthood and into old age. Men have a more pronounced decrease in SWS than women. Prolonged work hours, stress, and family obligations often lead to self-imposed sleep restriction, resulting in decreased total sleep time. Chronic medical conditions that develop in adulthood may negatively impact sleep. The incidence of many adult sleep disorders increases in this age group. Chronic medical conditions impact the quantity and quality of sleep and the prevalence of sleep disorders, particularly toward middle age. As a person's overall wellness declines, even in the absence of a diagnosed condition, sleep is affected. Insufficient physical activity, obesity, and alcohol and cigarette consumption can negatively impact sleep.

Sleep and Aging

Sleep patterns continue to change in the elderly. The NSF defines older adults as those 65 and older. A pronounced loss of N3, particularly in men, occurs. By age 70, men have approximately 5.5% N3, whereas women have about 17% N3 sleep (12). REM also decreases, but only by 2% to 3% from middle age (12). An increase in N1 sleep occurs as does the incidence of arousals and awakenings from sleep. Sleep efficiency decreases from greater than 90% in early adulthood to about 79% in those over 70 (12). The elderly experience increased difficulty with phase-shifting. Bedtime and rise times tend to remain fairly constant, but when traveling or changing bedtimes, sleep becomes difficult. Napping is common, which may interfere with nighttime sleep. Phase advancing, causing early bed and rise times, is prevalent. Newspapers are often delivered in over 55 communities by 5 a.m. to avoid customer complaints. The elderly often spend more hours in bed than needed, reducing sleep efficiency and leading to sleep complaints. Incidence of sleep disorders is high in this population. Insomnia and sleep-related breathing disorders are prevalent, as are restless legs syndrome and periodic limb movement disorder. Common chronic conditions such as heart disease, chronic obstructive pulmonary disease, diabetes, Alzheimer disease, and dementia negatively impact sleep and contribute to sleep disorders. Medications to treat these conditions may also disturb sleep. Chronic pain causes short sleep durations and fragmented sleep. The NSF recommends 7 to 8 hours of sleep for optimal health for older adults (2).

SUMMARY

Sleep begins in fetal life and changes throughout the life span. The first year of life sees many changes, both in the wake and in the sleep patterns of babies. At birth, babies spend the majority of a 24-hour period asleep, in short bouts of sleep interspersed with short periods of wakefulness. As infants age, sleep consolidates, the sleep cycle lengthens, and a clear day–night pattern emerges. Sleep patterns and needs continue to change, particularly in adolescence and throughout teenage years, when intrinsic phase delays often conflict with early school start times. Sleep in the middle aged, and certainly in the elderly population, can be of sufficient duration and quality but is often disturbed by underlying chronic conditions and physiologic changes associated with aging.

Patients often ask their sleep technologist about sleep quality and quantity. An understanding of the sleep needs, patterns, and cycles of patients throughout the life span prepares technologists to advise patients on their sleep needs and behaviors. The importance of a good night's sleep cannot be overemphasized.

REFERENCES

1. Paruthi, S., Brooks, L. J., D'Ambrosio, C., et al. (2016). Recommended amount of sleep for pediatric populations: A consensus statement of the American Academy of Sleep Medicine. *Journal of Clinical Sleep Medicine, 12*(6), 785–786.
2. Dement, W. (1999). *The promise of sleep.* New York, NY: Random House.
3. Jenni, O. G., & Carskadon, M. A. (2007). Sleep behavior and sleep regulation from infancy through adolescence: Normative aspects. *Sleep Medicine Clinics, 2,* 321–329.
4. Hirshkowitz, M., Whiton, K., Albert, S. M., et al. (2015). National Sleep Foundation's sleep time duration recommendations: Methodology and results summary. *Sleep Health, 1,* 40–43.
5. American College of Obstetricians and Gynecologists. (2013). Committee opinion no. 579: Definition of term pregnancy. *Obstetrics and Gynecology, 122,* 1139–1140.
6. Berry, R. B., Albertario, C. L., Harding, S. M., et.al; for the American Academy of Sleep Medicine. (2018). *The AASM Manual for the scoring of sleep and associated events: Rules, terminology and technical specifications* [Version 2.5]. Darien, IL: American Academy of Sleep Medicine.
7. Mindell, J., & Owens, J. (2015). *Pediatric sleep* (pp. 9–36). Philadelphia, PA: Wolters Kluwer.
8. Weisman, O., Magori-Cohen, R., Louzoun, Y., et al. (2011). Sleep-wake transitions in premature neonates predict early development. *Pediatrics, 128,* 706–714.
9. Sheldon, S. H., Ferber, R., & Kryger, H. (2005). *Principles and practice of pediatric sleep medicine* (p. 56). New York, NY: Elsevier.
10. Carskadon, M. A., Keenan, S., & Dement, W. C. (1987). Nighttime sleep and daytime sleep tendency in preadolescents. In C. Guilleminault (Ed.), *Sleep and its disorders in children* (pp. 43–52). New York, NY: Raven Press.
11. Carskadon, M. A., & Dement, W. C. (2011). Monitoring and staging human sleep. In M. H. Kryger, T. Roth, & W. C. Dement (Eds.), *Principles and practice of sleep medicine* (5th ed., p. 16). St. Louis, MO: Elsevier Saunders.
12. Bliwise, D. L. (2005). Normal aging. In M. H. Kryger, T. Roth, & W. C. Dement (Eds.), *Principles and practice of sleep medicine* (4th ed., pp. 24–36). St. Louis, MO: Elsevier Saunders.

Sleep Disorders and Disorders That Affect Sleep

chapter 12

Obstructive Sleep Apnea

ELISE A. MAHER   LAWRENCE J. EPSTEIN

LEARNING OBJECTIVES

On completion of this chapter, the reader should be able to:

1. List the symptoms, risk factors, and associated comorbid conditions seen with obstructive sleep apnea (OSA).
2. Define the polysomnographic patterns associated with sleep-disordered breathing.
3. Describe the major treatments used for OSA.

KEY TERMS

Apnea
Arrhythmias
Craniofacial structure
Excessive daytime sleepiness (EDS)
Hypopnea
Continuous positive airway pressure (CPAP)
Obstructive sleep apnea
Pharynx
Sleep-disordered breathing (SDB)
Snoring
Surgical treatment of OSA
Upper airway resistance syndrome (UARS)

Obstructive sleep apnea (OSA) is a repetitive pattern of upper airway obstruction that occurs during sleep and is associated with sleep fragmentation and/or oxygen desaturation. The combination of sleep fragmentation, oxygen desaturation, and the other pathophysiologic changes causes daytime impairment, particularly excessive daytime sleepiness (EDS), and cardiovascular disease. The disorder was first clinically described as recently as (1). There is a gradient of airway closure in OSA ranging from mild and partial obstruction to a complete and sustained blockage of the upper airway. An event with complete obstruction is called an "apnea," whereas the one with partial obstruction is called a "hypopnea." A milder respiratory disturbance called a respiratory effort–related arousal (RERA) fragments sleep with even minimal increases in upper airway resistance.

The clinical syndrome has variously been called OSA, the obstructive sleep apnea syndrome, and the obstructive sleep apnea/hypopnea syndrome (OSAHS). The current terminology recommended by the *International Classification of Sleep Disorders*, 3rd edition (2), and used in this chapter, is OSA. Partial obstruction or hypopnea is frequently seen in the syndrome and so the term OSAHS is used interchangeably with OSA.

Mild obstruction of the upper airway causes turbulent airflow that leads the tissues to vibrate and creates snoring, and sometimes choking, sounds. The sound levels resulting from snoring range from soft to decibel levels loud enough to be considered unsafe in the workplace (>80 dB). Obstructive events can last from 10 seconds to as long as 2 minutes, after which a brief central nervous system arousal from sleep restores the patency (opening or unblocking) of the airway. Severity is defined by the number of breathing disruptions per hour, or apnea–hypopnea index (AHI). Some authors use the term "respiratory disturbance index" (RDI) interchangeably with AHI; however, the American Academy of Sleep Medicine (AASM) Manual for the Scoring of Sleep and Associated Events defines RDI as the number of apneas + hypopneas + RERAs per hour of sleep. An AHI below 5 is considered normal in adults. Mild OSA is in the range of 5 to 14, moderate 15 to 30, and severe more than 30. The number of times that a patient's oxygen level drops below the minimum normal saturation of 88% to 90% is another indicator of severity, with greater stress on the cardiovascular system and increased risk of cardiovascular disorders related to the more frequent and larger desaturation.

SLEEP AND BREATHING

Most body systems slow down during sleep. The breathing rate slows, and tidal volume is reduced as breaths become shallower, resulting in mild hypoventilation (2 to 8 mm Hg increase in $PaCO_2$). At the same time, the heart rate slows down, and oxygenation levels dip a little below waking levels. Muscles relax and the airway narrows, leading to an increase in upper airway resistance in the pharynx (the soft tissue pathway starting from the nasal and oral airways that leads down to the larynx; Fig. 12-1). The anatomic and neuromuscular systems

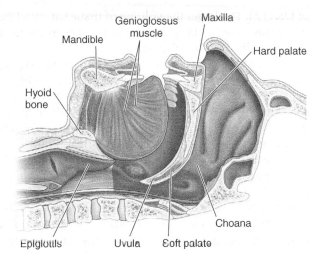

Figure 12-1 This is a sagittal section through the pharyngeal airway of a normal human. The opening to the nose is just above the **maxilla**. The other structures of the airway include the **mandible**, **hard palate**, **soft palate**, and **uvula**. The body of the tongue is the **genioglossus muscle**. Pharyngeal collapse in apneic patients occurs somewhere between the **choana** and the **epiglottis**, usually behind the uvula and the soft palate, behind the tongue, or some combination of these sites. In humans, the hyoid bone is not firmly attached to bony structures, thus increasing dependency on the upper airway muscles to keep the airway open. (Modified with permission from Moore, K. L., Dalley, A. F., & Agur, A. M. R. (2013). *Clinically oriented anatomy* [7th ed., Figure 7.83]. Baltimore, MD: Lippincott Williams & Wilkins/Wolters Kluwer.)

Labels on figure: Mandible, Genioglossus muscle, Maxilla, Hard palate, Hyoid bone, Choana, Epiglottis, Uvula, Soft palate

that keep the airway open for normal breathing during wakefulness are not as active during sleep and can fail to compensate for the changes that occur in sleep.

The human airway is anatomically at greater risk than other animals. The hyoid bone that anchors the pharyngeal muscles is not rigidly attached in humans as it is in other mammals, which allows us wide-ranging vocalizations needed for speech. However, this feature makes the upper airway more collapsible when the many muscles responsible for dilating and maintaining the airway are not fully functioning during sleep. The areas of obstruction differ considerably, depending on body position, craniofacial structure, and weight distribution. It has been shown that obese patients tend to have collapse of the velopharynx (soft palate and side-walls of the pharynx), whereas nonobese patients with a recessed chin showed collapse in the oropharynx and velopharynx (3).

The typical reclining sleeping posture causes a gravitational effect on the soft tissue of the upper airway, promoting collapse. This positional effect is at its worst when patients are sleeping on their back (supine). Patients sometimes unknowingly self-treat their OSA by preferring to sleep propped up with extra pillows or in a recliner. In rapid eye movement (REM) sleep, the upper airway can collapse further when dilator muscle activation, reduced the greatest amount compared with waking levels, is chemically blocked.

There are two general types of breathing disturbances in sleep: central and obstructive. Central breathing events are caused by a malfunction in the respiratory control system, leading the person to not take a breath, whereas obstructive events are caused by a physical block of the airway that prevents airflow despite efforts to breathe. Central and obstructive apneas represent a complete lack of airflow, obstructive hypopneas (and less commonly described central hypopneas) represent a partial obstruction to airflow, and both of these can cause fragmented sleep and oxygen desaturation. On the mildest end of the spectrum is the RERA. The limitation of airflow from mild obstruction requires more muscle effort to breathe, like having to suck harder through a narrow straw. This increased effort can cause a brief arousal from sleep or RERA. Taken altogether, these patterns of abnormal breathing—snoring, RERAs, hypopneas, and apneas—are called sleep-disordered breathing (SDB).

EPIDEMIOLOGY

It is difficult to accurately determine the prevalence of OSA in the population because of the various ways that breathing obstructions in sleep are defined and measured, how individuals are screened, and how they are tested. A widely referenced study found that the occurrence of more than five obstructive events per hour during sleep is high, reported at 24% in men and 9% in women aged 30 to 60 years. The same study found the prevalence of OSA, defined as more than five obstructive events per hour *and* symptoms of sleepiness, was 2% in women and 4% in men aged 30 to 60 years (4). This seminal study was published in 1993 and likely underestimates the prevalence of OSA because of the rapid increase in obesity in the general population since that time. More recent studies suggest prevalence rates of 5% in women and 14% in men, with higher rates associated with older age and higher weight (5).

RISK FACTORS

There are multiple and often intertwined risk factors that predispose to OSA. Longitudinal studies have found that the most significant independent risk factor for OSA is being overweight (5–7). There is a 4-fold risk for OSA associated with a body mass index (BMI) increase of one standard deviation (this amount of change in BMI is approximately the difference between normal and overweight or between overweight and obese) (1).

Even a 10% weight reduction can lower the AHI by an average of 26% (6). For patients with mild OSA, AHI may be objectively reduced to normal levels after significant weight loss. In a 2009 study that had patients follow a very low-calorie diet, the AHI was brought below 5 when patients lost an average of 10.6% of initial weight (8).

Gender plays a large role in the relative expression of OSA symptoms and health consequences, with males having a reported 2:1 or 3:1 prevalence over females. Hormones and fat distribution both predispose males toward a more collapsible airway. Interestingly, the ratio of males to females who present to the sleep center for testing is closer to 8:1. Males may tend to be identified more readily by primary care doctors as being candidates for OSA or may be prompted more often by female partners to seek treatment (9). The gender difference in prevalence starts to equalize postmenopause.

There is a linear relationship between age and risk for OSA, which starts in middle age and plateaus at about age 65 (10). In women, there is a marked increase in OSA after menopause when the protective effects of progesterone on the respiratory system diminish (11). Although the incidence of OSA is higher in old age than in middle age, at 70% for men and 56% for women, the symptoms and risk factors are different (12). The AHI is not as strongly correlated with obesity (10), EDS, cognitive dysfunction, or hypertension (13, 14) in older individuals. Snoring, one of the main complaints in middle age, subsides in old age. This could be because of hearing loss or because a central component to respiration emerges (15).

Race is a risk factor for OSA although not as widely researched as weight, gender, age, or other factors. African Americans younger than 25 and older than 65 have an elevated risk over African American males between 25 and 65 or males of other races (16, 17). Asians have similar rates of OSA as those in Western cultures. However, BMI rates are lower, and craniofacial features may be the determining factor. Chinese males, for example, have a shorter cranial base, maxilla (upper jaw), and mandible (lower jaw), causing more crowding of the airway (18).

Craniofacial features can have a large impact on the airway, particularly during sleep when muscle relaxation, body position, and gravity can compromise the airway patency of susceptible individuals. There are two types of features that impact potential upper airway obstruction: soft tissue and bone structure. Soft tissue from large turbinates, a deviated septum, occluded sinuses, polyps, a large tongue or uvula, enlarged tonsils or adenoids, or an elongated soft palate can crowd the oronasal airway and cause obstruction and reduced airflow. A large neck size (>17 inches in men and >16 inches in women) is one of the most predictive features

of OSA (2). The larger the volume of tissue surrounding the airway, whether fatty or muscular, the more prone it is to partially or fully collapse.

A receding (retrognathic) or small (micrognathic) chin or narrow/high arched palate can be problematic and cause OSA in nonobese patients. Congenital conditions that impact facial bones and soft tissue of the upper airway are associated with increased risk for OSA that can be especially difficult to treat. Features of Down syndrome include a large tongue (macroglossia), small chin, narrow airway, and generalized hypotonia. In a 2009 study, 94% of Down syndrome patients were found to have at least mild OSA and 69% were in the severe range (19). Pierre Robin, Marfan syndrome, and achondroplasia are some of the other genetic disorders that result in decreased airway size and predispose for OSA.

Familial incidence of OSA increases the risk to an individual for OSA. There is a direct increase in risk for OSA with each diagnosed family member (20). This may be because of a combination of genetic and environmental factors. For instance, obesity is an independent risk factor and can be affected by familial lifestyle and dietary factors.

Smoking and sedative use (including alcohol), particularly near bedtime, are additional predisposing factors. Smoking may affect the function of upper airway tissue because of inflammation and toughening from prolonged smoke exposure. One study showed that active smokers are three times more likely to have OSA than nonsmokers (21). Sedatives act as muscle relaxants and also reduce reactivity in the respiratory control system. Sedatives can induce apneas and snoring in people without OSA and worsen respiratory events in symptomatic patients (22–24).

Other clinical conditions that affect airway size or airway muscle function are risk factors for OSA, including polycystic ovary syndrome, hypothyroidism, and pregnancy. Although hormones can have a protective effect on the airway in sleep, gestational weight gain and pressure on the thoracic cavity can cause or increase snoring and apneas. Apneas during pregnancy that are associated with hypoxemia can be associated with low fetal birth weight and lower Apgar scores (25).

CARDIOVASCULAR DISEASE

Cardiac disease and progression frequently coexist with OSA. Patients with OSA are at increased risk for hypertension, arrhythmias, myocardial infarction (MI), coronary artery disease, pulmonary hypertension, stroke, and sudden cardiac death. Cardiac arrhythmias are more common in patients with OSA as a result of sympathetic nervous system activation (which causes vasoconstriction and increased blood pressure), hypoxia (low oxygen levels), hypercapnia (elevated carbon dioxide levels), and increased fluctuations in intrathoracic pressure. The increase in negative intrathoracic pressure during an obstructive event negatively affects left ventricular function and decreases stroke volume and cardiac output. Many patients with OSA develop a brady-tachy heart rate pattern in which bradycardia occurs during the apneic phase and tachycardia occurs when breathing returns (26).

Of note, the Sleep Heart Health Study (SHHS) showed that hypopneas accompanied by an oxyhemoglobin desaturation of more than or equal to 4% were associated with prevalent cardiovascular disease independently of confounding covariates (27). In contrast, no association was observed between cardiovascular disease and hypopneas associated with milder desaturation or arousals.

Hypertension

Analysis of data from more than 6,000 adults participating in the SHHS showed that those in the upper quartile of AHI (≥11.0 events per hour) had 42% greater odds of cardiovascular disease than those in the lowest quartile (AHI <1.3 events per hour) (28). Patients with hypertension have an increased incidence of OSA (30%) and 50% of patients with OSA have hypertension (29, 30). Hypertension is strongly associated with OSA, even when mild (31).

The SHHS showed a linear relationship between increasing AHI and incidence of hypertension. Prevalence rates of hypertension in increasing AHI categories were 43% (<1.5 per hour), 53% (1.5 to 4.9 per hour), 59% (5 to 14.9 per hour), 62% (15 to 29.9 per hour), and 67% (≥30 per hour) (32). It is likely that hypertension itself increases the risks of other types of cardiac disease.

Arrhythmias

Arrhythmias are more common in patients with OSA, even in the absence of structural or electrical heart conduction problems. The higher incidence of abnormal rhythms is most likely caused by a combination of hypoxemia, the vagal response to obstructed breathing, increased sympathetic activation, acute increases in blood pressure, and rapid changes in intrathoracic pressure.

Cardiac variability is commonly seen in OSA patients with repetitive alternations between bradycardia and tachycardia in synchrony with obstructive events. Bradycardia is caused by the vagal response to apnea and is followed by an overshoot to tachycardia during the hyperpneic (recovery) phase of breathing. Decreased heart rate variability in response to repetitive apneas is a marker for subsequent development of hypertension because of excessive sympathetic activity and potential loss of vagal control (33).

Other bradycardic patterns, including second- and third-degree atrioventricular (AV) blocks and sinus pauses, are frequently seen in OSA patients. In the absence of any electrophysiologic abnormalities of the sinus or AV node, heart block was found in 10% of patients with OSA. The blocks included AV block type II (Mobitz), third-degree block, and sinus pauses and occurred more often in REM sleep and during 4% or greater oxygen desaturations (34). Sinus pauses of up to 12 seconds can be seen in REM sleep and during long apneas with desaturation.

Ventricular ectopy is also frequently seen in patients with OSA and increases in frequency along with increasing AHI. Individuals with SDB had three times the odds of nonsustained ventricular tachycardia and almost twice the odds of complex ventricular ectopy (nonsustained ventricular tachycardia with bigeminy, trigeminy, or quadrigeminy) (35). In a study of 400 OSA patients conducted by Guilleminault et al. (1), premature ventricular contractions were noted in 193 (48%) of subjects. The common arrhythmias seen in patients with OSA without known cardiac history often occur during sleep (35, 36). Positive airway pressure (PAP) therapy has been shown to decrease ventricular ectopy in patients with heart failure and OSA (37).

There is a 4-fold increase in atrial fibrillation in patients with OSA (35). There is also a higher recurrence of atrial fibrillation after cardioversion in patients with untreated SDB and atrial fibrillation than in patients without a known SDB diagnosis (38).

Congestive Heart Failure

Congestive heart failure (CHF) is strongly associated with Cheyne–Stokes respiration, a type of central sleep apnea (CSA). However, many patients with CSA also have an obstructive component, and there is increased risk of heart failure with OSA as well. In a sample of 81 male patients with CHF, 40% had CSA and 11% had OSA (39). Patients with OSA were heavier, on average, than those with CSA. There is a high frequency of atrial fibrillation and ventricular arrhythmias in patients with both OSA and CHF. The SHHS reported that OSA is associated with a relative odds ratio of 2.38 for heart failure, independent of other known risk factors (28, 40).

Coronary Artery Disease

There is increased risk for MI in patients with OSA, reported to be about four times greater than in those without OSA (41–43). Additionally, OSA patients may be at higher risk for subsequent cardiovascular events after an MI, possibly because of hypoxemia (44).

Stroke

There is a high incidence of OSA in stroke patients (45, 46). In the SHHS, there was a positive relationship between the history of stroke and the AHI (28). Prospective studies have shown an increased risk of stroke in patients with OSA, with an increased hazard ratio of 2.5 in those with OSA (47).

Sudden Cardiac Death

Although sudden cardiac death tends to occur between 6 and 11 a.m. in the general population, there is 2.5 times the risk of sudden cardiac death between 12 and 6 a.m. for patients with known OSA (48). Increased nocturnal arrhythmias in patients with OSA could be a contributing factor to nocturnal sudden cardiac death (35).

ENDOCRINE DYSFUNCTION

Over the past decade, a strong relationship between diabetes mellitus, other metabolic syndromes, and OSA has been increasingly defined. Although obesity is a common comorbidity in both OSA and diabetes mellitus, OSA is independently associated with altered glucose metabolism and may predispose to the eventual development of type 2 diabetes mellitus (49). The repetitive effects of cortical arousal and hypoxia can worsen insulin sensitivity and glucose tolerance (50, 51).

There is evidence of an increased risk of OSA in patients with diabetes mellitus also. One in four patients diagnosed with diabetes with autonomic neuropathy also have OSA (52, 53). Neuropathy may contribute to the collapsibility of the upper airway. Given the surge in diabetes mellitus in the population, it is becoming more important to treat for OSA in order to help control the negative health consequences. Metabolic syndrome is a cluster of health concerns that includes obesity, hyperlipidemia (high low-density lipoprotein cholesterol), hypertension, and insulin resistance. Of these conditions, insulin resistance is considered to be the core dysfunction. Metabolic syndrome, also known as Syndrome X, has become so closely associated with OSA that the term "Syndrome Z" has been proposed for patients diagnosed with both conditions (54).

Hypothyroidism is caused by reduced production of thyroid hormone and is another endocrine system dysfunction that increases the risk of OSA. This is due mainly to associated weight gain, soft tissue (especially the tongue) and facial swelling, and myopathy.

NEUROLOGIC DYSFUNCTION

Recent studies have explored a relationship between OSA and Alzheimer disease (AD). A meta-analysis of published clinical data on the overlap of OSA and AD indicates a 5-fold increased risk of AD patients presenting with OSA when compared with cognitively nonimpaired subjects of similar age (55). A 2016 study found that 50% of patients with OSA had elevated levels of amyloid beta, a peptide that is the main component of amyloid plaques found in the brains of AD patients, and individuals who experienced more apneas throughout their normal sleep period had increased levels of amyloid beta (56). These and other studies suggest that OSA may be a risk factor for AD and the possible importance of assessing older adults for OSA.

CLINICAL SYMPTOMS

The most common symptoms that OSA patients experience are habitual snoring, pauses in breathing, gasping and choking during sleep, frequent urination, and feeling excessively sleepy during the day even after adequate sleep time. Other nighttime symptoms include difficulty falling or staying asleep, sleep fragmentation, gastric disturbance, excessive sweating, and movement during sleep. Daytime symptoms are not as obviously associated with OSA. Patients with untreated OSA often suffer from cognitive and behavioral dysfunction and can be more depressed, forgetful, impatient, irritable and suffer from morning headaches, daytime gastric reflux, and sexual dysfunction.

The primary symptom is often EDS that interferes with work, leisure activities, and relationships. However, there is not a clear relationship between the severity of OSA and subjective or objective measures of sleepiness. Many patients are unaware of the profound impact of OSA on their attentiveness and performance. There may be genetic phenotypes that make some patients more resilient against sleep disturbance. Conversely, some patients with very mild OSA can suffer from EDS and benefit from treatment. Snoring is often the reason for patients seeking treatment, and bed partners play a large role in discovering the patterns of obstructed breathing and supporting testing and treatment.

COGNITIVE AND BEHAVIORAL SYMPTOMS

There are various components to cognitive function: attention, psychomotor response, vigilance, memory, decision making, and executive function. Deficits in cognitive function are thought to be caused by sleep fragmentation and changes in cerebral blood flow from low oxygen levels (57). Executive function and vigilance have been found to be impaired in clinic-based samples of OSA patients. In a study of newly diagnosed OSA patients, 25% showed neuropsychological dysfunction on a battery of cognitive indexes that assessed constructive ability, deductive thinking, verbal attainment, and immediate memory (58). Several studies have shown that memory is impaired in untreated OSA, but improves with PAP treatment (59, 60). Sustained attention may be the function most impacted by daytime sleepiness. These decreased functions have significant consequences when OSA patients are responsible for public safety, as in commercial transportation.

There is a strong association between OSA and mood disorders, particularly depression (61–63). A 2005 study of over 4 million veterans showed that 3% had sleep apnea, and more than 21% of those with OSA also had comorbid depression (64). In a recent community-based sample of 18,900 survey respondents in Europe, 17.6% of those meeting criteria for SDB also met the criteria for major depression (65). It may be clinically important to understand how many patients with depression also have OSA. Because many patients with depression are treated pharmacologically with sedative hypnotics, there could be a worsening of nighttime breathing that could compound depressive symptoms. Both depression and OSA have the symptoms of sleepiness and fatigue in common, and it can be difficult to pull apart which is primary.

Quality of life (QOL) is a subjective self-assessment of a spectrum of factors such as standard of living, life satisfaction, health, job status, and the ability to carry out daily activities. Patients with severe OSA may be the most affected in terms of QOL (66), but even those with mild OSA report difficulties. In the SHHS, an inverse relationship between OSA severity and scores on "vitality/energy" was shown, but only when oxygen desaturation was part of the severity determination (15).

CLINICAL EVALUATION

The signs and symptoms of OSA are easily recognizable by health professionals if patients are forthcoming about them or if clinicians ask the right questions (Table 12-1). Snoring, pauses in breathing, gasping or choking, restlessness, and EDS are indicators that a patient should be evaluated for OSA. Evaluation requires a careful review of medical history, sleep habits and problems, related daytime symptoms, and a physical examination. The physical examination includes a review of respiratory, cardiovascular, and neurologic systems, with a focus on evaluation of BMI, neck size, and the anatomy of the upper airway. Physicians use the Mallampati classification to rate the size of the airway opening at the back of the throat. Scores range from I to IV, with IV being the most occluded and ≥III having an increased risk of OSA (67).

Sleep testing should be performed when moderate-to-severe OSA is suggested by the presence of EDS and at least two of the following three criteria: habitual loud snoring, witnessed apnea or gasping or choking, or diagnosed hypertension. Patients with EDS

Table 12-1	OSA Symptoms That Should Be Evaluated during a Comprehensive Sleep Evaluation
Witnessed apneas
Snoring
Gasping/choking at night
Excessive sleepiness not explained by other factors
Nonrefreshing sleep
Total sleep amount
Sleep fragmentation/maintenance insomnia
Nocturia
Morning headaches
Decreased concentration
Memory loss
Decreased libido
Irritability

OSA, obstructive sleep apnea.
From Epstein, L. J., Kristo, D., Strollo, P. J., Jr., et al. (2009, June 15). Clinical guideline for the evaluation, management and long-term care of obstructive sleep apnea in adults. Adult obstructive sleep apnea task force of the American Academy of Sleep Medicine. *Journal of Clinical Sleep Medicine, 5*(3), 263–276.

who report falling asleep at the wheel or having had a motor vehicle accident should be expedited for testing and treatment. Preoperative evaluation is important for risk reduction because of increased collapsibility of the upper airway during anesthesia and sedation.

Patients with conditions that are closely associated with OSA should also be proactively screened (Table 12-2). Because obesity is one of the most predictive risk factors for OSA, anyone with a BMI of more than 35 should be evaluated, as well as patients undergoing bariatric surgery. Endocrine disorders associated with excess weight, like hypothyroidism or diabetes mellitus, will also increase the risk of OSA. Certain types of cardiovascular disease and arrhythmias are increased in patients with OSA. Likewise, patients who have had cardiovascular events like stroke or MI have a much higher risk of OSA and should be screened.

Research on the relationship of OSA and cancer is starting to suggest that patients with OSA have a higher risk of dying from cancer (68). In the Wisconsin Sleep Cohort Study, a 4-fold increase in cancer mortality was found in OSA patients compared with matched patients without OSA (69). It may be important in the future to test for and treat OSA to prescreen for cancer and slow progression of established cancer.

Table 12-2 **Patients at High Risk for OSA Who Should Be Evaluated for OSA Symptoms**

Obesity (BMI >35)
Congestive heart failure
Atrial fibrillation
Treatment refractory hypertension
Type 2 diabetes
Nocturnal dysrhythmias
Stroke
Hypertension
High-risk driving populations
Preoperative for bariatric surgery

BMI, body mass index; OSA, obstructive sleep apnea.
From Epstein, L. J., Kristo, D., Strollo, P. J., Jr., et al. (2009). Clinical guideline for the evaluation, management and long-term care of obstructive sleep apnea in adults. Adult obstructive sleep apnea task force of the American Academy of Sleep Medicine. *Journal of Clinical Sleep Medicine, 5*(3), 263–276.

DIAGNOSTIC TESTING

Testing for OSA is usually performed in a sleep center, where multiple systems (brain activity, cardiac activity, breathing, and movements) are comprehensively monitored and can be correlated in time. The channels for standard polysomnography (PSG) required by AASM standards are comprehensive enough to definitively rule OSA in or out (70). To expedite diagnosis and treatment, a split-night study is often ordered, during which the first part of the night is diagnostic for SDB and the second part introduces PAP therapy when indicated. When a PAP titration is incomplete after a split-night study, the patient can return to the lab for an all-night titration or be set up on an auto-titrating PAP device at home to determine optimal therapeutic pressure.

When there is the likelihood of OSA in the absence of a set of comorbidities (moderate-to-severe pulmonary disease, neuromuscular disease, CHF, history of stroke and chronic opiate medication use) or other potential sleep disorders, a limited-channel portable test can be done at home or in other settings outside the sleep center. These tests have been variously labeled "out-of-center sleep tests," portable monitoring, limited-channel tests, and home sleep tests. The AASM recommends the term "home sleep *apnea* test" (HSAT) to emphasize that home testing is indicated only in evaluating obstructed breathing (presumed to be during sleep), as sleep markers are generally not recorded. Evaluation by a sleep specialist for suitability for HSAT is required to appropriately

order and interpret these tests. HSATs can underestimate SDB, especially when a patient primarily or exclusively has arousals rather than desaturations associated with hypopneas. In addition, total recording time is used to calculate the AHI rather than total sleep time because sleep is not measured, which can artificially reduce the AHI. These factors can cause a false-negative result in an estimated 17% of tests, and patients with a high pretest likelihood of OSA should be retested with in-lab PSG if their HSAT is negative for OSA (71). The accuracy of the diagnostic method, convenience, cost, patient preference, physical/cognitive ability for self-administration, and wait time and access issues may all be considered when choosing between home and attended sleep apnea testing. When evidence of nonobstructive SDB, such as CSA, is suggested by HSAT, full PSG should be performed.

Effectiveness of treatment for OSA on sleepiness may be evaluated by a multiple sleep latency test to determine residual sleepiness or by a maintenance of wakefulness test to determine the ability to stay awake and resume work in safety-related jobs.

PSG FINDINGS

The specifications for scoring SDB are outlined in the *AASM Manual for the Scoring of Sleep and Associated Events: Rules, Terminology and Technical Specifications* (70). The breathing events that indicate OSA are apneas and hypopneas that last a minimum of 10 seconds in adults (at least two missed breaths in children). An obstructive apnea is defined by the absence of breathing in the oronasal thermal channel with continued respiratory effort throughout the event. Absence of breathing is further specified to be 90% reduced for 90% of the event's duration. The recommended hypopnea definition occurs when there is a minimum of 30% reduction in the nasal pressure transducer signal associated with a minimum of 3% oxygen desaturation and/or an associated arousal. An acceptable alternate definition requires the nasal pressure transducer signal to be reduced by at least 30% with an associated 4% or greater oxygen desaturation (70).

PSG recordings of patients with OSA reveal abnormal sleep patterns related to sleep fragmentation: decreased sleep efficiency, increased stage N1, decreased stage N3, reduced REM sleep, and increased stage changes and electroencephalogram (EEG) arousals. Oxygen desaturations and resaturations related to apneas and hypopneas may be seen, as well as elevated CO_2 levels (routinely monitored during pediatric sleep studies, but infrequently in adults).

With the modified lead II configuration of electrocardiogram (ECG) electrode placement used during

PSG, only certain types of arrhythmias can be accurately detected. However, heart rate and regularity can be assessed as well as irregular QRS formations. The ECG can be interpreted in correlation with sleep state and breathing patterns. A pattern of bradycardia is often seen during apneic events followed by tachycardia at the termination of the event or the hyperpneic phase of recovery breathing. Body position and body movements are recorded and can also be correlated with sleep stage and cardiorespiratory status.

Some patients have a pattern of sustained airflow limitation that can cause mild snoring and/or arousals from sleep. Some authors have called this breathing pattern, occurring along with daytime symptoms, the "upper airway resistance syndrome" (UARS). These patients have a low AHI and often a pattern of flattening or cupping of the nasal transducer signal that does not meet criteria for hypopnea. Airflow limitation can be termed a RERA when it lasts at least 10 seconds, shows progressively increasing or maintained respiratory effort, and ends in an arousal (69). RERAs are included in the RDI calculated in some sleep centers. The PSG in patients with UARS shows an AHI below 5 per hour, but there is a dominance of RERAs, resulting in an overall RDI above 5 per hour. SaO$_2$ is maintained to a minimum of 92%. Chronic insomnia tends to be much more common in these patients; they report nocturnal awakenings and find it difficult to return to sleep. Parasomnias are more frequently reported in younger subjects with UARS (72, 73).

TREATMENT

Behavioral Management

Patients should be educated about the causes, consequences, and treatment options for OSA. Behavioral measures can reduce risk factors and improve airway patency, including weight loss and avoidance of sedatives, alcohol, and smoking. It has been shown that alcohol near bedtime increases the duration and frequency of obstructions and significantly increases desaturations in the first hour of sleep (74). Weight loss can be curative in some cases or reduce the AHI and related symptoms. Weight loss after bariatric surgery has been shown to lower the AHI (75, 76).

In theory, PAP therapy would optimally correct sleep fragmentation, endocrine dysfunction, and other processes that impact energy balance and tendencies for weight gain. However, recent research shows that on average, patients on PAP therapy show a 0.4 kg increase in weight after 3 months (77). It is possible that the small uptick in weight could be explained by a reduced energy burden after the treatment of labored breathing,

resulting in fewer calories burned during sleep. More studies with better controls for PAP compliance, calorie intake, and OSA severity are warranted to further investigate the relationship between treating OSA with PAP and weight change. For some patients, treating OSA can give the energy and vitality to begin an effective weight loss program; however, counseling on weight reduction strategies should go hand in hand with PAP recommendations.

For patients with positional OSA, for whom obstruction occurs predominantly while supine, positional therapy that keeps them off their back can be a treatment option. Positional therapy is indicated only when positional apnea has been established during sleep testing. Some patients only have obstructed breathing when lying on their back. For this reason, it is essential that effort is made to get a sample of sleep in lateral and supine positions during in lab testing. One study showed that 55.8% of patients with OSA in a large sample had twice as many respiratory events in the supine position compared with the lateral position. These patients tended to have a lower BMI and were younger than those without a positional effect (78). There are various positioning products on the market now, but any object affixed to the back (tennis balls and backpack) that makes it difficult or uncomfortable to roll onto the back can reduce obstructive events for some patients.

PAP Therapy

PAP, which may be in the form of continuous PAP (CPAP), bilevel PAP (BPAP), or auto-titrating PAP (APAP), is the cornerstone of treatment. PAP is created by an air blower that generates airflow, increasing positive pressure in the airway, and keeping the airway inflated and open. CPAP was the first developed and, as the name implies, provides the same continuous pressure during both inspiration and exhalation. BPAP maintains the patency of the airway at a lower pressure during exhalation than the higher pressures that are triggered by inhalation, which can be more comfortable for some patients with OSA. APAP adjusts the pressure to the minimum needed to maintain an open airway in variable conditions (i.e., different positions and sleep stages, weight changes). The airflow of the various PAP modalities is delivered through a nasal or oral–nasal interface. The pressure level is predetermined by an attended PAP or APAP titration study performed to evaluate the lowest pressure that can prevent snoring and minimize obstructive events, desaturations, and flow limitation. PAP therapy can be utilized for all categories of OSA and represents first-line therapy for mild, moderate, and severe OSA. Treatment of nasal obstruction, use of lowest required pressure levels, attention to mask-fit issues, use of heated humidification for nasal dryness and nasal discomfort, patient education, and regular follow-up play important roles in acceptance and tolerance.

Improvement is dependent upon effective use of PAP. Compliance with the therapy consists of acceptance and adherence. Some patients will initially refuse to accept and use PAP therapy, and others have difficulty using PAP consistently night to night or for the duration of the sleep period. Most PAP devices have built-in compliance tracking monitors that determine nightly and average usage, leak rate, and AHI. Data from older machines are transferred through smart card, cable connectors, or modems to compliance software that tracks usage patterns. Increasingly, compliance data is updated almost continuously to cloud-based platforms and can be accessed wirelessly by providers. Patients may use web-based portals and phone apps to track their own patterns and access more information about their therapy.

Interventions to improve PAP compliance are based on patient education and behavioral principles of positive reinforcement and empowerment. These include education about OSA and the benefits of treatment, addressing patient-perceived problems, familial and/or group support, regular compliance checks, and clinic follow-ups.

Nonadherence to nasal PAP therapy can be attributed to noise, inconvenience, partner intolerance, mask leak, skin abrasions, claustrophobia, aerophagia, epistaxis, improper fit of equipment, and incomplete resolution of symptoms. Finding an interface that is well fitting, leak free, and maximally comfortable to the patient is critical to patient acceptance of PAP. Extra time should be taken to find the correct interface because a poor fitting, uncomfortable interface can cause a patient to refuse PAP therapy. Adding heated humidification has been shown to prevent discomfort and dryness and increase compliance while using nasal CPAP (79). It is important to maximize airflow through the nasal airway by treating allergies and congestion. Nasal swelling and secretions create narrowing and resistance to nasal airflow. The AHI in patients with chronic nasal congestion can be reduced with the use of topical corticosteroids (80, 81).

Effective PAP therapy reduces SDB and improves nocturnal oxygenation, sleep architecture, daytime sleepiness, neurocognitive performance, driving performance, and perceived health status (82, 83). Although oxygen therapy is sometimes used in conjunction with PAP therapy to address comorbid respiratory disorders, oxygen therapy alone is not an approved treatment for OSA. Although hypoxemia caused by SDB can improve from supplemental oxygen, hypercapnia can worsen in patients with respiratory disease. Additionally, the arousal response to SDB can be impeded, thus lengthening apneas (84). Cardiovascular endpoints, such as hypertension, cardiac arrhythmia, nocturnal ischemia, left ventricular function, and mortality, may also improve with PAP therapy (83). Health care utilization is also reduced in OSA patients on PAP therapy compared with untreated patients.

Oral Appliances

Oral appliances can be used in mild-to-moderate cases of OSA, with a success rate of up to 52% (85). Dentists and orthodontists who specialize in sleep medicine assess the patient for eligibility for the appliance by evaluating jaw and dental structure. The dental appliances are made after taking an impression of the bite. The appliances are worn during sleep and work by bringing the tongue and jaw forward to increase the posterior airway space and prevent airway collapse (86, 87). Adjustments are made to advance the jaw forward until the patient reports improvements in symptoms. Side effects may include jaw stiffness or significant temporomandibular joint pain. The devices require some original teeth in patients with dentures for proper fit. Elderly people who have fewer original teeth will have difficulty tolerating the appliances and may not be good candidates. Because of the variable success rate, patients should have a repeat sleep study after the final adjustment to ensure satisfactory therapeutic benefit (88).

Nasal Expiratory Resistance Devices

Nasal valves that build negative back pressure to maintain patency of the airway during expiration can be trialed on patients with mild-to-moderate OSA. These nasal expiratory resistance devices adhere to the nares and restrict expiratory airflow, increasing pressure in the airway during expiration to keep the airway open and reduce snoring. There are variable results from these devices; generally, an improvement in respiratory disturbance is seen, even without improvements in objective sleep quality. Some patients find the sensation of breathing against the nasal valves uncomfortable, but when tolerated, a lowered AHI and snoring reduction or elimination can be seen. There are no known predictors of patient types that will tolerate or respond well to the device, so trials of the device and follow-up on the efficacy of the device are indicated.

Surgical Management

Surgery can be considered when there is an anatomic obstruction that compromises the airway, when other effective treatments have failed (PAP, oral appliance), or when the patient cannot accept or tolerate other therapies. It is important that the airway is examined to determine if there are sites of possible surgical correction. The risks, potential side effects, complications, and success rates must be communicated to the patient considering surgical intervention. There are three main areas of obstruction that are amenable to surgical correction: the nose, soft tissue of the upper airway (tongue, uvula, and soft palate), and jaw.

Nasal Reconstruction

Deviated septum, nasal valve collapse, and turbinate enlargement can commonly produce resistance to airflow and are amenable to surgical correction. Radiofrequency treatment of the turbinate is a short outpatient procedure. The success rate for eliminating OSA with these procedures is low, but they can also be helpful for patients who are using PAP but have compromised nasal flow because of obstruction.

Pharyngeal Surgery

In children with sleep-related breathing, there is a high surgical success rate for adenotonsillectomy. Adults with enlarged tonsils and OSA may benefit from surgical removal, but the success rate is lower. Tonsils can be so large that they actually meet in the middle and can make PAP therapy unviable. If tonsils are still present in adulthood, they are usually removed as part of palate surgery.

The uvulopalatopharyngoplasty (UPPP), initially introduced for the treatment of snoring, is the most common OSA surgical procedure. It may also be a component of multistep procedures, which increase surgical effectiveness. The UPPP involves removal of the uvula, tonsils, and tonsillar pillars along with the lower part of the soft palate. Success rates are variable (up to 55%). Uvulopalatal flap is a more conservative surgery, with less pain during recovery (89).

Radiofrequency ablation (RFA) to reduce the size of the soft palate can be considered for patients with mild-to-moderate OSA to reduce the AHI. The average postprocedure AHI after RFA was 14.9, consistent with residual mild OSA. RFA studies have shown improvement in EDS and, in one study, QOL (90).

Genioglossus advancement and hyoid myotomy (GAHM) is a procedure that moves the tongue forward to enlarge the hypopharyngeal space. This surgery can be performed along with palatal surgery as part of phase I surgery in a multiphase process. In a study where just the GAHM was performed, 61% of patients were deemed successfully treated. If phase II is performed (maxillomandibular advancement [MMA]), the success rate rises to 97% (91).

Palatal implants are designed to stiffen the palate and reduce snoring. Dacron rods are inserted into the soft palate to make it more rigid. This procedure can be performed under local anesthesia. There are little data on the efficacy of this procedure.

Maxillomandibular Advancement

MMA is one of the most successful surgical interventions for OSA. It involves cutting and advancing the upper and lower jaw bones, which can enlarge the posterior airway space up to 12 mm. In an analysis of nine case studies following primary MMA surgery, there was an overall reduction in AHI of 87% with a mean postoperative AHI of 7.7 (91). MMA can also be considered for patients with OSA and craniofacial developmental abnormalities resulting in a small jaw (micrognathia and retrognathia).

Tracheotomy

Tracheotomy was once a primary treatment for OSA (before the invention of CPAP). According to the *AASM Practice Parameter for the Surgical Modifications of the Upper Airway for Obstructive Sleep Apnea in Adults*, "Tracheostomy has been shown to be an effective single intervention to treat OSA. This operation should be considered only when other options do not exist, have failed, are refused, or when this operation is deemed necessary by clinical urgency" (90).

Implantable Upper Airway Stimulation

An implanted nerve stimulator targeting the hypoglossal nerve has recently been introduced for the treatment of moderate-to-severe OSA. A lead in the chest monitors respiration and triggers mild stimulation of the hypoglossal nerve when inspiration is detected. This stimulation helps maintain airway patency by activating the genioglossus muscle. Presurgical evaluation includes phenotyping for the pattern of collapse that occurs during obstructed breathing, with complete concentric collapse at the soft palate a contraindication to this type of treatment. This device is considered a nonfirst-line OSA treatment and requires an ENT physician for placement and management of the device along with management by the sleep specialist. Patients must have tried and been intolerant of PAP therapy for at least 3 months to be candidates for the device, and it is generally recommended that ideal patients have a BMI of less than 32 (Sleep Review, February 2016). A multicenter, prospective, single-group cohort design study showed that upper airway stimulation led to significant objective and subjective improvements in OSA severity (92).

NEW AREAS OF RESEARCH

Research in OSA continues in many areas. One is understanding the impact of untreated OSA on health and well-being. Active areas of study include metabolic and neurologic consequences of SDB, impact of OSA on learning and development in children, and the role of SDB in the development of visual problems. Another area is new treatment options, including new surgeries and medications as well as refinements and improvements in current treatments such as PAP. Another exciting area is work on utilizing personalized medicine in sleep disorders. Multiple mechanisms contribute to airway collapse in OSA, including airway anatomy, muscle function, and individual responses to physiologic changes such as hypoxemia or hypercapnia. By identifying the specific mechanism, called "phenotyping," it will be possible to apply the precise treatment option to address that mechanism, thereby improving effectiveness and tolerance of therapy.

SUMMARY

OSA is a common disorder that has a huge impact on individual health and the public health system, but can be managed by sleep professionals to reduce a patient's risk of death, major cardiovascular morbidity, cerebrovascular events, and motor vehicle accidents and to reduce symptoms and improve QOL.

REFERENCES

1. Guilleminault, C., Tilkian, A., & Dement, W. C. (1976). The sleep apnea syndromes. *Annual Review of Medicine, 27*, 465–484.
2. American Academy of Sleep Medicine. (2014). *International classification of sleep disorders: Diagnostic and coding manual* (3rd ed.). Darien, IL: Author.
3. Watanabe, T., Isono, S., Tanaka, A., et al. (2002). Contribution of body habitus and craniofacial characteristics to segmental closing pressures of the passive pharynx in patients with sleep-disordered breathing. *American Journal of Respiratory and Critical Care Medicine, 165*, 260–265.
4. Young, T., Palta, M., Dempsey, J., et al. (1993). The occurrence of sleep-related breathing among middle-aged adults. *New England Journal of Medicine, 328*, 1230–1235.
5. Peppard, P. E., Young, T., Barnet, J. H., et al. (2013). Increased prevalence of sleep-disordered breathing in adults. *American Journal of Epidemiology, 177*(9), 1006–1014.
6. Redline, S. (1998). Epidemiology of sleep-disordered breathing. *Seminars in Respiratory and Critical Care Medicine, 19*, 113–122.
7. Peppard, P. E., Young, T., Palta, M., et al. (2000). Longitudinal study of moderate weight change and sleep-disordered breathing. *The Journal of the American Medical Association, 284*, 3015–3021.
8. Tuomilehto, H. P., Seppa, J. M., Partinen, M. M., et al.; Kuopio Sleep Apnea Group. (2009). Lifestyle intervention with weight reduction: First-line treatment in mild obstructive sleep apnea. *American Journal of Respiratory and Critical Care Medicine, 179*, 320–327.
9. Redline, S., Kump, K., Tishler, P. V., et al. (1994). Gender differences in sleep disordered breathing in a community-based sample. *American Journal of Respiratory and Critical Care Medicine, 149*, 722–726.
10. Young, T., Shahar, E., Nieto, F. J., et al. (2002). Predictors of sleep-disordered breathing in community dwelling adults: The Sleep Heart Health Study. *Archives of Internal Medicine, 162*, 893–900.
11. Bixler, E. O., Vgontzas, A. N., Lin, H. M., et al. (2001). Prevalence of sleep-disordered breathing in women: Effects of gender. *American Journal of Respiratory and Critical Care Medicine, 163*, 608–613.
12. Ancoli-Israel, S., Kripke, D. F., Klauber, M. R., et al. (1991). Sleep disordered breathing in community dwelling elderly. *Sleep, 14*(6), 486–495.
13. Ancoli-Israel, S., & Coy, T. (1994). Are breathing disturbances in elderly equivalent to sleep apnea syndrome? *Sleep, 17*, 77–83.
14. Young, T. (1996). Sleep-disordered breathing in older adults: Is it a condition distinct from that in middle-aged adults? *Sleep, 19*, 529–530.
15. Young, T., Peppard, P., & Gottlieb, D. (2002). Epidemiology of obstructive sleep apnea: A population health perspective. *American Journal of Respiratory and Critical Care Medicine, 165*, 1217–1239.
16. Redline, S., Tishler, P., Hans, M., et al. (1997). Racial differences in sleep-disordered breathing in African-Americans and Caucasians. *American Journal of Respiratory and Critical Care Medicine, 155*, 186–192.
17. Ancoli-Israel, S., Klauber, M. R., Stepnowsky, C., et al. (1995). Sleep-disordered breathing in African-American elderly. *American Journal of Respiratory and Critical Care Medicine, 152*, 1946–1949.
18. Lee, R. W., Vasudevan, S., Hui, D. S., et al. (2010). Differences in craniofacial structures and obesity in Caucasian and Chinese patients with obstructive sleep apnea. *Sleep, 33*(8), 1075–1080.
19. Trois, M. S., Capone, G. T., Lutz, J. A., et al. (2009). Obstructive sleep apnea in adults with Down syndrome. *Journal of Clinical Sleep Medicine, 15*, 317–323.
20. Redline, S., Tishler, P. V., Tosteson, T. D., et al. (1995). The familial aggregation of obstructive sleep apnea.

American Journal of Respiratory and Critical Care Medicine, 151, 682–687.

21. Wetter, D. W., Young, T. B., Bidwell, T. R., et al. (1994). Smoking as a risk factor for sleep-disordered breathing. *Archives of Internal Medicine, 154,* 2219–2224.

22. Taasan, V. C., Block, A. J., Boysen, P. G., et al. (1981). Alcohol increases sleep apnea and oxygen desaturation in asymptomatic men. *American Journal of Medicine, 71,* 240–245.

23. Krol, R. C., Knuth, S. L., & Bartlett, D., Jr. (1984). Selective reduction of genioglossal muscle activity by alcohol in normal human subjects. *American Review of Respiratory Disease, 129,* 247–250.

24. Scrima, L., Broudy, M., Nay, K. N., et al. (1982). Increased severity of obstructive sleep apnea after bedtime alcohol ingestion: Diagnostic potential and proposed mechanism of action. *Sleep, 5,* 318–328.

25. Sahin, F. K., Koken, G., Cosar, E., et al. (2008). Obstructive sleep apnea in pregnancy and fetal outcome. *International Journal of Gynecology and Obstetrics, 100*(2), 141–146.

26. Guilleminault, C., Connoly, S. J., & Winkle, R. A. (1983). Cardiac arrhythmia and conduction disturbances during sleep in 400 patients with sleep apnea syndrome. *American Journal of Cardiology, 52,* 490–494.

27. Punjabi, N. M., Newman, A., Young, T., et al. (2008). Sleep-disordered breathing and cardiovascular disease: An outcome-based definition of hypopneas. *American Journal of Respiratory and Critical Care Medicine, 177,* 1150–1155.

28. Shahar, E., Whitney, C. W., Redline, S., et al. (2001). Sleep-disordered breathing and cardiovascular disease: Cross-sectional results of the Sleep Heart Health Study. *American Journal of Respiratory and Critical Care Medicine, 163,* 19–25.

29. Bassiri, A., & Guilleminault, C. (2000). Clinical features and evaluation of obstructive sleep apnea-hypopnea syndrome. In M. Kryger, T. Roth, & W. Dement (Eds.), *Principles and practice of sleep medicine* (3rd ed., pp. 869–878). Philadelphia, PA: W.B. Saunders Company.

30. Somers, V., & Fletcher, E. (2002). Mechanisms of hypertension in obstructive sleep apnea. In A. Pack (Ed.), *Sleep apnea pathogenesis diagnosis and treatment* (pp. 353–376). New York, NY: Marcel Dekker.

31. Hla, K. M., Young, T. B., Bidwell, T., et al. (1994). Sleep apnea and hypertension. A population based study. *Annals of Internal Medicine, 120,* 382–388.

32. Nieto, F. J., Young, T. B., Lind, B. K., et al. (2000). Association of sleep-disordered breathing, sleep apnea, and hypertension in a large community-based study. *The Journal of the American Medical Association, 283,* 1829–1836.

33. Singh, J. P., Larson, M. G., Tsuji, H., et al. (1998). Reduced heart rate variability and new-onset hypertension: Insights into pathogenesis of hypertension: The Framingham Heart Study. *Hypertension, 32,* 293–297.

34. Koehler, U., Fus, E., Grimm, W., et al. (1998). Heart block in patients with obstructive sleep apnoea: Pathogenetic factors and effects of treatment. *The European Respiratory Journal, 11*(2), 434–439.

35. Mehra, R., Benjamin, E. J., Shahar, E., et al. (2006). Association of nocturnal arrhythmias with sleep-disordered breathing: The Sleep Heart Health Study. *American Journal of Respiratory and Critical Care Medicine, 173,* 910–916.

36. Harbison, J., O'Reilly, P., & McNicholas, W. T. (2000). Cardiac rhythm disturbances in the obstructive sleep apnea syndrome: Effects of nasal continuous positive airway pressure therapy. *Chest, 118,* 591–595.

37. Ryan, C. M., Usui, K., Floras, J. S., et al. (2005). Effect of continuous positive airway pressure on ventricular ectopy in heart failure patients with obstructive sleep apnoea. *Thorax, 60,* 781–785.

38. Kanagala, R., Murali, N. S., Friedman, P. A., et al. (2003). Obstructive sleep apnea and the recurrence of atrial fibrillation. *Circulation, 107,* 2589–2594.

39. Javaheri, S., Parker, T. J., Liming, J. D., et al. (1998). Sleep apnea in 81 ambulatory male patients with stable heart failure. Types and their prevalences, consequences, and presentations. *Circulation, 97,* 2154–2159.

40. Javaheri, S. (2003). Heart failure and sleep apnea. Emphasis on practical therapeutic options. *Clinics in Chest Medicine, 24*(2), 207–222.

41. D'Alessandro, R., Magelli, C., Gamberini, G., et al. (1990). Snoring every night as a risk factor for myocardial infarction: A case–control study. *British Medical Journal, 300,* 1557–1558.

42. Mooe, T., Rabben, T., Wiklund, U., et al. (1996). Sleep-disordered breathing in men with coronary artery disease. *Chest, 109,* 659–663.

43. Mooe, T., Rabben, T., Wiklund, U., et al. (1996). Sleep-disordered breathing in women: Occurrence and association with coronary artery disease. *The American Journal of Medicine, 101,* 251–256.

44. Kuniyoshi, F. H., Singh, P., Gami, A. S., et al. (2011). Post-myocardial infarction patients with obstructive sleep apnea exhibit impaired endothelial function. *Chest, 140*(1), 62–67.

45. Good, D. C., Henkle, J. Q., Gelber, D., et al. (1996). Sleep-disordered breathing and poor functional after stroke. *Stroke, 27,* 252–259.

46. Wessendorf, T. E., Dahm, C., & Teschler, H. (2003). Prevalence and clinical importance of sleep apnea in the first night after cerebral infarction. *Neurology, 60,* 1053.

47. Yaggi, H. K., Concato, J., Kernan, W. N., et al. (2005). Obstructive sleep apnea as a risk factor for stroke and death. *The New England Journal of Medicine, 353,* 2034–2041.

48. Gami, A. S., Howard, D. E., Olson, E. J., et al. (2005). Day-night pattern of sudden death in obstructive sleep apnea. *The New England Journal of Medicine, 352,* 1206–1214.

49. Punjabi, N. M., & Polotsky, V. Y. (2005). Disorders of glucose metabolism in sleep apnea. *Journal of Applied Physiology, 99,* 1998–2007.

50. Punjabi, N. M., Ahmed, M. M., Polotsky, V. Y., et al. (2003). Sleep-disordered breathing, glucose intolerance, and insulin resistance. *Respiratory Physiology and Neurobiology, 136,* 167–178.

51. Tasali, E., Mokhlesi, B., & Van Cauter, E. (2008). Obstructive sleep apnea and type 2 diabetes: Interacting epidemics. *Chest, 133,* 496–506.

52. Ficker, J. H., Dertinger, S. H., Siegfried, W., et al. (1998). Obstructive sleep apnoea and diabetes mellitus: The role of cardiovascular autonomic neuropathy. *The European Respiratory Journal, 11,* 14–19.

53. Bottini, P., Dottorini, M. L., Cristina, C. M., et al. (2003). Sleep-disordered breathing in nonobese diabetic subjects with autonomic neuropathy. *The European Respiratory Journal, 22,* 654–660.

54. Wilcox, I., McNamara, S. G., Collins, F. L., et al. (1998). "Syndrome Z": The interaction of sleep apnoea, vascular risk factors and heart disease. *Thorax, 53*(Suppl. 3), S25–S28.

55. Emamian, F., Khazaie, H., Tahmasian, M., et al. (2016). The association between obstructive sleep apnea and Alzheimer's disease: A meta-analysis perspective. *Frontiers in Aging Neuroscience, 8,* 78.

56. Beebe, D. W., & Gozal, D. (2002). Obstructive sleep apnea and the prefrontal cortex: Towards a comprehensive model linking nocturnal upper airway obstruction to daytime cognitive and behavioral deficits. *Journal of Sleep Research, 11,* 1–16.

57. Sharma, R. A., Varga, A. W., Bubu, O. M., et al. (2018). Obstructive sleep apnea severity affects amyloid burden in cognitively normal elderly: A longitudinal study. *American Journal of Respiratory and Critical Care Medicine, 197,* 933–943.

58. Naegele, B., Launois, S. H., Mazza, S., et al. (2006). Which memory processes are affected in patients with obstructive sleep apnea? An evaluation of 3 types of memory. *Sleep, 29,* 533–544.

59. Zimmerman, M. E., Arndt, J. T., Stanchina, M., et al. (2006). Normalization of memory performance and positive airway pressure adherence in memory-impaired patients with obstructive sleep apnea. *Chest, 130,* 1772–1778.

60. Borak, J., Cieslicki, J. K., Koziej, M., et al. (1996). Effects of CPAP treatment on psychological status in patients with severe obstructive sleep apnoea. *Journal of Sleep Research, 5,* 123–127.

61. Flemons, W. W., & Tsai, W. (1997). Quality of life consequences of sleep disordered breathing. *The Journal of Allergy and Clinical Immunology, 99,* S750–S756.

62. Millman, R. P., Fogel, B. S., McNamara, M. E., et al. (1989). Depression as a manifestation of obstructive sleep apnea: Reversal with nasal continuous positive airway pressure. *The Journal of Clinical Psychiatry, 50,* 348–351.

63. Reynolds, C. F., III, Kupfer, D. J., McEachran, A. B., et al. (1984). Depressive psychopathology in male sleep apneics. *The Journal of Clinical Psychiatry, 45,* 287–290.

64. Sharafkhaneh, A., Giray, N., Richardson, P., et al. (2005). Association of psychiatric disorders and sleep apnea in a large cohort. *Sleep, 28*(11), 1405–1411.

65. Ohayon, M. M. (2003). The effects of breathing-related sleep disorders on mood disturbances in the general population. *The Journal of Clinical Psychiatry, 64,* 1195–1200.

66. Finn, L., Young, T. B., Palta, M., et al. (1998). Sleep-disordered breathing and self-reported general health status in the Wisconsin Sleep Cohort Study. *Sleep, 21,* 701–706.

67. Mallampati, S., Gugino, S., Desai, S., et al. (1985). A clinical sign to predict a difficult tracheal intubation: A prospective study. *Canadian Anesthesiologists' Society Journal, 32,* 429–434.

68. Owens, R. L., Gold, K. A., Gozal, D., et al. (2016). Sleep and breathing . . . and cancer? *Cancer Prevention Research, 9,* 821–827.

69. Young, T., Finn, L., Peppard, P. E., et al. (2008). Sleep disordered breathing and mortality: Eighteen-year follow-up of the Wisconsin sleep cohort. *Sleep, 31,* 1071–1078.

70. Berry, R. B., Albertario, C. L., Harding, S. M., et al.; for the American Academy of Sleep Medicine. (2018). *The AASM manual for the scoring of sleep and associated events: Rules, terminology and technical specifications.* Version 2.5. Darien, IL: American Academy of Sleep Medicine.

71. Collop, N. A., Anderson, W. M., Boehlecke, B., et al.; Portable Monitoring Task Force of the American Academy of Sleep Medicine. (2007). Clinical guidelines for the use of unattended portable monitors in the diagnosis of obstructive sleep apnea in adult patients. *Journal of Clinical Sleep Medicine, 3,* 737–747.

72. Guilleminault, C., Kirisoglu, C., da Rosa, A. C., et al. (2006). Sleepwalking, a disorder of NREM sleep instability. *Sleep Medicine, 7*(2), 163–170.

73. Guilleminault, C., Palombini, L., Pelayo, R., et al. (2003). Sleepwalking and night terrors in prepubertal children: What triggers them? *Pediatrics, 111,* e17–e25.

74. Issa, F. Q., & Sullivan, C. E. (1982). Alcohol, snoring and sleep apnoea. *Journal of Neurology, Neurosurgery, and Psychiatry, 45,* 353–359.

75. Guardiano, S. A., Scott, J. A., Ware, J. C., et al. (2003). The long-term results of gastric bypass on indexes of sleep apnea. *Chest, 124,* 1615–1619.

76. Rasheid, S., Banasiak, M., Gallagher, S. F., et al. (2003). Gastric bypass is an effective treatment for obstructive sleep apnea in patients with clinically significant obesity. *Obesity Surgery, 13,* 58–61.

77. Drager, L. F., Brunoni, A. R., Jenner, R., et al. (2015). Effects of CPAP on body weight in patients with obstructive sleep apnoea: A meta-analysis of randomised trials. *Thorax, 70,* 258–264.

78. Jokic, R., Klimaszewski, A., Crossley, M., et al. (1999). Positional treatment vs continuous positive airway pressure in patients with positional obstructive sleep apnea syndrome. *Chest, 115,* 771–781.

79. Massie, C. A., Hart, R. W., Peralez, K., et al. (1999). Effects of humidification on nasal symptoms and compliance in sleep apnea. *Chest, 116,* 403–408.

80. Kiely, J. L., Nolan, P., & McNicholas, W. T. (2004). Intranasal corticosteroid therapy for obstructive sleep apnoea in patients with co-existing rhinitis. *Thorax, 59,* 50–55.

81. Joe, S., & Benson, A. (2005). Nonallergic rhinitis. In C. W. Cummings (Ed.), *Otolaryngology: Head neck surgery* (pp. 996–999). Philadelphia, PA: Mosby.

82. Weaver, T. (2002). Adherence to continuous positive airway pressure treatment and functional status in adult obstructive sleep apnea. In A. Pack (Ed.), *Sleep apnea pathogenesis diagnosis and treatment* (pp. 523–554). New York, NY: Marcel Dekker.

83. Roux, F., & Hilbert, J. (2003). Continuous positive airway pressure: New generations. *Clinics in Chest Medicine, 24*(2), 315–342.

84. Epstein, L. J., Kristo, D., Strollo, P. J., Jr., et al. (2009). Clinical guideline for the evaluation, management and long-term care of obstructive sleep apnea in adults. Adult obstructive sleep apnea task force of the American Academy of Sleep Medicine. *Journal of Clinical Sleep Medicine, 5*(3), 263–276.

85. Ferguson, K. A., Cartwright, R., Rogers, R., et al. (2006). Oral appliances for snoring and obstructive sleep apnea: A review. *Sleep, 29*(2), 244–262.

86. Lowe, A. (2000). Oral appliances for sleep breathing disorders. In M. Kryger, T. Roth, & W. Dement (Eds.), *Principles and practice of sleep medicine* (3rd ed., pp. 929–939). Philadelphia, PA: W.B. Saunders Company.

87. Lowe, A., & Schmidt-Nowara, W. (2002). Oral appliance therapy for snoring and sleep apnea. In A. Pack (Ed.), *Sleep apnea pathogenesis diagnosis and treatment* (pp. 555–573). New York, NY: Marcel Dekker.

88. Ramar, K., Dort, L. C., Katz, S. G., et al. (2015). Clinical practice guideline for the treatment of obstructive sleep apnea and snoring with oral appliance therapy: An update for 2015. *Journal of Clinical Sleep Medicine, 11*(7), 773–827.

89. Malhotra, A., Crowley, S., Pillar, G., et al. (2000). Age-related changes in pharyngeal structure and function in normal subjects [Abstract]. *Sleep, 161*(2), A42.

90. Aurora, R. N., Casey, K. R., Kristo, D., et al. (2010). Practice parameters for the surgical modifications of the upper airway for obstructive sleep apnea in adults. *Sleep, 33*(10), 1408–1413.

91. Caples, S. M., Rowley, J. A., Prinsell, J. R., et al. (2010). Surgical modifications of the upper airway for obstructive sleep apnea in adults: A systematic review and meta-analysis. *Sleep, 33*(10), 1396–1407.

92. Strollo, P. J., Jr., Soose, R. J., Maurer, J. T., et al.; STAR Trial Group. (2014). Upper-airway stimulation for obstructive sleep apnea. *New England Journal of Medicine, 370*(2), 139–149.

chapter 13
Central Sleep Apnea

LAURA A. LINLEY

LEARNING OBJECTIVES

On completion of this chapter, the reader should be able to:

1. Describe the clinical presentation of central sleep apnea (CSA).
2. Define the two different conditions contributing to CSA.
3. Explain the respiratory drive mechanisms of sleep.
4. Review physiologically normal apneic events.
5. Summarize the presentation of Cheyne–Stokes respiration, primary CSA, and treatment-emergent CSA.
6. Outline the patient evaluation procedure/differential diagnosis and workup.
7. Review the polysomnographic findings of CSA.
8. Cite the treatment goals and options for CSA.

KEY TERMS

Central sleep apnea
Treatment-emergent central sleep apnea
Hypercapnia
Hypoventilation
Cheyne–Stokes respiration
Congestive heart failure
Central nervous system (CNS) dysfunction
PAP therapy
Adaptive servo-ventilation

Central sleep apnea (CSA) is a disorder of decreased breathing rate or depth during the sleep period because of a transient reduction or withdrawal of central neural output to the respiratory muscles (the diaphragm and intercostal muscles) (1, 2). There is an instability of ventilation control at sleep onset, and respiratory irregularity and abnormal breathing patterns can arise during this time. The respiratory drive centers respond differently to levels of oxygen and carbon dioxide (CO_2) during sleep and wakefulness.

The prevalence of CSA in clinical practice is less than that of obstructive apnea, constituting 5% to 10% of all sleep apnea cases (except in very premature infants, in whom it is seen fairly commonly because of their relatively immature or underdeveloped central respiratory control centers) (1, 3). A few short central apneas (CAs) are not uncommon, particularly following a deep breath such as with a sigh or yawn.

Sleep apnea is described as an interruption of airflow for 10 seconds or more during sleep, associated with significant oxygen desaturation (2). In CSA, the patient's airway remains patent, and there are no accompanying chest and abdomen movements (1, 2).

SLEEP RESPIRATORY DRIVE MECHANISMS

Sleep respiratory function is driven by the bulbar respiratory center, which reacts to metabolic, mechanic, and behavioral influences. Metabolic regulation is exerted by changes in PO_2 and PCO_2: Increased PCO_2 stimulates the bulbar center, whereas a critical reduction in PCO_2 inhibits it. Ventilation drive is also increased with decreased levels of PO_2.

Mechanical (autonomic) regulation is under the control of pulmonary vagal receptors and can, if stimulated, give rise to reflex hyperventilation. Behavioral regulation of breathing is typical during the awake state. Behavioral regulation reacts to changing patterns of breathing such as seen during talking or with exercise. Ventilation will respond to behavioral inputs only during wake, not during nonrapid eye movement (NREM) sleep. It is thought that the reason for this is that the receptors for behavior regulation are in the forebrain and are not active during NREM sleep (4). PCO_2 during sleep decreases temporarily to below the critical level that is necessary to keep the respiratory rhythm normal.

There are many causes for loss of central respiratory impulse during sleep. Metabolic control and neuromuscular failure may cause chronic alveolar hypoventilation syndrome that worsens during sleep when the stimulating effect of wakefulness is absent (4, 5). CSA may also be caused by a transient instability of the respiratory drive that is otherwise undamaged: When the stimulating effect of wakefulness (neural wakefulness impulse) on respiration is lacking, then the apneic episode begins and continues until the PCO_2 critical level is reached (2).

Sleep affects respiration primarily at sleep onset when PCO_2 oscillates around the hypocapnic threshold (6, 7). Thus, CSA occurs with hypocapnia, and it ceases with arousal and hyperventilation. Subsequently recurring hypocapnia leads to a new apneic episode when sleep is resumed (8). Posthyperventilation CSA is less common during rapid eye movement (REM) sleep (9, 10).

RISK FACTORS

Several physiologic and pathologic factors increase the risk of CSA, including age, sex, and many medical conditions. The threshold for hypocapnic CSA is higher in males, and CSA is rare in premenopausal women (11). Disorders such as thyroid dysfunction, cerebrovascular disease, acromegaly, renal failure, congestive heart failure (CHF), and atrial fibrillation may increase susceptibility to the development of CSA in older patients (12, 13).

CSA comprises 40% of apneas that develop following a cerebrovascular accident (CVA). The brainstem is the primary center for ventilation control, so any damage occurring there or to the medullary area from a CVA could impact regular respiration during sleep (14).

Over the last decade, there has been a dramatic change in the way chronic pain has been managed. The American Academy of Pain Medicine (AAPM) and the American Pain Society issued a joint position statement in 1997 stating, "It is now accepted by practitioners of the specialty of pain medicine that respiratory depression induced by opioids tends to be a short-lived phenomenon, generally occurs only in the opioid-naive patient, and is antagonized by pain. Therefore, withholding the appropriate use of opioids from a patient who is experiencing pain on the basis of respiratory concerns is unwarranted" (15). Ever since this statement was made, there have been multiple studies demonstrating an association of opioids with sleep apnea. Opioid use for pain management has increased, resulting in a rise in opioid-associated morbidity and mortality. The AAPM updated its statement on the *Use of Opioids for the Treatment of Chronic Pain* (15). Position 3 of that statement indicates: "Physicians should be sensitive to and seek to minimize the risks of addiction, respiratory depression and other adverse effects, tolerance and diversion" (15). The statement cautions titration of opioid medications in patients with underlying diagnoses such as sleep apnea (specifically CSA) or end-stage respiratory disease due to the increased risk of cardiorespiratory events. CSA occurs in 30% of patients undergoing stable methadone (opioid) maintenance treatment (15). The concern is that some patients present with CSA without any apparent risk factors. In these cases of "idiopathic" CSA, increased chemoresponsiveness

or sleep state instability could be responsible for the irregularity in breathing patterns. Occasionally, these patients may have a theretofore undiagnosed metabolic or cardiac disorder (16, 17). Although CAs are commonly observed during initial polysomnography (PSG), they may be absent initially and appear during continuous positive airway pressure (CPAP) titration and present as treatment-emergent CSA. Central events that persisted with the use of CPAP or bilevel devices required more advanced therapy such as adaptive servo-ventilation (ASV) (18).

ETIOLOGY AND PATHOPHYSIOLOGY

There are two general categories of disorders that cause the central nervous system (CNS) respiratory control system to decrease output to the respiratory muscles:

1. Disorders that cause defects to the system itself (CSA with abnormal respiratory control system)
2. Disorders outside the system that cause a normal system to reduce its output (CSA with normal respiratory control system) (3)

The first condition leads to hypoventilation and CSA and is found in patients with diseases involving the brainstem, neuromuscular disorders, and central hypoventilation syndromes. These disorders involve a chemical or neural change that causes a normal control system to alternate between stimulating breathing and inhibiting breathing. Patients are not apneic while awake because the waking neural drive stimulates breathing. With sleep, loss of the CNS drive may cause apnea to occur. These apneas disappear as sleep becomes deeper. When the respiratory control system is impaired by brainstem disease or an abnormal chemical drive to breathe, withdrawal of the waking stimulus results in a profound decrease in neural drive. Transient apneas may occur upon initiation of sleep, when relative waking hypocapnia triggers a central apneic event.

The pathophysiology of CSA invokes two key mechanisms (9). One is a tendency for baseline hypoventilation with hypercapnia to place breathing controllers closer to the apneic threshold during NREM sleep. The second is delayed circulation time from the lung to the chemoreceptors in the carotid artery, with destabilization and overshoot of feedback control, seen in low cardiac output states. This may be associated with a destabilization of the feedback control of breathing with delayed overshoot in the ventilatory response to stimuli. Prolonged periods of CA or hypopnea (underbreathing in response to hypocapnic hyperventilation) alternate with exaggerated periods of ventilation (overbreathing and arousals in response to apnea), perpetuating a cycle of hyperventilatory overshoot and subsequent CAs.

In various studies of cardiac patients with an ejection fraction less than 45%, the prevalence of sleep apnea in patients undergoing PSG was 40% to 68%. The majority of these cardiac patients exhibited CSA with high levels of sleep disruption, repetitive oxygen desaturation episodes, and more nocturnal dysrhythmias than did nonapneic patients with similar levels of left ventricular dysfunction.

Excessive daytime sleepiness, as assessed by the Epworth Sleepiness Scale and by lower scores on multiple sleep latency testing, is a common problem for patients with repetitive CSA. Over the past decade, the diagnosis and management of obstructive sleep apnea (OSA) has received considerable attention in sleep medicine. Its impact on daytime cognitive function and cardiovascular health is increasingly recognized and its frequency in the adult population (2% to 4%) renders it the most common pathologic diagnosis in sleep centers. Cardiac patients with left ventricular dysfunction and Cheyne–Stokes respiration (CSR) with CSA are also prevalent. Mounting evidence suggests that this diagnosis may have important implications for the outcome and management of chronic CHF (19, 20).

Periodic CSR is present in about 30% to 40% of CHF patients, worsening their prognostic outcome. Its presence indicates a shorter survival compared with CHF patients who do not exhibit CSR. Pulmonary congestion in a recumbent position induces reflex hyperventilation, with critical reduction of PCO_2 that causes apneic episodes. Cessation of breathing increases blood PCO_2 stimulating bulbar centers and leads to resumption of breathing (21). The slowing of blood circulation contributes to CSR as a result of the delay of blood gas concentration information reaching the respiratory center. It is, however, unclear if CSR–CSA is simply a reflection of severely compromised cardiac function with elevated left ventricular filling pressure or if CSR–CSA itself exerts unique and independent pathologic effects on the failing myocardium. Regardless of its etiology, there is evidence that CSR–CSA may have detrimental physiologic effects on the failing heart (22).

In CSA, upper respiratory airways remain patent and apneic episodes end with a different mechanism than the arousal seen with OSA. In fact, arousals seen with CSA generally occur together with the recovery of breathing activity. Arousal occurs with hyperventilation and gives rise to a vicious circle.

Patients with OSA convert to CSA and vice versa. Deterioration of left ventricular contractile function because of OSA may create conditions that lead to the emergence of pathophysiologic CSR. In turn, CSA makes the CHF prognosis worse, even if the mechanism of this phenomenon is still not clear (23). See Figure 13-1 for an example of Cheyne–Stokes respirations.

The diagnosis of CSR requires overnight PSG performed in a sleep center. It has been reported that mortality over a 3-year period is 56% in CHF patients with CSA compared with 11% in patients without CSA, despite comparable left ventricular function. More recently, studies in 62 CHF patients with left ventricular

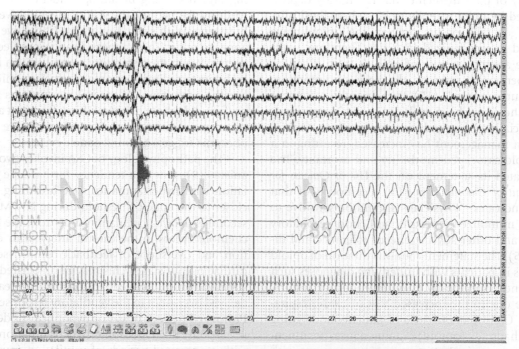

Figure 13-1 Cheyne–Stokes respirations. There is a crescendo–decrescendo breathing pattern during each breathing cycle, which drops the carbon dioxide levels below the "apnea threshold," causing central apnea.

dysfunction demonstrated that apnea–hypopnea index was the most powerful independent predictor of survival (24).

TREATMENT-EMERGENT CSA

Treatment-emergent CSA (formerly referred to as complex sleep apnea) is characterized by the combined phenomena of both OSA (respiratory drive and respiratory muscle activity are present, but airways are obstructed) and CSA. In many studies, treatment-emergent CA is defined as the development of CSA in the OSA patient during the initial CPAP titration. Patients with treatment-emergent CSA can have persistent sleep fragmentation and central events on CPAP treatment, predominately in N1 and N2 sleep while breathing normalizes in N3 and REM. Note that there have been reports of treatment-emergent CSA developing with other treatment modalities for OSA including tracheostomy,

maxillomandibular advancement, and oral appliance treatment (25). ASV is an advanced positive pressure therapy option for normalizing central events (26).

The pathophysiology of treatment-emergent CSA is not clearly defined. Treatment with excessive positive airway pressure (PAP) may trigger events in patients with a low arousal threshold where increased arousals destabilize breathing. Further study is needed to verify factors that predispose a patient to developing treatment-emergent CSA.

CLINICAL PICTURE

The clinical features of CSA are directly related in the cardiorespiratory and nervous systems. Figure 13-2 shows examples of CA events.

Frequent arousals cause frequent sleep disturbances. Both slow-wave sleep and REM sleep are reduced. CSA can be divided into two groups: hypercapnic CSA and nonhypercapnic CSA. Hypercapnic CSA with alveolar

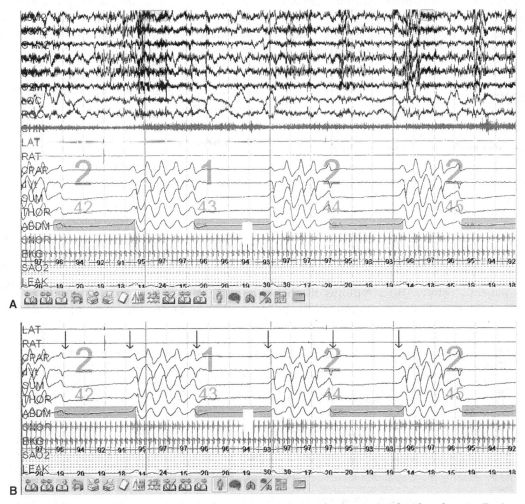

Figure 13-2 A: Central apnea. Notice the low oxygen saturation that is associated with each event. During a central apnea, there is a complete loss of diaphragmatic and intercostal activity, with resumption of activity when breathing begins. **B:** The arrows denote the beginning and end of the central apneic event.

hypoventilation is idiopathic and is caused by diseases in the brainstem or secondary to neuromuscular disorders, such as myopathies, motor neuron disorders, and neuromuscular junction disorders. People with idiopathic central alveolar hypoventilation have severe daytime hypoventilation without lung disease or any known lesions in the nervous system. Chemical control of breathing is absent in these patients. People with brainstem abnormalities have no control for breathing because of disorders in the medulla, such as infarction, tumor, or hemorrhage. These may cause a true hypoventilation syndrome.

Central hypoventilation (Fig. 13-3) is a disorder of decreased breathing rate or volume. This may cause daytime sleepiness and, if significant, may cause elevated blood pressure in the lungs (pulmonary hypertension) (21). There is a complete cessation of breathing during sleep with CSA. Individuals with Prader–Willi syndrome may be at increased risk for death because of a decreased neural drive for breathing.

Myopathies are neuromuscular disorders that include a large number of disorders such as muscular dystrophies and metabolic myopathies. Postpolio patients may become symptomatic 30 to 40 years after recovering. Some apparently healthy men may develop insomnia, which can stem from a nonhypercapnic CSA.

DIAGNOSIS

CSA diagnosis is based on technical documentation, PSG findings, and cardiorespiratory monitoring of apneic events. In this manner, it is possible to define sleep breathing characteristics and obtain indexes useful to quantify the gravity of the sleep-related clinical picture (24). These indexes, together with the underlying comorbidities, guide therapy (24).

Evaluation includes history, physical examination, and laboratory testing. Snoring, apneas, sleepiness, neurologic, cardiovascular, and renal history should be included in the patient's history. Also, symptoms of other disorders that cause sleepiness or insomnia, such as narcolepsy, periodic limb movements in sleep, insufficient sleep, and drug abuse or medication side effects, should be reviewed. During the physical examination, a general inspection of the skeletal structure of the face can be useful to observe if the upper or lower jaws are too far back (retrognathic) or too small (micrognathic). The nasal airway should also be examined for patency and for anatomic obstruction (deformity, deviation, polyps). Examination of the oral airway may give information about the size of tonsils, configuration of palate and uvula, and any other obstructing mass lesion. Cardiovascular examination can be useful to check for the presence of heart murmurs, peripheral blood hypertension, and cor pulmonale. Some tests may be needed to diagnose the medical disorders that may cause CSA, whereas others may be needed to document the location of a CNS lesion. Apnea itself can be confirmed by a sleep study. Other tests may include imaging, chest radiographs, pulmonary function tests, and blood gases.

The American Academy of Sleep Medicine (AASM) has updated the classification of sleep disorders in the *International Classification of Sleep Disorders*, 3rd edition (27). Within this classification, there is an expanded definition of CSA associated with other identifiable etiologies along with updated ICD-10-CM codes. These include the following:

R06.3 Central Sleep Apnea with Cheyne–Stokes Breathing

G47.37 Central Apnea Due to a Medical Disorder without Cheyne–Stokes Breathing

G47.32 Central Sleep Apnea Due to a High-Altitude Periodic Breathing

G47.39 Central Sleep Apnea Due to a Medication or Substance

G47.31 Primary Central Sleep Apnea

P28.3 Primary Central Sleep Apnea of Infancy

P28.4 Primary Central Sleep Apnea of Prematurity

G47.39 Treatment-Emergent Central Sleep Apnea

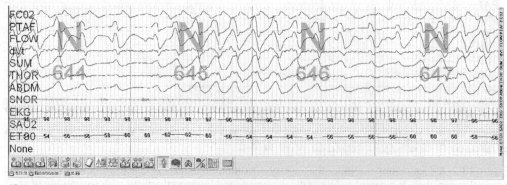

Figure 13-3 Hypoventilation verified by increasing end-tidal carbon dioxide levels.

PSG FINDINGS

CSA syndrome is characterized by a cessation or reduction of ventilatory effort and cessation of airflow during sleep and is usually associated with oxygen desaturation. Full PSG is required to properly diagnose CSA disorders. To adequately score a CA event, there must be no recorded respiratory effort. The recommended sensor for detection of respiratory effort is esophageal manometry, dual thoracoabdominal calibrated or uncalibrated respiratory inductance plethysmography (RIP) belts, or dual thoracoabdominal polyvinylidene fluoride. Piezo crystal belts are not recommended. If there is a complete lack of movement in the RIP channel, you can deduce that the event is central in nature (22, 27). If transitional central events seem to be inhibiting sleep onset, noting this in the technical observations is important. Figure 13-4 is an example of a sleep-onset CA.

The PSG montage should include the recording of electroencephalogram, body position, movement events, cardiac abnormalities, and respiratory events. Appropriate system calibrations, observation, and documentation by the technologist during the PSG are required. To be considered a clinical event in adults, a CA is defined as a minimum of 10 seconds of cessation of breathing effort and airflow. Scoring hypopneas as central is optional, although in patients with central syndromes this may be important. Many Medicare local coverage determinations require reporting a central apnea–hypopnea index in order to qualify a patient for an advanced respiratory assist device such as ASV therapy. To score a central hypopnea (Fig. 13-5), the event must have none of the following:

1. snoring,
2. increased inspiratory flattening of the nasal pressure or PAP device flow signal compared with baseline breathing, and
3. thoracoabdominal paradox during the event compared with pre-event breathing.

Reporting an occurrence of Cheyne–Stokes breathing (CSB) on the PSG report is required if repetitive CAs and/or central hypopneas are present. The *AASM Manual for Scoring of Sleep and Associated Events* (27) indicates scoring criteria for CSB (Fig. 13-2). Score CSB if both of the following criteria are met:

1. Three or more consecutive CAs and/or central hypopneas separated by a crescendo and decrescendo change in breathing amplitude with a cycle length of more than 40 seconds,
2. More than or equal to five CAs and/or central hypopneas per hours of sleep associated with the crescendo/decrescendo breathing pattern recoded over more than 2 hours of monitoring (27).

TREATMENT

Treatment of CSA can be difficult. In patients with CHF, optimize CHF treatment first. Among those with persistent CSR, various forms of CPAP have been advocated and some patients do respond well to PAP devices. The use of CPAP has been shown to improve cardiac function and quality of life and reduce the need for organ transplantation in patients with CHF. Overall, the goal is to normalize breathing patterns, so that patients will

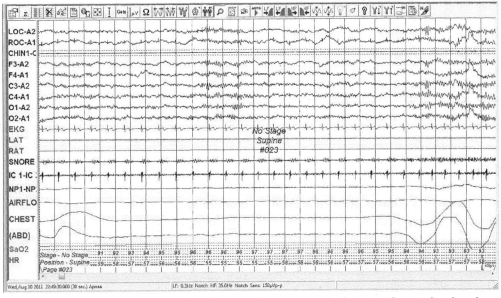

Figure 13-4 Sleep-onset central apnea. The central pauses seen in the example are related to sleep onset. The breathing pattern normalizes when the patient progresses to stage N2 sleep.

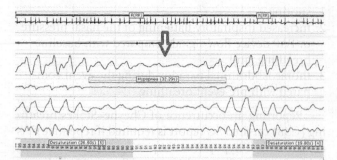

Figure 13-5 Central hypopnea.

have improved cardiac function and quality of life. Patients using PAP devices experience less fluctuation of blood gases, indicating that normalizing PCO_2 may normalize breathing drive. CPAP titration in these patients is usually more time-consuming, and these patients are fragile sleepers.

CSA may respond to nasal CPAP, especially if it is combined with OSA episodes. CPAP therapy showed positive reduction of CSA events, increasing overnight oxygen intake, lowering of norepinephrine levels, and improved cardiac ejection fraction (22). CPAP therapy corrects CSA in some patients even if it is not accompanied by OSA. In patients with hypocapnic CSA, CPAP may, however, increase hypocapnic status, worsening the clinical picture (25, 28).

Some patients with hypocapnic CSA may benefit from the use of bilevel positive airway pressure (BPAP). However, BPAP may also increase CSA caused by reduced PCO_2 levels. BPAP has also been used in patients with CHF or CSR–CSA with variable results. Further studies are necessary to better evaluate the role of BPAP treatment in these patients.

Servo-ventilation incorporates an automatic, minute ventilation or peak flow targeted device that performs breath-to-breath analysis and adjusts pressure settings accordingly. Depending on airflow, the device will automatically adjust the amount of pressure it delivers in order to reduce hyperpneas, hypopneas, and apneas (29). Further discussion and an outline of appropriate treatment for CSA syndromes can be found in Chapter 49 of this textbook.

REFERENCES

1. Franklin, K., Eriksson, P., Sahlin, C., et al. (1997). Reversal of central sleep apnea with oxygen. *Chest, 111,* 163–169.
2. Eckert, D. J., Jordan, A. S., Merchia, P., et al. (2007). Central sleep apnea: Pathophysiology and treatment. *Chest, 13*(2), 595–607.
3. Malhotra, A., & Owens, R. L. (2010). What is central sleep apnea? *Respiratory Care, 55*(9), 1168–1178.

4. Khoo, M. C., Kronauer, R. E., Strohl, K. P., et al. (1982). Factors inducing periodic breathing in humans: A general model. *Journal of Applied Physiology, 53,* 644–659.
5. Wellman, A., Malhotra, A., Fogel, R. B., et al. (2003). Respiratory system loop gain in normal men and women measured with proportional-assist ventilation. *Journal of Applied Physiology, 94,* 205–212.
6. Pack, A. I., Cola, M. F., Goldszmidt, A., et al. (1992). Correlation between oscillations in ventilation and frequency content of the electroencephalogram. *Journal of Applied Physiology, 72,* 985–992.
7. Dunai, J., Kleiman, J., & Trinder, J. (1999). Ventilatory instability during sleep onset in individuals with high peripheral chemosensitivity. *Journal of Applied Physiology, 87,* 661–672.
8. Safwan, B. (2009). Central sleep apnea in patients with congestive heart failure. *Heart Failure Reviews, 14,* 135–141.
9. Orem, J., Lovering, A. T., Dunin-Barkowski, W., et al. (2002). Tonic activity in the respiratory system in wakefulness, NREM and REM sleep. *Sleep, 25,* 488–496.
10. Orem, J. (1980). Neuronal mechanisms of respiration in REM sleep. *Sleep, 3,* 251–267.
11. Phillips, B. A., Berry, D. T., Schmitt, F. A., et al. (1992). Sleep-disordered breathing in the healthy elderly: Clinically significant? *Chest, 101,* 345–349. doi:10.1378/chest.101.2.345
12. Bixler, E. O., Vgontzas, A. N., Lin, H. M., et al. (2001). Prevalence of sleep-disordered breathing in women: Effects of gender. *American Journal of Respiratory and Critical Care Medicine, 163,* 608–613.
13. Wang, D., Teichtahl, H., Drummer, O., et al. (2005). Central sleep apnea in stable methadone maintenance treatment patients. *Chest, 128,* 1348–1356.
14. Grunstein, R. R., Ho, K. Y., Berthon-Jones, M., et al. (1994). Central sleep apnea is associated with increased ventilatory response to carbon dioxide and hypersecretion of growth hormone in patients with acromegaly. *American Journal of Respiratory and Critical Care Medicine, 150,* 496–502.
15. American Academy of Pain Medicine and the American Pain Society. (1997). The use of opioids for the treatment of chronic pain. A consensus statement from the American Academy of Pain Medicine and the American Pain Society. *The Clinical Journal of Pain, 13*(1), 6–8.
16. Xie, A., Rutherford, R., Rankin, F., et al. (1995). Hypocapnia and increased ventilatory responsiveness in patients with idiopathic central sleep apnea. *American Journal of Respiratory and Critical Care Medicine, 152,* 1950–1955.
17. Xie, A., Wong, B., Phillipson, E. A., et al. (1994). Interaction of hyperventilation and arousal in the

pathogenesis of idiopathic central sleep apnea. *American Journal of Respiratory and Critical Care Medicine, 150*, 489–495.

18. Javaheri, S., Malik, A., Smith, J., et al. (2008). Adaptive pressure support servoventilation: A novel treatment for sleep apnea associated with use of opioids. *Journal of Clinical Sleep Medicine, 4*, 305–310.

19. Naughton, M. T., Benard, D. C., Liu, P. P., et al. (1995). Effects of nasal CPAP on sympathetic activity in patients with heart failure and central sleep apnea. *American Journal of Respiratory and Critical Care Medicine, 152*, 473–479.

20. Franklin, K. A., Sandstrom, E., Johansson, G., et al. (1997). Hemodynamics, cerebral circulation, and oxygen saturation in Cheyne-Stokes respiration. *Journal of Applied Physiology, 83*, 1184–1191.

21. Trinder, J., Merson, R., Rosenberg, J. I., et al. (2000). Pathophysiological interactions of ventilation, arousals, and blood pressure oscillations during Cheyne-Stokes respiration in patients with heart failure. *American Journal of Respiratory and Critical Care Medicine, 162*, 808–813.

22. Saunders, M. H. (2005). Sleep breathing disorders/central sleep apnea. In M. Kryger, T. Roth, & W. Dement, (Eds.), *Principles and practice of sleep medicine* (4th ed.). Philadelphia, PA: Elsevier Saunders.

23. Farre, R., Montserrat, J. M., & Navajas, D. (2004). Noninvasive monitoring of respiratory mechanics during sleep. *European Journal of Respiration, 24*, 1052–1060.

24. Yumino, D., & Bradley, T. D. (2008). Central sleep apnea and Cheyne-Stokes respiration. *Proceedings of the American Thoracic Society, 5*, 226–236. doi:10.1513/pats.200708-129MG

25. Naughton, M. T., Liu, P. P., Benard, D. C., et al. (1995). Treatment of congestive heart failure and Cheyne-Stokes respiration during sleep by continuous positive airway pressure. *American Journal of Respiratory and Critical Care Medicine, 151*, 92–97.

26. Allam, J. S., Olson, E. J., Gay, P. C., et al. (2007). Efficacy of adaptive servoventilation in treatment of complex and central sleep apnea syndromes. *Chest, 132*, 1839–1846.

27. Berry, R. B., Albertario, C. L., Harding, S. M., et al.; for the American Academy of Sleep Medicine. (2018). *The AASM Manual for the Scoring of Sleep and Associated Events: Rules, Terminology and Technical Specifications.* Version 2.5. Darien, IL: American Academy of Sleep Medicine.

28. Lehman, S., Antic, N. A., Thompson, C., et al. (2007). Central sleep apnea: Commencement of continuous positive airway pressure in patients with a diagnosis of obstructive sleep apnea–hypopnea. *Journal of Clinical Sleep Medicine, 3*, 462–466.

29. Oldenburg, O., Schmidt, A., Lamp, B., et al. (2008). Adaptive servoventilation improves cardiac function in patients with chronic heart failure and Cheyne-Stokes respiration. *European Journal of Heart Failure, 10*, 581–586.

chapter 14

Hypoventilation Syndromes

JOYCE M. BLACK

LEARNING OBJECTIVES

On completion of this chapter, the reader will be able to:

1. Discuss the physiology of normal ventilation and respiration.
2. Describe sleep-disordered breathing identified during sleep studies.
3. Define hypoventilation and the associated pathophysiology.
4. Discuss the clinical significance of hypoventilation.
5. Describe how hypoventilation is identified during a sleep study.
   a. Explain the difference between hypopneas and hypoventilation.
   b. Review the process for a diagnostic study for patients with hypoventilation.
6. Review treatments for hypoventilation.

KEY TERMS

Ventilation
Respiration
Noninvasive ventilation (NIV)
Gas exchange
Tidal volume (Vt)
Minute ventilation (MV)
Pulmonary hypertension
Arterial blood gas (ABG)
Pulmonary function test (PFT)

INTRODUCTION

Hypoventilation is an impairment of the body's ability to breathe. Chronic hypoventilation may be the result of disorders that affect any part of the respiratory system. It may be caused by congenital disorders, brainstem disorders, neurologic disorders associated with signal communication from the brain through the spinal column, or neuromuscular disorders that compromise the signals in the nerves or muscles (1).

Before delving more deeply into hypoventilation, let's first discuss normal breathing and how the respiratory and circulatory systems work to deliver oxygen (O_2) to the cells of the body, and the other sleep-disordered breathing (SDB) events seen in the sleep laboratory during polysomnography (PSG).

PHYSIOLOGY OF NORMAL VENTILATION AND RESPIRATION

Ventilation or breathing is the process of moving air in and out of the lungs. Inhalation brings needed O_2 to the lungs and exhalation removes carbon dioxide (CO_2), the waste by-product of cell metabolism.

Inhalation is initiated when the brain signals the diaphragm (the major muscle of ventilation) to contract, making the thoracic cavity to expand. The expansion creates a pressure drop in the chest. It is a pressure gradient between the atmosphere and the chest that causes the air to pass through the nasal cavity, upper airway, bronchi and bronchioles, and ultimately to the alveoli. The alveoli are small sacks in the lungs that are surrounded by capillaries where respiration or gas exchange takes place (exchange of O_2 with CO_2).

The right side of the heart pumps blood to the lung's capillary bed where O_2 molecules, brought to the alveoli by the inhalation process, pass through the alveolar membrane and the capillary walls into the blood. Conversely, CO_2 passes through the capillary wall and the alveolar membrane into the alveoli where it is eliminated by exhalation. It is the concentration gradient between the gases in the alveoli and the capillaries that allow this gas exchange to take place through simple diffusion. Once the blood in the capillary bed surrounding the alveoli has less CO_2 and more O_2, the oxygenated blood is then pumped by the right side of the heart to the left side of the heart. The heart's left ventricle then pumps the oxygenated blood, through the arteries, to all the cells in the body.

The body's motivation to breathe (contract the diaphragm) is created by the amount of CO_2 in the blood. The CO_2 molecules, pumped to the brain by the heart, pass through capillaries into the spinal fluid that bathes the brain. Through a chemical process, the CO_2 molecule is turned to hydrogen ion and water. It is the hydrogen molecule that changes the spinal fluid pH, making it more acidic. The change in spinal fluid pH is detected in the hindbrain by the medulla oblongata and pons, which, in turn, signal the diaphragm to contract. CO_2 levels in the blood are the primary driver to breathe. This is the normal breathing process and how every cell in the body receives O_2 and maintains life (2).

Now let's discuss what occurs during sleep that may compromise or impair this process.

KEY TAKEAWAY: Physiology of Normal Breathing

- Normal breathing: CO_2 levels in the blood provide the primary drive to breathe. As CO_2 levels increase, the spinal fluid becomes more acidic and triggers the brain to send a signal to the diaphragm to contract and start the breathing process.
- Air is inhaled into the body when the diaphragm contracts, creating negative pressure in the lungs. A pressure gradient causes air to pass through the respiratory system into the alveoli.
- Gas exchange takes place between the alveoli and the blood in the capillary beds surrounding the alveoli—CO_2 is exchanged for O_2.
- The heart pumps the blood through the arteries to the entire body exchanging the O_2 for CO_2 (a by-product of cell metabolism) to keep cells alive.
- The veins carry the CO_2 from the cells back to the right side of the heart and into the lungs to exchange the CO_2 for O_2 and start the breathing process again.

SLEEP-DISORDERED BREATHING

A PSG monitors how well a person sleeps and how well the body functions while he or she is asleep. A PSG records the patient's brain activity using a modified electroencephalogram (EEG), eye movement using electrooculogram (EOG), muscle tone using electromyogram (EMG), and the heart and heart rate via a modified electrocardiogram (ECG). SDB is identified by monitoring airflow, respiratory effort, oxygen saturation, and, if possible, CO_2 levels in the blood (3).

SDB disrupts the normal breathing process during sleep. This may be caused by air not getting into the lungs because of airway obstructions, the drive to breathe being affected due to the diaphragm not receiving the signal to contract or it cannot contract, or a combination of both.

Table 14-1 summarizes the categories of SDB and how they are monitored, and includes short descriptions (4).

The treatment for SDB caused by airway blockage is continuous positive airway pressure (CPAP) or bilevel positive airway pressure (BPAP) if CPAP is not tolerated, applied to the airway via a mask to keep the airway open. The treatment for a patient who has diminished drive to breathe or no drive to breathe is usually a BPAP device that includes a spontaneous/timed backup mode (BPAP S/T) or more sophisticated noninvasive ventilation (NIV) if needed (5).

Table **14-1** Description of Sleep-Disordered Breathing Categories Seen during Polysomnography

SDB Categories	Airflow	Effort	Description
Obstructive sleep apnea (OSA)/hypopnea	No airflow or reduced airflow	Effort is noted	Airway blocked, can't get air into the lungs
Central sleep apnea (CSA)/hypopnea	No airflow or reduced airflow	No effort or reduced effort	Compromised drive to breathe
Mixed apnea	No airflow	No effort at beginning of event noted before airway opens	Starts with no drive to breathe, then airway is blocked
Cheyne–Stokes respirations (CSR)	Waxing and waning noted in the airflow channel	Waxing and waning noted in the effort channels	Drive to breathe is compromised—breathing cycles exhibit waxing and waning lasting 30 s–2 min duration
Complex sleep apnea	No airflow—central apneas appear with CPAP changes	No effort—as CPAP is increased, the obstructive apneas change to central apneas	Closure of airway is present, but the drive to breathe is compromised by the administration of CPAP, causing changes in CO_2 and decreased drive to breathe.
Hypoventilation	Airflow reduced for long periods of time—AASM rules state at least 10 min	Equal reduction in effort noted	Drive to breathe is compromised.

AASM, American Academy of Sleep Medicine; CPAP, continuous positive airway pressure; SDB, sleep-disordered breathing.

Cheyne-Stokes Respirations (CSR) are characterized by the appearance of a crescendo-decrescendo (waxing and waning) of the breathing pattern caused by changes in the partial pressures of oxygen and carbon dioxide. CSR may be caused by cardiac failure, renal failure, narcotic poisoning, and raised intracranial pressures. CSR displays periods of increased tidal volumes and respiratory rate (blowing off CO_2) caused by increases in CO_2 and a decrease in volume and rate often resulting in central apnea caused by decreases in CO_2.

Treating CSR and complex sleep apnea with conventional BPAP S/T may overventilate the patient and knock out the drive to breathe even more. Servo-ventilation is the treatment of choice for these patients. By identifying the patient's peak flow or minute ventilation and applying supplemental pressure support, the patient gets only the flow that he or she needs without overventilation (8).

KEY TAKEAWAY: Sleep-Disordered Breathing

- PSG monitors and records how well the body is working during rest and while asleep.
- SDB is identified during a PSG using airflow, effort, oximetry, and, in some cases, CO_2 monitors.
- The most common SDB identified during PSG is obstructive sleep apnea (OSA), which does not let air enter the lungs. The treatment of choice for OSA is CPAP therapy.
- Other types of SDB may be secondary to a diminished or absent drive to breathe. This can be caused by compromises in the signal to breathe: the brain not identifying the need to breathe, the signal being interrupted and not reaching the lungs, or the muscles not responding to the signal. The most common therapy is some form of BPAP or, if necessary, NIV.

HYPOVENTILATION AND ASSOCIATED PATHOPHYSIOLOGY

Hypoventilation is a state in which there is a reduced amount of air entering the alveoli that causes an increase in CO_2 levels in the blood. The primary function of the lungs is to inhale O_2 and exhale CO_2. When we discuss the needed amount of air that a person breathes, we often refer to it in terms of tidal volume (Vt) or minute ventilation (MV). The Vt is the amount of air inhaled or exhaled during a normal breathing cycle. In a normal young adult, it is approximately 500 mL per inspiration or 7 mL per kg of body mass. The MV is found by multiplying the Vt by the respiratory rate (Fig. 14-1).

Some normal variables influence our Vt and therefore our MV—issues such as stress, exercise, and sympathetic nervous system activation (fight or flight). These can cause Vt and respiratory rates to increase. Conversely, when we relax by reading a book or watching TV, our Vt and respiratory rate may decrease and still be able to maintain adequate oxygenation for the body.

Another variable is the normal increase in CO_2 retention that occurs when we transition from wakefulness to sleep. There is an additional increase in CO_2 retention when we transition from nonrapid eye movement to rapid eye movement (REM) sleep. All of these are normal occurrences that elicit a decrease or increase in Vt, and all are done without conscious effort (1).

The body uses the Vt to adequately oxygenate and eliminate CO_2. In normal adults, it is not unusual for the CO_2 level to increase by 7 mm Hg from wake to sleep and to fluctuate by 10 mm Hg throughout the sleep stages. These variables should still be no higher than 50 mm Hg. This normal variability is maintained by the body taking deeper or shallower breaths as well as increasing or decreasing the respiratory rate. In addition, diminished muscle tone develops during REM sleep, which may further exacerbate hypoventilation secondary to reduced respiratory effort.

Now let's discuss what happens when the body can't maintain adequate ventilation. A very short and concise definition of hypoventilation is an increase in CO_2 and decrease in O_2. Hypoventilation is a complicated breathing pattern caused by breathing that is too shallow, too slow, or has diminished lung function.

The body/brain tries to maintain adequate ventilation. Think about it when you exercise. First, you try to take deeper breaths, then you breathe faster—you don't do this consciously, the brain knows it needs to do this to keep you oxygenated. At some point, your body says enough, and you stop exercising to catch your breath. You breathe fast and deep until you reach an equilibrium and start breathing normally.

This type of breathing (fast rate, deep volume) is what happens in the body during sleep if the patient's CO_2 level increases and they try to blow off the CO_2 and get more O_2. This also occurs in patients with lung disorders that cause them to breathe with accessory muscles during the day. They increase their lung volume by raising their shoulders (to pull in more O_2) and use purse lip breathing while exhaling, to keep oxygen in their lungs longer. When they lay down, gravity puts additional stress on their diaphragm and accessory muscles and muscle tone is decreased. The patient's airflow and effort decreases and their O_2 level will slowly decrease over time. During REM sleep, the patient will often have central apneas due to the lack of muscle tone–they can no longer use the accessory muscles. The patient will often have very short periods of REM (since they cannot use accessory muscles during this time–central apneas are longer) and spend most of their sleep time in N-REM sleep.

Remember, the brain is trying to move enough air in and out of the lungs to keep the body alive and oxygenated. These compromised breathing periods may last for a very long time. The American Academy of Sleep Medicine (AASM) states that they should be at least 10 minutes in duration for scoring purposes, but they may last much longer.

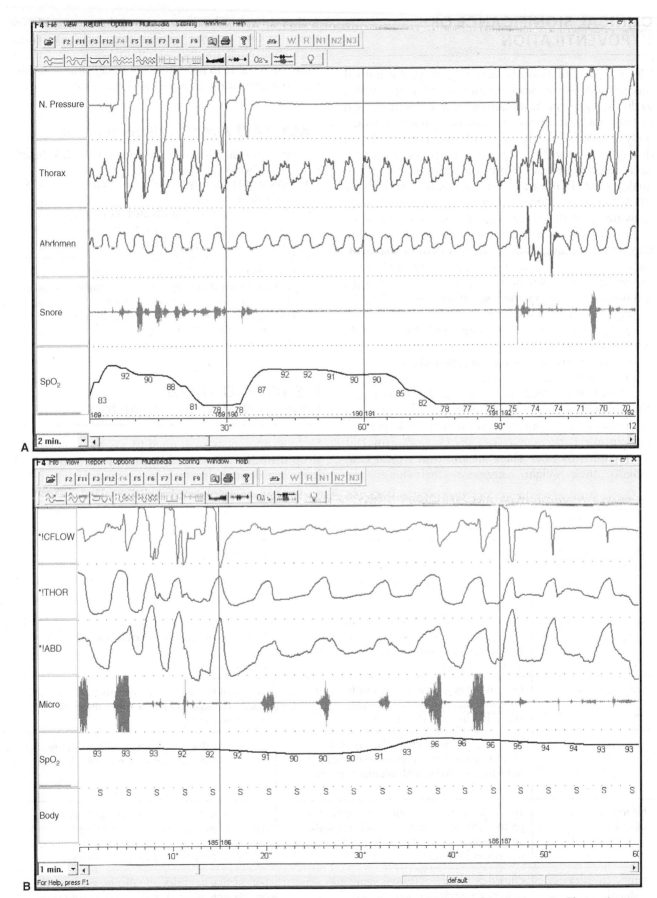

Figure 14-1 A: Obstructive apnea—no airflow, effort, snoring noted when airway is open, desaturations. **B:** Obstructive hypopnea—decreased airflow, effort, and snoring noted as well as desaturations.

CLINICAL SIGNIFICANCE OF HYPOVENTILATION

When hypoventilation occurs during sleep, the normal mechanisms to maintain adequate ventilation are not able to do their job. The lungs cannot breathe deeply enough or fast enough to maintain adequate ventilation, so the body starts to accumulate CO_2. Chronic hypoventilation during sleep may be associated with excessive daytime sleepiness, frequent awakenings resulting in poor sleep quality, enuresis, insomnia, fatigue, nightmares, morning headaches, and reduced exercise capacity. These symptoms are due to the increases in CO_2 and decreases in O_2.

What happens when there is a chronic condition that affects the lungs? The ventilatory control system attempts to compensate by increasing the drive to breathe to keep the CO_2 level in normal range (35 to 45 mm Hg). It is done by increasing the respiratory rate and decreasing the Vt (decreased flow) (9).

Sleep-related hypoventilation may be an early symptom of chronic disorders.

The disorders most often associated with hypoventilation are summarized in Table 14-2.

Obesity hypoventilation syndrome (OHS) is a condition that is often seen in the sleep laboratory. OHS is defined as a combination of obesity (BMI 30 kg per m^2) and chronic hypercapnia (i.e., $PaCO_2$ >45 mm Hg) accompanied by SDB. These are not your typical OSA patients; their weight compresses their lungs and makes it hard to breathe, and they have extra adipose tissue in their tongue, airway, and neck. The added intra-abdominal or visceral fat makes these patients more susceptible to pulmonary hypertension, heart disease, diabetes, some cancers, and death (10).

KEY TAKEAWAY: Hypoventilation

- Hypoventilation is an impairment of the body's ability to breathe normally.
- Hypoventilation may be defined as an increase in CO_2 and decrease in O_2.
- Hypoventilation is a complicated breathing pattern caused by breathing that is too shallow, too slow, or has diminished lung function.
- Chronic hypoventilation may be the result of disorders that affect any part of the respiratory system.
- Chronic hypoventilation may be associated with excessive daytime sleepiness, poor sleep quality, enuresis, fatigue, nightmares, and morning headaches.
- OHA makes the patient more susceptible to OSA and sleep disturbances.

IDENTIFICATION OF HYPOVENTILATION DURING PSG

Sleep technologists are trained to recognize all types of sleep disorders. They can identify a patient with OSA, insomnia, central sleep apnea (CSA), narcolepsy, REM

Table 14-2 Types of Hypoventilation with Short Descriptions

Type of Disorder	Description	Diseases/Conditions
OHS	BMI >30 with weight accumulated in the thoracic region putting stress on the functionality of the lungs	OHS may also be associated with obstructive apneas and central apneas during sleep
Congenital disorders	Genetic form of sleep apnea: Patient stops breathing when falling asleep—if undiagnosed, death may occur	Central hypoventilation syndrome, formerly known as Ondine's curse, kyphoscoliosis, or chest wall deformities
Brainstem disorders	Issue in the brainstem that controls the normal breathing process resulting in inadequate ventilation and increased levels of CO_2	Causes of brainstem disorders include stroke, tumor, trauma, and medical conditions such as meningitis, etc.
Neurologic disorders	Disorders that affect either the signals to breathe or the signal transmission from the brain through the spinal column to the nerves in the body	Neurologic disorders include Parkinson disease, memory disorders, multiple sclerosis, ALS, etc.
Neuromuscular disorders	Typical features are a reduced forced vital capacity, reduced respiratory muscle strength, and, in some cases, malfunction of the neurons that control breathing	Disorders that compromise the signals in the nerves or muscles such as myasthenia gravis, Guillain–Barré syndrome, poliomyelitis, muscular dystrophy, and Duchenne muscular dystrophy
Drug or medication induced	Caused by drugs that depress ventilatory drive or impair muscle function	Long-acting narcotics, anesthetics, sedatives, muscle relaxants, alcohol, and chronic opioid usage

ALS, amyotrophic lateral sclerosis; BMI, body mass index; OHS, obesity hypoventilation syndrome.

behavior disorder, and all types of parasomnias. They can identify if a patient is having a seizure or some other medical emergency during the PSG, and they know what to do. They work all night monitoring their patients and make sure the information that is collected is complete and accurate. As Dr. German Nino Murcia said, "Sleep techs are the eyes and ears of the physician."

Most of the patients who are diagnosed using PSG have OSA and the sleep recordings verify this diagnosis. The events recorded are obstructive apneas and hypopneas with associated oxygen desaturations and EEG arousals. These events happen all night long and are worse when the patient is in the supine sleeping position and/or in REM sleep.

Apnea events need to be at least 10 seconds in duration for scoring purposes but will often last longer. Some sleep laboratories have a general rule that if an event lasts longer than 60 to 90 seconds with associated desaturations, the patient should be awakened and started on therapy (Fig. 14-1A).

According to the AASM scoring guidelines, an obstructive hypopnea is scored if there is a reduction of airflow by 30%, the reduced airflow lasts for at least 10 seconds, and there is a 3% or greater drop in oxygen saturation. Any of the following should also be noted (Fig. 14-1B):

1. snoring during the event
2. flattening of the nasal pressure signal
3. paradoxical thoracoabdominal movement

Sleep technologists may see central apneas in patients who are diagnosed with neurologic or neuromuscular disorders, severe OSA, or complex sleep apnea. These events are at least 10 seconds in duration and are associated with no airflow and no drive to breathe (flat respiratory effort signals). Central hypopneas are identified by the same criteria as obstructive hypopneas for reduction in flow and duration, but a central hypopnea must include (Fig. 14-2A, B) the following:

1. no snoring
2. no inspiratory flattening of the flow signal compared with baseline
3. no associated thoracoabdominal paradoxical movement during the event

Please see the specific criteria for event scoring in the current version of the AASM Manual for Scoring of Sleep and Associated Events (11).

In addition to sleep disorders that are diagnosed easily with a PSG, there are patients who have sleep studies because they have a condition that makes

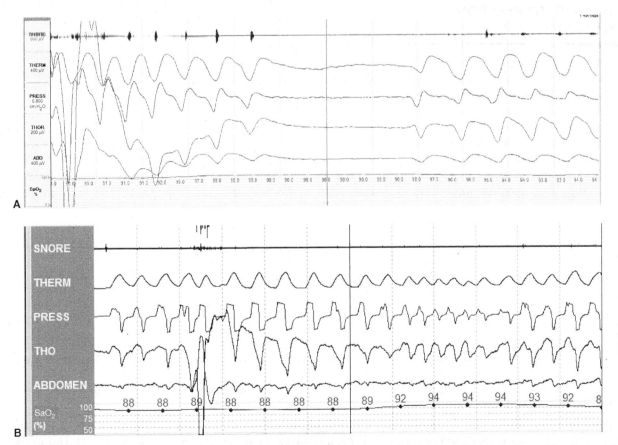

Figure 14-2 **A:** Central apnea 60-second epoch—no airflow, no effort. **B:** Central hypopnea (30-second epoch)—decreased airflow, decreased effort, no snoring, no squaring off of airflow signal, and no paradoxical movement.

breathing during sleep difficult or impossible. These are the patients who mainly have central events and may have hypoventilation.

As previously mentioned, diseases that cause the patient to have hypoventilation and difficulty breathing when they are sleeping include central hypoventilation syndrome (Ondine's curse), neurologic conditions (amyotrophic lateral sclerosis, postpolio syndrome, etc.), OHS, narcotic abuse, etc. Often, these patients have an exacerbation of their condition and are placed on NIV in the emergency room or intensive care unit. Once they are stable, the physician may order a PSG to verify the need for NIV and to validate the settings.

A second patient population includes those who have not been diagnosed with a disease that causes hypoventilation but have difficulty breathing while they are sleeping. The physician may suspect that these patients have OSA or some type of CSA and study them to better understand their symptoms and identify the cause. These patients may have been diagnosed with chronic obstructive pulmonary disease or some underlying lung problem and come into the sleep laboratory to be evaluated for excessive daytime sleepiness or fatigue upon exertion. The technologist and physician may anticipate OSA or identify some type of overlap syndrome (12).

DIAGNOSTIC PSG FOR HYPOVENTILATION

When a patient arrives in the sleep laboratory, a review of his or her chart is imperative. The technologist needs to understand why the patient is having a PSG. Does the physician suspect OSA, insomnia, or some type of parasomnia, or does the patient have a condition that may cause hypoventilation? The technologist reviews the patient's comorbidities and the types of diagnostic tests the latter has had, such as arterial blood gas (ABG), stress tests, pulmonary function test (PFT), and so on.

Some of the test results that may be helpful for the sleep technologist in identifying the possibility of hypoventilation include the following:

- ABG shows the patient's PaO_2 is decreased and $PaCO_2$ is increased. If the patient's blood is compensating for the increased CO_2, high levels of bicarbonate (HCO_3) and increased pH acidity will be noted (13).
- Blood cell count shows an elevated hematocrit level (increased red blood cells)—the body does this to carry more O_2 and CO_2 to compensate for hypoventilation.
- PFT shows a measurement of maximal inspiratory and expiratory pressures, which may be useful in screening for respiratory muscle weakness and neuromuscular disorders.

For the PSG, the patient will be set up with traditional recording parameters: EEG, EOG, EMG, ECG airflow, abdominal and thoracic effort, oximetry, and CO_2 monitoring if available. During the daytime and while up and about, the patient that has chronic obstructive pulmonary disease (COPD) or some other breathing disorder will use accessory muscles to breathe. When they lay down, gravity plays a negative role and results in accessory muscles not able to support adequate respirations. This causes the patient's breathing ability to deteriorate especially if the bed is in the flat position. At home, the patient may have compensated for this deterioration in the ability to breathe by having his or her head of the bed elevated or by using multiple pillows to be in a sitting position. If questioned the patient may admit that they sleep in a lounge chair with the head elevated.

A simple description of hypoventilation is inadequate ventilation leading to an increase in CO_2 and decrease in O_2. Sleep reduces MV in healthy adults, and it is much more pronounced in patients with diseases that affect lung function. Therefore, sleep-related hypoventilation may be an early manifestation of chronic hypoventilation (Fig. 14-3) (1).

With sleep onset, the patient may exhibit central apneas and central hypopneas. This will last for a few

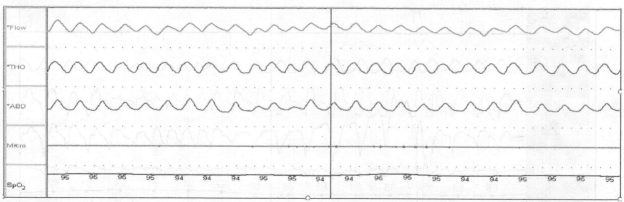

Figure 14-3 One-minute excerpt of hypoventilation showing decreased airflow, decreased effort, slight decrease in SpO_2 (as the time increases, the SpO_2 will decrease more), and increased respiratory rate 26 breaths per minute. This breathing pattern lasted for over 15 minutes, with the SpO_2 declining to 83%.

minutes, then the patient may start taking deep breaths with shorter pauses. The pauses are often too short to technically be called a central event. Eventually when the patient goes into deeper sleep stages, the deep breathing may be replaced with shallow breaths and an increase in the respiratory rate—very consistent with hypoventilation.

It is not unusual to see hypoventilation occurring in patients who have not yet been diagnosed with some type of disorder that causes hypoventilation. The disorders are often not respiratory based but have respiratory ramifications. If CO_2 is not being monitored, a decrease in airflow and effort with slow desaturations may be noted along with increased respiratory rates.

Remember, central hypopneas show decreased airflow, decreased effort, and associated oxygen desaturations. The difference between central hypopneas and hypoventilation is the length of time before the patient takes a deep breath or begins to breathe normally. The duration of a hypopnea is at least 10 seconds but usually not more than 60 to 90 seconds. According to AASM guidelines, hypoventilation should be at least 10 minutes in duration and is often of much longer duration.

The most recent revision of the AASM scoring criteria (11) suggests scoring sleep-related hypoventilation if

- there is an increase in the arterial PCO_2 to a value greater than 55 mm Hg for greater than or equal to 10 minutes or
- there is an increase in arterial PCO_2 during sleep (in comparison with an awake supine value) to a value greater than 50 mm Hg for greater than or equal to 10 minutes.

Hypoventilation is usually associated with long-term oxygen desaturation, so that an oxygen saturation of less than 90% for greater than 5 minutes with a nadir of less than or equal to 85% may also indicate hypercapnia and should warrant a further diagnostic workup (1).

Many of the patients who have hypoventilation syndrome may also have OSA. During the PSG, you may see obstructive apneas, central apneas, and hypoventilation. Look at the airflow and the effort. If they are both reduced and the condition lasts for 10 minutes, you are seeing hypoventilation. After the patient changes position or uses the bathroom and sleep is reinitiated, central apneas resume, changing to deep breaths with long pauses until the reduced flow and effort is displayed, indicating hypoventilation. Typically, desaturations are very slow and no additional respiratory effort is apparent, with hypoventilation.

If a CO_2 monitor is not used, the patient cannot be diagnosed with hypoventilation, but a strong indication that hypoventilation is occurring can and should be made known to the physician. There needs to be a protocol available in the event that hypoventilation is suspected that indicates how and when it should be treated.

Hypoventilation puts additional stress on the body. Patients with hypoventilation are at increased risk for congestive heart failure, cor pulmonale, pulmonary hypertension, angina, etc. When possible, the cause of hypoventilation should be treated by controlling weight, decreasing the intake of opioids, etc., and ventilatory support should be administered expeditiously in the interim (14).

KEY TAKEAWAY: PSG and Hypoventilation

- Hypoventilation may initially be identified or suspected during a PSG.
- At the start of the PSG, patients who have hypoventilation may have central apneas and hypopneas because of an inability to use accessory muscles effectively while lying down.
- Central hypopneas and hypoventilation have some of the same properties, but central hypopneas are usually no longer than 60 to 90 seconds, whereas hypoventilation, as defined by the AASM, must be at least 10 minutes in duration.
- Patients with OHS are unable to move enough air in and out of the lungs because of their increased girth and therefore breathe very shallow, causing decreased levels of O_2 and increased levels of CO_2.
- Hypoventilation is a complicated breathing pattern that makes the patient at risk for congestive heart failure, cor pulmonale, pulmonary hypertension, and the like.

TREATMENTS FOR HYPOVENTILATION

As stated throughout this chapter, hypoventilation is a breathing disorder that may be seen and diagnosed during a PSG. The causes vary from OHS and drug use to physiologic disorders, but the result is that the patient has difficulty breathing sufficiently while sleeping.

Treating the underlying condition by undertaking weight loss methods or weaning off opioids is the primary goal. In OHS, CPAP may be sufficient to treat the patient until sufficient weight loss is achieved. There is a subset of OHS patients for whom CPAP is not viable, and they need NIV to support their breathing during the weight loss process.

Many of the underlying conditions causing hypoventilation do not have a cure, and therefore, the symptom itself needs to be addressed. A few years ago, the only option was a tracheostomy and volume ventilation. Since the mid-1990s, NIV with BPAP using a mask has been a very strong treatment option.

During the diagnostic PSG, the patient may present with hypoventilation, central apneas, and obstructive apneas. All these need to be considered when treating the patient. NIV is

Table 14-3 BPAP Titration Process for OSA and Ventilation

BPAP Setting	Titration for OSA (15)	Titration for Ventilation (16)
EPAP	Increase for apneas	Increase to open airway; airway closure may be seen at the end of a central event or may be seen by decreased or lack of flow with delivered breaths. Also used to increase oxygenation (increases the time oxygen is held in the lungs)
IPAP	Increase for hypopneas, desaturations, EEG arousals, snoring	Increase to ensure sufficient tidal volume delivered on each breath—verified by watching SpO_2 and CO_2
Backup rate	Used if central events are noted on diagnostic PSG. Rate identified by the physician or should be 2–3 breaths below the patient's respiratory rate.	Backup rate set to deliver mechanical breaths during central events (the rate is usually recommended by the physician and may be around 8–10 breaths/min with the option to increase as needed to keep the oxygen and CO_2 at acceptable levels)
Volume-assured pressure support	Not used for OSA	Tidal volume delivered via pressure support so that if the patient's condition deteriorates, the set Vt is still maintained

BPAP, bilevel positive airway pressure; EEG, electroencephalogram; EPAP, expiration positive airway pressure; IPAP, inspiration positive airway pressure; OSA, obstructive sleep apnea; PSG, polysomnography; Vt, tidal volume.

the treatment of choice for hypoventilation. This is initially delivered by using a BPAP unit with BPAP S/T or volume-assured pressure support. The settings on the device that the technologist uses during the titration support ventilation instead of only keeping the airway open (see Table 14-3).

NIV has proven to improve quality of sleep, nocturnal oxygen saturation, diurnal and nocturnal $PaCO_2$, and quality of life in a broad spectrum of chronic hypoventilation disorders. Moreover, NIV may improve patients' survival. In addition, untreated OHS patients are more likely to require invasive ventilation and have prolonged hospital stays.

When observing central apneas, be aware of the machine-driven breaths. If an obstructive component is present during a central apnea, the machine breath cannot be delivered or is restricted as in a hypopnea. See Figure 14-4 for examples.

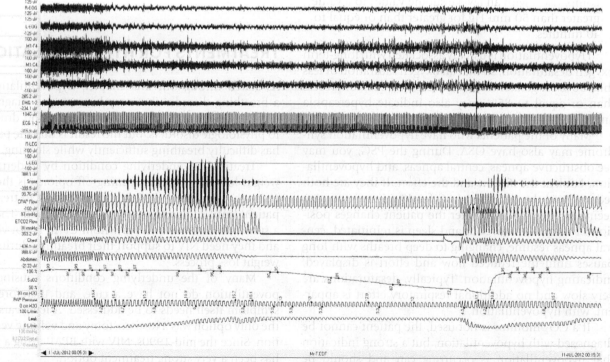

Figure 14-4 There is no effort recorded during the central events. The machine-driven breaths are indicated by the absence of flow in the end-tidal CO_2 flow channel. To correct this issue, the expiration positive airway pressure needs to be increased.

In summary, if a patient has a PSG because of excessive sleepiness or reduced functionality during the day and the study is to rule out OSA, the diagnosis of a disease process causing hypoventilation may not yet have been made. The sleep technologist may be the first to identify that the patient has hypoventilation. Everything the technologist sees needs to be well documented so that the physician can take the next step with an assurance that the information gathered is accurate.

Remember, the technologist is the eyes and the ears of the physician. This role is especially important when a patient with hypoventilation has a PSG. This may be a condition that has already been diagnosed and the physician is gathering baseline information and verifying the therapy setting, or it may be part of a new diagnosis.

ACKNOWLEDGMENT

I would like to thank David Glowark, RRT, Ed Bredel RRT, RPSGT and Dawn Penrod, RPSGT for assistance in review and suggestions for this document.

REFERENCES

1. Böing, S., & Randerath, W. J. (2015). Chronic hypoventilation syndromes and sleep-related hypoventilation. *Journal of Thoracic Disease, 7*(8), 1273–1285.
2. Egan, D. F. (1990). *Eagan's fundamentals of respiratory care* (5th ed). St. Louis, MO: Mosby.
3. Carskadon, M. A., & Rechtschaffen, A. (2000). Monitoring and staging human sleep. In M. Kryger, T. Roth, & W. Dement (Eds.), *Principles and practice of sleep medicine* (3rd ed., pp. 1197–1214). Philadelphia, PA: WB Saunders Company.
4. Kryger, M. (2000). Monitoring respiratory and cardiac function. In M. Kryger, T. Roth, & W. Dement (Eds.), *Principles and practice of sleep medicine* (3rd ed., pp. 1217–1229). Philadelphia, PA: WB Saunders Company.
5. Sullivan, C., Issa, F., Berthon-Jones, M., & Eves, L. (1981). Reversal of obstructive sleep apnea by continuous positive airway pressure applied through the nares. *Lancet, 1,* 862–865.
6. Sanders, M.H., & Kern, N. (1990). Obstructive sleep apnea treated by independently adjusted inspiratory and expiratory positive airway pressures via nasal mask; physiologic and clinical implications. *Chest, 98*(2), 317–324.
7. Kushida, C. A., Littner, M. R., Hirshkowitz, M., et.al. (2006). Practice parameters for the use of continuous and bilevel positive airway pressure devices to treat adult patients with sleep-related breathing disorders. *Sleep, 29*(3), 375–380.
8. Javaheri, S., Brown, L. K., & Randerath, W. J. (2014). Clinical applications of adaptive servoventilation devices part 2. *Chest, 146*(3), 858–868.
9. Piper, A. J., & Yee, B. J. (2014). Hypoventilation syndromes. *Comprehensive Physiology, 4*(4), 1639–1676.
10. Balachandran, J. S., Masa, J. F., & Mokhlesi, B. (2014). Obesity hypoventilation syndrome epidemiology and diagnosis. *Sleep Medicine Clinic, 9*(3), 341–347.
11. Berry, R. B., Albertario, C. L., Harding, S. M., et al.; for the American Academy of Sleep Medicine. (2018). *The AASM Manual for the Scoring of Sleep and Associated Events: Rules, Terminology and Technical Specifications.* Version 2.5. Darien, IL: American Academy of Sleep Medicine.
12. Eckert, D. J., Jordan, A. S., Merchia, P., et al. (2007). Central sleep apnea: Pathophysiology and treatment. *Chest, 131*(2), 595–607.
13. Malley, W. J. (1990). *Clinical blood gases.* Philadelphia, PA: WB Saunders Company.
14. Ozsancak, A., D'Ambrosio, C., & Hill, N. S. (2008). Nocturnal noninvasive ventilation. *Chest, 133*(5), 1275–1286.
15. AASM Task Force. (2008). Clinical guidelines for the manual titration of positive airway pressure in patients with obstructive sleep apnea. *Journal of Clinical Sleep Medicine, 4*(2), 157–171.
16. NPPV Titration Task Force of AASM. (2010). Best clinical practices for the sleep center adjustment of noninvasive positive pressure ventilation (NPPV) in stable chronic alveolar hypoventilation syndromes. *Journal of Clinical Sleep Medicine, 6*(5), 491–509.

chapter 15

Insomnia

ROBERT N. TURNER

LEARNING OBJECTIVES

On completion of this chapter, the reader should be able to:

1. Summarize the complexity of insomnia.
2. Describe the prevalence, types, and potential causes of insomnia.
3. Describe the sleep history and relevant self-report techniques used in the assessment of insomnia.

KEY TERMS

Depression
Hyperarousal
Insomnia
Pittsburgh Sleep Quality Index
Polysomnography
Psychological testing
Sleep diary
Sleep history
Sleep hygiene

Difficulties with initiating and/or maintaining sleep have been described for centuries, yet significant progress in the understanding of these problems has occurred only within the past 60 years or so. Some cultures believed that disturbed sleep and dreams were associated with evil spirits and ghosts. Others have suggested that the gods determined poor sleep and the severity of the condition was in proportion to one's sinful deeds. As significant mysticism surrounded the complaint of sleep disturbances, remedies for these troubles included religious practices as well as assorted other rituals and various compounds. Disturbed sleep has long been associated with a wide variety of medical and psychological conditions. Chronic and acute pain, allergies, and various other disease processes have certainly disturbed the sleep of many throughout the centuries. In addition, psychiatric conditions and insomnia have long been described. An early study with groups of good and poor sleepers suggested a biologic basis for insomnia,

with greater physiologic arousal, including higher electromyogram levels and a faster heart rate, among poor sleepers (1). These differences were noted both during wakefulness and during sleep.

ISSUES OF DEFINITION

What Is Insomnia?

From our own lifetime experiences, most of us intuitively understand what is meant by the term "insomnia." There are criteria for diagnosis provided by the American Academy of Sleep Medicine (AASM). Short-term insomnia is considered a transient disturbance, typically lasting a few days to a few weeks, and typically not requiring treatment. Chronic insomnia persists for months or even years. The *International Classification of Sleep Disorders*, 3rd edition *(ICSD-3)* (2) requires that adults and children diagnosed with insomnia report one or more of the following:

1. Difficulty initiating sleep
2. Difficulty maintaining sleep
3. Waking up earlier than desired
4. Resistance to going to bed on an appropriate schedule
5. Difficulty sleeping without parent or caregiver intervention

In the past, subtypes of insomnia were described, but patients often failed to fit into a single category. Multiple sleep symptoms are more common than any single symptom, with symptoms occurring simultaneously or switching from one to another over time. In addition, patients with insomnia often overestimate the time taken to fall asleep and underestimate sleep duration, indicating an altered perception of sleep (3).

Patients with insomnia vary in the amount of sleep per night. Some people may feel alert, refreshed, and energized with only 6 hours of sleep, whereas other individuals may feel "horrible" after such a "poor" night's sleep. In addition, some regularly require more than an hour to initiate sleep, awaken four or more times during the sleep episode, and generally sleep about 6 hours per night, yet do not complain of insomnia. Others may awaken early in the morning. They may not complain of poor sleep. However, some may experience sleep-onset problems when requiring longer than 15 minutes to fall asleep, complain of insomnia with one or two brief awakenings during the sleep episode, and/or describe disturbed sleep if awakened earlier than usual. How do we make clinical sense of this?

First, the subjective experience of insomnia may have little to do with currently utilized objective sleep-electroencephalogram (EEG) parameters. Considerable variability obviously exists between one's perception and impression of sleep and laboratory findings (sleep latency and sleep duration). There exists a possibility that several other important measures of physiologic functioning, both during wakefulness and during sleep, which are not routinely employed in clinical evaluation settings, may more accurately reflect the subjectively experienced complaint of insomnia. As such, our current view of insomnia remains limited and only a partial view of the entire problem is understood.

Second, people with other sleep–wake disorders may incorrectly perceive that their problem is insomnia. Consider the middle-aged, moderately overweight, "stressed-out" male who snores and awakens frequently. He may believe that his problem is insomnia, yet obstructive apnea is one of his significant problems. Another example is a 50-year-old married female with a history of recurrent depression, migraine headaches, fibromyalgia, and asthma. Upon polysomnographic evaluation, snoring with repetitive arousals and stereotypic movements of the lower extremities are observed. Diagnoses may include upper airway resistance syndrome, periodic limb movement sleep disorder, and major depressive disorder. Both patients complain of insomnia, yet objective evaluation reveals other causes, likely promoting the experience of inadequate, nonrefreshing sleep.

Third, *people may have disorders comorbid with insomnia*. In other words, the patients described previously may have obstructive apnea *and* insomnia, or perhaps most commonly, depression *and* insomnia. In the past, primary insomnia was intended to represent discrete conditions, predicated upon conditioning factors, sleep-wake processes, and other matters as well. Secondary insomnia referred to the disturbance as a symptom associated with other variables, such as personality styles, numerous illnesses and disease, and a variety of psychiatric disorders. However, the cause-and-effect relationships of these factors have been difficult to determine. The most recent version of the *ICSD* (2) uses the term "comorbid" instead of secondary, reflecting a complex interaction between insomnia and other disorders. This is evident in a variety of medical disorders, especially those associated with pain; many psychiatric disorders, especially depression; and in interactions between sleep and medications used to treat comorbid disorders.

Fourth, circadian and aging factors also require consideration. In general, variations in core body temperature are correlated with the timing and duration of sleep and alertness. Older people may exhibit a lower amplitude of temperature rhythms and may also advance the sleep-alertness phase to an earlier time than younger people. Older patients may also report more frequent awakenings during the major sleep episode and complain of sleep-maintenance insomnia, whereas younger patients may describe sleep-onset insomnia. Both circadian and aging issues require consideration of normal sleep and rhythmic processes across the life span.

Fifth, in order to meet *ICSD-3* criteria for diagnosis (2), some degree of distress *must* be associated with the complaint. It has long been known that poor sleep can be associated with decrements in mood and performance. Consequences of poor sleep can be described in terms of interpersonal, emotional, cognitive, vocational, and/or other areas of general functioning. Resultant sleepiness during normal waking hours may or may not occur. Although these troubles can be merely annoying with short-term insomnia, data suggest the potential medical consequences of persistent difficulties initiating and/or maintaining sleep.

Sixth, chronic insomnia may be conceptualized as a disorder of hyperarousal. It is essential that one is aware of the potential 24-hour overactivation of the hypothalamic–pituitary–adrenal (HPA) axis and/or other systemic physiologic processes, because these may be primary etiologic factors. As mentioned, hyperarousal is typically present throughout the day and night (1).

To summarize, numerous factors, characteristics, and consequences are associated with insomnia. These sleep–wake disturbances require careful consideration of many potential medical/psychiatric factors in the complaint of insomnia, as well as environmental factors, primary sleep–wake pathologies, and numerous other variables.

EPIDEMIOLOGY

Early epidemiologic studies indicated that approximately one-third of respondents to surveys described sleep difficulties over the previous year and at least 50% reported the experience of insomnia at some time during their lives. Severe or constant sleep troubles were reported by about 10% to 30% and an estimated 6% meet criteria for the diagnosis of insomnia (4). The most frequent type of disturbance was sleep-maintenance insomnia, whereas sleep-onset insomnia and early-morning awakening insomnia were less common. Importantly, some individuals reported a combination of these troubles.

More recent studies have documented daytime consequences of insomnia. Patients with insomnia reported memory problems and attention/concentration impairments, as well as mood decrements and less positive experiences with interpersonal relationships. Katz and

McHorney (5) found that insomnia was associated with a worsened quality of life among a variety of patients with various illnesses. Collectively, evidence indicates that insomnia is widely prevalent, associated with daytime consequences, correlated with medical and mental health conditions, and associated with a reduced quality of life.

SHORT-TERM INSOMNIA

Short-term insomnia, or a brief episode of trouble falling and/or remaining asleep, affects almost everyone from time to time. Short-term insomnia is defined as a sleep problem lasting less than 3 months. During periods of stress or change (such as the loss of a loved one), individuals may exhibit time-limited difficulties with sleep. Sparingly studied through empirical methods, much remains unknown about this common problem within the general population.

According to the *ICSD-3* (2), the diagnosis of short-term insomnia requires that a sleep disturbance occurs for less than 3 months and represents a clear change from the person's typical sleep–wake patterns and habits.

Numerous external factors may promote short-term insomnia. Environmental disturbances, such as light and noise, stress, problematic interpersonal circumstances, and other matters, can initiate the problem. Changing one's typical circadian sleep–wake pattern and drug initiation and/or withdrawal are also possible contributors to short-term insomnia. Other external events, internal circumstances (e.g., medical problems), and short-duration pain or discomfort can also promote short-term insomnia. It is important to keep in mind that this time-limited, usually resolvable, problem can become a very significant issue in people's lives. It is well known that numerous factors can activate short-term insomnia. Personality style, genetic makeup, vulnerability to psychiatric illness, medical problems, and other issues can make the patient susceptible to persistent insomnia.

CHRONIC INSOMNIA

Criteria for the diagnosis of chronic insomnia are provided in *ICSD-3* (2). These problems must occur for 3 months or longer, and some degree of daytime impairment or distress is essential. The new classification system makes the diagnosis a binary decision—yes or no. Previous insomnia subcategories may have some value in tailoring treatment plans to address primary complaints, but no longer have an influence on whether or not the diagnosis is made.

A common thread in the diagnosis of chronic insomnia provided by research is the role of neuroendocrine dysregulation. Twenty-four-hour HPA axis activation has been reported among a small sample of subjects, as assessed by plasma levels of adrenocorticotropic hormone and cortisol (6). Shaver et al. (7) found elevations of morning urine cortisol levels among women with psychophysiologic insomnia. These studies suggest HPA overactivation among a proportion of insomnia patients.

A useful model of insomnia has been provided by Spielman and colleagues (see the review by Espie in reference [8]). The model proposes predisposing, precipitating, and perpetuating factors as key to the development of chronic insomnia. The predisposing factors would include HPA activation and other biologic contributors to insomnia. Precipitating events typically lead to short-term insomnia, which can evolve into chronic insomnia when perpetuating factors are present. Evaluating these factors is no longer a necessary part of the diagnostic process, but can be key to the choice of effective treatment options.

Previous Insomnia Subcategories

In earlier editions of ICSD, several subcategories of insomnia were listed. The current *ICSD-3* (2) has chosen to eliminate these categories because it is difficult to reliably distinguish between them, and their validity is questionable. Many of these classifications are, however, illustrative of the scope of the problem and help in framing issues with chronic insomnia. Only a brief, introductory description of selected subcategories will be presented here.

Psychophysiologic Insomnia

People with psychophysiologic insomnia tend to be absorbed with their troubles initiating and/or maintaining sleep. This condition is manifested by agitation, somatized tension, and conditioning factors, which prevent sleep from occurring. Both anticipatory and performance anxiety can be significant components. Most work to fall asleep, feel frustrated and anxious, become more aroused, and subsequently experience increased trouble falling and remaining asleep. Polysomnographic studies can reveal increased wakefulness, reduced sleep efficiency, and prolonged sleep latency. This form of conditioned or learned insomnia appears to perpetuate itself.

Paradoxical Insomnia

People with paradoxical insomnia are seen to sleep normally on measures observed by routine sleep-EEG measures. However, they report a reduced amount of, or a complete lack of, sleep. Older terminologies referred to this condition as "pseudoinsomnia" or sleep state misperception disorder, because objective measures did not parallel the patient's subjective complaint. Occasionally, patients report a complete lack of sleep and will passionately debate objective, sleep-EEG data when it is presented to them. One patient described the sleep study report as a good read but a work of complete fiction. Primary psychiatric disorders apparently are not clearly causative.

Hypnotic-Dependent Sleep Disorder

Because people can become tolerant of the effects of sedative-hypnotics, higher dosages may be required in order to achieve the same effect (an insomnia patient may need more and more medication to fall and/or remain asleep). Following abrupt cessation of hypnotic use, severe insomnia can result. Nervousness, intense dreams or nightmares, fragmented sleep, and other physiologic symptoms (nausea and tension) can be experienced. This is sometimes called "drug-withdrawal insomnia" and is particularly common following the withdrawal of benzodiazepines with short half-lives (<4 hours).

Inadequate Sleep Hygiene

Some people engage in behavioral patterns that are inconsistent with sleeping well. Consumption of caffeine, irregular sleep–wake timing, various poor presleep habits, and numerous other factors will promote trouble falling and remaining asleep. This is seen when these variables are the most significant factors underlying the patient's insomnia.

Idiopathic Insomnia

Idiopathic insomnia is a condition characterized by lifelong difficulties initiating and maintaining sleep. It seems to begin during infancy or early childhood and causes ongoing functional impairment or distress. Unusual sleep spindles can be seen during stage N2 sleep, and rapid eye movement (REM) sleep can contain few eye movements. Although its etiology is not completely understood, an underlying neurologic abnormality is suspected. Severity can range from mild to severe, and daytime consequences often include attention/concentration problems, irritability, depressed or anxious mood, daytime fatigue, and, perhaps, memory impairment. The course of this condition is chronic and is not better explained by another sleep, neurologic, medical, psychiatric, or substance abuse disorder.

Circadian Rhythm Disorders and Chronic Insomnia

Circadian rhythm disorders can initially present as insomnia. Difficulty initiating or maintaining sleep may be perceived by the patient as the primary complaint. However, patients with advanced or delayed sleep phase sleep relatively normally when time constraints are removed. Chronic insomnia may include an element of chronobiologic dysfunction (8), and patients may or may not achieve diagnostic criteria for circadian rhythm sleep disorders as defined in *ICSD-3* (2).

Other Associated Disorders

Previously, a distinction of insomnia associated with other conditions was referred to as "secondary insomnia." The current *ICSD-3* has eliminated these distinctions. It argues that even when other disorders are treated, there is often a residual insomnia that must be addressed. Nevertheless, other disorders can, and do, impact insomnia and are valuable to discuss.

Psychiatric Disorders

Virtually any psychiatric disorder can be associated with comorbid insomnia. Most notably, generalized anxiety disorder, acute stress disorder, posttraumatic stress disorder, dysthymia, major depression, bipolar disorder, and schizoaffective disorder are all associated with sleep-alertness disorders. Abbreviated REM sleep latencies, delta sleep abnormalities (usually decreases in slow-wave sleep), increased REM densities (especially during the first third of the night), and sleep continuity disturbances can be found among patients with major depressive disorder. However, these sleep-EEG characteristics may also be found among patients with other psychiatric syndromes and personality disorders. Diagnostic and research issues with sleep and depression were discussed by Buysse (3). The interaction between insomnia and depression is complex, and the comorbidity of the two makes treatment challenging.

Medical Conditions

Many medical conditions or disease processes may promote secondary insomnia. Pain syndromes, asthma, chronic obstructive pulmonary disease, fibromyalgia, migraine and cluster headaches, gastroesophageal reflux disease, peptic ulcers, and scores of other medical problems can be associated with chronic disturbances of sleep initiation and/or sleep maintenance. Neurologic conditions, such as Parkinson disease and dementia, can also contribute to insomnia. Sleep research data are limited or simply not available for many medical conditions, and the impact of insomnia on patients with these problems has not been fully explored.

Medications and Insomnia

Virtually any medication can potentially promote problems falling or remaining asleep. These therapeutic agents target the treatment of medical or psychiatric conditions, but sleeplessness can be an undesirable side effect of the given compound. Stimulants and antidepressants with inhibition of serotonin uptake are known to promote insomnia in some patients. Corticosteroids, bronchodilators, and some antihypertensives can have the same effect. Insomnia can also be caused by the abrupt discontinuation of hypnotics and anxiolytics.

Other Sleep Disorders

Many other sleep–wake disorders can facilitate disturbances initiating and/or maintaining sleep. Restless legs syndrome and periodic limb movement sleep disorder, central sleep apnea, and some types of parasomnias can be associated with complaints of chronic insomnia. Even patients with narcolepsy can present with complaints of insomnia. As indicated previously, a robust kinship between any primary sleep disorder and the complaint of trouble falling and/or remaining asleep may exist.

EVALUATION

Evaluation of insomnia requires several steps in order to effectively assess the problem and determine appropriate treatment strategies. Establishing a diagnosis of chronic insomnia is relatively straightforward, but because chronic difficulties initiating and maintaining sleep may be a symptom of other medical/psychiatric problems, a sleep history, a full medical history, a family history of disease, a family history of sleep disorders, and a physical examination are always indicated. Specific sleep questionnaires and sleep diaries, as well as psychological assessment measures, are also important in describing the characteristics and consequences of the patient's sleep problem(s). It is important to note that, at this writing, a standardized manner of data collection has not been clearly established and procedures may vary from setting to setting. Some evaluation and treatment programs prefer the completion of questionnaires and other forms before the first visit, whereas others initiate the consultation first and then obtain self-report measures.

Sleep History

The initial, absolutely crucial step in the evaluation of disturbed sleep (insomnia, sleep apnea, or any sleep–wake disorder) includes one-on-one consultation with the sleep specialist. This first appointment serves several very important purposes, including information gathering and providing an environment for the description of wakefulness and/or sleep problems. Importantly, the first contact often fosters alliance with the sleep specialist, promoting a sense of security and also implying that the patient's complaint will (finally!) be taken seriously. Because the patient may or may not be aware of certain features of the disturbance, a family member or bed partner can accompany him or her during this visit.

In this manner, sleep specialists work to build rapport, promoting a calm, trusting environment for addressing and expounding upon relevant issues and complaints.

Flexibility in obtaining subjective information pertaining to the patient's sleep–wake disorder is important. Other related procedures, such as a mental status examination and general psychological evaluation interview, can be completed along with the consultation. What follows is only a general overview of some parameters assessed during the first visit. Table 15-1 describes the core elements of the sleep history.

The sleep consultation includes both open-ended questions and opportunities for straightforward, concrete "yes" or "no" responses to inquiries. Starting the interview with basic demographic information (name, date, referral source, age, birth date, and telephone number) followed by the patient's description of the reason for referral initiates the process smoothly. It is imperative that the interviewer listen carefully to the patient's perception of the problem, because *his or her view of the problem* will be very important to integrate later with acquired clinical information. In addition, this preliminary information can aid in establishing a reasonable

Table 15-1 Core Elements of a Sleep History Consultation

- Ask about and define the patient's sleep–wake problem
- Determine the duration and course of the condition(s)
- Assess sleep–wake patterns, habits, and daytime sleepiness
- Address symptoms of sleep-related breathing disorders, parasomnias, narcolepsy, and movement disorders
- Discuss both prescription and over-the-counter drug use, as well as alcohol and other substance use
- Address weight loss/gain, as well as cardiac, pulmonary, neurologic, psychiatric, and other system illnesses
- Evaluate current medication schedule, current medical problems, and medical–surgical history
- Assess other subjective characteristics of sleep-alertness disorders
- Assess family medical and sleep disorder histories and social history
- Review obtained information with the patient
- Explain tentative diagnoses to the patient
- Describe further testing and/or treatment strategies
- Offer follow-up visit

treatment plan and may also provide clues to potential compliance issues.

Following the patient's open-ended response to the "Why are you here today?" inquiry, it is useful to ask about the duration of the problem as well as sleep–wake habits (bedtime, time in bed, perceived sleep latency, the frequency and duration of awakenings, and customary arising time). Thereafter, one may choose to ask about the tendency to arise immediately following awakenings and how he or she feels at that time. These data are essential in describing sleep–wake rhythms, as well as to document variations in habits and potential physiologic disturbances.

An assessment of circadian functioning is useful. Simply asking about the patient's "best time of day," if any, will allow the interviewer to ascertain whether the patient's "peak time" corresponds with established patterns and habits. An assessment of daytime sleepiness follows, determining the likelihood of sleeping while driving, at work, during social situations, at home, or during other quiet activities. An evaluation of the consequences of sleepiness is also helpful, because hypersomnia may negatively impact familial, occupational, social, and leisure functions. Additionally, problems with attention and concentration, memory functions (especially recent memory), and stability of mood are also worth exploring.

Because insomnia can be comorbid to a variety of sleep disorders, questions pertaining to snoring and sleep apnea are also necessary. Awakening with chest pain, brady-tachycardia episodes, and/or respiratory distress are all significant. A determination of whether apneic events have been observed by others is likewise important. An inquiry regarding sleep position preference is also helpful.

An assessment of vital signs, the physical examination, and a brief medical history may follow. The patient may report current weight and height, whether he or she has gained or lost weight over the past year, and if substantial changes in weight have occurred during the previous years. Patients may be asked about hypertension, as well as a medical history that includes cardiac, pulmonary, thyroid, kidney, liver, diabetes, or other diseases. Psychiatric history and associated past treatments, including therapies for sleep disturbance, are also discussed. An evaluation of the patient's current medication schedule, as well as a history of sedative–hypnotic and other psychotropic drug use, is important. A review of current medical problems, as well as medical/surgical history, is necessary. A discussion of alcohol, caffeine, and other substance use is also indicated. Finally, a determination of when the patient last visited his or her doctor is essential.

An evaluation of parasomnias, movement disorders, and narcolepsy should be done. A review of the occurrence of sleepwalking, nightmares, enuresis, sleep terrors,

significant somniloquy, and other potential unusual behavioral disorders of sleep is helpful. Symptoms of restless legs syndrome or periodic limb movement sleep disorder require exploration. Furthermore, addressing other potential medical conditions and sleep (gastroesophageal reflux disease, nocturnal headache, etc.) is necessary. Finally, a discussion of intentional and unintentional nap episodes, cataplexy, sleep paralysis, and both hypnagogic and hypnopompic hallucinations is essential.

Toward the end of the sleep history consultation, the authors have found it beneficial for patients to describe the last time they slept well and felt alert throughout the following day. The patient's view of the severity of his or her problem (mild, moderate, or severe), as well as any previous treatment gains and preferences, is also important. A family medical history, addressing cardiac, neurologic, pulmonary, thyroid and other diseases, as well as diabetes and hypertension, is also necessary. The family sleep disorders history, detailing snoring, insomnia, parasomnias, and so on, is also described. In concluding the interview, the patient's relational, academic, and occupational histories should round out the initial consultation.

These data provide the sleep specialist with a reasonable amount of information to assign preliminary diagnoses, as well as justify the need for confirmatory testing or treatment implementation. Polysomnograms and/or multiple sleep latency tests are necessary if significant symptoms of sleep apnea, narcolepsy, or other primary sleep–wake disorders are likely on the basis of historical data. If physiologic evaluation of sleep and/or wakefulness is not clearly indicated, an individualized sleep diary can be written with the patient. Other questionnaires and psychological evaluations can also be completed.

Before ending the consultation, it is helpful for the patient to review obtained information, discuss diagnoses, and address steps that will be taken in his or her evaluation and treatment. The latter is an essential part of the initial process, because this provides objective reasons for further assessment, serves to inform about procedures involved (including polysomnography and psychological testing), and establishes the groundwork for interventions. It is also important for the interviewer to respond openly and directly to patient inquiries and to do so in an appropriate fashion. Neglecting or minimizing this last portion of the initial assessment can lead to patient dissatisfaction, compliance problems, and, unfortunately, numerous other evaluation and treatment problems.

Questionnaires/Self-Monitoring Materials Associated with Sleep and Alertness

Many questionnaires and other self-report inventories are currently available that purportedly assess the subjective aspects of disordered sleep and wakefulness. Some clinics and sleep centers may use assessment instruments that have been authored by staff members. Although these may possess some degree of validity (measure what they are intended to measure) and reliability (consistency or stability), they may not adequately describe symptoms, associated problems, or the nature and the impact of the condition upon an individual's functioning. In addition, the use of inventories and/or questionnaires as a "substitute" for the more time-intensive sleep history consultation is suboptimal because interview and questionnaire procedures actually serve different, complementary purposes. At worst, many significant aspects of the ongoing sleep–wake disorder are neglected. Therefore, these self-report instruments need to be integrated with the sleep disorder consultation findings.

Two widely used assessment instruments, developed within sleep research, have been subject to psychometric evaluation. The Pittsburgh Sleep Quality Index (9), a brief clinically useful self-report inventory, evaluates subjective sleep quality and disturbance over the previous month. The Epworth Sleepiness Scale (10) measures subjective sleepiness. Reliability and validity measures have been acceptable for both. Together, these provide additional subjective information, which may support the patient's perception of the sleep–wake disturbance and provide evidence to support the diagnostic criteria. However, these instruments may not strongly correlate with objective physiologic findings and do not substitute for polysomnograms or multiple sleep latency tests in the diagnosis of other sleep disorders.

Mood and Personality Assessment

Although there are numerous purposes for psychological assessment, these procedures generally concern themselves with utilizing various techniques and specific psychological tests in evaluating an individual's cognitive, emotional, interpersonal, and behavioral functioning, as well as providing recommendations for appropriate treatment interventions. A large number of instruments are available, focusing upon several different domains of professional practice. Many self-report tests have not been used in clinical sleep medicine, but focused psychological testing can be quite valuable in clarifying areas of problematic functioning. In addition, some brief inventories or scales provide objective scores in measuring or determining the severity of depression, anxiety, anger, irritability, and other mood states or traits. Longer or more involved procedures, such as personality or neuropsychological assessment, focus upon broader ranges of the person's cognitive abilities, strengths and weaknesses, emotional and adaptive functioning, interpersonal style, and behavioral tendencies. The collaborating psychologist usually

determines which tests are most appropriate for use with individual patients.

As with inventories assessing sleep quality and disturbances, self-report instruments have been administered to clinical and research samples of patients. Dozens of these brief, symptom-oriented questionnaires are available, and many possess adequate validity and reliability. A few have been routinely used in sleep disorder clinics. The Beck Depression Inventory (11) is a multiple choice, 21-item device, which detects the presence of depression and accurately rates its severity. This and other scales are useful for evaluation of patients in sleep disorder clinics.

Assessment of psychopathology and personal adjustment generally requires the use of clinical interviews and structured, standardized psychological tests. This typically falls outside of the purview of the sleep center evaluation.

POLYSOMNOGRAPHY AND ACTIGRAPHY

In the absence of symptoms of sleep apnea or movement disorders, the AASM recommends that "Polysomnography and daytime multiple sleep latency testing (MSLT) are not indicated in the routine evaluation of chronic insomnia, including insomnia due to psychiatric or neuropsychiatric disorders" (12). An overnight sleep study may be indicated if the patient fails treatment or if the diagnosis is uncertain. Actigraphy provides an indication of sleep timing and duration, as estimated from periods of reduced movement. "Actigraphy is indicated as a method to characterize circadian rhythm patterns or sleep disturbances in individuals with insomnia, including insomnia associated with depression" (12).

REFERENCES

1. Monroe, L. (1967). Psychological and physiological differences between good and poor sleepers. *Journal of Abnormal Psychology, 72*(3), 255–264.
2. American Academy of Sleep Medicine. (2014). *International classification of sleep disorders* (3rd ed.). Darien, IL: Author.
3. Buysse, D. J. (2013). Insomnia. *JAMA, 309*, 706–716.
4. Roth, T. (2007). Insomnia: Definition, prevalence, etiology, and consequences. *Journal of Clinical Sleep Medicine, 3*, S7–S10.
5. Katz, D. A., & McHorney, C. A. (2002). The relationship between insomnia and health-related quality of life in patients with chronic illness. *Journal of Family Practice, 51*, 229–235.

6. Vgontzas, A. N., Bixler, E. O., Lin, H., et al. (2002). Chronic insomnia is associated with nyctohemeral activation of the hypothalamic-pituitary-adrenal axis: Clinical implications. *The Journal of Clinical Endocrinology and Metabolism, 86*(8), 3787–3794.

7. Shaver, J. L., Johnston, S. K., Lentz, M. J., et al. (2002). Stress exposure, psychological distress, and physiological stress activation in midlife women with insomnia. *Psychosomatic Medicine, 64*, 793–802.

8. Espie, C. A. (2002). Insomnia: Conceptual issues in the development, persistence, and treatment of sleep disorder in adults. *Annual Review of Psychology, 53*(1), 215–243.

9. Buysse, D. J., Reynolds, C. E., Monk, T. H., et al. (1989). The Pittsburgh Sleep Quality Index: A new instrument for psychiatric practice and research. *Psychiatry Research, 28*, 193–213.

10. Johns, M. W. (1997). A new method for measuring daytime sleepiness: The Epworth Sleepiness Scale. *Sleep, 14*(6), 540–545.

11. Beck, A. T., Ward, C. H., Mendelson, M., et al. (1961). An inventory of measuring depression. *Archives of General Psychiatry, 4*, 561–571.

12. Schutte-Rodin, S., Broch, L., Buysse, D., et al. (2008). Clinical guideline for the evaluation and management of chronic insomnia in adults. *Journal of Clinical Sleep Medicine, 4*(5), 487–504.

chapter 16

Central Disorders of Hypersomnolence

RUI M. DE SOUSA   TAMARA KAYE SELLMAN

LEARNING OBJECTIVES

On completion of this chapter, the reader should be able to:

1. Describe the two different types of narcolepsy.
2. Name and describe the narcoleptic tetrad.
3. Explain the role of hypocretin in sleep.
4. Define hypersomnia.
5. Describe sleep drunkenness.
6. Name the three salient features of Kleine–Levin syndrome.
7. Name medical disorders that may cause hypersomnia.
8. Name drugs or substances that may cause hypersomnia.
9. Name psychiatric disorders that may cause hypersomnia.

KEY TERMS

Actigraphy
Advanced sleep phase syndrome (ASPS)
Areflexia
Atonia
Cataplexy
Conversion disorder
CSF hypocretin-1
Differential diagnosis
Delayed sleep phase syndrome (DSPS)
Excessive daytime sleepiness (EDS)
Epworth Sleepiness Scale (ESS)
γ-aminobutyric acid (GABA)
Human leukocyte antigen (HLA)
Hyperphagia
Hypersexuality
Hypnagogic and hypnopompic hallucinations
Hypocretin/orexin
Idiopathic
Insufficient sleep syndrome
Kleine–Levin syndrome (KLS)
Long sleep
Mazindol

Menstrual-related hypersomnia
Modafinil
Multiple sleep latency test (MSLT)
Maintenance of wakefulness test (MWT)
Narcolepsy tetrad
Narcolepsy types 1 and 2
Objective versus subjective tests
Oxford Sleep Resistance Test (OSLER)
Pitolisant
Periodic limb movement disorder (PLMD)
Posttraumatic hypersomnia
Rapid eye movement (REM) related
Seasonal affective disorder (SAD)
Sedating substances
Short sleep
Sleep debt
Sleep diary
Sleep drunkenness
Sleep hygiene
Sleep inertia
Sleeping Beauty syndrome
Sodium oxybate
Sleep-onset REM period (SOREMP)
Stanford Sleepiness Scale (SSS)

CENTRAL DISORDERS OF HYPERSOMNOLENCE—INTRODUCTION

The primary hypersomnias:
- Narcolepsy
  - Narcolepsy type 1
  - Narcolepsy type 2
- Idiopathic hypersomnia (IH)
- Recurrent hypersomnia (Kleine–Levin syndrome [KLS])
  - Subtype: Menstrual-related hypersomnia

The secondary hypersomnias:
- Hypersomnia due to a medical disorder
- Hypersomnia due to a medication or substance
- Hypersomnia due to a psychiatric disorder
- Insufficient sleep syndrome (ISS)

Normal variant: Long sleeper (1)

Introduction

Hypersomnia, derived from the Greek *hyper* (over, above, too much) and the Latin *somnus* (sleep), literally refers to the condition of sleeping too much. However, in current medical terminology, both *hypersomnia* and the related word *hypersomnolence* are used more broadly and interchangeably to indicate long sleep duration, excessive daytime sleepiness (EDS), or both.

Hypersomnolence, the state of being excessively sleepy when a person should be alert, is one of the most common sleep-related complaints that patients mention to their doctors. The *International Classification of Sleep Disorders* (*ICSD-3*) describes eight central disorders of hypersomnolence. Although the *ICSD-3* does not explicitly divide these eight sleep disorders into two categories, we can discern two basic groups of hypersomnias: the *primary hypersomnias* (not caused by another condition) and *secondary hypersomnias* (caused by or related to a different condition).

The four primary hypersomnias are those occurring independently of any other condition or effect. They include the two types of narcolepsy, IH, and recurrent hypersomnia.

The most salient feature of primary hypersomnia is an extreme, overwhelming sleepiness during periods when the patient should be alert and awake (usually the daytime hours). Even though the patient's nighttime sleep may seem to be of normal quality and timing, patients still feel sleepy and lethargic during the day.

A vast array of conditions can cause secondary hypersomnias. They aren't limited to just other sleep disorders like obstructive sleep apnea (OSA) or periodic limb movement disorder (PLMD), but extend to other medical conditions, disorders, and diseases. For example, drugs (prescribed or not) and other substances will often have side effects that cause extreme sleepiness in those who take them. Hypersomnia is also often noted in psychiatric disorders.

In addition, people sometimes curtail their normal nocturnal sleep on a regular basis, resulting in inappropriate daytime sleepiness.

EDS is the primary concern for many patients presenting with sleep complaints. EDS is a significant public health problem, with prevalence in the community estimated to be anywhere from 4% (2), 18% (3), or almost 28% (4). Yet, because it is an invisible condition, hypersomnolence is linked to social stigmas which often prevent patients from seeking help. Patients who are excessively sleepy are also at greater risk for psychosocial problems, behavioral disorders, motor vehicle and workplace accidents, and obesity (5).

There are several tools, both objective and subjective, that can be used to assess and diagnose sleepiness and disorders of hypersomnolence:
- Polysomnography (PSG), the multiple sleep latency test (MSLT), and the maintenance of wakefulness test (MWT) are used to objectively measure sleep and propensity to sleep.
- In some cases, actigraphy is an adequate proxy in the absence of PSG.
- Scaled questionnaires such as the Epworth Sleepiness Scale and the Stanford Sleepiness Scale that provide subjective information to measure sleepiness.
- Self-reported sleep diaries and detailed medical histories are also crucial tools when diagnosing or treating hypersomnia.

Some significant changes were made to the *ICSD* between the second and third edition that deserve mention here:
- The narcolepsies are no longer divided by the presence or absence of a symptom (narcolepsy with cataplexy vs. narcolepsy without cataplexy [6]); they are now divided by their inferred pathogenesis:
  - narcolepsy type 1 (absent or low hypocretin levels)
  - narcolepsy type 2 (normal hypocretin levels [7])
- IH was also streamlined, from IH (with and without long sleep time) to a more simplified diagnosis of IH.
- The recurrent hypersomnias were also combined into just one major concern: KLS and a subtype related to menstruation.

The rest of this chapter will mirror the general blueprint of the hypersomnia disorders as outlined in the *ICSD-3*.

CENTRAL DISORDERS OF HYPERSOMNOLENCE—NARCOLEPSY

Introduction

Narcolepsy is a rare, chronic, neurologic sleep disorder with no known cure. This lifelong condition is characterized by EDS and deterioration in the brain's ability to control sleep–wake cycles.

There are two subtypes, *narcolepsy type 1*, with extremely low concentration of hypocretin, and *narcolepsy type 2*, with near-normal hypocretin levels.

The Narcolepsy Tetrad

Although the severity and range of symptoms may vary, narcolepsy is generally characterized by a tetrad of symptoms:

1. **Excessive daytime sleepiness:** EDS is the most common feature of narcolepsy. It can manifest as difficulty staying awake, irresistible microsleeps, increased napping, memory loss, cognitive problems, and struggles in work, school, or personal life. This sleepiness usually persists throughout the day, irrespective of the quality or quantity of sleep during the night. Naps are characteristically short but refreshing, although the normal wakefulness state between naps will not typically last. The narcoleptic will soon return to a sleepy state after a nap.

2. **Cataplexy:** This is a symptom in which strong emotion or laughter causes a person to suffer sudden physical collapse caused by an abrupt loss of voluntary muscle tone (atonia). It is characterized by the preservation of consciousness and memory and occurs for a short duration (less than a few minutes). It is believed that in cataplexy, the processes that produce paralysis during rapid eye movement (REM) sleep become inappropriately active during times of wakefulness.

Typical examples of cataplexy include simple buckling of the knees, head dropping, facial muscle drooping, sagging of the jaw, or weakness in the arms. Slurred speech or a complete inability to speak may also be observed. At times, these "drop attacks" or "sleep attacks" can escalate into episodes of complete muscle paralysis lasting up to several minutes. However, the patient often has sufficient warning of cataplexy and can sit or lay down in time to prevent falls or injury. Episodes may occur several times per day or a few times per year. Longer episodes can sometimes evolve into sleep, often with hypnagogic hallucinations.

Cataplexy usually develops within a few months of EDS symptoms, but may develop 10 to 30 years later. Cataplexy has been reported to improve with age, likely after the patient has learned to better control his or her emotions (7). In rare cases, withdrawal from certain antidepressant or anticataplectic drugs can result in *status cataplecticus*, a state in which the patient is cataplectic for a prolonged time, often hours (7, 8).

The importance of cataplexy for the diagnosis of narcolepsy has been recognized since its first connection with narcolepsy. Historically, narcolepsy was divided into the presence or absence of cataplexy. More recently, however, this approach has been abandoned for a different model focusing on underlying disease processes rather than witnessed symptoms. The *ICSD-3* now divides narcolepsy into two distinct subgroups:
- Those having narcolepsy with very low levels of hypocretin in the cerebrospinal fluid (CSF), often manifesting as cataplexy
- Those having narcolepsy with near-normal concentrations of hypocretin, which does not result in cataplexy (1)

3. **Hypnagogic and hypnopompic hallucinations:** Hallucinations are a common characteristic of narcolepsy. They occur either as the patient is falling asleep (hypnagogic) or right as he or she is waking up (hypnopompic). Although the majority of hallucinations are visual, they can also be auditory or tactile (8).

The hallucinations are often unpleasant, tinged with an underlying current of fear or threat (7). Common themes are hallucinations of an intruder in the room or a sensation of floating. Hypnagogic hallucinations are often associated with sleep attacks (cataplexy). Like cataplexy, these hallucinations are believed to be REM-related phenomena (dreams) intruding into the wake state.

4. **Sleep paralysis:** Sleep paralysis is a state in which a person is physically immobile, but fully conscious before or following a period of sleep. This symptom has been reported in 20% to 50% of narcoleptics. Patients with cataplexy experience an inability to move their limbs or lift their head, or describe difficulty breathing. Sleep paralysis is often distressing because it may last up to a few minutes. It is usually interrupted by noise or other stimuli (7). Just like cataplexy and hallucinations, sleep paralysis is likewise believed to be a particular feature of REM-related atonia manifesting into wakefulness. It is also more commonly noted with hypnagogic hallucinations.

It is also important to note that sleep paralysis and hypnagogic hallucinations are not specific for narcolepsy. These symptoms can occur in 15% of otherwise normal persons and can often be precipitated by sleep loss, schedule change, or alcohol consumption. These symptoms can also occur in IH. Narcoleptic hallucinations are sometimes misdiagnosed as schizophrenic ones (7, 8). However, most of the narcolepsy-related hallucinations tend to be visual, whereas the schizophrenic ones are more likely to be auditory.

The presentation of this tetrad is variable in symptoms and intensity across patients and over time. Only about 10% of patients concurrently exhibit all components (9). Other characteristic features outside the narcolepsy tetrad include objective differences in REM sleep (namely, a short latency to REM sleep and REM episodes during short naps), fragmented nocturnal sleep, automatic behavior, loss of concentration and memory, and blurred vision (1, 10).

Presently, treatment for both forms of narcolepsy is tailored to the individual and focused on managing symptoms with various medications and lifestyle changes.

Literature Review and a History of Narcolepsy

A case study by Gélineau (1880) is recognized for giving narcolepsy its name and for recognizing the disorder as a specific clinical entity.

However, Gélineau did not differentiate episodes of muscle weakness and "sleep attacks" triggered by emotions. The first descriptions of narcolepsy–cataplexy were reported in Germany by Westphal (1877) and Fisher (1878). They both reported irresistible sleepiness and episodes of muscle weakness triggered by excitement (11).

Following WWII, as a result of the prevailing psychoanalytic influence, sleep researchers were pressured to describe and treat narcolepsy as a psychosomatic disorder. However, work by Kleitman and Daniels refocused research to investigate an organic cause to narcolepsy (11).

In 1960, Vogel was the first to report REM sleep at sleep onset in a narcoleptic patient, which was confirmed and then extended and expanded by Rechtschaffen and Dement a few years later. These observations were the basis that led to the hypothesis that narcolepsy and REM were associated. This also led to the development of the MSLT test, discussed in further detail later. The first narcolepsy clinic was opened in Stanford University in 1964 by Dement.

The first epidemiologic studies by Solomon (1945) concluded a prevalence rate of 20 per 100,000 (12). Subsequent studies by Roth (13), Dement (14, 15), and Honda (16) estimate the prevalence from 40 to 160 per 100,000. These numbers are the most commonly quoted even today.

In the early 1900s, ephedrine was used as a treatment for EDS in narcolepsy until Prinzmetal and Bloomberg introduced amphetamines in 1935. In 1959, Yoss and Daly used methylphenidate to treat narcolepsy, and in 1960, Akimoto, Honda, and Takahashi used imipramine (a tricyclic antidepressant) in the treatment of human cataplexy, establishing the stimulant/antidepressant model used to treat narcolepsy to this date (11).

In the mid-1990s, research into the neurogenesis of narcolepsy by two separate and independent teams of researchers revealed the role of a new neuropeptide simultaneously named both *hypocretin* and *orexin*. Today, both terms are used interchangeably to reference the same neuropeptide (17, 18).

Prevalence of Narcolepsy

Prevalence of narcolepsy is estimated to be between 0.02% and 0.16% of the general population, with possible ethnic or genetic factors influencing the observed variance in rates (19).

Symptoms usually appear in the middle of adolescence, but diagnosis is typically made later in life. A second, although smaller, peak is observed in the mid-30s. Although the prevalence of narcolepsy type 2 in first-degree relatives of patients with narcolepsy is only 1% to 2%, this still represents a 10 to 40 times higher relative risk of getting narcolepsy compared with the general population (19, 20).

Genetic Determinants of Narcolepsy

Genetic predisposition is suspected because of narcolepsy's strong association with the human leukocyte antigen (HLA), leading the first investigators to believe that narcolepsy was an autoimmune disorder. Early genetic research into narcolepsy showed a relation with the HLA genes, more specifically, the subtypes DR2/DRB1*1501 and DQB1*0602. Other HLA subtypes have shown a weaker association with narcolepsy.

Current research focuses on the HLA DQB1*0602 allele, present in over 90% of narcoleptic patients.

However, because about 20% of the population carries this allele and only 0.05% of the population develops narcolepsy, this association is not specific (21).

Although the HLA research is most well known, there are many studies that point to other genetic links with narcolepsy, including polymorphisms in the T-cell receptor-α (TCRA) locus on chromosome 14, TNFSF4 (also called OX40L), Cathepsin H (CTSH), the purinergic receptor P2RY11, the DNA (cytosine-5)-methyltransferase 1, and carnitine palmitoyltransferase (CPT1B) (20).

Despite the genetic evidence in narcolepsy, the picture is complex and incomplete. In fact, even with monozygotic (identical) twins, chances are that narcolepsy is not shared between the two, with reported concordance rates of between 25% and 31% (22). Genetic expression is also likely influenced by environmental factors.

Environmental Factors in Narcolepsy

The nature of possible environmental triggers is unknown; nevertheless, onset of narcolepsy is frequently associated with environmental factors. These include head trauma, stroke, and change in the sleep–wake cycle (22). Recent studies have also shown an association with streptococcal infection (23, 24), influenza A virus subtype H_1N_1 (swine flu) infection (as well as vaccination in European countries) (25), and exposure to heavy metals, insecticides, and weed killers (26). Table 16-1 lists the etiologic factors associated with narcolepsy.

Narcolepsy: A Tale of Two Types
Narcolepsy Type 1

Diagnostic criteria for narcolepsy type 1 (1).
Criteria A and B must be met:

a. The patient has daily periods of irrepressible need to sleep or daytime lapses into sleep occurring over a period greater than or equal to 3 months.
b. The presence of one or both of the following:
1. Cataplexy and a mean sleep latency of less than or equal to 8 minutes and greater than or equal to two sleep-onset REM periods (SOREMPs) on an MSLT performed according to standard techniques. A SOREMP (within 15 minutes of sleep onset) on the preceding nocturnal polysomnogram may replace one of the SOREMPs on the MSLT.
2. CSF hypocretin-1 concentration, measured by immunoreactivity, is either less than or equal to 110 pg per mL or less than one-third of mean values obtained in normal subjects with the same standardized assay.

To diagnose narcolepsy type 1, the patient must present with irresistible sleep attacks and either cataplexy or decreased hypocretin levels.

Narcolepsy type 1 was previously known as *narcolepsy with cataplexy*. Narcolepsy type 2 was previously known as *narcolepsy without cataplexy*. This underlies the role that cataplexy has had in the history of narcolepsy and its diagnosis. However, with the discovery of the neuropeptide *hypocretin* (also known as *orexin*), which plays an important role in diagnosing narcolepsy, the *ICSD-3* elected to categorize narcolepsy by the absence (type 1) or presence (type 2) of hypocretin, rather than using cataplexy in the diagnostic criteria.

Narcolepsy Type 1: The Role of Hypocretin

Hypocretin is a hypothalamic neuropeptide that is involved in the regulation of arousal, wakefulness, and appetite. Using immunoassay techniques, hypocretins were first discovered in 1998 (17), when their roles in sleep regulation became immediately evident. Narcolepsy type 1 is caused by a lack (or significant reduction) of this neuropeptide in the brain due to destruction of the cells that produce it.

Hypocretins are measured in the CSF, collected via a lumbar puncture (spinal tap). When testing for narcolepsy type 1, CSF concentration of hypocretin is either less than 110 pg per mL or less than one-third of mean values of normal subjects (1).

In the healthy population (those with well-regulated sleep), hypocretins are released when awake to target neurons that promote wakefulness and suppress REM sleep. In people who have narcolepsy type 1, up to 95% of these neurons die off (20, 27). Other neurologic insults may also reduce hypocretin concentrations, such as hypothalamic lesions or injuries to the brain characterized as vascular, inflammatory, or traumatic in nature (see Table 16-1). These insults can affect hypocretin levels either permanently or temporarily (28). The consequent lack of hypocretins results in prolonged sleepiness and poor control of REM sleep. REM sleep can become so poorly regulated that the paralysis or dreaming that normally occurs only in REM sleep can intrude upon wakefulness, causing cataplexy and dreamlike hallucinations.

Table 16-1 Known Primary and Secondary Etiologies of Narcolepsy

Hypocretin deficiency
Hypothalamic lesions
Inherited disorders (e.g., Niemann–Pick disease type C)
Brain tumors
Craniocerebral trauma
Cerebrovascular disorders
Encephalomyelitis
Neurodegenerative diseases
Demyelinating disorders

Data from American Academy of Sleep Medicine. (2014). *International classification of sleep disorders* (3rd ed.). Darien, IL: Author. Copyright © American Academy of Sleep Medicine.

Although low levels of hypocretin can assist in diagnosing narcolepsy, one must be aware that low levels can also be observed in other neurologic disorders, such as Guillain–Barré syndrome, Miller Fisher syndrome, advanced forms of Parkinson disease (PD), and other neurologic conditions associated with lesion or dysfunction of the lateral hypothalamus (29).

Lower levels of hypocretin aren't the only concern for those with narcolepsy type 1. Cataplexy and sleep paralysis are states in which the processes that produce paralysis during REM sleep become activated during wakefulness. During REM sleep, most muscles are temporarily paralyzed by processes controlled by the lower brainstem. The release of the neurotransmitters norepinephrine and serotonin is typically blocked by the brainstem during wakefulness in those experiencing cataplexy or sleep paralysis. Along with reduced levels of hypocretins, levels of these other neurotransmitters may also be lower, permitting abnormal periods of paralysis even during wakefulness. This observation provides a basis for treating cataplexy with antidepressants, which serve to increase brain levels of norepinephrine and serotonin.

The role of hypocretins may also explain how cataplexy may be triggered by strong emotions. The amygdala and prefrontal cortex, brain regions that regulate emotional responses, connect with the paralysis pathways in the brainstem. Neurons in the amygdala and prefrontal cortex have been found to be active during cataplexy.

Researchers have also learned that deactivating either of these regions reduces cataplexy in mice with narcolepsy. As these triggering pathways become better understood, it may be possible to target them with new medications (30).

Narcolepsy Type 2

Diagnostic criteria narcolepsy type 2 (1). Criteria A to E must be met:

a. The patient has daily periods of irrepressible need to sleep or daytime lapses into sleep occurring over a period greater than or equal to 3 months.
b. A mean sleep latency of less than or equal to 8 minutes and greater than or equal to two sleep-onset REM periods (SOREMPs) is found on an MSLT performed according to standard techniques. A SOREMP (within 15 minutes of sleep onset) on the preceding nocturnal PSG may replace one of the SOREMPs on the MSLT.
c. Cataplexy is absent.
d. Either CSF hypocretin-1 concentration has not been measured or CSF hypocretin-1 concentration measured by immunoreactivity is more than 110 pg per mL or greater than one-third of mean values obtained in normal subjects with the same standardized assay.
e. The hypersomnolence and/or MSLT findings are not better explained by other causes such as insufficient sleep, OSA, delayed sleep phase disorder, or the effect of medication or substances or their withdrawal.

As mentioned previously, the *ICSD-3* no longer divides narcolepsy by symptom (i.e., presence or absence of cataplexy), but rather by hypocretin levels.

Between 15% and 25% of all narcolepsy cases present without cataplexy. Of these, about 24% will present with abnormally low CSF hypocretin-1 levels, and almost all of these subjects will test positive for the HLA DQB1*0602 antigen (1). These noncataplectic narcoleptics share more in common with narcolepsy type 1 and should be classified as such.

However, because the lumbar puncture procedure is not common, nor recommended, in diagnosing simple narcolepsy, it is possible that some narcolepsy cases may go misdiagnosed as narcolepsy type 2 (noncataplexy) rather than narcolepsy type 1 (which shows low hypocretin concentrations). If so, an estimated 10% of type 2 narcoleptics may go on to develop cataplexy as their disease progresses, necessitating a revised diagnosis to narcolepsy type 1.

Because of the nonspecific nature of the HLA DQB1*0602 test (25% test HLA positive in the general population), it is not recommended as a diagnostic tool for narcolepsy. However, virtually all narcolepsy type 1 cases test positive for the HLA DQB1*0602 antigen. Consequently, a negative HLA test can be a useful shortcut for eliminating a narcolepsy type 1 diagnosis in a known narcoleptic patient with questionable, borderline, or mild cataplexy before a lumbar puncture is performed (1).

The HLA test is safer and less invasive than lumbar puncture. If the HLA test result is positive, then narcolepsy type 1 cannot be ruled out and the lumbar puncture can be performed to definitively test for CSF hypocretin concentration if the test is deemed of necessary value.

Diagnosis

The first step in the diagnosis of narcolepsy is a complete and thorough sleep history from the patient and, if possible, from partners, relatives, and friends.

The physical examination should be normal unless the patient is having an attack of cataplexy. In this case, muscle atonia and areflexia (the absence of reflexes) would be noted, lasting from a few seconds to a couple of minutes.

The sleep history should reflect all or part of the narcoleptic tetrad, most notably EDS, throughout the day, with possible episodes of sleep attacks, varying severity and frequency of cataplexy, possible hypnagogic or hypnopompic hallucinations, and probable sleep paralysis.

The frequency and number of the narcoleptic tetrad markers vary from patient to patient, although EDS is its most persistent symptom.

Because EDS is the most salient feature of narcolepsy, it is crucial that it be measured as accurately as possible. To this end, there are a number of subjective and objective tests at our disposal.

Subjective Scales of Sleepiness

Two widely used subjective measures are the Epworth Sleepiness Scale (ESS) and the Stanford Sleepiness Scale (SSS). The major advantages of both of these scales are that they are rapidly taken, easily scored, and inexpensive to administer.

The Epworth Sleepiness Scale

The ESS is a self-administered questionnaire in which patients rate their likelihood of falling asleep in eight different life situations. Each situation is scored from 0 to 3 and the total score varies from 0 to 24 (see Fig. 16-1). Deceptively simplistic and rudimentary, it has been validated across different clinical situations and various languages (31). Internal consistency and external validity are well established.

Epworth scores can be interpreted as follows:

- 0 to 5 lower normal daytime sleepiness
- 6 to 10 higher normal daytime sleepiness
- 11 to 12 mild EDS
- 13 to 15 moderate EDS
- 16 to 24 severe EDS

The Stanford Sleepiness Scale

The SSS is a subjective instrument (see Fig. 16-2) that rates EDS according to subjects' perceptions of sleepiness/alertness at a particular time. When averaged throughout the day, scores are found to correlate highly with performance tasks known to be sensitive to moderate amounts of sleep (32). The SSS may provide useful information on sleep loss, drug effects, and clinical states in sleep disorders.

Objective Tools for Assessing Sleepiness

Other kinds of tests can be used to collect scientific data that more objectively measure sleepiness as an aid in diagnosing narcolepsy. These include the PSG, the MSLT, genetic testing (HLA), and immunoassay testing (CSF hypocretin-1 levels).

Note that these subjective scales and the objective tests do not always correlate highly with each other, and appropriate clinical judgment and a detailed medical history must be considered as well.

Polysomnogram

PSG is used to reveal other possible causes of EDS, thus possibly ruling out narcolepsy as a cause of daytime sleepiness. It is also used to investigate other features of narcolepsy, such as sleep-onset REM and fragmented sleep. The PSG is most often performed the night before the MSLT.

The Multiple Sleep Latency Test

The MSLT is the standard diagnostic test for narcolepsy (33). It is a diurnal sleep test, with designated nap times every 2 hours.

The Epworth Sleepiness Scale

How Sleepy Are You?

How likely are you to doze off or fall asleep in the following situations? You should rate your chances of dozing off, not just feeling tired. Even if you have not done some of these things recently, try to determine how they would have affected you. For each situation, decide whether or not you would have:

- No chance of dozing = 0
- Slight chance of dozing = 1
- Moderate chance of dozing = 2
- High chance of dozing = 3

Situation	Chance of Dozing
Sitting and reading	
Watching TV	
Sitting inactive in a public place (e.g., theater or meeting)	
As a passenger in a car for an hour without a break	
Lying down in the afternoon when circumstances permit	
Sitting and talking to someone	
Sitting quietly after a lunch without alcohol	
In a car while stopped for a few minutes in traffic	

Total Score = _____

Interpretation of Scores:
0–5: Lower Normal Daytime Sleepiness
6–10: Higher Normal Daytime Sleepiness
11–12: Mild Excessive Daytime Sleepiness
13–15: Moderate Excessive Daytime Sleepiness
16–24: Severe Excessive Daytime Sleepiness

Figure 16-1 The Epworth Sleepiness Scale. (From Johns, M. W. (1991). A new method for measuring daytime sleepiness: The Epworth sleepiness scale. *Sleep, 14*(6), 540–545.)

Each nap can last from 20 to 35 minutes, and 4 or 5 scheduled naps, 2 hours apart, are run during the day. Patients are required to stay awake between each nap opportunity and asked to try and sleep during the 20-minute nap window.

Various measures are recorded; of particular interest are sleep latency (the length of time it takes one to fall asleep) and the presence of SOREMPs in each nap window. SOREMPs are more common in narcolepsy than in the general population.

In the MSLT, a SOREMP is defined as a REM period during the first 15 minutes following sleep onset. A mean sleep latency of less than or equal to 8 minutes and greater than or equal to two SOREMPs should be found on an MSLT in order to confirm a narcolepsy

diagnosis. A SOREMP found on the preceding nocturnal PSG may replace one of the SOREMPs on the MSLT (1).

A mean sleep latency of less than 5 minutes is indicative of significant EDS; when longer than 10 minutes, it is considered within normal levels of alertness. Approximately 90% of narcoleptics have a mean sleep latency of 8 minutes or less; however, SOREMPs remain a more specific predictor of narcolepsy (1).

Genetic Testing (HLA)

Although narcolepsy (HLA DQB1*0602) genotyping may help rule out narcolepsy when clinical history and sleep studies are inconclusive, it is not diagnostic by itself and should be used only to help when clinical tests

Stanford Sleepiness Scale

Using the 7-point scale below pick what best represents how you are feeling and note the corresponding number on the chart below.

Degree of Sleepiness	Scale Rating
Feeling active, vital, alert, or wide awake	1
Functioning at high levels, but not fully alert	2
Awake, but relaxed; responsive but not fully alert	3
Somewhat foggy, let down	4
Foggy; losing interest in remaining awake; slowed down	5
Sleepy, woozy, fighting sleep; prefer to lie down	6
No longer fighting sleep, sleep onset soon; having dream-like thoughts	7
Asleep	X

Figure 16-2 Stanford Sleepiness Scale. (From Hoddes, E., Zarcone, V., Smythe, H., et al. (1973). Quantification of sleepiness: A new approach. *Psychophysiology, 10*(4), 431–436.)

and past medical history are inconclusive. Although this allele is present in a very high percentage of narcoleptic patients, its low specificity limits the diagnostic strength of this test.

Immunoassay Testing (CSF Hypocretin-1 Levels)
Immunoassay testing of hypocretin-1 concentration in the CSF is a valid and reliable way to test for narcolepsy type 1. In short, a low concentration of hypocretin in the CSF meets diagnostic criteria for narcolepsy type 1, even in the absence of cataplexy. Low concentration is defined as less than or equal to 110 pg per mL or less than one-third of mean values obtained in normal subjects.

Differential Diagnosis

One of the biggest challenges in diagnosing hypersomnias relates to arriving at a differential diagnosis, because so many symptoms are shared between this family of sleep disorders. By definition, daytime sleepiness is the most common symptom underlying all hypersomnias. Although IH may present with the extreme EDS that afflicts narcoleptics, people with IH do not have cataplexy (separating them from narcolepsy type 1). Mean sleep latency may be similar in the MSLT; however, IH patients have fewer than two SOREMPs. Meanwhile, sleep efficiency tends to

be higher in IH patients, and overall sleep for them is better consolidated. Daytime naps also tend to be longer and less refreshing than naps of narcoleptic patients.

Sleepiness may also be secondary to other sleep disorders, such as OSA, delayed sleep phase syndrome (DSPS), ISS, or PLMD. Sleepiness may also be a direct result of shift work, or the use or abuse of prescribed medications, illicit drugs, environmental toxins, or other substances. Other medical conditions, such as chronic fatigue syndrome, multiple sclerosis, congestive heart failure, depression, and malingering, should also be ruled out.

In short, all of these variables need to be addressed and other disorders or influences ruled out before a diagnosis of narcolepsy can be declared.

Treatment

There is presently no cure for narcolepsy. Treatment involves controlling and improving symptoms, especially daytime sleepiness and cataplexy.

Scheduling several short naps throughout the day (under 20 minutes) has been shown to reduce EDS, both subjectively and objectively, but it is not recommended as the only course of treatment. Other lifestyle strategies include keeping a consistent sleep schedule by going to sleep and waking up at the same time every day, including weekends. Getting regular exercise and avoiding the use of tobacco, alcohol, or drugs may also help increase energy during the day. These strategies should improve sleep consolidation during the night and could lead to more daytime alertness. However, pharmacologic interventions are currently the most effective way to manage narcolepsy (see Table 16-2).

First-line drug therapy for the management of EDS is currently modafinil (Provigil) and armodafinil (Nuvigil) (20). Although not as widely used anymore, occasional use of dextroamphetamine (Dexedrine), amphetamine/dextroamphetamine (Adderall), and methylphenidate (Ritalin, Concerta) is still warranted in patients who do not respond adequately to first-choice options.

The current first-line therapy for the treatment of cataplexy and EDS is γ-hydroxybutyrate (GHB), also known as sodium oxybate (Xyrem). There is some evidence that sodium oxybate may also improve hypnagogic hallucinations and sleep paralysis (20).

Various antidepressants are still prescribed as alternatives to, or in conjunction with, the above-mentioned medications, albeit less commonly than in the past:

- Venlafaxine (Effexor), a serotonin–norepinephrine reuptake inhibitor
- Fluoxetine (Prozac) and sertraline (Zoloft), selective serotonin reuptake inhibitors
- Imipramine (Tofranil) and clomipramine (Anafranil), tricyclic antidepressants (20)

Future Directions

With our deeper understanding of narcolepsy comes a renewed and exciting search for novel medications. The discovery of the role of hypocretin/orexin focuses new research on hypocretin-based therapies, and new immunotherapies aim to prevent hypocretin loss. Various hypocretin replacement therapies have been pursued, including cell transplantation (from one area of the brain to another), peptide replacement (doses of hypocretin-1), and gene replacement therapy. So far, only gene replacement therapy has shown promise, although it's still a long way from coming to market (20).

Pitolisant (Wakix), a histamine inverse-agonist, is currently approved to treat EDS in narcolepsy and is now in phase III clinical trials for treating cataplexy symptoms (34).

Mazindol (Sanorex) is a tricyclic nonamphetamine stimulant. Although used as an appetite suppressant, recent evidence indicates an improvement in EDS and cataplexy in patients taking mazindol (35, 36).

Conclusion

Narcolepsy is a life-long sleep disorder. It is often characterized by EDS, cataplexy, hypnagogic hallucinations, sleep paralysis, and fragmented nocturnal sleep. Although there is no known cure, for many, it can be relatively well controlled with medication and personalized lifestyle adjustments. New research into its etiology and the novel treatments that arise may one day lead to a cure for narcolepsy.

Table 16-2 Current Medication for Narcolepsy

For Cataplexy, Hypnogogic Hallucinations, and Sleep Paralysis	For Excessive Daytime Sleepiness
First-Line Therapy	
Sodium oxybate (Xyrem)	Modafinil (Provigil)
	Armodafinil (Nuvigil)
Second-Line Therapy	
Venlafaxine (Effexor)	Methylphenidate three forms:
Atomoxetine (Strattera)	1. Immediate release (Methylin, Ritalin)
Fluoxetine (Prozac)	2. Extended release (Metadate CD, Ritalin LA, Concerta)
Sertraline (Zoloft)	3. Sustained release (Ritalin LA)
Protriptyline (Vivactil)	Dextroamphetamine (Dexedrine, Dextrostat)
Clomipramine (Anafranil)	Amphetamine/dextroamphetamine (Adderall)
	Pitolisant (Wakix)
	Mazindol (Sanorex, Mazanor)

CENTRAL DISORDERS OF HYPERSOMNOLENCE—IDIOPATHIC HYPERSOMNIA

Diagnostic criteria (1)
Criteria A to F must be met:

a. The patient has daily periods of irrepressible need to sleep or daytime lapses into sleep occurring over a period of at least 3 months.
b. Cataplexy is absent.
c. An MSLT shows fewer than two sleep-onset REM periods or no sleep-onset REM periods if the REM latency on the preceding PSG was less than or equal to 15 minutes.
d. At least one of the following is present:
   1. The MSLT shows a mean sleep latency of less than or equal to 8 minutes.
   2. Total 24-hour sleep time is more than or equal to 660 minutes (typically 12 to 14 hours) on 24-hour PSG monitoring (after correction of chronic sleep deprivation), or by wrist actigraphy in association with a sleep log (averaged over at least 7 days with unrestricted sleep).
e. ISS is ruled out.
f. The hypersomnolence and/or MSLT findings are not better explained by another sleep disorder, other medical or psychiatric disorders, or the use of drugs or medications.

Introduction

IH is a rare sleep disorder of unknown etiology. Evaluation of the prevalence of IH in the general population is difficult because of the limited number of patients with IH and the difficulty of making a definitive diagnosis. It has been reported to occur 6 to 10 times less frequently than narcolepsy (37, 38), suggesting a prevalence in the general population between 1 in 10,000 and 1 in 50,000.

As the name suggests, IH is characterized by EDS, and the patient often wakes up with difficulty, feeling disoriented or confused, seemingly "drunk" with sleep (sleep drunkenness). This sleepiness is pervasive and lasts all day. The severity of sleepiness, though, may fluctuate from person to person and from day to day.

Unlike narcolepsy, however, there is no evidence of cataplexy with IH, and SOREMPs in the PSG and MSLT together are rare (maximum 1 SOREMP combined). Also, unlike narcolepsy, naps in IH tend to last longer, sometimes hours, and are usually unrefreshing (2, 39).

There is some recent research that suggests that IH and narcolepsy type 2 (without cataplexy, HLA negative) may be related pathophysiologically. This is especially evident after criteria for diagnosing narcolepsy were divided into types 1 and 2 in the *ICSD-3*.

Narcolepsy type 1 can easily be differentiated from both narcolepsy type 2 and IH because narcolepsy type 1 has clear and easily observed symptoms (i.e., cataplexy and/or very low hypocretin concentrations). However, the differences between narcolepsy type 2 and IH are less distinct. Both are genetically similar (HLA negative, with normal or near-normal hypocretin levels) and clinical observations show equivalent severity of hypersomnia (40–42).

Despite the similarities between narcolepsy type 2 and IH, there are still some significant features that help differentiate them:
- an absence of multiple SOREMPs on the MSLT
- the presence of long habitual sleep periods, long unrefreshing naps, and sleep inertia; and
- a high sleep efficiency on the overnight PSG (2, 43)

Literature Review and a History of Idiopathic Hypersomnia

The term *idiopathic hypersomnia* was used as early as 1829 by Schindler ("die idiopathische chronische Schlafsucht") for EDS of undetermined origin. Narcolepsy was then described in the literature by Gélineau in 1880.

By 1928, Wilson had described several "narcolepsies" and often used the term *narcolepsy* to refer to any condition characterized by irresistible sleepiness (37). The discovery of REM sleep in 1953 by Aserinsky, Kleitman, and Dement helped establish the premise that true narcolepsy could be diagnosed by analyzing the REM sleep of the patient (44).

Subsequent work in the development of the MSLT in the mid-1980s by Carskadon provided objective evidence to separate narcolepsy (which had REM-related features) and hypersomnia (which did not) (33).

It wasn't until the 1976 paper by Roth that IH was described in its modern definition. Roth reviewed almost 650 personal cases of "narcolepsies" and classified them according to etiology, clinical form, and suspected pathophysiology. At that time, Roth divided hypersomnias into symptomatic and functional groups (45, 46). Subsequently, he described a large cohort of patients distinct from those with narcolepsy with EDS. These patients had significant sleepiness, often with prolonged nocturnal sleep but without clinical or electrophysiologic features of REM sleep disturbance. That is, no cataplexy was noted and the MSLT did not show significant SOREMPs during naps.

Roth further classified these patients as *monosymptomatic* (having normal nighttime sleep period with EDS) and *polysymptomatic* (having prolonged sleep time with sleep drunkenness and EDS) (45, 46). These forms were eventually described as *idiopathic hypersomnia with long sleep time* and *idiopathic hypersomnia without long sleep time,* respectively, in the original *ICSD* (47) in 1979. IH was then defined as a central nervous system disorder associated with a normal or prolonged major sleep episode (nighttime sleep) and excessive sleepiness consisting of prolonged (1- to 2-hour) episodes of NREM sleep during daytime naps.

Today, the *ICSD-3* has since eliminated these diagnostic classifications because recent research shows there is no significant pathophysiologic or therapeutic difference between either. A comparison of patients with more than or equal to 10 hours of sleep with those with less than 10 hours shows no differences in ESS scores, MSLT mean sleep latencies, sleep drunkenness, unrefreshing naps, hypnagogic hallucinations, or sleep paralysis.

The only reported differences are that the group with long sleep is somewhat marginally younger and thinner (1). IH patients also tend to overestimate their total sleep time by an average of an hour. For this reason, taking a detailed medical history will be subject to these perceptual inconsistencies, which can make criterion of sleep time (long vs. short) almost meaningless. As research using objective measures like actigraphy becomes more commonplace, these criteria may yet be revisited. For now, however, one may continue to note sleep duration as an important clinical feature, but not consider it diagnostic or defining. Separating IH into distinct conditions must await further research and a better understanding of its underlying pathophysiology (1).

Salient Features

EDS is the essential feature of all hypersomnias, but it is especially prominent in IH. The sleepiness is pervasive, lasting throughout the day. The disorder has significant debilitating impact on social, family, scholastic, and occupational life (39, 48).

Naps, when taken, are long in duration, often an hour or longer, and the patient wakes up still tired and feeling unrefreshed. Unlike narcoleptic sleep attacks (cataplexy), the IH subject can usually hold off from napping until a more convenient time. Also, sleep paralysis (5% of patients) and hypnagogic/hypnopompic hallucinations (5% to 10%) are rare for those with IH (46, 49).

Waking up is very difficult for someone with IH. The subject is overwhelmed by a sense of extreme grogginess or confusion. *Sleep drunkenness* is the clinical term for the state after awakening defined by extreme difficulty arousing, with confusion, disorientation, automatic behaviors, and poor coordination occurring. The transition from sleep to wakefulness can be long and difficult

(45, 46). Often, the subject just returns to sleep rather than waking up. The majority of IH patients will report sleep drunkenness (46, 49).

Other salient features of IH (although the same may be said for someone deeply sleep deprived) are motor hyperactivity (constantly active, talking a lot), cognitive dysfunction (memory, attention, and concentration problems), hallucinations, sleep paralysis, and headaches (1, 39).

The major sleep period (usually at night) is well consolidated and may even show elevated deep (N3) sleep in those with IH. This major sleep period may be very long, or within normal parameters, but the overall sleep time in a 24-hour cycle is always elevated. To meet diagnostic criteria for IH, total sleep time over the 24-hour period must be minimum 660 minutes (11 hours) (1). PSG testing typically indicates low sleep fragmentation and relatively high sleep efficiency, typically in the 90th percentile for this population.

There seems to be a small, but positive, family history tied to IH (45, 49). Gender ratio for IH is unknown. It is believed to be equal between males and females, although one study has reported 65% female patients in its dataset (49). Age of onset has been reported to be in the middle to late teens; average age of diagnosis is in the low 30s (46, 49). The diagnosis of IH is complicated by the fact that differentiating between excessive versus long sleep, or normal versus abnormal wakefulness, is often difficult in this population. Consequently, patients must deal with IH an average of 10 to 12 years before a diagnosis is made and effective treatment commenced.

The symptoms of IH tend to remain stable over many years, but up to 11% of patients in one study had spontaneous remission of their symptoms (46) and another more recent study showed 14% to 25% spontaneous remission. Note that narcolepsy, on the contrary, has no history of remission and is considered a lifelong disorder (48).

Diagnosis

The pathophysiology of IH is not well understood, and diagnosis requires the exclusion of other more common causes of excessive sleepiness. The *ICSD-3* lists six criteria that must be met before a diagnosis of IH can be considered. First, the symptoms of excessive and irrepressible sleepiness must have persisted every day for a minimum of 3 months. Unlike narcolepsy, there is no evidence of cataplexy or SOREMPs. In fact, when the MSLT is performed, a maximum of one SOREMP can be observed. And at least one of the following must be present: a mean sleep latency on the MSLT of less than or equal to 8 minutes, or more than or equal to 660 minutes of total sleep in a 24-hour period as measured by 24-hour PSG monitoring or wrist actigraphy averaged over 7 consecutive days.

Other tools and techniques that complement the above-mentioned diagnostic markers are available to the clinician to clarify the clinical impact of the disorder on the patient.

A sleep diary may be used to complement the actigraphy data. Although self-reported impressions of total sleep time are notoriously overestimated (49), a sleep diary may give other important information that may impact the amount and quality of sleep, like sleep hygiene. Sleep diaries can record the timing and length of naps, the episodes of sleep drunkenness, and other essential features of IH. Although not necessarily diagnostic, these are helpful in tracking indicators of IH.

The ESS can help quantify sleepiness in certain situations, and a minimum score of 10 can signify someone suffering from EDS and fighting to stay awake (50). Studies have shown a median ESS score in the 16 to 17 range (46, 49). Although the ESS is not diagnostic for IH, such a high score is rare and, in the absence of other obvious sleep disorders, can be a good clinical indicator for IH. A high score in the ESS is always noted, regardless of whether the subject had an extended nocturnal sleep period or if it was within normal parameters (46).

A comprehensive medical history and a battery of medical and personality tests should be performed in order to rule out ISS and other sleep, medical, or psychiatric disorders. A toxicology screen can also be ordered to rule out drug use or certain medications. A nocturnal PSG followed by an MSLT the next day will rule out narcolepsy, especially narcolepsy type 2, which closely mimics IH. OSA and PLMD must also be ruled out because the fragmented sleep they cause will often result in EDS and fatigue.

Other objective measures that may complement the MSLT are the MWT and the Oxford Sleep Resistance test (see Glossary). Like the ESS, these tests are not diagnostic, but they may help the clinician to more accurately diagnose IH (51, 52).

Differential diagnosis is important in correctly diagnosing IH because IH is primarily a diagnosis of exclusion. When a patient presents with symptoms of EDS, all other known contributors to EDS must be excluded before a diagnosis of IH can be contemplated. Given the exclusionary nature of diagnosing IH, its prevalence could be overestimated because it is very difficult to always rule out all other possible contributors to daytime somnolence (2).

Treatment

Because the underlying cause of IH is unknown, the goal of treatment is symptom relief and improvement in the quality of life. When a diagnosis of IH is established, treatment is largely pharmacologic with generally good, but somewhat variable, results.

Stimulants such as modafinil (Provigil), armodafinil (Nuvigil), methylphenidate (Ritalin), or other amphetamine-like compounds are effective in reducing the sleepiness felt during the wake period, but other symptoms such as sleep inertia or sleep drunkenness persist (2). If amphetamine-like stimulants are prescribed, tolerance and dependence should be closely monitored as possible complications.

Self-medication is common in patients with IH because of the long gap between the onset of symptoms and eventual diagnosis and treatment. Case histories reveal excessive intake of caffeine, energy drinks, and other stimulants, which are often used to help the subject achieve a minimum level of awareness during the day.

Behavioral therapies are typically not effective for treating IH. Nocturnal sleep is already well consolidated, and improving sleep hygiene should show very little improvement of daytime function. The daytime hypersomnolence observed in IH is independent of the length or quality of nocturnal sleep.

Scheduling naps is likewise not very helpful because patients with IH do not recover energy from napping. They wake up as tired as before the nap. However, it has been reported that some patients with IH have found cognitive behavioral therapy to be helpful for learning coping skills (53).

Diagnosis and treatment of coexisting circadian disorders or sleep apnea must also be addressed.

Although not strictly a treatment, support for the patient and family through organized patient advocacy and support groups is often reported by patients to be helpful in providing information and combating the negative public perception of those who are excessively sleepy (47).

Future Directions

With IH, research seems to suggest that the brain may overproduce a small molecule that acts like a sleeping pill. The exact composition of this molecule is yet to be determined, but it is known to interact with γ-amino-butyric acid (GABA), which plays a major role in the brain mechanisms that promote sleep. In the presence of this compound, the inhibitory and sleep-promoting actions of GABA are enhanced at the receptors (54). Other new medications in use with narcolepsy may prove to be useful for IH in the future. Pitolisant stimulates histamine release and promotes wakefulness. It has been used with some success in patients with treatment-resistant IH (43).

As mentioned earlier, historically, there were two categories of IH. Because of the lack of evidence for therapeutic or pathophysiologic differences between the two groups, the *ICSD-3* has combined them into the single disorder known as IH. However, some researchers are now dividing IH into three possible subgroups, pending more evidence.

Subgroup I is defined by IH with a positive family history. Associated clinical symptoms suggest dysfunction of the autonomic nervous system. Symptoms may include headache, syncope, orthostatic hypotension, and peripheral vasoconstriction (cold hands and feet).

Subgroup II is characterized by an initial viral infection associated with neurologic symptoms, such as Guillain–Barré syndrome, infectious mononucleosis, or atypical viral pneumonia. Even after their infectious disease resolves, these patients continue to require significantly more total sleep and continue to feel very tired and sleepy in the day, often napping. An analysis of CSF demonstrates moderate lymphocytosis (30 to 50 cells per μL with mild-to-moderate elevation in protein).

Subgroup III suggests that some patients do not have a positive family or viral infection history, making the cause of this disorder truly idiopathic. To what extent these subgroups will define the future of IH is unknown and in need of further validation (55).

Despite current understanding that narcolepsy type 2 and IH are separate and independent sleep disorders, there are some researchers who believe they are closer in nature than what we currently understand. Symptoms of narcolepsy type 2 and IH can often overlap significantly, and there are few fundamental differences between these two disorders, prompting some to hypothesize that they are the same sleep disorder, or different aspects of the same disorder (54, 56). More research is being done to better understand this relationship.

CENTRAL DISORDERS OF HYPERSOMNOLENCE—RECURRENT PRIMARY HYPERSOMNIA

Diagnostic criteria (1)
Criteria A to E must be met:

a. The patient experiences at least two recurrent episodes of excessive sleepiness and sleep duration, each persisting for 2 days to 5 weeks.
b. Episodes recur usually more than once a year and at least once every 18 months.
c. The patient has normal alertness, cognitive function, behavior, and mood between episodes.

d. The patient must demonstrate at least one of the following during episodes:
   1. Cognitive dysfunction
   2. Altered perception
   3. Eating disorder (anorexia or hyperphagia)
   4. Disinhibited behavior (such as hypersexuality)
e. The hypersomnolence and related symptoms are not better explained by another sleep disorder; other medical, neurologic, or psychiatric disorders (especially bipolar disorder); or the use of drugs or medications.

Introduction

Recurrent hypersomnias, as the name suggests, are sleep disorders that alternate between active and inactive phases. Periods of remission are characterized by relatively normal sleep. Social, scholastic, and occupational impairment are observed during the active phase of the disorder.

The *ICSD-3* has streamlined the definition of recurrent hypersomnias to include a single sleep disorder, Kleine-Levin syndrome (KLS), and its subtype (menstrual-related hypersomnia). This is based on data suggesting that the condition is fairly homogeneous and that there is a lack of absolute evidence for other major subcategories of the disorder (1).

KLS, often referred to as "Sleeping Beauty syndrome," presents in recurring cycles of severe hypersomnia with associated cognitive (memory, language), psychiatric (mood, delusions, hallucinations), and behavioral (hyperphagia, hypersexuality) disturbances. These cycles are followed by remission periods of relatively average sleep and normalized associated features.

Although the cause of KLS is unknown, it follows a benign clinical course with eventual spontaneous remission of all symptoms with no (or very few and mild) direct lingering effects. Patients typically experience less frequent and less intense episodes toward the end of the disease course. They are considered cured if they do not experience an episode for 6 or more years (57). Because of the typical age of the patient at disease onset, scholastic impairment may be long term.

Literature Review and a History of KLS

The first account in the literature of a person with recurrent sleep episodes was reported by William Oliver in 1705 (58). The first case of quite possibly KLS to appear in the literature was in 1815, when Satterley presented the case of a 16-year-old male with hypersomnia and hyperphagia following a short period of fever and headache. This was followed by another case in 1862 by Brierre de Boismont (57). A literature review counted a total of only 12 cases with similar features published between 1786 and 1924 (59).

Multiple cases of recurrent hypersomnia were first collected and reported in Germany by Willi Kleine (60). Max Levin emphasized the association of periodic somnolence with morbid hunger in 1929 and 1936 (61, 62). Critchley was the first to name this sleep disorder Kleine-Levin syndrome (KLS) in 1942 (63). By 1962, Critchley had developed the fundamental features that we recognize as KLS today. He described a triad of symptoms, highlighting periodic hypersomnia, excessive and compulsive eating, and abnormal behavior. He also noted that young adolescent males are predominantly affected, and that the syndrome will spontaneously disappear (59, 63, 64).

In 1990, the diagnostic criteria for KLS were codified in the ICSD, where it was defined as a syndrome composed of recurring episodes of undue sleepiness lasting some days, which may or may not be associated with hyperphagia and abnormal behavior (65).

Prevalence/Etiology

The etiology of this disorder is not known or fully understood. Although many (39%) KLS patients reported no precipitating factors before their first episode, others (42%) had reported feeling sick with an infection or fever 3 to 5 days before their initial episode. Alcohol or marijuana use, head trauma, sleep deprivation, or menses/lactation accounted for a further 13% of the cases (1, 66, 67). Interestingly, an infection or fever preceded almost 9% of recurring episodes.

This evidence has led to speculation that KLS may be the result of a viral or postinfectious autoimmune response. Subsequently, the HLA subtype DQB1*0201 has been identified and implicated in this disease (68). The authors concluded that these findings, together with the relatively young age of disease onset, the recurrence of symptoms, and the frequency of infectious precipitating factors, suggest an autoimmune etiology for KLS.

Inflammatory lesions in the thalamus, diencephalon, and midbrain have been described in some postmortem case reports, also suggesting a viral infection as a potential cause of, or association with, KLS (69, 70).

The other proposed causes of KLS are hypothalamic dysfunction, because hypothalamic and third ventricle tumors have symptoms similar to those of KLS (71), or a neurotransmitter imbalance, because some abnormalities in serotonin and dopamine metabolism have been reported in these cases (72, 73).

Although population-based studies reporting on KLS prevalence are not readily available, it is generally considered an exceptionally rare disorder, affecting approximately 1 in 1 to 1.5 million (57). By 2014, approximately 500 cases had been reported worldwide in the literature (1).

KLS usually starts in the mid-teens (median age is 15 years) and affects mostly males (2:1 to 3:1) (55, 66). Approximately 80% of KLS cases were first observed during the second decade, and the syndrome will last, on average, 8 to 10 years, with only a small fraction still exhibiting symptoms after 20 years (see Fig. 16-3).

Interestingly, there is a link between duration of the disorder and hypersexuality, with KLS patients without hypersexuality suffering on average 10 years and those with hypersexuality suffering upward of 20 years.

Although some have reported no correlation between age at onset and resolution of the disease (57, 66), the ICSD-3 reports there may indeed be a link between adult-onset KLS and prolonged disease duration (1).

The episodes recur a few times per year and last, on average, 10 days. Women tended to have longer active phases and a longer overall duration of the disorder. It is very rare for an active episode to last beyond 4 weeks, and remission periods very rarely last 12 to 15 months (see Fig. 16-4) (66).

Although reported worldwide, KLS seems to be somewhat more frequent in Israel and in American Ashkenazi Jews (59, 74, 75). The preponderance of cases in this patient demographic suggests a genetic component in the disorder.

However, familial KLS is rarely encountered, with a low risk for occurrence in first-degree relatives (59). A recent study examining 260 patients from the United States and France (76) concluded that in familial cases, KLS tends to be present within the same generation (14 of 21 familial KLS patients). Out of a total of 249 families, 10 (4%) were found to contain at least two family members who were either first- or second-degree familial relation. This is in keeping with previous estimates of 5% familial cases (75). And although the symptoms for the groups (familial KLS vs. isolated KLS) were clinically similar, familial KLS patients tended to have less severe symptoms than their nonfamilial counterparts (76).

It is likely that KLS is caused by the interplay of some environmental factors acting on a susceptible genetic background.

Neurophysiologic Evidence

PSG and MSLT studies were performed on 19 patients. Slow-wave sleep (SWS) was markedly reduced during the first half of the active episode, with eventual return to normal amounts in the second half of the episode. By the last days of the episode, SWS had been at near-normal levels (when KLS is inactive). This improvement in SWS amount had no effect on the persistence and severity of KLS symptoms.

REM sleep also changed as the days progressed during the active phase of the disorder. REM remained normal, or near-normal, in the first half of the episode, but subsequently decreased as the days progressed. The statistical

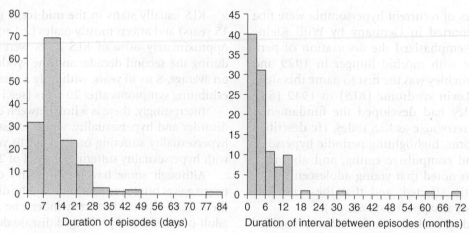

Figure 16-3 Histogram of the duration of Kleine–Levin syndrome episodes, in days (left), with a median of 10 days, and of the duration of the interval between episodes, in months (right), with a median of 3 months. (Reprinted with permission from Arnulf, I., Zeitzer, J. M., File, J., et al. (2005). Kleine-Levin syndrome: a systematic review of 186 cases in the literature. *Brain, 128,* 2763–2776.)

differences between the first and second half of episodes were significant for SWS and REM sleep (57, 77).

Meanwhile, results of the MSLT were ambiguous and difficult to interpret because they were highly dependent on the willingness and motivation of the patient to comply with the procedure.

Electroencephalography (EEG) showed a general slowing of background EEG activity in about 70% of reported cases. Half- to 2-second paroxysmal bursts of bisynchronous, generalized, moderate- to high-voltage (5 to 7 Hz) waves were also observed (57, 66, 78).

Salient Features

People with KLS suffer from a variety of unusual symptoms (see Box 16-1).

Hypersomnia

Hypersomnia is present in 100% of KLS cases during the active phase of the disorder. The patients have recurrent episodes of severe hypersomnia, which are often associated with compulsive overeating and hypersexuality (55, 79).

Each individual sleep period is extremely long, ranging from 12 to 24 hours (mean + 18.62 hours) (57, 66). The active phase of KLS can last for days to weeks at a time (averaging 10 days, ranging between 2.5 and 80 days) (1) and can recur several times a year. Often, the patients remain arousable, waking up only to void and eat. Despite the prolonged sleep time, incontinence is not observed.

Patients can become irritable or aggressive when they do awaken or are prevented from sleeping. It has

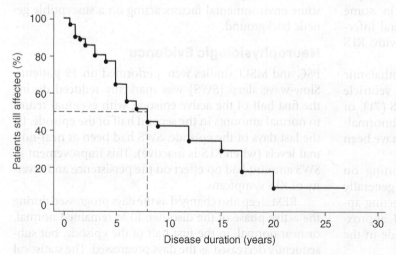

Figure 16-4 Duration of Kleine–Levin syndrome (KLS) (*n* = 110 patients, 41% censored), presented as a Kaplan–Meier analysis. On the *x*-axis is the total duration of the disease (years), on the *y*-axis is the cumulative decreasing percentage of patients still presenting with a KLS episode. The median duration of the disease (dotted line) is 8 years. (Reprinted with permission from Arnulf, I., Zeitzer, J. M., File, J., et al. (2005). Kleine-Levin syndrome: A systematic review of 186 cases in the literature. *Brain, 128,* 2763–2776.)

BOX 16-1: Symptoms during Episodes of Kleine–Levin Syndrome

Hypersomnia
Cognitive disorders
    Abnormal speech
    Confusion
    Amnesia
    Derealization
    Hallucinations
    Delusions
Eating behavior disorders
    Megaphagia
    Craving for sweets
    Increased drinking
    Binge eating
    Decreased appetite
    Food utilization behavior
Depression
Irritability
Other behavior disorders
    Hypersexuality
    Compulsions to sing, write, pace

also been reported in some cases that a short period of insomnia may be present as the active phase ends and a normal period of sleep is about to commence.

Between these symptomatic periods, the disorder will enter a time of remission whereby patients will have relatively normal sleep without EDS (57).

Hypersomnia itself may also change as the disorder progresses. In the early years, it can be more intense and longer lasting, whereas in later years, it may be described as a "heavy fatigue," with feelings of being "in a zone" between wakefulness and sleep (57).

Cognitive Disturbances

During an active episode, most of the patients often report feelings of confusion and difficulty with concentration, attention, and memory (57, 66).

Abnormal speech has also been reported in the majority of cases. Going beyond simple slurred speech, examples include periods of being mute or going without spontaneous speech, using monosyllabic or short sentences with limited vocabulary, incoherent speech, childish stereotypical language, slowness in speech itself or in its comprehension, and the practice of echoing questions. Occasionally, amnesia is reported, with patients often not remembering events that occurred during an episode. When awake for a few hours every day, patients will report feeling exhausted, generally confused, anxious at being left alone, or otherwise apathetic.

During the remission period between active episodes, the overwhelming majority of patients reported normalized sleep and cognitive functioning. In some patients, a mild but long-lasting cognitive decline was observed, even years after the final episode (57).

Eating Disorders

The vast majority of KLS patients ate larger amounts of food than were considered normal (megaphagia). A preference for sweets was noted in some cases. The increase in food could be mild to severe, with some patients eating up to three times their normal amounts. Increased drinking was also noted, but never in isolation. A minority of patients ate less food than normal in a few episodes, but then once more overindulged in subsequent episodes (57, 80). The changes in appetite and eating were normalized after each episode.

Changes in Mood

Another common feature of KLS is the accompanying change in mood during an episode. Depressed mood was observed in half of the patients, particularly in women. Approximately 15% of the patients reported suicidal thoughts in one study, and 2 of 186 patients attempted suicide (66).

Interestingly, just as insomnia is sometimes noted at the end of an episode, hypomania (elevated mood) is also occasionally observed at this time. A few patients report flattened affect, irritability, anxiety, and feelings of panic. Irritability and, sometimes, severe aggressive behavior were observed (although rare) when sleep, sexual, or food drive was impeded. All mood phenomena were transient and normalized after each episode (57).

Compulsive Behaviors

Another salient feature of KLS is the presence of compulsions. They are defined as behaviors that result from an abnormal and uncontrollable need to perform a particular action. If the impulse is resisted, there is intense anxiety. The action is often repetitive and ritualized.

The most common of these compulsions in KLS involves sexual activity. This hypersexuality is much more common in males than in females. It can range from increased or overt masturbation, exposing oneself, or making unwanted and inappropriate sexual advances. Obscene language is also common, as is compulsive singing, body rocking, lips chewing, writing on walls, and even setting fires (57). Interestingly, it has been reported that 53% of all patients are hypersexual, with the majority being males, and 53% of all patients are depressed, with the majority being women (1). Hypersexuality and other compulsions subside after each episode.

Perceptual Anomalies

Defined as a feeling that one's surroundings are not real (especially as a symptom of mental disturbance), derealization is a common feature in the subjective experience of the KLS patient. Almost all patients report a feeling of "unreality" or "disconnected thinking." Surroundings seem wrong somehow, distorted or unreal, as in a dream. Perception is described as strange, detached, or different. Objects are often seen to be "far away," with the sounds of voices seeming "distant, bizarre, wrong, or unpleasant." Some patients experience visual or auditory hallucinations (57).

Normality during Remission

As noted previously, KLS is characterized by recurring periods when the hypersomnia and other characteristic symptoms are present and longer periods when all symptoms are absent. During these periods of remission, the patient is essentially "back to normal," with all or most of the clinical symptoms absent.

KLS will eventually disappear spontaneously after a number of years (average range 8 to 12 years) for most people. Some patients may develop symptoms of irritability, impulsive behavior, hallucinations, depression, confusion, and memory problems, which may linger for years after the final episode (55, 81).

Diagnosis

Despite the typical and salient features of KLS, there is still no defining symptom or test that provides a positive diagnosis. Currently, KLS is a diagnosis of exclusion, after all other possible conditions are ruled out. The diagnosis is completely based on a thorough clinical history, because there is currently no test that will diagnose KLS.

Close attention must be paid to other disorders that may closely mimic KLS. Severe depression will share periods of somnolence, overeating, and social withdrawal. The occasional brief period of hypomania (elevated energy) at the end of some episodes of KLS may also mimic a manic episode of bipolar disorder. Some characteristic mood or perceptual disturbances may mimic primary psychiatric disorders.

Narcolepsy, Klüver–Bucy syndrome, and temporal lobe epilepsy may also produce symptoms that are similar to those of KLS. Metabolic encephalopathies should also be ruled out (57), as well as the use of drugs and exposures to toxins.

Treatment

Treatment of KLS is not standardized and is mostly pharmacologic. The goal is symptom relief and improvement in quality of life.

As of 2016, there have not been any randomized, placebo-controlled studies for KLS treatments (82). This is likely due to the rare nature of the disorder, making larger studies difficult.

A myriad of drugs have been used to mitigate the severity of the symptoms with varying degrees of efficacy, from stimulant medications, antidepressants, antiepileptics, antivirals, benzodiazepines, levodopa, and lithium. Stimulant therapy was effective in treating the hypersomnia, especially once the episodes had decreased in severity, but failed to improve cognitive function, mood, or other symptoms of KLS. Approximately 40% of the patients responded to lithium, improving abnormal behaviors and reducing the duration of episodes.

Medications such as flumazenil, chlorpromazine, levomepromazine, trifluoperazine, haloperidol, thioridazine, clozapine, and risperidone have also been used and found to be ineffective. Electroconvulsive therapy similarly had no effect on KLS symptoms and, in fact, seemed to increase the confusion already present in KLS (57).

During the remission phase, mood stabilizers such as lithium, carbamazepine, valproate, phenytoin, and phenobarbital have been tried. Only lithium was shown to improve mood (57).

Special Mention

Menstrual-related hypersomnia is diagnosed when EDS occurs on a periodic basis over a few days preceding menstruation (55). It is assumed that the symptoms follow hormonal changes, but the etiology of the syndrome, as well as its prevalence and course, is virtually unknown. Menstrual-related hypersomnia is considered an extremely rare disorder, with only 18 cases reported worldwide in the literature by 2014 (1).

In cases of KLS, women had a longer disease course than men, despite a comparable age at onset. Women had the same frequency of megaphagia and psychotic symptoms as that of men, but a lower frequency of hypersexuality and cognitive impairment (57). Women were more likely to report symptoms of depression than men (1).

Although menstrual-related hypersomnia is currently considered a variant of KLS, a positive response to estrogen and progesterone therapy may indicate a reproductive endocrine abnormality (1).

Future Directions

Current studies are investigating the relationship between flu-like symptoms and onset of episodes and may shed some light on the autoimmune or inflammatory processes involved in KLS (83). Recent evidence suggests encephalopathy during episodes of KLS, with thalamic, temporal, and frontal lobe involvement. The causes have yet to be determined, but may be genetic, autoimmune, inflammatory, or metabolic (1, 81, 84, 85).

More stringent, multicentered, double-blind, placebo-controlled, randomized drug studies need to be conducted in order to uncover the most effective therapies to treat KLS.

Conclusion

KLS is a rare and little understood sleep disorder with a cyclical pattern of hypersomnia and normalized episodes. Although the clinical features are well defined and readily observed, the causes and prevalence are not well-known. It is seen mostly in males, and in the second decade of life. The disorder spontaneously goes away after about 10 to 15 years in most people, with little or no lingering effects. Treatment is given for symptom relief and consists mostly of stimulants or lithium. Most other medications are deemed ineffective.

Improving social support and patient education may be an effective way to reduce the stress of KLS. Setting up contingencies during times when KLS is active and reassuring the family that this is usually a benign disorder that will eventually disappear go a long way to helping patients cope with the anxiety and mystery associated with their affliction. Involvement of the school, teacher, or employer will also help mitigate long-term adverse effects. Special dispensation and a more flexible workload at school may reduce the educational burden seen when KLS patients are still students.

CENTRAL DISORDERS OF HYPERSOMNOLENCE— HYPERSOMNIA DUE TO A MEDICAL DISORDER

Diagnostic criteria (1)
Criteria A to D must be met:

a. The patient has daily periods of irrepressible need to sleep or daytime lapses into sleep occurring over a period of at least 3 months.
b. The daytime sleepiness occurs as a consequence of a significant underlying medical or neurologic condition.
c. If an MSLT is performed, the mean sleep latency is less than or equal to 8 minutes, and fewer than two sleep-onset REM periods (SOREMPs) are observed.
d. The symptoms are not better explained by another untreated sleep disorder, a mental disorder, or the effects of medications or drugs.

Notes

1. In the subtype of residual hypersomnolence after treatment of OSA, the MSLT mean latency may be more than 8 minutes.
2. Should criteria for narcolepsy be fulfilled, a diagnosis of narcolepsy type 1 or type 2 due to a medical condition should be used rather than hypersomnia due to a medical disorder.
3. In patients with severe neurologic or medical disorders in whom it is not possible or desirable to perform sleep studies, the diagnosis can be made by clinical criteria.

Introduction

This collection of disorders identifies patients who experience hypersomnia secondary to a preexisting medical or neurologic disorder. Hypersomnia may take the form of prolonged nocturnal sleep, EDS, or excessive napping. EDS may be of variable severity and may resemble that of narcolepsy (e.g., refreshing naps) or IH (e.g., long periods of nonrestorative sleep).

Narcolepsy due to a Medical Condition

This condition is diagnosed when an underlying comorbid medical disorder is the direct cause of narcolepsy. The medical condition may feature involvement of the areas of the brain responsible for REM sleep, such as the hypothalamus and pons, in hypothalamic pituitary pathology (86), head trauma and brain tumors (87), hypothalamic sarcoidosis, multiple sclerosis, and myotropic dystrophy (88).

Along with EDS, other features of narcolepsy may be present, such as sleep paralysis, hypnagogic hallucinations, or automatic behaviors, but if the patient also has cataplexy, or the MSLT shows two or more SOREMPs, or CSF hypocretin-1 levels are low, then narcolepsy (type 1 or type 2) due to a medical condition should be diagnosed (1).

Hypersomnia Secondary to Parkinson's Disease (PD)

Some patients with Parkinson's Disease (PD) have reported significant hypersomnolence as documented by the MSLT. The hypersomnia may be due to inadequate control of nocturnal symptoms, resulting in insufficient or poor sleep and consequent EDS. If this is the case, then the diagnosis should be an insomnia disorder.

Although dopaminergic drugs are an effective treatment for PD, they are known to have side effects that include hypersomnolence. In this case, the diagnosis should be hypersomnia due to a medication or substance. Patients with PD with a disease profile consistent with narcolepsy should be diagnosed as narcolepsy due to a medical condition. All other cases of hypersomnia in a PD patient should be diagnosed as hypersomnia secondary to PD (1).

Posttraumatic Hypersomnia

Mild-to-moderate traumatic brain injury (TBI) often results in hypersomnia (89). The most common causes of TBI are falls, vehicle-related collisions (cars, motorcycles, bicycles, pedestrians), violence/gun shots, sports injuries, and explosive blasts/combat injuries (89).

In a study of 87 TBI patients, 11% were diagnosed with posttraumatic hypersomnia, a further 6% with narcolepsy, and 25% were found to have objectively quantified EDS as measured by an average MSLT sleep latency of less than 10 minutes (90).

Because of the nature of TBI, varying symptoms will manifest depending on where the injury took place. This may impact other sleep disorders (e.g., sleep apnea, if control of breathing centers were affected by the TBI), consequently resulting in hypersomnia.

Studies have shown that sleepiness is common following TBI, with more severe injuries often resulting in greater sleepiness. Although sleepiness improves in many patients, about a quarter of TBI subjects remained sleepy up to 1 year after injury (91). Care must be taken to eliminate any other sleep disorders or circadian dysrhythmia sometimes noted in TBI survivors that may be causing hypersomnia (92).

Genetic Disorders Associated with Primary Central Nervous System Somnolence

Many genetic disorders and diseases have been associated with daytime sleepiness. Niemann–Pick type C disease and Norrie disease (myotonic dystrophy), Moebius syndrome, Fragile X syndrome, and Prader–Willi syndrome are known to result in EDS.

Care must be taken to account for some genetic disorders that are also associated with sleep-disordered breathing (SDB), such as myotonic dystrophy and Prader–Willi syndrome. Hypersomnia due to a medical disorder should be diagnosed only after adequate treatment of SDB. Smith–Magenis syndrome is a neurodevelopmental disorder characterized by a circadian reversal in melatonin secretion, where melatonin levels are high during the day and low at night, resulting in daytime sleepiness (1).

Hypersomnia Secondary to Brain Tumors, Infections, or Other Central Nervous System Lesions

Brain tumors, infections, strokes, or neurodegenerative lesions in the brain can result in disturbances in sleep, including daytime somnolence, depending where the assault was localized. Damage to the hypothalamus,

pons, or rostral midbrain may produce daytime sleepiness (87). In patients with brain tumors, the sleepiness may be due to the tumor itself or the effects of treatment, in which case the diagnosis should be hypersomnia due to a medication or substance (1).

Hypersomnia Secondary to Endocrine Disorder

Hypothyroidism is the most recognized example of this condition (1). Case studies have shown a positive response to the administration of low-dose levothyroxine (25 μg per day) in some cases of hypersomnia in subclinical or mild hypothyroidism. Not only were overall sleep times reduced, but overall sleepiness was significantly improved as measured by the ESS (93).

Hypersomnia Secondary to Metabolic Encephalopathy

Not all hypersomnias are caused by neurologic or structural abnormalities within the brain or brainstem. Before diagnosing a primary hypersomnia, care should be taken to eliminate toxic metabolic encephalopathies. A number of disorders caused by systemic illness—such as adrenal or pancreatic insufficiency, liver disease, renal failure, heart failure, exposure to toxins, and certain inherited metabolic disorders in childhood—may also cause hypersomnia (1, 94).

Residual Hypersomnia in Patients with Adequately Treated OSA

Some patients with SDB report persistent daytime sleepiness despite documented treatment success and adequate sleep.

Before a diagnosis is made, the patient should be treated for at least 3 months, and treatment success evaluated objectively by assessment of continuous positive airway pressure (CPAP) (or other PAP modality) data demonstrating optimal compliance (at least 7 hours per night). An overnight sleep study demonstrating the elimination of essentially all SDB may also be warranted (1).

Proposed mechanisms for continued daytime sleepiness include persistent arousals from emergent PLMD or other sleep disorders (95), previously undiagnosed obesity hypoventilation syndrome (OHS) (96), or possible structural or physical damage to wake neurons (97).

Hypoventilation, through OHS or other chronic obstructive lung disease, will result in continued hypercapnia, which can cause EDS. Brainstem dysfunction may be the underlying cause behind a lack of both alertness and cardiovascular control (96). The possible cause of this dysfunction is unknown. However, in animal models, prolonged exposure to hypoxia-reoxygenation cycling (similar to that seen in severe OSA patients) has been shown to irreversibly damage catecholaminergic wake neurons. Catecholamines (epinephrine/adrenaline, norepinephrine/noradrenaline, dopamine, etc.) are also involved in the arousal response, and excessive arousals over many years may cause damage to these neurons.

It is likely that, even after successful PAP therapy, patients may have subtle cardiac dysrhythmia and EDS because of damage to the brainstem (97).

CENTRAL DISORDERS OF HYPERSOMNOLENCE—HYPERSOMNIA DUE TO A MEDICATION OR SUBSTANCE

Diagnostic criteria (1)
Criteria A to C must be met:

a. The patient has daily periods of irrepressible need to sleep or daytime lapses into sleep.
b. The daytime sleepiness occurs as a consequence of current medication or substance use or withdrawal from a wake-promoting medication or substance.
c. The symptoms are not better explained by another untreated sleep disorder, medical or neurologic disorder, or mental disorder.

Introduction

These disorders occur in patients who have hypersomnia secondary to sedating medications, alcohol, or drugs of abuse. This diagnosis also includes hypersomnolence associated with withdrawal from amphetamines and other drugs (1).

Hypersomnia due to Sedating Medications

Sedation is a common side effect of many prescription medications, such as benzodiazepines, nonbenzodiazepine hypnotics, opioids, barbiturates, anticonvulsants, antipsychotics, anticholinergics, and some antidepressants and antihistamines. Sleepiness can also occur with some dopamine agonists such as pramipexole or ropinirole, and with many antiepileptic medications.

Although less common, sleepiness may occur with nonsteroidal anti-inflammatory drugs, some antibiotics, antispasmodics, antiarrhythmics, and beta blockers. Over-the-counter supplements, such as valerian and melatonin, can produce sedation (1, 98). Natural herbs and plants such as kava kava, passionflower, poppies, hops, Jamaican dogwood, marijuana, chamomile, lavender, and valerian can also have powerful sedating effects.

Elderly patients are especially susceptible to sleepiness induced by sedating substances. Some of the drowsy side effects of these drugs may be further amplified when used in combination with other medications, complicating the managed care of patients who are treating multiple comorbidities. Tolerance to these sedative substances can also develop over time.

Hypersomnia due to Substance Abuse

Daytime sleepiness can occur as a result of the abuse of alcohol, benzodiazepines, barbiturates, GHB, opiates, and cannabis.

Hypersomnia due to Stimulant Withdrawal

A sudden discontinuation of stimulants can result in an increased total sleep time, including daytime napping and general sleepiness, lasting for up to 3 weeks after their withdrawal. Despite the longer sleep time, sleep itself may be more fragmented and nonrestorative.

Milder and briefer periods of sleepiness, fatigue, and inattentiveness can also occur when caffeine is withdrawn from regular coffee drinkers. It is also possible that some residual sleepiness can last for years after the discontinuation of stimulants (1).

Before a diagnosis can be made, a thorough medical history and toxicology screen should be considered to eliminate the possible presence of sedating medications in the patient.

CENTRAL DISORDERS OF HYPERSOMNOLENCE—HYPERSOMNIA DUE TO A PSYCHIATRIC DISORDER

Diagnostic criteria (1)
Criteria A to C must be met:

a. The patient has daily periods of irrepressible need to sleep or daytime lapses into sleep occurring over a period of at least 3 months.
b. The daytime sleepiness occurs in association with a concurrent psychiatric disorder.
c. The symptoms are not better explained by another untreated sleep disorder, a medical or neurologic disorder, or the effects of medications or drugs.

Introduction

These disorders of hypersomnolence occur in patients who experience hypersomnia that is secondary to a psychiatric disorder, such as depression, bipolar disorder, posttraumatic disorders, and panic disorder (99–101).

In the case of all other secondary hypersomnias, the excessive sleepiness is a direct causal result of the associated medical disorder, drugs used in its treatment, or its potential short habitual sleep times.

However, in psychiatric disorders, the link to hypersomnia is not quite as clear. The hypersomnolence observed is not necessarily caused by the psychiatric disorder. For example, a patient diagnosed with depression and hypersomnia will have both depression and hypersomnia, but whether the depression caused the hypersomnia or the hypersomnia caused the depression, or whether the two are related in some other way is neither known nor implied.

Patients may report sleeping in excess during the night, napping often or at length during the day, sleep inertia, or EDS or fatigue (99). Fatigue is not usually relieved by increased sleep and may be unrelated to sleep quantity or quality. Many will also feel that sleep itself is nonrestorative, or of poor quality, often waking up just as tired, or more tired, than before bedtime. Often, patients will have poor attendance at work or at school. They often spend days in bed several times a week. Patients may experience social withdrawal, apathy, and feelings of low energy (1).

Hypersomnia associated with a psychiatric disorder accounts for an estimated 5% to 7% of all hypersomnolence cases. Women are more susceptible than men, and the typical age range is between 20 and 50 years (1). In some psychiatric disorders, hypersomnia may predict a different disease outcome (1, 102).

Before a diagnosis can be made, a thorough medical history and psychiatric consult should be considered to eliminate possible psychiatric disorders that may have hypersomnia as a symptom. In these disorders, the diagnosis should be hypersomnia associated with mood disorder or conversion disorders (somatic symptom disorder).

Hypersomnia Associated with Mood Disorder

Hypersomnolence is a common feature of depression. Patients may sleep too much or have little energy during the day. Daytime function at school, at work, or in social situations is often impaired.

Similar symptoms are noted during the depressive episodes in bipolar disorder and in seasonal affective disorder (SAD), a mood disorder in which people exhibit symptoms of depression at the same time of year, most commonly in the winter (1).

Depending on how it is defined, hypersomnolence can occur at a rate between 5% and 50% in patients with diagnosed major depression (1). Sleep complaints are very common in patients diagnosed with major depression. Up to 92% report sleep problems.

The prevalence of insomnia alone is reported as 48%, hypersomnia alone at 14%, and the co-occurrence of both is 30% (98, 99). In fact, co-occurring insomnia and hypersomnia are associated with more severe symptoms of major depression (102).

With major depression, hypersomnolence may persist even after the depressive episode improves, and persistent hypersomnolence is associated with an increased risk of recurrent depression (1).

A reported 29% of bipolar disorder patients have hypersomnia. As opposed to symptoms of insomnia, these patients are more likely to be younger and to have shorter illness duration (103). Hypersomnolence also affects more than 50% of patients with SAD (1).

Hypersomnia Associated with a Conversion Disorder (Somatic Symptom Disorder)

Conversion disorder, also referred to as *somatic symptom disorder*, is a psychiatric condition in which a person has blindness, paralysis, or other neurologic symptoms that cannot be explained by medical evaluation.

In relevant cases, patients will show symptoms of IH, narcolepsy, or cataplexy, without the objective support and confirmation of diagnostic testing. When this occurs, pseudohypersomnia or pseudonarcolepsy, sometimes with pseudocataplexy, may be described.

CENTRAL DISORDERS OF HYPERSOMNOLENCE—ISS

Diagnostic criteria (1)
Criteria A to F must be met:

a. The patient has daily periods of irrepressible need to sleep or daytime lapses into sleep; or, in the case of prepubertal children, there is a complaint of behavioral abnormalities attributable to sleepiness.
b. The patient's sleep time, established by personal or collateral history, sleep logs, or actigraphy, is usually shorter than expected for age.
c. The curtailed sleep pattern is present most days for at least 3 months.
d. The patient curtails sleep time by such measures as an alarm clock or being awakened by another person and generally sleeps longer when such measures are not used, such as on weekends or vacations.
e. Extension of total sleep time results in resolution of the symptoms of sleepiness.
f. The symptoms are not better explained by other untreated sleep disorders, the effects of medications or drugs, or other medical, neurologic, or mental disorders.

Notes

1. If there is doubt about the accuracy of personal history or sleep logs, then actigraphy should be performed, preferably for at least 2 weeks.
2. In the case of long sleepers, reported habitual sleep periods may be normal on the basis of age. However, these sleep periods may be insufficient for these patients.

Introduction

ISS describes a condition caused by the patient's voluntary curtailment of his or her normal sleep on a regular basis. This behavior eventually leads to severe sleepiness during the day.

Reasons for reducing the patient's sleep periods vary, but typically include work or school commitments, social obligations, or personal choice (such as overnight binge-watching of movies). Sleep debt accumulates over many nights as a result, leading to the deterioration of daytime function and extreme sleepiness.

Prevalence

A reported 2% of all sleep lab cases are diagnosed as ISS (104). In one study, 7% of all EDS patients were diagnosed as ISS (105), but in studies of adolescents, 10% of Norwegian teens (106), 12% of Japanese teens (107), and 18% of Korean teens (108) were reported to have ISS.

Although ISS affects all ages and sexes, it seems to be more frequent in adolescence when intrinsic sleep need is higher, yet social and scholastic pressures prompt these patients to curtail total sleep time. Homework and studying may result in later bedtimes, and sports/extracurricular activities may require earlier wakeup times. ISS is also noted in young adults starting new jobs. Working long hours and taking on extra work may be seen as a desirable trait in the employee wanting to advance in the corporate environment.

In addition, female patients may experience additional pressures in the home even after a full day of work. Childrearing and housekeeping continue to tax working parents, especially mothers. This can result in later bedtimes and/or earlier wakeup times that lead to ongoing sleep loss.

Cultural influences may also contribute to ISS. In countries where napping, or the siesta, is commonplace, ISS may lead to enhanced nighttime alertness, delaying bedtime or sleep onset.

A factor that is especially salient to the sleep technologist: those who perform shift work may be particularly susceptible to ISS. Often, chores and errands are run during daytime hours, when the shift worker should be asleep. Many times there is no choice but to conform to daytime business hours; this means cutting sleep time by going to bed later than normal or waking up sooner than usual. This is especially true for long-shift workers (10 to 12 hours), when the demands of a 12-hour shift leave less time to manage obligations and still acquire sufficient sleep. Many times these errands are one-off occurrences and, therefore, not truly ISS. Sometimes, however, they are regular everyday events, such as taking children to and from school, lengthy commute times, or trips to the gym.

Salient Features

The primary symptom is daytime somnolence. The patient's ability to initiate and maintain sleep is within normal parameters. There is a noted discrepancy between the amount of sleep needed to maintain normal levels of alertness and wakefulness and the amount of sleep the patient reports getting nightly. The patient is often unaware that his or her daytime sleepiness is affected by poor sleeping choices (1). When sleep time is increased during the holidays, weekends, or vacation, daytime sleepiness is improved immediately.

If voluntary sleep restriction is severe enough, the patient may experience sleep paralysis and/or hypnagogic hallucinations (1). Other features include personality changes, irritability, lack of motivation, fatigue, restlessness, and problems with memory, motor coordination, concentration, and attention (1).

Other researchers have noted an increase in obesity, depressed mood, increased anxiety, decline in school performance, and adolescent suicidal ideation (107, 108). Suicidal ideation was noted independent of depression, daytime sleepiness, snoring, or insomnia. In fact, the greater the sleep restriction (as measured by longer weekend "oversleep"), the higher the suicidality scores (108).

Also of significance is the finding that people with severe ISS are at higher risk for getting into motor vehicle accidents (105). Short sleep, defined as lasting 4 to 7 hours, also increases the risk for heart disease, stroke, type 2 diabetes, obesity/weight gain, workplace injuries, depression, and mortality (109).

No other medical reason is readily apparent for the complaint of daytime sleepiness for those with true ISS.

Diagnosis

Diagnosis is made via a detailed medical history and elimination of other possible disorders.

Actigraphy can be used in combination with sleep diaries for 2 to 3 weeks until a pattern emerges. Results would show a curtailed total time in bed, short sleep latency, short total sleep time, and high sleep efficiency. The PSG and the MSLT are not indicated in the diagnosis of ISS. After a sleep history via actigraphy and sleep diary is complete, a trial period with longer times in bed is tried. If the symptoms are alleviated, then the diagnosis of ISS is made.

Differential Diagnosis

DSPS may mimic the habits of ISS patients who go to bed late. Although the ISS patient chooses to stay up late, the DSPS patient is simply not sleepy because of delays in his or her intrinsic circadian rhythms. When a patient has an endogenous (internally regulated) circadian period that is more than 24 hours, he or she will not feel sleepy until later in the evening. Often, such patients set their alarms for specific wakeup times (for school or for work) that aren't ordinarily flexible. This results in a persistent late bedtime with an earlier-than-desired wakeup time.

Similarly, advanced sleep phase syndrome results in a constant early rise time. A patient with this syndrome may go to bed at a "normal" hour (which for his or her circadian rhythm may already be late), but then wake up too early as a result. These patients may lose out on work opportunities and social time with friends and family because of their inability to stay awake in the early evening.

ISS may also mimic insomnia, but it is distinctly different. ISS patients maintain the ability to sleep normally, with sleep latency and sleep duration within normal parameters. They simply choose not to. Insomnia patients do not consciously choose to stay up late or curtail their sleep. Sleep initiation and consolidation of sleep are impaired beyond their control. ISS patients sleep "normally" on vacation, holidays, or the weekend, whereas insomnia sufferers continue to experience sleep troubles during these times.

A note about so-called "long sleepers." These individuals have natural sleep requirements that range significantly longer than the average 7 to 8 hours. In these patients, getting average amounts of sleep (e.g., 7 hours per night) may not be enough. Social pressures (work, school, family) and stigma (laziness) may prevent these patients from sleeping enough hours, leading to chronic sleep deprivation. In this case, ISS should be diagnosed even if the patient reports an "average" full night's sleep of 7 or 8 hours.

Treatment

A therapeutic trial of a longer major sleep period can reverse the symptoms of ISS. If so, treatment would be to maintain that sleep schedule indefinitely. Sleep hygiene is also an effective tool to treat ISS. Education and adherence to proper sleep hygiene procedures will help increase total sleep time.

Conclusion

A sufficient amount of sleep is essential for optimal physical health, immune function, mental health, and cognitive function. Adults should sleep 7 to 8 or more hours per night on a regular basis for optimal sleep health. Infants, children, and teenagers require substantially more sleep than adults. However, societal, familial, entertainment, scholastic, and work-related pressures often demand more time of us than there are hours in the day. One of the first things to be sacrificed is sleep time.

To deal with this epidemic of sleep debt, we must continue to emphasize the need for, and benefits of, a full night of uninterrupted sleep. The health costs of reduced sleep put a burden not only on the patients themselves, but on society as a whole.

CENTRAL DISORDERS OF HYPERSOMNOLENCE—NORMAL VARIANT: THE LONG SLEEPER

Introduction

As alluded to earlier in the chapter, long sleepers are people with natural sleep requirements significantly longer than average; typically, they sleep between 10 and 12 hours nightly. Their sleep, although long, is normal in architecture and physiology and is reportedly of a good quality, refreshing, and consistent throughout the years. It is simply much longer than what most people need (1). Long sleepers are often stigmatized as lazy or depressed. However, there is no definite link between long sleepers and adverse long-term or chronic health problems (110, 111).

Prevalence

An estimated 2% of men and 1.5% of women subjectively identify as long sleepers, reporting sleeping 10 hours per night or more. There seems to be a strong genetic heritability (44%) and a high concordance with monozygotic twins. Genome studies indicate an involvement of circadian clock and other related genes (1).

Salient Features

Long sleepers have longer than normal primary sleep periods, but are not excessively sleepy in the daytime, nor are they more likely to nap. Sleep efficiency is on par with normal sleepers, as is arousal index, total slow-wave time, and REM sleep percentage. Apnea and PLM indices are also comparable to those of average sleepers.

In general, long sleepers tend to go to bed earlier and wake up later than average sleepers (112). Long sleepers will often function on near-average sleep times, sleeping 9 hours per night, then catch up on the weekends, sometimes sleeping 12 hours or more (1).

ISS may be common among long sleepers because of societal expectations to conform to the sleep times of average adults. Although average sleep times may be 8 hours for most people, this amount of sleep time would still be inadequate for the long sleeper.

Diagnosis

Before diagnosing a patient as a long sleeper, one must first rule out any of the myriad of sleep disorders that could cause a patient to feel the need to sleep longer times, such as sleep apnea, any one of the hypersomnia disorders, some psychiatric disorders, physical illnesses, or drug effects. These are the limitations to previous research studying long sleep.

Although previous studies have sometimes found an increased mortality, higher body mass index, and greater prevalence of type 2 diabetes or coronary heart disease, research is still unclear whether most subjects were true long sleepers or had disorders resulting in an elevated need for sleep (1). This may explain the often contradictory studies that sometimes show long sleepers at higher risk for health problems; more recent studies show long sleepers are completely normal without additional health risks. These studies relied on objective measures of sleep (PSG and actigraphy) and semiobjective measures, such as the sleep diary, as opposed to subjective questionnaires and self-reporting over telephone interviews. Consequently, because of inherent limitations in the subjectivity of reported sleep times (112), it is suggested that patients keep an accurate sleep diary or use actigraphy to get a more accurate portrait of their sleep schedules.

A diagnosis of a long sleeper can be confidently made after other medical conditions have been ruled out and objective measures record at least 10 hours of sleep over a minimum of seven nights (1). These longer sleep times should be consistent throughout most of the individual's life, and must be considered relatively of high quality, with the subject waking up refreshed and not feeling sleepy during the day.

Treatment

There is no treatment for long sleep because this is not, strictly speaking, a sleep disorder. However, care should be taken to ensure that these patients acquire adequate sleep in spite of pressure to curtail it.

Conclusion

Long sleepers do not importantly differ in their sleep from those reporting normal sleep times other than in the increased amount of time they spend in bed while asleep. Health outcomes are normal, and no long-term adverse consequences are expected because of this longer-than-average sleep drive. Long sleepers presumably represent the high end of the normal sleep duration continuum.

REFERENCES

1. American Academy of Sleep Medicine. (2014). *International classification of sleep disorders* (3rd ed.). Darien, IL: Author.

2. Dauvilliers, Y., & Buguet, A. (2005). Hypersomnia *Dialogues in Clinical Neuroscience, 7*(4), 347–356.

3. Slater, G., & Steier, J. (2012). Excessive daytime sleepiness in sleep disorders. *Journal of Thoracic Disease, 4*(6), 608–616.

4. Ohayon, M. M., Dauvilliers, Y., & Reynolds, C. F. (2012). Operational definitions and algorithms for excessive sleepiness in the general population: Implications for DSM-5 nosology. *Archives of General Psychiatry, 69*(1), 71–79.

5. de Mello, M. T., Narciso, F. V., Tufik, S., et al. (2013). Sleep disorders as a cause of motor vehicle collisions. *International Journal of Preventive Medicine, 4*(3), 246–257.

6. American Academy of Sleep Medicine. (2005). *International classification of sleep disorders: Diagnostic and coding manual* (2nd ed.). Westchester, IL: Author.

7. Nishino, S. (2007). Clinical and neurobiological aspects of narcolepsy. *Sleep Medicine, 8*(4), 373–399.

8. Flygare, J., & Parthasarathy, S. (2015). Narcolepsy: Let the patient's voice awaken us! *American Journal of Medicine, 128*(1), 10–13.

9. Morrish, E., King, M. A., Smith, I. E., et al. (2004). Factors associated with a delay in the diagnosis of narcolepsy. *Sleep Medicine, 5*(1), 37–41.

10. Nobili, L., Beelke, M., Besset, A., et al. (2001). Nocturnal sleep features in narcolepsy: A model-based approach. *Revue neurologique (Paris), 157*(11, Pt. 2), S82–S86.

11. Mignot, E. (2001). A hundred years of narcolepsy research. *Archives Italiennes de Biologie, 139*(3), 207–220.

12. Hublin, C., Partinen, M., Kaprio, J., et al. (1995). Epidemiology of narcolepsy. *Sleep, 17*, S7–S12.

13. Roth, B. (1980). *Narcolepsy and hypersomnia* (pp. 1–301). Basel, Switzerland: Karger.

14. Dement, W., Zarcone, W., Varner, V., et al. (1972). The prevalence of narcolepsy [abstract]. *Journal of Sleep Research, 1*, 148.

15. Dement, W. C., Carskadon, M., & Ley, R. (1973). The prevalence of narcolepsy II [abstract]. *Journal of Sleep Research, 2*, 147.

16. Honda, Y. (1979). Census of narcolepsy, cataplexy and sleep life among teenagers in Fujisawa city [abstract]. *Journal of Sleep Research, 8*, 191.

17. de Lecea, L., Kilduff, T. S., Peyron, C., et al. (1998). The hypocretins: Hypothalamus-specific peptides with neuroexcitatory activity. *Proceedings of the National Academy of Sciences of the United States of America, 95*, 322–327.

18. Sakurai, T., Amemiya, A., Ishii, M., et al. (1998). Orexins and orexin receptors: A family of hypothalamic neuropeptides and G protein-coupled receptors that regulate feeding behavior. *Cell, 92*, 573–585.

19. Nishino, S., Okura, M., & Mignot, E. (2000). Narcolepsy: Genetic predisposition and neuropharmacological mechanisms. *Sleep Medicine Reviews, 4*(1), 57–99.

20. Abad, V. C., & Guilleminault, C. (2017). New developments in the management of narcolepsy. *Nature and Science of Sleep, 9*, 39–57.

21. Lammers, G. J., & Overeem, S. (2005). Hypocretin/orexin and sleep. In L. de Lecea, & J. G. Sutcliffe (Eds.), *Hypocretins* (pp. 279–290). Boston, MA: Springer.

22. Mignot, E. (1998). Genetic and familial aspects of narcolepsy. *Neurology, 50*(2 Suppl. 1), S16–S22.

23. Aran, A., Lin, L., Nevsimalova, S., et al. (2009). Elevated anti-streptococcal antibodies in patients with recent narcolepsy onset. *Sleep, 32*(8), 979–983.

24. Longstreth, W. T. Jr., Ton, T. G., & Koepsell, T. D. (2009). Narcolepsy and streptococcal infections. *Sleep, 32*(12), 1548.

25. Dauvilliers, Y., Montplaisir, J., Cochen, V., et al. (2010). Post-H_1N_1 narcolepsy-cataplexy. *Sleep, 33*(11), 1428–1430.

26. Ton, T. G., Longstreth, W. T. Jr., & Koepsell, T. D. (2010). Environmental toxins and risk of narcolepsy among people with HLA DQB1*0602. *Environmental Research, 110*(6), 565–570.

27. Thannickal, T. C., Moore, R. Y., Nienhuis, R., et al. (2000). Reduced number of hypocretin neurons in human narcolepsy. *Neuron, 27*(3), 469–474.

28. Bourgin, P., Zeitzer, J. M., & Mignot, E. (2008). CSF hypocretin-1 assessment in sleep and neurological disorders. *The Lancet Neurology, 7*(7), 649–662.

29. Bourgin, P., & Dauvilliers, Y. (2005). Hypocretin in neuropsychiatric disorders. In L. de Lecea, & J. G. Sutcliffe (Eds.), *Hypocretins* (pp. 263–277). Boston, MA: Springer.

30. Schwartz, S., Ponz, A., Poryazova, R., et al. (2008). Abnormal activity in hypothalamus and amygdala during humour processing in human narcolepsy with cataplexy. *Brain, 131*(Pt. 2), 514–522.

31. Akintomide, G. S., & Rickards, H. (2011). Narcolepsy: A review. *Neuropsychiatric Disease and Treatment, 7*, 507–518.

32. Hoddes, E., Zarcone, V., Smythe, H., et al. (1973). Quantification of sleepiness: A new approach. *Psychophysiology, 10*(4), 431–436.

33. Carskadon, M. A., Dement, W. C., Mitler, M. M., et al. (1986). Guidelines for the multiple sleep latency test (MSLT): A standard measure of sleepiness. *Sleep, 9*(4), 519–524.

34. Szakács, Z., Dauvilliers, Y., Mikhaylov, V., et al. (2017). Safety and efficacy of pitolisant on cataplexy in patients with narcolepsy: A randomised, double-blind, placebo-controlled trial. *The Lancet Neurology, 16*(3), 200–207.

35. Iijima, S., Sugita, Y., Teshima, Y., et al. (1986). Therapeutic effects of mazindol on narcolepsy. *Sleep, 9*(1, Pt. 2), 265–268.

36. Nittur, N., Konofal, E., Dauvilliers, Y., et al. (2013). Mazindol in narcolepsy and idiopathic and symptomatic hypersomnia refractory to stimulants: A long-term chart review. *Sleep Medicine, 14*(1), 30–36.

37. Bassetti, C., & Aldrich, M. S. (1997). Idiopathic hypersomnia: A series of 42 patients. *Brain, 120*, 1423–1435.

38. Billiard, M., & Dauvilliers, Y. (2001). Idiopathic hypersomnia. *Sleep Medicine Reviews, 5*, 351–360.

39. Billiard, M., & Šonka, K. (2016). Idiopathic hypersomnia. *Sleep Medicine Reviews, 29*, 23–33.

40. Sasai, T., Inoue, Y., Komada, Y., et al. (2009). Comparison of clinical characteristics among narcolepsy with and without cataplexy and idiopathic hypersomnia without long sleep time, focusing on HLA-DRB1(*)1501/DQB1(*)0602 finding. *Sleep Medicine, 10*(9), 961–966.

41. Hong, S. C., Lin, L., & Jeong, J. H. (2006). A study of the diagnostic utility of HLA typing, CSF hypocretin-1 measurements, and MSLT testing for the diagnosis of narcolepsy in 163 Korean patients with unexplained excessive daytime sleepiness. *Sleep, 29*(11), 1429–1438.

42. Vernet, C., & Arnulf, I. (2009). Narcolepsy with long sleep time: A specific entity? *Sleep, 32*(9), 1229–1235.

43. Leu-Semenescu, S., Nittur, N., Golmard, J.-L., et al. (2014). Effects of pitolisant, a histamine H3 inverse agonist, in drug-resistant idiopathic and symptomatic hypersomnia: A chart review. *Sleep Medicine, 15*(6), 681–687.

44. Aserinsky, E., & Kleitman, N. (1953). Regularly occurring periods of eye motility, and concomitant phenomena, during sleep. *Science, 118*(3062), 273–274.

45. Roth, B. (1976). Narcolepsy and hypersomnia: Review and classification of 642 personally observed cases. *Schweizer Archiv für Neurologie, Neurochirurgie und Psychiatrie, 119*, 31–41.

46. Anderson, K., Phil, D., Pilsworth, S., et al. (2007). Idiopathic hypersomnia: A study of 77 cases. *Sleep, 30*(10), 1274–1281.

47. Roth, T. (2007). Introduction: Narcolepsy and excessive daytime sleepiness: From the bench to the bedside. *The Journal of Clinical Psychiatry, 68*(Suppl. 13), 4.

48. Khan, Z., & Trotti, L. M. (2015). Central disorders of hypersomnolence: Focus on the narcolepsies and idiopathic hypersomnia. *Chest, 148*(1), 262–273.

49. Ali, M., Auger, R., Slocumb, N. L., et al. (2009). Idiopathic hypersomnia: Clinical features and response to treatment. *Journal of Clinical Sleep Medicine, 5*(6), 562–568.

50. Johns, M. W. (1994). Sleepiness in different situations measured by the Epworth Sleepiness Scale. *Sleep, 17*, 703–710.

51. Alakuijala, A., Maasilta, P., & Bachour, A. (2013). The Oxford Sleep Resistance test (OSLER) is sensitive in showing modifications in vigilance with CPAP therapy in sleep apnea patients. *Sleep Medicine, 14*, e57.

52. Alakuijala, A., Maasilta, P., & Bachour, A. (2014). The Oxford Sleep Resistance test (OSLER) and the multiple unprepared reaction time test (MURT) detect vigilance modifications in sleep apnea patients. *Journal of Clinical Sleep Medicine, 10*(10), 1075–1082.

53. Mignot, E. (2012). A practical guide to the therapy of narcolepsy and hypersomnia syndromes. *Neurotherapeutics, 9*, 739–752.

54. Gupta, D., & Chatterjee, T. (2017). Idiopathic hypersomnia. *Research & Reviews: Neuroscience, 1*(2), 1–5.

55. Preda, A. (n.d.). Primary hypersomnia. *eMedicine Psychiatry*, Updated November 3, 2009. Retrieved May 15, 2018, from http://www.academia.edu/550258/Primary_Hypersomnia

56. Šonka, K., Šusta, M., Billiard, M. (2015). Narcolepsy with and without cataplexy, idiopathic hypersomnia with and without long sleep time: A cluster analysis. *Sleep Medicine, 16*(2), 225–231.

57. Ramdurg, S. (2010). Kleine-Levin syndrome: Etiology, diagnosis, and treatment. *Annals of Indian Academy of Neurology, 13*(4), 241–246.

58. Billiard, M. (2015). Kleine–Levin syndrome. In S. Chokroverty, & M. Billiard (Eds.), *Sleep Medicine*. New York, NY: Springer.

59. Gadoth, N., & Oksenberg, A. (2017). Kleine-Levin syndrome: An update and mini-review. *Brain and Development, 39*(8), 665–671.

60. Kleine, W. (1925). Periodische schlafsucht. *Monatsschrift fur Psychiatrie und Neurologie 57*, 285–320.

61. Levin, M. (1929). Narcolepsy (Gélineau's syndrome) and other varieties of morbid somnolence. *Archives of Neurology & Psychiatry, 22*, 1172–1200.

62. Levin, M. (1936). Periodic somnolence and morbid hunger: A new syndrome. *Brain, 59*, 494–504.

63. Critchley, M. (1962). Periodic hypersomnia and megaphagia in adolescent males. *Brain, 85*, 627–656.

64. Critchley, M., & Hoffman, H. L. (1942). The syndrome of periodic somnolence and morbid hunger (Kleine-Levin syndrome). *British Medical Journal, 1*, 137–139.

65. Thorpy, M. J. (1990). *International classification of sleep disorders: Diagnostic and coding manual*. Rochester, MN: American Sleep Disorders Association.

66. Arnulf, I., Zeitzer, J., Farber, N., et al. (2005). Kleine-Levin syndrome: A systematic review of 186 cases in the literature. *Brain, 128*(12), 2763–2776.

67. Russel, J., & Grunstein, R. (1992). Kleine-Levin syndrome: A case report. *The Australian and New Zealand Journal of Psychiatry, 26*(1), 119–123.

68. Dauvilliers, Y., Mayer, G., Lecendreux, M., et al. (2002). Kleine-Levin syndrome: An autoimmune hypothesis based on clinical and genetic analyses. *Neurology, 59*, 1739–1745.

69. Fenzi, F., Simonati, A., Crosato, F., et al. (1993). Clinical features of Kleine-Levin syndrome with localized encephalitis. *Neuropediatrics, 24*, 292–295.

70. Salter, M. S., & White, P. D. (1993). A variant of Kleine-Levin syndrome precipitated by both Epstein-Barr and varicella-zoster virus infections. *Biological Psychiatry, 33*, 388–390.

71. Haugh, R. M., & Markesbery, W. R. (1983). Hypothalamic astrocytoma. Syndrome of hyperphagia, obesity, and disturbances of behaviour and endocrine and autonomic function. *Archives of Neurology, 40*, 560–563.

72. Chesson, A., Levine, S., Kong, L. S., et al. (1991). Neuroendocrine evaluation in Kleine-Levin syndrome: Evidence of reduced dopaminergic tone during periods of hypersomnolence. *Sleep, 14*, 226–232.

73. Koerber, R. K., Torkelson, R., Haven, G., et al. (1984). Increased cerebrospinal fluid 5-hydroxytryptamine and 5-hydroxyindoleacetic acid in Kleine-Levin syndrome. *Neurology, 34*, 1597–1600.

74. Arnulf, I., Lin, L., Gadoth, N., et al. (2008). Kleine-Levin syndrome: A systematic study of 108 patients. *Annals of Neurology, 63*, 482–493.

75. Miglis, M. G., & Guilleminault, C. (2014). Kleine-Levin syndrome: A review. *Nature and Science of Sleep, 6*, 19–26.

76. Nguyen, Q. T., Groos, E., Leclair-Visonneau, L., et al. (2016). Familial Kleine-Levin syndrome: A specific entity? *Sleep, 39*, 1535–1542.

77. Huang, Y. S., Lin, Y. H., & Guilleminault, C. (2009). Polysomnography in Kleine-Levin syndrome. *Neurology, 70*, 795–801.

78. Goswami, M., Thorpy, M. J., & Pandi-Perumal, S. R. (2016). *Narcolepsy: A clinical guide*. Switzerland: Springer International Publishing.

79. Guilleminault, C. (1985). Disorders of excessive sleepiness. *Annals of Clinical Research, 17*(5), 209–219.

80. Poppe, M., Friebel, D., Reuner, U., et al. (2003). The Kleine-Levin syndrome—Effects of treatment with lithium. *Neuropediatrics, 34*, 113–119.

81. Landtblom, A. M., Dige, N., Schwerdt, K., et al. (2003). Short-term memory dysfunction in Kleine-Levin syndrome. *Acta Neurologica Scandinavica, 108*, 363–367.

82. de Oliveira, M. M., Conti, C., & Prado, G. F. (2016). Pharmacological treatment for Kleine-Levin syndrome. *Cochrane Database of Systematic Reviews, 5*, CD006685.

83. Kleine Levin Syndrome Foundation (n.d.). *Stanford's KLS research program seeking volunteers for a viral study*. Retrieved May 15, 2018, from https://klsfoundation.org/stanfords-kls-research/

84. Engström, M., Vigren, P., Karlsson, T., et al. (2009). Working memory in 8 Kleine-Levin syndrome patients: An fMRI study. *Sleep, 32*(5), 681–688.

85. Engström, M., Hallböök, T., Szakács, A., et al. (2014). Functional magnetic resonance imaging in narcolepsy and the Kleine-Levin syndrome. *Frontiers in Neurology, 5*, 105.

86. Malik, S., Boeve, B. F., Krahn, L. E., et al. (2001). Narcolepsy associated with other central nervous system disorders. *Neurology, 57*, 539–541.

87. Guilleminault, C., Yuen, K. M., Gulevich, M. G., et al. (2000). Hypersomnia after head-neck trauma: A medico-legal dilemma. *Neurology, 54*, 653–659.

88. Martinez-Rodriguez, J. E., Lin, L., Iranzo, A., et al. (2003). Decreased hypocretin-1 (Orexin-A) levels in the cerebrospinal fluid of patients with myotonic dystrophy and excessive daytime sleepiness. *Sleep, 26*, 287–290.

89. Mayo Clinic. (2018, January 17). *Traumatic brain injury*. Retrieved March 2, 2018, from https://www.mayoclinic.org/diseases-conditions/traumatic-brain-injury/symptoms-causes/syc-20378557

90. Castriotti, R. J., Wilde, M. C., Lai, J. M., et al. (2007). Prevalence and consequences of sleep disorders in traumatic brain injury. *Journal of Clinical Sleep Medicine, 3*, 349–356.

91. Watson, N. F., Dikmen, S., Machamer, J., et al. (2007). Hypersomnia following traumatic brain injury. *Journal of Clinical Sleep Medicine, 3*(4), 363–368.

92. Hong, C. T., Wong, C. S., Ma, H. P., et al. (2015). PERIOD3 polymorphism is associated with sleep quality recovery after a mild traumatic brain injury. *Journal of the Neurological Sciences, 358*(1–2), 385–389.

93. Shinno, H., Inami, Y., Inagaki, T., et al. (2009). Successful treatment with levothyroxine for idiopathic hypersomnia patients with subclinical hypothyroidism. *General Hospital Psychiatry, 31*(2), 190–193.

94. Butterworth, R. F. (1999). Metabolic encephalopathies. In G. J. Siegel, B. W. Agranoff, R. W. Albers, S. K. Fisher, & M. D. Uhler (Eds.), *Basic neurochemistry: Molecular, cellular and medical aspects* (6th ed.). Philadelphia, PA: Lippincott-Raven.

95. Vernet, C., Redolfi, S., Attali, V., et al. (2011). Residual sleepiness in obstructive sleep apnoea: Phenotype and related symptoms. *European Respiratory Journal, 38*(1), 98–105.

96. Castiglioni, P., Lombardi, C., Cortelli, P., et al. (2012). Why excessive sleepiness may persist in OSA patients receiving adequate CPAP treatment. *European Respiratory Journal, 39*(1), 226–227; author reply 227–228.

97. Zhu, Y., Fenik, P., Zhan, G., et al. (2007). Selective loss of catecholaminergic wake active neurons in a murine sleep apnea model. *Journal of Neuroscience, 27*, 10060–10071.

98. Shimazaki, M., & Martin, J. L. (2007). Do herbal agents have a place in the treatment of sleep problems in long-term care? *Journal of the American Medical Directors Association, 8*(4), 248–252.

99. Dauvilliers, Y., Lopez, R., Ohayon, M., et al. (2013). Hypersomnia and depressive symptoms: Methodological and clinical aspects. *BMC Medicine, 11*, 78.

100. Waldrop, E. A., Back, S. E., Sensenig, A., et al. (2008). Sleep disturbances associated with posttraumatic stress disorder and alcohol dependence. *Addictive Behaviors, 33*(2), 328–335.

101. Staner, L. (2003). Sleep and anxiety disorders. *Dialogues in Clinical Neuroscience, 5*(3), 249–258.

102. Soehner, A. M., Kaplan, K. A., & Harvey, A. G. (2014). Prevalence and clinical correlates of co-occurring insomnia and hypersomnia symptoms in depression. *Journal of Affective Disorders, 167*, 93–97.

103. Steinan, M. K., Scott, J., Lagerberg, T. V., et al. (2016). Sleep problems in bipolar disorders: More than just insomnia. *Acta Psychiatrica Scandinavica, 133*(5), 368–377.

104. Hublin, C., Kaprio, J., Partinen, M., et al. (2001). Insufficient sleep—A population-based study in adults. *Sleep, 24*(4), 392–400.

105. Komada, Y., Inoue, Y., Hayashida, K., et al. (2008). Clinical significance and correlates of behaviorally induced insufficient sleep syndrome. *Sleep Medicine, 9*(8), 851–856.

106. Pallesen, S., Saxvig, I. W., Molde, H., et al. (2011). Brief report: Behaviorally induced insufficient sleep syndrome in older adolescents: Prevalence and correlates. *Journal of Adolescence, 34*(2), 391–395.

107. Morita, Y., Sasai-Sakuma, T., Asaoka, S., et al. (2015). Prevalence and correlates of insufficient sleep syndrome in Japanese young adults: A web-based cross-sectional study. *Journal of Clinical Sleep Medicine, 11*(10), 1163–1169.

108. Lee, Y. J., Cho, S. J., Cho, I. H., et al. (2012). Insufficient sleep and suicidality in adolescents. *Sleep, 35*(4), 455–460.

109. Kecklund, G., & Axelsson, J. (2016). Health consequences of shift work and insufficient sleep. *British Medical Journal, 355*, i5210.

110. Lauderdale, D. S., Knutson, K. L., Rathouz, P. J., et al. (2009). Cross-sectional and longitudinal associations between objectively measured sleep duration and body mass index: The CARDIA Sleep Study. *American Journal of Epidemiology, 170*, 805–813.

111. van den Berg, J. F., Knvistingh Neven, A., Tulen, J. H., et al. (2008). Actigraphic sleep duration and fragmentation are related to obesity in the elderly: The Rotterdam Study. *International Journal of Obesity (Lond), 32*(7), 1083–1090.

112. Patel, S. R., Blackwell, T., Ancoli-Israel, S., et al. (2012). Sleep characteristics of self-reported long sleepers. *Sleep, 35*(5), 641–648.

chapter 17

Circadian Rhythms and Circadian Rhythm Sleep–Wake Disorders

CHAD WHITTLEF   KATHERINE M. SHARKEY

LEARNING OBJECTIVES

On completion of this chapter, the reader should be able to:

1. Define and give examples of circadian rhythms.
2. Define the common terms used to describe circadian physiology.
3. Describe the neurobiology of the circadian clock and the effects of light, darkness, and other factors on circadian function.
4. Identify the clinical features of circadian rhythm sleep–wake disorders (CRSWD).
5. Describe circadian rhythm measurements used for clinical diagnosis of CRSWD.
6. Explain laboratory assessments of circadian rhythms.
7. Discuss the most common treatments for CRSWD.
8. Appreciate the potential risks associated with shift work in the sleep laboratory.

KEY TERMS

Advanced sleep–wake phase disorder
Chronotherapy
Circadian rhythms
Circadian rhythm sleep–wake disorders
Constant routine
Delayed sleep–wake phase disorder
Dim light melatonin onset
Entrainment
Forced desynchrony
Free running
Infradian
Irregular sleep–wake rhythm
Jet lag disorder
Light therapy
Masking
Melatonin
Phase
Phase response curve
Phase shift

Shift-work disorder
Sleep–wake diaries
Suprachiasmatic nuclei
Ultradian
Wrist actigraphy
Zeitgeber

FUNDAMENTALS OF CIRCADIAN RHYTHMS

Throughout history, scientists have observed that most living things have physiologic rhythms that parallel the 24-hour cycle of day and night. These are called "circadian rhythms" from the Latin "circa," meaning about, and "diem," meaning day, a term coined by Franz Halberg in 1959 (1). Circadian rhythms are found in virtually all living things, including one-celled animals and plants. The sleep–wake cycle, rhythm of core body temperature, and hormonal rhythms (e.g., melatonin) fluctuating across the 24-hour period are examples of human circadian rhythms. Circadian rhythms are so foundational to physiology and behavior that the scientists whose work unraveled the molecular mechanisms of circadian rhythms, Jeffrey Hall, Michael Rosbash, and Michael Young, were awarded the 2017 Nobel Prize in Physiology or Medicine for their contributions to science (2).

In addition to circadian rhythms, there are other oscillations that are present in humans and animals. *Ultradian rhythms* are rhythms shorter than 24 hours, for instance, the rapid eye movement–nonrapid eye movement (REM–NREM) cycles that are observed in sleep. The term *infradian rhythms* refers to oscillations that are longer than 24 hours. As an example, the menstrual cycle approximates 28 days.

Typically, circadian rhythms are represented by a sine wave (Fig. 17-1). Various terms are used to describe different aspects of the rhythm. The *period*, also referred to as *tau*, is the length of the rhythm. This is usually very

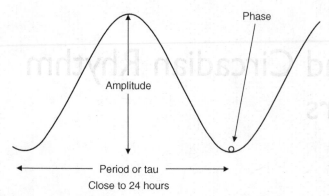

Figure 17-1 Circadian rhythms are schematically represented by a sine wave.

close to 24 hours. The *amplitude* is the magnitude of the rhythm from its peak to nadir. The amplitude of different circadian rhythms is variable and can be affected by age, sex, sleep state, and so on. The *phase* refers to the circadian position at any specific instant of time. Depending on what rhythm is measured, different phase markers are used. For instance, when the circadian rhythm of core temperature is measured, the temperature minimum or maximum is commonly used as a marker of phase. When hormonal rhythms are measured—most commonly melatonin—the onset, offset, or peak of hormone secretion is used as a phase marker.

NEUROBIOLOGIC BASIS OF THE INTERNAL CIRCADIAN CLOCK

Circadian rhythms are endogenously driven by a master circadian clock located in the suprachiasmatic nuclei (SCN) of the anterior hypothalamus (3–5). Information about the lighting conditions of the external environment is conveyed to the SCN from the retina through the retinohypothalamic tract (6, 7) (Fig. 17-2). The cells in the retina responsible for conveying information about light and dark are called intrinsically photosensitive retinal ganglion cells (8); these ganglion cells differ from the conventional ganglion cells that transmit rod and cone input to the brain for visual image formation.

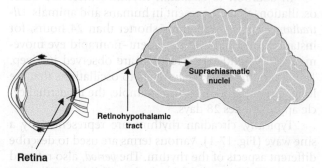

Figure 17-2 Diagram of the retinohypothalamic tract.

The SCN also receive input from the intergeniculate leaflet of the thalamus and the midbrain raphe nuclei. These two pathways are thought to transmit both photic (light) and nonphotic information to the circadian clock (6).

Most SCN projections stay within the hypothalamus, although a small fraction of SCN neurons terminate in the basal forebrain and midline thalamus (7). Secondary efferents from these three areas project to many brain regions, including the neocortex, hippocampus, basal ganglia, anterior pituitary, hypothalamus, reticular formation, and pineal gland. It is through this expansive network that the SCN exert control over many physiologic functions, including endocrine regulation, body temperature, the sleep–wake cycle, metabolism, autonomic regulation, psychomotor and cognitive performance, attention, memory, and emotion (7).

Recent progress in circadian biology has demonstrated that circadian physiology is driven by a hierarchical multioscillator system where the SCN serves as the central circadian clock orchestrating peripheral clocks in the various organ systems throughout the body (8). These peripheral clocks are responsive to, and integrate, information from input outside of the SCN. For instance, circadian rhythms of liver function and metabolism are influenced by a food-entrainable oscillator located in brain regions outside the SCN.

Circadian rhythm researchers measure physiologic rhythms that are downstream outputs of the endogenous clock to infer the phase position of the circadian rhythms. The circadian rhythms of the hormone melatonin and core body temperature are common measures of circadian phase in humans.

EFFECTS OF THE LIGHT–DARK CYCLE ON CIRCADIAN RHYTHMS

As mentioned, sensory receptors in the retina provide information about the light–dark cycle to the master circadian clock in SCN. The light–dark cycle helps the organism remain synchronized or entrained to the 24-hour day of the external environment (Fig. 17-3). In the absence of a light–dark cycle and other time cues, circadian rhythms "free run" at a rate not equal to 24 hours, but equal to the endogenous period length, or tau. The period (tau) is close to, but not exactly, 24 hours. Free running is observed in humans when they have no photic (light) stimuli, for instance in people with blindness and no photoreception (9–12), or when the light–dark cycle to which they are exposed is outside of the time range of possible biologic entrainment, as occurs in orbiting astronauts, for instance.

Wever and colleagues (13) performed some of the initial experiments using bright light to entrain human

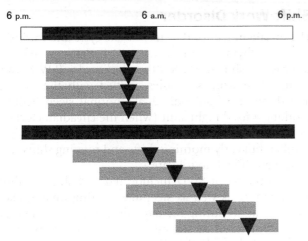

Figure 17-3 Examples of entrainment and free running. The gray bars represent time when the body temperature is low and the triangles represent the temperature minimum. The black and white bars represent the lighting conditions. The top half of the figure depicts entrainment. When a changing light–dark cycle is present, the internal circadian clock uses the photic cues to synchronize or entrain to the 24-hour light–dark cycle. The bottom half of the figure depicts free running. When there is no change in the light–dark cycle, the circadian rhythms free-run at a period length (tau) determined by the endogenous circadian clock. In this case, the period length is longer than 24 hours, which causes the circadian rhythms to delay (move later) because each day starts and ends at a slightly later clock time than the previous day.

circadian rhythms, confirming an important principle of human circadian rhythms: the light–dark cycle is one of the most powerful synchronizers of the endogenous circadian pacemaker in humans. More recent studies have tested various intensities of light (14) and have shown that in humans, as in animals, the brighter the light is, the stronger it is as an entraining stimulus. More recent studies suggest that the circadian system is most sensitive to short-wavelength (blue-green spectrum) light (15–17).

Whether free running or entrained, circadian rhythms can be reset to a new time. This process is called "phase shifting." Humans are frequently faced with situations in which their circadian rhythms are misaligned with the environmental light–dark cycle. This can be a result of jet lag, daylight savings time, or night shift work. In these situations, circadian rhythms may (but do not always) phase-shift to adapt to the new light–dark cycle. Various external stimuli, called *zeitgebers* (from the German "time giver"), act as time cues and can affect the internal clock, causing a resetting or phase shifting of circadian rhythms. Photic information about the light–dark cycle is the strongest stimulus for resetting the biologic clock (18). Phase shifts differ in direction and magnitude depending on where in the circadian cycle (at what circadian phase) the zeitgeber is administered.

PHASE-SHIFTING EFFECTS OF LIGHT AND LIGHT PHASE RESPONSE CURVES

The relationships between circadian rhythms, phase shifting, and various time cues or zeitgebers are described using phase response curves (PRCs). A PRC is derived by administering a stimulus at many different circadian phases and measuring the resulting shifts in the circadian clock. The multiple phase-shift data points are then plotted to predict the magnitude and direction of a phase shift given a particular stimulus at a specific circadian phase.

Several PRCs describing how humans respond to light exposure have been published (13, 19–21). A schematic PRC (22) for light is shown in Figure 17-4. When humans are exposed to light at the end of the

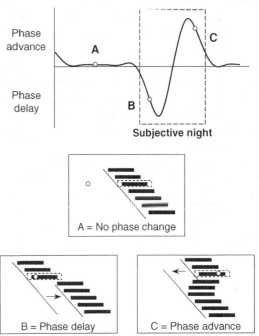

Figure 17-4 Schematic light phase response curve (PRC). The horizontal black bars in A, B, and C indicate circadian measures that occur at night, such as low core temperature or high melatonin levels. Within each inset, the effect of a single stimulus (e.g., a light pulse in otherwise constant darkness) on free-running circadian measures is shown. The effects of stimuli (open circles) presented during the subjective day (**A**), the early part of the subjective night (**B**), and late in the subjective night (**C**) are shown. Note the very different effects that these identical stimuli have at those different phases. Those results are then plotted at the corresponding points (labeled A, B, and C) in the central diagram, which is a PRC. The boxed area represents the subjective night of the organism, and the remaining area represents subjective day. (Adapted from Czeisler, C. A., Richardson, G. S., Coleman, R. M., et al. (1981). Chronotherapy: Resetting the circadian clocks of patients with delayed sleep phase insomnia. *Sleep, 4*, 1–21, used with permission.)

day and beginning of the night, circadian rhythms shift to a later time, which is called a "phase delay." In contrast, when light exposure occurs at the end of the night and early part of the day, circadian rhythms shift to an earlier time, which is called a "phase advance." Minimal phase shifting occurs when humans are exposed to light in the middle of the day. Shifts in circadian phase elicited by light are dependent not only on the timing and duration of the exposure (14, 19, 23) but also on the intensity of light, which decreases as distance from the light source increases (17), and the wavelength of light (24–26).

PHASE-SHIFTING EFFECTS ON NONPHOTIC STIMULI

In addition to light, other nonphotic stimuli have been shown to affect circadian rhythms. For instance, exogenous administration of the hormone melatonin can lead to phase shifts in the circadian clock. Lewy and colleagues (27, 28) produced a PRC for melatonin that demonstrates that circadian phase delays are produced when melatonin is administered in the later hours of sleep and in the morning, and phase advances are produced when melatonin is administered in the afternoon and early evening.

Physical activity or exercise has also been shown to phase-shift the human circadian clock (29–32). Phase advances in circadian rhythms occur after exercise in the evening, and phase delays are produced with exercise in the middle of the night (30). The magnitude of the circadian phase shifts produced with exercise appears to be related to the duration and intensity of the physical activity.

TYPES OF CIRCADIAN RHYTHM SLEEP–WAKE DISORDERS

Before describing the types of circadian rhythm sleep–wake disorders (CRSWD), it is important to note that by influencing the timing of virtually all physiologic and behavioral phenomena, circadian rhythms have an impact on health and safety that extends far beyond CRSWD. Examples of circadian variation include the timing and severity of clinical symptoms unrelated to sleep disorders and the daily pattern of critical events in the population, such as stroke, myocardial infarction, and motor vehicle accidents. In addition, the outcomes of clinical experiments, diagnostic tests, and treatments can all vary as a function of administration time. Clearly, the influence of circadian rhythms needs to be appreciated throughout the biomedical sciences.

Shift-Work Disorder

The misalignment of the sleep–wake cycle and intrinsic circadian rhythms seen in CRSWD is demonstrated in the case of shift work. Shift-work disorder (SWD) can occur when work schedules conflict with the timing and duration of an individual's normal sleep period. Working a fixed night shift (when the circadian clock is programmed for sleep) is a primary example of such a conflict, but early morning shifts and rotating shifts can be just as difficult to tolerate.

Symptoms of SWD include reduced sleep quality and quantity as well as sleepiness during time awake. Sleep duration during the day following a night shift is typically reduced by several hours (33, 34). Subjective sleep quality can be impaired, and sleep is nonrestorative. Impairments of sleep quality during shift work include prolonged sleep latencies, sleep maintenance difficulties, and early termination of the sleep period. Owing in part to this reduction in sleep quality and quantity, an individual typically experiences excessive sleepiness during the time of day in which they are attempting to remain awake and work. Another major factor contributing to sleepiness during a night shift is the acute reduction in alertness that usually occurs in the early morning hours (35). This early morning nadir of alertness is a circadian phenomenon, occurring independent of accumulated sleep loss. At the end of a night shift, sleepiness is typically high because of this reduced alerting effect in tandem with the long period of wakefulness that has elapsed since the last sleep period. This can potentially place night shift workers in a dangerous position during the commute home (36).

A number of other disturbances unrelated to sleep may be reported by shift workers (37, 38). A common complaint is increased gastrointestinal disturbance. Cardiovascular disease, as well as several major risk factors for this disease—smoking, high cholesterol, hypertension, and obesity—have been found to be more prevalent among shift workers (39, 40). Reproductive difficulties such as menstrual irregularities and increased time to conception may be more prevalent in female shift workers (41–43). Night shift work has repeatedly been associated with increased risk of developing cancer and has been classified as a "probable carcinogen" by the International Agency for Research on Cancer (44). The psychosocial consequences of shift work can include disturbances of family and marital relationships (45).

Although SWD may be transient in that resuming a daytime work/nighttime sleep schedule will attenuate its symptoms, adaptation to late night, early morning, and rotating shifts is difficult to achieve, and in most cases does not occur. Adaptation to a nighttime work and daytime sleep schedule, however, is possible if appropriate steps are taken to reinforce a nocturnal lifestyle. This is rare among most shift workers because environmental zeitgebers, such as light, as well as social and domestic responsibilities, reinforce a diurnal schedule, preventing significant adaptation from occurring. In addition, maintaining a nocturnal lifestyle is not a priority for most individuals, suggesting that not only is circadian adaptation difficult, but that it may be undesirable. Figure 17-5 shows the activity of a shift worker over a several-week period, and Figure 17-6G depicts a typical phase relationship between the temperature minimum and the sleep period for a night shift worker.

A number of individual differences mediate tolerance to shift work (46, 47). One of the most important determinants of shift-work tolerance is commitment to the work schedule. Individuals who are able and choose to alter their sleep–wake pattern by adhering to a light–dark schedule to assist in phase shifting are much more likely to adapt to shift work than those who disregard the diurnally oriented zeitgebers. Older individuals typically tolerate night shift work less well than younger individuals. Those with a short sleep requirement, as well as a relatively delayed circadian rhythm (night owls), typically tolerate night work better than those needing more sleep or who are relatively phase advanced (morning larks).

A proactive way for employers to address the increased risks associated with shift work is through the implementation of specific policies aimed at mitigating those risks. Because all sleep laboratories utilize shift work, having fatigue management policies in place should be considered a matter of professional integrity.

Jet Lag Disorder

Jet lag disorder is identified by difficulty initiating or maintaining sleep following the rapid crossing of time zones, which occurs in air travel in the east or west direction (34, 48). The cause of these symptoms is a misalignment of the endogenous circadian system with the environmental time cues of the new time zone (Fig. 17-6F). For example, airline flights from North America may land during the morning hours in Europe. This morning arrival time corresponds to nighttime hours in North America, and the travelers are thus presented with European day at a time when their bodies are primed for night and sleep. Furthermore, when the European night arrives, the traveler may have difficulty initiating sleep because the biologic clock remains entrained to North American time, where it is afternoon. Secondary to this misalignment, as well as sleep loss that comes about because of the misalignment, excessive sleepiness and decreases in alertness may

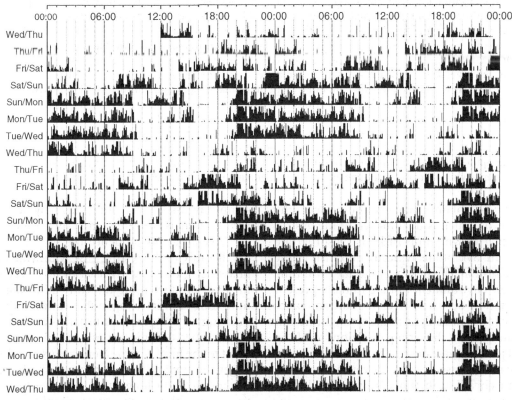

Figure 17-5 Double plot of wrist actigraphy from a middle-aged man working four consecutive night shifts. Note that when this individual is not working the night shift, he reverts to a diurnal schedule. Shift-work disorder becomes chronic because the circadian rhythms do not have enough time to fully entrain to either the weekend or the work schedule.

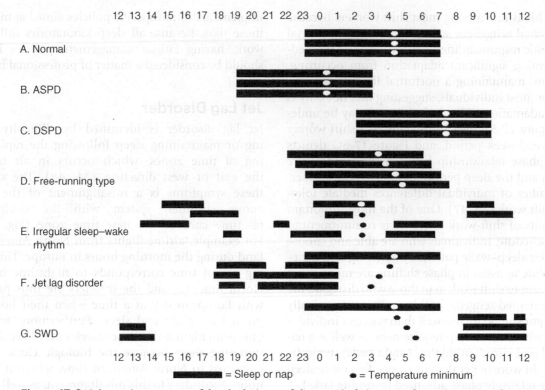

Figure 17-6 Schematic summary of the clock times of sleep periods in normal entrainment and circadian rhythm sleep–wake disorder, as well as typical phase relationships between sleep period and the temperature minimum (Tmin), which is an approximate time of peak sleep propensity. **A:** Normally entrained sleep. Tmin occurs 2 to 3 hours before habitual wake time. **B:** Advanced sleep phase disorder (ASPD). Preferred sleep onset and waking times occur at substantially earlier clock times than conventional sleep and wake times. **C:** Delayed sleep phase disorder (DSPD). Preferred sleep onset and wake times occur at substantially later clock times than conventional sleep and wake. **D:** Free-running type. Sleep and wakefulness occur at a progressively later clock time each successive day. **E:** Irregular sleep–wake rhythm. The normal periodicity of the sleep–wake cycle is attenuated or absent. **F:** Jet lag disorder. After an initial night of normal sleep, rapid transmeridian travel (as illustrated, eastward across six time zones) results in an abrupt shift of the attempted sleep period to an earlier time, and subsequent misalignment of circadian rhythms and environmental time. Tmin occurs after the scheduled wake time in the new time zone, giving rise to symptoms of sleepiness. **G:** Shift-work disorder (SWD). After an initial night of normal sleep, night shift workers typically attempt to work through the night during the time of peak sleep propensity, and sleep during the daytime, when increased circadian alerting can fragment and curtail sleep.

ensue. Somatic complaints may also be present, the most common of which is disturbance of the gastrointestinal tract. The symptoms of jet lag disorder are usually transient. Symptoms typically diminish as the endogenous circadian rhythms adapt to the local time cues of the new environment but are initially present because adaptation occurs slowly. In addition, exposure to time cues such as light at the wrong time can cause reentrainment in the wrong direction, resulting in prolonged jet lag. Phase delays are believed to occur more rapidly than phase advances because the length of the human circadian rhythms is typically slightly more than 24 hours. This makes it easier for an individual to stay up for a period longer than 24 hours before initiating the next sleep period (delaying) than to initiate a sleep period before 24 hours have elapsed since the previous bedtime (advancing). The

symptoms associated with jet lag may become chronic for individuals who frequently fly across time zones.

Several factors influence the severity of this disorder. Because of the relative ease with which individuals phase delay, traveling in the eastward direction (advancing) can produce more difficulty adjusting to the new time zone than traveling in the westward direction. The duration of symptoms is usually commensurate with the number of time zones crossed. Because entrainment to the local environment occurs at a slow pace, the larger the time difference between the home and new environment, the longer the symptoms may be expected to persist. Although the overly simple rule of thumb is that reentrainment occurs at a rate of approximately one time zone per day, conflicting timing of light exposure and other zeitgebers can slow this adjustment and prolong jet lag symptoms.

Non–24-Hour Sleep–Wake Rhythm Disorder

Non–24-hour sleep–wake rhythm disorder occurs when circadian rhythms of an individual persist with a periodicity of more than 24 hours despite living in society and being exposed to the time cues that normally entrain the rhythms (34) to the 24-hour day (Figs. 17-6D and 17-7). The symptoms of this disorder result from the conflict that arises when a person with free-running rhythms attempts to adhere to a normal diurnal schedule in which sleep and wake times are relatively fixed from day to day. As the endogenous rhythms progressively shift around the clock, some nighttime sleep periods will occur when there is a normal phase relationship between the sleep period and body rhythms. On other days, attempts to initiate nighttime sleep periods at the usual environmental time will conflict with the current phase of the biologic clock. During these times of desynchronization between the circadian clock and the environment, the quality and quantity of sleep may be reduced, with accompanying increases in daytime sleepiness. In this way, free running can manifest as periodically recurring symptoms of insomnia and sleepiness.

Although the disorder has been observed in sighted individuals (49), most non–24-hour sleep–wake rhythm disorder patients have some degree of blindness (50). This is because light is the most important environmental time cue for the entrainment of circadian rhythms in humans. Enucleated patients, totally blind patients, or patients with disrupted transmission of light information to the brain are most susceptible to free-running circadian rhythms and non–24-hour sleep–wake rhythm disorder. However, visual blindness is not necessarily associated with attenuated circadian responses because the photoreceptors mediating conscious vision are not necessary for the entrainment of circadian rhythms. Nonconscious ocular light perception occurring through distinct pathways may be sufficient for photic entrainment to occur.

Irregular Sleep–Wake Rhythm Disorder

Irregular sleep–wake rhythm disorder is a rare syndrome in which total sleep time within each 24-hour day may remain roughly equal to the amount that would be obtained if sleep was obtained in a single sleep period,

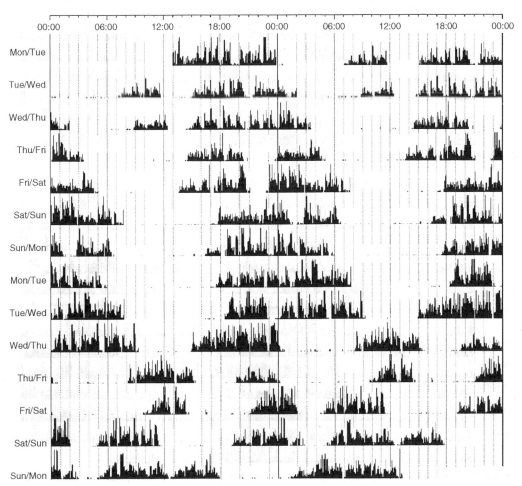

Figure 17-7 Double plot of wrist actigraphy of a patient with free-running type disorder. Note that the activity onset (the time of awakening) trends progressively later each successive day.

but the sleep is distributed throughout the day and night in multiple short episodes (34) (Fig. 17-6E). This disorder is commonly observed in patients with neurologic diseases, such as children with neurodevelopmental disorders and elderly patients with dementia. Irregular sleep–wake patterns can also be observed in individuals not suffering from brain disease. In these rare cases, the disorder may be precipitated by a disregard for social and environmental zeitgebers. An erratic, self-perpetuating pattern of sleep and wakefulness can develop, in which nocturnal wakefulness instigates daytime naps, which then exacerbate nocturnal insomnia.

Delayed/Advanced Sleep–Wake Phase Disorders

There is variation in the times of day that any given person prefers to sleep and to be awake. Night owls feel most alert and have a relatively easy time functioning late in the day, into the evening and night, and may also experience a more difficult time awakening early in the morning. In contrast, morning larks prefer to awaken early in the morning, feel most alert early

in the day, and have a relatively difficult time staying awake late at night.

Not everyone has a strong morning or evening preference. The range of preferences can be thought of as a continuum, with strong evening types on one end and strong morning types on the other end. In between are degrees of each, including those who have a slight morning or evening preference, or those who have no preference at all. At the extreme ends of this continuum are those patients whose morning or evening preference comes into conflict with conventional sleep–wake schedules. This conflict is the basis of both delayed sleep–wake phase disorder (DSWPD) and advanced sleep–wake phase disorders (ASWPD) (34).

Delayed Sleep–Wake Phase Disorder

DSWPD results when a patient's biologic clock naturally begins and ends the sleep–wake period at a time of day significantly later than what is considered normal. The sleep period is typically initiated between the hours of 2:00 and 6:00 a.m. (Fig. 17-8). Sleep has normal quality and duration when the patient is allowed to maintain the late schedule preferred by the biologic clock.

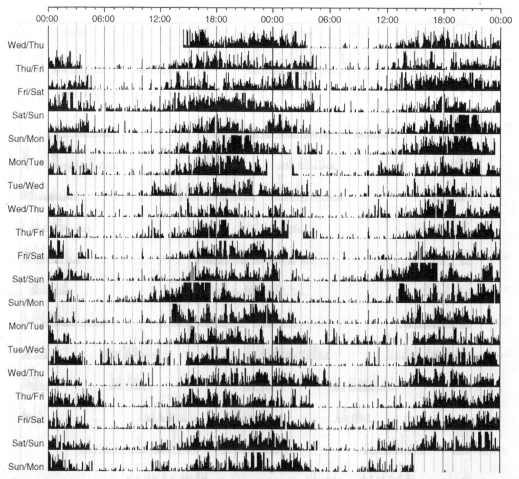

Figure 17-8 Double plot of wrist actigraphy on a patient with delayed sleep phase disorder. Note that the bedtime typically occurs from 2:00 to 4:00 a.m., with wake times in the early afternoon.

In DSWPD, sleep problems and the resulting difficulties occur when a person with a late sleep–wake period attempts to adhere to a conventional (earlier) sleep–wake schedule.

The symptoms of DSWPD result from the misalignment of biologically preferred and socially conventional rhythms. When attempting to initiate the sleep period at a conventional bedtime, complaints of sleep onset insomnia are prevalent. Often, sleep onset occurs at the same (late) clock time—the time at which the circadian system allows sleep to occur—regardless of the time at which a person attempts to go to sleep. Extreme difficulty awakening in the morning at a conventional time is a second prominent symptom. When awakening for work or school, individuals with DSWPD are trying to prepare for the day at a time when their circadian alerting system is at or near its minimum. For a person who copes well with a 9-a.m.-to-5-p.m. work schedule, this is akin to awakening for the day at around 3:30 or 4:00 a.m., while maintaining the same bedtime.

Excessive sleepiness during the daytime occurs in DSWPD for two reasons. First, when attempting to maintain a conventional schedule, those with DSWPD will become sleep deprived. Second, levels of sleepiness will be high during the morning hours because the circadian system is not yet producing its alerting effects. In essence, the biologic clock of a person with DSWPD is telling the body to be asleep during the morning hours.

The sleepiness caused by this type of misalignment can cause difficulty in work, school, and domestic settings. DSWPD is most common in adolescence and young adulthood.

Advanced Sleep–Wake Phase Disorder

At the other end of the morning–evening continuum are the extreme morning larks. In some cases, the morning preference is so strong and is in conflict with conventional sleep times to such an extent that an individual is diagnosed with an ASWPD. In ASWPD, a patient has a biologic predisposition for the sleep period to occur at a time that is significantly earlier than for the average adult. The intrinsically preferred bedtime will occur in the early evening, and a person may experience difficulty sleeping later than the very early morning hours. Consequently, the circadian alerting system often awakens a person with ASPD between 2:00 and 4:00 a.m. (Fig. 17-9).

As in DSWPD patients, there appears to be nothing inherently wrong with the sleep of an individual with ASWPD. If sleep occurs at the biologically preferable (early) time, it is usually of normal duration and quality. The conflict again arises because the early sleep period is misaligned with the socially acceptable sleep period. In the case of ASWPD, patients experience pressure to remain awake in the evening hours, often for social or domestic reasons, when the biologic clock has reduced

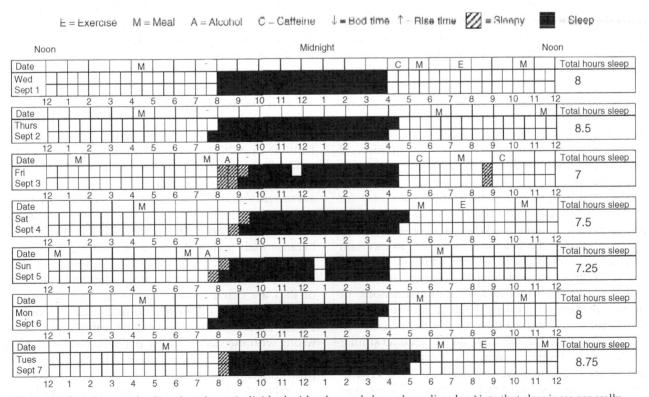

Figure 17-9 A sleep–wake diary kept by an individual with advanced sleep phase disorder. Note that sleepiness generally ensues in the early evening hours, whereas spontaneous awakenings typically occur from 4:00 to 5:00 a.m.

its alerting influence, resulting in an increasing drive to sleep. In addition, early morning awakenings occur because of increased circadian alerting, resulting in wakefulness at times when most people are asleep. Therefore, patients with ASWPD can become sleep deprived and develop excessive sleepiness during their waking hours. Contrary to the occupational and academic conflicts occurring in the morning hours in DSWPD, the misalignment of circadian rhythms and social cues in ASWPD is often a source of social and family conflict, because the evening hours are typically a time one spends with family and friends. Advanced circadian rhythms are more prominent in older individuals and have also been associated with premature birth. Finally, there is evidence that human diurnal preference, including DSWPD and ASWPD, is associated with specific genetic variants (51–53).

EVALUATION OF CRSWD

Clinical evaluation of CRSWD typically begins with a patient history by a qualified clinician (54). A thorough patient history includes examination of the intrinsic and extrinsic factors that may combine to precipitate the symptoms of CRSWD. Other medical or psychological problems that present with fatigue and insomnia can masquerade as CRSWD. Similar symptoms can also occur secondary to certain medical treatments or following neurologic damage and are frequently seen in other sleep disorders, such as narcolepsy, idiopathic hypersomnia, insufficient sleep syndrome, and insomnia.

Evaluation of CRSWD often involves analysis of the patient's sleep–wake diary (Fig. 17-9). Sleep–wake diaries provide useful and inexpensive information that, together with the patient history, can lead to a quick diagnosis. Typically, the patient maintains a sleep–wake diary for at least 2 weeks. Several parameters are documented, including the timing and duration of sleep, wakefulness, and time in bed, along with a record of medication, caffeine, alcohol, and other drug intake. Well-designed sleep–wake diaries are easy for the patient to use and contain designated space for the patient's daily comments. When a sleep–wake diary is collected from the patient, it is helpful to ascertain whether the information is representative, accurate, and understandable. Potential inaccuracies due to the patient's neglect, misunderstanding of instructions, or sleep-state misperception are the main shortcomings of the sleep–wake diary. The subjective data obtained from sleep–wake diaries can be analyzed in a manner similar to objective polysomnography (PSG) data. In reporting the results, ranges and averages can be utilized to summarize bedtimes, sleep latencies, total sleep times, and other relevant parameters. In addition, it is important to note the interaction of work hours and the sleep–wake schedule as well as weekend variations and other patterns that emerge. In addition to data from a sleep–wake diary, wrist actigraphy can be valuable for the diagnosis of CRSWD. Wrist actigraphy is an unobtrusive and relatively inexpensive method for collecting objective activity data, usually over the course of 2 weeks or more (Figs. 17-5, 17-7, and 17-8). Daily patterns of rest and activity normally correlate with the sleep–wake cycle, providing a useful objective measure of sleep and wakefulness that can be compared with the subjective information in sleep–wake diaries. It should be recognized that wrist actigraphy may not reliably differentiate between sleep and motionless wakefulness. Thus, activity data are less reliable in the presence of insomnia or, conversely, in the presence of frequent sleep-related movements that can appear as wakefulness. Nevertheless, wrist actigraphy and sleep–wake diaries often provide ample information to detect and characterize CRSWD.

PSG and the multiple sleep latency test (MSLT) are of limited value in the diagnosis of CRSWD because they usually provide only a snapshot of a single sleep–wake cycle. The results of PSG in each of the different CRSWD will vary depending on the clock time and the day of PSG administration. For example, PSG performed on a patient with SWD on a day off or during a vacation may be normal, because SWD is not a problem with the patient's sleep per se, but a clash between the attempted sleep schedule and the circadian clock. A daytime PSG performed after a night of shift work may show reduced total sleep time, increased wake after sleep onset, and relatively low sleep efficiency. These findings are due to the daytime alerting influence of the circadian clock, which does not change its orientation in most shift workers and disrupts and curtails daytime sleep.

PSG findings in patients with DSWPD and ASWPD reflect the altered timing of sleep in these disorders. Although PSG is not usually performed to diagnose DSWPD or ASWPD, these syndromes can coexist with other sleep disorders and may result in PSG data that require additional interpretation. If PSG is performed at conventional times, patients with DSWPD are likely to have long sleep latencies, whereas patients with ASWPD are likely to exhibit early morning awakenings because their preferred sleep and wake times are later and earlier, respectively, relative to conventional sleep and wake times. In contrast, if the start and end times of PSG are determined by the preference of patients with DSWPD and ASWPD, normal results would be expected because there is typically nothing inherently wrong with the sleep of these patients, but the conflict arises when their preferred sleep and wake times differ from conventional times.

PSG is clearly warranted when the possibility of other sleep disorders exists. When performing PSG in patients with CRSWD, it is recommended that the start time be adjusted to match the patient's routine bedtime. Likewise, MSLT schedules can be altered to begin 2 to 3 hours after the habitual rise time. This technique is particularly useful in the evaluation of SWD. In such cases, it may be clinically relevant to record PSG during the day and extend the MSLT schedule to cover times corresponding to both the night shift and the commute home.

MEASURING CIRCADIAN RHYTHMS

Circadian rhythms are measured with more precision in research situations. For instance, if a circadian phase-shift intervention is planned, the baseline circadian phase is determined in order to time the intervention correctly. Similarly, the rhythms are measured after the intervention to measure the magnitude of the shift in circadian rhythms. Rhythms are also measured when a researcher wants to demonstrate that an intervention did not affect circadian rhythms.

In humans, the master circadian clock (SCN) cannot be monitored directly; thus, marker rhythms that are controlled by this master clock are used to estimate circadian phase. Several markers are employed in studies of human circadian rhythms, including the rhythm of core body temperature, rest-activity rhythms, and hormonal rhythms (e.g., melatonin, cortisol). Each of these has its advantages and disadvantages with respect to cost, invasiveness, precision, labor intensity, influences of confounding variables, and duration of monitoring.

One difficulty in measuring circadian rhythms is that rhythms can be affected by other physiologic variables and by the techniques used to measure the rhythms. This is called *masking*. For instance, as shown in Figure 17-10, human core body temperature has a robust circadian rhythm—it is high during the day, peaks in the midafternoon, and becomes lower at night, with a nadir about 2 hours before wakefulness. However, core body temperature varies because of things other than the circadian cycle. Sleep and wakefulness, activity, drugs, fever, and menstrual phase are a few of the factors that can alter the "true" circadian rhythm of core body temperature. These factors obscure or "mask" the endogenous temperature rhythm produced by the circadian pacemaker. There is extensive literature on mathematical and statistical techniques that can be used to "demask" data, so that other physiologic variables do not interfere with measuring the "true" circadian rhythm (31, 55–61). As with many physiologic variables, it can be difficult to measure circadian rhythms without also affecting the rhythm you are attempting to measure.

Another method for estimating circadian phase is to derive it from rhythms of hormone secretion. The onset of melatonin secretion recorded in dim light, that is, the

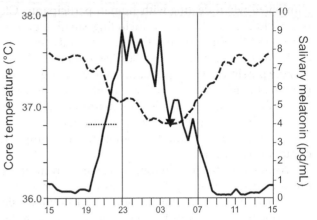

Figure 17-10 Circadian rhythms of core body temperature and salivary melatonin in a young adult male recorded in constant conditions. As shown in the solid line, temperature is high during the daytime hours and low at night. Melatonin (depicted in the dashed line) is low during the day and high at night. Two circadian phase markers are shown: the fitted temperature minimum, indicated by the black triangle, and the dim light melatonin onset (DLMO) (with DLMO threshold set at 4 pg per mL), indicated by the dotted black line.

dim light melatonin onset, is used frequently as a circadian phase marker (see Fig. 17-10), and the peak of cortisol also has been used as a measure of circadian phase. These hormonal measures, particularly melatonin, are quite reliable. Nevertheless, hormonal secretion is also subject to masking. For instance, stress can increase the amplitude of the circadian rhythm of cortisol, and light can attenuate or eliminate the circadian rhythm of melatonin. In addition, hormonal measures require assays that can be expensive and require specialized training and equipment to perform. Hormonal measures can also be invasive depending on which body fluid (saliva, serum, or urine) is used to determine the hormone levels. Another disadvantage to measuring circadian phase using hormonal rhythms is that there is usually a time delay between data collection and determination of phase. The masking effects on circadian rhythms can be reduced by the use of constant routine (CR) protocols (62). The purpose of a CR is to attenuate factors that can influence the circadian rhythm(s) being measured, or when this is not possible, evenly distribute them across a circadian cycle. For example, because light exposure can mask (suppress) the circadian rhythm of melatonin, CRs typically involve dim and/or longer wavelength light, which does not appreciably influence the melatonin rhythm. Also, because body temperature decreases during sleep and increases with physical activity, CRs may incorporate constant wakefulness with recumbent posture to eliminate the masking influence of sleep and activity when the circadian temperature rhythm is being measured. In most situations, other factors such as eating and drinking cannot ethically be reduced or eliminated when dealing with human participants. CR protocols deal with this by including small identical snacks and liquid portions at regular intervals (e.g., every hour) or by using intravenous feeding methods, so that the possible influence of eating and drinking on the rhythms being measured is distributed evenly over the circadian cycle. CR protocols for determining circadian phase position are usually used in a research setting in which participants stay in the laboratory for a complete circadian cycle or more.

Another circadian rhythm research technique is the forced desynchrony (FD) protocol. FD protocols are utilized to separate the circadian and homeostatic components to a variable being measured. For example, sleep and alertness are influenced by both circadian and homeostatic factors, such that the homeostatic drive for sleep increases across the normal waking day and dissipates when sleep occurs at night, whereas the circadian drive for sleep is low across the normal waking day and increases when sleep occurs at night. During a normal day and night, the homeostatic and circadian contributions to sleep interact in a coordinated manner, producing consolidated wakefulness during the day and consolidated sleep at night. During an FD protocol, individuals stay in the laboratory for several circadian cycles, and the laboratory light–dark cycle is manipulated in such a way that the internal circadian clock cannot adjust (or entrain). For example, an FD protocol could involve 20-hour "days," in which a participant stays awake for 13.3 hours and then has a 6.7-hour sleep opportunity. A 20-hour "day" is outside the "range of entrainment" of the internal biologic clock, meaning that the clock cannot adjust to a schedule that is so different in cycle length from its own, and instead the internal clock will continue to drive circadian rhythms at its endogenous cycle length, which is typically about 24 hours. When this occurs, the imposed sleep–wake rhythm (20 hours) becomes dissociated (or desynchronized) from the endogenous circadian rhythms (~24 hours), and each persists with its own cycle length. As this desynchronization persists over the course of days or weeks, the time of scheduled sleep and wakefulness is eventually distributed across all circadian phases. This permits dependent variables (e.g., sleepiness, performance, or mood) to be measured with respect to either factor, while controlling for the other. For example, performance on a reaction time task can be measured upon awakening from every sleep episode. Because each sleep episode ends at a different circadian phase, the circadian influence on performance can be assessed while controlling for the homeostatic drive for sleep. The homeostatic drive for sleep is thought to be held relatively constant because the sleep opportunity preceding each performance test is thought to satiate the homeostatic sleep drive. FD protocols thus provide paradigms that can separate

the circadian and homeostatic modulation of behavior and physiology to examine specific research questions.

Many of these specialized circadian rhythm measurement techniques fall outside the range of most clinical sleep disorders services, but it is important to be aware of them. The correct interpretation of these data is dependent on accurate and valid sampling techniques in the setting of a strictly controlled environment, as well as an understanding of statistical techniques for analyzing circadian rhythms data. For unusual cases of CRSWD that warrant additional testing, referral to a specialized laboratory may be advisable.

TREATMENT OF CRSWD

In most cases, the key to treating CRSWD is the correct utilization of PRCs (54). According to the 2015 Clinical Practice Guideline for the Treatment of Intrinsic Circadian Rhythm Sleep–Wake Disorders published by the American Academy of Sleep Medicine, administration of light therapy in accordance with the PRC is the preferred first-line treatment for ASWPD and irregular sleep-wake rhythm disorder (ISWRD) (63) (Fig. 17-4). CRSWD treatment may also involve controlled exposure to light, darkness, and other time cues. A patient might be given a "prescription" to actively seek and avoid light at appropriate times. In appropriate climates and weather conditions, artificial therapeutic light sources may be unnecessary. For example, a regular walk outside in sunlight immediately upon awakening could benefit a patient with DSWPD because bright light exposure at that time would likely fall on the phase advance portion of their light PRC, resetting the circadian clock to a relatively earlier time. Conversely, bright light exposure in the evening and the first half of the night, falling on the phase delay portion of the light PRC, would exacerbate a delayed sleep schedule. Thus, actively seeking morning light and avoiding bright evening light are behavioral strategies used to treat delayed sleep phase disorder (DSPD). On the contrary, avoiding early morning light and seeking bright light in the evening can help patients with ASWPD.

Light exposure at inappropriate times can prevent phase shifts in a desired direction or even induce shifts in the opposite direction. In individuals working night shifts, wearing low-transmission, blue-blocking sunglasses during the morning commute and avoidance of light during the daytime sleep period by the installation of blackout shades for bedroom windows can promote phase delays (64). These practices reduce morning light exposure, which is beneficial if adaption to the night shift is desired because morning light typically falls on the phase advance portion of the light PRC and will thus hinder any phase delays that might occur when working consecutive night shifts. Jet lag sufferers can be directed to printed resources (48, 65-68) or websites that provide customized instructions for the manipulation of zeitgebers to promote entrainment to the new time zone.

PRCs for exogenous melatonin (27, 61, 69, 70) are also utilized therapeutically. For example, in patients with DSWPD, it is recommended that melatonin administration occur in the late afternoon or early evening, when it is expected to promote a phase advance. Appropriately timed melatonin administration is recommended in the AASM Clinical Practice Guidelines for the Treatment of Intrinsic Circadian Rhythm Sleep–Wake Disorders for DSWPD, N24, and treatment of ISWPD in children and adolescents with neurologic disorders (63). Because of scant evidence for benefit and possible increases in depressed mood, however, melatonin for ISWPD is not recommended in demented elderly patients. Consumption of morning melatonin produces a phase delay, but this approach is less well studied and may have limited clinical utility because melatonin may have a soporific effect in diurnal mammals such as humans. Exogenous melatonin is particularly useful in some blind or enucleated patients with free-running type disorder as a nonphotic method of achieving circadian entrainment to the 24-hour day (71). In the United States, melatonin is classified as a dietary supplement and available without prescription in a wide range of doses, many of which produce melatonin concentrations much higher than normal endogenous levels. There is little evidence indicating that larger doses of melatonin produce a larger phase shift. To the contrary, data from blind patients indicate that high doses of exogenous melatonin may attenuate the size of a phase shift and that a lower dose can result in a larger net phase shift of the circadian clock (72). The routine use of melatonin for unsound reasons should be discouraged. Long-term safety data for melatonin are sparse, and in many countries, the drug is available only by prescription.

Chronotherapy is another technique utilized for treating highly motivated patients with DSPD. This technique utilizes the relative ease with which individuals are able to progressively delay their sleep periods by 1 or 2 hours per day. Over the course of several days, the sleep period is shifted around the clock until the desired bedtime is reached and a rigid sleep schedule is introduced. After the desired sleep schedule has been reached, bright light upon awakening in the morning is utilized to maintain entrainment to the earlier schedule.

Several other treatments are available for CRSWD. Hypnotics and stimulants are used to treat the symptoms of CRSWD, yet these treatments do not address the cause of the disorder, which is circadian misalignment. In some cases, the best solution to CRSWD is accommodation of the patient's circadian tendencies through lifestyle adaptation.

SUMMARY

Circadian rhythms are internally generated daily cycles in physiology and behavior that are characteristic of life on earth. In time isolation, human circadian rhythms normally persist with a period slightly more than 24 hours. Examples of circadian rhythms include such diverse phenomena as hormone secretion, body temperature, alertness, and performance. The circadian rhythms most commonly recorded in the clinical sleep laboratory are those of sleep and activity.

Normally, circadian rhythms are synchronized with the 24-hour terrestrial day by continuously adjusting in response to time cues known as zeitgebers. The process of resetting circadian time is known as entrainment. Light is the most effective zeitgeber for the entrainment of circadian rhythms in sighted humans. Other potential zeitgebers include physical activity and social cues. Administration of exogenous melatonin has also been shown to influence the timing of circadian rhythms. The change in circadian timing elicited by a zeitgeber is known as a phase shift. The magnitude and direction of a phase shift evoked by a zeitgeber varies with the time of day. This relationship is expressed in a PRC.

When circadian rhythms are disrupted, the resulting symptoms of insomnia and/or excessive daytime sleepiness may be categorized as a CRSWD. In most cases, CRSWDs arise from a combination of intrinsic and extrinsic factors. The types of CRSWDs are summarized in Figure 17-6. Clinical sleep laboratories routinely collect and analyze the data necessary for the diagnosis and treatment of CRSWDs, primarily through sleep diaries and wrist actigraphy. PSG and MSLT are used less frequently in the diagnosis of CRSWD, primarily for the detection of comorbid sleep disorders. Some specialized sleep laboratories record additional circadian parameters, such as body temperature and melatonin concentration. The most common treatments for CRSWD include carefully timed light therapy, exogenous melatonin administration, and lifestyle adaptation.

ACKNOWLEDGMENT

Special thanks to Mark R. Smith, PhD, for his contributions to earlier editions of this chapter.

REFERENCES

1. Moore-Ede, M. C., Sulzman, F. M., & Fuller, C. A. (1982). *The clocks that time us: Physiology of the circadian timing system.* Cambridge, MA: Harvard University Press.

2. Burki, T. (2017). Nobel Prize awarded for discoveries in circadian rhythm. *Lancet, 390*(10104), e25.

3. Lydic, R., Schoene, W. C., Czeisler, C. A., et al. (1980). Suprachiasmatic region of the human hypothalamus: Homolog to the primate circadian pacemaker? *Sleep, 2,* 355–361.

4. Moore, R. Y. (1979). The anatomy of central neural mechanisms regulating endocrine rhythms. In D. T. Krieger (Ed.), *Endocrine rhythms* (pp. 63–87). New York, NY: Raven Press.

5. Rusak, B., & Zucker, I. (1979). Neural regulation of circadian rhythms. *Physiological Reviews, 59,* 449–526.

6. Hastings, M. H., Best, J. D., Ebling, F. J. P., et al. (1996). Entrainment of the circadian clock. In R. M. Buijs, A. Kalsbeek, H. J. Romijn, et al. (Eds.), *Progress in brain research* (pp. 147–174). Amsterdam, The Netherlands: Elsevier Sciences.

7. Moore, R. Y. (1997). Circadian rhythms: Basic neurobiology and clinical applications. *Annual Review of Medicine, 48,* 253–266.

8. Honma, S. (2018). The mammalian circadian system: A hierarchical multi-oscillator structure for generating circadian rhythm. *The Journal of Physiological Sciences, 68,* 207–219.

9. Arendt, J., Aldhous, M., & Wright, J. (1988). Synchronisation of a disturbed sleep–wake cycle in a blind man by melatonin treatment. *Lancet, 1,* 772–773.

10. Sack, R. L., Lewy, A. J., Blood, M. L., et al. (1991). Melatonin administration to blind people: Phase advances and entrainment. *Journal of Biological Rhythms, 6,* 249–261.

11. Sack, R. L., Stevenson, J., & Lewy, A. J. (1990). Entrainment of a previously free-running blind human with melatonin administration. *Journal of Sleep Research, 19,* 404.

12. Tzischinsky, O., Pal, I., Epstein, R., et al. (1992). The importance of timing in melatonin administration in a blind man. *Journal of Pineal Research, 12,* 105–108.

13. Wever, R. A. (1989). Light effects on human circadian rhythms. A review of recent experiments. *Journal of Biological Rhythms, 4,* 161–185.

14. Boivin, D. B., Duffy, J. F., Kronauer, R. E., et al. (1996). Dose–response relationships for resetting of human circadian clock by light. *Nature, 379,* 540–542.

15. Brainard, G. C., Hanifin, J. P., Greeson, J. M., et al. (2001). Action spectrum for melatonin regulation in humans: Evidence for a novel circadian photoreceptor. *Journal of Neuroscience, 21*(16), 6405–6412.

16. Thapan, K., Arendt, J., & Skene, D. J. (2001). An action spectrum for melatonin suppression: Evidence for a novel non-rod, non-cone photoreceptor system in humans. *Journal of Physiology, 535*(Pt. 1), 261–267.

17. Wright, H. R., & Lack, L. C. (2001). Effect of light wavelength on suppression and phase delay of the melatonin rhythm. *Chronobiology International, 18,* 801–808.

18. U.S. Congress, Office of Technology Assessment. (1991). *Biological rhythms: Implications for the worker.* Washington, DC: U.S. Government Printing Office.

19. Czeisler, C. A., Kronauer, R. E., Allan, J. S., et al. (1989). Bright light induction of strong (type 0) resetting of the human circadian pacemaker. *Science, 244,* 1328–1333.

20. Honma, K., & Honma, S. (1988). A human phase response curve for bright light pulses. *Japanese Journal of Psychiatry and Neurology, 42,* 167–168.

21. Minors, D. S., Waterhouse, J. M., & Wirz-Justice, A. (1991). A human phase–response curve to light. *Neuroscience Letters, 133,* 36–40.

22. Czeisler, C. A., Richardson, G. S., Coleman, R. M., et al. (1981). Chronotherapy: Resetting the circadian clocks of patients with delayed sleep phase insomnia. *Sleep, 4,* 1–21.

23. Czeisler, C. A., Duffy, J. F., Shanahan, T. L., et al. (1999). Stability, precision, and near-24-hour period of the human circadian pacemaker. *Science, 284,* 2177–2181.

24. Lockley, S. W., Brainard, G. C., & Czeisler, C. A. (2003). High sensitivity of the human circadian melatonin rhythm to resetting by short wavelength light. *Journal of Clinical Endocrinology and Metabolism, 88,* 4502–4505.

25. Gooley, J. J., Rajaratnam, S. M., Brainard, G. C., et al. (2010). Spectral responses of the human circadian system depend on irradiance and duration of exposure to light. *Science Translational Medicine, 2,* 31ra33.

26. Zeitzer, J. M., Dijk, D. J., Kronauer, R. E., et al. (2000). Sensitivity of the human circadian pacemaker to nocturnal light: Melatonin phase resetting and suppression. *Journal of Physiology, 526,* 695–702.

27. Lewy, A. J., Ahmed, S., Jackson, J. M. L., et al. (1992). Melatonin shifts human circadian rhythms according to a phase–response curve. *Chronobiology International, 9,* 380–392.

28. Lewy, A. J., Bauer, V. K., Ahmed, S., et al. (1998). The human phase response curve (PRC) to melatonin is about 12 hours out of phase with the PRC to light. *Chronobiology International, 15,* 71–83.

29. Baehr, E. K., Fogg, L. F., & Eastman, C. I. (1999). Intermittent bright light and exercise to entrain human circadian rhythms to night work. *American Journal of Physiology, 277,* R1598–R1604.

30. Buxton, O. M., Lee, C. W., L'Hermite-Baleriaux, M., et al. (2003). Exercise elicits phase shifts and acute alterations of melatonin that vary with circadian phase. *American Journal of Physiology, 284,* R714–R724.

31. Eastman, C. I., Hoese, E. K., Youngstedt, S. D., et al. (1995). Phase-shifting human circadian rhythms with exercise during the night shift. *Physiology and Behavior, 58,* 1287–1291.

32. Van Reeth, O., Sturis, J., Byrne, M. M., et al. (1994). Nocturnal exercise phase delays circadian rhythms of melatonin and thyrotropin secretion in normal men. *American Journal of Physiology, 266,* E964–E974.

33. Akerstedt, T. (1995). Work hours, sleepiness, and the underlying mechanisms. *Journal of Sleep Research,* 2(Suppl. 2), 15–22.

34. Sateia, M. (Ed.). (2005). *International classification of sleep disorders: Diagnostic and coding manual* (2nd ed.). Westchester, IL: American Academy of Sleep Medicine.

35. Akerstedt, T. (1988). Sleepiness as a consequence of shift work. *Sleep,* 11(1), 17–34.

36. Akerstedt, T., Czeisler, C., Dinges, D. F., et al. (1994). Accidents and sleepiness: A consensus statement from the international conference of work hours, sleepiness, and accidents, Stockholm, 8–10 September 1994. *Journal of Sleep Research, 3,* 195.

37. Scott, A. J. (1990). Shift work and health. *Occupational and Environmental Medicine,* 27(4), 1057–1078.

38. Harrington, J. M. (1994). Shift work and health: A critical review of the literature on working hours. *Annals of Academy of Medicine Singapore, 23,* 699–705.

39. Boggild, H., & Knutsson, A. (1999). Shift work, risk factors, and cardiovascular disease. *Scandinavian Journal of Work and Environmental Health, 25,* 85–99.

40. Karlsoon, B., Knutsoon, A., & Lindahl, B. (2001). Is there an association between shift work and having a metabolic syndrome? Results from a population based study of 27285 people. *Occupational and Environmental Medicine, 58,* 747–752.

41. Nurminen, T. (1998). Shift work and reproductive health. *Scandinavian Journal of Work and Environmental Health,* 3(Suppl. 4), 28–34.

42. Davis, S., Mirick, D. K., & Stevens, R. G. (2001). Night shift work, light at night, and risk of breast cancer. *Journal of the National Cancer Institute, 93,* 1557–1562.

43. Shernhammer, E. S., Laden, F., Speizer, F. E., et al. (2001). Rotating night shifts and risk of breast cancer in women participating in the nurses' health study. *Journal of the National Cancer Institute, 93,* 1563–1568.

44. International Agency for Research on Cancer. (2010). Painting, firefighting, and shiftwork. *IARC Monographs on the Evaluation of Carcinogenic Risks in Humans, 98,* 1–818.

45. Scott, A. J., & LaDou, J. (1990). Shiftwork: Effects on sleep and health with recommendations for medical surveillance and screening. *Occupational Medicine,* 5(2), 273–299.

46. Harma, M. (1993). Individual differences in tolerance to shiftwork: A review. *Ergonomics, 36,* 101–109.

47. Monk, T. H. (2000). Shift work. In M. Kryger, T. Roth, & W. Dement (Eds.), *Principles and practice of sleep medicine* (pp. 600–605). Philadelphia, PA: W.B. Saunders Company.

48. Arendt, J., Stone, B., & Skene, D. (2000). Jet lag and sleep disruption. In M. Kryger, T. Roth, & W. Dement (Eds.), *Principles and practice of sleep medicine* (pp. 600–605). Philadelphia, PA: W.B. Saunders Company.

49. Hayakawa, T., Uchiyama, M., Kamei, Y., et al. (2005). Clinical analyses of sighted patients with non-24-hour sleep–wake syndrome: A study of 57 consecutively diagnosed cases. *Sleep, 28,* 945–952.

50. Sack, R. L., & Lewy, A. J. (2001). Circadian rhythm sleep disorders: Lessons from the blind. *Sleep Medicine Reviews, 5,* 189–206.

51. Katzenberg, D., Young, T., Finn, L., et al. (1998). A clock polymorphism associated with human diurnal preference. *Sleep, 21,* 569–576.

52. Ebisawa, T., Uchiyama, M., Kajimura, N., et al. (2001). Association of structural polymorphisms in the human period3 gene with delayed sleep phase syndrome. *European Molecular Biology Organization Reports, 2,* 342–346.

53. Jones, C. R., Campbell, S. S., Zone, S. E., et al. (1999). Familial advanced sleep phase syndrome: A short period circadian variant in humans. *Nature Medicine, 5,* 1062–1065.

54. Morgenthaler, T. I., Lee-Chiong, T., Alessi, C., et al. (2007). Practice parameters for the clinical evaluation and treatment of circadian rhythm sleep disorders. *Sleep, 30,* 1445–1459.

55. Barrett, J., Lack, L., & Morris, M. (1993). The sleep-evoked decrease of body temperature. *Sleep, 16,* 93–99.

56. Carrier, J., & Monk, T. H. (1997). Estimating the endogenous circadian temperature rhythm without keeping people awake. *Journal of Biological Rhythms, 12,* 266–277.

57. Eastman, C. I., Stewart, K. T., Mahoney, M. P., et al. (1994). Dark goggles and bright light improve circadian rhythm adaptation to night-shift work. *Sleep, 17,* 535–543.

58. Folkard, S. (1989). The pragmatic approach to masking. *Chronobiology International, 6,* 55–64.

59. Martin, S. K., & Eastman, C. I. (1998). Medium-intensity light produces circadian rhythm adaptation to simulated night-shift work. *Sleep, 21,* 154–165.

60. Mitchell, P. J., Hoese, E. K., Liu, L., et al. (1997). Conflicting bright light exposure during night shifts impedes circadian adaptation. *Journal of Biological Rhythms, 12,* 5–15.

61. Sharkey, K. M., & Eastman, C. I. (2002). Melatonin phase shifts human circadian rhythms in a placebo-controlled simulated night-work study. *American Journal of Physiology, 282,* R454–R463.

62. Duffy, J. F., & Dijk, D. J. (2002). Getting through to circadian oscillators: Why we use constant routines. *Journal of Biological Rhythms, 17,* 4–13.

63. Auger RR, Burgess HJ, Emens JS, Deriy LV, Thomas SM, Sharkey KM. Clinical practice guideline for the treatment of intrinsic circadian rhythm sleep-wake

disorders:advanced sleep-wake phase disorder (ASWPD), delayed sleep-wake phase disorder (DSWPD), non-24-hour sleep-wake rhythm disorder (N24SWD), and irregular sleep-wake rhythm disorder (ISWRD). An update for 2015. *J Clin Sleep Med* 2015;11(10):1199–1236.

64. Crowley, S. J., Lee, C., Tseng, C. Y., et al. (2003). Combinations of bright light, scheduled dark, sunglasses, and melatonin to facilitate circadian entrainment to night shift work. *Journal of Biological Rhythms, 18*, 513–523.

65. Burgess, H. J., Crowley, S. J., Gazda, C. J., et al. (2003). Preflight adjustment to eastward travel: 3 days of advancing sleep with and without morning bright light. *Journal of Biological Rhythms, 18*, 318–328.

66. Eastman, C. I., Gazda, C. J., Burgess, H. J., et al. (2005). Advancing circadian rhythms before eastward flight: A strategy to prevent or reduce jet lag. *Sleep, 28*, 33–44.

67. Revell, V. L., Burgess, H. J., Gazda, C. J., et al. (2006). Advancing human circadian rhythms with afternoon melatonin and intermittent bright light. *Journal of Clinical Endocrinology and Metabolism, 91*, 54–59.

68. Revell, V. L., & Eastman, C. I. (2005). How to trick mother nature into letting you fly around or stay up all night. *Journal of Biological Rhythms, 20*, 353–365.

69. Burgess, H. J., Revell, V. L., & Eastman, C. I. (2008). A three pulse phase response curve to three milligrams of melatonin in humans. *Journal of Physiology, 586*, 639–647.

70. Burgess, H. J., Revell, V. L., Molina, T. A., et al. (2010). Human phase response curves to three days of melatonin: 0.5 mg versus 3.0 mg. *Journal of Clinical Endocrinology and Metabolism, 95*, 3325–3331.

71. Lewy, A. J., Emens, J. S., Bernert, R. A., et al. (2004). Eventual entrainment of the human circadian pacemaker by melatonin is independent of the circadian phase of treatment initiation: Clinical implications. *Journal of Biological Rhythms, 19*, 68–75.

72. Lewy, A. J., Emens, J. S., Sack, R. L., et al. (2002). Low, but not high, doses of melatonin entrained a free-running blind person with a long circadian period. *Chronobiology International, 19*, 649–659.

chapter 18
Parasomnias

SONYA ABERCROMBIE   JOSEPH W. ANDERSON

LEARNING OBJECTIVES

On completion of this chapter, the reader should be able to:

1. Express a basic understanding of nonrapid eye movement and rapid eye movement parasomnias.
2. Recognize clinical presentation to enhance documentation procedures.
3. Recognize issues that require a technologist response.
4. Identify a parasomnia that occurs during the polysomnographic recording.
5. Describe the processes related to responding to the patient exhibiting a parasomnia event during the sleep study.
6. Differentiate between parasomnias that usually occur in children or in adults or in both.

KEY TERMS

Parasomnia
Arousal
REM sleep
NREM sleep

Parasomnias are undesirable physical phenomena that occur predominantly or exclusively during the sleep period (1, 2). Classification by the *International Classification of Sleep Disorders*, 3rd edition (*ICSD-3*) is as follows (Fig. 18-1):

1. During nonrapid eye movement (NREM) sleep.
2. Associated with rapid eye movement (REM) sleep.
3. During the transition from wakefulness to sleep and from sleep to wakefulness.

The pathogenesis of the various parasomnias remains incompletely understood. It is believed that the simultaneous occurrence or rapid oscillation of the various state-determining variables of wakefulness, NREM or N3 sleep, and REM sleep may give rise to the intrusion of elements of one state into another. Therefore, a combination of wakefulness and NREM sleep produces disorders of arousal (DOA), and persistence of REM sleep and elements of wakefulness result in REM behavior disorder (RBD) (3). Parasomnias are, thus, especially likely to emerge during the transition periods from one state to another and may consist of complex seemingly purposeful behaviors. These behaviors may not be recalled by the patient upon awakening. These actions are often termed automatisms, apparently without any conscious motivation or control. Patients may have more than one parasomnia, and overlapping features of parasomnias can make it difficult to differentiate between the parasomnias and seizure (4).

DISORDERS OF AROUSAL (FROM NREM SLEEP)

DOA occur primarily out of NREM sleep, particularly stage N3 sleep, and are more prevalent during the first third of the night. There is often a strong familial pattern. These disorders are most commonly encountered during childhood, and their frequency often diminishes with increasing age as stage N3 sleep declines. These disorders are believed to result from abnormal arousal processes, when motor activity is restored without full consciousness.

Confusional Arousals

Confusional arousals, also termed "sleep drunkenness," are seen more commonly during the first third of the night, when NREM stage N3 sleep is most prevalent. Confusional arousals are characterized by diminished vigilance, excessive sleep inertia, unclear thoughts, and slowed speech. Behaviors tend to demonstrate lack of

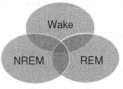

Figure 18-1 Human consciousness is traditionally categorized into three distinct states: wake, nonrapid eye movement (NREM), and rapid eye movement (REM) sleep. As humans transition from one state of consciousness into another, there exists a state that is not fully declared. This temporary and unstable period is known as the *state of dissociation* (dark intersection). Parasomnias are often a result of this period of sleep, which is a combination of one or more states of consciousness.

orientation to the environment. The person may react inappropriately, be resistive, and even violent. Episodes may last minutes or hours. Consoling the person can cause even more agitation. These arousals may be associated with behaviors that are inappropriate, violent, resistive, or otherwise bizarre. These episodes may also occur during morning awakening (1).

Confusional arousals may be caused by sleep deprivation, the use of central nervous system (CNS) depressants, neurologic disorders, or forced awakenings from deep sleep. They are most prevalent in young children and are less common among adults. There is no gender difference (4). During an episode of confusional arousal, polysomnographic (PSG) recordings may demonstrate an alpha rhythm, repetitive microsleeps, or stage N1 sleep activity.

Treatments may include sleep extension, scheduled awakenings, avoidance of sleep deprivation, psychotherapy, or drug therapy (e.g., tricyclic antidepressants or benzodiazepines) (5). Treatment for children may not be required because time may be all that is required for the arousals to disappear (4).

Sexsomnia

Sexsomnia is an NREM parasomnia in which the patient has atypical sexual manifestations during sleep, such as masturbation, fondling, and sexual intercourse followed by morning amnesia (1, 6). PSG data demonstrate sudden spontaneous arousals from non-REM slow-wave (N3) sleep (6). The *ICSD-3* considers sexsomnia a "confusional arousal." Terms used in the literature are "atypical sexual behavior during sleep," "sexsomnia," or "sleep sex." Sexsomnia is a recently reported variation of NREM arousal parasomnias (1, 4). These behaviors often occur during confusional arousals and have been reported during somnambulism (somnambulistic sexual behavior) (1). Most people reporting sexsomnia have had past episodes of sleepwalking (6). Sleepwalking does not present with sexual arousal; however, sexsomnia is associated with engorgement of the sexual organs, lubrication, and ejaculation. Confusional arousals are different, in that movement is related to the person's agitation and confusion with crying and screaming and there is no sexuality to it. Males are described as being more physical, with sexual fondling and intercourse often occurring, whereas females are more likely to present with masturbation and vocalization of a sexual nature (6).

This parasomnia can be quite disturbing, making relationships difficult as both partners suffer utterly different emotions about themselves and yet must muster empathy for the other. This can strain marriages and cause relationships much hardship. The medicolegal ramifications can also be substantial.

There is some evidence that alcohol and drug abuse may be factors in some cases in addition to stress and sleep deprivation. Past trauma may also be a factor. PSG performed to capture these episodes may need to be repeated in order to capture an episode. Home sleep testing may be of benefit in these patients. Home studies also allow the patient to mimic behaviors seen at home that are not allowed in the lab: same sleeping partner, alcohol use, and so on.

Treatments for this parasomnia include serotonin reuptake inhibitors, benzodiazepines (e.g., clonazepam), and antidepressant medications (5, 6). Sleep hygiene issues should be addressed with these patients, and stress management for those with depression or anxiety is often indicated.

Parasomnias Because of Medications or Substances

Association between medications or other substances and the induced parasomnias is increasingly recognized. Parasomnias may be associated with the use or withdrawal of a substance, often a medication, and the associated nonconscious behaviors can occur during NREM or REM sleep. The *ICSD-3* does not list substances that cause this specific disorder. The literature does cite cases and this is a cursory overview of some of these cases.

The newer "Z drugs" are being seen in the literature with often bizarre consequences. Zolpidem (Ambien), zaleplon (Sonata), and eszopiclone (Lunesta) are benzodiazepine receptor agonists that react with $\alpha1$ γ-aminobutyric acid (GABA)$_A$ receptors, thought to eliminate sedative, amnesic, and motor impairment actions associated with benzodiazepines that react at other GABA receptor sites (7). Zolpidem states, on its packaging materials, that alcohol or other CNS depressants when taken together may increase the risk of associated parasomnias. The behaviors or automatisms involved, such as sleep driving and sleep shopping, are parasomnias associated with DOA, RBD, or parasomnia overlap disorder (4, 7). Sexsomnia, somnambulism, and sleep-eating can also be seen as a result of medication or substance use. These topics are covered under their own headings.

Somnambulism was reported in a case study where bupropion's use may have initiated somnambulism episodes; when the medication was discontinued, the sleepwalking was curtailed (8). The bupropion (a noradrenaline and dopamine reuptake inhibitor) was prescribed for use during smoking cessation; however, because of nicotine withdrawal, bupropion could not be assumed causal in this case (8). Another case report describes a patient prescribed bupropion for depression, who about 2 weeks later was discovered to be leaving her bed, making phone calls, and bringing back food that she hid under her pillow. Bupropion was stopped, and that night so did the parasomnia. Months later, another physician prescribed bupropion and the parasomnia returned in about 2 weeks. Again, the parasomnia went away the first night she stopped taking the bupropion. Bupropion increases slow-wave sleep and also REM total duration, density, and latency (8).

Patient medications and other substances used by patients tend to present problems in the study of parasomnias and also in their treatment. New classes of sleep medications and substances that have been around for years (e.g., alcohol) can be the cause of parasomnias. The use of these substances is increasing, and more reporting has indicated a likely relationship between their use and some parasomnias.

Although we would normally expect to see a short amount of time between starting a new medication and seeing a reaction to it, many medications take weeks for their full effects to be established. Polypharmacy presents confounding evidence of what medication may be causing a parasomnia. The drug or drugs used to treat an original disorder may cause the problem, but it may also be an interaction between several medications that is the cause. Patients can be taking large numbers of drugs for comorbid and morbid conditions unrelated to sleep. It has been postulated that parasomnias, such as sexsomnia, may emerge because of medication initiation or withdrawal (4).

These parasomnias may be quite dangerous and yet unknown to the patient for a time before he or she or his or her physician is able to put the pieces together and identify that he or she has a sleep disorder. RBD, discussed later in this chapter, can be associated with the use of medications and biologic substances and is an example of a disorder that can be dangerous to the patient or others in the proximity of the patient having an episode.

Treatment of these parasomnias may consist of removal of the offending medication or substance. Changes in dosage and timing of medication may also prove beneficial.

Sleepwalking

Sleepwalking or somnambulism refers to ambulation that occurs during sleep. Somnambulism is considered a DOA and is most commonly seen in the first third of the night, when NREM stage N3 sleep is more prominent. The episode will often start with the person sitting up in bed, followed by walking or running. The sleepwalker may return to bed without waking or wake somewhere else. Behaviors may occasionally be inappropriate, such as driving a car over long distances. It is associated with diminished arousability and inappropriate behaviors, sometimes highly elaborate, and amnesia for the event. The sleepwalker's eyes are usually wide open, but attempts to communicate are usually unsuccessful. Episode duration varies widely from several minutes to an hour. It is most prevalent in young children and is less common in adults (9, 10). Familial occurrence is common (11, 12).

Episodes generally follow an arousal from N3 sleep. PSG patterns seen in adults with injurious sleepwalking and sleep terrors include (1) diffuse, rhythmic delta activity, (2) diffuse delta and theta activities, and (3) prominent alpha and beta activities. Abrupt heart rate acceleration may be noted postarousal (13).

Treatment may include hypnosis, scheduled awakenings, or medication (e.g., tricyclic antidepressants or benzodiazepines) (5). In children, time and protection from harm may be all that is required for these events to resolve (4).

Sleep Terrors

Sleep terrors, also referred to as "night terrors or pavor nocturnus," are one of the most dramatic forms of arousal disorders. Sleep terrors are seen most often in the first third of the night, when stage N3 sleep is more prevalent. The parasomnia occurs more commonly in children. Among adults, sleep terrors may occur throughout the night. They are characterized by crying or loud screaming and a general sense of fear. Autonomic responses, such as tachycardia, tachypnea, diaphoresis, and increased muscle tone, can be noted. Patients are inconsolable and have amnesia of the event.

PSG features include a reduction in sleep efficiency, more frequent arousals, and greater wake time after sleep onset. There is often a decrease in NREM stage N2 sleep and an increase in stage N3 sleep.

Therapy may include sleep extension, avoidance of sleep deprivation, scheduled awakenings, hypnosis, or medications (e.g., benzodiazepines or L-5-hydroxytryptamine) in children (5). In children, treatment may not be required because the disorder will often resolve over time (4). Consideration of other sleep disorders, such as obstructive sleep apnea (OSA), that might be causing the night terrors is always appropriate and may lead the physician to identify and treat an underlying disorder first (4).

Parasomnias Usually Associated with REM Sleep
REM Sleep Behavior Disorder

RBD was formally identified as a sleep disorder by Schenck et al. in 1986 (14, 15). It is characterized by the intermittent absence of muscle atonia during REM sleep, with dream mentation and motor activity. Episodes are more common during the second half of the night (early morning hours), when REM sleep is most common. Complex behaviors associated with RBD range from simple motions to highly elaborate performances (screaming, punching, kicking, or running). These dream-enacting behaviors can result in sleep disruption or injury to the sleeper or bed partner (16). Dream content can be altered or unpleasant (17). The episode ends with a rapid awakening and full alertness. The eyes are usually closed, in contrast to the case of the sleepwalker, whose eyes are open during the episode. RBD most often occurs in the sixth or seventh decade of life and is most prevalent in males. Neurologic disorders (dementia, Parkinsonism, or narcolepsy) are predisposing factors.

PSG is routinely performed to establish the diagnosis of RBD. PSG can demonstrate an augmentation of electromyographic (EMG) activity and the presence of body movements during REM sleep. Mild RBD may present with nothing more than arm movement or flailing; however, more violent activities such as slapping, punching, kicking, leaping from the bed, and running have been documented during PSG. Walking is uncommon. Time-synchronized video recording is essential and more than a single study may be required in order to capture an episode. Additional EMG monitoring of the upper extremity muscles (flexor digitorum) is useful.

The technologist must consider the safety of the patient and others when studying these patients. Treatment may include assuring a safe sleeping environment and treatment with melatonin and/or clonazepam (4, 5).

Recurrent Isolated Sleep Paralysis

Sleep paralysis manifests as an inability to perform voluntary movements either at sleep onset (hypnagogic) or upon waking from sleep (hypnopompic). There is a generalized transient paralysis of the head, body, and extremities, with sparing of the ocular and respiratory muscles. Paralysis may last several seconds to several minutes. Consciousness is unaffected and dream imagery may be recalled. Onset is often during adolescence, with both genders affected equally. Most cases are identified in an isolated form; others occur in a familial form or in persons with narcolepsy (17). Lack of sleep and poor sleep hygiene are predisposing factors.

PSG recordings are characterized by abundant alpha electroencephalogram (EEG) activity and persistence of muscle atonia into wakefulness (18). Treatment may include REM sleep suppression with medication (e.g., antidepressants) (4).

Nightmare Disorder

Nightmares are unpleasant and frightening dreams that occur during REM sleep. Episodes typically occur in the latter half of the night when REM sleep is more prevalent. Dream content is disturbing and often relates to imminent physical danger to the patient. The patient can often describe the nature of the nightmare upon waking and there is little, if any, confusion, which differentiates nightmare disorder from night terrors. Nightmares

often occur after periods of REM sleep deprivation and can be precipitated by illness, traumatic experiences, acute alcohol ingestion, and certain medications (19). Occasional nightmares are not uncommon during childhood. Nightmares generally become less frequent during adulthood (20). Recurring nightmares can result in insomnia, sleep avoidance because of fear of falling asleep, excessive daytime sleepiness, and anxiety.

PSG demonstrates abrupt awakenings from REM sleep. REM sleep abnormalities, including a reduction in REM sleep latency, an increased REM density, and an increased percentage of REM sleep, may be observed. Treatment may include sleep hygiene, comfort, image rehearsal, psychotherapy, and medications for REM suppression (5).

Other Parasomnias

Sleep-Related Dissociative Disorders

Dissociative disorder can emerge throughout the sleep period (1). Nighttime episodes can consist of violent or sexualized behavior, self-mutilation, screaming, running, eating, or driving a car. There is generally amnesia for the event. Dissociative disorders can result in injuries. The disorder is more prevalent in females, and episodes may be sporadic or slowly increase across time (4). Patients also usually present with daytime dissociative disorders, and these may be associated with a history of trauma, physical abuse, or sexual abuse (4).

PSG reveals sustained EEG wakefulness during these episodes. Treatment may require psychiatric intervention because this parasomnia is often associated with past traumatic events (4).

Sleep Enuresis

Sleep enuresis (SE) is recurrent, involuntary bed-wetting occurring during sleep in a child older than 5 years. Most children achieve bladder control at night by 3 years of age. Although it can arise throughout the night, enuresis tends to occur most commonly early during sleep in the first third of the evening. There are two classifications of enuresis: primary and secondary. In primary enuresis, bladder control has not been realized by 5 years of age. Children with primary enuresis often have a positive family history among their siblings or parents. Spontaneous cure rate in children with primary SE is estimated at 15% annually. In secondary cases, enuresis begins after at least a 6-month period of being dry. Secondary SE can occur at any age and accounts for approximately 5% to 10% of cases. SE can be seen during adolescence and also in about 1% to 3% of adult patients with primary nocturnal enuresis (4).

PSG typically demonstrates normal sleep architecture. Treatment may include "bed-wetting alarms," bladder training, medications (e.g., desmopressin, oxybutynin, or imipramine) (4, 5). In secondary SE, the physician must diagnose and treat any underlying cause that may be present before treating the SE.

Sleep-Related Groaning (Catathrenia)

Sleep-related groaning (catathrenia) is defined as groaning during exhalation in sleep (mostly during REM sleep). The person with this disorder is often unaware of the episodes; however, the bed partner is often disturbed because of the loud vocalizations. PSG may demonstrate episodes of bradypnea, and loud expiratory groaning sounds occurring in clusters that recur several times throughout the night. Sleep architecture and oxygen saturation are normal.

Exploding Head Syndrome

Exploding head syndrome is characterized by a sudden, loud imagined noise or explosion in the head occurring during the transition between wakefulness and sleep. A flash of light, myoclonic jerk, and sense of fear or concern may accompany the experience. The frequency of attacks varies significantly among individuals. Frequent attacks can give rise to complaints of insomnia.

PSG features of the disorder are sudden arousals occurring during the sleep–wake transition, with the EEG demonstrating alpha and theta activity. Treatment is not required because of the benign nature of the disorder and the fact that these episodes often resolve over time (4).

Sleep-Related Eating Disorder

Sleep-related eating disorder demonstrates episodes of recurrent drinking and eating during arousals from sleep. This disorder often manifests when the individual is experiencing severe stress, has discontinued smoking, or is recovering from alcohol or substance abuse. Affected individuals are unaware or only partly conscious of the abnormal behavior. Episodes can be observed anytime during sleep, and episodes may occur many times every night. In many instances, the awakenings appear to be triggered by learned behavior and not by real hunger or thirst.

PSG may show multiple arousals, typically from NREM stage N3 sleep but occasionally from REM sleep as well. Treatment may include treating an underlying sleep disorder that is causing sleep fragmentation, for example, leg movements and OSA (4).

Sleep-Related Hallucinations

Hallucinations can occur during sleep–wake transitions, either at sleep onset (hypnagogic hallucinations) or during awakening (hypnopompic hallucinations). These hallucinatory experiences can take a variety of forms, including visual, auditory, or tactile phenomena. These may be associated with sleep paralysis and are more common in patients with narcolepsy, but can be experienced by anyone.

PSG demonstrates events occurring predominantly during sleep-onset REM periods, but these episodes can also arise during NREM sleep. Hypnagogic and hypnopompic hallucinations may be normal for some individuals, but narcolepsy should be considered in patients presenting with these symptoms because it may be the underlying cause, and treatment of narcolepsy would be indicated (4).

Parasomnia Because of Medical Condition

This diagnosis is indicated when a parasomnia (e.g., RBD) is associated with an underlying neurologic or medical condition. Sleep paralysis and sleep hallucinations may also be related to ongoing neurologic disorders.

Parasomnia, Unspecified

When a parasomnia cannot be classified in any of the known parasomnia categories, the physician may use unspecified parasomnia as a temporary diagnosis. This is often appropriate when a psychiatric condition may be the cause, but the actual condition is still elusive. If a psychiatric condition is established, that becomes the diagnosis; however, if a psychiatric condition is not established, the diagnosis remains unspecified parasomnia.

EVALUATION OF PARASOMNIAS

Clinical evaluation of a patient presenting with a possible parasomnia involves an interview with the patient, the spouse, and other family members. A comprehensive sleep questionnaire is valuable (Fig. 18-2). Neurologic and psychiatric examinations and complete psychological testing may also be indicated using psychological measurement tools such as the Minnesota Multiphasic Personality Inventory or Beck Depression Inventory.

During a sleep study, if a parasomnia event occurs, the sleep technologist should record the time and describe the event. For direct observation of the event, the technologist might need to go into the patient's room and do the following: document whether the eyes are open or closed, and whether the eyes appear alert or "glassy," whether the patient appears to be asleep in a dreaming or nondreaming state or awake, and the level of consciousness during the event. The technologist should ask the patient about dream recall associated with the parasomnia event if he or she awakens and note the emotional state of the patient.

The sleep technologist must be prepared to intervene immediately and enter the room if the patient exhibits behavior that may cause injury. Simultaneous

Please answer the following questions using this scale. (Consult bed partner.)

0 = never; 1 = rarely; 2 = sometimes; 3 = often; 4 = frequently; 5 = always

0 1 2 3 4 5	I have been told that I walk in my sleep
0 1 2 3 4 5	I wet the bed as an adult
0 1 2 3 4 5	I move my arms, legs, and/or body during sleep
0 1 2 3 4 5	I have been told that I act out my dreams
0 1 2 3 4 5	I cannot tell dreams from reality
0 1 2 3 4 5	I make loud, unusual sounds during my sleep
0 1 2 3 4 5	I have been told that I talk, shout, or groan in my sleep
0 1 2 3 4 5	I have unusual behaviors during my sleep
0 1 2 3 4 5	I have vivid dream-like scenes upon falling asleep
0 1 2 3 4 5	I have experienced violent behaviors during my sleep
0 1 2 3 4 5	I hurt myself or my bed partner during my sleep
0 1 2 3 4 5	I have experienced night terrors with shouting or loud screaming
0 1 2 3 4 5	I eat or drink during my sleep
0 1 2 3 4 5	I have awakened in the morning feeling bloated, sick to my stomach and do not want to eat breakfast
0 1 2 3 4 5	I have initiated unusual or hurtful sexual behaviors during my sleep, either by myself or with my bed partner
0 1 2 3 4 5	I have had episodes of muscle paralysis while falling asleep or waking up
0 1 2 3 4 5	I have recurrent nightmares
0 1 2 3 4 5	I have now or in the past had seizures during my sleep

Figure 18-2 Parasomnia questionnaire.

digital video recording is available on many acquisition systems and should be utilized during the sleep study. This provides the ability to correlate the parasomnia event with activity on the PSG tracing. When video recording is performed with a separate recording device,

the use of a time stamp system, close observation, and detailed documentation by the sleep technologist are required. PSG features of the various parasomnias are described in Table 18-1. Indications for PSG are outlined in Table 18-2.

Table 18-1 Polysomnographic Features of Parasomnias

Parasomnia	Observation
Confusional arousals	Arise while in the bed from SWS, REM with apnea, often sitting up in bed looking around confused
Sexsomnia	Arousals seen in transitions between sleep–wake or between differing sleep stages, SWS
Parasomnias due to medications or substances	Altered motor control during sleep, arousals
Sleepwalking	Persistence of sleep while leaving the bed, arousal from SWS, ambulation, normal muscle atonia in REM, amnesia for event, automatic behaviors that are inappropriate, disoriented with slow speech
Sleep terrors	Arousal from SWS, screaming, autonomic activation, RBD, and seizures need to be ruled out; adults may have overlap with other arousal disorders
RBD	Loss of atonia in REM, excessive submental EMG activity in REM, disruptive or abnormal REM sleep behaviors ranging from mild limb movements in REM to getting out of bed and acting out dreams
Recurrent isolated sleep paralysis	REM sleep atonia continuing into wake, alpha intrusion into REM sleep, EMG shows atonia during the paralysis

Table 18-1 Polysomnographic Features of Parasomnias (*continued*)

Parasomnia	Observation
Nightmare disorder	Nightmares generally in REM, little confusion, there is dream recall usually with fear or anxiety, return to sleep may be difficult, occur in the latter half of the night
Sleep-related dissociative disorders	Emerge from sustained EEG of wakefulness, self-mutilation, repeated injury of self or others
Sleep-related groaning	Groaning recorded during (predominantly) REM sleep
Exploding head syndrome	Patient perceives sudden loud noise (explosion) in his or her head during wake–sleep or sleep–wake transitions, absence of significant pain
Sleep-related eating disorder	Waking concurrent EEG pattern, multiple confusional arousals with various levels of consciousness achieved
Sleep-related hallucinations	Hallucinations before sleep onset or awakening, usually visual

EEG, electroencephalogram; EMG, electromyogram; OSA, obstructive sleep apnea; PSG, polysomnography; RBD, REM behavior disorder; REM, rapid eye movement; SWS, slow-wave sleep.

Table 18-2 Indications for Polysomnography

Parasomnia Type	When Disorder Is Uncomplicated and Noninjurious	Forensic Considerations, Injury or Atypical Behavior, Age, Time, Duration, Frequency, or Motor Patterns
Confusional arousals	No	Yes
Sexsomnia	No	Yes
Confusional arousals	No	Yes
Sexsomnia	No	Yes
Parasomnia due to medications or substances	No	Yes
Sleepwalking	No	Yes
Sleep terrors	No	Yes
REM behavior disorder	Yes	Yes
Recurrent isolated sleep paralysis	No	Yes
Nightmare disorder	No	Yes
Sleep-related dissociative disorders	No	Yes
Sleep-related groaning	No	Unusual
Exploding head syndrome	No	Unusual
Sleep-related hallucinations	No	Yes
Sleep-related eating disorder	No	Unusual

REM, rapid eye movement.

SUMMARY

Parasomnias are common clinical complaints. Formal sleep evaluation including PSG is indicated for parasomnias that are injurious, disruptive to the bed partner or other household members, associated with daytime sleepiness, or related to medical, psychiatric, or neurologic disorders (2). The initial assessment usually starts with the patient interview and discussion of the presenting sleep complaint and a patient history. Often, more information may be obtained through further discussions with the bed partner, caregivers, or others familiar with the sleep problem. Parasomnias must be distinguished from nocturnal seizures, both of which may manifest as unusual and inappropriate movements and behaviors.

REFERENCES

1. American Academy of Sleep Medicine. (2014). *International classification of sleep disorders* (3rd ed.). Darien, IL: Author.
2. Mahowald, M. W. (2002). Arousal and sleep-wake transition parasomnias. In T. L. Lee-Chiong, M. J. Sateia, & M. A. Carskadon (Eds.), *Sleep medicine* (pp. 207–213). Philadelphia, PA: Elsevier.
3. Mahowald, M. W. (2004). Parasomnias. *Medical Clinics of North America, 88*(3), 669–678.
4. Thorpy, M. J., & Plazzi, G. (2010). *The parasomnias and other sleep-related movement disorders.* New York, NY: Cambridge University Press.
5. Lee-Chiong, T. (2010). *Somnology.* Seattle, WA: On-Demand Publishing LLC.
6. Bejot, Y., Juenet, N., Garrouty, R., et al. (2010). Sexsomnia: An uncommon variety of parasomnia. *Clinical Neurology and Neurosurgery, 112*(1), 72–75.
7. Gibson, C. E., & Caplan, J. P. (2011). Zolpidem-associated parasomnia with serious self-injury: A shot in the dark. *Psychosomatics, 52*(1), 88–91.
8. Oulis, P., Kokras, N., Papadimitriou, G. N., et al. (2010). Bupropion-induced sleepwalking. *Journal of Clinical Psychopharmacology, 30*(1), 83–84.
9. Ohayon, M. M., Guilleminault, C., & Priest, R. G. (1999). Night terrors, sleepwalking, and confusional arousals in the general population: Their frequency and relationship to other sleep and mental disorders. *Journal of Clinical Psychiatry, 60,* 268–276.
10. Joncas, S., Zadra, A., Paquet, J., et al. (2002). The value of sleep deprivation as a diagnostic tool in adult sleepwalkers. *Neurology, 58*(6), 936–940.
11. Kales, A., Soldatos, C. R., Bixler, E. O., et al. (1980). Hereditary factors in sleepwalking and night terrors. *British Journal of Psychiatry, 137,* 111–118.
12. Abe, K., Amatomi, M., & Oda, N. (1984). Sleepwalking and recurrent sleep talking in children of childhood sleepwalkers. *American Journal of Psychiatry, 141,* 800–801.
13. Schenck, C. H., Pareja, J. A., Patterson, A. L., et al. (1998). Analysis of polysomnographic events surrounding 252 slow-wave sleep arousals in thirty-eight adults with injurious sleepwalking and sleep terrors. *Journal of Clinical Neurophysiology, 15*(2), 159–166.
14. Schenck, C. H., Bundlie, S. R., Ettinger, M. G., et al. (1986). Chronic behavioral disorders of human REM sleep: A new category of parasomnia. *Sleep, 9,* 293–308.
15. Schenck, C. H., Bundlie, S. R., Patterson, A. L., et al. (1987). Rapid eye movement sleep behavior disorder: A treatable parasomnia affecting older adults. *Journal of the American Medical Association, 257,* 1786–1789.
16. Olson, E. J., Boeve, B. F., & Silber, M. H. (2000). Rapid eye movement sleep behaviour disorder: Demographic, clinical and laboratory findings in 93 cases. *Brain, 123*(Pt. 2), 331–339.
17. Buzzi, G., & Cirignotta, F. (2000). Isolated sleep paralysis: A web survey. *Sleep Research Online, 3*(2), 61–66.
18. Takeuchi, T., Miyasita, A., Sasaki, Y., et al. (1992). Isolated sleep paralysis elicited by sleep interruption. *Sleep, 15*(3), 217–225.
19. Pagel, J. F., & Helfter, P. (2003). Drug induced nightmares—An etiology based review. *Human Psychopharmacology, 18*(1), 59–67.
20. Germain, A., & Nielsen, T. A. (2003). Sleep pathophysiology in posttraumatic stress disorder and idiopathic nightmare sufferers. *Biological Psychiatry, 54*(10), 1092–1098.

chapter 19

Restless Legs Syndrome and Periodic Limb Movement Disorder

JOSEPH W. ANDERSON

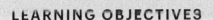

LEARNING OBJECTIVES

On completion of this chapter, the reader should be able to:

1. Define the clinical syndrome of restless legs syndrome (RLS).
2. Identify the characteristic polysomnographic features of periodic limb movement disorder (PLMD).
3. Differentiate between periodic limb movements and movements related to respiratory and other sleep-related events.
4. Recognize the relationship and differences between PLMD and RLS.

KEY TERMS

Periodic limb movement disorder (PLMD)
Restless legs syndrome (RLS)
Fasciculations
Sensorimotor
Physiologic
Accelerometry
Myoclonus
Impedance
Augmentation

Restless legs syndrome (RLS), sometimes called *Willis–Ekbom disease*, and periodic limb movement disorder (PLMD) are associated with each other; however, they remain as two separate clinical entities. RLS is a neurosensory motor disorder that occurs during wakefulness and may significantly impact sleep onset in the first half of the night as patients often must stretch, move, or walk to provide relief, resulting in a significant disruption to sleep quality. RLS is reported by about 10% of North American and northern European adults, with 2% to 3% having moderate-to-severe RLS (1). Periodic limb movements of sleep (PLMS) are physiologic signals that represent rhythmic movement of the lower extremity that are measured during sleep, which may or may not have clinical relevance. Periodic limb movements can also present in the upper extremities during sleep.

RLS is diagnosed through interview and appropriate questionnaires. A polysomnogram is not a requirement for diagnosis. In contrast, PLMD requires not only a patient interview confirming clinical sleep disturbances but also monitoring via a polysomnogram of specific limb movement activity. By convention, periodic electromyographic (EMG) activity recorded from bilateral anterior tibialis muscles defines PLMS. Movements of the upper limbs may also be sampled, if clinically indicated. Other techniques such as accelerometry of the toe, foot, or leg have also been used to measure movements in sleep. PLMS can be monitored in numerous muscle groups, including extensors and flexors of the toe, foot, knee, hip, finger, hand, elbow, and shoulder. The EMG of the anterior tibialis muscle provides a robust signal, and it was chosen by earlier researchers for measurement of limb movement activity, thereby becoming the standard.

The recording technologist must recognize that movements during sleep arise from multiple factors and that clinical relevance of a movement is based on the degree of arousal, which is usually defined by a 3-second or longer abrupt shift in electroencephalograph (EEG) frequency, although new research has additionally focused on cardiovascular measures of autonomic arousal from PLMS.

BRIEF HISTORY OF RLS AND PLMD

The first known medical description of RLS and PLMD was by Sir Thomas Willis in 1672 (". . .arms and legs, leapings and contractions of the tendons ensued . . . [making the bed into] a place of the greatest torture") (2). In 1945, Karl-Axel Ekbom (1907 to 1977) provided a detailed and comprehensive report of this condition in his doctoral thesis and a subsequent publication (3).

The first published report of periodic movements in sleep was by Symonds in 1953 (4). He used the term *nocturnal myoclonus* in describing the movements, but the term is best avoided because the characteristic movement of myoclonus is different from that of PLMS. Lugaresi and colleagues (5) in Italy described the association between PLMD and RLS in 1965. Coleman (6), working at Stanford University, described the technique for recording and scoring of PLMS in 1982 that continues to be utilized (with modification) today.

Various investigators have shown that PLMS predominate during the first half of the night and tend to increase in frequency over each decade of life, with children under 10 years rarely having PLMS and many adults of age 60 or older having more than 15 limb movements per hour of sleep (7) Zucconi et al. (8) at the National Institutes of Health demonstrated that PLMS arise from regulatory motor neurons in the spine.

The reader should be aware that generalized body movements and limb movements during sleep can have multiple causes, including sleep-disordered breathing. In particular, limb movements presenting 0.5 seconds before or after increased upper airway resistance and subsequent respiratory effort–related arousals may be misinterpreted as PLMS. Conversely, PLMS, or other sleep-related movements, may cause changes in breathing patterns or create artifacts in the respiratory channels that can resemble sleep-disordered breathing. A careful examination of all relevant polysomnographic (PSG) data is essential for differentiating PLMS from other sleep-related events. Current consensus identifies PLMS as a relatively infrequent cause of insomnia or hypersomnia, the clinical symptoms that are required to arrive at a diagnosis of PLMD.

OVERVIEW OF MOVEMENTS IN SLEEP

Motor activity in sleep is common, as any arousing event may cause movement. Movement represents the primary reason for abrupt changes in any PSG signal. Isolated movements of the arms and legs typically occur 50 to 100 times during 7 to 8 hours of sleep. Axial changes of body position occur five to seven times during an average night and will often cluster in the 10 minutes before or after rapid eye movement (REM) sleep. During REM sleep, muscle twitching is common and may be recorded as brief fasciculations in the limb EMG channels.

Generalized movements in sleep may be exacerbated by a wide variety of sleep-related disorders such as physical pain or discomfort, psychological disturbances, and environmental factors. In contrast to these, PLMS exhibit a stereotypical pattern of independent limb movements that meet specific criteria as described in the Movement Rules section of the *AASM (American Academy of Sleep Medicine) Manual for the Scoring of Sleep and Associated Events: Rules, Terminology and Technical Specifications*, version 2.5 (9).

RLS often causes patients to shift and move as they attempt to relax into sleep. The confinement of the recording environment in the sleep center may heighten the sensation of restlessness and the urge to move the legs. Normally,

patients will be able to report to the technologist that their legs are making it "difficult to settle." Some patients show heightened anxiety as RLS symptoms increase.

It occasionally proves to be a challenge for the technologist to decide whether anxiety is the principal reason for difficulty with sleep onset or whether the restriction of movement in the RLS patient is worsening their anxiety. It is common to observe periodic limb movements of wakefulness (PLMW) appearing in a regular fashion in the anterior tibialis recording as the RLS patient falls asleep.

In some sleep centers, an average of five or more independent periodic leg movements per hour of sleep can be seen in 25% to 40% of adult patients undergoing clinical PSG. Only one-tenth to one-fifth of these PLMS lead to EEG-defined arousals of 3 or more seconds. Frequently, limb movements with arousals are secondary to the termination of breathing-related events.

DEFINITION OF RLS AND PLMS

The *International Classification of Sleep Disorders*, third edition lists three clinical criteria for the diagnosis of RLS (10). Testing to establish the diagnosis is not required. The patient must provide a history of an urge to move the legs that may or may not include an abnormal sensation in the affected limb(s), (1) begins or worsens at rest, is partially or completely relieved by movement, and occurs predominantly or exclusively in the evening or night; (2) the symptoms are not related to another condition; and (3) they must cause distress, sleep disruption, or functional impairment. All three criteria must be met, and differentiation from similar disorders such as leg cramps, peripheral neuropathy, and habitual foot tapping among others is important.

To assist in the recall of the primary criteria for the diagnosis of RLS, the acronym URGE is suggested:

U—urge to move

R—rest worsens the urge

G—gyration (movement) relieves the urge

E—evening or night worsening of the urge

PLMS are defined as a burst of EMG activity in the anterior tibialis muscle with a duration of at least 0.5 seconds but not longer than 10 seconds. Quantitatively, the burst should be 8 μV greater than the resting baseline EMG amplitude. Periodicity is defined when there are four or more consecutive movements that occur with intermovement intervals of between 5 and 90 seconds. The movement onset is defined as the starting point of the movement that produces an 8 μV increase above resting EMG, and the movement offset is defined as the decline of EMG to less than 2 μV of resting EMG. Leg movements occurring in both legs that are separated by less than 5 seconds between movement onsets are counted as a single leg movement (9).

Traditionally, a mean total of five or more PLMS per hour of sleep has been considered abnormal, especially if the movements are accompanied by an EEG arousal. The European Sleep Society and the International Restless Legs Syndrome Study Group reviewed the methodology and clinical relevance of PLMS, proposing that the normal number of PLMS may be as high as 15 per hour in the elderly (7).

To score an EEG arousal associated with a limb movement, the movement must be accompanied by an abrupt shift in EEG frequency of at least 3 seconds duration, occurring within the 2 seconds before or after the limb movement.

METHODOLOGY AND RECORDING TECHNIQUES

PLMS are monitored during clinical PSG. Proper skin preparation of the recording site over the body of the anterior tibialis muscle is essential for a quality recording. Preparation is similar to that for an EEG recording. The prepped area for each electrode should be no larger than the size of the electrode used to monitor for PLMS. To assure quality signals, excess hair may need to be shaved over the monitoring site to prevent electrode slippage throughout a full night of monitoring. A standard EEG electrode should be used and taped over the body of the muscle to be monitored, with strain relief loop.

To define the body of the muscle, instruct the patient to flex the foot and then place the electrodes over the middle of the anterior tibialis muscle 2 to 3 cm apart or 1/3 the length of the muscle, whichever is shorter. Impedance below 5,000 Ω is ideal, but impedance of less than 10,000 Ω will generally allow for an adequate signal. The EMG channel should be filtered according to the standard EMG configurations, typically with a low-frequency filter setting of 10 Hz and a high-frequency filter setting of 100 Hz. Of equal importance is to complete bio-calibrations by asking the patient to flex each foot/raise the toes on each foot separately, five times, to confirm adequate signal before lights off (see Fig. 19-1).

Recording of PLMS can be done in two ways:

1. The recommended method is to use two electrodes on each leg that are referenced to each other by placing them longitudinally and symmetrically across each anterior tibialis muscle; this allows for two separate leg channels and is the preferred recording method.

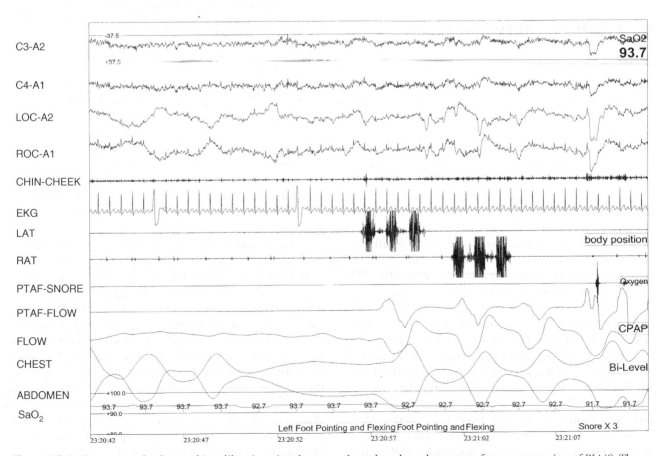

Figure 19-1 Thirty seconds. Correct biocalibration signals are used as a benchmark measure for proper scoring of PLMS. The patient's EEG shows wakefulness, as he follows the technologist's instruction to flex the left foot three times, then the right foot three times.

2. Two electrodes on each leg muscle with the signals "tied" to one channel. The "tied" method can be used to conserve channels; however, this may result in a change in the number of limb movements that are detected.
3. Movements of the upper limbs may be sampled, if clinically indicated. The recommended upper limb muscles include the flexor digitorum superficialis and the extensor digitorum communis.

EXAMPLES OF INDEPENDENT AND SECONDARY PLMS

- Proper bio-calibration signals for left and right limb movements (Fig. 19-2)
- Periodic limb movements without arousal (Fig. 19-2A, B)
- Periodic limb movements with arousal (Figs. 19-3 and 19-4)
- Muscle fasciculations and other movements that do not meet criteria for PLMS (Figs. 19-5 to 19-7)
- Leg movements secondary to obstructive apneas or hypopneas (Fig. 19-8A, B)
- Other movements (Figs. 19-9 to 19-12)

RELATIONSHIP BETWEEN PLMD AND RLS

RLS and PLMD are independent medical disorders, although RLS has a strong association with PLMS. PLMS do not establish the diagnosis of RLS, although they can support the clinical diagnosis.

In contrast, 80% or more of patients with RLS will have five or more PLMS per hour of sleep on a single night of testing (10), and most of the limb movements will be seen in the first half of the night. Although an EEG arousal, as defined by the AASM arousal rule, results in limited sleep disturbances from PLMS, the majority of PLMS in RLS patients are arousing when other definitions of arousal are used, such as delta EEG spectrum enhancement and heart rate or other cardiovascular variables. RLS can be diagnosed only by patient interview (11).

Most cases of RLS are primary, meaning that the cause is unknown. A genetic predisposition is suggested in situations where several family members carry the diagnosis before the age of 40. Secondary RLS develops as a result of other conditions such as pregnancy, renal failure, and iron deficiency. Given that iron deficiency can contribute to RLS, measurement of serum ferritin level and iron studies are recommended (11). Also of note is that certain medications, such as antinausea medications and antidepressants, may contribute to RLS. It is also of importance to consider renal disease, myelopathy, and pregnancy as a cause to avoid misdiagnosis.

An electrophysiologic monitoring technique, termed the Suggested Immobilization Test, can be used to measure PLMW in the 1 hour prior to beginning a polysomnogram (12). The patient sits up in bed with legs outstretched and is instructed to remain still during the recording ("Please do not move during the test."). EMG is recorded over the bilateral anterior tibialis muscles. Every 5 minutes during the 1-hour test, the patient is asked to document the severity of any urge to move their legs.

Most patients with RLS discover that the urge to move increases in the last 30 minutes of the test. Occasionally, the most severe patients will terminate the study before 60 minutes of recording has been completed. PLMW are periodic in presentation, but the motor activity recorded by the EMG may last for up to 10 seconds. Patients will often report that the "jerking" is involuntary. Control subjects without RLS have fewer than 5 PLMW per hour, whereas RLS patients with moderate or severe disease show 10 or more PLMW per hour. A higher PLMW rate is seen in more severe cases of RLS.

TREATMENT OF RLS AND PLMD

Treatment options for RLS and PLMD are similar (12). Published guidelines from the AASM (13) and the Medical Advisory Board of the RLS Foundation (13) support the use of dopaminergic agents as the first-line treatment in most patients. The approved agents considered "standard of care" for the treatment of RLS include ropinirole (Requip) and pramipexole (Mirapex). Other treatment options considered within the "guidelines" of the AASM practice parameters include gabapentin enacarbil (Horizant) and levodopa. Although clonazepam (Klonopin), opioids, and clonidine have been used for many years, it is recommended that these potentially addictive agents be closely monitored and used only after first-line therapy with Food and Drug Administration–approved medications have failed.

Dopaminergic therapy infrequently causes side effects such as nausea or vomiting, excessive sleepiness, muscle or joint achiness, headaches, light-headedness, edema, or impulsive behaviors (i.e., gambling), thereby limiting their continued usage. One of the long-term risks of dopaminergic therapy is the development of augmentation, a worsening of RLS symptoms. After some months of therapy, patients who develop augmentation report that they need increasing amounts of the dopaminergic medication because of increased RLS symptoms that present earlier in the day, sometimes including a spread of symptoms into the arms or other body parts. There is no specific recommendation for pharmacotherapy for PLMD alone (14).

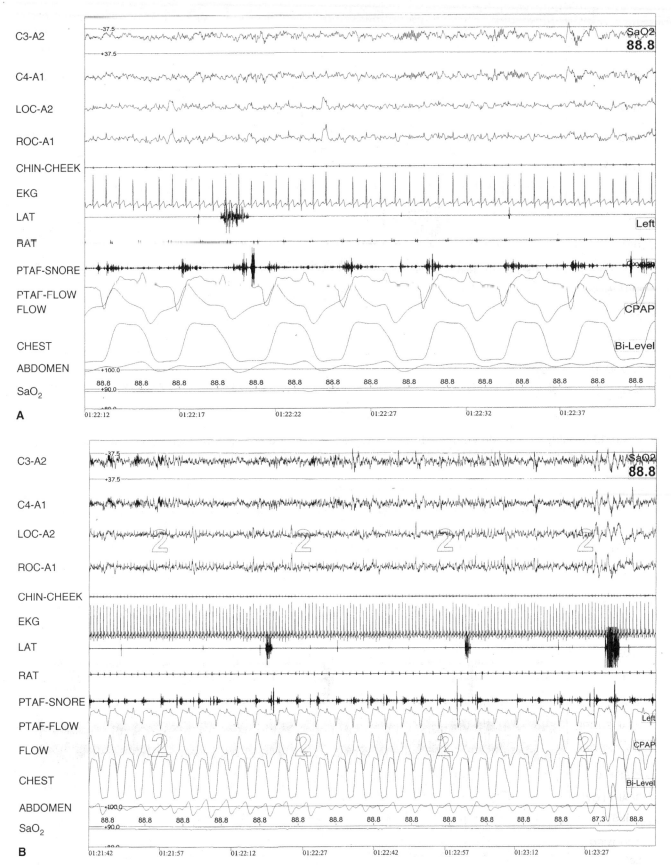

Figure 19-2 Sequence of periodic limb movements recorded in the left anterior tibialis (LAT) channel without evidence of cortical arousal in the EEG. A: 30 seconds; B: 120 seconds.

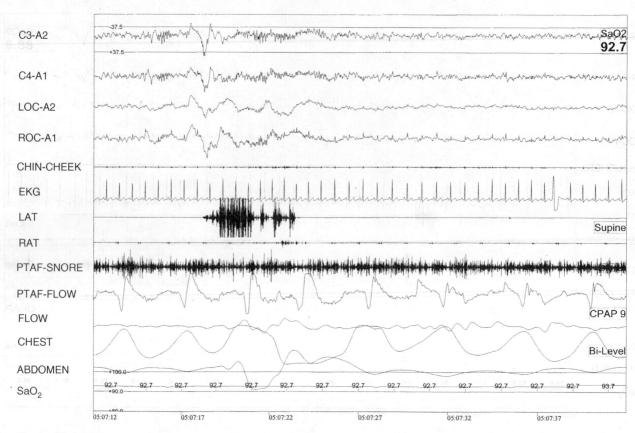

Figure 19-3 Thirty seconds. Movement in the LAT EMG channel, followed by an at least 3-second arousal, demonstrated by increased alpha activity in the EEG following an initial K complex (a "K-arousal").

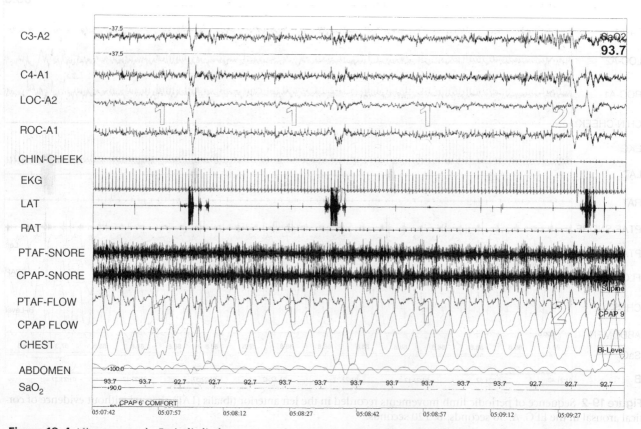

Figure 19-4 Ninety seconds. Periodic limb movements occurring at 40- to 60-second intervals with arousal.

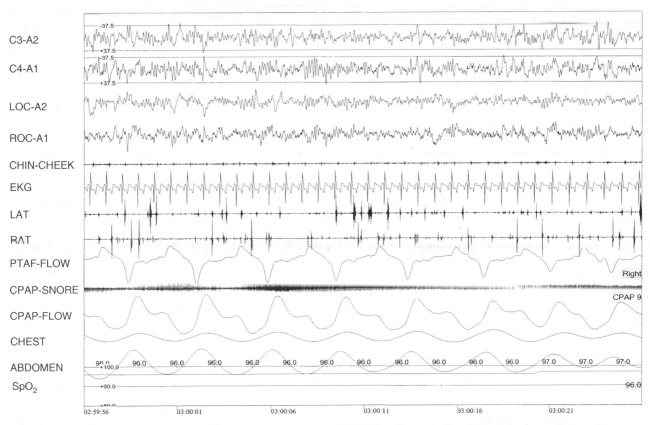

Figure 19-5 Thirty seconds. Muscle twitching activity is present in both leg channels, but these do not meet the requirements for scoring PLMS.

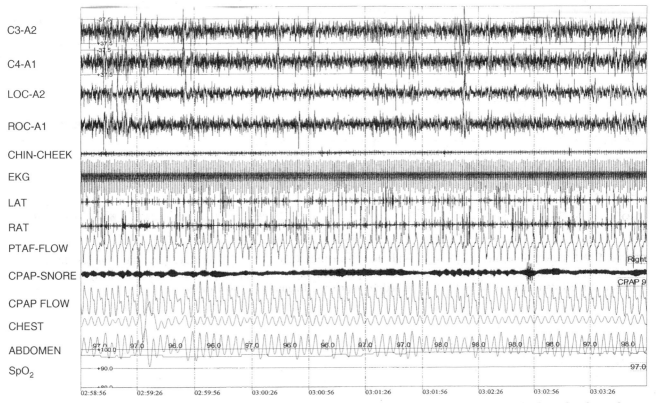

Figure 19-6 Three hundred seconds. Muscle twitching recorded throughout the printout. The patient had insulin-dependent diabetes and a history of peripheral neuropathy.

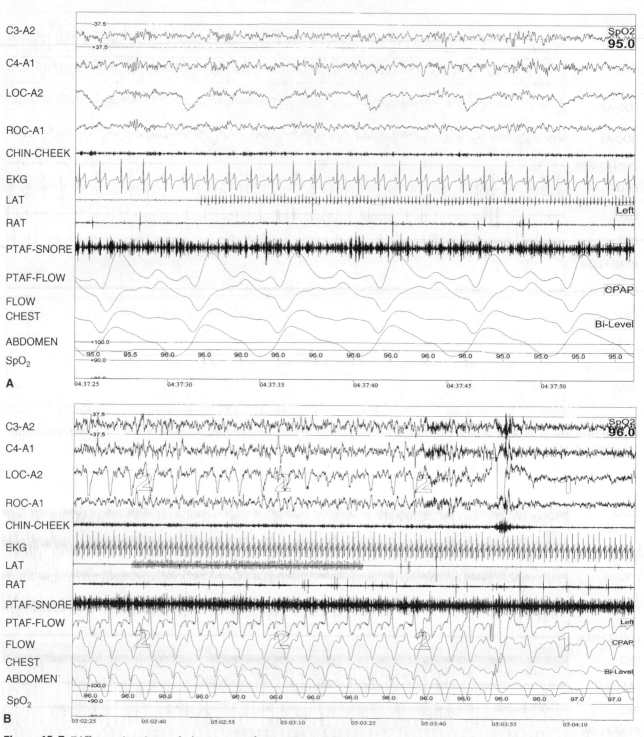

Figure 19-7 Different time intervals (A: 30 seconds; B: 120 seconds; C:300 seconds), recorded from the same patient of sustained motor bursts that last over 30 seconds and then repeat. Although these appear periodic the EMG activity continues far too long to meet standard criteria for PLMS. This activity represents fragmentary myoclonus.

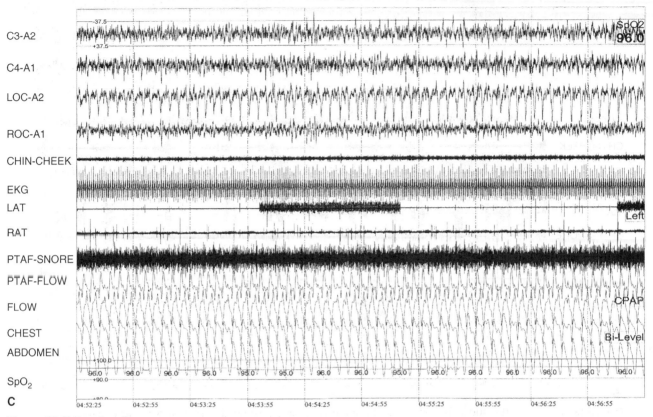

Figure 19-7 (*continued*)

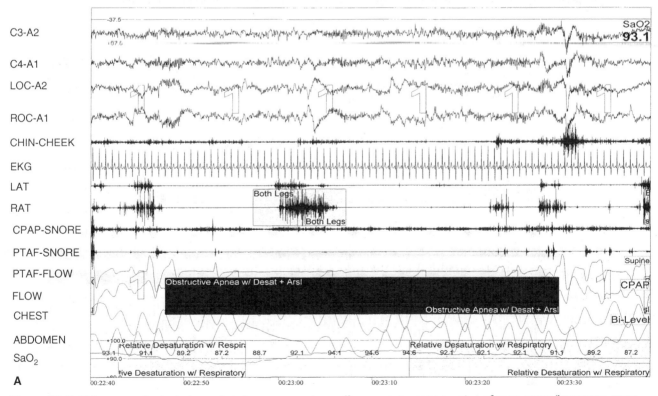

Figure 19-8 Thirty seconds. An independent leg movement as well as a movement occurring after an apnea/hypopnea event. It is important to avoid scoring leg movements that occur at the end of respiratory events as PLMS.

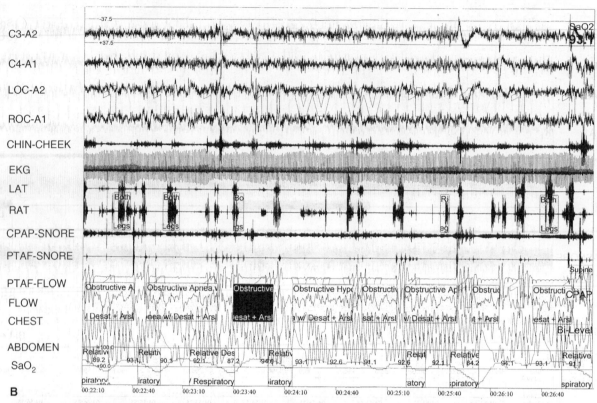

Figure 19-8 (*continued*) A 300-second recording from the same patient shows the respiratory events causing leg movements at the termination of the apnea or hypopnea events. In the middle of the obstructive respiratory events, note the presentation of independent limb movements, only a few of which are associated with arousal.

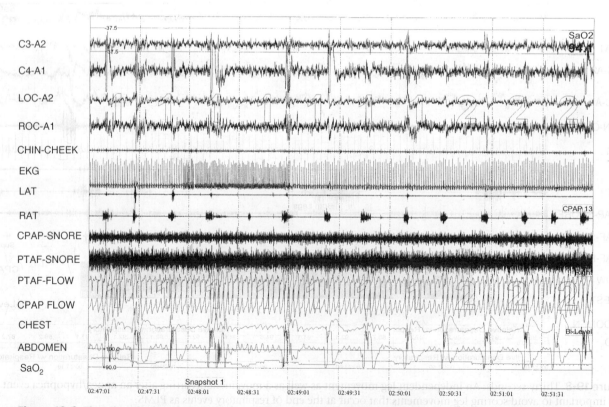

Figure 19-9 Three hundred seconds. Patient on CPAP at 13 cm H₂O. PLMS are seen in the RAT channel, but there are also minor changes in the respiratory belt and airflow channels, with mild O₂ desaturations. The limb movements were scored as PLMS, along with intermittent respiratory events. The limb movements did not appear to be related to the respiratory events because increased CPAP levels, as high as 10 cm H₂O, did not change the limb movements.

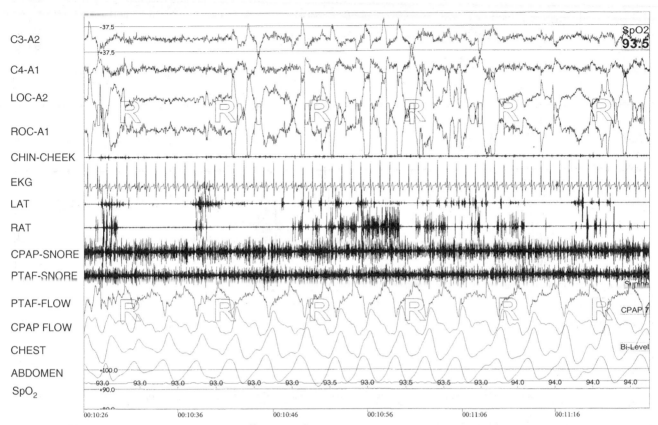

Figure 19-10 Sixty seconds. Patient effectively treated with CPAP at 7 cm H_2O who had REM sleep rebound. Increased motor activity is seen during REM sleep, but the movements do not appear to be stereotypical PLMS.

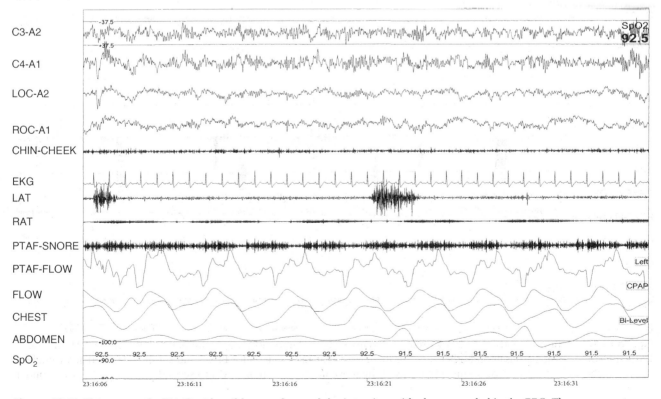

Figure 19-11 Thirty seconds. PLMS with mild to moderate alpha intrusion with sleep recorded in the EEG. The movements were classified as non-arousing events, even with the occurrence of aloha activity because the alpha activity did not change in frequency or amplitude with the anterior tibialis movements.

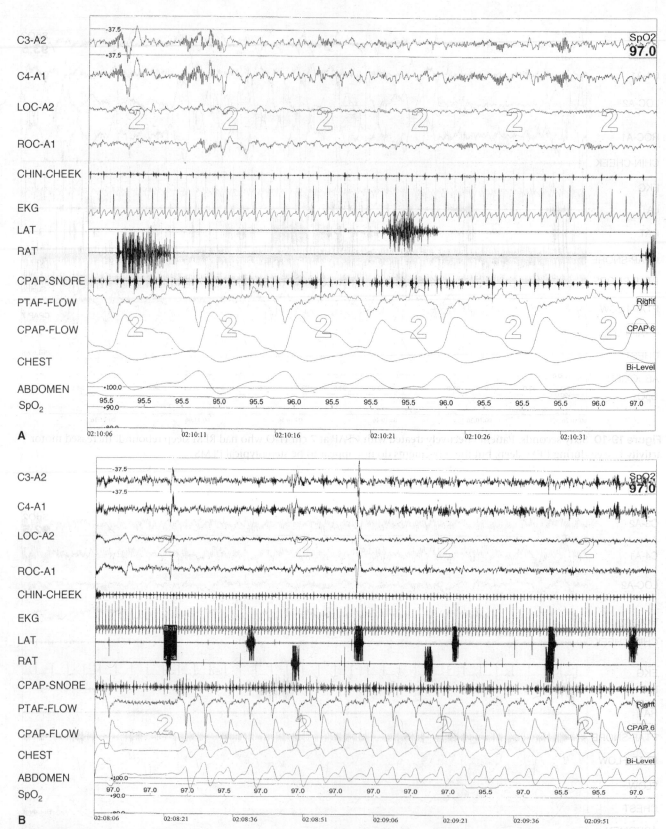

Figure 19-12 A: Thirty seconds. B: One hundred and twenty seconds. Limb movements alternating between the LAT and the RAT, with some causing arousals and others not. All the movements meet criteria for PLMS and should be scored accordingly. In B, note the difference in intermovement intervals of the movements seen on the LAT (15 seconds) and the RAT (25 seconds).

SUMMARY

RLS and PLMS are common, affecting up to 10% of adults. Although they are two separate disorders, RLS patients usually have PLMS, but an individual with PLMS on a PSG probably does not have RLS. Because a PSG is commonly recorded in older individuals, PLMS may occur in 25% or more of those undergoing PSG. To determine whether PLMS are significant, EEG must be simultaneously recorded to identify movements that result in significant EEG disturbances.

Ongoing research is underway that may determine whether PLMS have cardiovascular consequences, including higher rates of hypertension. The clinical relevance of PLMS continues to be studied, although current opinion suggests that symptoms of insomnia or hypersomnia do not frequently become clinically significant when other sleep disorders such as apneas are excluded. Dopamine agonists are considered to be the first-line treatment for RLS and will also reduce PLMS.

REFERENCES

1. Allen, R. P., Picchietti, D., Hening, W. A., et al. (2003). Restless legs syndrome: Diagnostic criteria, special considerations, and epidemiology: A report from the restless legs syndrome diagnosis and epidemiology workshop at the National Institutes of Health. *Sleep Medicine, 4*(2), 101–119.
2. Coccagna, G., Vetrugno, R., Lombardi, C., et al. (2004). Restless legs syndrome: An historical note. *Sleep Medicine, 5*(3), 279–283.
3. Ekbom, K. A. (1945). Restless legs syndrome. *Acta Medica Scandinavica, 158* (Suppl.), 122.
4. Symonds, C. P. (1953). Nocturnal myoclonus. *Journal of Neurology, Neurosurgery Psychiatry, 16*(3), 166–171.
5. Ambrosetto, C., Lugaresi, E., Coccagna, G., et al. (1965). Clinical and polygraphic remarks in the syndrome of restless legs. *Rivista Patologia Nervosa Mentale, 86*(2), 244–252.
6. Coleman, R. M., Bliwise, D. L., Sajben, N., et al. (1982). Daytime sleepiness in patients with periodic movements in sleep. *Sleep, 5*(Suppl. 2), S191–S202.
7. Zucconi, M., Ferri, R., Allen, R., et al. (2006). The official World Association of Sleep Medicine (WASM) standards for recording and scoring periodic leg movements in sleep (PLMS) and wakefulness (PLMW) developed in collaboration with a task force from the International Restless Legs Syndrome Study Group (IRLSSG). *Sleep Medicine, 7*(2), 175–183.
8. Bara-Jimenez, W., Aksu, M., Graham, B., et al. (2000). Periodic limb movements in sleep: State-dependent excitability of the spinal flexor reflex. *Neurology, 54*(8), 1609–1616.
9. Michaud, M., Paquet, J., Lavigne, G., et al. (2002). Sleep laboratory diagnosis of restless legs syndrome. *European Neurology, 48*(2), 108–113.
10. American Academy of Sleep Medicine. (2014). *International classification of sleep disorders* (3rd ed.). Darien, IL: Author.
11. Montplaisir, J., Boucher, S., Nicolas, A., et al. (1998). Immobilization tests and periodic leg movements in sleep for the diagnosis of restless leg syndrome. *Movement Disorders, 13*(2), 324–329.
12. Littner, M. R., Kushida, C., Anderson, W. M., et al. (2004). Practice parameters for the dopaminergic treatment of restless legs syndrome and periodic limb movement disorder. *Sleep, 27*(3), 557–559.
13. Vignatelli, L., Billiard, M., Clarenbach, P., et al. (2006). EFNS Task Force: EFNS guidelines on management of restless legs syndrome and periodic limb movement disorder in sleep. *European Journal of Neurology, 13*(10), 1049–1065.
14. Aurora, R. N., Kristo, D. A., Bista, S. R., et al. (2012). The treatment of restless legs syndrome and periodic limb movement disorder in adults—An update for 2012; Practice parameters with an evidence-based systematic review and meta-analysis. *Sleep, 35*(8), 1039–1062.

chapter 20
Movement Disorders

MATTHEW LEE UHLES   RAMAN K. MALHOTRA

LEARNING OBJECTIVES

On completion of this chapter, the reader should be able to:

1. Possess a practical understanding and classification of different motor events, behaviors, or phenomena that may occur in sleep.
2. Describe the polysomnographic findings of these conditions and their utility in diagnosis and differential diagnosis.
3. Define the importance of video-polysomnography and the use of other laboratory tests.

KEY TERMS

Polysomnography (PSG)
Video polysomnography (VPSG)
Movement disorders

In recent years, there has been a growing awareness and interest in sleep-related problems. It is being increasingly recognized that there are several different kinds of movements, behaviors, or phenomena that may occur in sleep. These can range from a variety of physiologic to pathologic conditions with a wide variety of manifestations. Some behaviors or movements are more likely to be associated with a specific state or stage of sleep. This chapter includes a basic approach to a patient who presents with abnormal events or behaviors in sleep. It focuses predominantly on the roles of polysomnography (PSG) or video-polysomnography (VPSG) and the technologist in the differential diagnostic process of "motor events in sleep."

APPROACH TO A PATIENT WITH MOVEMENT DISORDER IN SLEEP

Because many of the disorders associated with motor movements during sleep are sporadic in nature, accurate identification and diagnosis can be clinically challenging. As a result, a detailed sleep and medical history including general medical, neurologic, psychiatric, social, and family history all form the foundation in the assessment of patients with complaints of movement disorders during sleep. Particular attention should be given to the age of onset, time of night, pattern, duration, and frequency of the abnormal motor movement or behavior (1). In most cases, the patient is asleep and unaware during the time of the motor event; therefore, it is often beneficial to include the patient's bed partner or parent (in case of a child) at the time of the clinical interview. Often, the observer can provide more detailed observations regarding the motor event and the patient's state of mind immediately following the event. With the wide availability of personal video recorders, capable of low light recording, home recording may be used for the purpose of providing the clinician with a detailed illustration of the motor event within the patient's home. Vignatelli et al. reported that trained observers were able to correctly identify nocturnal frontal lobe epilepsy (NFLE) associated with major body movements using video recording alone, but video recording alone lacked the specificity in those cases associated with brief or minor body movements (2).

The *International Classification of Sleep Disorders*, 3rd edition (*ICSD-3*) lists 10 core categories of parasomnias with only one, rapid eye movement (REM) behavior disorder (RBD), requiring VPSG as an essential diagnostic requirement (3). VPSG is useful in distinguishing parasomnias such as sleepwalking or RBD from disorders such as NFLE or potentially injurious or atypical behaviors (i.e., unusual age of onset, duration, frequency, or occurrence) (1, 4). Fois et al. demonstrated that the utility of VPSG in these types of presentations was as high as 40% (5). Therefore, VPSG should be considered for patients with unusual nocturnal events that are potentially harmful or suggestive of another underlying disorder (6). If the patient is taking benzodiazepines or antidepressants, VPSG may need to be conducted after they are appropriately weaned from these medications as they may inhibit clinical manifestations during the testing (5).

Correlation of an event with the time of the night and the correct sleep stage is essential for correct diagnosis of motor events. For example, arousal disorders typically occur in the first third of the night during stage

N3 slow-wave sleep (SWS); RBD occurs during REM sleep usually in the last half to third of the night; epileptic seizures are more common during nonrapid eye movement (NREM) sleep; rhythmic movement disorder usually occurs during sleep–wake transitions; and in dissociative disorders, patients may appear to be asleep, but the PSG reflects an electroencephalographic (EEG) pattern of wakefulness.

Today, most commercially available PSG systems provide digital video recording synchronized with the PSG signals, which helps time-lock the motor events to the PSG signals. It also allows for a segment of PSG to be reviewed at varying paper speeds (window durations), filters, sensitivities, and montages, which help in the detection of abnormalities and differentiation from artifacts. The infrared camera is useful for recording nighttime events. Double cameras may be used to capture the face and body simultaneously. The camera should be mounted on the wall or ceiling across from the head end of the bed. An intercom with a microphone near the patient must be available for audio recordings. The monitoring station should have a remote control, which can zoom or tilt the camera for adequate viewing. Video recordings can be played back in real time or at a slower speed to better visualize and analyze the section of interest. Digital video recordings are the preferred method for synchronized PSG and video data storage for later recall and review. Although the minimum required by the American Academy of Sleep Medicine (AASM) is 1 frame per second, the digital video should be recorded with sufficient resolution and frame rate to allow for adequate visualization during review to differentiate subtle movements and establish proper temporal relationship (3). The standard indications for PSG are outlined in the published guidelines by the AASM. Table 20-1 lists the indications for VPSG (7).

In routine PSG recordings, most laboratories utilize six EEG channels (F3-M2, F4-M1, C3-M2, C4-M1, O1-M2, and O2-M1) with electrodes placed in these locations according to the International 10-20 System of Electrode Placement (3). Although the EEG electrodes routinely used in PSG are typically insufficient to accurately identify and localize abnormal EEG activity, abnormal motor activity is often observed in cases where the patient's clinical history did not indicate the possibility of this activity. In these cases, it may be helpful to re-reference from the standard contralateral derivation (F3 referenced to M2) to ipsilateral deviations (F3-M1). This allows for better verification and possible localization of the epileptiform activity. Extending scalp leads to include the full 10 to 20 EEG is typically required to better differentiate patients whose motor movements are due to epileptiform activity arising from other etiologies.

VPSG combines video recording with an extended EEG montage, PSG monitoring, and at times additional electromyographic (EMG) electrodes. It is superior to

Table 20-1	Indications for Video-Polysomnography
• Unusual and complex arousal disorders
• Complex behaviors suspicious of RBD but not absolutely certain based on the history
• Behavior and motor events at night suggesting possible nocturnal seizure disorder
• Excessive daytime sleepiness in patients with epilepsy to determine if excessive sleepiness is due to repeated nocturnal seizures, an undesirable side effect of antiepileptic medications, or an associated sleep disorder (e.g., sleep apnea)
• Suspected psychogenic dissociative disorder
• Other motor parasomnias which may be mistaken for nocturnal seizures, for example, rhythmic movement disorder, bruxism
• Involuntary diurnal movement disorder persisting during sleep
• Coexisting second sleep disorder, for example, narcolepsy, RBD, obstructive sleep apnea, or sleepwalking
• For medicolegal purposes, when the patient presents with violent behavior during sleep, video-polysomnography studies are mandatory to evaluate such patients for making a correct diagnosis of parasomnias or seizure disorders

RBD, REM behavior disorder.
Reprinted from Chokroverty, S. (2003). Polysomnography and related procedures. In M. Hallett (Ed.), *Handbook of clinical neurophysiology: Movement disorders* (Vol. 1, 1st ed., p. 145). Amsterdam, The Netherlands: Elsevier. Copyright © 2003 Elsevier. With permission.

conventional PSG for the evaluation of parasomnias, nocturnal seizures, and other motor events in sleep because of the increased capability to identify and localize EEG abnormalities and to correlate the observed motor behavior with EEG and PSG variables (8). Watember et al. demonstrated that adding video recording to routine EEGs increases the diagnostic yield of routine EEGs in children with frequent paroxysmal events (9). The specific montage used varies depending on the indication for the study, the number of channels available for EEG, and the need to record additional PSG parameters. Table 20-2 lists a few sample recording montages that can be further customized as required (10). Foldvary et al. showed that seizure detection was better using 7 and 18 channels (sensitivity of 82% and 86%, respectively) rather than 4 EEG channels (sensitivity of 67%) in patients with temporal lobe seizures; the same was not true for frontal lobe seizures, in which accuracy was similar regardless of the number of EEG channels available (11). A follow-up study by Foldvary et al., exploring accuracy of the 8-channel montage recommended by the American

Table 20-2 Sample Electroencephalographic–Polysomnographic Montages

Indication	Montage
Arousal disorder, possible nocturnal seizures (36 channels)	F3-M2, F4-M1, C3-M2, C4-M1, O1-M2, O2-M1, Fp1-F7, F7-T3, T3-T5, T5-O1, Fp1-F3, F3-C3, C3-P3, P3-O1, Fp2-Fp8, F8-T4, T4-T6, T6-O2, Fp2-F4, F4-C4, C4-P4, P4-O2, Fz-Cz, Cz-Pz, LEOG-M2, REOG-M1, Chin EMG, LAT EMG, RAT EMG, snoring, PTAF, thermistor, thoracic effort, abdominal effort, ECG, SaO$_2$
RBD, possible nocturnal seizures (28 channels)	F3-M2, F4-M1, C3-M2, C4-M1, O1-M2, O2-M1, Fp1-F7, F7-T3, T3-T5, T5-O1, Fp2-Fp8, F8-T4, T4-T6, T6-O2, LEOG-M2, REOG-M1, Chin EMG, LAT EMG, RAT EMG, LED EMG, RED EMG, snoring, PTAF, thermistor, thoracic effort, abdominal effort, ECG, SaO$_2$
RBD, possible nocturnal seizures (38 channels)	F3-M2, F4-M1, C3-M2, C4-AM1, O1-M2, O2-M1, Fp1-F7, F7-T3, T3-T5, T5-O1, Fp1-F3, F3-C3, C3-P3, P3-O1, Fp2-Fp8, F8-T4, T4-T6, T6-O2, Fp2-F4, F4-C4, C4-P4, P4-O2, Fz-Cz, Cz-Pz, LEOG-M2, REOG-M1, Chin EMG, LAT EMG, RAT EMG, LFD EMG, RFD EMG, snoring, PTAF, thermistor, thoracic effort, abdominal effort, ECG, SaO$_2$
PLMS, extended limb coverage (24 channels)	F3-M2, F4-M1, C3-M2, C4-M1, O1-M2, O2-M1, LEOG-M2, REOG-M1, Chin EMG, LAT EMG, RAT EMG, LPT EMG, RPT EMG, LED EMG, RED EMG, LFD EMG, RFD EMG, snoring, PTAF, thermistor, thoracic effort, abdominal effort, ECG, SaO$_2$

ECG, electrocardiogram; EMG, electromyogram; EOG, electrooculogram; L, left; LAT, left anterior tibialis; LED, left extensor digitorum; LFD, left flexor digitorum; LPT, left posterior tibialis; R, right; RAT, right anterior tibialis; RED, right extensor digitorum; RFD, right flexor digitorum; RPT, right posterior tibialis; PTAF, pressure transducer airflow.
Modified from Malow, B. A., & Aldrich, M. S. (2003). Polysomnography. In S. Chokroverty, W. A. Hening, & A. S. Walters (Eds.), *Sleep and movement disorders* (1st ed., p. 128). Philadelphia, PA: Butterworth-Heinemann. Copyright © 2003 Elsevier. With permission.

Clinical Neurophysiology Society (addition of T3 and T4 to standard PSG EEG electrodes), showed the abbreviated 8-channel montage was only slightly inferior to the 18-channel montage regarding interpreter agreement distinguishing seizure activity from nonepileptic activity (78% agreement for 8 channel and 84% agreement for 18 channel) (12). The 8-channel montage, however, was not as effective in localizing the seizure activity as the 18-channel montage (27% and 49%, respectively), especially in the temporal and parieto-occipital regions.

Adjunct EMG channels to record from additional muscles are recommended in special situations. In patients with preliminary diagnosis of RBD, adding electrodes over the forearm flexor and extensor muscles aids in detecting upper extremity movements. These electrodes are placed 2 to 3 cm apart in line with the lateral edge of the belly of the forearm flexor (outside of the underside of the forearm) and belly of the forearm extensor (center of the topside of forearm) (Figs. 20-1 and 20-2) (13). Proper localization of these muscle groups can be verified by asking the patient to bend only at the base of the fingers, avoiding bending at the distal joints, and extend the fingers backward without moving the wrists, to identify the flexor and extensor muscles, respectively (3). Although bruxism can be accurately identified with standard chin EMG derivations recording mentalis and submentalis muscles, the addition of at least one masseter electrode aids in accurately identifying sleep bruxism (SB). The masseter

muscle is best located by palpating the belly of the muscle several centimeters in front of the ear while the patient clenches the teeth. The recording pair can be either a single electrode placed over the center of the belly of the masseter referenced to one of the standard chin EMG leads or two masseter electrodes placed 2 to 3 cm apart in line with the direction of the muscle fibers referenced to one another (3, 13). In cases of propriospinal myoclonus (PSM), additional EMG electrodes (sternocleidomastoid, intercostal, deltoid, orbicularis oculi, and rectus abdominis) to record the progression of muscle activation can be useful to

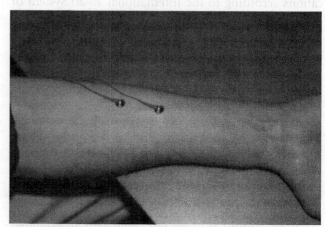

Figure 20-1 Proper placement of electrodes on the forearm flexors, 2 to 4 cm apart in line to the lateral edge of the belly of the forearm flexor (outside of the underside of the forearm).

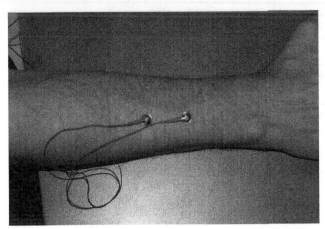

Figure 20-2 Proper placement of electrodes on the forearm extensors for evaluation of parasomnia during a sleep study.

differentiate between organic and psychogenic etiologies (14, 15). Finally, placing a pair of electrodes along the back of the neck over the paraspinal muscles may be useful when rhythmic movement disorder is suspected (3).

VPSG may help define and classify abnormal nocturnal motor events and behaviors into different diagnostic entities, as listed in Table 20-3. Frequently, many nocturnal motor events may be mistaken for seizures on the basis of history alone, for example, confusional arousals, sleep terrors, bruxism, rhythmic movement disorder, or RBD. These conditions can be diagnosed and differentiated from one another on the basis of characteristic clinical features combined with the use of VPSG. The major disadvantage of VPSG is the cost of the study: the technologist time needed to place an extended EEG montage and then continuously observe the patient throughout the study. Interpretation of PSG with video and extended EEG montage requires skills in both sleep medicine and seizure recognition.

INDICATIONS FOR VPSG

Observation of the EEG and EMG patterns preceding, during, and following the events is important to enhance accurate diagnosis. Unfortunately, because of their sporadic and unpredictable occurrence, nocturnal motor spells are difficult to capture within the controlled environment of the sleep center. The chance of capturing a motor event increases with the increasing frequency of home occurrence of the abnormal motor event. For these reasons, as well as the alterations in naturally occurring sleep patterns of "first night effect," it has been suggested that one night in the sleep center is insufficient for diagnostic purposes for suspected nocturnal motor events. Therefore, some sleep centers schedule patients for two consecutive nights to maximize the

yield of recording an event. Alternatively, a few reports have suggested that one night is sufficient to confirm a diagnosis (5, 16).

Several studies have reported increasing the likelihood of capturing a nocturnal motor spell during VPSG by priming the patient using a variety of different means, including sleep deprivation, medication, alcohol, noise, and baiting (17). Sleep deprivation has long been a standard tool in increasing the yield of documenting abnormal EEG activity in seizure patients. With the high correlation of sleepwalking associated with stage N3 sleep, coupled with the SWS rebound observed on nights following sleep deprivation, several researchers have experimented with sleep deprivation to prime sleepwalking patients. Several studies with sleep deprivation periods of 24, 25, and 38 hours significantly increased the number of sleepwalking episodes in sleepwalkers (18–21). Only one study failed to show an increase in sleepwalking episodes after 36 hours of sleep deprivation (22). Most of these studies involved recovery sleep periods occurring during daytime hours in patients who habitually slept at night. Given that REM rebound is often observed following sleep deprivation, this technique may also increase the likelihood of observing an RBD episode in the sleep center. Although there are no controlled studies to date using medications or alcohol to elicit motor events, there are published reports of medications and/or alcohol associated with sleepwalking (17, 23). Presentation of a loud sound during stage N3 sleep for NREM motor events and during REM for REM-related motor events has been reported to trigger motor events (17). Pilon et al. even combined the use of a loud stimulus with 25 hours of sleep deprivation to elicit sleepwalking spells in 100% of the 10 patients, in which they attempted this technique (19). In the case of sleep-related eating disorder (SRED), placing a table with the patient's preferred food and drink beside the bedside was demonstrated to evoke episodes of documented sleep eating in 26 out of 35 patients (24).

TECHNICAL CONSIDERATIONS

Patient Safety

The increased risk of injury in patients with unexplained nocturnal motor activity requires that appropriate precautions be incorporated to ensure the safety of the patient during a PSG (25). The greatest risk of patient injury is from a sudden motor movement with the patient leaping or falling out of bed. The monitoring technologist should remain alert and attentive throughout the recording, remaining vigilant to intervene immediately if he or she perceives a potential risk to the patient. To reduce response time, it is recommended to locate the patient in the room closest to the technologist monitoring

Table 20-3 Movement Disorders Stage and Characteristics

Disorder	Stage of Sleep	Other Characteristics
Confusional arousals	Predominantly N3, but any NREM	↑ Arousal out of N3/N1 theta/poorly reactive alpha
Sleep terrors	Predominantly N3, but any NREM	↑ Arousal out of N3/often associated with ≠ heart and respiratory rate. Limited recall.
Sleepwalking	Predominantly N3, but any NREM	↑ Arousal out of N3/N1 theta/poorly reactive alpha. Limited recall.
Nightmare	REM sleep	↑ REMs and mild ≠ heart and respiratory rate. Often associated dream recall.
REM behavior disorder	REM sleep	↑ Tonic or phasic activity during REM. Often associated dream recall.
Dissociative disorder	Wakefulness	Wakefulness before, during, and after event
Sleep-related eating disorder	Predominantly N3, also NREM/REM	↑ Arousal out of N3
Bruxism	All stages	Typical electromyographic artifact/audible tooth grinding
Rhythmic movement disorder	Typically transitional sleep, but any stage	Repetitive/stereotyped rhythmic movement
Epileptic seizures	NREM > REM	Sharps, spikes, or slow waves on EEG
Pseudoseizures	Wakefulness	No epileptiform activity noted
Propriospinal myoclonus	Sleep onset	Muscular jerks during transition from wakefulness to sleep
Excessive fragmentary myoclonus	All stages	Brief myoclonic potentials lasting >10 min
Sleep starts	Sleep onset	Sudden, brief, simultaneous contractions
Hypnagogic foot tremor	Sleep onset, N1 and N2	Rhythmic movement of feet and toes
Alternating leg muscle activation	All stages	Brief alternating leg movements
Myoclonus of infancy	All stages	Bilateral large myoclonic jerks in infants
Panic attacks	Typically transition from N2 to N3	↑ Sleep latency, ↑ wake after sleep onset, accompanied by other panic attack symptoms
Posttraumatic stress disorder	All stages	↓ Total sleep time, ↑ awakenings, ↓ sleep efficiency
		↓ REM and ↑ REM density

EEG, electroencephalography; NREM, nonrapid eye movement; REM, rapid eye movement.
↑=increase in designated measurement or observation; ↓=decrease in designated measurement or observation.

area. It is not always feasible for the technologist to react in time to prevent an injury to the patient. Therefore, universal seizure precautions are recommended. These precautions include keeping the bed as low to the floor as possible, removing any unnecessary equipment from the room, and maintaining constant observation. Some sleep centers recommend the use of bed rails or pillows to restrict the mobility of the patient during a nocturnal spell. Although these measures can impede the patient from leaving the bed, they can also trip the patient or (in case of bed rails) even increase the height from which the patient jumps out of bed. Thus, in some instances, these safety precautions may actually increase the likelihood of a patient injury (26). Individual sleep centers will need to develop their own policy regarding the use of rails or pillows. Patient injuries from striking sharp corners of furniture can be minimized by padding them with foam corners commercially available for nurseries. Any breakable room decorations (lamps, vases, etc.) that may injure the patient should be removed from the room. In extreme cases such as with a history of the patient diving out of bed, padding or a second mattress placed on the floor next to the patient's bed may further reduce the risk of injury.

Technologist Interactions

It is imperative for the technologist to provide detailed notes regarding his or her direct observation of the motor event. The observation notes should document the stage of sleep in which the event occurred and whether it was elicited or preceded by an arousal or any other stimulus. The technologist should refrain from drawing any conclusions in the notes but should objectively describe the observed behavior. It is helpful to describe the onset, progression, and duration of the event. Describing if the movement was repetitive, stereotypical, or unique is also helpful. If time allows, adjusting the camera to further isolate and highlight the motor event can facilitate classification. Because motor movement cases are sometimes associated with injuries to others, these cases sometimes result in medical–legal issues. Often, the sleep evaluation may precede the injury by months or even years. Therefore, the technologist should approach documentation in these cases with the same detail and rigor as if every case is a forensic one.

Often, the technologist's assessment and documentation of the patient's conscious state after the motor event is the key diagnostic component in accurately differentiating one motor event from another. Immediately following a motor event, the technologist should assess and document the patient's mental status and awareness without posing leading questions that may alter the patient's self-report. For example, following a motor event, the technologist should not ask "What were you dreaming about?" Instead the technologist could ask the more open-ended question "What thoughts or images were you just thinking before I entered the room?"

CHARACTERISTIC PSG FINDINGS IN "MOTOR EVENTS IN SLEEP"

PSG Findings in Motor Parasomnias
Disorders of Arousal (from NREM Sleep)

Disorders of arousal (DOA); confusional arousals, sleepwalking, and sleep terrors typically occur during stage N3 sleep, most commonly in the first third of nocturnal sleep, but can also occur later in the night and from other NREM sleep stages—even during daytime naps (27–30). Although diagnosis of a DOA is typically based only on clinical criteria, VPSG is often indicated if the patient has a history of nocturnal injury or to differentiate them from RBD or nocturnal seizures. Patients suffering from DOA do not typically have any recollection of their motor activity and do not usually report dream content correlating with their motor activity during sleep. Complex motor activity such as talking, eating, driving, and sexual activity has been shown to occur during NREM sleep parasomnias. Eyes are usually open during the event, although the patient may appear clumsy and confused (3).

Many times during a DOA, the EEG will be difficult to interpret secondary to artifact from movement, although the event in question should be preceded by NREM sleep. If the EEG is readable, it can continue to show a slow-wave pattern (delta waves) (Fig. 20-3). The EEG may also show NREM stage N1 theta patterns, repeated microarousals, or diffuse, slow, poorly reactive alpha rhythm, all indicating incomplete awakening (see Fig. 20-4) (27, 31–33). Sleep deprivation (the night before study) and forced awakenings during stage N3 sleep have been used by some to increase the chance of precipitating an episode during an overnight sleep study (19).

Sleep terrors are sudden episodes of terror occurring out of NREM sleep initiated by a cry or loud scream and accompanied by fear, confusion, and autonomic symptoms (rapid heart rate, rapid respiratory rate, and sweating). On PSG, sleep terror, in particular, is associated with tachycardia and increased respiratory rate in addition to the above-mentioned EEG findings, which can also be found in other arousal disorders.

Even if the typical episode of motor activity does not occur during the attended sleep study, a PSG is still helpful for identifying arousal disorders by displaying NREM sleep instability or long blocks of stage N3 sleep ending in spontaneous arousals (34). Lopez et al. recently published a quantified measurement of Slow Wave Sleep Fragmentation Index (SWSFI) (35). The SWSFI is the sum of SWS interruptions per hour of SWS. They demonstrated that 6.8 or more SWS interruptions per hour correlated with a diagnosis of DOA. The PSG is also useful in evaluating for possible underlying sleep disorders (obstructive sleep apnea and periodic limb movement disorder [PLMD]) that could be fragmenting sleep and precipitating the arousal disorder (Fig. 20-5).

Parasomnias Usually Associated with REM Sleep

RBD is characterized by abnormal motor behaviors appearing during REM sleep that lead to sleep disruption or even injury to the patient or bed partner. RBD typically occurs during the second half of nocturnal sleep when REM sleep is more prevalent. Many times the patient will remember dream content related to the

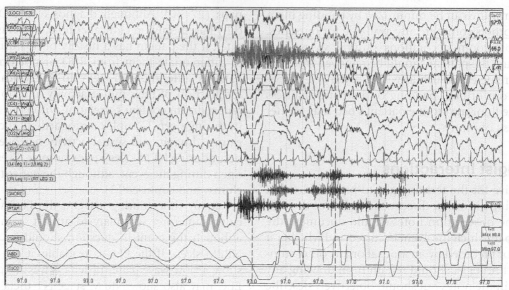

Figure 20-3 A 26-year-old female with a chief complaint of increase in episodes of sleepwalking, later found to be related to exacerbating factors of stress, sleep deprivation, and drug use. During overnight polysomnography (PSG), an event is captured where she awakens from stage N3 sleep and sits up in bed before later trying to get out of bed to walk. This 30-second PSG fragment is an example of electroencephalogram (EEG) findings that can be seen during a sleepwalking episode. Delta slowing on EEG is seen before the event and persists even as the patient is sitting up in bed and getting ready to sleepwalk.

motor activity displayed. The episodes are typically brief with rapid return to alertness or sleep. The characteristic abnormal behavior emerges from REM sleep, and the video may capture excessive limb movements, which may be rhythmic or arrhythmic. Common RBD actions during sleep include laughing, yelling, swearing, grabbing, punching, kicking, jumping, or running during

sleep. The eyes are usually closed during the event, and the patient rarely leaves the bedroom during an event. Episodes can vary in frequency from once every several months to as many as several times during the night (3).

A PSG may document an excessive amount of sustained EMG activity (tonic activity) in the chin or limbs when there is an epoch of REM sleep with at least 50%

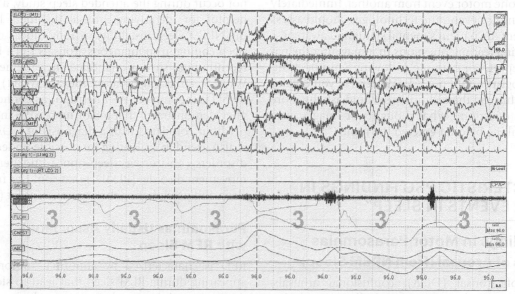

Figure 20-4 This 30-second video-polysomnography fragment is taken from a 30-year-old with a history of confusional arousals. Electroencephalogram during this episode of confusional arousal shows a change from preceding delta slowing to a mixed theta and alpha rhythm during the event, which can also be seen in arousal disorders.

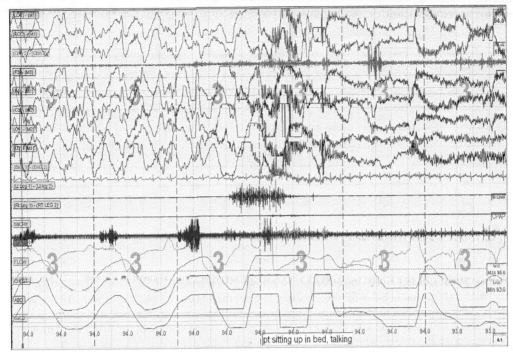

Figure 20-5 This is a 30-second video-polysomnography fragment of a 24-year-old patient with a history of sleepwalking and snoring. It displays an obstructive respiratory event (respiratory effort–related arousal) leading to arousal from stage N3 sleep and subsequent sleep talking and motor activity. Once the obstructive sleep apnea was treated with continuous positive airway pressure, sleepwalking events disappeared in this patient.

chin EMG amplitude greater than the minimum amplitude seen in NREM sleep (Fig. 20-6). Other times tonic activity is normal, but excessive transient muscle activity (phasic activity) in REM sleep is abnormally high (Fig. 20-7). This is defined when at least 50% of "mini-epochs" (3 seconds in duration) contain bursts of muscle activity lasting 0.1 to 5 seconds in duration, with EMG being at least four times higher than background EMG activity (3). Some patients almost exclusively have arm and hand movements during REM sleep, indicating the need for both upper extremity and lower extremity EMG monitoring for complete evaluation of RBD. The anterior tibialis, extensor digitorum, and forearm flexor muscles are typically used when measuring EMG from four limbs.

In order to meet criteria for RBD, the above-mentioned PSG findings must be in addition to either a clinical history of dream enactment behavior or complex motor behaviors noted during an overnight attended sleep study. When suspicious PSG findings without the aforementioned clinical history or complex behaviors are noted during the recording, it is consistent with REM sleep without atonia, also referred to as "subclinical" or "preclinical" RBD. Many of these patients (at least 25%) will eventually develop RBD (3). The use of antidepressants such as serotonin reuptake inhibitors and tricyclic antidepressants can cause PSG findings of REM sleep without atonia. REM sleep percentage and latency are usually preserved, although

many RBD patients have a higher percentage of stage N3 sleep. Autonomic nervous system activation is uncommon during REM sleep in RBD. Approximately 75% of RBD patients have periodic limb movements in sleep (PLMS) during NREM sleep (3).

A PSG during a nightmare may reveal increased amounts of REM and EMG twitches during REM sleep. There may also be a mild increase in heart rate or respiratory rate, but the marked tachycardia/tachypnea noted during a sleep terror is absent. In addition, patients with nightmares often have recollection of the event or dream, in contrast to amnesia for events typical of night terrors (3).

Status dissociatus manifests as an extreme form of state dissociation without identifiable sleep stages but with sleep and dream-related behaviors that closely resemble RBD. Parasomnia overlap disorder consists of RBD combined with a DOA (3). Diagnostic criteria for both RBD and a DOA must be met.

Other Parasomnias

Sleep-Related Dissociative Disorders

Dissociation is a defense mechanism whereby some elements are disconnected from other elements of the conscious experience. For instance, during a severe trauma, a person may dissociate the "observing self" from the "experiencing self," as if he or she were watching another

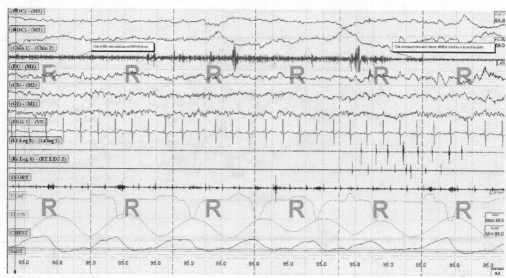

Figure 20-6 This is a 30-second video-polysomnography fragment of a 62-year-old complaining of dream enactment behavior during sleep. During this epoch of rapid eye movement (REM) sleep, there is sustained increased chin electromyogram (EMG) activity for over 50% of the epoch when compared with EMG tone during NREM sleep. This is an example of increased tonic muscle activity during REM sleep, which can be seen in patients with REM sleep behavior disorder.

person experience the trauma (31). A dissociative disorder is defined in the *Diagnostic and Statistical Manual of Mental Disorders*, 5th edition (*DSM-V*) as a disturbance in the integrated organization of consciousness, memory, identity, emotion, perception, body representation, motor control, and behavior. Some examples include dissociative identity disorder and dissociative amnesia with and without fugue. Sleep-related dissociative disorders

emerge throughout the sleep period during well-established wakefulness, either at the transition from wakefulness to sleep or within several minutes after an awakening from NREM or REM sleep (3). During the sleep period, patients with sleep-related dissociative disorders can scream, walk, run, and engage in self-mutilating and other violent behaviors. The episodes last several minutes to an hour or longer, often involving behaviors that represent

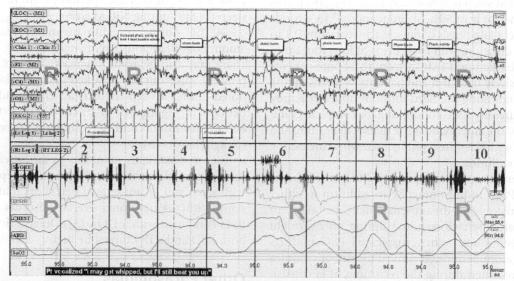

Figure 20-7 This is a 30-second video-polysomnography fragment from a 58-year-old with dream enactment behavior and vocalizations during sleep. There is an increase in excessive transient muscle activity during rapid eye movement (REM) sleep noted in this epoch consistent with increased phasic muscle activity during REM sleep, which can be seen in patients with REM sleep behavior disorder. Electromyogram (EMG) tone was greater than four times the background EMG tone accompanied by vocalizations from the patient. The epoch has been segmented into 10 (3 seconds) fragments for better visualization of the scoring rules.

reenactments of previous physical and sexual abuse situations. EEG wakefulness is present before, during, and after episodes. It is important to note that abnormal behaviors emerging shortly after an arousal from NREM sleep are not necessarily a dissociative disorder because DOA may also demonstrate an alpha rhythm during the event. The distinction between the two on a PSG can be made by recognizing the lag time of at least approximately 15 to 60 seconds between EEG arousal and behavior activation in dissociative disorder, as opposed to behaviors appearing immediately after the EEG arousal in DOA. In addition, the DOA typically have a shorter duration.

Sleep-Related Eating Disorder

SRED consists of recurrent episodes of involuntary eating and drinking during arousals from sleep with problematic consequences. This is currently listed as a separate diagnosis in the *ICSD-3*, whereas in past editions it was placed under sleepwalking or confusional arousal. Episodes can be triggered by stress, medical disorders, or drug use or withdrawal. Common characteristics include eating high-calorie foods, binge eating, and sloppy preparation. It can also include eating peculiar combinations of food or even toxic or inedible substances. The most common PSG findings are multiple confusional arousals, with or without eating, arising predominantly from stage N3 sleep but also from all stages of NREM sleep and rarely from REM sleep (3). Sleep architecture is generally preserved, although reduced sleep efficiency has been reported (24). PSG evaluations have been diagnostic of a primary sleep disorder in 80% of SRED cases. The sleep disorders most commonly associated with SRED are NREM sleep parasomnias (sleepwalking, sleep terrors, confusional arousals), obstructive sleep apnea syndrome (OSAS), restless legs syndrome (RLS), and PLMD. Another possible trigger is the use of hypnotics such as zolpidem (36–38). Primary SRED is associated with younger patients with a higher trend toward total amnesia of the episode as opposed to medication-induced episodes (39). SRED needs to be distinguished from night eating syndrome (NES), which occurs out of wakefulness, with full recollection of the events by the patient. However, a patient may have both SRED and NES.

PSG Findings in Sleep-Related Movement Disorder
Sleep-Related Bruxism

SB is defined in the *ICSD-3* as the presence of regular or frequent tooth-grinding sounds occurring during sleep with the presence of either abnormal tooth wear consistent with teeth grinding or transient morning jaw muscle pain or fatigue, headache, or jaw locking upon awakening (3). It can also cause sleep disturbance for both the patient and the bed partner, as the tooth-grinding sounds can be loud. There is high individual variability in the intensity and length of bruxism during sleep, although the intensity and frequency do not correlate with clinical signs and symptoms such as headaches or jaw pain. There is evidence suggesting a correlation between bruxism and stress and anxiety of the patient in both adults and children. Caffeine or cigarette use in the hours before sleep also increases the chance of bruxism. Bruxism is more common in childhood (14% to 17%) and decreases in prevalence over the life span. SB does tend to run in families, with 20% to 50% of affected individuals having at least one direct family member affected.

The diagnosis of SB is based on history and an orofacial examination, but a PSG may be indicated to demonstrate the disorder or exclude associated respiratory disturbance, RBD, night terrors, faciomandibular myoclonus, or epilepsy. In routine PSG recordings, bruxism is suggested by a typical EMG artifact recorded on EEG derivations, especially those referred to ear or mastoid electrodes. In addition to the routine chin EMG leads placed, masseter EMG electrodes may be added to better identify bruxism.

Traditionally, in routine PSG recordings, bruxism episodes have not been quantified but instead were reported by the technologist comments and description. Consistent objective scoring criteria for bruxism was not established until the publication of *The AASM Manual for the Scoring of Sleep and Associated Events: Rules, Terminology and Technical Specifications* in 2007 (40), and these scoring rules have been updated since then. Current criteria define bruxism events as either phasic (brief) or tonic (sustained) increases in the chin EMG activity, which is at least double the existing background activity of the chin EMG channel. If the events are phasic in nature, there must be at least three bursts of increased activity, each 0.25 to 2 seconds in duration. These phasic events are also referred to as "rhythmic masticatory muscle activity" (Fig. 20-8). For tonic bruxism episodes, the chin EMG activity must be maintained for at least 2 seconds in duration (3). Care should be given to distinguish sustained increases in chin EMG because of bruxism events as opposed to sustained chin EMG activity as a result of arousals. The technologist can further clarify by documenting audio or video verification of teeth grinding. Whether they are phasic or tonic bruxism events, the criteria require at least 3 seconds of stable reduced EMG activity before scoring another episode of bruxism. Bruxism can be scored reliably by audio in combination with a PSG by at least two audible tooth-grinding episodes per night in the absence of epilepsy. SB can occur during all sleep stages but is most common in stages N1 and N2 sleep (41, 42). There is sometimes an increase in the amplitude

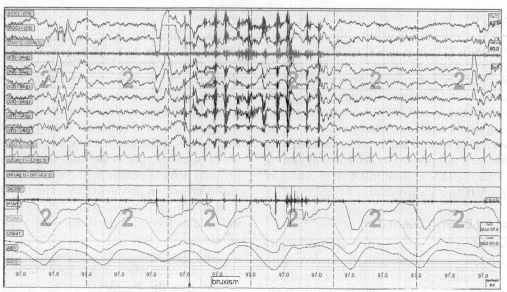

Figure 20-8 A 30-second video-polysomnography fragment showing rhythmic masticatory muscle activity of bruxism. There are several bursts of increased chin electromyogram activity, each lasting 0.25 to 2 seconds in duration. Audible teeth grinding was noted by the technician.

of respiration preceding the bruxism (43). Monitoring SB with ambulatory recordings has also been described (44).

Sleep-Related Rhythmic Movement Disorder

This disorder consists of repetitive, stereotyped, and rhythmic motor behaviors (not tremors) that involve large muscle groups and occur predominantly during drowsiness or sleep (3). In susceptible individuals, they may also occur during quiet relaxation. It is typically seen in infants and children and usually resolves by 10 years of age. It can persist in older individuals, especially those with developmental disabilities or other neurologic disorders, and has been associated with attention deficit disorder. There is a male predominance and a childhood prevalence of 5% to 15%. It comprises several subtypes, for example, body rocking, head banging, or head rolling. Leg-banging and leg-rolling types are also described along with combinations of the above-mentioned subtypes. Body rocking consists of whole body or torso rocking when the individual is on his or her hands and knees or sitting. Head banging occurs with the individual prone, repeatedly lifting the head and often banging the head on a pillow, mattress, or headboard. Head rolling usually occurs while the patient is supine with side-to-side movements of the head. These may rarely result in severe injuries including fractures, subdural effusions, and eye injuries (45). The behaviors are usually more disruptive to family members or bed partners because of the noise and disruption

to their sleep. The movements usually occur near sleep onset, although they may occur at other times of quiet wakefulness during the day.

The movements occur in clusters, with rhythmic movements repeating at a frequency of 0.5 to 2.0 per second with a minimum amplitude of two times the background EMG activity. There must be a minimum of four individual movements to make a cluster. A cluster usually lasts for less than 15 minutes (Fig. 20-9). If head banging is suspected, surface EMG electrodes can be placed on the paraspinal muscles on the back of the neck. Subjects are usually unresponsive during the episodes and amnestic of their occurrence on awakening. Diagnosis rests on the clinical presentation. In infants and very young children, it may need to be differentiated from bruxism or thumb sucking. Rarely, PLMD produces similar features. Sleep-related rhythmic movement disorder needs to be differentiated from seizures, which can be difficult by history alone. A PSG recording, first reported by Gastaut and Broughton and later by others, shows the presence of rhythmic movement artifact primarily in the immediate presleep period and during light NREM sleep stages, particularly in association with stage N2 sleep (27, 46, 47). The activity rarely has also been recorded in stage N3 sleep and REM sleep (48, 49). These diagnoses can be confirmed by VPSG recording. Underlying sleep-disordered breathing may also contribute to RMD, and treatment with continuous positive airway pressure may reduce the motor activity (50). RMD can also be seen in patients with RLS as a means to help relieve leg discomfort or in narcoleptic patients who are trying to end episodes of sleep paralysis.

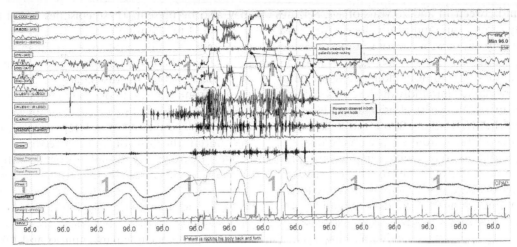

Figure 20-9 This is a 30-second video-polysomnography fragment in a 45-year-old male patient with a history of snoring and daytime sleepiness. The tracing displays one of many episodes of the patient rocking back and forth during brief arousals from sleep. These episodes were noted to occur out of stage N1, N2, and even rapid eye movement sleep. Episodes typically lasted from 3 to 15 seconds, although there were longer periods of rocking associated with prolonged wake periods.

PSG Findings in Epileptic and Nonepileptic (Pseudoseizure) Seizures

Epileptic Seizures

The close relationship between sleep and epilepsy has long been realized. Langdon-Down and Brain first classified seizures according to the time of the occurrence into diurnal, nocturnal, and diffuse types. In the late 19th century, Gowers documented that 21% of epilepsy patients had seizures exclusively during sleep, and 37% had a combination of diurnal and nocturnal epilepsies (51, 52). Several mechanisms have been proposed to explain this relationship and include the widespread neuronal synchronization in NREM sleep, which is conducive to the generation and propagation of discharges, the arousal mechanisms that may facilitate seizures by exacerbation of cortical hyperexcitability (as seen in juvenile myoclonic epilepsy and generalized tonic–clonic seizures on awakening, where seizures occur shortly after awakening), and finally the role of the anatomic substrate (e.g., in frontal lobe epilepsy patients, most seizures occur in sleep, whereas in temporal lobe epilepsy patients, most seizures occur in wakefulness).

Description of Different Types of Seizures

Benign Epilepsy of Childhood with Centrotemporal Spikes (Benign Rolandic Epilepsy)

Benign epilepsy of childhood is the most common partial epilepsy in children (53). Seizures begin around 7 years of age, are seen predominately in drowsiness and NREM sleep, are characterized by focal clonic twitchings, and often are preceded by perioral paresthesias. Consciousness is usually preserved. EEG reveals characteristic centrotemporal spike and wave discharges.

The spike activity is enhanced by sleep and in approximately 30% may be present only in sleep. The prognosis is excellent, and seizures generally stop by 15 to 20 years of age without neurologic sequelae.

Primary Generalized Tonic–Clonic Seizures (Grand Mal Epilepsy)

These seizures may occur only during sleep, may occur only during daytime, or may be diffusely distributed. Nocturnal seizures occur almost exclusively in NREM sleep, most frequently 1 to 2 hours after sleep onset and between 5 and 6 a.m., and disappear in REM sleep. Interictal discharges similarly increase in NREM sleep and disappear in REM sleep.

Juvenile Myoclonic Epilepsy

The typical presentation consists of generalized tonic–clonic seizures, which often occur in the first 1 or 2 hours after awakening. Seizures may also occur on awakening from sleep but are rare at other times of the day. Bilaterally synchronous myoclonic jerks occur frequently, particularly on awakening, although patients may not easily notice them (54). The age of onset is usually between 12 and 18 years. The characteristic EEG abnormality consists of generalized 4-to-6-Hz spike-wave and polyspike-wave complexes that occur increasingly at sleep onset and following awakening but are virtually nonexistent during the rest of the sleep cycle.

Nocturnal Frontal Lobe Epilepsy

NFLE presents a spectrum of clinical manifestations currently subgrouped into three seizure patterns, namely, paroxysmal arousals (PAs), nocturnal paroxysmal dystonia (NPD), and episodic nocturnal wandering (ENW). NFLE predominates in males. The age of onset centers around infancy or adolescence, but seizures become more frequent between 14 and 20 years of age. Seizures are frequently cryptogenic, and nearly 40% have a positive family history of one or more parasomnias. Seizures occur mainly during stages N1 and N2 sleep. Marked autonomic activation is a common finding during seizures. Patients display marked intraindividual stereotypy in the pattern of seizures. PAs consist of brief and sudden motor paroxysmal behavior lasting 2 to 20 seconds characterized by sudden arousal from sleep with eye opening, head raising, sitting up in bed with a frightened expression, and even utterance of a scream. NPD consists of a sudden arousal associated with complex motor dystonic–dyskinetic features lasting 20 seconds to 2 minutes. The associated complex motor behavior is characterized by movement of legs and arms, including kicking, cycling, rocking, ballistic flailing limb movements, dystonic posturing, or choreoathetoid movements of limbs and trunk. ENW episodes consist of stereotyped agitated somnambulism characterized by sudden ambulation from sleep, often with agitated behavior, talking, or screaming with a frightened expression. Dystonic movements of the limbs

may also be present. These episodes are of the longest duration (1 to 3 minutes).

The most challenging aspect of diagnosing NFLE is the fact that the ictal and interictal EEGs frequently fail to reveal epileptiform discharges because of the deep mesial frontal location of generated source. They are frequently misdiagnosed as parasomnias (confusional arousals, sleepwalking, and sleep terrors), particularly in children. The onset of episodes between 3 and 6 years of age, rare frequency (usually <1 per month), long duration of episodes (usually longer than 5 minutes), and disappearance before age 16 to 18 years are main features characterizing sleepwalking and sleep terrors as opposed to NFLE (55). The other differential diagnostic considerations include panic attacks and RBD. VPSG is mandatory to confirm the diagnosis (Fig. 20-10).

Continuous Spikes and Waves in Sleep

Continuous spikes and waves during slow-wave sleep (CSWS) is a syndrome originally called "electrical status epilepticus of sleep." It is characterized by generalized

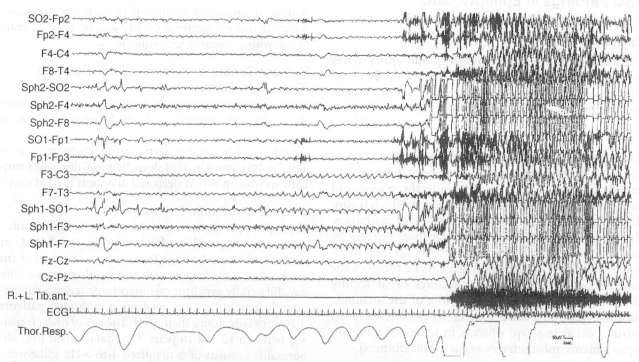

Figure 20-10 Nocturnal paroxysmal dystonia in nocturnal frontal lobe epilepsy. A 14-year-old girl presented with nocturnal episodes since age 12, characterized by head rising and complex motor automatism involving legs, arms, and trunk with dystonic postures. Seizures recurred several times a night, two to three times per month. Video-polysomnography recordings showed that at the beginning of the seizure, the patient opens her eyes, presents a deep inspiration while raising her head, then abducts her hyperextended upper limbs and presents rhythmic movements of limbs and trunk with back arching. The polysomnographic tracing shows this seizure arising from stage N2 sleep. The motor manifestation is preceded for 10 to 15 seconds by repetitive sharp waves on left anterior electroencephalogram (EEG) channels; then paroxysmal EEG activity is almost completely masked by muscle artifacts. During the seizure, tachycardia and modification of respiration occur. R. + L. Tib. Ant., right and left tibialis anterior; SO, supraorbital electrode; Sph, sphenoidal electrode; Thor. Resp, thoracic respiration. (Reprinted from Zucconi, M., Montagna, P., & Chokroverty, S. (2005). Sleep and epilepsy. In S. Chokroverty, R. Thomas, & M. Bhatt (Eds.), *Atlas of sleep medicine* (1st ed., p. 213). Philadelphia, PA: Butterworth-Heinemann. Copyright © 2005 Elsevier. With permission.)

spike–wave complexes at 2 to 2.5 Hz present for 85% to 90% of SWS and relatively suppressed during REM sleep and wakefulness. Seizures may have a variable presentation manifesting as nocturnal focal motor, generalized tonic–clonic, atypical absence, or myoclonic seizures. Emergence of CSWS is associated with neuropsychological regression, and disappearance of CSWS is associated with an improvement in neuropsychological function. The disorder may be cryptogenic or result from a variety of central nervous system lesions. These seizures are usually responsive to antiepileptic drugs and remit by middle teenage years.

Nonepileptic Seizures (Pseudoseizures)

Nonepileptic seizures occur most commonly in young adults and are three times more common in women than in men. The episodes are typically characterized by uncoordinated nonsynchronous bizarre motor movements, for example, pelvic thrusting, side-to-side head movements, and opisthotonic posturing. Screaming or talking during episodes may also occur. The spells are commonly emotionally triggered with a gradual onset and termination, may last for several minutes or even hours, and may lack the postictal confusion seen in epileptic seizures. Nonepileptic seizures are not common during sleep but may rarely occur on awakening from sleep at night. It is important to realize that certain features suggestive of autonomic activation and normally associated with epileptic seizures may also accompany nonepileptic seizures, for example, pupillary dilatation, Babinski responses, autonomic cardiorespiratory changes, injury, and urinary and fecal incontinence.

Interictal EEG recordings have limited utility in the diagnosis or exclusion of nonepileptic seizures. EEG recording during a spell is useful in documenting the absence of epileptiform discharges associated with the movements and the absence of postictal slowing. However, frequently, the EEG may be obscured because of muscle and movement artifacts. Long-term video-EEG recording is usually necessary to properly evaluate nonepileptic spells. Frequently, epileptic and nonepileptic seizures may coexist in the same person, and definite diagnosis requires video-EEG of all seizure types experienced by the patient. Furthermore, malingering and factitious seizures may present similarly and need to be differentiated with the help of history.

PSG Findings in Other Sleep-Related Disorders

Obstructive Sleep Apnea Syndrome

Patients with OSAS may have flailing and jerking limb and body movements in association with repeated apneas and hypopneas. Sometimes respiratory-related leg movements following apneas and hypopneas may occur in a repeated manner resembling PLMS. OSA-induced arousal from NREM sleep with complex or violent behaviors may be indistinguishable from primary DOA (confusional arousals, sleepwalking, and sleep terrors), nocturnal complex seizures, nocturnal dissociative states, or RBD (pseudo-RBD) (56, 57). Time-synchronized VPSG is essential for accurate diagnosis. OSA is also an increasingly recognized precipitant of sleepwalking (58). Nasal positive airway pressure therapy for OSA may result in SWS rebound with emergent confusional arousals, sleepwalking, or sleep terrors (59). OSA-induced arousals from NREM (or occasionally REM) sleep may trigger repeated episodes of SRED (37).

Fatal Familial Insomnia

Fatal familial insomnia is an autosomal dominant prion disease. It is a progressive disorder characterized by initial difficulties in falling asleep and maintaining sleep, spontaneous lapses from quiet wakefulness into a sleep state with enacted dreams, and loss of SWS features. Progressive autonomic hyperactivity with pyrexia, salivation, tachycardia, tachypnea, myoclonus, and tremor-like muscle activity are present (60). The 24-hour EEG recording shows progressive deterioration. In advanced cases, patients spend most of the recorded time in a nonwake/nonsleep-like state characterized by a combination of alpha and theta EEG activity, also defined as "subwakefulness." On PSG, there is severe disorganization of the cyclic sleep pattern, REM sleep may reveal a loss of muscle atonia and may occur abruptly, often associated with oneiric behavior (61, 62). NREM sleep may eventually be lost completely with loss of spindles and SWS. In the final stages of the disorder, the EEG becomes unreactive and progressively attenuated until death occurs. The disorder is fatal, usually within 8 to 72 months.

Drug-Related Nocturnal Dyskinesias

Dyskinesias are choreic movements seen in selected circumstances, such as drug side effect or toxicity. They are less intense and more frequent at night than during the day. When present at night, they generally occur during transitions from sleep to wakefulness and in light NREM sleep. The most frequent dyskinesia is related to levodopa (LD) use in patients with Parkinson disease (PD). Violent kicking and flailing limb movements in sleep are also reported with a high intake of LD. They tend to be associated with other behaviors like yelling and screaming and may need to be differentiated from RBD, sleep-related dissociative state, other parasomnias, and seizures (63). LD also enhances nocturnal myoclonus in patients with PD. Similarly, other dopaminergic drugs can produce involuntary movements in sleep. Myoclonus may be induced by a toxic serum level of lithium and the use of opiates or amitriptyline in PD patients. Neuroleptics are also well known to cause akathisia. Tics may be induced by neuroleptics, LD, stimulants, and anticonvulsants.

PSG Findings in Other Sleep-Related Issues

Propriospinal Myoclonus at Sleep Onset

PSM at sleep onset consists of sudden muscular jerks occurring in the relaxation period during transition from wakefulness to sleep, mainly involving the abdomen, neck, and trunk (64, 65). Owing to their association with sleep onset, these movements can result in insomnia or be associated with RLS (14, 66). PSG demonstrates brief myoclonic EMG bursts recurring nonperiodically, with alpha activity present on the EEG. The jerks disappear with onset of stage N2 sleep or with mental activation. PSG has demonstrated that the jerks arise first in the spinal-innervated muscles (usually thoracic or cervical spinal segments) and then spread to more rostral and caudal muscles according to a propriospinal pattern of propagation. Back-averaging of the EEG does not show any jerk-locked cortical activity. Interestingly, it has been shown in a recent study that the polymyographic patterns of PSM can be voluntarily mimicked and therefore additional studies, such as jerk-locked cortical potential, may be required to confirm the diagnosis of true PSM and distinguish it from movements that are functional or psychogenic in origin (67). Magnetic resonance imaging (MRI) of the spine in these patients can be abnormal in up to 20% of patients showing focal abnormalities.

Excessive Fragmentary Myoclonus

Excessive fragmentary myoclonus (EFM) is characterized by small movements of the fingers, toes, or corners of the mouth, or small muscle twitches resembling fasciculations that do not cause gross movement across a joint space. These movements are typically too small to be visible. Episodes of these myoclonic potentials typically last from 10 minutes to several hours. They often appear at sleep onset, continue through the NREM stages, and persist during REM sleep. On PSG, the motor activity consists of recurrent, brief (75 to 150 milliseconds) EMG potentials in various muscles of the face, trunk, arms, and legs, occurring asynchronously and asymmetrically on the two sides in a sustained manner. Electromyographically, they resemble physiologic phasic REM twitches but occur irregularly and not in clusters. More than five potentials per minute must be sustained for at least 20 minutes of NREM sleep (3, 68). The clinical significance of EFM remains uncertain as there are no consistently reported clinical consequences, and it can

be seen in patients with a variety of sleep disorders and in normal individuals. Recent data suggest that it may be a sign of peripheral nerve pathology, requiring patients to undergo neurophysiologic evaluation (nerve conduction studies/EMG) (69). It may occur in isolation or may be associated with other sleep disorders (70). EFM is typically differentiated from PLMS by a significantly shorter duration and lack of stereotypical periodicity, which defines PLMS. REM-related phasic twitches are confined to REM sleep, whereas EFM is observed during a minimum of 20 minutes of NREM sleep. Scoring and documentation of EFM is considered optional by AASM standards.

Sleep Starts (Hypnic Jerks)

Sleep starts are sudden, brief, simultaneous contractions of the body or one or more body segments occurring at sleep onset. They are of very common occurrence in the normal population, reported in as high as 70% of the general population, and are considered normal physiologic events (3). They may become more frequent with stimulant use, sleep deprivation, or emotional or physical stress. Occasionally, these are intensified in frequency or magnitude sufficiently to impair sleep onset or maintenance, which is considered pathologic, and termed "intensified hypnic jerks" (71). They may be accompanied by sensory feelings of falling into a void, flash of light, unexplained fear, and electric shock–like sensation or a dream. Purely sensory sleep starts in the absence of a body jerk have been described (72). The EEG correlates were initially described by Oswald in 1959. Gastaut and Broughton in 1965 described the surface EMG correlates (27). On PSG, superficial EMG recordings of the involved muscles show brief, myoclonic (generally 75 to 250 milliseconds), high-amplitude potentials, either singly or in succession. The EEG typically shows stage N1 sleep, sometimes accompanied by a vertex sharp wave. Sleep starts may be mistaken for epileptic myoclonus, EFM, PSM, startle disease, or PLMS. Hypnic jerks can be differentiated from EFM, in that EFM consists of repetitive brief jerks that occur not only at sleep onset but also throughout other sleep stages. The motor movements associated with PLMS are typically longer in duration and occur with the periodicity associated with PLMS observed during sleep. Purely sensory hypnic jerks may lead to an erroneous diagnosis of epileptic seizures or a psychiatric disorder. History of occurrence limited to sleep onset and PSG evaluation are helpful in differentiation.

Hypnagogic Foot Tremor and Alternating Leg Muscle Activation

Hypnagogic foot tremor (HFT) is a rhythmic movement of feet or toes (similar to nervous jiggling of foot with legs crossed) that occurs at the transition between wake and sleep or during light NREM sleep (stages N1 and N2). HFT may be relatively common and can be a normal finding. One study (73) reported a prevalence of at least 7.5% in patients obtaining a sleep study. In HFT, the leg movements cannot be better explained by any other sleep disorder.

Alternating leg muscle activation (ALMA) is a PSG pattern with unknown clinical significance. ALMA consists of brief activation of the tibialis anterior muscle in one leg in alternation with similar activation in the other leg during sleep or arousals from sleep (3). The pattern in ALMA is as if the patient was marching, left right, left right, and so on. Owing to the alternating pattern in ALMA, it is mandatory to record left and right leg EMG independently. As shown in Figure 20-11, ALMA is usually associated with arousals, occurring either immediately before or after the arousal (3). ALMA, however, may occur during any stage of sleep, independent of arousals, and is seen more often in patients taking antidepressants. HFT and ALMA are considered together because of the similarities in a number of their features. Scoring for both HFT and ALMA is considered optional by AASM standards.

In HFT, PSG demonstrates trains of recurrent 0.3-to-4-Hz EMG potentials or movements in one or both feet (3). In ALMA, PSG demonstrates a pattern of brief, repeated activation of the anterior tibialis in one leg alternating with similar activation in the other leg, occurring at a frequency of 0.5 to 3 Hz (usually 1 to 2 Hz). Similar to PLMS, both HFT and ALMA have a minimum series of at least four muscle bursts. In contrast with PLMS, both HFT and ALMA have a much shorter

interval between individual movements. Their maximum intervals of 3.3 and 2 seconds, respectively, are shorter than the minimum 5-second interval associated with PLMS. Their minimum intervals are almost equal at 0.25 seconds for HFT and 0.3 seconds for ALMA.

Summary of PSG Findings in Movement Disorders

Motor Event	Minimum No. in Series	Interval between Movements (seconds)	Duration of Movement (seconds)	Scoring
PLMS	4	5–90 (0.01–0.2 Hz)	0.5–10	Recommended
RBD	50%	3	0.1–5	Recommended
HFT	4	0.2–1	0.25 3	Optional
Bruxism	3	3	0.5–2	Recommended
RMD	4	2	0.5–2	Recommended
HFT	4	0.25–3.3 (0.3–4 Hz)	0.25–1	Optional
ALMA	4	0.3–2 (0.5–3 Hz)	0.1–0.5	Optional

Benign Sleep Myoclonus of Infancy

Benign sleep myoclonus of infancy is characterized by repetitive myoclonic jerks that occur during sleep in infants. The jerks are often bilateral and massive, typically involving large muscle groups, and they occur exclusively

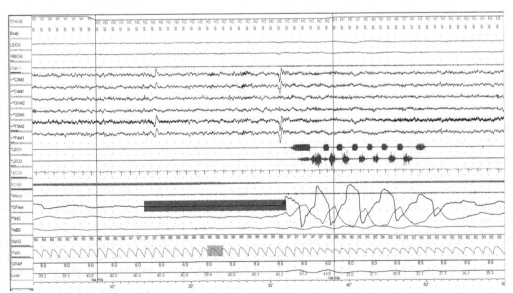

Figure 20-11 A 60-second video-polysomnography fragment showing a period of alternating leg muscle activation with electromyographic activity alternating between the left and right legs during arousal as a result of an apnea. The leg movements cease once the patient returns to sleep.

in sleep. Onset is usually between birth and 1 month of age and resolves in the vast majority by 1 year of age. VPSG has shown paroxysmal muscle activity without ictal or interictal EEG abnormalities. It occurs predominantly during NREM sleep but may also be present during REM sleep. The jerks are usually seen in clusters of four or five jerks per second, each jerk lasting 40 to 300 milliseconds. Awakening the infant leads to prompt, abrupt, and consistent cessation of the movements. Benign sleep myoclonus of infancy must be distinguished from myoclonic seizures, as misdiagnosis can lead to unnecessary treatment.

PSG Findings in Psychiatric Etiologies
Sleep-Related Panic Attacks

Sleep-related panic attacks are characterized by discrete periods of intense fear or discomfort upon awakening from sleep, associated with symptoms such as palpitations, sweating, trembling, shaking, shortness of breath, choking, chest pain, nausea, dizziness, fear of dying, tingling, or hot flashes. The panic attacks occur typically during transition from stage N2 to stage N3 sleep but can occur during any stage of sleep (74). Nocturnal panic attacks typically mirror episodes that occur during the day. Most patients with panic attacks during the day will have at least one sleep-related panic attack. Episodes last up to 10 minutes with preservation of memory of the event. A PSG may reveal a delay in sleep onset, increased wake after sleep onset, reduced sleep efficiency, and increased movement time (75). Unlike posttraumatic stress disorder (PTSD), there is no increase in REM density (76). Panic attacks may need to be differentiated from nightmares, sleep terrors, and epileptic nocturnal seizures, where VPSG plays an important role. Tachycardia and tachypnea (rapid respiratory rate) may be noted once the panic attack begins.

Posttraumatic Stress Disorder

PTSD is an anxiety disorder characterized by recurrent stereotypical anxiety dreams occurring in the aftermath of a psychological traumatic stressor (77). Frequent nightmares in NREM and REM sleep are typical of PTSD. Patients may strike out violently, make swinging limb movements, or even run out of bed during the reenactment of past traumatic events. Although disturbed sleep is a common complaint in patients with PTSD, PSG findings have failed to reveal consistent evidence of objective sleep disturbance. The reported PSG findings include decreased total sleep time, increased awakenings, reduced sleep efficiency, and reduced REM sleep and increased REM density (78–81), whereas others have reported no significant differences in PSG parameters between PTSD and non-PTSD patients (82, 83), postulating altered sleep perception rather than sleep disturbance per se. Unlike nightmares, motor behavior

associated with PTSD commonly appears out of NREM sleep, primarily stage N3 sleep.

PSG Findings in Diurnal Involuntary Movement Disorders

PD is a motor disorder characterized by resting tremor, rigidity, slow movements, and unsteady gait. The resting tremor associated with PD persists in stages N1 and N2 sleep but is typically absent in stage N3 or REM sleep. Sleep dysfunction in PD is reported in 70% to 90% of PD patients. Patients with PD have been found to have decreased stage N3 sleep and REM sleep along with increased sleep fragmentation (84). RBD is found in as many as half of PD patients (3).

Gilles de la Tourette syndrome is a condition involving multiple motor tics with vocalization that usually starts in childhood or adolescence. PSG shows increased body movements and motor tics during all sleep stages, most prominently in stages N1 and N2 sleep (85). Tourette patients have been reported to have impaired sleep with frequent awakenings, increased incidence of sleepwalking, and sleep terrors (86).

Hemifacial spasm is a synchronous, usually repetitive contraction of one side of face, thought to arise from damage to the facial nerve or nucleus. It persists during sleep, progressively decreasing as sleep gets deeper and becoming 80% less frequent in stage N3 and REM sleep (87).

Changes in sleep can be found early in *Huntington chorea* with deterioration with disease progression (88). Findings include sleep fragmentation and reduced sleep efficiency with mild reduction in REM sleep. Persistence of the involuntary movements in stages N1 and N2 sleep and reemergence during REM sleep may also be seen. Sleep spindles are increased and amplified in density (89).

OTHER DIAGNOSTIC TESTS

Ambulatory PSG

In laboratory attended VPSG is the accepted and gold standard test in the evaluation of patients with motor events in sleep. Utility of ambulatory PSG is also under consideration, given the lower cost. Ambulatory PSG systems are available today that can record extended EEG–PSG with synchronized video recordings. The major disadvantage of ambulatory VPSG is the absence of a technologist. The technologist is unable to make the necessary technical adjustments as may be required during the study for complete and meaningful data acquisition. In addition, the technologist is unable to document the clinical aspects of the motor event or behavior and assess the patient's status after the event which, as previously discussed, can significantly aid in the diagnostic process.

Actigraphy

Actigraphy is a technique of motion detection used to record activity during sleep and waking. It is very useful in the diagnosis of circadian rhythm sleep disorders, insomnias, and sometimes PLMS (90, 91). Actigraphy allows the continuous recording of rest/activity for extended periods. The limitations of actigraphy are the relative inability to differentiate between resting wakefulness and sleep periods, and the inability to discriminate and differentiate between the origins of various motor movements in sleep, for example, those resulting from PLMS, seizures, or dyskinesias. Current AASM Clinical Practice Guidelines do not recommend the use of actigraphy for evaluation of sleep-related movement disorders or parasomnias (92).

24-Hour Ambulatory EEG Recording

Ambulatory EEG recordings allow 24 hours of continuous EEG recording during a subject's routine activities. Recordings can be extended to 48 or 72 hours as necessary. Extended recording increases the possibility of capturing abnormal epileptiform activity. The major disadvantage is the absence of video documentation and clinical description in the event of a seizure.

Long-Term Video-EEG Recordings

Long-term video-EEG recordings provide clinical and EEG documentation of ictal events with video recordings performed in a monitored environment. This is the most definitive method of documenting the presence of true seizure or to confirm there are nonepileptic spells (93).

Neuroimaging

A neuroimaging study, in particular, MRI of the brain, is indicated when a neurologic illness or structural lesion is suspected as the underlying cause of abnormal motor events in sleep. All adults with new-onset seizures and children without characteristic epilepsy syndromes typically require a brain MRI to exclude the possibility of structural brain disorders. If someone presents with an abrupt-onset motor activity or has other concerning symptoms or signs on examination suggestive of a central nervous system lesion (headaches, focal weakness, or sensory findings), imaging is indicated.

CONCLUSION

Abnormal movements, behaviors, or events in sleep pose a challenge to clinicians because of a frequent lack of adequate information from patients who may themselves be unaware or amnestic of the events. This is further compounded when there is a lack of testimonial information from a bed partner or eyewitness. Such events, therefore, frequently remain misdiagnosed or undiagnosed and untreated or incorrectly treated for a long time. The use of digital VPSG has revolutionized the field and has brought new light to the subject. VPSG provides an opportunity to obtain an audio–video recording of the event in addition to simultaneous and synchronous measurement of other PSG features, for example, extended EEG, EMG, and cardiorespiratory parameters.

This chapter has outlined an approach to a patient with abnormal movements and behaviors in sleep, provided a practical classification for motor events in sleep, and discussed the utility of VPSG and related tests in the diagnosis and differential diagnosis of these conditions.

REFERENCES

1. Kushida, C. A., Littner, M. R., Morgenthaler, T., et al. (2005). Practice parameters for the indications for polysomnography and related procedures: An update for 2005. *Sleep, 28*(4), 499–521.
2. Vignatelli, L., Bisulli, F., Provini, F., et al. (2007). Interobserver reliability of video recording in the diagnosis of nocturnal frontal lobe seizures. *Epilepsia, 48*(8), 1506–1511.
3. American Academy of Sleep Medicine. (2014). *International classification of sleep disorders: Diagnostic and coding manual* (3rd ed.). Darien, IL: Author.
4. Lamm, C. I., Zak, R. S., Kristo, D. A., et al. (2012). Practice parameters for the non-respiratory indications for polysomnography and multiple sleep latency testing for children. *Sleep, 35*(11), 1467–1473.
5. Fois, C., Wright, M.-A. S., Sechi, G., et al. (2015). The utility of polysomnography for the diagnosis of NREM parasomnia: An observational study over 4 years of clinical practice. *Journal of Neurology, 262,* 385–393.
6. Zucconi, M., & Ferini-Strambi, L. (2000). NREM parasomnia: Arousal disorders and differentiation from nocturnal frontal lobe epilepsy. *Clinical Neurophysiology, 111,* S129–S135.
7. Chokroverty, S. (2003). Polysomnography and related procedures. In M. Halett (Ed.), *Handbook of clinical neurophysiology: Movement disorders* (Vol. 1, p. 145). Amsterdam, The Netherlands: Elsevier.
8. Aldrich, M. S., & Jahnke, B. (1991). Diagnostic value of video EEG polysomnography. *Neurology, 41*(7), 1060–1066.
9. Watemberg, N., Tziperman, B., Dabby, R., et al. (2005). Adding video recording increases the diagnostic yield of routine electroencephalograms in children with frequent paroxysmal events. *Epilepsia, 46*(5), 716–719.

10. Malow, B. A., & Aldrich, M. S. (2003). Polysomnography. In S. Chokroverty, W. Hening, & A. Walters (Eds.), *Sleep and movement disorders* (p. 128). Philadelphia, PA: Butterworth-Heinemann.

11. Foldvary, N., Caruso, A. C., Mascha, E., et al. (2000). Identifying montages that best detect electrographic seizure activity during polysomnography. *Sleep, 23*(2), 221–229.

12. Foldvary-Schaefer, N., DeOcampo, J., Mascha, E., et al. (2006). Accuracy of seizure detection using abbreviated EEG during polysomnography. *Journal of Clinical Neurophysiology, 23*(1), 68–71.

13. Criswell, E. (2011). *Cram's introduction to surface electromyography*. Mississauga, ON: Jones & Bartlett Learning.

14. Khoo, S., Tan, J., Shi, D., et al. (2009). Propriospinal myoclonus at sleep onset causing severe insomnia: A polysomnographic and electromyographic analysis. *Sleep Medicine, 257*, 686–688.

15. Van der Salm, S., Koelman, J., Hennecke, S., et al. (2010). Axial jerks: A clinical spectrum ranging from propriospinal to psychogenic myoclonus. *Journal Neurology, 257*, 1349–1355.

16. Zhang, J., Lam, S. P., Ho, C., et al. (2008). Diagnosis of REM sleep behavior disorder by video-polysomnographic study: Is one night enough? *Sleep, 31*(8), 1179–1185.

17. Pressman, M. (2007). Factors that predispose, prime and precipitate NREM parasomnias in adults: Clinical and forensic implications. *Sleep Medicine Review, 11*, 5–30.

18. Joncas, S., Zadra, A., Paquet, J., et al. (2002). The value of sleep deprivation as a diagnostic tool in adult sleepwalkers. *Neurology, 58*, 936–940.

19. Pilon, M., Montplaisir, J., & Zadra, A. (2008). Precipitating factors of somnambulism. Impact of sleep deprivation and forced arousals. *Neurology, 70*, 2284–2290.

20. Zadra, A., Pilon, M., & Montplaisir, J. (2008). Polysomnographic diagnosis of sleepwalking effects of sleep deprivation. *Annals Neurology, 63*, 513–519.

21. Perrault, R., Carrier, J., Desautels, A., et al. (2013). Slow wave activity and slow oscillations in sleepwalkers and controls: Effects of 38 h of sleep deprivation. *Journal of Sleep Research, 22*, 430–433.

22. Guilleminault, C., Leger, D., Philip, P., et al. (1998). Nocturnal wandering and violence: Review of a sleep clinic population. *Journal Forensic Science, 43*, 158–163.

23. Stallman, H. M., Kohler, M., & White, J. (2018). Medication induced sleepwalking: A systematic review. *Sleep Medicine Reviews, 37*, 105–113.

24. Vertugno, R., Manconi, M., Ferini-Strambi, L., et al. (2006). Nocturnal eating: Sleep-related eating disorder or night eating syndrome? A videopolysomnographic study. *Sleep, 29*(7), 949–954.

25. Baran, A. S., & Chervin, R. D. (2009). Approach to the patient with sleep complaints. *Seminars in Neurology, 29*(4), 297–304.

26. Capezuti, E., Maislin, G., Strumpf, N., et al. (2002). Side rail use and bed-related fall outcomes among nursing home residents. *Journal of the American Geriatric Society, 50*(1), 90–96.

27. Gastaut, H., & Broughton, R. (1965). A clinical and polygraphic study of episodic phenomena during sleep. *Recent Advances in Biological Psychiatry, 7*, 197.

28. Brought, R. (1968). Disorders of sleep: Disorders of arousal? *Science, 59*, 1070.

29. Fisher, C., Kahn, E., Edwards, A., et al. (1973). A psychophysiological study of nightmares and sleep terrors. *Journal of Nervous and Mental Disease, 157*(2), 75–98.

30. Jacobson, A., Kales, A., Lehmann, D., et al. (1965). Somnambulism: All night electroencephalography studies. *Science, 148*, 975–977.

31. Jacobson, J. L., & Jacobson, A. L. (2001). *Psychiatry secrets* (2nd ed.). Philadelphia, PA: Hanley & Belfus.

32. Halasz, P., Ujszaszi, J., & Gadoros, J. (1985). Are microarousals preceded by electroencephalographic slow wave synchronization precursors of confusional awakenings? *Sleep, 8*(3), 231–238.

33. Schneck, C. H., Pareja, J. A., Patterson, A. L., et al. (1998). Analysis of polysomnographic events surrounding 252 slow-wave sleep arousals in thirty-eight adults with injurious sleepwalking and sleep terrors. *Journal of Clinical Neurophysiology, 15*(2), 159–166.

34. Brought, R. (1991). Phasic and dynamic aspects of sleep: A symposium review and synthesis. In M. G. Tarzano, P. Halasz, A. C. Declerck (Eds.), *Phasic events and the dynamic organization of sleep* (p. 185). New York, NY: Raven.

35. Lopez, R., Shen, Y., Chenini, S., et al. (2018). Diagnostic criteria for disorders of arousal: A video-polysomnographic assessment. *Annals of Neurology, 83*(2), 341–351.

36. Schenck, C. H., Hurwitz, T. D., O'Connor, K. A., et al. (1993). Additional categories of sleep-related eating disorders and the current status of treatment. *Sleep, 16*(5), 457–466.

37. Schenck, C. H., & Mahowald, M. W. (1994). Review of nocturnal sleep-related eating disorders. *The International Journal of Eating Disorders, 15*(4), 343–356.

38. Winkelman, J. W. (1998). Clinical and polysomnographic features of sleep-related eating disorder. *The Journal of Clinical Psychiatry, 59*(1), 14–19.

39. Komada, Y., Takaesu, Y., Matsui, K., et al. (2016). Comparison of clinical features between primary and drug-induced sleep-related eating disorder. *Neuropsychiatric Disease and Treatment, 12*, 1275–1280.

40. Iber, C., Ancoli-Israel, S., Chesson, A. L., et al. (2007). *The AASM manual for scoring of sleep and associated*

events. Westchester, IL: American Academy of Sleep Medicine.

41. Reding, G. R., Zepelin, H., Robinson, J. E., et al. (1968). Nocturnal tooth-grinding: All night psychophysiological studies. *Journal of Dental Research, 47*, 786–797.

42. Ware, J. C., & Rugh, J. (1988). Destructive bruxism: Sleep stage relationship. *Sleep, 11*, 172–181.

43. Khoury, S., Rouleau, G. A., Rompre, P. H., et al. (2008). A significant increase in breathing amplitude precedes sleep bruxism. *Chest, 134*(2), 332–337.

44. Gallo, L. M., Lavigne, G., Rompre, P., et al. (1997). Reliability of scoring EMG orofacial events: Polysomnography compared with ambulatory recordings. *Journal of Sleep Research, 6*(4), 259–263.

45. Hoban, T. (2003). Rhythmic movement disorder in children. *CNS Spectrums, 8*, 135–138.

46. Oswald, I. (1964). Rocking at night. *Electroencephalography and Clinical Neurophysiology, 16*, 577.

47. Dyken, M. E., Lin-Dyken, D. C., & Yamada, T. (1997). Diagnosing rhythmic movement disorder with video-polysomnography. *Pediatric Neurology, 16*(1), 37–41.

48. Kempenaers, C., Bouillon, E., & Mendlewicz, J. (1994). A rhythmic movement disorder in REM sleep: A case report. *Sleep, 17*(3), 274–279.

49. Gagnon, P., & de Koninck, J. (1985). Repetitive head movements during REM sleep. *Biological Psychiatry, 20*(2), 176–178.

50. Gharagozlou, P., Seyffert, M., Santos, R., et al. (2009). Rhythmic movement disorder associated with respiratory arousals and improved by CPAP titration in a patient with restless legs syndrome and sleep apnea. *Sleep Medicine, 10*(4), 501–503.

51. Langdon-Down, M., & Brain, W. R. (1929). Time of day in relation to convulsions in epilepsy. *Lancet, 2*, 1029.

52. Passouant, P. (1991). Historical aspects of sleep and epilepsy. In R. Degen, E. A. Rodin (Eds.), *Epilepsy, sleep, and sleep deprivation* (2nd ed., p. 19). Amsterdam, The Netherlands: Elsevier.

53. Chabolla, D. R. (2002). Characteristics of the epilepsies. *Mayo Clinic Proceedings, 77*(9), 981–990.

54. Sirven, J. I. (2002). Classifying seizures and epilepsy: A synopsis. *Seminars in Neurology, 22*(3), 237–246.

55. Zucconi, M. (2003). Sleep differential diagnosis and evaluation of unknown motor disorders during sleep. In S. Chokroverty, W. A. Hening, A. S. Walters (Eds.), *Sleep and movement disorders* (pp. 222–223). Philadelphia, PA: Butterworth-Heinemann.

56. Espa, F., Dauvilliers, Y., Ondze, B., et al. (2002). Arousal reactions in sleepwalking and night terrors in adults: The role of respiratory events. *Sleep, 25*(8), 871–875.

57. Iranzo, A., & Santamaria, J. (2005). Severe obstructive sleep apnea/hypopnea mimicking REM sleep behavior disorder. *Sleep, 28*(2), 203–206.

58. Guilleminault, C., Kirisoglu, C., Bao, G., et al. (2005). Adult chronic sleepwalking and its treatment based on polysomnography. *Brain, 128*(5), 1062–1069.

59. Millman, R. P., Kipp, G., & Carskadon, M. A. (1991). Sleepwalking precipitated by treatment of sleep apnea with nasal CPAP. *Chest, 99*(3), 750–751.

60. Lugaresi, E., Medori, R., Montagna, P., et al. (1986). Fatal familial insomnia and dysautonomia with selective degeneration of thalamic nuclei. *The New England Journal of Medicine, 315*(16), 997–1003.

61. Sforza, E., Montagna, P., Tinuper, P., et al. (1995). Sleep-wake cycle abnormalities in fatal familial insomnia: Evidence of the role of the thalamus in sleep regulation. *Electroencephalography and Clinical Neurophysiology, 94*(6), 398–405.

62. Montagna, P., Gambetti, P., Cortelli, P., et al. (2003). Familial and sporadic fatal insomnia. *Lancet Neurology, 2*(3), 167–176.

63. Riley, D. E., & Lang, A. E. (1993). The spectrum of levodopa-related fluctuations in Parkinson's disease. *Neurology, 43*(8), 1459–1464.

64. Montagna, P., Provini, F., Plazzi, F., et al. (1997). Propriospinal myoclonus upon relaxation and drowsiness: A cause of severe insomnia. *Movement Disorders, 129*(10), 66–72.

65. Vetrugno, R., Provini, F., Meletti, S., et al. (2001). Propriospinal myoclonus at the sleep-wake transition: A new type of parasomnia. *Sleep, 24*(7), 835–843.

66. Vetrugno, R., Provini, F., Plaxxi, G., et al. (2005). Propriospinal myoclonus: A motor phenomenon found in restless legs syndrome different from periodic limb movements during sleep. *Movement Disorders, 20*(10), 1323–1329.

67. Kang, S., & Sohn, Y. (2006). Electromyography patterns of propriospinal myoclonus can be mimicked voluntarily. *Movement Disorders, 21*(8), 1241–1244.

68. Lins, O., Castonguay, M., Dunham, W., et al. (1993). Excessive fragmentary myoclonus: Time of night and sleep stage distributions. *Canadian Journal of Neurological Sciences, 20*(2), 142–146.

69. Raccagni, C., Loscher, W. N., Stefani, A., et al. (2016). Peripheral nerve function in patients with excessive fragmentary myoclonus during sleep. *Sleep Medicine, 22*, 61–64.

70. Vetrugno, R., Plazzi, G., Provini, F., et al. (2002). Excessive fragmentary hypnic myoclonus: Clinical and neurophysiological findings. *Sleep Medicine, 3*(1), 73–76.

71. Mitchell, S. (1890). Some disorders of sleep. *International Journal of Medicine, 100*, 109.

72. Sander, H., Geisse, H., Quinto, C., et al. (1998). Sensory sleep starts. *Journal of Neurology, Neurosurgery & Psychiatry, 64*(5), 690.

73. Wichniak, A., Tracik, F., Geisler, P., et al. (2001). Rhythmic feet movements while falling asleep. *Movement Disorders, 16*(6), 1164–1170.

74. Mellman, T. A., & Uhde, T. W. (1989). Electroencephalographic sleep in panic disorder: A focus on sleep-related panic attacks. *Archives of General Psychiatry, 46*(2), 178–184.

75. Hauri, P. J., Friedman, M., & Ravaris, C. L. (1989). Sleep in patients with spontaneous panic attacks. *Sleep, 12*(4), 323–337.

76. Uhde, T. W., Roy-Byrne, P., Gillin, J. C., et al. (1984). The sleep of patients with panic disorder: A preliminary report. *Psychiatry Research, 12*(3), 251–259.

77. Ross, R. J., Ball, W. A., Sullivan, K. A., et al. (1989). Sleep disturbance as the hallmark of posttraumatic stress disorder. *The American Journal of Psychiatry, 146*(6), 697–707.

78. Ross, R. J., Ball, W. A., Dinges, D. F., et al. (1994). Rapid eye movement sleep disturbance in posttraumatic stress disorder. *Biological Psychiatry, 35*(3), 195–202.

79. Mellman, T. A., Kulick-Bell, R., Ashlock, L. E., et al. (1995). Rapid eye movement sleep disturbance in posttraumatic stress disorder. *The American Journal of Psychiatry, 152*(1), 110–115.

80. Mellman, T. A., Nolan, B., Hebding, J., et al. (1997). A polysomnographic comparison of veterans with combat-related PTSD, depressed men, and non-ill controls. *Sleep, 20*(1), 46–51.

81. Ross, R. J., Ball, W. A., Sanford, L. D., et al. (1999). Rapid eye movement sleep changes during the adaptation night in combat veterans with posttraumatic stress disorder. *Biological Psychiatry, 45*(7), 938–941.

82. Hurwitz, T. D., Mahowald, M. W., Kuskowski, M., et al. (1998). Polysomnographic sleep is not clinically impaired in Vietnam combat veterans with chronic posttraumatic stress disorder. *Biological Psychiatry, 44*(10), 1066–1073.

83. Klein, E., Koren, D., Arnon, I., et al. (2002). No evidence of sleep disturbance in post-traumatic stress disorder: A polysomnographic study in injured victims of traffic accidents. *The Israel Journal of Psychiatry and Related Sciences, 39*(1), 3–10.

84. Thorpy, M. J., & Adler, C. H. (2005). Parkinson disease and sleep. *Neurologic Clinics, 23*(4), 1187–1208.

85. Glaze, D. G., Frost, J. D., Jr., & Jankovic, J. (1983). Sleep in Gilles de la Tourette syndrome: Disorder of arousal. *Neurology, 33*(5), 586–592.

86. Wand, R. R., Matazow, G. S., Shady, G. A., et al. (1993). Tourette syndrome: Associated symptoms and most disabling features. *Neuroscience and Biobehavioral Reviews, 17*(3), 271–275.

87. Montagna, P., Imbriaco, A., Zucconi, A., et al. (1986). Hemifacial spasm in sleep. *Neurology, 36*(2), 270–273.

88. Goodman, A. O., & Rogersm, L. (2011). Asymptomatic sleep abnormalities are a common early feature in patients with Huntington's disease. *Current Neurology and Neuroscience Reports, 11*(2), 211–217.

89. Goodman, A. O., & Barker, R. A. (2010). How vital is sleep in Huntington's disease? *Journal of Neurology, 257*(6), 882–897.

90. Kemlink, D., Pretl, M., Kelemen, J., et al. (2005). Periodic limb movements in sleep: Polysomnographic and actigraphic methods for their detection. *Casopis Lekaru Ceskych, 144*(10), 689–691.

91. Sforza, E., Johannes, M., & Claudio, B. (2005). The PAM-RL ambulatory device for detection of periodic leg movements: A validation study. *Sleep Medicine, 6,* 407–413.

92. Morgenthaler, T., Alessi, C., Friedman, L., et al. (2007). Practice parameters for the use of actigraphy in the assessment of sleep and sleep disorders: An update for 2007. *Sleep, 30*(4), 519–529.

93. Cascino, G. (2002). Clinical indications and diagnostic yield of video-electroencephalographic monitoring in patients with seizures and spells. *Mayo Clinic Proceedings, 77*(10), 1111–1120.

chapter 21
Sleep and Respiratory Disorders

ALESHIA L. DORST

LEARNING OBJECTIVES

On completion of this chapter, the reader should be able to:

1. Define and describe the definition, prevalence, etiology, pathophysiology, diagnosis, treatment, and prognosis of patients with chronic obstructive pulmonary disease (COPD).
2. Describe the changes in cardiopulmonary function in COPD patients during sleep.
3. Define and describe the prevalence, etiology, pathophysiology, diagnosis, treatment, and prognosis of patients with asthma.
4. Describe overlap syndrome.
5. Describe restrictive disease.

KEY TERMS

Asthma
Chronic obstructive pulmonary disease
Hyperventilation
Hypoventilation
Noninvasive ventilation
Obstructive sleep apnea
Overlap syndrome (COPD and OSA)
Positive airway pressure
Pulmonary function test (PFT)
Restrictive lung disease
Neuromuscular disease

TYPE OF RESPIRATORY DISORDERS—RESTRICTIVE VERSUS OBSTRUCTIVE CLASSIFICATIONS

There are several different types of respiratory disorders that can primarily be described as either restrictive or obstructive. Obstructive disorders are more common than restrictive and share the characteristics of blocked airways. With a restrictive disorder, such as cystic fibrosis, the person would show an inability to expand the lungs to the needed volume to properly ventilate. Restrictive disorders can also be a consequence of pulmonary scarring because of diseases such as idiopathic pulmonary fibrosis, which will result in failure of lung expansion. Restrictive disorders typically have a lower survival rate. Diseases that would be considered obstructive include chronic obstructive pulmonary disease (COPD), asthma, and bronchitis. There are some similarities noted with obstructive and restrictive disorders such as symptoms, signs, diagnosis, and treatment methods (1).

There are a wide variety of restrictive lung diseases that range in severity and have fluctuating treatments. Conditions that lead to lung restriction include, but are not limited to, neuromuscular disease, obesity hypoventilation syndrome, kyphoscoliosis, interstitial lung disease, and pregnancy. People with restrictive lung diseases such as interstitial lung disease are noted to have increased sleep difficulties, which often present as obstructive sleep apnea (OSA) (1). Treatment for OSA as well as restrictive lung diseases does frequently correlate because of the mechanisms that affect both diagnoses and the benefits of noninvasive ventilation or continuous positive airway pressure in these patients. Given the prevalence of OSA as well as restrictive lung diseases, it is not uncommon to see them in association with each other. The unfortunate consequences of both diagnoses increase the severity of these diseases and, in turn, could lead to higher morbidity and mortality rates. With treatment, it is possible to reduce the long-term consequences of OSA and restrictive lung disease.

OSA is the most common form of sleep apnea and is an obstructive respiratory disorder (2). There are several sleep disorders that have been identified using polysomnography (PSG). OSA has shown negative consequences on a person's health because it affects his or her ability to properly perform gas exchange—carbon dioxide (CO_2) and oxygen, while asleep. Although someone may have no trouble breathing during the day, the shift that the body makes from wake to sleep reduces the muscle tension throughout the body. During an apneic event, there is a reduction in the airway when the pharynx collapses, resulting in reduced airflow (hypopnea) or a completely obstructed airway (apnea). The frequency and the severity of these events are typically dependent on anatomic and neural factors. When there is a reduction or cessation of airflow, the oxygen provided to the body is reduced, which will notify the body's neurochemical receptors that the body has gone into a hypoxic state and this leads to hypercapnia because of inefficient exchange of gases. Generally, when these events show a cyclic pattern, it increases the severity. The negative effects of sleep apnea are notable for the importance of diagnosis and treatment. A person presenting with sleep apnea commonly shows adverse effects on all body systems that could result in the following: hypertension, coronary artery disease, stroke, cardiac arrhythmias, and pulmonary hypertension. Patients with OSA often report daytime sleepiness, concentration problems, memory loss, and less commonly studied but noteworthy anxiety and depression. There are many contributors to OSA such as obesity, altitude, gender, age, anatomic features, genetics, smoking status, and other lung diseases (2).

DIAGNOSING RESTRICTIVE AND OBSTRUCTIVE DISORDERS USING PULMONARY FUNCTION TESTING (PFT)

Diagnosis of lung disorders is similar in restrictive and obstructive disorders. A person presenting with symptoms of cough, wheezing, and shortness of breath would have spirometry testing. Spirometry is relatively quick and inexpensive. Spirometers measure how much air someone can breathe out and how quickly. How well the lungs deliver oxygen to the blood can also be measured by simply breathing into a spirometer. Other means of diagnosing and marking the severity of lung disorders are by checking arterial blood gases or by performing a chest x-ray or computed tomography of the chest to evaluate signs of damage and determine from where these are originating. In cases of severe restrictive disorders such as cystic fibrosis, genetic testing may reveal a gene mutation resulting in the disorder.

ICSD CLASSIFICATION OF SLEEP-RELATED HYPOVENTILATION

Sleep-related hypoventilation is described as insufficient sleep-related ventilation that results in hypercapnia or increased partial pressure of carbon dioxide ($PaCO_2$). This is the result of slow and shallow breaths that are inadequate for proper gas exchange. Sleep-related hypoventilation is not always in association with other lung or airway diseases and does not require associated disorders for diagnosis. Sleep-related hypoventilation is diagnosed by monitoring $PaCO_2$ during a PSG using transcutaneous or end-tidal CO_2 monitoring. OSA is often present in these situations, and treatment of OSA can reduce the severity of sleep-related hypoventilation. Because of the presence of hypercapnia and hypoxia, these patients commonly develop pulmonary hypertension,

heart failure, cardiac arrhythmias, and neurocognitive dysfunction. Sleep-related hypoventilation is worsened by the use of sedatives, alcohol, and depressants (3).

SLEEP PROBLEMS IN COPD PATIENTS

COPD can increase the severity of OSA in patients because of the decrease in cardiopulmonary function during sleep. Both diseases result in insufficient exchange of oxygen and CO_2. Patients with COPD have increased severity of oxygen desaturations and they typically occur more frequently, thus resulting in increased work on the heart (4). Unlike patients with OSA alone, those who are diagnosed with OSA and COPD show effects on the respiratory system during the day as well. Approximately 1% of adults have been diagnosed with overlapping OSA and COPD (5).

Typically, during sleep, the parasympathetic nervous system controls breathing, resulting in deep breaths, which ensures adequate tidal volume and gas exchange. In patients with OSA and COPD, the sympathetic nervous system is activated during sleep, causing slow and shallow breathing (hypoventilation), often in association with mouth breathing (4). Because of sympathetic hyperactivity in these patients, often, proper gas exchange is difficult to achieve. Because of the association of these disorders, the likelihood of increased cardiovascular, autonomic, and functional deficiencies is high (4). In a study designed to test different treatments on patients with COPD and OSA, it was found that those who shared the two diagnoses presented with a higher apnea–hypopnea index (AHI) and a higher oxygen desaturation index. Patients with COPD alone still showed longer periods of low saturations classified as below 90% and 80%, showing the correlation between increased nocturnal hypoxemia and COPD (6).

Because of hypercapnia and hypoxia, it is not uncommon to see central apneas in COPD patients. When the body's chemoreceptors identify a drop in oxygen levels and a rise in CO_2, the brain will wake from sleep and trigger hyperventilation to increase oxygen levels. The hyperventilation then blows off too much CO_2, and when the body drifts back to sleep, the brain does not trigger the lungs to expand. Therefore, with the cessation of airflow, the CO_2 rises again, whereas the oxygen drops and continues the vicious cycle of overcompensation and undercompensation, otherwise known as the "loop gain model." Because of the constant struggle for the body to breathe and because of frequent awakenings, these patients commonly present with symptoms of insomnia, hypoxemia, and restless legs syndrome. In fact, a study revealed that sleep efficiency was notably lower (<82%) in patients with COPD versus patients without COPD, resulting in 27.3% of patients having a high prevalence of insomnia disorder (7).

SLEEP PROBLEMS IN OVERLAP SYNDROME—OSA + COPD

Factors of COPD That Predispose to OSA

COPD is a progressive disease that affects the ability to breathe. COPD is also known as "emphysema," which is diagnosed when the walls between alveoli are damaged. Chronic bronchitis is diagnosed when the walls of the airway are constantly irritated and inflamed, typically resulting in thick mucus in the airways. Most people with COPD present symptoms of both emphysema and bronchitis. COPD is commonly associated with smoking; other causes include smoke exposure or exposure to other irritants such as air pollution, chemical fumes, and dust. There have been findings linking one genetic marker known as α1-antitrypsin (AAT) to COPD when there is a deficiency in AAT (3). COPD is the leading cause of disability and the fourth leading cause of death in the United States. An estimated 16 million people are diagnosed, according to the National Heart Lung and Blood Institute (3).

COPD is a result of air sacs and blood capillaries not exchanging oxygen and CO_2 efficiently because of a lack of elasticity or damage to the air sacs. Thick and inflamed walls of airways will also result in reduced airflow. This can also result in too much mucus being produced; mucus production is a means of protection for the airway (3).

Because of the pathophysiology of COPD and asthma, these patients have a higher chance of having OSA. A study performed at the Clinical Research Center of Lam Dong Medical College in Vietnam showed that patients who present with both asthma and COPD had higher AHIs than patients who presented with asthma or COPD alone (8).

Although COPD and OSA are not always associated, the increase of mucus production and coughing in COPD patients appear to be factors that contribute to the severity of sleep disorders. Other contributing symptoms are hypercapnia, resulting in increased sympathetic activity similar to OSA which, with the presence of both diagnoses, can increase the negative effects of both (7). There are documented adverse effects of having both COPD and insomnia; with the addition of an OSA, this diagnosis can have long-term negative consequences without treatment.

Treating COPD and Overlap Syndrome

In all cases of respiratory disorders and diseases, the first suggestion to reduce symptoms is to quit smoking and reduce smoke exposure along with exposure to other irritants. The treatment goals for COPD are to manage COPD and reduce admissions due to exacerbations. COPD does not have a cure. Some medications that have been used to alleviate symptoms include bronchodilators and steroids. Surgery may be an option as well. A bullectomy can be performed to remove large bullae from the lungs, or lung volume reduction surgery can be done to remove damaged tissue. In severe cases, a lung transplant could be considered (3). Oral steroids and oxygen therapy can improve symptoms of COPD and improve sleep quality (7).

Oxygen therapy has been shown to reduce symptoms associated with COPD and increase day and night oxygen levels. A trial of home oxygen therapy and home mechanical ventilation therapy revealed longer periods before readmission due to exacerbations and prolonged mortality from 1.4 to 4.3 months (9). When both OSA and COPD are present, the effects of noninvasive ventilation (NIV) therapy have been shown to significantly reduce symptoms.

NIV therapy will help increase mechanical drive, lessen hypercapnia, and reduce the work of breathing. Randomized trials have shown that oxygen, in addition to NIV therapy, has increased the positive effects of NIV and also daytime $PaCO_2$ and oxygen levels. Although there are not enough data to reveal how this would resolve overlap syndrome, these trials do show an increase in a patient's ability to properly ventilate (9).

ASTHMA AND OSA

Asthma is defined as a chronic inflammatory disorder of the airways. Asthma presents in various forms, which include intermittent, persistent, exercise-associated, aspirin-sensitive, or severe. Although there are various forms of asthma, the disease is typically categorized as acute or chronic. Asthma patients present with symptoms such as wheezing, breathlessness, chest tightness, and coughing. These symptoms are a result of the body overreacting to foreign substances or allergens. The airway can be irritated by a number of outside factors: air pollution, postnasal drip, gastroesophageal reflux disease, smoke, dandruff or pet dander, and many others.

An "asthma attack" is, in fact, a series of complex interactions between inflammatory cells and mediators in reaction to the irritants mentioned in the previous paragraph. More specifically, when an irritant is introduced to the body, the body starts an immune response by producing antibodies called "immunoglobulin E" (IgE) (10). The IgE will seek out the mast cell to release histamine; the histamine responds strongly and results in swelling of the airway and glands overproducing mucus.

Patients with asthma often experience airway constriction as a result of bronchoconstriction in response to exposure to stimuli. Airway edema can result from long-term inflammation to the airway and progression of asthma. Someone with asthma has an airway with thickened muscle walls as well as a swollen mucus layer and increased mucus production, which results in a smaller lumen, reducing airflow. All of these symptoms can make life with asthma painful.

The treatment for asthma can depend on the status of acute versus chronic as well as the patient's lifestyle. The most common treatments are bronchodilators to reduce bronchoconstriction and avoid irritants. Asthma is very prevalent in society and managed through medications as well as lifestyle changes. In the long term, asthma can cause airway remodeling or permanent structural changes such as thickening of the sub-basement membrane and airway smooth muscle hypertrophy and hyperplasia (10).

SLEEP DISORDERS IN NEUROMUSCULAR DISORDERS

Neuromuscular disease is a progressive disorder in which the patient will present with symptoms of muscle weakness in addition to stiffness and cramping in extremities and demonstrate problems with speech, swallowing, and occasionally breathing. According to the National Institute for Health and Care Excellence, shortness of breath being present at diagnosis will shorten life expectancy. These symptoms are commonly noticed initially as unexplained instances of falls or tripping when the patient is truly suffering from increased muscle weakness. Neuromuscular disease (NMD) is associated with a high mortality rate. The most common form of this disease is amyotrophic lateral sclerosis. The cause of NMD is unknown, although a correlation in family history has been recognized (11).

Diagnosis of a neuromuscular disease needs to come from a neurologist. Common routes of assessing neuromuscular disease would involve oximetry testing, forced vital capacity, and sniff nasal inspiratory pressure to obtain a respiratory baseline for the patient. Once a patient is diagnosed with NMD, several levels of care are initiated. Medications can be given to alleviate muscle cramps and pain. Not only will patients need help with the physical effects of the diagnosis, but the emotional effects of the diagnosis will require additional support (11).

NIV can also be offered as a treatment for patients showing increased breathing difficulty. Although NIV treatment can improve symptoms of respiratory distress and decrease mortality rate in patients with NMD, there is unfortunately no cure at this time. The main goal of treatment of NMD is to increase quality of life and maintain functional ability (11).

TREATING SLEEP-DISORDERED BREATHING IN NEUROMUSCULAR DISEASE PATIENTS

The diagnosis and care of patients with neuromuscular disease is determined by the physician caring for them. This can result in the start of NIV, which typically follows a process of acclimation to treatment and increased hours of use as needed.

SLEEP-RELATED HYPOXEMIA

Sleep-related hypoxemia is classified as sustained periods of low oxygen during sleep. Low oxygen levels can be a result of hypoventilation, ventilation–perfusion mismatch, low partial pressure of oxygen, and a combination of multiple factors. These symptoms can be increased by alcohol, depressants, and sedatives as we see in other respiratory disorders. Patients with severe respiratory diseases (COPD, morbid obesity) are at a higher risk of developing pulmonary hypertension and cor pulmonale. Sleep-related hypoxemia can result from decreased end-expiratory lung volume and reduced ventilatory drive, which will also increase hypocapnia. All of these factors increase the chances of upper airway resistance (3).

REFERENCES

1. *Restrictive Lung Disease.* Retrieved May 21, 2016, from https://www.alpfmedical.info/obstructive-sleep/restrictive-lung-disease.html
2. Dempsey, J. A., Veasey, S. C., Morgan, B. J., et al. (2010). Pathophysiology of sleep apnea. *Physiological Reviews, 90*(1), 47–112. doi:10.1152/physrev.00043.2008
3. Sateia, M. J. (2014). International classification of sleep disorders—third edition. *Chest, 146*(5), 1387–1394.
4. Du, W., Liu, J., Zhou, J., et al. (2018). Obstructive sleep apnea, COPD, the overlap syndrome, and mortality: Results from the 2005–2008 National Health and Nutrition Examination Survey. *International Journal of Chronic Obstructive Pulmonary Disease, 13*, 665–674. doi:10.2147/COPD.S148735
5. McNicholas, W. T., Verbraecken, J., & Marin, J. M. (2013). Sleep disorders in COPD: The forgotten dimension. *European Respiratory Review, 22*(129), 365–375.
6. Economou, N.T., Ilias, I., Velentza, L., et al. (2018). Sleepiness, fatigue, anxiety and depression in chronic obstructive pulmonary disease and obstructive sleep apnea-overlap-syndrome, before and after continuous positive airways pressure therapy. *PLOS One, 13*(6), e0197342. doi:10.1371/journal.pone.0197342
7. Budhiraja, R., Siddiqi, T. A., & Quan, S. F. (2015). Sleep disorders in chronic obstructive pulmonary disease: Etiology, impact, and management. *Journal of Clinical Sleep Medicine, 11*(3), 259–270.
8. Boing, S., & Randerath, W. J. (2014). Sleep disorders in asthma and chronic obstructive pulmonary disease (COPD). *Therapeutische Umschau, 71*, 301–308.
9. Murphy, P. B., Rehal, S., Arbane, G., et al. (2017). Effect of home noninvasive ventilation with oxygen therapy vs oxygen therapy alone on hospital

readmission or death after an acute COPD exacerbation: A randomized clinical trial. *The Journal of American Medical Association, 317*(21), 2177–2186. doi:10.1001/jama.2017.4451

10. Sundborn, F., Janson, C., Malinovschi, A., et al. (2018). Effects of coexisting asthma and obstructive sleep apnea on sleep architecture, oxygen saturation, and systemic inflammation in women. *Journal of Clinical Sleep Medicine, 14*(2), 253–259.

11. Dawoud, D., & Guideline Development Group. (2016, February). *NICE Motor neuron disease: Assessment and management.* NICE guideline [NG42]. Retrieved December 12, 2018, from https://www.nice.org.uk/guidance/ng42

chapter 22

Impact of Vascular Disorders on Sleep

JENNIFER PARR-CHRISTMAS   MONICA M. HENDERSON   JAMES D. GEYER   PAUL R. CARNEY

LEARNING OBJECTIVES

On completion of this chapter, the reader should be able to:

1. Explain the autonomic physiology of sleep.
2. Explain the relationship between sleep and hypertension.
3. Describe the relationship between sleep and stroke.
4. Explain the relationship between sleep and heart failure.
5. Describe the effect of treatment with positive airway pressure on vascular disease.

KEY TERMS

Myocardial infarction
Heart failure
Metabolic syndrome
Sympathetic
Parasympathetic
Hypertension
Arrhythmia
CPAP
ECG
Catecholamines

VASCULAR DISORDERS AND SLEEP

Vascular diseases, including myocardial infarction, stroke, cerebrovascular disease, heart failure (HF), and cardiac arrhythmias, are the most common causes of morbidity and mortality in industrialized countries. Sleep-related breathing disorders are also widespread and increasing in prevalence because of the obesity epidemic, with approximately 20 million Americans (1) suffering from obstructive sleep apnea. Given the frequency of the two diseases, sleep disorders and vascular disorders, it is not surprising that they often coexist. The interactions between obstructive sleep apnea/hypopnea syndrome and vascular diseases are much more complex than originally thought, and their comorbidity is more than mere coexistence. Sleep-related breathing disorders, insomnia, and even normal autonomic changes associated with rapid eye movement (REM) sleep can adversely affect vascular diseases. This chapter will review the normal autonomic processes that are seen in sleep and discuss the role that sleep disorders play in heart disease, hypertension, and stroke.

NORMAL AUTONOMIC PHYSIOLOGY OF SLEEP

The autonomic nervous system regulates the involuntary, automatic functions of the visceral organs. It comprises the parasympathetic and sympathetic divisions, two opposing systems, the balance of which determines autonomic function. The sympathetic system has a stimulant effect and is responsible for the "fight or flight" response. Its primary neurochemical mediator is noradrenaline, an adrenaline-like substance that produces an increased heart rate, increased respiratory rate, vasoconstriction of blood vessels in visceral organs with vasodilatation of blood vessels in skeletal muscles, increased blood pressure, pupillary dilatation, plus inhibition of digestion, urination, and defecation. In contrast, the parasympathetic system counterbalances these effects. Its primary neurotransmitter is acetylcholine and its effects include slowing of the heart rate and respiration, vasodilatation of visceral organs with decreased blood pressure, pupillary constriction, increased peristalsis, plus emptying of the bladder and the rectum. Because vasoconstriction and hypertension are major contributors to myocardial infarction and stroke, it is useful to examine the body's normal sympathetic and parasympathetic responses during sleep.

In general, at sleep onset, there is a reduction in sympathetic tone and a concomitant increase in parasympathetic tone, which causes a lowering of the heart rate, blood pressure, respiration rate, and tidal volume which continues during non-REM (NREM) sleep (2). With the transition to tonic REM sleep, the parasympathetic activity continues to increase and the sympathetic activity is further suppressed. During phasic REM sleep, there are bursts of sympathetic activity (2). Heart rate variation during NREM sleep follows a sinusoidal pattern (2).

A normal respiratory sinus arrhythmia is produced by the normal respiratory activity coupled with cardiorespiratory center activity. During normal inspiration, the heart rate has a brief acceleration in order to accommodate venous return and increased cardiac output (2). During expiration, there is a progressive decrease in heart rate. This normal cardiac rhythm variability is a marker for cardiac health and its absence is associated with increasing age and possible cardiac disease. During REM sleep, it is normal for the heart rate to become increasingly variable, with episodes of moderate tachycardia and bradycardia. Respiratory patterns are also irregular and may result in mild oxygen desaturations. The neurons controlling the principal diaphragmatic respiratory muscles typically are not inhibited during REM sleep, but accessory muscles in the ribcage (the intercostal muscles) and neck may have partial muscle atonia. This causes the diaphragm to bear most of the load of respiration, which leads to partial diaphragmatic fatigue, hypoventilation, and decreased oxygenation over a period of several minutes in duration. These episodes are referred to as REM sleep hypoventilation episodes and should be scored as hypopneas if they produce an oxygen desaturation of 4% or greater over a period of time of 10 seconds or more (2).

There may be a transient 35% increase (3) in the baseline heart rate especially during phasic REM sleep because of a burst of sympathetic activation. Beta-blockers such as atenolol tend to reduce this phenomenon. Increased parasympathetic activity during NREM sleep contributes to cardiac electrical stability and helps decrease cardiac metabolic activity, reducing the risk of cardiac arrhythmia. The decreased blood pressure produced by the parasympathetic system during NREM sleep, however, can contribute to decreased blood flow to the coronary arteries and result in myocardial hypoperfusion, increasing the risk of infarction in patients with significant coronary atherosclerosis (2). The surges in autonomic activity and increased heart rate during REM sleep increase the risk for ventricular arrhythmias. Sympathetic activity not only results in increased oxygen consumption by the cardiac muscle but also produces coronary vasoconstriction, decreasing the blood flow to the heart, thus increasing the risk of cardiac ischemia. It has been documented that a significant number of myocardial infarctions occur in the early morning hours, upon awakening, or shortly after awakening; however, the relationship among sleep state, cardiac ischemia, and myocardial infarction is incompletely understood at this time.

Cerebral blood flow is closely linked to cardiac output, and the factors described earlier also impact blood flow to the brain. During REM sleep, there is an increase in blood flow to the limbic system and the brainstem, with circulation to these structures decreasing during NREM sleep. As brain activity increases during REM sleep, the cerebral requirements for glucose and oxygen both increase, and there is a compensatory increase in oxygenated hemoglobin delivery accompanying the transition from NREM sleep to REM sleep. Mild hypercapnia develops during NREM sleep and appears to counteract the circulatory effect of the decreased cerebral metabolic rate during NREM sleep. $PaCO_2$ is an important determinant of respiration and hence cerebral blood flow during sleep in obstructive sleep apnea and other related disorders (2).

VASCULAR PATHOLOGY AND SLEEP

Hypertension

The Sleep Heart Health Study was designed as a prospective cohort study to investigate obstructive sleep apnea and other sleep-disordered breathing as a risk factor for the development of hypertension and cardiovascular disease (4). The results of the study suggest that the elevated sympathetic activity associated with sleep-related breathing disorders likely represents the primary mechanism in the pathogenesis of developing subsequent hypertension. This would typically begin as a loss of nocturnal dipping, the normal drop in blood pressure which occurs during sleep (5). Following the loss of nocturnal dipping, some patients develop elevated nocturnal arterial blood pressure, which can then progress to an elevated daytime blood pressure. Obstructive sleep apnea is an independent risk factor for the development of both nocturnal and daytime arterial hypertension (6). There appears to be a linear association between the severity of obstructive sleep apnea and the likelihood of developing subsequent hypertension. According to the Wisconsin Sleep Cohort Study, a patient with an apnea/hypopnea index greater than 15 events per hour has a 2.9-fold relative risk of developing hypertension compared with the normal patient population. This implies that many patients thought to have essential hypertension actually have hypertension secondary, at least in part, to obstructive sleep apnea.

The Joint National Committee on Prevention, Detection, Evaluation, and Treatment of High Blood Pressure has recommended that obstructive sleep apnea be excluded as a contributing cause of medically refractory hypertension. With the new tighter controls recommended for hypertension, screening for these contributing causes becomes increasingly important, especially in patients who have already had a heart attack or stroke.

Nasal continuous positive airway pressure (CPAP) in hypertensive patients with moderate-to-severe obstructive sleep apnea leads to a significant reduction in the arterial blood pressure (7–11). The effect of CPAP on hypertension is more pronounced in patients with severe obstructive sleep apnea. Patients with only a 50% reduction in apnea on the apnea–hypopnea index did not have a significant reduction in blood pressure. This underscores the importance of good control of apnea and hypopnea followed by excellent patient compliance with CPAP.

Heart Failure

HF occurs when cardiac dysfunction requires the body to make compensatory changes to maintain adequate cardiac output. The failure of the heart to pump effectively results in venous congestion, which produces many of the symptoms of HF. The clinical features include dyspnea on exertion, orthopnea (dyspnea when lying down), and paroxysmal nocturnal dyspnea (sudden episodes of shortness of breath during sleep). Patients with HF have a significantly increased risk of sleep-disordered breathing, with obstructive sleep apnea occurring in 11% to 37% of patients, and patients with obstructive sleep apnea often have coexisting central sleep apnea (12, 13). Central apnea, periodic breathing, and Cheyne–Stokes breathing are also frequently associated with HF. The Sleep Heart Health Study identified a 2.38-fold increased relative risk for the development of HF in patients with obstructive sleep apnea, which was independent of all other recognized risk factors for HF. Symptoms classically associated with HF such as paroxysmal nocturnal dyspnea may in fact be related, in part, to obstructive sleep apnea.

Central sleep apnea occurs more frequently in patients with severe HF and in some cases contributes to the progression of the HF. Patients with HF and central sleep apnea have higher levels of catecholamines such as adrenaline than patients with HF without central sleep apnea. This catecholamine effect has further negative effects on cardiac function.

In patients with HF, aggressive treatment of concomitant obstructive sleep apnea results in both a reduction in systolic blood pressure and an improvement in left ventricular function. Treatment of obstructive sleep apnea with CPAP in patients with HF can improve the left ventricular ejection fraction and the left ventricular end systolic diameter, and augment the heart's stroke volume (14). Furthermore, the risk of ventricular tachycardia reduces, as does the frequency of premature ventricular contractions.

Cardiac Arrhythmias

Tachyarrhythmias commonly occur with obstructive sleep apnea, usually occurring at the end of an apnea or hypopnea episode during the period of hyperpneic breathing and often in association with an electroencephalogram

(EEG) arousal. Several studies have indicated that the frequency of atrial fibrillation is increased in patients with obstructive sleep apnea and other sleep-related breathing disorders (15). Ventricular tachycardia becomes more likely as oxygen saturation falls below 60% (2).

Bradyarrhythmias are also frequently associated with obstructive sleep apnea. Sinus bradycardia, which can be severe, is common during apnea or hypopnea. Patients rarely develop sinus arrest or atrioventricular block. Patients with nocturnal bradycardia should be screened for obstructive sleep apnea.

COAGULATION AND PLATELET ACTIVITY

Thrombus formation is the most common clinical event that leads to myocardial infarction and plays a significant role in stroke. The process of clot formation is a complex one, which involves the interaction of platelets, circulating coagulation factors, and the surface of endothelial cells which line blood vessels. When a blood vessel is injured, circulating platelets adhere to the wall, forming a loose aggregate which occludes the lumen of the vessel. The platelet aggregate then activates the coagulation cascade, resulting in the production of fibrin, a molecular "glue" which strengthens the loose aggregate, thereby forming a thrombus (blood vessel blockage). The tendency for platelets to aggregate increases with obstructive sleep apnea, at least in part mediated by the increased levels of catecholamines in these patients (16, 17). Furthermore, these patients may also have abnormally increased daytime levels of fibrinogen, the precursor to fibrin.

Hematocrit is defined as the volume percent of erythrocytes, or red blood cells, in whole blood. The higher a patient's hematocrit, the more red cells are in circulation. Although plasma, or the liquid component of blood, can flow freely, the cellular components of blood produce increased blood viscosity with a decreased rate of flow, especially in small blood vessels and in arteries narrowed by atherosclerotic plaque. As the rate of flow decreases, the tendency to form circulating platelet aggregates increases, increasing the risk of thrombosis. When patients with moderate-to-severe obstructive sleep apnea experience chronic nocturnal hypoxia, the body tries to compensate by producing more erythrocytes and increasing the oxygen-carrying capacity of the blood. This produces a state of hyperviscosity when coupled with the increased tendency to produce platelet aggregates, placing these patients at greatly increased risk of heart attack and stroke.

There is evidence that treatment of obstructive sleep apnea with CPAP can improve the nocturnal hypoxemia and decrease hematocrit and blood viscosity. Furthermore, lessening the episodes of catecholamine release would reduce the relative increase in platelet aggregation. CPAP may also reduce the activity of some circulating clotting factors.

METABOLIC SYNDROME X

Metabolic syndrome X is a recently recognized constellation of metabolic abnormalities which are associated with an increased risk of vascular diseases. The symptoms include central obesity with fat deposits centered around the abdomen, glucose intolerance/insulin resistance, hypertension, hypercholesterolemia, and abnormalities in the clotting of blood. Although syndrome X is not a vascular disease, it greatly increases a patient's risk of heart attack and stroke and is therefore included for discussion in this chapter. We have previously discussed the possible role sleep-related breathing disorders may have on hypertension with an increased tendency to form blood clots. We will now examine the possible role of sleep disorders and two of the other components of the syndrome: glucose intolerance and obesity.

Obstructive sleep apnea has been shown to produce glucose intolerance, with the severity of the apnea correlating with the degree of insulin resistance (18, 19). Obstructive sleep apnea is associated with higher blood glucose, higher insulin levels, and higher glycosylated hemoglobin levels, a laboratory finding that is seen in poorly controlled diabetes (20). Unfortunately, treatment of obstructive sleep apnea with CPAP has not resulted in consistent improvement of glucose tolerance. Further study of the exact metabolic effects of CPAP is needed.

There may also be an association between obstructive sleep apnea and obesity. Leptin is a hormone produced by fat cells, which is seen in increased levels in obese patients. Males with obstructive sleep apnea have relatively higher levels of leptin than males without obstructive sleep apnea. This may be secondary to leptin resistance. Leptin may increase the production of platelet aggregation and may serve as an independent marker for the risk of vascular disease. Studies have shown that leptin levels fall following treatment with CPAP, and therapy for obstructive sleep apnea may not only improve the patient's difficulty with weight gain but also reduce the risk of heart attack and stroke by minimizing the tendency of platelet aggregation (21).

ISCHEMIC HEART DISEASE

Obstructive sleep apnea and coronary artery disease frequently coexist, with at least 50% of patients with heart disease having significant obstructive sleep apnea. Obstructive sleep apnea is an independent risk factor for myocardial infarction similar to hypertension and smoking. The sympathetic activity of the autonomic nervous system during normal REM sleep increases blood pressure and heart rate with a concomitant increase in cardiac oxygen consumption (22–24). Significant oxygen desaturations in a patient with obstructive sleep apnea further contribute to nocturnal angina and nocturnal ischemic changes in the electrocardiogram (ECG).

Treatment of obstructive sleep apnea with CPAP has been shown to improve ECG changes. There is also evidence of fewer incidences or a lesser degree of nocturnal angina, but large clinical trials are lacking. Outcome following myocardial infarction is worse in patients with obstructive sleep apnea, with a higher mortality in patients with untreated obstructive sleep apnea and coronary artery disease, 38% in patients with cardiac disease, and 9% in patients without obstructive sleep apnea.

CEREBROVASCULAR DISEASE

Annually, more than 750,000 strokes occur in the United States, with approximately 150,000 fatalities (25). Tremendous resources are required to care for the over 3 million stroke survivors in the United States alone. Numerous studies have demonstrated that 31% to 54% of strokes occur during sleep, and the most common time of onset during wakefulness is in the first several hours following awakening. The Sleep Heart Health Study identified an increase in the prevalence of strokes in patients with concomitant obstructive sleep apnea, and other studies have shown the frequency of coexisting sleep apnea and stroke in 62.5% to 80% of stroke patients (26–30).

Cerebral autoregulation is the process by which the brain attempts to control intracranial blood pressure to maintain adequate blood flow. Obstructive sleep apnea interferes with this process. Although the change has not been shown to cause stroke, the inability of the brain to change pressures to ensure adequate circulation may produce decreased cerebral perfusion and result in enlargement of an acute stroke that originated from other causes. Treatment of obstructive sleep apnea with CPAP results in improvement of the cerebral autoregulation and overall cerebral blood flow measured by transcranial Doppler ultrasound.

The sleepiness and snoring associated with obstructive sleep apnea are frequently the presenting symptoms, and those with which the patients are most concerned. Sleep apnea has a major impact on a variety of vascular disorders. Identification and aggressive treatment of sleep-related breathing disorders not only reduces vascular risk but also improves functional status. This medical information can also be used to encourage the patient toward better CPAP adherence. Given the importance of effective treatment, patient adherence with CPAP therapy should be monitored closely.

REFERENCES

1. Young, T., Palta, M., Dempsey, J., et al. (1993). The occurrence of sleep-disordered breathing among middle-aged adults. *New England Journal of Medicine, 328,* 1230–1235.

2. Carney, P., Berry, R., & Geyer, J. (Eds.). (2005). *Clinical sleep disorders.* Philadelphia, PA: Lippincott, Williams & Wilkins.

3. Kirby, D. A., & Verrier, R. L. (1989). Differential effects of sleep stage on coronary hemodynamic function. *American Journal of Physiology, 256,* H1378–H1383.

4. Punjabi, N. M., Shahar, E., Redline, S., et al. (2004). Sleep disordered breathing, glucose intolerance, and insulin resistance: The Sleep Heart Health study. *American Journal of Epidemiology, 160*(6), 521–530.

5. Ancoli-Israel, S., Stepnowsky, C., Dimsdale, J., et al. (2002). The effect of race and sleep-disordered breathing on nocturnal BP "dipping": Analysis in an older population. *Chest, 122*(4), 1148–1155.

6. Phillips, C., Hedner, J., Berend, N., et al. (2005). Diurnal and obstructive sleep apnea influences on arterial stiffness and central blood pressure in men. *Sleep, 28*(5), 604–609.

7. Doherty, L. S., Kiely, J. L., Swan, V., et al. (2005). Long-term effects of nasal continuous positive airway pressure therapy on cardiovascular outcomes in sleep apnea syndrome. *Chest, 127*(6), 2076–2084.

8. Dhillon, S., Chung, S. A., Fargher, T., et al. (2005). Sleep apnea, hypertension, and the effects of continuous positive airway pressure. *American Journal of Hypertension, 18*(5, Pt. 1), 594–600.

9. Dursunoglu, N., Dursunoglu, D., Cuhadaroglu, C., et al. (2005). Acute effects of automated continuous positive airway pressure on blood pressure in patients with sleep apnea and hypertension. *Respiration, 72*(2), 150–155.

10. Borgel, J., Sanner, B. M., Keskin, F., et al. (2004). Obstructive sleep apnea and blood pressure: Interaction between the blood pressure-lowering effects of positive airway pressure therapy and antihypertensive drugs. *American Journal of Hypertension, 17*(12, Pt. 1), 1081–1087.

11. Becker, H. F., Jerrentrup, A., Ploch, T., et al. (2003). Effect of nasal continuous positive airway pressure treatment on blood pressure in patients with obstructive sleep apnea. *Circulation, 107*(1), 68–73.

12. Naughton, M. T. (2005). The link between obstructive sleep apnea and heart failure: Underappreciated opportunity for treatment. *Current Cardiology Report, 7*(3), 211–215.

13. Kenchaiah, S., Narula, J., & Vasan, R. S. (2004). Risk factors for heart failure. *Medical Clinics of North America, 88*(5), 1145–1172.

14. Weinstein, M. D. (2003). Continuous positive airway pressure in patients with heart failure. *New England Journal of Medicine, 349*(1), 93–95; author reply 93–95.

15. Kanagala, R., Murali, N. S., Friedman, P. A., et al. (2003). Obstructive sleep apnea and the recurrence of atrial fibrillation. *Circulation, 107*(20), 2589–2594.

16. Guardiola, J. J., Matheson, P. J., Clavijo, L. C., et al. (2001). Hypercoagulability in patients with obstructive sleep apnea. *Sleep Medicine, 2*(6), 517–523.

17. Geiser, T., Buck, F., Meyer, B. J., et al. (2002). In vivo platelet activation is increased during sleep in patients with obstructive sleep apnea syndrome. *Respiration, 69*(3), 229–234.

18. Babu, A. R., Herdegen, J., Fogelfeld, L., et al. (2005). Type 2 diabetes, glycemic control, and continuous positive airway pressure in obstructive sleep apnea. *Archives of Internal Medicine, 165*(4), 447–452.

19. Harsch, I. A., Hahn, E. G., & Konturek, P. C. (2005). Insulin resistance and other metabolic aspects of the obstructive sleep apnea syndrome. *Medical Science Monitor, 11*(3), RA70–RA75.

20. Svatikova, A., Wolk, R., Gami, A. S., et al. (2005). Interactions between obstructive sleep apnea and the metabolic syndrome. *Current Diabetes Report, 5*(1), 53–58.

21. Larkin, E. K., Elston, R. C., Patel, S. R., et al. (2005). Linkage of serum leptin levels in families with sleep apnea. *International Journal of Obesity, 29*(3), 260–267.

22. Phillips, B. (2005). Sleep-disordered breathing and cardiovascular disease. *Sleep Medicine Review, 9*(2), 131–140.

23. Nelson, C. A., Wolk, R., & Somers, V. K. (2005). Sleep-disordered breathing: Implications for the pathophysiology and management of cardiovascular disease. *Comprehensive Therapy, 31*(1), 21–27.

24. Parish, J. M., & Somers, V. K. (2004). Obstructive sleep apnea and cardiovascular disease. *Mayo Clinic Proceedings, 79*(8), 1036–1046.

25. Thorvaldsen, P., Kuulasmaa, K., Rajakangas, A. M., et al. (1997). Stroke trends in the WHO MONICA project. *Stroke, 28,* 500–506.

26. Culebras, A. (2004). Cerebrovascular disease and sleep. *Current Neurology and Neuroscience Report, 4*(2), 164–169.

27. Diaz, J., & Sempere, A. P. (2004). Cerebral ischemia: New risk factors. *Cerebrovascular Disease, 17*(Suppl. 1), 43–50.

28. Nachtmann, A., Stang, A., Wang, Y. M., et al. (2003). Association of obstructive sleep apnea and stenotic artery disease in ischemic stroke patients. *Atherosclerosis, 169*(2), 301–307.

29. Yaggi, H., & Mohsenin, V. (2003). Sleep-disordered breathing and stroke. *Clinics in Chest Medicine, 24*(2), 223–237.

30. Bassetti, C., & Aldrich, M. S. (1999). Sleep apnea in acute cerebrovascular diseases: Final report on 128 patients. *Sleep, 22*(2), 217–223.

chapter 23
Sleep and Other Medical Disorders

THERESA A. KRUPSKI

LEARNING OBJECTIVES

On completion of this chapter, the reader should be able to:

1. Describe the bidirectional influences of various respiratory, neurologic, gastrointestinal, endocrine, rheumatologic, renal, and infectious diseases on sleep and sleep disorders.

KEY TERMS

Asthma
Chronic obstructive pulmonary disease
Cystic fibrosis
Endocrine disorders
Fibromyalgia
Gastrointestinal disorders
Infectious diseases
Neuromuscular disorders
Renal disease
Rheumatologic disorders

RESPIRATORY DISORDERS

Asthma

Asthma is an inflammatory disease of the airways that occurs in about 5% of the population. It is characterized by episodic dyspnea and wheezing, reversible episodes of bronchoconstriction, and airway hyperreactivity to a variety of specific and nonspecific stimuli.

In a survey of asthmatic patients, 74% of subjects reported nocturnal awakenings at least once weekly, and 64% had one at least three times a week (1). In another group of asthmatic patients, nocturnal symptoms occurred less than once a week in 16% to 23% and at least once a week in 5% to 15% of subjects (2).

Patients with nocturnal asthma experience poor sleep quality and frequent arousals, resulting in sleep deprivation, irritability, and fatigue (1). Worsening of asthma at night or in the early morning occurs in over two-thirds of asthmatics, indicating nighttime bronchoconstriction (3). Besides normal sleep-related decreases in functional residual capacity (FRC), minute ventilation, and tidal volume, asthmatics have further abnormal reductions in these parameters during sleep that are attributed to increased airway responsiveness, increased airway secretions, and circadian changes in vagal tone, body temperature, cortisol, epinephrine, and inflammatory mediators (4, 5). Bronchoalveolar lavage fluid in patients with nocturnal asthma may show an increase in total leukocyte count, neutrophils, and eosinophils (6).

Polysomnographic (PSG) features of asthmatic subjects demonstrate increased wake time, less total sleep time, reduced sleep efficiency, increased number of awakenings, and greater wake time after sleep onset compared with normal subjects (7, 8). Nocturnal asthmatics who snore or have obstructive sleep apnea (OSA) show increased frequency of nocturnal asthma attacks. Although they are two distinct disease processes, nocturnal asthma and OSA often share overlapping symptoms of choking, coughing, and dyspnea. Continuous positive airway pressure (CPAP) therapy has been shown to improve asthma control and increase peak expiratory flow rate in this group of patients (9, 10).

Chronic Obstructive Pulmonary Disease

Chronic obstructive pulmonary disease (COPD) (also called "chronic obstructive lung disease") is a disease state characterized by airflow limitation that is relatively irreversible. The airflow limitation is usually associated with an abnormal inflammatory response of the lungs to noxious particles or gases and is progressive in nature (11). The inflammatory response of the lungs results in pathologic changes in the small airways and alveoli. Emphysema results when there is a predominance of alveolar destruction, whereas chronic bronchitis is the result of progressive airway narrowing because of excessive secretions blocking the lumen of the airways. Dyspnea and chronic cough are the chief complaints with which COPD patients usually present. Respiratory failure can complicate advanced cases, with hypoxemia and hypercapnia occurring during both wakefulness and sleep. The World Health Organization predicts that COPD will be the fifth most prevalent disease (currently 12th) and the third most common cause of death (currently sixth) by 2020 (12).

Clinicians distinguish between two subtypes of COPD patients: blue bloaters and pink puffers. Blue bloaters have lower baseline arterial oxygen saturation (SaO_2), hence their blood will be bluer and they will experience larger falls in SaO_2 (especially during rapid eye movement [REM] sleep), more episodes of oxygen desaturation, and longer durations of oxygen desaturation while asleep than will pink puffers.

Patients with COPD sleep poorly compared with healthy subjects (13–15). The incidence of sleep complaints is related to the rates of respiratory symptoms in COPD patients. In the Tucson Epidemiologic Study of Chronic Lung Diseases, 28% of asymptomatic COPD subjects reported insomnia and 9% reported daytime sleepiness. Among subjects with one respiratory symptom, either cough or wheezing, 39% reported insomnia and 12% reported daytime sleepiness. When both cough and wheezing were present as respiratory symptoms, sleep complaints increased in patients, with 52% of them reporting insomnia and 22% reporting daytime sleepiness (16).

PSG features show reduced total sleep time, increased sleep stage changes, and increased arousal frequency. Arousals may or may not be related to hypoxemia. Fleetham et al. showed that reversal of hypoxemia with supplemental oxygen did not diminish arousal frequency. Oxygen therapy may or may not affect sleep quality (17, 18).

During sleep, COPD patients may develop significant oxygen desaturation, with the most severe desaturations occurring during REM sleep (14, 19–21). Sleep-related hypoxemic episodes are more common among blue bloaters than among pink puffers and occur during periods of hypoventilation, typically during REM sleep, because of the relative atonia of the intercostal muscles that occurs during REM sleep (20, 22, 23). Ventilatory abnormalities associated with decreased lung volumes (because, for instance, of obesity) also contribute to hypoxemia during sleep (24).

Overlap syndrome, also referred to as OLDOSA (obstructive lung disease and obstructive sleep apnea), is a term used for patients with coexisting COPD and/or asthma and OSA. A more severe course of sleep-disordered breathing is noted in subjects with coexisting COPD (25). Sleep studies are usually indicated in COPD when there is a possibility of sleep apnea or obesity-hypoventilation syndrome (26–28). A triad of respiratory alterations contributes to the physiologic derangements seen in overlap syndrome:

1. Increase in upper airway resistance: in addition to the excessive soft tissue and oropharyngeal anomalies seen in OSA, upper airway luminal narrowing may be further compromised by COPD processes such as mucosal inflammation, chronic rhinitis and bronchitis, and reduced cough reflex.
2. Sleep alterations in lung volumes: REM skeletal muscle atonia, thoracic restrictions related to body position, and consequent tidal volume reduction result in FRC reduction, even in normal subjects. In patients with COPD, functional lung volumes are further compromised by alveolar air trapping or hyperinflation.
3. Changes in central mediators of respiratory effort: during wakefulness, chemoreceptor responses to hypoxemia and hypercapnia regulate respiratory rate and depth. These chemoreceptor responses are blunted during sleep, impacting both ventilatory and arousal responses.

Several studies have shown that patients with COPD and OSA have more profound nocturnal oxygen desaturations and sleep disturbances compared with either disease alone. Additionally, reports from observational studies suggest increased mortality in overlap syndrome compared with COPD and OSA alone (Table 23-1) (30).

Although supplemental oxygen is the mainstay for COPD and sleep-associated desaturation alone, positive airway pressure, either CPAP or bilevel positive airway pressure (BPAP), combined with supplemental oxygen, is required for the overlap syndrome (31, 32). Some patients may respond better to BPAP than to CPAP (33).

Table 23-1 The Cardinal Symptoms of COPD and OSA (29) with Potential Overlapping Symptoms Highlighted in the Center

OSA Symptoms	COPD Symptoms
Snoring	Wheezing
Respiratory pauses	Sputum production
Daytime sleepiness	Dyspnea
Overlapping Symptoms Poor sleep quality Insomnia Nocturnal cough/gasp Persistent fatigue Mood changes	

COPD, chronic obstructive pulmonary disease; OSA, obstructive sleep apnea.
Adapted from Mieczkowski, B., & Ezzie, M. E. (2014). Update on obstructive sleep apnea and its relation to COPD. *International Journal of Chronic Obstructive Pulmonary Disease, 9,* 349–362. doi:10.2147/COPD.S42394

Cystic Fibrosis

Cystic fibrosis (CF) is a multisystem genetic disorder that primarily affects Caucasian infants, children, and young adults. It is characterized by abnormal transport of sodium and chloride across the epithelium in all exocrine tissues, leading to an increase in sweat sodium and chloride concentration. This inability to move salt and chloride in and out of cells results in thick viscous secretions in the lungs, pancreas, intestine, liver, and reproductive tract. Consequently, CF patients develop bronchiectasis and progressive lung disease, exocrine pancreatic insufficiency, intestinal dysfunction, abnormal sweat gland function, and urogenital dysfunction (34–38).

CF patients have poor sleep quality (39). Nonetheless, sleep latency and sleep efficiency are often normal in CF patients despite poor sleep quality (39). Exacerbations of lung disease in adults with CF adversely affect sleep and neurobehavioral performance regardless of underlying disease severity (40). A study of 40 children with CF in stable condition showed an early occurrence of OSA associated with a mild level of sleep disruption. Early routine nocturnal respiratory monitoring is advised in children with CF (41).

Cough, sleep fragmentation, medication side effects such as β-agonists, increased work of breathing, and hypoxemia have all been documented during sleep in CF patients. Episodic nocturnal hypoxia may lead to the development of pulmonary hypertension and cor pulmonale. Poor daytime function and quality of life have also been reported (42, 43). Noninvasive ventilation has been proposed as a means to temporarily reverse or slow the progression of worsening respiratory failure in CF (44).

Restrictive Lung Diseases

Restrictive lung diseases are characterized by reduced lung volumes, either because of an alteration in the lung parenchyma or because of diseases of the chest wall, pleura, or neuromuscular apparatus. In the early stages, the patient may be totally asymptomatic, but with disease progression, exertional dyspnea, followed by dyspnea at rest, is commonly encountered. Restrictive lung diseases commonly associated with sleep-disordered breathing are obesity, kyphoscoliosis, interstitial lung disease, and pregnancy (45).

Patients with restrictive lung disease exhibit a wide range of respiratory and oxygenation abnormalities during sleep. The combination of restrictive severity (intrapulmonary as well as extrapulmonary) and confounding factors, such as obesity, age, and gender, determines the degree of disturbed nocturnal physiology (46). These patients often complain of disrupted sleep and excessive daytime sleepiness, often even before waking respiratory symptoms become discernible. Other sleep-related symptoms include apneas, awakenings, choking, unrefreshing sleep, and morning headaches (47).

PSG suggests that OSA is present in more than 50% of patients with restrictive lung diseases and nocturnal hypoventilation in more than 29% of severely obese individuals (48–50). REM sleep percentage and sleep efficiency are decreased in obese patients, but sleep-onset latency and REM latency can remain normal (48).

In patients with kyphoscoliosis, a spectrum of breathing abnormalities can be found, ranging from no abnormalities to obstructive apneas/hypopneas and central apneas (51–53). Patients with interstitial lung disease often demonstrate transient or sustained nocturnal desaturation during REM sleep, disturbances in sleep quality, increase in stage N1 sleep, reduction in REM sleep, and an increase in the number of arousals (54–57). During pregnancy, sleep quality is poor, with reduced sleep efficiency, increased nocturnal awakenings, increased stage N1 sleep, reduced REM sleep, increased daytime fatigue, and louder or more frequent snoring (58–62).

NEUROMUSCULAR DISORDERS

The neuromuscular disorders most commonly associated with sleep-disordered breathing are muscular dystrophy (MD), myotonic dystrophy (DM), amyotrophic lateral sclerosis (ALS), poliomyelitis, and myasthenia gravis. Neuromuscular disorders may be caused by defects in the neurons or the muscle itself. Motor neurons extend from the brain to the spinal cord (upper motor neurons) and from the spinal cord reach muscle fibers throughout the body (lower motor neurons). In neuromuscular disorders, the neurons are damaged and are unable to relay neural information or innervate muscle activity. The damage may occur in the brain, along the axon, or at the axon terminals (neuromuscular junctions). The principal consequence of a neuromuscular dysfunction in a sleeping individual is compromise of the ventilatory mechanism (i.e., lower motor neuron, neuromuscular junction, or muscle) (63). Nocturnal breathing abnormalities or sleep-related breathing disorders frequently precede respiratory failure during wakefulness by months or even years (64).

Subjective sleep complaints include air hunger, intermittent snoring, orthopnea (difficulty breathing except when in an upright position), cyanosis (a bluish or purplish discoloration of the skin due to deficient oxygenation of the blood), restlessness, and insomnia. Daytime symptoms such as morning drowsiness, frequent morning headaches, and excessive daytime sleepiness have been described in patients with neuromuscular diseases (65).

MD is a group of genetic diseases characterized by progressive weakness and degeneration of skeletal muscles. Age of onset, extent and distribution of weakness, and rate of progression vary by MD type. Duchenne MD (DMD) is the most common form of MD and seen primarily in boys. It is caused by the absence of the protein dystrophin. Dystrophin is found in muscle cell membrane and facilitates muscle cell self-repair. Muscle degeneration leads to loss of ambulation in adolescence and progresses to respiratory impairment, eventually requiring ventilatory support. The PSG of patients with DMD may reveal an increased number of arousals during the night, reduced REM sleep, and both central and obstructive apneas (66–70). Nocturnal noninvasive ventilation may improve daytime respiratory muscle function.

Patients with DM have disrupted sleep, apneic as well as hypopneic events, and hypoventilatory oxygen desaturation during REM sleep (71–74). Central nervous system (CNS) lesions may contribute to the hypersomnia without an accompanying sleep-disordered breathing or decrease in central respiratory drive (75).

ALS is a progressive and ultimately fatal neurodegenerative disorder, which affects neurons in the brain and spinal cord, eventually causing neural cell death. Loss of muscle-activating impulses and consequent muscle function leads to muscle weakness and eventual muscle atrophy. The diaphragm and chest wall muscles are not spared, and when they fail to function adequately, mechanical ventilatory support is required. Patients with ALS may have obstructive apneic and hypopneic events, with the majority of respiratory events occurring during REM sleep (76–78). Patients with ALS and diaphragmatic dysfunction have significant nocturnal desaturation secondary to hypoventilation as well as reduced REM sleep compared with those patients with preserved diaphragmatic function (79).

Poliomyelitis is an infectious viral disease mainly affecting young children. It is preventable through vaccination but not curable. The manifestations may be subclinical, nonparalytic, or paralytic. The enterovirus enters the body through the fecal–oral route, begins an alimentary phase, enters the bloodstream, and may eventually cross the blood–brain barrier, invading the nervous system. Polio is a lower motor neuron disease, which can involve the motor nuclei of the brainstem and respiratory motor nuclei, resulting in respiratory muscle dysfunction and/or paralysis, including that of the diaphragm. These patients may develop sleep-disordered breathing, including obstructive apneic and hypopneic events, nocturnal hypoventilation, reduced sleep efficiency, increased arousals, increased stage N1 sleep, and reduced REM sleep (80–82).

Decades after surviving paralytic poliomyelitis, survivors may develop symptoms of postpolio syndrome (PPS): fatigue, heat or cold intolerance, slowly progressive muscle weakness/atrophy, fasciculations, and muscle and joint pain. Although the cause of PPS is unknown, it is believed that excessive metabolic stress on those muscles initially damaged results in the loss of nerve terminals and eventually of motor neurons themselves (83). The stressors include illness, weight gain, and the aging process. Patients with PPS may suffer from weakness of the diaphragm and respiratory muscles sufficient to cause resting and/or exertional dyspnea and hypercapnia. PSG should be used to rule out obstructive, central, and mixed apneas as well as nocturnal hypoxemia and hypercapnia. Nocturnal noninvasive ventilation may improve sleep quality, symptoms of daytime fatigue, and daytime respiratory muscle function.

Myasthenia gravis is a chronic autoimmune disease characterized by varying degrees of skeletal muscle weakness. It is caused by a defect in the transmission of nerve impulses across the neuromuscular junction to the target muscles. The neurotransmitter acetylcholine is blocked from binding to the muscle by the body's own antibodies. Patients with myasthenia gravis have a higher incidence of both central and obstructive apneas and hypopneas that are associated with significant oxygen desaturation and that occur predominantly during REM sleep (84–86).

DM is a genetic multisystemic disease characterized by progressive muscular weakness, myotonia, and involvement of the CNS, eyes, heart, respiratory function, and endocrine systems (87). There are two major forms: DM1, also known as Steinert disease, which may have congenital, juvenile, or adult onset, and DM2, which presents in adulthood and is often less severe. DM1 is more prevalent.

The manifestations of DM1 include neuromuscular, behavioral, emotional, and cognitive disturbances. The daily activities and social roles of this population are compromised and life expectancy is shortened. Respiratory failure results from respiratory muscle weakness and myotonia, culminating in alveolar hypoventilation, and chronic hypercapnia and hypoxemia.

Diaphragm Paralysis

The diaphragm is the primary muscle of ventilation. When contracted, the diaphragm descends downward, increasing thoracic volume while decreasing intrapleural pressure. The change in intrapleural pressure creates a pressure gradient and allows air to flow into the lungs. A single anatomic structure, the diaphragm has two halves individually innervated by branches of the phrenic nerve. The individual nerve supply allows each half to function independently of the other, although in normal diaphragmatic function, both halves move synchronously.

The most common causes of bilateral diaphragmatic paralysis are high spinal cord injury, thoracic trauma, multiple sclerosis, anterior horn disease, and MD. Unilateral paralysis of the diaphragm is much more common than is bilateral paralysis and may be caused by phrenic nerve damage because of trauma, surgery, radiation, tumor, or neuropathy. Unilateral diaphragmatic paralysis is associated with nocturnal hypoxemia but, in the absence of systemic lung disease, it does not generally lead to chronic respiratory failure or cor pulmonale (88).

During REM sleep in normal persons, ventilation depends primarily on diaphragm function. In patients with diaphragm dysfunction, during both REM sleep and wakefulness, electromyographic activity of the extradiaphragmatic respiratory muscles is higher than normal as a compensation for diaphragm weakness (89). Patients with diaphragmatic paralysis have reduced REM and stage N3 sleep. Patients with unilateral diaphragm dysfunction are at risk of developing sleep disordered breathing during REM sleep (89). Bilateral diaphragmatic paralysis can be associated with sleep apnea (90). Watanabe et al. (91) reported a case of central sleep apnea (CSA) accompanied by bilateral paralysis of the diaphragm after pediatric cardiac surgery. Hoffstein and Taylor described a rapid development of OSA following hemidiaphragmatic and unilateral vocal cord paralysis as a complication of mediastinal surgery (92).

It had been hypothesized that patients with bilateral diaphragmatic paralysis might not be able to sustain REM sleep. However, Bennett et al. (93) observed that patients with bilateral diaphragmatic paralysis had a normal quantity of REM sleep achieved by inspiratory recruitment of extradiaphragmatic muscles in both tonic and phasic REM, suggesting brainstem reorganization.

GASTROINTESTINAL DISORDERS

Gastroesophageal Reflux

Gastroesophageal reflux (GER) is caused by a backflow of gastric acid and other gastric contents into the esophagus because of incompetent barriers at the gastroesophageal junction. The pathogenesis of GER is multifactorial, involving transient lower esophageal sphincter (LES) relaxation as well as other LES pressure abnormalities. Other factors contributing to the pathophysiology of GER include the presence of a hiatal hernia, poor esophageal clearance, delayed gastric emptying, and impaired mucosal defensive factors (94).

Regurgitation of gastric contents into the mouth and heartburn are the characteristic symptoms of GER. Reflux of acidic stomach contents into the pharynx, larynx, and tracheobronchial tree can cause chronic cough, bronchoconstriction, pharyngitis, laryngitis, bronchitis, or pneumonia. Morning hoarseness may be noted. Recurrent pulmonary aspiration can cause aspiration pneumonia, pulmonary fibrosis, or chronic asthma. Reflux in the sleeping horizontal person is exacerbated by delayed acid clearance secondary to decreased esophageal motility, and reduced salivation and swallowing.

Several studies have reported an association between OSA and GERD. On the one hand, GERD may play a role in the development of OSA by causing upper airway inflammation and obstruction. Acid suppression with proton pump inhibitors resulted in improvement of the apnea index in OSA patients in a small nonrandomized study. On the other hand, OSA may lead to GERD because of increased intrathoracic pressure, and treatment with CPAP has been shown to improve nocturnal heartburn and regurgitation, as well as distal esophageal acid exposure and frequency of acid reflux episodes (95).

The negative impact on quality of life may be greater in nocturnal GER than in daytime GER. In a large nationwide telephone survey in the United States, 79% of respondents reported having heartburn symptoms at night, of which 75% stated that their sleep was affected by heartburn, and 63% noted that heartburn had an impact on their ability to sleep well (96). Farup et al. (97) found a prevalence of 10% for nocturnal GER, with 74% of respondents who reported frequent GER symptoms having nocturnal GER.

GER is estimated to be present in 50% to 60% of asthmatic children and 60% to 80% of adult asthmatics (98). A study conducted by Wasilewska and colleagues reported a possible association between nocturnal GER and sleep-related breathing disorders in children. Higher numbers of apneas and hypopneas during REM sleep were found in children with nocturnal GER (99). Demeter et al. (100–102) noted that in patients with severe OSA, erosive reflux disease is more frequent, and a positive correlation between severity of reflux disease and sleep apnea has been reported by some, but not all, investigators.

PSG findings in GERD patients include an increased arousal index and decreased duration spent in the deeper stages of sleep (103).

Functional Bowel Disorders

Functional bowel disorders are characterized by chronic gastrointestinal tract symptoms without significant anatomic, metabolic, or infectious abnormalities. They can affect the entire digestive tract. These disorders include functional dyspepsia (FD), diarrhea, constipation, abdominal bloating, abdominal pain syndrome, and irritable bowel syndrome (IBS).

Patients with functional bowel disorders have a high incidence of sleep complaints as well as abnormalities of autonomic functioning. The measurement of autonomic functioning during sleep can differentiate the patients with functional bowel disorders from normal controls (104, 105). Patients reported significantly more dissatisfaction with their sleep quality and increased daytime fatigue as a result of both insomnia-type symptomatology and nonrestful sleep (106, 107).

A significant proportion of patients, particularly those with IBS and dyspepsia, reported nighttime gastrointestinal symptoms (106). In a study on patients with functional bowel disorders by Fass et al. (107), sleep disturbances were reported by 68% of those with FD, 50.2% with IBS, 71% with IBS and FD, and 55% of normal subjects. Vege et al. (108) reported that in patients who suffered from sleep disorders, there was a prevalence of 33.3% for IBS and 21.3% for FD. Although both IBS and FD are prevalent in those with self-reported sleep disturbance, the presence of objective sleep abnormalities may be more difficult to detect. Elsenbruch et al. (109) observed no significant differences in PSG parameters, such as sleep efficiency, sleep latency, number of arousals, and percentage of N3 sleep in patients with IBS compared with controls. In another study, women with IBS and significant depressive symptoms had increased sleep latency (110).

ENDOCRINE DISORDERS

Sleep Deprivation and Hormonal Alterations

Sleep deprivation has been linked to a wide variety of hormonal and metabolic alterations. The onset and severity of diabetes, hypertension, and obesity may be impacted by chronic sleep loss (111). Hormonal release by the pituitary is profoundly affected by sleep and may be either activated or inhibited through two pathways: the hypothalamic–pituitary axes and the autonomic nervous system. Modulation of hypothalamic releasing or inhibiting factors controls pituitary function, affecting growth hormone (GH) and corticotropin. The autonomic pathway impacts the hormonal control of carbohydrate metabolism. With chronic partial sleep loss, the body's ability to secrete and respond to insulin is reduced, causing alterations in glucose metabolism and is a characteristic early marker of diabetes. Sleep loss alters the ability of leptin, a satiety hormone, and ghrelin, an appetite-stimulating hormone, to accurately signal caloric need (112) and appetite control. Poor appetite control, altered glucose metabolism, and insulin resistance are predisposing factors for obesity and diabetes. In a study of 11 healthy young men over 16 consecutive nights, sleep deprivation was found to dampen the secretion of thyroid-stimulating hormone and increase blood levels of cortisol, especially during the afternoon and evening (113).

Hypothyroidism and Hyperthyroidism

The two main hormones produced by the thyroid, T3 (triiodothyronine) and T4 (thyroxine), are metabolism-regulating hormones essential for growth and development, and maturation of the body's nervous system. Hypothyroidism refers to an underactive thyroid that produces insufficient levels of thyroid hormone. The effect is metabolic lowering, which leads to symptoms of weight gain and fatigue. Marked reduction in slow-wave sleep (SWS) has been seen in patients, which is reversible with treatment (114). OSA has been reported to occur frequently in patients with untreated hypothyroidism, especially when myxedema (dry skin and hair, loss of mental and physical vigor) is present. Pathogenesis appears to involve both myopathy and upper airway edema (115). Unfortunately, indices of sleep apnea severity do not diminish significantly in all patients following attainment of a euthyroid state (normal thyroid hormone levels). In addition, therapy of hypothyroidism with thyroxine in this patient group may be complicated by the development of nocturnal angina and ventricular arrhythmias (116).

In contrast, thyroid overactivity results in excessive thyroid hormone production. Symptoms of hyperthyroidism include fatigue but difficulty sleeping, mood impairment, difficulty concentrating, muscle weakness, tachycardia, and heat intolerance.

Acromegaly

Acromegaly is a chronic metabolic disorder in which there is excessive GH production after the skeleton and other organs have finished growing. The abnormal GH release is caused by pituitary gland dysfunction, usually a pituitary adenoma. Symptoms include enlarged facial bones, feet, hands, sebaceous glands, tongue (macroglossia), and jaw (prognathism). Somnolence and sleep apnea are part of the clinical spectrum in patients with acromegaly.

OSA is common in acromegaly, with prevalence rates ranging from 13.2% to 75% in this population (117, 118). Sleep apnea is more likely to occur with greater severity of acromegaly, older age, greater neck circumference, greater initial tongue volume, alterations in craniofacial dimensions (predominantly of the mandible), and upper airway narrowing because of changes in pharyngeal soft tissues (118, 119). Other factors that could contribute to the development of OSA are facial bone deformity, mucosal edema, hypertrophy of the pharyngeal and laryngeal cartilages, and the presence of nasal polyps (120, 121). There appears to be no correlation between OSA and biochemical parameters of disease activity such as GH and insulin-like growth factor 1 (IGF-1) levels (122). Improvements in the indices of OSA severity have been reported following therapy of acromegaly with bromocriptine, octreotide (a long-acting somatostatin analog), and pituitary surgery (adenomectomy or hypophysectomy). Nonetheless, OSA may still persist despite normalization of GH levels during therapy (123–127). In one report, the frequency of sleep apnea in patients with treated acromegaly was estimated to still be at least 21% (128).

CSA is also common and is associated with higher random GH and IGF-1 levels than in OSA (129). Possible mechanisms for the development of CSA in patients with acromegaly include central respiratory control dysfunction, reflex inhibition of the respiratory center as a result of upper airway narrowing, or an increase in the ventilatory carbon dioxide response of the respiratory center (120, 130).

PSG features of acromegaly include a reduction in REM sleep and delta sleep, both of which can increase following normalization of GH levels (131).

Cushing Syndrome

Patients with Cushing syndrome (CS) have an excess of adrenocorticosteroid hormones, usually the hormone cortisol. Cortisol is normally released in response to stress and controls metabolism of carbohydrates, fats, and proteins. The most common cause is long-term use of exogenous corticosteroid medication, often prescribed for its anti-inflammatory effects in rheumatoid arthritis, transplant organ rejection, lupus, and asthma. Endogenous cortisol excess may be due to the overproduction of cortisol by the adrenal gland or the overproduction of the cortisol-regulating adrenocorticotropic hormone. These dysregulations are often caused by tumors of the adrenal or pituitary glands, respectively.

Symptoms include progressive obesity with hallmark fatty depositions between the shoulders (buffalo hump), on the face (moon face), midsection, and upper back. Skin changes often seen are acne, skin thinning with easy bruising, and dark purple-red striae on the abdomen, thighs, and breasts.

Sleep complaints are common, including an increased incidence of sleep apnea of approximately 32% in patients with CS and Cushing disease (CD). Parapharyngeal fat deposition may be contributory to the pathogenesis of OSA. In addition, patients without sleep apnea may present with snoring or may have changes in sleep architecture including more fragmented sleep, poorer sleep continuity, shortened REM latency, and an increased REM density (132, 133).

Addison Disease

Addison disease is a rare, chronic disorder caused by adrenal gland failure resulting in insufficient production of adrenal hormones, including cortisol, aldosterone, androgens (male), and estrogen (female). Patients with primary adrenal insufficiency or Addison disease may present with complaints of weakness, fatigue, anorexia, gastrointestinal symptoms, weight loss, hyperpigmentation, and hypotension. Owing to the nonspecific and slowly progressive nature of the symptoms, the disease is usually not apparent until the adrenal cortex is severely damaged. Hormone replacement therapy is the treatment for Addison disease.

In one study, weekly sleep disturbances were reported in 34% of patients with Addison disease, including difficulties falling asleep (13%), repeated awakenings (14%), and early morning awakenings (20%) (134). Bedtime administration of hydrocortisone in patients with Addison disease can lead to a significant reduction in REM latency, an increase in REM sleep time, and greater wake time after sleep onset (135).

RHEUMATOLOGIC DISORDERS

Acute and Chronic Pain Syndromes

Rheumatologic disorders are chronic debilitating diseases of the muscles, tendons, connective tissue, bones, and joints causing stiffness, pain, and limited mobility. There is a multitude of such disorders, with the most common being gout, juvenile arthritis, fibromyalgia (FM), osteoarthritis, and rheumatoid arthritis.

Acute and chronic pain can disrupt sleep, and poor sleep can magnify perceived pain intensity, leading to a vicious cycle of increasing pain and increasing sleep disturbances. Pain can give rise to insomnia, including sleep-onset insomnia, multiple awakenings (sleep fragmentation), and early morning awakenings (waking up too early and not being able to fall back to sleep) (136, 137). PSG studies of patients with acute pain may reveal shortened and fragmented sleep, reduced SWS, and reduced REM sleep. In one study, depressive symptoms were predictive of the severity of sleep disturbances in patients with chronic pain (138).

Fibromyalgia

FM has been defined by the American College of Rheumatology as the presence of widespread pain in combination with tenderness at 11 or more of 18 specific tender point sites (139). There may be complaints of tension headaches, fatigue, sleep, memory, and mood issues. Unlike other rheumatologic disorders in which pain is caused by tissue inflammation, the painful tissues in FM are not inflamed. As a result, FM does not cause tissue/organ damage or joint deformity. It is more prevalent among women than men. Symptoms may be precipitated by a single triggering event such as infection, psychological stress, or physical trauma, or they may gradually accumulate over time.

Sleep complaints, including insomnia, early morning awakenings, less satisfying sleep, and nonrestorative sleep have been reported. A relationship between poor sleep quality, pain intensity, and perception of pain may exist in FM patients; among patients with FM, poorer sleepers tend to report significantly more pain, and more daytime pain leads to poorer nighttime sleep (140).

PSG features of FM include an increased number of electroencephalogram (EEG) arousals, increased stage N1 sleep, fewer sleep spindles in stage N2 sleep, reduced SWS, and reduced REM sleep (141–143).

An alpha frequency rhythm, referred to as an alpha–delta sleep anomaly, has been described. Alpha activity (8 to 13 Hz), which is typically present only during relaxed wakefulness and brief arousals, is superimposed onto the delta waves of nonrapid eye movement (NREM) sleep. There are three patterns of alpha EEG sleep in patients with FM: phasic alpha (simultaneous with delta activity), tonic alpha (continuous throughout the low voltage, mixed EEG patterns of NREM sleep), and low alpha activity. A phasic alpha sleep activity has been correlated with poor sleep, less total sleep time, lower sleep efficiency, less SWS, worsening of pain after sleep, a postsleep increase in the number of tender points, and a longer duration of FM pain compared with the other patterns of alpha intrusion (144). The alpha-NREM sleep anomaly has also been observed in other patient groups, including those with chronic pain syndromes and depression. Furthermore, not only is the alpha-NREM sleep anomaly nonspecific for FM, it is not universally present in all patients with FM. Some investigators doubt that the alpha-NREM sleep anomaly is abnormal. Mahowald et al. (145) suggest that the alpha–delta NREM sleep EEG pattern is nonspecific and might actually represent a "sleep maintaining process," although others believe it to be a sign of poor quality, nonrestorative sleep.

RENAL DISEASE

Chronic Renal Failure (End-Stage Renal Disease)

The kidneys' functions are to regulate blood composition by removing toxic waste such as urea, ammonia, and drugs from the blood, preserve blood pressure by regulating water volume, and maintain the body's acid/base levels.

During metabolism, far more acids are produced than bases. Acids break down into hydrogen ions, are filtered through the kidneys, and excreted. The concentration of hydrogen ions (pH) in the blood is a balance of hydrogen ions, H^+, and sodium bicarbonate, HCO_3. Carbon dioxide (CO_2), a by-product of cellular respiration, combines with water to form carbonic acid, H_2CO_3, which separates into $H^+ + HCO_3$:

$$CO_2 + H_2O \Leftrightarrow H_2CO_3 \Leftrightarrow H^+ + HCO_3$$

The equation is bidirectionally driven on the basis of an excess of CO_2 or HCO_3. The renal response to excess CO_2 as seen in hypoventilation (respiratory acidosis) is to increase blood plasma levels of HCO_3. Conversely, an excess of HCO_3 (metabolic alkalosis) results in CO_2 retention in order to maintain a neutral pH level of 7.4. The respiratory response to metabolic alkalosis is hypoventilation, whereas metabolic acidosis is compensated through hyperventilation.

As renal failure progresses, the kidneys lose their ability to effectively maintain a normal blood pH and filter metabolic wastes, causing toxic accumulation in the blood. Chronic renal failure occurs with the gradual and usually permanent loss of kidney function over time. This failure may be caused by primary diseases of the kidneys, but the major causes are diabetes and hypertension. Chronic renal failure is incurable and will progress until dialysis or kidney transplantation is needed. Proper dietary management may help slow the progression and reduce complications.

Sleep disturbances are reported by up to 80% of patients on dialysis for end-stage renal disease (ESRD), with sleep apnea, restless legs syndrome (RLS), and periodic limb movement disorder (PLMD) being more prevalent than in the general population. PSG features include reduced total sleep times and sleep efficiency (146).

In one study, 63% of patients on maintenance hemodialysis (HD) for ESRD reported sleep disturbances, including diminished sleep efficiency and more fragmented sleep (147). In another report, 83.3% of patients on chronic HD had sleep–wake complaints, with 51% reporting disturbed sleep, 46% having delayed sleep onset, and 35% describing frequent awakenings (148). There appear to be no differences in the characteristics of sleep problems between HD and continuous peritoneal dialysis.

Excessive daytime sleepiness is an important problem. Excessive daytime sleepiness in patients with ESRD can be caused by sleep apnea, PLMD, metabolic disturbances including uremia, dialysis treatments (with accompanying changes in serum electrolytes, osmolarity, and acid–base balance), and the production of somnogenic substances, such as interleukin-1 and tumor necrosis factor alpha during dialysis (149).

Sleep apnea is estimated to be 10 times more prevalent in patients with ESRD than in the general population and is improved by HD (149). There is also a higher prevalence of RLS and PLMD in this patient population. In a study by Winkelman et al., 23% of patients with ESRD reported moderate-to-severe RLS symptomatology. Symptoms of RLS were associated with premature discontinuation of dialysis (150). Improvements in sleep quality have been reported in ESRD patients with RLS and anemia treated with recombinant human erythropoietin (a hormone-like substance that stimulates the formation of red blood cells). Correction of anemia was associated with reductions in the number of arousing periodic limb movements and sleep fragmentation (151).

INFECTIOUS DISEASES

Human Immunodeficiency Virus Infection

Sleep disturbances, including complaints of insomnia, recurrent nighttime arousals, and excessive daytime sleepiness, are among the most commonly reported sleep-related symptoms in human immunodeficiency virus (HIV)–seropositive patients (152–164). An estimated 35% of HIV-infected subjects have alterations in their sleep–wake patterns (153).

Sleep quality was related to a number of variables, including duration of HIV disease and HIV-related symptoms, depression, state anxiety, daytime sleepiness, fatigue, pain, functional status, and environmental factors. The prevalence of insomnia is higher in those with cognitive impairment, an acquired immunodeficiency syndrome–defining illness, drug use, or depression (154). Psychological morbidity is a major determinant of insomnia in HIV infection (155). Impaired functional status and longer duration of living with HIV disease were associated with worse sleep quality (156, 157). Immune status among HIV-seropositive patients may influence sleep quality, because lower T-cytotoxic/suppressor (CD3$^+$/CD8$^+$) cell counts are associated with greater sleep disturbances (162).

Sleep fragmentation is commonly seen in advanced HIV disease (159). There is an increase in the total percentage of SWS, SWS in the later sleep cycles, stage N1 shifts, REM periods and arousals, and a reduction in sleep latency and total percentage of stage N2 sleep (160, 161).

Antiviral therapy used for HIV infection can also give rise to sleep disruption. Efavirenz therapy produces a number of neuropsychiatric adverse reactions, such as abnormal dreams, nocturnal awakenings, and insomnia (163). Patients receiving efavirenz have been reported to have longer sleep latencies and shorter duration of deep sleep (164). Antiretroviral regimens may cause lipodystrophy, leading to fat deposition in the neck that impinges on the airway, as well as fat deposition in the thorax and abdomen, increasing respiratory effort. Evidence has also demonstrated higher rates of sleep apnea with the use of opioid medications; many of these patients may be on opioids for chronic pain or for the treatment of opioid dependence (i.e., methadone maintenance therapy) (165).

Lyme Disease

Lyme disease is a tick-borne spirochetal illness with clinical symptoms of fatigue, headache, chills, torticollis, nausea, and vomiting (166). Left untreated, Lyme disease can cause chronic joint inflammation, neurologic symptoms of facial palsy and neuropathy, impaired memory and other cognitive defects, and cardiac arrhythmias. Patients with Lyme disease typically report sleep disturbances (167). Sleep-related complaints include sleep-onset insomnia, frequent awakenings, excessive daytime sleepiness, and restless legs/nocturnal leg jerking. PSG may demonstrate increased sleep latency, reduced sleep efficiency, increased arousals, and greater sleep fragmentation. Alpha wave intrusion into NREM sleep may be observed in some patients. Mean sleep-onset latency during multiple sleep latency test is typically normal (168). Sleep difficulty may persist for several years in patients with previous Lyme disease, particularly those with facial palsy who did not receive antibiotics for acute neuroborreliosis (169).

Sleeping Sickness

Sleeping sickness, or human African trypanosomiasis, is a parasitic disease caused by trypanosomes and is endemic in intertropical Africa. Following the bite of a tsetse fly, human disease evolves through two stages. Diverse clinical features such as fever, cervical adenopathy, skin lesions, facial edema, and cardiac symptoms with arrhythmia characterize the first hemolymphatic stage. This is followed by increasing neurologic symptoms in the meningoencephalitic stage with excessive daytime sleepiness, headaches, sensory deficits, and abnormal reflexes and movements. If untreated, the infection culminates in altered consciousness, cachexia, and death.

Insomnia is not uncommon. Nocturnal PSG recordings have demonstrated reduced REM sleep latency with sleep-onset REM periods. The scarcity of vertex sharp waves, sleep spindles, and K-complexes may give rise to difficulties in scoring sleep stages. Sleep disturbances can be reversed by successful antiparasitic therapy (170, 171).

SLEEP IN THE INTENSIVE CARE UNIT

Sleep is characterized by a variety of physiologic, behavioral, and EEG changes and is necessary for the restoration of cognitive, mood, and physiologic functions (172). Physiologic changes that occur during sleep play an important role in homeostasis, growth, and cellular repair. Sleep disruption in the critically ill patient may negatively impact the treatment and recovery outcomes of the underlying illness or injury. Sleep deprivation, sleep-disordered breathing, and circadian misalignment are believed to have endocrine, metabolic, and cardiovascular implications (173). Sleep deprivation may also be a risk factor for delirium in critically ill patients, linking it to higher morbidity, mortality, and length of intensive care unit (ICU) stay (174).

Normal sleep architecture is divided into two distinct states: NREM sleep and REM sleep. NREM is composed of three distinct stages on the basis of EEG criteria. Stages N1 and N2 are considered to reflect light sleep followed by stage N3 deep SWS. SWS is an anabolic state and is considered the most restorative stage of sleep for physiologic repair. REM sleep is thought to be necessary for memory consolidation (172).

In adults, approximately 50% of ICU sleep occurs during the daytime hours, with a marked shift toward light stages of sleep (175). Compared with healthy adults, studies characterizing sleep disturbances in ICU patients using PSG have demonstrated prolonged sleep latency, sleep fragmentation, reduced sleep efficiency, numerous arousals, a preponderance of stage N2 sleep, reduced or absent stage N3 ("deep") sleep, and reduced or absent REM sleep (175).

The circadian rhythm or "internal biologic clock" controls the timing and duration of daily sleep–wake cycles and influences important body functions such as hormone release, body temperature, and digestion. Exposure to light has a controlling influence on circadian regulation, synchronizing sleep–wake cycles with daily external solar light and dark cycles. Alterations in circadian rhythmicity may impair recovery by disrupting the coordinated activity of normal physiologic processes. Most immunologic functions, from leukocyte numbers, activity, and cytokine secretion, undergo circadian variations, which might affect susceptibility to infections (176).

Normal physiologic alterations that occur during sleep are particularly significant in patients with unstable hemodynamics, impaired defense mechanisms, and limited physiologic reserve (177). Body temperature and thermoregulation are regulated, in part, by sleep and circadian rhythms. During sleep, voluntary control of respiration is lost and hypoxic and hypercapnic ventilatory drives are reduced. Responsiveness to low oxygen and high carbon dioxide levels is lowest during REM compared with NREM sleep. Dynamic cardiovascular fluctuations in blood flow and electrical activity occur and have been associated with life-threatening arrhythmias and ischemic events in patients with underlying heart disease. GH and prolactin, anabolic hormones necessary for cell differentiation and proliferation, follow the sleep–wake cycle and are suppressed during sleep restriction (177). Sleep deprivation alters neuroendocrine control systems and has been shown to cause increases in thyroid hormone, norepinephrine, and cortisol levels with decreases in GH levels and insulin resistance (175).

Delirium is an acute state of confusion that has been shown to occur in up to 80% of critically ill patients and to be an independent predictor of adverse

ICU outcomes, including increased risk of death, longer hospital stay, and higher costs (174). In healthy volunteers, sleep deprivation has been shown to impair memory, attention, response time, and other aspects of neurologic function (175).

Numerous studies have confirmed that the development of delirium during a hospital course is associated with worse physical and cognitive status upon discharge and for at least 12 months thereafter, and a higher mortality (174). Sleep disturbance and delirium in the ICU are frequently related, in part, to the shared etiology of sleep loss because of interruptions and sedatives. An imbalance in neurotransmitters and an alteration in melatonin production may contribute to the pathogenesis of both delirium and sleep disturbances (178). The relationship between sleep deprivation and delirium in the ICU is currently unproven. However, because sleep deprivation affects cognitive function, a connection between delirium and sleep deprivation in critically ill patients may exist (175).

In addition to the effect of preexisting sleep disorders and chronic medical disorders, patients admitted to the ICU are exposed to additional risk factors for sleep disruption such as environmental stimuli (light and noise), medications that affect sleep quality and architecture, patient-care activities (lab draws, imaging, vital signs), pain, and mechanical ventilation (Fig. 23-1).

The Environmental Protection Agency recommends maximum hospital noise levels of 45 dB during

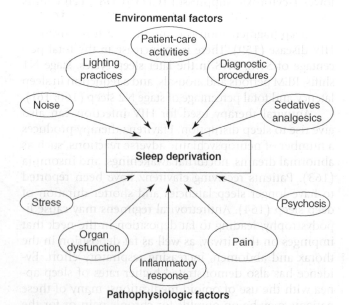

Figure 23-1 Factors related to sleep deprivation in critically ill patients. (Reprinted with permission of the American Thoracic Society. Copyright © 2019 American Thoracic Society. From Pisani, M. A., Friese, R. S., Gehlbach, B. K., et al. (2015). Sleep in the intensive care unit. *American Journal of Respiratory and Critical Care Medicine, 191*(7), 731–738. The *American Journal of Respiratory and Critical Care Medicine* is an official journal of the American Thoracic Society.)

the day and 35 dB at night. In the ICU setting, peak daytime and nighttime noise levels routinely exceed 80 dB, the threshold associated with sleep disruption in critically ill patients (172, 177). Noise, particularly staff talking and patient-care activities, are clearly contributing factors and represent 40% of the source of sleep disruption (172).

Approximately 60% of patients complain of disturbed sleep related to being on a ventilator; 30% stated they felt panic and anxiety, which directly inhibited their ability to rest and sleep (172). Improper ventilator settings, mode of ventilation, and patient-ventilator dyssynchrony are factors that may contribute to sleep disruption (172, 177). Noxious factors associated with mechanical ventilation, such as endotracheal tube discomfort, ventilator alarms, suctioning, positioning, and frequent assessments, likely contribute to sleep disruption as well, but these have not been studied (177).

Sedation is often used in ICU patients, to increase patient comfort, reduce anxiety and agitation, and promote amnesia and sleep, particularly in those requiring mechanical ventilation (177, 179). Any agent that acts on or through sleep regulatory neurotransmitters, modulators, or their receptors can impact sleep architecture (172). Despite their sedative, anxiolytic, and analgesic properties, benzodiazepines and opiates are potentially disruptive to sleep (177). Benzodiazepines provide sedation through gamma-aminobutyric acid-ergic pathways but increase stage N2 and reduce stage N3 sleep at low doses in healthy participants. Opiates such as fentanyl and morphine promote sleep onset in healthy adults, but inhibit REM, profoundly suppress stage N3 sleep, provoke nocturnal awakenings, and can precipitate central apneas. Both benzodiazepines and opiates are associated with delirium in critically ill patients, even at low doses (177). In critically ill patients, propofol has been shown to suppress REM sleep and to

Table 23-2 Strategies to Improve Sleep in ICU Patients

Barriers to Sleep in the ICU	Strategies to Optimize Sleep in the ICU
Noise	Limit unnecessary noise, phones, and television If possible, liberalize alarm system and add central alarm personnel Keep patients' door closed, when possible Post signs regarding minimizing conversations at or near the bedside Enforce visiting hours At night, encourage staff to switch beepers/electronic devices to vibrate Limit the number of visitors at once, and/or consider ear plugs Add background, low-level, white noise Consider monitoring decibel levels, particularly at night
Patient-care activities	At night, minimize bathing, dressing, room changes, and other wakeful activities Regularly review nighttime orders regarding monitoring (vital checks, blood draws, fingersticks, etc.)
Circadian rhythm	Encourage daytime brighter light exposure (lights on, open curtains) Turn off lights by 10 p.m.
Medications/substances	Minimize the use of benzodiazepines for sleep; consider melatonin Consider short-acting intravenous agents, such as propofol Avoid starting multiple medications at one time; minimize the use of sleep-disrupting medications
Discomfort	Maximize pain management, particularly with procedures Evaluate the patient for anxiety as a source of sleep disruption and treat accordingly with reorientation to the environment; nightmares, dyssynchrony with ventilator, medication effects, etc.
Ventilator	Adjust settings and the mode of ventilator to maximize patient-ventilator synchrony; avoid hyperventilation Provide nocturnal O_2, NIPPV as appropriate; if the patient is receiving NIPPV, assess the mask fit and comfort and maximize synchrony with the ventilator

ICU, intensive care unit; NIPPV, noninvasive positive pressure ventilation.
Adapted from Hardin, K. A. (2009). Sleep in the ICU: Potential mechanisms and clinical implications. *Chest*, 136(1), 284–294.

worsen sleep quality. Inotropic medications can affect sleep through their effects on adrenergic receptors. Beta blockers, which are a frequently used medication in the ICU, can negatively affect sleep and may cause insomnia and nightmares because of suppressed REM sleep (175).

The use of PSG in the ICU setting is met with numerous challenges. This expensive, labor-intensive test requires skilled personnel to apply equipment and interpret the dispersion of sleep in critically ill patients throughout both day and night to study sleep in the ICU (175, 180).

Traditional scoring rules are difficult to apply in ICU patients (175). Renal failure, hepatic dysfunction, and sedative and analgesic use, each common among ICU patients, can be associated with significant EEG changes that make PSG interpretation problematic. Sedative-induced beta EEG activity, for example, may lead to an overestimation of wake or stage N1 sleep (180).

Alternatively, actigraphy is a device worn on the wrist or ankle and is a valid tool to measure rest–wake patterns and total rest time (175). Actigraphy measures a patient's movement to study sleep and has been successfully used in ICU patients to show loss of circadian rhythm and sleep disruption. Actigraphy cannot, however, be considered an accurate tool to measure sleep time in ICU patients whose movement may be restricted by neuromuscular weakness, sedatives, or restraints (180).

Patient and nurse assessments of sleep using questionnaires can be unreliable. The accuracy of patient self-reporting may be impacted by sedation and/or delirium. Nurse-derived assessments of sleep overestimate total sleep time and sleep efficiency and underestimate the number of awakenings compared with PSG (175). There are a number of strategies to improve sleep for patients in the ICU (Table 23-2).

MISCELLANEOUS

Fatal Familial Insomnia

Fatal familial insomnia is a rare, hereditary prion-protein disease characterized by progressive sleep disturbances including refractory insomnia, autonomic dysregulation, and neurologic abnormalities. Caused by a genetic mutation affecting intracellular protein structure, it is similar in nature to other human prion diseases such as Creutzfeldt–Jakob. Clinical features include disrupted sleep, vivid dreaming, and increasingly frequent lapses into a dreamlike (oneiric) state with motor activity as the disease progresses.

PSG features vary depending on the stage of the disease. EEG may be normal in early stages, changing to a pattern of monomorphic flat activity with occasional 1 to 2 Hz sharp waves; absent sleep spindles, K-complexes, and delta activity; and reduced and fragmented REM sleep. REM sleep may occur without muscle atonia reminiscent of REM behavior disorder. There is no known specific treatment. The condition is rapidly progressive and is uniformly fatal (181, 182). For further information on fatal familial insomnia, see Chapter 20.

REFERENCES

1. Turner-Warwick, M. (1988). Epidemiology of nocturnal asthma. *The American Journal of Medicine*, *85*(1B), 6–8.
2. Bellia, V., Pistelli, R., Filippazzo, G., et al. (2000). Prevalence of nocturnal asthma in a general population sample: Determinants and effect of aging. *The Journal of Asthma*, *37*(7), 595–602.
3. Connolly, C. K. (1979). Diurnal rhythms in airway obstruction. *British Journal of Diseases of the Chest*, *73*(4), 357–366.
4. Ballard, R. D., Irvin, C. G., Martin, R. J., et al. (1990). Influence of sleep on lung volume in asthmatic patients and normal subjects. *Journal of Applied Physiology*, *68*(5), 2034–2041.
5. Martin, R. J. (1993). Nocturnal asthma: Circadian rhythms and therapeutic interventions. *The American Review of Respiratory Disease*, *147*(6, Pt. 2), S25–S28.
6. Martin, R. J., Cicutto, L. C., Smith, H. R., et al. (1991). Airways inflammation in nocturnal asthma. *The American Review of Respiratory Disease*, *143*(2), 351–357.
7. Kales, A., Beall, G. N., Bajor, G. F., et al. (1968). Sleep studies in asthmatic adults: Relationship of attacks to sleep stage and time of night. *Journal of Allergy*, *41*(3), 164–173.
8. Montplaisir, J., Walsh, J., & Malo, J. L. (1982). Nocturnal asthma: Features of attacks, sleep and breathing patterns. *The American Review of Respiratory Disease*, *125*(1), 18–22.
9. Chan, C. S., Woolcock, A. J., & Sullivan, C. E. (1988). Nocturnal asthma: Role of snoring and obstructive sleep apnea. *The American Review of Respiratory Disease*, *137*(6), 1502–1504.
10. Ciftci, T. U., Ciftci, B., Guven, S. F., et al. (2005). Effect of nasal continuous positive airway pressure in uncontrolled nocturnal asthmatic patients with obstructive sleep apnea syndrome. *Respiratory Medicine*, *99*(5), 529–534.
11. Global Initiative for Chronic Obstructive Lung Disease. Retrieved from https://goldcopd.org
12. Murray, C. J., & Lopez, A. D. (1997). Global mortality, disability, and the contribution of risk factors:

Global Burden of Disease Study. *Lancet, 349*(9063), 1436–1442.

13. Cormick, W., Olson, L. G., Hensley, M. J., et al. (1986). Nocturnal hypoxaemia and quality of sleep in patients with chronic obstructive lung disease. *Thorax, 41*(11), 846–854.

14. Fleetham, J., West, P., Mezon, B., et al. (1982). Sleep, arousals, and oxygen desaturation in chronic obstructive pulmonary disease: The effect of oxygen therapy. *The American Review of Respiratory Disease, 126*(3), 429–433.

15. Klink, M. E., & Quan, S. F. (1987). Prevalence of reported sleep disturbances in a general adult population and their relationship to obstructive airway diseases. *Chest, 91*(4), 540–546.

16. Klink, M. E., Dodge, R., & Quan, S. F. (1994). The relation of sleep complaints to respiratory symptoms in a general population. *Chest, 105*(1), 151–154.

17. Calverley, P. M., Brezinova, V., Douglas, N. J., et al. (1982). The effect of oxygenation on sleep quality in chronic bronchitis and emphysema. *The American Review of Respiratory Disease, 126*(2), 206–210.

18. Plywaczewski, R., Sliwinski, P., Nowinski, A., et al. (2000). Incidence of nocturnal desaturation while breathing oxygen in COPD patients undergoing long-term oxygen therapy. *Chest, 117*(3), 679–683.

19. Fletcher, E. C., Gray, B. A., & Levin, D. C. (1983). Nonapneic mechanisms of arterial oxygen desaturation during rapid-eye-movement sleep. *Journal of Applied Physiology, 54*(3), 632–639.

20. Douglas, N. J., Calverley, P. M., Leggett, R. J., et al. (1979). Transient hypoxaemia during sleep in chronic bronchitis and emphysema. *Lancet, 1*(8106), 1–4.

21. George, C. F., West, P., & Kryger, M. H. (1987). Oxygenation and breathing pattern during phasic and tonic REM in patients with chronic obstructive pulmonary disease. *Sleep, 10*(3), 234–243.

22. Catterall, J. R., Douglas, N. J., Calverley, P. M., et al. (1983). Transient hypoxemia during sleep in chronic obstructive pulmonary disease is not a sleep apnea syndrome. *The American Review of Respiratory Disease, 128*(1), 24–29.

23. DeMarco, F. J., Jr., Wynne, J. W., Block, A. J., et al. (1981). Oxygen desaturation during sleep as a determinant of the "Blue and Bloated" syndrome. *Chest, 79*(6), 621–625.

24. Hudgel, D. W., Martin, R. J., Capehart, M., et al. (1983). Contribution of hypoventilation to sleep oxygen desaturation in chronic obstructive pulmonary disease. *Journal of Applied Physiology, 55*(3), 669–677.

25. Bednarek, M., Plywaczewski, R., Jonczak, L., et al. (2005). There is no relationship between chronic obstructive pulmonary disease and obstructive sleep apnea syndrome: A population study. *Respiration, 72*(2), 142–149.

26. Fanfulla, F., Cascone, L., & Taurino, A. E. (2004). Sleep disordered breathing in patients with chronic obstructive pulmonary disease. *Minerva Medica, 95*(4), 307–321.

27. Connaughton, J. J., Catterall, J. R., Elton, R. A., et al. (1988). Do sleep studies contribute to the management of patients with severe chronic obstructive pulmonary disease? *The American Review of Respiratory Disease, 138*(2), 341–344.

28. Weitzenblum, E., & Chaouat, A. (2004). Sleep and chronic obstructive pulmonary disease. *Sleep Medicine Reviews, 8*(4), 281–294.

29. Mieczkowski, B., & Ezzie, M. E. (2014). Update on obstructive sleep apnea and its relation to COPD. *International Journal of Chronic Obstructive Pulmonary Disease, 9*, 349–362. doi:10.2147/COPD.S42394

30. Owens, R. L., Macrea, M. M., & Teodorescu, M. (2017). The overlaps of asthma or COPD with OSA: A focused review. *Respirology, 22*, 1073–1083.

31. Brown, L. K. (1998). Sleep-related disorders and chronic obstructive pulmonary disease. *Respiratory Care Clinics of North America, 4*(3), 493–512.

32. de Miguel, J., Cabello, J., Sanchez-Alarcos, J. M., et al. (2002). Long-term effects of treatment with nasal continuous positive airway pressure on lung function in patients with overlap syndrome. *Sleep and Breathing, 6*(1), 3–10.

33. Resta, O., Guido, P., Picca, V., et al. (1998). Prescription of nCPAP and nBIPAP in obstructive sleep apnoea syndrome: Italian experience in 105 subjects. A prospective two centre study. *Respiratory Medicine, 92*(6), 820–827.

34. Rosenstein, B. J. (1998). What is a cystic fibrosis diagnosis? *Clinics in Chest Medicine, 19*(3), 423–441.

35. Bye, M. R., Ewig, J. M., & Quittell, L. M. (1994). Cystic fibrosis. *Lung, 172*(5), 251–270.

36. Conway, S. (1996). Cystic fibrosis in teenagers and young adults. *Archives of Disease in Childhood, 75*(2), 99–101.

37. Balistreri, W. F. (1990). Spectrum of liver disease in patients with CF. *Pediatric Pulmonology, 5*, 71–73.

38. Dodge, J. A. (1995). Male fertility in cystic fibrosis. *Lancet, 346*(8975), 587–588.

39. Jankelowitz, L., Reid, K. J., Wolfe, L., et al. (2005). Cystic fibrosis patients have poor sleep quality despite normal sleep latency and efficiency. *Chest, 127*(5), 1593–1599.

40. Dobbin, C. J., Bartlett, D., Melehan, K., et al. (2005). The effect of infective exacerbations on sleep and neurobehavioral function in cystic fibrosis. *American Journal of Respiratory and Critical Care Medicine, 172*(1), 99–104.

41. Spicuzza, L., Sciuto, C., Leonardi, S., et al. (2012). Early occurrence of obstructive sleep apnea in infants

and children with cystic fibrosis. *Archives of Pediatrics and Adolescent Medicine, 166*(12), 1165–1169.

42. Milross, M. A., Piper, A. J., Dobbin, C. J., et al. (2004). Sleep disordered breathing in cystic fibrosis. *Sleep Medicine Reviews, 8*(4), 295–308.

43. Milross, M. A., Piper, A. J., Norman, M., et al. (2002). Subjective sleep quality in cystic fibrosis. *Sleep Medicine, 3*(3), 205–212.

44. Moran, F., Bradley, J. M., & Piper, A. J. (2009). Non-invasive ventilation for cystic fibrosis. *Cochrane Database of Systematic Reviews,* (1), CD002769. doi:10.1002/14651858.CD002769.pub3

45. Kurtz, D. (1990). Changes in sleep and night respiration in asthma and obstructive or restrictive lung diseases [in French]. *Presse medicale, 19*(40), 1857–1861.

46. George, C. F., & Kryger, M. H. (1987). Sleep in restrictive lung disease. *Sleep, 10*(5), 409–418.

47. Resta, O., Foschino-Barbaro, M. P., Bonfitto, P., et al. (2003). Low sleep quality and daytime sleepiness in obese patients without obstructive sleep apnoea syndrome. *Journal of Internal Medicine, 253*(5), 536–543.

48. Resta, O., Foschino-Barbaro, M. P., Legari, G., et al. (2001). Sleep-related breathing disorders, loud snoring and excessive daytime sleepiness in obese subjects. *International Journal of Obesity and Related Metabolic Disorders, 25*(5), 669–675.

49. Sergi, M., Rizzi, M., Comi, A. L., et al. (1999). Sleep apnea in moderate—Severe obese patients. *Sleep and Breathing, 3*(2), 47–52.

50. Weitzenblum, E., Kessler, R., & Chaouat, A. (2002). Alveolar hypoventilation in the obese: The obesity-hypoventilation syndrome [in French]. *Revue de Pneumologie Clinique, 58*(2), 83–90.

51. Mezon, B. L., West, P., Israels, J., et al. (1980). Sleep breathing abnormalities in kyphoscoliosis. *The American Review of Respiratory Disease, 122*(4), 617–621.

52. Guilleminault, C., Kurland, G., Winkle, R., et al. (1981). Severe kyphoscoliosis, breathing, and sleep: The "Quasimodo" syndrome during sleep. *Chest, 79*(6), 626–630.

53. Sawicka, E. H., & Branthwaite, M. A. (1987). Respiration during sleep in kyphoscoliosis. *Thorax, 42*(10), 801–808.

54. Perez-Padilla, R., West, P., Lertzman, M., et al. (1985). Breathing during sleep in patients with interstitial lung disease. *The American Review of Respiratory Disease, 132*(2), 224–229.

55. Shea, S. A., Winning, A. J., McKenzie, E., et al. (1989). Does the abnormal pattern of breathing in patients with interstitial lung disease persist in deep, non-rapid eye movement sleep? *The American Review of Respiratory Disease, 139*(3), 653–658.

56. Bye, P. T., Issa, F., Berthon-Jones, M., et al. (1984). Studies of oxygenation during sleep in patients with interstitial lung disease. *The American Review of Respiratory Disease, 129*(1), 27–32.

57. Hira, H. S., & Sharma, R. K. (1997). Study of oxygen saturation, breathing pattern and arrhythmias in patients of interstitial lung disease during sleep. *The Indian Journal of Chest Diseases and Allied Sciences, 39*(3), 157–162.

58. Prodromakis, E., Trakada, G., Tsapanos, V., et al. (2004). Arterial oxygen tension during sleep in the third trimester of pregnancy. *Acta Obstetricia et Gynecologica Scandinavica, 83*(2), 159–164.

59. Santiago, J. R., Nolledo, M. S., Kinzler, W., et al. (2001). Sleep and sleep disorders in pregnancy. *Annals of Internal Medicine, 134*(5), 396–408.

60. Edwards, N., Middleton, P. G., Blyton, D. M., et al. (2002). Sleep disordered breathing and pregnancy. *Thorax, 57*(6), 555–558.

61. Brownell, L. G., West, P., & Kryger, M. H. (1986). Breathing during sleep in normal pregnant women. *The American Review of Respiratory Disease, 133*(1), 38–41.

62. Guilleminault, C., Querra-Salva, M. A., Chowdhari, S., et al. (2000). Normal pregnancy, daytime sleeping, snoring and blood pressure. *Sleep Medicine, 117*, 137–141.

63. Culebras, A. (2005). Sleep disorders and neuromuscular disease. *Seminars in Neurology, 25*(1), 33–38.

64. Piper, A. (2002). Sleep abnormalities associated with neuromuscular disease: Pathophysiology and evaluation. *Seminars in Respiratory and Critical Care Medicine, 23*(3), 211–220.

65. Barthlen, G. M. (1997). Nocturnal respiratory failure as an indication of noninvasive ventilation in the patient with neuromuscular disease. *Respiration, 64*(Suppl. 1), 35–38.

66. Barbé, F., Quera-Salva, M. A., McCann, C., et al. (1994). Sleep-related respiratory disturbances in patients with Duchenne muscular dystrophy. *The European Respiratory Journal, 7*(8), 1403–1408.

67. Khan, Y., & Heckmatt, J. Z. (1994). Obstructive apnoeas in Duchenne muscular dystrophy. *Thorax, 49*(2), 157–161.

68. Takasugi, T., Ishihara, T., Kawamura, J., et al. (1995). Respiratory disorders during sleep in Duchenne muscular dystrophy [in Japanese]. *Nihon Kokyuki Gakkai Zasshi, 33*(8), 821–828.

69. Redding, G. J., Okamoto, G. A., Guthrie, R. D., et al. (1985). Sleep patterns in nonambulatory boys with Duchenne muscular dystrophy. *Archives of Physical Medicine and Rehabilitation, 66*, 818–821.

70. Hukins, C. A., & Hillman, D. R. (2000). Daytime predictors of sleep hypoventilation in Duchenne muscular dystrophy. *American Journal of Respiratory and Critical Care Medicine, 161*, 166–170.

71. Guilleminault, C., Cummiskey, J., Motta, J., et al. (1978). Respiratory and hemodynamic study during

wakefulness and sleep in myotonic dystrophy. *Sleep, 1*(1), 19–31.

72. Cirignotta, F., Mondini, S., Zucconi, M., et al. (1987). Sleep-related breathing impairment in myotonic dystrophy. *Journal of Neurology, 235*(2), 80–85.

73. Coccagna, G., Mantovani, M., Parchi, C., et al. (1975). Alveolar hypoventilation and hypersomnia in myotonic dystrophy. *Journal of Neurology, Neurosurgery and Psychiatry, 38*, 977–984.

74. Ververs, C. C., Van der Meche, F. G., Verbraak, A. F., et al. (1996). Breathing pattern awake and asleep in myotonic dystrophy. *Respiration, 63*(1), 1–7.

75. Zifko, U., Remtulla, H., Power, K., et al. (1996). Transcortical and cervical magnetic stimulation with recording of the diaphragm. *Muscle Nerve, 19*, 614–620.

76. Gay, P. C., Westbrook, P. R., Daube, J. R., et al. (1991). Effects of alterations in pulmonary function and sleep variables on survival in patients with amyotrophic lateral sclerosis. *Mayo Clinic Proceedings, 66*(7), 686–694.

77. Ferguson, K. A., Strong, M. J., Ahmad, D., et al. (1996). Sleep-disordered breathing in amyotrophic lateral sclerosis. *Chest, 110*(3), 664–669.

78. Santos, C., Braghiroli, A., Mazzini, L., et al. (2003). Sleep-related breathing disorders in amyotrophic lateral sclerosis. *Monaldi Archives for Chest Disease, 59*(2), 160–165.

79. Arnulf, I., Similowski, T., Salachas, F., et al. (2000). Sleep disorders and diaphragmatic function in patients with amyotrophic lateral sclerosis. *American Journal of Respiratory and Critical Care Medicine, 161*(3, Pt. 1), 849–856.

80. Steljes, D. G., Kryger, M. H., Kirk, B. W., et al. (1990). Sleep in postpolio syndrome. *Chest, 98*(1), 133–140.

81. Hsu, A. A., & Staats, B. A. (1998). "Postpolio" sequelae and sleep-related disordered breathing. *Mayo Clinic Proceedings, 73*(3), 216–224.

82. Dean, A. C., Graham, B. A., Dalakas, M., et al. (1998). Sleep apnea in patients with postpolio syndrome. *Annals of Neurology, 43*(5), 661–664.

83. Bridgens, R., Sturman, S., & Davidson, C; British Polio Fellowship's Expert Panel. (2010). Post-polio syndrome—Polio's legacy. *Clinical Medicine, 10*(3), 213–214.

84. Stepansky, R., Weber, G., & Zeitlhofer, J. (1997). Sleep apnea and cognitive dysfunction in myasthenia gravis. *Acta Medica Austriaca, 24*(3), 128–131.

85. Amino, A., Shiozawa, Z., Nagasaka, T., et al. (1998). Sleep apnoea in well-controlled myasthenia gravis and the effect of thymectomy. *Journal of Neurology, 245*(2), 77–80.

86. Gajdos, P., & Quera Salva, M. A. (2001). Respiratory disorders during sleep and myasthenia. *Revue Neurologique, 157*(11, Pt. 2), S145–S147.

87. Kaminsky, P., Poussel, M., Pruna, L., et al. (2011). Organ dysfunction and muscular disability in myotonic dystrophy type 1. *Medicine, 90*(4), 262–268.

88. Patakas, D., Tsara, V., Zoglopitis, F., et al. (1991). Nocturnal hypoxia in unilateral diaphragmatic paralysis. *Respiration, 58*(2), 95–99.

89. Steir, L., Jolley, C. J., Seymour, J., et al. (2008). Sleep-disordered breathing in unilateral diaphragm paralysis or severe weakness. *European Respiratory Journal, 32*, 1479–1487.

90. Stradling, J. R., & Warley, A. R. (1988). Bilateral diaphragm paralysis and sleep apnoea without diurnal respiratory failure. *Thorax, 43*(1), 75–77.

91. Watanabe, Y., Kumon, K., Yahagi, N., et al. (1998). A case of central sleep-apnea syndrome accompanied by bilateral paralysis of the diaphragm after pediatric cardiac surgery. *Masui, 47*(6), 714–719.

92. Hoffstein, V., & Taylor, R. (1985). Rapid development of obstructive sleep apnea following hemidiaphragmatic and unilateral vocal cord paralysis as a complication of mediastinal surgery. *Chest, 88*(1), 145–147.

93. Bennett, J. R., Dunroy, H. M., Corfield, D. R., et al. (2004). Respiratory muscle activity during REM sleep in patients with diaphragm paralysis. *Neurology, 62*(1), 134–137.

94. Castell, D. O., Murray, J. A., Tutuian, R., et al. (2004). Review article: The pathophysiology of gastro-oesophageal reflux disease—Oesophageal manifestations. *Alimentary Pharmacology and Therapeutics, 20*(Suppl. 9), 14–25.

95. Vela, M. F., Kramer, J. R., Richardson, P. A., et al. (2014). Poor sleep quality and obstructive sleep apnea in patients with GERD and Barrett's esophagus. *Neurogastroenterology and Motility, 26*(3), 346–352.

96. Shaker, R., Castell, D. O., Schoenfeld, P. S., et al. (2003). Nighttime heartburn is an under-appreciated clinical problem that impacts sleep and daytime function: The results of a Gallup survey conducted on behalf of the American Gastroentero-logical Association. *The American Journal of Gastroenterology, 98*(7), 1487–1493.

97. Farup, C., Kleinman, L., Sloan, S., et al. (2001). The impact of nocturnal symptoms associated with gastroesophageal reflux disease on health-related quality of life. *Archives of Internal Medicine, 161*(1), 45–52.

98. Sontag, S. J. (2000). Gastroesophageal reflux disease and asthma. *Journal of Clinical Gastroenterology, 30*(Suppl. 3), S9–S30.

99. Wasilewska, J., & Kaczmarski, M. (2004). Sleep-related breathing disorders in small children with nocturnal acid gastrooesophageal reflux. *Roczniki Akademii Medycznej w Bialymstoku, 49*, 98–102.

100. Demeter, P., Vardi, V. K., & Magyar, P. (2004). Correlations between gastroesophageal reflux disease

and obstructive sleep apnea [in Hungarian]. *Orvosi hetilap, 145*(37), 1897–1901.

101. Demeter, P., Visy, K. V., & Magyar, P. (2005). Correlation between severity of endoscopic findings and apnea-hypopnea index in patients with gastroesophageal reflux disease and obstructive sleep apnea. *World Journal of Gastroenterology, 11*(6), 839–841.

102. Kim, H. N., Vorona, R. D., Winn, M. P., et al. (2005). Symptoms of gastro-oesophageal reflux disease and the severity of obstructive sleep apnoea syndrome are not related in sleep disorders center patients. *Alimentary Pharmacology and Therapeutics, 21*(9), 1127–1133.

103. Guda, N., Partington, S., & Vakil, N. (2004). Symptomatic gastrooesophageal reflux, arousals and sleep quality in patients undergoing polysomnography for possible obstructive sleep apnoea. *Alimentary Pharmacology and Therapeutics, 20*(10), 1153–1159.

104. Orr, W. C. (2001). Gastrointestinal functioning during sleep: A new horizon in sleep medicine. *Sleep Medicine Reviews, 5*(2), 91–101.

105. Thompson, J. J., Elsenbruch, S., Harnish, M. J., et al. (2002). Autonomic functioning during REM sleep differentiates IBS symptom subgroups. *The American Journal of Gastroenterology, 97*(12), 3147–3153.

106. Elsenbruch, S., Thompson, J. J., Harnish, M. J., et al. (2002). Behavioral and physiological sleep characteristics in women with irritable bowel syndrome. *The American Journal of Gastroenterology, 97*(9), 2306–2314.

107. Fass, R., Fullerton, S., Tung, S., et al. (2000). Sleep disturbances in clinic patients with functional bowel disorders. *The American Journal of Gastroenterology, 95*(5), 1195–2000.

108. Vege, S. S., Locke, G. R., III, Weaver, A. L., et al. (2004). Functional gastrointestinal disorders among people with sleep disturbances: A population-based study. *Mayo Clinic Proceedings, 79*(12), 1501–1506.

109. Elsenbruch, S., Harnish, M. J., & Orr, W. C. (1999). Subjective and objective sleep quality in irritable bowel syndrome. *The American Journal of Gastroenterology, 94*(9), 2447–2452.

110. Robert, J. J., Orr, W. C., & Elsenbruch, S. (2004). Modulation of sleep quality and autonomic functioning by symptoms of depression in women with irritable bowel syndrome. *Digestive Diseases and Sciences, 49*(7/8), 1250–1258.

111. University of Chicago Medical Center. (1999, October 25). Lack of sleep alters hormones, metabolism, simulates effects of aging. *Science News.* Retrieved from https://www.sciencedaily.com/releases/1999/10/991025075844.htm

112. Van Cauter, E., Knutson, K., Leproult, R., et al. (2005). The impact of sleep deprivation on hormones and metabolism. *Medscape Neurology, 7*(1). Retrieved March 4, 2012, from http://www.medscape.org/viewarticle/502825

113. Spiegel, K., Leproult, R., & Van Cauter E. (1999). Impact of sleep debt on metabolic and endocrine function. *Lancet, 354,* 1435–1439.

114. Grunstein, R. (2000). Endocrine disorders. In M. H. Kryger, T. Roth, & W. C. Dement (Eds.), *Principles and practice of sleep medicine* (p. 1108). Philadelphia, PA: W.B. Saunders.

115. Rosenow, F., McCarthy, V., & Caruso, A. C. (1998). Sleep apnoea in endocrine diseases. *Journal of Sleep Research, 7*(1), 3–11.

116. Grunstein, R. R., & Sullivan, C. E. (1988). Sleep apnea and hypothyroidism: Mechanisms and management. *The American Journal of Medicine, 85*(6), 775–779.

117. Mestron, A., Webb, S. M., Astorga, R., et al. (2004). Epidemiology, clinical characteristics, outcome, morbidity and mortality in acromegaly based on the Spanish Acromegaly Registry (Registro Espanol de Acromegalia, REA). *European Journal of Endocrinology, 51*(4), 439–446.

118. Weiss, V., Sonka, K., Pretl, M., et al. (2000). Prevalence of the sleep apnea syndrome in acromegaly population. *Journal of Endocrinological Investigation, 23*(8), 515–519.

119. Herrmann, B. L., Wessendorf, T. E., Ajaj, W., et al. (2004). Effects of octreotide on sleep apnoea and tongue volume (magnetic resonance imaging) in patients with acromegaly. *European Journal of Endocrinology, 151*(3), 309–315.

120. Fatti, L. M., Scacchi, M., Pincelli, A. I., et al. (2001). Prevalence and pathogenesis of sleep apnea and lung disease in acromegaly. *Pituitary, 4*(4), 259–262.

121. Dostalova, S., Sonka, K., Smahel, Z., et al. (2001). Craniofacial abnormalities and their relevance for sleep apnoea syndrome aetiopathogenesis in acromegaly. *European Journal of Endocrinology, 144*(5), 491–497.

122. Blanco Perez, J. J., Blanco-Ramos, M. A., Zamarron Sanz, C., et al. (2004). Acromegaly and sleep apnea [in Spanish]. *Archivos de bronconeumologia, 40*(8), 355–359.

123. Ziemer, D. C., & Dunlap, D. B. (1988). Relief of sleep apnea in acromegaly by bromocriptine. *The American Journal of the Medical Sciences, 295*(1), 49–51.

124. Grunstein, R. R., Ho, K. K., & Sullivan, C. E. (1994). Effect of octreotide, a somatostatin analog, on sleep apnea in patients with acromegaly. *Annals of Internal Medicine, 121*(7), 478–483.

125. Buyse, B., Michiels, E., Bouillon, R., et al. (1997). Relief of sleep apnoea after treatment of acromegaly: Report of three cases and review of the literature. *The European Respiratory Journal, 10*(6), 1401–1404.

126. Pekkarinen, T., Partinen, M., Pelkonen, R., et al. (1987). Sleep apnoea and daytime sleepiness in acromegaly: Relationship to endocrinological factors. *Clinical Endocrinology, 27*(6), 649–654.

127. Mickelson, S. A., Rosenthal, L. D., Rock, J. P., et al. (1994). Obstructive sleep apnea syndrome and acromegaly. *Otolaryngology—Head and Neck Surgery, 111*(1), 25–30.

128. Rosenow, F., Reuter, S., Deuss, U., et al. (1996). Sleep apnoea in treated acromegaly: Relative frequency and predisposing factors. *Clinical Endocrinology, 45*(5), 563–569.

129. Grunstein, R. R., Ho, K. Y., & Sullivan, C. E. (1991). Sleep apnea in acromegaly. *Annals of Internal Medicine, 115*(7), 527–532.

130. Grunstein, R. R., Ho, K. Y., Berthon-Jones, M., et al. (1994). Central sleep apnea is associated with increased ventilatory response to carbon dioxide and hypersecretion of growth hormone in patients with acromegaly. *American Journal of Respiratory and Critical Care Medicine, 150*(2), 496–502.

131. Astrom, C., Christensen, L., Gjerris, F., et al. (1991). Sleep in acromegaly before and after treatment with adenomectomy. *Neuroendocrinology, 53*(4), 328–331.

132. Shipley, J. E., Schteingart, D. E., Tandon, R., et al. (1992). Sleep architecture and sleep apnea in patients with Cushing's disease. *Sleep, 15*(6), 514–518.

133. Shipley, J. E., Schteingart, D. E., Tandon, R., et al. (1992). EEG sleep in Cushing's disease and Cushing's syndrome: Comparison with patients with major depressive disorder. *Biological Psychiatry, 32*(2), 146–155.

134. Lovas, K., Husebye, E. S., Holsten, F., et al. (2003). Sleep disturbances in patients with Addison's disease. *European Journal of Endocrinology, 148*(4), 449–456.

135. Garcia-Borreguero, D., Wehr, T. A., Larrosa, O., et al. (2000). Glucocorticoid replacement is permissive for rapid eye movement sleep and sleep consolidation in patients with adrenal insufficiency. *The Journal of Clinical Endocrinology and Metabolism, 85*(11), 4201–4206.

136. Wilson, K. G., Watson, S. T., & Currie, S. R. (1998). Daily diary and ambulatory activity monitoring of sleep in patients with insomnia associated with chronic musculoskeletal pain. *Pain, 75*(1), 75–84.

137. Roehrs, T., & Roth, T. (2005). Sleep and pain: Interaction of two vital functions. *Seminars in Neurology, 25*(1), 106–116.

138. Palermo, T. M., & Kiska, R. (2005). Subjective sleep disturbances in adolescents with chronic pain: Relationship to daily functioning and quality of life. *The Journal of Pain, 6*(3), 201–207.

139. Wolfe, F., Smythe, H. A., Yunus, M. B., et al. (1990). The American College of Rheumatology 1990 Criteria for the Classification of Fibromyalgia: Report of the Multicenter Criteria Committee. *Arthritis and Rheumatism, 33*(2), 160–172.

140. Affleck, G., Urrows, S., Tennen, H., et al. (1996). Sequential daily relations of sleep, pain intensity, and attention to pain among women with fibromyalgia. *Pain, 68*(2–3), 363–368.

141. Harding, S. M. (1998). Sleep in fibromyalgia patients: Subjective and objective findings. *The American Journal of the Medical Sciences, 315*(6), 367–376.

142. Anch, A. M., Lue, F. A., MacLean, A. W., et al. (1991). Sleep physiology and psychological aspects of the fibrositis (fibromyalgia) syndrome. *Canadian Journal of Psychology, 45*(2), 179–184.

143. Landis, C. A., Lentz, M. J., Rothermel, J., et al. (2004). Decreased sleep spindles and spindle activity in midlife women with fibromyalgia and pain. *Sleep, 27*(4), 741–750.

144. Roizenblatt, S., Moldofsky, H., Benedito-Silva, A. A., et al. (2001). Alpha sleep characteristics in fibromyalgia. *Arthritis and Rheumatism, 44*(1), 222–230.

145. Mahowald, M. L., & Mahowald, M. W. (2000). Nighttime sleep and daytime functioning (sleepiness and fatigue) in less well-defined chronic rheumatic diseases with particular reference to the alpha-delta NREM sleep anomaly. *Sleep Medicine, 1*(3), 195–207.

146. Parker, K. P. (2003). Sleep disturbances in dialysis patients. *Sleep Medicine Reviews, 7*(2), 131–143.

147. Strub, B., Schneider-Helmert, D., Gnirss, F., et al. (1982). Sleep disorders in patients with chronic renal insufficiency in long-term hemodialysis treatment [in German]. *Schweizerische Medizinische Wochenschrift, 112*(23), 824–828.

148. Walker, S., Fine, A., & Kryger, M. H. (1995). Sleep complaints are common in a dialysis unit. *American Journal of Kidney Diseases, 26*(5), 751–756.

149. Hanly, P. (2004). Sleep apnea and daytime sleepiness in end-stage renal disease. *Seminars in Dialysis, 17*(2), 109–114.

150. Winkelman, J. W., Chertow, G. M., & Lazarus, J. M. (1996). Restless legs syndrome in end-stage renal disease. *American Journal of Kidney Diseases, 28*(3), 372–378.

151. Benz, R. L., Pressman, M. R., Hovick, E. T., et al. (1999). A preliminary study of the effects of correction of anemia with recombinant human erythropoietin therapy on sleep, sleep disorders, and daytime sleepiness in hemodialysis patients (The SLEEPO study). *American Journal of Kidney Diseases, 34*(6), 1089–1095.

152. Davis, S. (2004). Clinical sequelae affecting quality of life in the HIV-infected patient. *The Journal of the Association of Nurses in AIDS Care: JANAC, 15*(Suppl. 5), 28S–33S.

153. Diaz-Ruiz, O., Navarro, L., Mendez-Diaz, M., et al. (2001). Inhibition of the ERK pathway prevents HIVgp120-induced REM sleep increase. *Behavioural Brain Research, 913*(1), 78–81.

154. Rubinstein, M. L., & Selwyn, P. A. (1998). High prevalence of insomnia in an outpatient population with HIV infection. *Journal of Acquired Immune Deficiency Syndromes and Human Retrovirology, 19*(3), 260–265.

155. Reid, S., & Dwyer, J. (2005). Insomnia in HIV infection: A systematic review of prevalence, correlates,

and management. *Psychosomatic Medicine, 67*(2), 260–269.

156. Nokes, K. M., & Kendrew, J. (2001). Correlates of sleep quality in persons with HIV disease. *The Journal of the Association of Nurses in AIDS Care: JANAC, 12*(1), 17–22.

157. Robbins, J. L., Phillips, K. D., Dudgeon, W. D., et al. (2004). Physiological and psychological correlates of sleep in HIV infection. *Clinical Nursing Research, 13*(1), 33–52.

158. Franck, L. S., Johnson, L. M., Lee, K., et al. (1999). Sleep disturbances in children with human immunodeficiency virus infection. *Pediatrics, 104*(5), e62.

159. Darko, D. F., Mitler, M. M., & White, J. L. (1995). Sleep disturbance in early HIV infection. *Focus, 10*(11), 5–6.

160. Norman, S. E., Chediak, A. D., Kiel, M., et al. (1990). Sleep disturbances in HIV-infected homosexual men. *AIDS, 4*(8), 775–781.

161. Norman, S. E., Chediak, A. D., Freeman, C., et al. (1992). Sleep disturbances in men with asymptomatic human immunodeficiency (HIV) infection. *Sleep, 15*(2), 150–155.

162. Cruess, D. G., Antoni, M. H., Gonzalez, J., et al. (2003). Sleep disturbance mediates the association between psychological distress and immune status among HIV-positive men and women on combination antiretroviral therapy. *Journal of Psychosomatic Research, 54*(3), 185–189.

163. Lochet, P., Peyriere, H., Lotthe, A., et al. (2003). Long-term assessment of neuropsychiatric adverse reactions associated with efavirenz. *HIV Medicine, 4*(1), 62–66.

164. Gallego, L., Barreiro, P., del Rio, R., et al. (2004). Analyzing sleep abnormalities in HIV-infected patients treated with Efavirenz. *Clinical Infectious Diseases, 38*(3), 430–432.

165. Taibi, D. M. (2013). Sleep disturbances in persons living with HIV. *The Journal of the Association of Nurses in AIDS Care: JANAC, 24*(1 Suppl.), S72–S85.

166. Jaffe, S. E. (2000). Sleep and infectious disease. In M. H. Kryger, T. Roth, & W. C. Dement (Eds.), *Principles and practice of sleep medicine* (p. 1099). Philadelphia, PA: W.B. Saunders.

167. Kaplan, R. F., & Jones-Woodward, L. (1997). Lyme encephalopathy: A neuropsychological perspective. *Seminars in Neurology, 17*(1), 31–37.

168. Greenberg, H. E., Ney, G., Scharf, S. M., et al. (1995). Sleep quality in Lyme disease. *Sleep, 18*(10), 912–916.

169. Kalish, R. A., Kaplan, R. F., Taylor, E., et al. (2001). Evaluation of study patients with Lyme disease, 10–20-year follow-up. *The Journal of Infectious Diseases, 183*(3), 453–460.

170. Buguet, A., Gati, R., Sevre, J. P., et al. (1989). 24 hour polysomnographic evaluation in a patient with sleeping sickness. *Electroencephalographic and Clinical Neurophysiology, 72*(6), 471–478.

171. Sanner, B. M., Buchner, N., Kotterba, S., et al. (2000). Polysomnography in acute African trypanosomiasis. *Journal of Neurology, 247*(11), 878–879.

172. Hardin, K. A. (2009). Sleep in the ICU: Potential mechanisms and clinical implications. *Chest, 136*(1), 284–294.

173. Sharma, S., & Kavuru, M. (2010). Sleep and metabolism: An overview. *International Journal of Endocrinology, 2010*, 12.

174. Weinhouse, G. L., Schwab, R. J., Watson, P. L., et al. (2009). Bench-to-bedside review: Delirium in ICU patients—Importance of sleep deprivation. *Critical Care, 13*(6), 234.

175. Pisani, M. A., Friese, R. S., Gehlbach, B. K., et al. (2015). Sleep in the intensive care unit. *American Journal of Respiratory and Critical Care Medicine, 191*(7), 731–738.

176. Paganelli, R., Petrarca, C., Di Gioacchino, M. (2018). Biologic clocks: Their relevance to immune-allergic diseases. *Clinical and Molecular Allergy, 16*, 1.

177. Kamdar, B. B., Needham, D. M., & Collop, N. A. (2012). Sleep deprivation in critical illness: Its role in physical and psychological recovery. *Journal of Intensive Care Medicine, 27*(2), 97–111.

178. Matthews, E. E. (2011). Sleep disturbances and fatigue in critically ill patients. *AACN Advanced Critical Care, 22*(3), 204–224.

179. Parthasarathy, S., & Tobin, M. J. (2004). Sleep in the intensive care unit. *Intensive Care Medicine, 30*(2), 197–206.

180. Watson, P. L. (2007). Measuring sleep in critically ill patients: Beware the pitfalls. *Critical Care, 11*(4), 159.

181. Cortelli, P., Gambetti, P., Montagna, P., et al. (1999). Fatal familial insomnia: Clinical features and molecular genetics. *Journal of Sleep Research, 8*(Suppl. 1), 23–29.

182. Polnitsky, C. A. (2006). Fatal familial insomnia. In T. Lee-Chiong (Ed.), *Encyclopedia of sleep medicine* (pp. 111–115). New York, NY: John Wiley & Sons.

chapter 24
Seizures and Sleep

AMY KORN-REAVIS   DAVID A. DAVIS

LEARNING OBJECTIVES

On completion of this chapter, the reader should be able to:

1. Describe the causes and classifications of seizures.
2. Recognize clinical signs of seizure activity.
3. Review the treatment options available for people who have seizures.
4. Discuss how sleep relates to the identification and control of seizures.
5. Identify seizure activity on the electroencephalogram.
6. Describe the appropriate response to a seizure and when to activate Emergency Medical Services.

KEY TERMS

Sleep
Seizure
Epileptiform discharges
Patient's safety

A seizure is a sudden abnormal discharge of electrical activity in the brain, usually affecting how a person acts or feels for a short time. These involuntary actions or sensations can range from a brief muscle twitch to a distorted vision to a staring spell to complete loss of consciousness with tonic–clonic activity (see Table 24-1). One in 10 Americans will have a seizure at some point in their lifetime, with 3% of those developing epilepsy, or seizure disorder, by the age of 80 (1). Epilepsy is defined as two or more unprovoked seizures (2), and is the third most common brain disorder after Alzheimer disease and stroke (3). Epilepsy affects 50 million people worldwide (3). The chances of having a seizure are greatest during early childhood or after the age of 65, with men slightly more at risk than women.

The known causes of seizures include birth trauma, brain injury, brain tumor, cerebral hemorrhage, anoxic event, brain infection (meningitis or encephalitis), stroke, cerebral palsy, mental handicap, high fever, toxins (lead), and illegal drug use (cocaine). When no underlying cause is found for the seizure, which happens in 7 out of 10 people (3), it is referred to as idiopathic.

"EEGs are known to capture approximately 50% of people with seizures however with repeat recording and recordings that include sleep the capture rate increases to 80% to 90% range" (4). It therefore becomes important to record patients during sleep. Many of the symptoms that are indications for a sleep study such as sleep paralysis, memory loss, confusional arousals, and fatigue are also symptoms of seizures. This can bring to the sleep laboratory patients who may not be aware they are having seizures. Therefore, it is essential for the technologist to be familiar with seizure activity and how

Table 24-1 Terminology

Aura	A sensation experienced by some people with epilepsy before a seizure. Commonly described auras include copper taste, distorted vision, burning sensation, dizziness, headache, déjá vu, and jamais vu (5)
Déjá vu	A feeling that you have experienced something before (5)
Jamais vu	The familiar seems unfamiliar (5)
Ictal	During the time a seizure is occurring (6)
Interictal	The time between seizures (6)
Preictal	The time before a seizure occurs (6)
Postictal	The time after a seizure occurs (6)
Spike	Transient electroencephalography wave with pointed peak and duration of 20–70 ms (5)
Polyspikes	Multiple spike complexes (5)
Sharp wave	Same morphology as a spike but with duration of >70 and <200 ms (5)
Spike and slow wave	Spike followed by a high-amplitude slow wave (5)

to identify it on electroencephalogram (EEG) and with video recording (5, 6).

CLINICAL OBSERVATIONS

Clinical observations during a seizure will vary depending on the location and size of the seizure focus (area of the brain where the seizure originates) and how the seizure is classified (Table 24-2) (7–9).

Location

Functions of the *frontal lobe* include speech and language skills, reasoning, and problem solving (7). Seizure activity in this area may present with difficulty speaking, hollering profanities, or laughing inappropriately. *Parietal lobe* functions are perception of stimuli (touch, pressure, and taste), recognition, orientation, and motor control (7). Presentation may include face or upper extremity numbness or twitching. Visual processing is the primary function of the *occipital lobe* of the brain (6). Clinical presentation may include distorted vision or visual hallucinations. Functions of the *temporal lobe* include recognition of auditory stimuli, memory, language skills, and emotional responses (6). Impairments during a seizure may include not being able to respond to auditory stimuli, impaired memory, or fear. The functions of each lobe of the brain are specific, and the clinical observations indicated are simplistic and may represent other medical conditions.

Standard Nomenclature for the Description of EEG Discharges

The American Clinical Neurophysiology Society provides specific nomenclature for documentation of discharges seen in the EEG. They are defined by the area that is affected: generalized, lateralized, bilateral independent, and multifocal. When describing discharges, document

Table 24-2 Seizure Classifications

Generalized seizures	Event begins as widespread epileptiform activity over both hemispheres of the brain associated with sudden movement or loss of consciousness (6–8).
• Tonic–clonic	Occurs without warning with loss of consciousness, can be associated with injury (tongue biting or from initial fall), usually lasts up to 2–3 min, consciousness returns slowly, respirations may be absent during the tonic phase and may be labored during the clonic phase. Confusion, sleepiness, agitation, headache, and nausea all can be present postictal (6).
• Absence	Most commonly seen in children aged 4–14, has a duration of 5–15 s, begins and ends abruptly, described as a blank stare, appears to be daydreaming, and can be associated with rapid eye blinking (6).
• Myoclonic	Abnormal brief jerk-like movements involving both sides of the body lasting a second or two (8).
• Atonic (drop attack)	Complete loss of muscle tone, including falling to the ground, usually associated with injury and often noticed by head drop (8).
Partial seizures	Event begins as an electrical discharge over a localized area of the brain (one hemisphere). Note: Partial seizures can evolve, spreading to involve both hemispheres (6–8).
• Simple partial	Consciousness is not impaired, memory remains intact, awareness is preserved, may exhibit face twitching, eye blinking, odd smiling, or unexplained emotions (6).
• Complex partial	At least one of the following is present: impaired consciousness, memory, or awareness. Presents with trance-like appearance, may appear afraid and exhibit random undirected movements like walking, lip smacking, or picking at clothing (8).
Psychogenic nonepileptic seizures	These events are defined as clinical events that appear to be an epileptic seizure without correlating electroencephalogram changes. Other terminology used in the past for this type of activity has been pseudoseizure, psychological, or psychosomatic. It is important to recognize that many precipitating factors can lead to this diagnosis including past or present abuse, depression, and mental disorders (9).

which lobes are predominant and whether the discharges are symmetrical or asymmetrical. In addition, describe the frequency and pattern of the discharge, such as rhythmic discharges, periodic discharges, or spike-and-wave discharges. The morphology and the shape of the discharge should also be described. Discharges can consist of sharp waves 70 to 200 ms, spikes 20 to 70 ms, sharp- and slow-wave complexes, and multiple spike- and slow-wave complexes that are similar to spike and slow wave but include multiple spikes associated with one or more slow waves (10), and paroxysmal slow-wave discharges.

It can be difficult to identify these discharges using a 30-second epoch; utilize a 10-second page to assist with identification. It can also be difficult to identify interictal epileptiform discharges (IEDs). Some normal variants can be mistaken for IEDs. An example is Mu rhythm, which is a rhythmic discharge of 8 to 11 Hz that has a sharp and comb-like shape. Mu rhythm can be suppressed with movement of the contralateral limb. Positive sharp transients of sleep are 4 to 6 Hz discharges seen in the occipital region. These can be confused with IEDs. However, most IEDs are of negative polarity (4). Electrocardiogram (ECG) artifact can also be mistaken for spikes. If a technologist is suspicious that a wave looks like a spike, one of the first steps would be to rule out artifact.

The technologist should also be aware of interictal changes that can be seen in the EEG such as voltage attenuation or augmentation, burst-suppression activity, or electrocerebral inactivity. These patterns can occur as well and should be documented (11).

EEG and patient activity (video) must be recorded. IEDs can be either electroclinical in nature or purely electrographic; therefore, the behavior of the patient and what occurred pre- and postevent must be clearly documented.

SLEEP AND EPILEPSY OVERVIEW

The sleep–wake cycle significantly affects the frequency of interictal epileptiform activity (IEA) as well as epileptic seizures. The two neurophysiologic states that characterize sleep (nonrapid eye movement [NREM] and rapid eye movement [REM]) have opposite consequences on both. According to most studies, generalized discharges and clinical seizures mostly occur in NREM sleep (12), which may be considered a natural "convulsive agent" (13), when brain activity is relatively more synchronous. The majority of EEG discharges are seen in stage N2, whereas REM sleep, with its asynchronous cell discharge patterns and atonia, is resistant to epileptic EEG potentials (14). NREM sleep activates IEDs in both partial and generalized syndromes (15).

For a patient with epilepsy presenting with EDS, several possible causes need to be considered.

These include, but are not limited to, nocturnal seizure activity, side effects from medications used for seizure control, an underlying sleep disorder fragmenting sleep, or poor sleep hygiene (16). If multiple causes are present, one can feed off the other and the patient can be caught in a vicious cycle. For example, untreated obstructive sleep apnea is associated with increased arousals, increased NREM sleep, and decreased REM sleep. All of these lower the threshold for the appearance of seizure discharges and seizures during sleep. The disruption in sleep quality leads to daytime symptoms, which can include sleepiness, increased frequency of seizures, and memory impairment.

EPILEPTIFORM DISCHARGES DURING SLEEP IN GENERALIZED EPILEPSY

Primary Generalized Tonic–Clonic Seizures

Sleep has a well-documented influence on this class of seizure that tends to occur during NREM sleep (17, 18). Generalized IEA increases in NREM (18–20) and is most prominent at sleep onset and during the first part of the night. Interestingly, the morphology of IEA changes during sleep (21). In NREM sleep, generalized bursts of spike–wave complexes may become fragmented, polyspikes may appear, and the discharges may occur in a focal distribution (usually in a frontocentral region; Fig. 24-1).

One of the concerns with generalized tonic–clonic seizures (GTCS) is the suppression that occurs postictally. This suppression of brain waves can also lead to suppression of respirations and, finally, asystole. This occurs more frequently in nocturnal GTCS and can lead to sudden death (22).

Primary Generalized Myoclonus

Primary generalized myoclonic seizures are the typical awakening seizures that occur shortly after awakening in 88% to 96% of patients (19, 23). Myoclonus occurs during both spontaneous and provoked arousals. IEA is characterized by generalized polyspike and polyspike-wave discharges, more commonly at the onset of sleep and during nocturnal arousals than during awakenings. Induced arousals from NREM sleep and spontaneous morning awakening activate epileptiform abnormalities. IEA decreases markedly during REM sleep.

Juvenile Myoclonic Epilepsy

These seizures are myoclonic or generalized tonic–clonic with an onset in adolescence or in early childhood and are idiopathic in nature. They usually occur in the

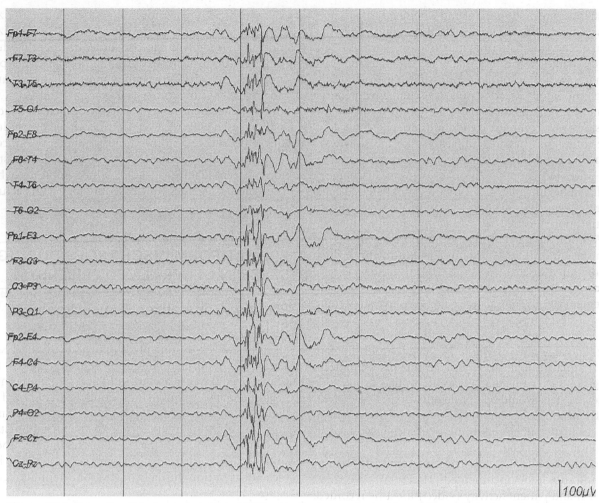

Figure 24-1 Polyspike. This is a typical generalized polyspike in a patient with an idiopathic (primary) generalized epilepsy. Note that the discharge is followed by about 2 seconds of delta activity. This aftergoing slow activity indicates substantial disruption of the background and is a significant argument to consider this discharge pathologic and not a normal variant. (From Benbadis, S. R. (2006). Introduction to sleep electroencephalography. In T. L. Lee-Chiong (Ed.), Sleep: *A comprehensive handbook* (1st ed., p. 1013). Hoboken, NJ: John Wiley and Sons. Copyright © 2006 by John Wiley & Sons, Inc. Reprinted by permission of John Wiley & Sons, Inc.)

morning during the first 1 to 2 hours after awakening. Some may occur on awakening from a nap, but rarely at other times during the day (24). The EEG will show spike-and-wave complexes, typically polyspike and wave complexes. The epileptiform discharges in juvenile myoclonic epilepsy (JME) increase markedly at sleep onset and on awakening, but are virtually absent in NREM and REM sleep and during the waking state. A high proportion of patients with JME (30% to 42%) demonstrate photosensitivity, which is an increase in IEA with photic stimulation (rhythmic flashing of a strobe light).

Absence Epilepsy

Absence seizures usually develop in the first decade of life and are characterized by the abrupt onset of unresponsiveness and behavioral arrest, usually lasting 5 to 15 seconds, followed by an abrupt return to

consciousness. These seizures may occur multiple times per day and may be activated by arousals from drowsiness or sleep. Clinical absence seizures are only detectable in the waking state and are usually precipitated by photic stimulation or hyperventilation. The activation of IEA is most marked in the first sleep cycle during NREM sleep (25). The typical EEG abnormality consists of 3-Hz spike–wave complexes in a generalized distribution (Fig. 24-2). Absence-appearing seizures can also be simple partial seizures.

West Syndrome

This syndrome, with a peak age of onset at 3 to 6 months, is characterized by the triad of infantile spasms, psychomotor retardation, and EEG hypsarrhythmia, which is a typical EEG pattern consisting of multifocal and at times generalized high-voltage spikes superimposed

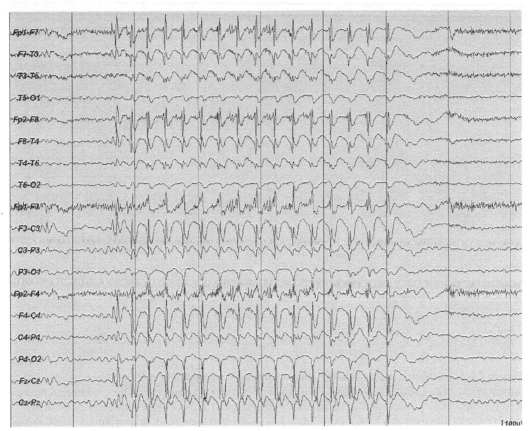

Figure 24-2 Three-Hertz spike–wave complexes. This shows typical 3-Hz spike–wave complexes in a patient with an idiopathic (primary) generalized epilepsy. This patient likely has absence seizures. If tested with a clicker, a discharge of this duration (about 4.5 seconds) is likely associated with a brief impairment of awareness. (From Benbadis, S. R. (2006). Introduction to sleep electroencephalography. In T. L. Lee-Chiong (Ed.), *Sleep: A comprehensive handbook* (1st ed., p. 1014). Hoboken, NJ: John Wiley and Sons. Copyright © 2006 by John Wiley & Sons, Inc. Reprinted by permission of John Wiley & Sons, Inc.)

on a disorganized and chaotic background. The infantile spasms occur infrequently during sleep (<5% of the cases). The hypsarrhythmic pattern shows a striking variation during sleep. The EEG abnormalities tend to increase in NREM sleep, and the spike–slow-wave discharges tend to become grouped, at times having a periodic appearance. During REM sleep, there is a marked attenuation or disappearance of the hypsarrhythmia pattern (26, 27). In some cases, the hypsarrhythmia is observed only during sleep.

Lennox–Gastaut Syndrome

This syndrome is characterized by intractable seizures (generalized tonic–clonic, tonic, atonic, myoclonic, and atypical absence seizures), mental retardation, and the presence of generalized slow spike–wave complexes at a frequency of 2.5 Hz or less (Fig. 24-3). An increased quantity of bursts of slow spike–wave complexes is observed in NREM sleep. The morphology of EEG discharges may change, with polyspikes becoming more prominent; also, runs of polyspikes and rhythmic

bursts of rapid activity (10 to 20 Hz) may be observed. There may also be a burst-suppression-like pattern (high-amplitude discharges separated by very low voltage activity).

EPILEPTIFORM DISCHARGES DURING SLEEP IN FOCAL SEIZURES

Temporal Lobe Epilepsy

Studies have shown that nocturnal seizures in patients with temporal lobe epilepsy (TLE) are infrequent and usually do not cluster (24, 25). Most studies of TLE have observed an increase in epileptiform discharges in NREM sleep with a decrease in REM sleep (28–30). The spike frequency is generally highest in the deep NREM sleep (N3). Morphology and distribution of IEA are often affected by sleep. Contralateral focal discharges that facilitate the secondary generalization of focal discharges may appear during NREM sleep. Secondary generalization occurs when a focal epileptiform discharge

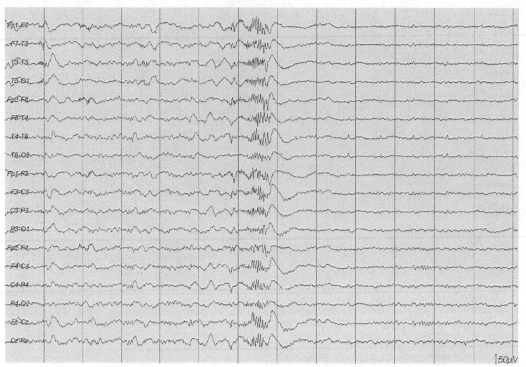

Figure 24-3 Generalized paroxysmal fast activity followed by attenuation (electrodecrement) in a patient with a symptomatic generalized epilepsy of the Lennox–Gastaut type. This could be an inter-ictal (asymptomatic) discharge, but could also be an ictal pattern associated with a tonic–atonic seizure. (From Benbadis, S. R. (2006). Introduction to sleep electroencephalography. In T. L. Lee-Chiong (Ed.), *Sleep: A comprehensive handbook* (1st ed., p. 1015). Hoboken, NJ: John Wiley and Sons. Copyright © 2006 by John Wiley & Sons, Inc. Reprinted by permission of John Wiley & Sons, Inc.)

spreads broadly to both hemispheres. Isolated spikes seen during wakefulness in patients with neocortical foci may be replaced by high-frequency bursts of spikes during NREM sleep (20). Sleep has different effects on temporal and frontal lobe seizures (Fig. 24-4).

Frontal Lobe Epilepsy

It is well known that seizures originating from the frontal lobe show a tendency to occur preferentially during sleep. They tend to have prominent motor manifestations and are likely to be recognized by the parents or bed partners. Three major clinical forms of epilepsy may be distinguished: benign focal epilepsy of childhood, supplementary sensorimotor epilepsy, and nocturnal frontal lobe epilepsy (NFLE).

Benign Focal Epilepsy of Childhood

This syndrome is also referred to as benign rolandic epilepsy or benign childhood epilepsy. Benign focal epilepsy of childhood with centrotemporal spikes is a common form of childhood epilepsy, accounting for 15% to 25% of childhood epilepsy (31). Approximately 75% of these seizures occur during sleep (30). The EEG is characterized by slow spikes or sharp waves recorded

simultaneously over frontal, central, and midtemporal areas. These often appear in small clusters and may be seen in children without epilepsy. The IEA is activated by sleep; during NREM sleep, there is a marked increase in the frequency and amplitude of the interictal spike discharges, with no change in morphology. The IEA is maximal during N3 sleep. REM sleep is associated with a decrease in both the frequency and the amplitude of the spikes. Despite an increased frequency of both seizures and IEA during sleep, the sleep profile of these children is usually normal (31–33).

Supplementary Sensorimotor Area Epilepsy

This form refers to epilepsy originating from the supplemental sensorimotor area. The typical seizures are characterized by abrupt tonic posturing of the extremities. The upper extremities are usually asymmetrically involved with the abduction at the shoulders, flexion of the elbow on one side, and extension in the other extremity. The head is turned to one side as though looking toward the flexed arm (fencing posture). The lower extremities are involved in the tonic posture, with abduction at the hips and flexion or extension at the knees. There may be associated vocalization and kicking with

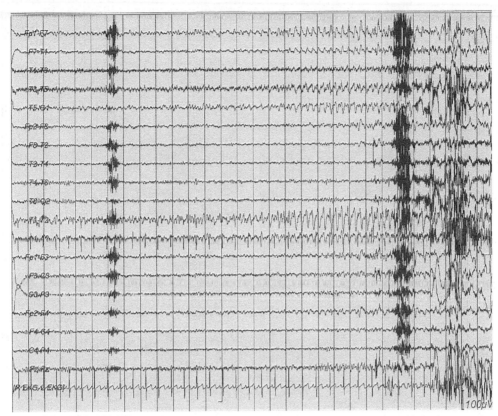

Figure 24-4 Focal seizure. Left temporal seizure (singular), showing the typical rhythmic activity that evolves (buildup). (From Benbadis, S. R. (2006). Introduction to sleep electroencephalography. In T. L. Lee-Chiong (Ed.), *Sleep: A comprehensive handbook* (1st ed., p. 1015). Hoboken, NJ: John Wiley and Sons. Copyright © 2006 by John Wiley & Sons, Inc. Reprinted by permission of John Wiley & Sons, Inc.)

preserved responsiveness (34). Somatosensory (lateralized or diffuse) symptoms may precede the tonic contraction and consist of a feeling of pulling or heaviness or a limb sensation of moving (34).

The seizures tend to occur predominantly during sleep. Interictal sharp waves are usually found at the midline, maximum at the vertex, or just adjacent to the midline in the frontocentral region. It is fundamentally important to distinguish epileptiform discharges from vertex sharp transients of sleep. The appearance of sharp waves during the waking state aids discrimination between them. The ictal EEG pattern is characterized by a high-amplitude slow transient or sharp wave at the vertex, followed by low-amplitude fast activity, or an electrodecremental pattern (34, 35) (Fig. 24-5). Following this pattern, there is a high-amplitude slowing in the frontocentral regions distributed bilaterally.

Nocturnal Frontal Lobe Epilepsy

A distinct form of clear-cut attacks originating from epileptic foci located in the frontal lobe (in particular, in the mesial and orbital cortex) and emerging almost exclusively from sleep has been described (36, 37).

Seizures are characterized by a wide spectrum of clinical features: assumption of postures; rhythmic and repetitive movements of arms and legs; rapid uncoordinated movements, with dystonic or dyskinetic components; complex motor activities (deambulation, wandering, and pelvic thrusting); and sudden elevation of the trunk and head associated with expression of fear and vocalization. There are three subgroups of NFLE:

1. Paroxysmal arousals: Characterized by a brief (<20 seconds) abrupt arousal from sleep with vocalization and motor activity consisting of head movements, sudden eye opening, head raising, or sitting up in bed, often with a frightened expression (38).
2. Nocturnal paroxysmal dystonia: Characterized by episodes of intermediate duration (20 seconds to 2 minutes) beginning as a paroxysmal arousal, but subsequently associated with complex movements including rhythmic movements of the trunk and pelvis, dystonic posturing, and vocalization (38).
3. Episodic nocturnal wandering: Characterized by episodes of longer duration (1 to 3 minutes) with stereotyped, paroxysmal ambulation, accompanied by screaming and bizarre, dystonic movements (38).

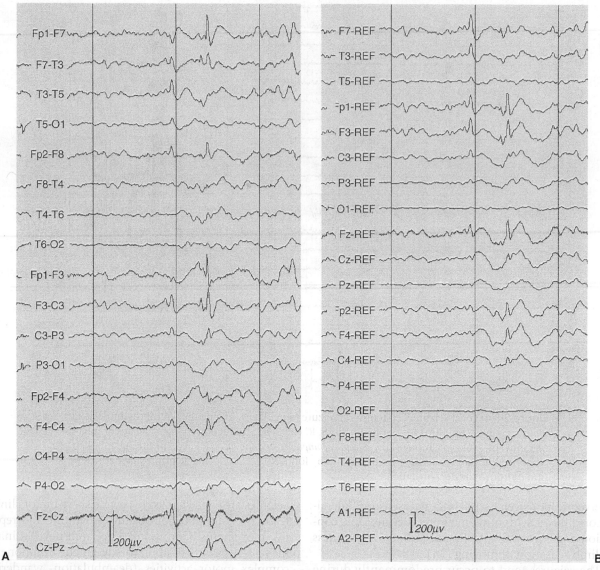

Figure 24-5 Left frontal spike in a patient with left frontal lobe epilepsy. **A:** Double banana. **B:** Referential montage showing the same sample. There are two different spikes: the first is maximum at F7 and the second at Fp1. (From Benbadis, S. R. (2006). Introduction to sleep electroencephalography. In T. L. Lee-Chiong (Ed.), *Sleep: A comprehensive handbook* (1st ed., p. 1012). Hoboken, NJ: John Wiley and Sons. Copyright © 2006 by John Wiley & Sons, Inc. Reprinted by permission of John Wiley & Sons, Inc.)

Surface EEG during the attacks and interictally is often normal, uninformative, or not interpretable because of the presence of muscle artifacts (39). Deep (intracranial, sphenoidal) electrode recordings can identify ictal and/or interictal discharges (36, 40). Various ictal EEG patterns may be observed: background flattening, rhythmic theta/delta activity, or sharp wave on the frontal regions.

Treatment for these types of seizures only results in a partial reduction of seizure activity, with events occurring most commonly during NREM sleep. This causes subsequent sleep disturbance due to recurrence of both major seizures and more subtle arousal activities (41).

Electrical Status Epilepticus of Sleep

This syndrome is also known as epilepsy with continuous spike waves during stage N3 sleep and refers to the occurrence of continuous epileptiform activity for at least 85% of slow-wave sleep (42). The EEG is characterized by generalized spike–wave complexes at 2 to 2.5 Hz, and there is a marked attenuation of the pattern during REM sleep and in the wake state. With the onset of electrical status epilepticus of sleep (ESES), there is an associated decline in cognitive function, with improvement once the ESES has resolved (43). Seizures may manifest as nocturnal focal motor or generalized tonic–clonic seizures or as atypical absence or myoclonic seizures.

Landau–Kleffner Syndrome

This syndrome is a childhood disorder occurring in previously normal children, characterized by the association of loss of language skills with acquired verbal auditory agnosia and multifocal spikes and spike-and-wave discharges mainly localized over the centrotemporal regions (44, 45). There is dramatic activation of the epileptic discharges during sleep, with discharges occurring for more than 85% of slow-wave sleep, similar to ESES (46). However, the occurrence of seizures is relatively rare. There is usually remission of seizures and epileptiform EEG discharges by the age of 15 years.

TREATMENT OPTIONS

Antiepileptic drugs (AEDs) are the most commonly used treatment for seizure control (47). As with any medication, there is a risk of both side effects and adverse reactions. Side effects include, but are not limited to, nausea, vomiting, weight gain, weight loss, headaches, clumsiness, and vision change. AEDs also have an effect on sleep. For the most part, older AEDs decrease sleep latency, decrease REM sleep, and increase daytime drowsiness (48).

Newer AEDs appear to have less of an effect on sleep, and some increase REM sleep. Insomnia has been associated with lamotrigine, zonisamide, ethosuximide, and felbamate. Their effect on daytime sleepiness is still not well known. Keeping in mind that multiple medications are sometimes necessary for seizure control, the effects on sleep architecture from a combination of AEDs could not be found.

Commonly used medications to control seizures include carbamazepine (Carbatrol/Tegretol), valproate/valproic acid (Depakote/Depakene), phenytoin (Dilantin), felbamate (Felbatol), tiagabine (Gabitril), levetiracetam (Keppra), clonazepam (Klonopin), lamotrigine (Lamictal), pregabalin (Lyrica), primidone (Mysoline), gabapentin (Neurontin), topiramate (Topamax), oxcarbazepine (Trileptal), ethosuximide (Zarontin), and Zonegran zonisamide (Lyrica).

Cannabinoids, including selective cannabinoid receptor 1 antagonists, appear to prevent seizures and are currently being researched for treatment of seizures (49). Much of this research came from the effects of Cannabis on seizures and generalized convulsions.

A *vagal nerve stimulator* is also a treatment option. This is an implantable stimulator that is usually recommended when seizures cannot be adequately controlled with AEDs or the side effects cannot be tolerated. Using the pathway of the vagus nerve, the device (which is surgically implanted on the left side of the neck) delivers mild electrical pulses to the brain (47).

Surgical intervention with removal of a small specific area of the brain where the seizure activity originates is an option for some patients where other forms of treatment have not been successful.

Independent of which treatment path is being followed, maintaining regular sleep cycles, avoiding stress, and regular follow-up with physicians are important too.

GENERAL GUIDELINES FOR SEIZURE MONTAGES

Current polysomnographic (PSG) standards, in regard to assisting in the diagnosis of sleep-related seizure activity, do not mandate a specific recording montage to be used. The minimum channels required include sleep scoring channels (EEG, electrooculogram [EOG], and chin electromyogram [EMG]), EEG using an expanded bilateral montage, and EMG for body movements (anterior tibialis or extensor digitorium) (50). Audiovisual recording and documented technologist observations during the period of study are also essential (50).

The purpose of monitoring additional EEG channels is to not only identify IEA but also to be able to define the seizure focus if possible. With standard PSG monitoring, a referential montage is recorded. Incorporating a full EEG longitudinal bipolar montage can be useful in localizing seizure activity. This would require adding 12 electrodes and recording 16 channels, which is not always feasible. An abbreviated longitudinal bipolar montage is an option. Additional electrodes commonly utilized to record an abbreviated longitudinal bipolar montage include Fp1, Fp2, T3, and T4. Four additional EEG channels could be recorded: Fp1-T3, T3-O1, Fp2-T4, and T4-O2.

EMG should be recorded from all four limbs and should be performed for clinical correlation of tonic–clonic activity. If possible, each limb should be monitored independently. An alternative would be to place one electrode on each extremity and record EMG channels using left arm to right arm and left leg to right leg.

Reviewing the patient history and considering any information the patient may share with the technologist, and acquiring additional EEG data using a seizure montage may be prudent. Circumstances in which the technologist should consider using an expanded EEG montage include a diagnosis of epilepsy, any known cause of seizures with ongoing symptoms, witnessed rhythmic movements during sleep with nocturnal incontinence, and injury (tongue biting). As always, protocols specific to each sleep center must be followed. Be proactive for the patient, even if it means taking the time to seek approval to do additional monitoring.

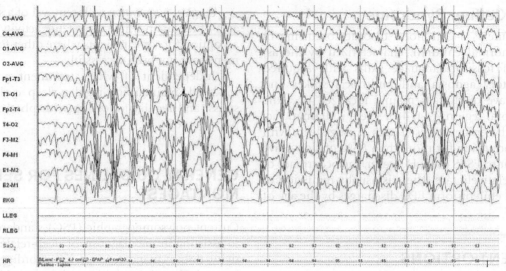

Figure 24-6 Generalized interictal epileptiform activity on a 10-second epoch.

VISUAL DIFFERENCES OF EPILEPTIFORM ACTIVITY ON 10- AND 30-SECOND EPOCHS

Morphology of epileptiform activity on a 10-second epoch has been documented in all previous figures. During a PSG when viewing IEA on a 30-second epoch, an abnormal burst of electrical activity is apparent, although not clearly defined until viewed on a 10-second epoch (Figs. 24-6 to 24-9).

GENERAL GUIDELINES FOR RESPONDING TO IEA

The patient's safety is always top priority when seizure activity is recognized by the technologist. If the epileptiform discharges are prolonged or frequent, it is certainly appropriate for the technologist to assess the patient and determine whether any further intervention may be required. Keeping in mind that there is a balance, that data need to be recorded to confirm a diagnosis, and

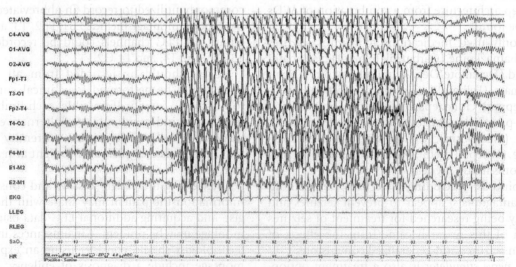

Figure 24-7 Generalized interictal epileptiform activity depicted in Figure 24-6 but on a 30-second epoch.

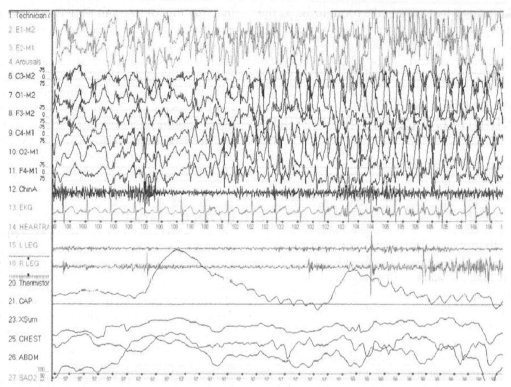

Figure 24-8 Generalized interictal epileptiform activity on a 10-second epoch.

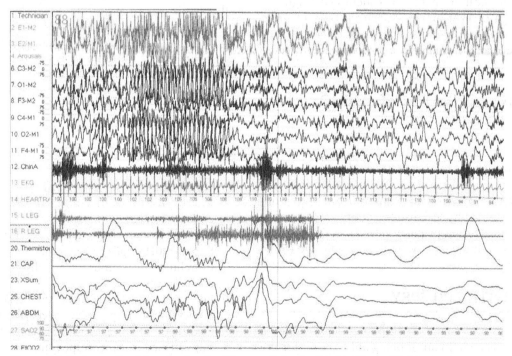

Figure 24-9 Generalized interictal epileptiform activity depicted in Figure 24-8 but on a 30-second epoch.

therefore, knowing when to enter the room to assess the patient is a judgment call. A review of the patient's history will aid in making these decisions; and protocols specific to each sleep center must be followed as well.

GENERAL GUIDELINES FOR RESPONDING TO A CLINICAL SEIZURE

- *Remain calm and (51) continue recording.*
- *Protect the patient from harm (51)*—ensure the patient does not fall out of bed, shield from hard or sharp objects, loosen anything that could become tight around the neck (clothing or electrodes) and to maintain the airway either positioning the patient laterally or turning the head to one side.
- *Time* how long the seizure lasts (51).
- *Do not* attempt to stop any clonic movements (51).
- *Do not* place objects in the patient's mouth (51).
- *Stay with the patient (51).* With return of consciousness, the patient will need to be reassured and reoriented. During the postictal period, reorientation may need to be repeated as necessary.
- *Document* the event including the date, time, and duration of the occurrence; a description of the event; and the actions taken by the technologist. Include a list of notifications made, the patient's vital signs following the event, and the time it took for "baseline level of consciousness" to return. All specific sleep center protocols would need to be followed as well.

WHEN TO ACTIVATE EMERGENCY MEDICAL SERVICES

The following situations are medical emergencies: seizures lasting longer than 5 minutes; a second seizure starting soon after the first one has ended; consciousness not returning after clonic movements have subsided; or signs of physical distress, injury, or pregnancy (51). A seizure during pregnancy can be a symptom of eclampsia and immediate evaluation is indicated (51).

LIVING WITH EPILEPSY

The ability to understand the impact epilepsy has on a person's life is a vital part of being able to care for the person when seizures occur. Seizures are frightening and unknown to many, and sadly, even in today's society, a stigma still surrounds epilepsy.

Sometimes it can be a lengthy process from the initial seizure to the diagnosis and eventual management and treatment of seizures. Although AEDs are effective

in a majority of cases, finding the correct medication(s) and dosage may take time. Meanwhile, employment issues, isolation, medication side effects, the possibility of invasive procedures, and loss of independence will be but a few of the hurdles these patients face. For instance, in some states, driving privileges are restricted until a person is "seizure free" for 6 months. Technologists should be aware that each patient presenting to the sleep center may be dealing with any or all of the aforementioned processes and adjust the care offered to seizure patients accordingly.

CONCLUSION

The role of the sleep technologist encompasses more than placing electrodes on a patient and recording data. Depending on patient population, nocturnal seizure activity may rarely be seen at some sleep facilities. Despite this, all sleep professionals need to understand the relationship between sleep and sleep disorders with seizure control. Reviewing the patient history may lead a technologist to question if recording additional EEG channels is warranted. Familiarity with commonly used AEDs, recognition of epileptiform activity on the EEG, and knowing how to keep a patient safe in the event of a seizure while in the sleep center are all necessary skills. All patients deserve a well-trained technologist treating them with respect and compassion. Patients put at ease by a knowledgeable technologist and comfortable sleeping environment quite possibly are more apt to share information, which may aid the physician in rendering a diagnosis and offering an improved individualized treatment plan.

REFERENCES

1. Centers for Disease Control and Prevention. (2011). *Epilepsy fast facts*. Retrieved from http://www.cdc.gov/epilepsy/basics/fast_facts.htm
2. National Institute of Neurological Disorders and Stroke. (2011). *Epilepsy information page*. Retrieved from http://www.ninds.nih.gov/disorders/epilepsy/epilepsy.htm
3. Epilepsy Foundation. (2011). *About epilepsy: The basics*. Retrieved from http://www.epilepsyfoundation.org
4. Medscape. (2017). *Epileptiform discharges*. Retrieved from https://emedicine.medscape.com/article/1138880-overview
5. The Internet Stroke Center. (2011). *Glossary of neurological terms*. Retrieved from http://www.strokecenter.org/education/glossary.html#a
6. U.S. National Library of Medicine–National Institutes of Health. (2018). *Medical encyclopedia: MedlinePlus*.

Retrieved from https://vsearch.nlm.nih
.gov/vivisimo/cgi-bin/query-meta?&v:project=
medlineplus&v:sources=medlineplus-bundle&
query=ictal&binning-state=group%3d%3d
Medical%20Encyclopedia&

7. National Institute of Neurological Disorders and
Stroke. (2018). *Brain basics: Know your brain*. Re-
trieved from https://www.ninds.nih.gov/Disorders/
Patient-Caregiver-Education/Know-Your-Brain

8. Kammerman, S., & Wasserman, L. (2001). Seizure
disorders: Part 1. Classification and diagnosis. *Western
Journal of Medicine, 175*(2), 99–103.

9. Lesser, R. P. (2003). Treatment and outcome of psychogenic nonepileptic seizures. *Epilepsy Currents, 3*(6),
198–200.

10. American Clinical Neurophysiology Society. (2012).
*American Clinical Neurophysiology Society Standard ICU
EEG Nomenclature v. 2012*. Retrieved from https://
www.acns.org/pdf/guidelines/Guideline-14-pocket-
version.pdf

11. Tatum, W. O., Olga, S., Ochoa, J. G., et al. (2016).
American Clinical Neurophysiology Society Guideline 7:
Guidelines for EEG Reporting. *Journal of Clinical Neu-
rophysiology, 33*(4), 328–332.

12. Parrino, L. (2011). *Impact of sleep on epileptic manifestations*. Retrieved from https://www.medlink.com/
MedLinkContent.asp

13. Passouant, P. (1991). Historical aspects of sleep and
epilepsy. In R. Degen & E. A. Rodin (Eds.), *Epilepsy,
sleep and sleep deprivation* (2nd ed., pp. 19–22). Amsterdam, The Netherlands: Elsevier Science.

14. Shouse, M. N., Langer, J., King, A., et al. (1995). Paroxysmal microarousals in amygdale-kindled kittens: Could
they be subclinical seizures? *Epilepsia, 36,* 290–300.

15. Kellaway, P. (1985). Sleep and epilepsy. *Epilepsia, 26,*
15–30.

16. Vaughn, B. (2011). *Sleep and epilepsy*. Retrieved from
https://www.medlink.com/MedLinkContent.asp

17. Passouant, P., Besset, A., Carrier, A., et al. (1974).
Night sleep and generalized epilepsies. In W. P. Koella
& P. Levin (Eds.), *Sleep research* (pp. 185–196). Basel,
Switzerland: S. Karger.

18. Besset, A. (1982). Influence of generalized seizures on
sleep organization. In M. B. Sterman, M. N. Shouse, &
P. Passouant (Eds.), *Sleep and epilepsy* (pp. 339–346).
New York, NY: Academic Press.

19. Billiard, M. (1982). Epilepsy and the sleep-wake cycle
in man. In M. B. Sterman, M. N. Shouse, & P. Passouant (Eds.), *Sleep and epilepsy* (pp. 269–272). New
York, NY: Academic Press.

20. Montplaisir, J., Laverdiere, M., & Saint-Hiliare, J. M.
(1985). Sleep and epilepsy. In J. Gotman, J. R. Ives, &
P. Gloor (Eds.), *Long term monitoring in epilepsy* (EEG
supplement no. 37) (pp. 215–239). Amsterdam, The
Netherlands: Elsevier.

21. Broughton, R. J. (1984). Epilepsy and sleep: A synopsis
and prospectus. In R. Degen & E. Niedrmeyer (Eds.),
Epilepsy and sleep and sleep deprivation (pp. 317–346).
Amsterdam, The Netherlands: Elsevier Science
Publishers.

22. Peng, W., Danison, J. L., & Seyal, M. (2017). Postictal
generalized EEG suppression and respiratory dysfunction following generalized tonic-clonic seizures in
sleep and wakefulness. *Epilepsia, 58*(8), 1409–1414.
doi:10.1111/epi.13805

23. Janz, D. (1962). The grand mal epilepsies and the
sleep-waking cycle. *Epilepsia, 3,* 69–109.

24. Dinner, D. S., Luders, H., Morris, H. H., et al. (1987).
Juvenile myoclonic epilepsies. In H. Luders & R. P.
Lesser (Eds.), *Epilepsy: Electro-clinical syndromes* (clini-
cal medicine and the nervous system series). London,
UK: Springer-Verlag.

25. Ross, J. J., Johnson, L. C., & Walter, R. D. (1966).
Spike and wave discharges during stages of sleep. *Annals of Neurology, 14,* 399–407.

26. Gomez, M. R., & Klass, D. W. (1983). Epilepsies
of infancy and childhood. *Annals of Neurology, 13,*
113–124.

27. Jeavons, P. M., & Bower, B. D. (1961). The natural
history of infantile spasms. *Archives of Disease in the
Child, 36,* 17–21.

28. Rowan, A. J., Veldhuisen, R. J., & Nagelkerke, N. J. D.
(1982). Comparative evaluation of sleep deprivation
and sedated sleep EEG as a diagnostic aid in epilepsy.
Electroencephalography & Clinical Neurophysiology, 54,
357–364.

29. Rossi, G. F., Colicchio, G., & Pola, P. (1984). Interictal
epileptic activity during sleep: A stero-EEG study in
patients with partial epilepsy. *Electroencephalography &
Clinical Neurophysiology, 58,* 97–106.

30. Sammaritano, M., Gigli, G., & Gotman, J. (1991). Interictal spiking during wakefulness and sleep and the
localization of foci in temporal lobe epilepsy. *Neurology, 4,* 290–297.

31. Lerman, P., & Kivity, S. (1975). Benign focal epilepsy
in childhood. *Archives of Neurology, 32,* 261–264.

32. Gregory, D. L., & Wong, P. K. (1984). Topographical
analysis of the centrotemporal discharges in benign
rolandic epilepsy in childhood. *Epilepsia, 25,*
705–711.

33. Dalla Bernardina, B., & Beghini, G. (1976). Rolandic
spikes in children with and without epilepsy (20 subjects polygraphically studied during sleep). *Epilepsia,
17,* 161–167.

34. Morris, H., III, Dinner, D., Luders, H., et al. (1988).
Supplementary motor seizures: Clinical and electroencephalographic findings. *Neurology, 38,* 1075–1082.

35. Bleasel, A., So, N., Van Ness, P., et al. (1993). The clinical syndrome of seizures arising from supplementary
motor area. *Epilepsia, 34*(Suppl. 6), S54.

36. Tinuper, P., Cerullo, A., & Cirignotta, F. (1990). Nocturnal paroxysmal dystonia with short-lasting attacks: Three cases with evidence for an epileptic frontal lobe origin of seizures. *Epilepsia, 31*, 549–556.

37. Plazzi, G., Tinuper, P., Montagna, P., et al. (1985). Epileptic nocturnal wanderings. *Sleep, 18*, 749–756.

38. Derry, C. (2011). *Autosomal dominant sleep-related hypermotor epilepsy.* Retrieved from http://www.medlink.com/article/autosomal_dominant_sleep-related_hypermotor_epilepsy

39. Zucconi, M., & Ferini-Strambi, L. (2000). NREM parasomnias: Arousal disorders and differentiation from nocturnal frontal lobe epilepsy. *Clinical Neurophysiology, 111*(Suppl. 2), 129–135.

40. Godbout, R., Montplaisir, J., & Rouleau, I. (1985). Hypnogenic paroxysmal dystonia: Epilepsy or sleep disorder? A case report. *Clinical EEG, 16*, 136–142.

41. De Paolis, F., Colizzi, E., Milioli, G., et al. (2013). Effects of antiepileptic treatment on sleep and seizures in nocturnal frontal lobe epilepsy. *Sleep Medicine, 14*(7), 597–604. doi:10.1016/j.sleep.2013.02.014

42. Tassinari, C. A., Rubboli, G., Volpi, L., et al. (2000). Encephalopathy with electrical status epilepticus during slow sleep or ESES syndrome including the acquired aphasia. *Clinical Neurophysiology, 111*(Suppl. 2), S94–S102.

43. Jayakar, R. B., & Seshia, S. S. (1991). Electrical status epilepticus during slow-wave sleep: A review. *Journal of Clinical Neurophysiology, 8*, 299–311.

44. Landau, W., & Kleffner, F. R. (1957). Syndrome of acquired aphasia with convulsive disorder in children. *Neurology, 7*, 523–530.

45. Fejerman, N. (n.d.). *Landau–Kleffner syndrome.* Retrieved from https://www.medlink.com/MedLinkContent.asp

46. Tassinari, C. A., Bureau, M., Dravet, C., et al. (1992). Epilepsy with continuous spikes and waves during slow sleep—Otherwise described as ESES. In J. Roger, M. Bureau, & C. Dravet (Eds.), *Epileptic syndromes in infancy, childhood and adolescence* (2nd ed., pp. 245–256). London, UK: John Libbey.

47. National Library of Medicine–National Institutes of Health. (2011). *Epilepsy.* MedlinePlus. Retrieved from http://www.nlm.nih.gov/medlineplus/epilepsy.html#cat3

48. Epilepsy.com. (2018). *Antiepileptic drugs and sleep? Epilepsy and seizure information for patients and health professionals.* Retrieved from https://www.epilepsy.com/learn/challenges-epilepsy/sleep-and-epilepsy

49. Malyshevskaya, O., Aritake, K., Kaushik, M. K., et al. (2017). The relationship between sleep, cannabinoids and seizures. *Sleep Medicine, 40*(Suppl. 1), e207–e208. doi:10.1016/j.sleep.2017.11.607

50. American Academy of Sleep Medicine. (2005). Practice parameters for the indications for polysomnography and related procedures. *Sleep, 28*(4), 512.

51. Centers for Disease Control and Prevention. (2011). *Epilepsy–First aid.* Retrieved from http://www.cdc.gov/epilepsy/basics/first_aid.htm

chapter 25

Impact of Degenerative Disorders on Sleep

MONICA M. HENDERSON   JENNIFER PARR-CHRISTMAS   JAMES D. GEYER   PAUL R. CARNEY

LEARNING OBJECTIVES

On completion of this chapter, the reader should be able to:

1. Discuss degenerative neurologic diseases.
2. Describe the impact of degenerative neurologic diseases on polysomnography and sleep.
3. Explain patient management issues in the sleep laboratory.

KEY TERMS

Alzheimer disease
Dementia with Lewy bodies
Pick disease
Vascular dementia
Restless legs syndrome
Parkinson disease
Multiple system atrophy
Progressive supranuclear palsy
Rapid eye movement (REM) sleep behavior disorder
Nocturnal stridor

DEGENERATIVE DISORDERS AND SLEEP

Degenerative neurologic disorders encompass a broad range of diseases. They include common entities such as dementia and rare diseases such as amyotrophic lateral sclerosis (ALS, or Lou Gehrig disease). The incidence of such diseases in the general population increases with advancing age. Given the increasing age of the demographically large baby-boom generation, sleep technologists can expect to deal with patients with these degenerative diseases on an increasingly frequent basis.

Neurologic disorders and sleep disorders are linked in a complex fashion. For most of the syndromes, little is known about how the disorders affect normal sleep, because the typical clinical description of patients with degenerative diseases has largely reflected data gathered during wakefulness, with little attention given to the manifestations of these disorders during sleep. There has been even less attention focused on the effects that preexisting sleep disorders have on the neurologic function during wakefulness of patients affected with these disorders. This chapter will examine the relationship of sleep and some of the more common neurologic disorders as well as a few rare but more well-known conditions. We have also included practical information to help sleep technologists to establish guidelines to address effectively the physical needs of the neurologically impaired patient.

GENERAL PATIENT MANAGEMENT ISSUES

The sleep technologist must be aware of the potential cognitive and physical limitations of each patient. A demented patient may have difficulty following directions and may not be compliant with standard monitoring protocols. Patients with physically debilitating diseases may need assistance turning or ambulating. It is not uncommon for patients with degenerative neurologic conditions to have previously undiagnosed parasomnias, which may disrupt sleep monitoring. Patient safety is paramount. Once the sleep study has been initiated, the technologist may choose to limit interruptions of monitoring once the patient is asleep, even if electrodes are not making good electrical contact. A recording with the loss of some electrophysiologic signals can still provide clinically important data.

DEGENERATIVE NEUROLOGIC DISORDERS

The relationships between sleep-related breathing disorders, especially obstructive sleep apnea/hypopnea, neurobehavioral and cognitive function, and dementia are incompletely defined and are the subject of frequent study and debate. The relationships are even less well described for the degenerative movement disorders. We have attempted to present the most current information available, while keeping unproven theories to a minimum.

Dementia

Dementia, including all of its subtypes, is one of the most common and debilitating degenerative neurologic disorders. It is frequently undiagnosed in the elderly, with the symptoms dismissed as normal aging. There are numerous subtypes which are categorized on the basis of etiology and pathologic findings; however, they often have similar effects on sleep. Dementia is defined as a syndrome characterized by deterioration of baseline mental function in multiple cognitive/intellectual areas with little or no disturbance of perception or consciousness. Dementia is not necessarily an irreversible condition. Although most common types of dementia are permanent and progressive, some forms are treatable and reversible, such as those caused by thiamine deficiency, hypothyroidism, and long-standing untreated sleep apnea.

Dementia should not be confused with delirium, a transient confusional state which is characterized by an inability to think with proper speed, clarity, and coherence, and which is associated with disorientation, reduced attention and concentration, impaired immediate recall, and diminution of all mental activity. Delirium has a variety of causes, the most common of which include infection, medication side effects, alcoholic or other drug intoxication, acute drug withdrawal in a substance abuser, and metabolic abnormalities, which complicate liver failure, renal failure, etc. In comparison, the more common types of dementia arise from primary changes occurring within the brain cells. Although the symptoms of most types of dementia develop over the course of months to years, delirium typically arises over hours to a few days and may last several weeks. The initial signs and symptoms of delirium usually include reduced concentration, irritability, tremulousness, insomnia, and poor appetite. The patient will typically describe vivid and unpleasant dreams, which are further complicated by transient illusions and hallucinations during wakefulness. Seizures are relatively common, occurring in approximately one-third of cases. Later in the course of the condition, patients may experience paranoia, tremor, and autonomic hyperactivity. Unlike dementia, recovery from delirium is usually complete and heralded by increased lucid intervals and sound sleep.

In contrast, dementia is conventionally said to involve impairment in memory and at least one other cognitive sphere (language, praxis or the ability to perform simple tasks, calculation, judgment, visuospatial orientation, abstract thinking, or concentration). There may be behavioral abnormalities and personality changes with little or no disturbance of consciousness or perception. Delirium and dementia may coexist, and because of diminished brain function, patients with dementia are at increased risk of developing delirium from minor infections, changes in medication, etc.

Alzheimer Disease

Alzheimer disease (AD) is the most common cause of degenerative dementia and is estimated to be the etiology in 60% to 80% of patients with dementia. The figures are not exact because a definite diagnosis of AD requires detection of characteristic lesions on postmortem examination of brain tissue. For this reason, clinical trials and studies of AD have likely contained significant numbers of patients with other dementia subtypes.

AD occurs with equal frequency in men and women and usually begins after 60 years of age. Risk factors include advanced age, family history, Down syndrome (essentially all patients with Down syndrome who are over 35 years of age have AD), low educational level, chromosomal mutations on chromosomes 1, 14, and 21, apolipoprotein E ε4 genotype, and a history of brain injury. Regardless of the cause, AD is characterized by decreased levels of the neurotransmitter acetylcholine in the hippocampus and neocortex because of loss of cholinergic projections from the nucleus basalis of Meynert. The clinical features of AD include a gradual decline of intellectual function, poor short-term memory with relative sparing of long-term memory in the early stages of the disease, visuospatial disorientation, language/speech problems, and personality changes. Patients develop difficulty performing simple tasks, including activities of daily living such as eating, drinking, and walking. New-onset seizures occur in approximately 10% of Alzheimer patients.

More recently, obstructive sleep apnea syndrome has been related to AD. The degree of the impact of obstructive sleep apnea syndrome on the development and progression of AD continues to be a topic of research.

Dementia with Lewy Bodies

Dementia with Lewy bodies (DLB) is the second most common cause of degenerative dementia, representing approximately 15% to 20% of cases. It occurs twice as often in men as in women. The onset of symptoms typically begins between 50 and 80 years of age. The hallmark pathologic feature in brain tissue is Lewy bodies, which are inclusions seen within neurons. The clinical features of DLB include dementia, psychosis, and mild extrapyramidal symptoms such as spasticity. The presenting symptoms are usually personality changes and behavioral problems, followed by deterioration of memory over months to years. Hallucinations and delusions are common.

Pick Disease

Pick disease is one of the dementias that is associated with loss of neurons in the frontotemporal region of the brain. It is a rare degenerative dementia occurring in less than 10% of the patients with dementia. Unlike DLB, it occurs more frequently in women than in men. The onset of symptoms is typically in the sixth decade of life.

The hallmark pathologic features of Pick bodies are cytoplasmic inclusion bodies which are present in affected neurons. Similar to DLB, the clinical features of Pick disease include personality changes and behavioral problems usually associated with poor judgment. There is a gradual decline of intellectual function and poor short-term memory. Patients may develop Kluver–Bucy syndrome, which is characterized by hypersexuality, hyperorality, and docile behavior.

Vascular Dementia

Vascular dementia is the cause of approximately 10% of cases of dementia. It occurs in patients with a history of stroke and cerebrovascular disease. As with other types of atherosclerotic vascular disease, it is more common in men. Because stroke and cerebrovascular disease are so common, vascular factors may also complicate other dementia subtypes. Vascular dementia can be caused by ischemic stroke, cerebral hemorrhage, anoxic/ischemic brain injury, or vasculitis. Unlike AD, which has a gradual cognitive decline, there is typically a stepwise progression of symptoms associated with each new vascular event.

Sleep Disorders Associated with Dementias

Dementia patients have the same risk of developing sleep disorders as the general population. There is speculation that sleep-related breathing disorders may be one of the underlying factors contributing to vascular dementia, but definitive data regarding this relationship are lacking at present. In general, the effect of restful sleep versus unrefreshing sleep on the dementias is poorly understood. Untreated or inadequately treated obstructive sleep apnea/hypopnea in the general population causes excessive daytime somnolence, depressed mood, reduced quality of life, and subsequent cognitive dysfunction. Treatment of obstructive sleep apnea can improve this cognitive dysfunction (1–4). Treatment with positive airway pressure (PAP) in neurologically intact individuals improves attention, speed of thinking, short-term memory, and general cognitive status (3–5). There are limited data regarding the effect of sleep apnea treatment on the cognitive status of patients with degenerative dementia, yet our experience has been that many patients will receive some benefit. An important consideration is that treatment of sleep disorders improves the bed partner's (and usually the primary caregiver's) quality and amount of sleep (6). Theoretically, improvement in the quality of sleep can result in some improvement in the patient's level of cognitive function, so diagnosis and correction of any underlying sleep disorder is desirable for the benefit of both the patient and his or her bed partner.

Patients with DLB appear to have a greater risk of rapid eye movement (REM) sleep behavior disorder (RBD), although the prevalence is not yet known (7–9). RBD is so common that it is now regarded as a supportive feature for the diagnosis of DLB (10). RBD typically begins years before the onset of other symptoms of the dementia. The differential diagnosis for the abnormal behaviors includes RBD as well as epileptic seizures and wandering, behaviors that commonly occur in the demented population. Episodes of wandering are usually less violent, do not appear to be associated with REM sleep, and are often of longer duration than a typical REM period. Polysomnography with video monitoring, a full electroencephalogram (EEG) montage, and additional electromyography leads on all four extremities can help confirm the diagnosis of RBD. Clonazepam is the drug of choice in treating RBD and is effective in the majority of cases (11). If clonazepam proves ineffective or is not tolerated, alternative treatments include melatonin, carbamazepine (12), donepezil (13), and dopamine agonists. Aggressive treatment of any underlying sleep-related breathing disorder is extremely important in the management of RBD.

The epidemiology of restless legs and periodic limb movements (PLMs) in patients with degenerative neurologic disorders is not well understood. Restless legs syndrome (RLS) is quite common, occurring in at least 10% of the population who are generally affected by degenerative cognitive disorders.

Restless legs may occur as a genetic disorder, or may be secondary to arthritis, peripheral vascular disease, peripheral neuropathy, or relative iron deficiency. A number of medications have shown efficacy for the treatment of restless legs, including ropinirole, carbidopa/levodopa (L-dopa), pramipexole, benzodiazepines, opiates, pregabalin, and gabapentin enacarbil, but some of these medications should be used cautiously in the demented population. L-Dopa has been associated with augmentation of symptoms, a paradoxical worsening of the frequency and severity of symptoms related to the medication itself, as well as an increased risk of psychosis and insomnia. Dopamine agonists (pramipexole and ropinirole) have a lesser risk of augmentation but can be associated with an increased risk of psychosis, insomnia, and the possibility of inappropriate sleepiness. As sedatives or central nervous system depressants, benzodiazepines and opiates can help overcome restlessness but may have unacceptable cognitive consequences in patients with dementia. Likewise, the antiepileptic medications can also have adverse cognitive side effects. Patients who have decreased levels of serum ferritin may experience a sufficient reduction in symptoms with iron replacement such that medication may be unnecessary. It is uncommon for patients without RLS to experience PLMs during wakefulness; however, PLMs occur during sleep in about 80% of patients with RLS. PLMs are more common in the normal elderly population (14) than in younger individuals. PLMs without associated sleep disruption should not be treated, especially in patients with dementia who are more likely to have adverse medication side effects.

Hypersomnolence is also common among patients with degenerative neurologic disorders, although the etiology is unknown. The sleepiness can result from a number of underlying factors, including sleep apnea/hypopnea, nocturnal movement disorders, circadian rhythm disorders, and medication side effects. The patient should be screened for treatable underlying sleep disorders. When all identified instigating factors are remedied, residual sleepiness typically responds to proalerting medications such as armodafinil or modafinil. Traditional stimulants such as amphetamines may also be of some benefit. Behavioral complications caused by these stimulant medications are rare but may occur, and the patient's behavior should be monitored for agitation and worsening of cognitive function.

The origin of insomnia in patients with degenerative neurologic disorders is poorly understood (15, 16). The patient with dementia and insomnia should be evaluated for medical causes including medication side effects before symptomatic treatment is initiated. Many of the medications traditionally used for treatment of dementia conditions can result in a paradoxical worsening of insomnia, with subsequent decline of cognitive function and a worsening of undesirable behaviors. Circadian dysrhythmia is an abnormal fragmentation of the normal sleep–wake cycle that is common in patients with dementia (15, 16) and is often associated with wandering behavior. Degeneration of the suprachiasmatic nucleus of the hypothalamus is most likely the basis for circadian dysrhythmia in this population. Supplemental melatonin and phototherapy are the two primary treatment modalities. Melatonin may improve sleep architecture and continuity with an increase in the total sleep time; however, it should be used with caution. Because melatonin is classified as a supplement rather than a medication, its production is not regulated by the Food and Drug Administration, and it has not undergone rigorous testing for long-term detrimental side effects. Phototherapy may also be beneficial, but a standardized treatment protocol has not been established.

Patient Management

In the setting of the sleep center, it is useful to keep in mind that patients with degenerative dementias show a broad range of cognitive dysfunction and coexisting psychiatric symptoms, so the approach to each patient should be tailored to his or her individual needs. Some patients may seem "a little forgetful" and have some degree of confusion upon awakening in a strange environment. "Sundowning" is a relatively common phenomenon in which the patient's functional status deteriorates in the late afternoon and evening and may complicate monitoring with increasing confusion or agitation. Other patients may have paranoid tendencies, which limit their ability to cooperate with the sleep technologist. These affected patients have lost the ability to process complex instructions and explanations, and, as a result, respond to the actions and tone of the voice of the technologist rather than the content of the explanations that are given. Their confusion may result in combativeness. The technologist should maintain a calm, reassuring demeanor because arguing with a patient with dementia will likely worsen the agitation and aggressive behavior. As an added precaution, the sleep center should establish a policy for dealing with violent patients. It is best to limit patient interaction to reduce external stimuli. Benzodiazepines and similar sedative hypnotic medications should be avoided, as these drugs can worsen the degree of confusion. Alternative medications that should be used with combative or difficult patients include the antipsychotics, such as quetiapine and risperidone. It is important that home medications be administered routinely, because missed doses may further compound cognitive symptoms.

Nocturnal wandering may occur, and patients should be carefully monitored to prevent falls. Patients should be gently redirected back to bed, and medications used as needed. Insomnia, sundowning, and wandering can be extremely disruptive (15), both at home and in the sleep center. Because AD is associated with an increased incidence of seizures, monitoring should be performed with standard seizure precautions in place. Surprisingly, many patients with dementia tolerate continuous positive airway pressure (CPAP) therapy quite well. For those patients who find the mask intolerable, positional treatment of sleep apnea may be an acceptable alternative in the appropriate patient.

Urinary incontinence is commonly seen in patients with degenerative neurologic disorders. Family members should be discreetly asked about the use of adult diapers at home.

Although some demented patients may seem quite difficult and unpleasant to the sleep center staff, it is important that the staff understand that this is part of the patient's disease process and cannot be controlled by the patient.

Technical Aspects of Recording

There are no specific technical requirements for recording patients with degenerative neurologic disorders. Degenerative dementias may be associated with slowing of the alpha rhythm. There may be increased delta activity in the EEG even during wakefulness, making sleep staging difficult.

MOVEMENT DISORDERS

Movement disorders are a diverse group of neurologic diseases, which share some symptoms while differing in many other respects. As a group, they have more diverse clinical manifestations than the dementias previously discussed. What the syndromes share is a progressive downhill course which leads in many patients to death from aspiration pneumonia or complications of falls. The more common diseases and those that have a known association with sleep disorders are discussed in the following paragraphs. Given the scope of this textbook, the discussion is not exhaustive, and other less common entities such as Huntington disease, Wilson disease, and tic disorders have been excluded.

Parkinson Disease

Parkinson disease is one of the more common and well-known progressive degenerative movement disorders. Its hallmark features include resting tremor, bradykinesia (slowness of movement), rigidity, and gait disturbance. In contrast, Parkinsonism is a syndrome that occurs in patients without Parkinson disease who develop some but not all of the Parkinsonian symptoms, usually consisting of tremor, bradykinesia, and rigidity. It frequently occurs as a side effect of medications such as antipsychotic and antiemetic drugs, although a number of other neurologic disorders may result in Parkinsonism. As with the dementias, little is known about the interaction between sleep and most movement disorders.

Parkinson disease affects about 1% of the population over 50 years of age and occurs slightly more often in men than in women. The age of onset for Parkinson disease is quite broad, ranging from 20 to 80 years, with a peak in the sixth decade of life. The symptoms are typically slowly progressive over a course of years, but some sleep abnormalities may arise in the presymptomatic phase.

The pathophysiology of Parkinson disease is dominated by a loss of pigmented neurons in the substantia nigra of the basal ganglia and locus ceruleus, which results in decreased levels of dopamine in the brain. The four characteristic clinical features of Parkinson disease are rigidity with cogwheeling (increases in muscle tone with alternating catches and release), bradykinesia (slowness of movement), resting tremor (often described as a pill-rolling movement), and postural instability (difficulty maintaining standing posture, resulting in a tendency to fall forward). Patients may also have a stooped posture, reduced blinking, an unusually quiet voice, difficulty writing, and drooling. Depression is a common complicating factor. Approximately 30% of afflicted patients will develop dementia.

A number of treatments are available for Parkinson disease and its associated complications. L-dopa or its most common clinical form, Sinemet (carbidopa/L-dopa), crosses the blood–brain barrier and is metabolized to dopamine. Side effects include nausea, vomiting, orthostatic hypotension, dyskinesias (increased involuntary movements), restlessness, and hallucinations. Many of these side effects are dose related and are sometimes reversible. Sleep-related side effects include insomnia, nightmares, and anxiety. Monoamine oxidase inhibitors such as Selegiline are used less often. These drugs have a stimulant effect and must be given early in the day to avoid insomnia at night. Dopamine agonists, drugs that can bind to the cell's dopamine receptor and act in a dopaminergic fashion, include bromocriptine (Parlodel), pergolide (Permax), ropinirole (Requip), and pramipexole (Mirapex). The dopamine agonists can be used to delay the need for L-dopa and can be combined with L-dopa to allow a reduction in the dosage of L-dopa, which reduces medication side effects. The dopamine agonists have side effects similar to those of L-dopa, including orthostatic hypotension, nausea, hallucinations, and dyskinesias. Sleep-related side effects include drowsiness and sleep attacks.

Multiple System Atrophy

Multiple system atrophy (MSA) is present in 10% of the patients with Parkinsonian features. MSA is a neuropathologic term that encompasses several overlapping disorders, which are known as the Parkinson plus syndromes. A Parkinson plus syndrome should be suspected when the patient has Parkinsonism plus one or more of the following non-Parkinsonian symptoms: prominent dysautonomia (abnormal autonomic control of blood pressure and heart rate), ataxia (unstable gait), corticospinal tract findings (including weakness, increased muscle tone, and increased reflexes), bilateral, symmetrical onset of symptoms (both arms with the same degree of increased tone), lack of resting tremor, or a poor response to L-dopa treatment.

Progressive Supranuclear Palsy

Progressive supranuclear palsy (Steele–Richardson–Olszewski syndrome) is a Parkinsonian syndrome with typically less tremor and poor response to Parkinson medication. It is commonly misdiagnosed as Parkinson disease. Similar to Parkinson disease, it occurs more frequently in men, with an onset of symptoms typically occurring after 40 years and with a peak in the sixth decade of life.

The clinical features of progressive supranuclear palsy include reduced balance and falling, typically backward compared with the forward direction of falls usually seen in patients with Parkinson disease, supranuclear gaze palsy (reduced ability to produce voluntary vertical eye movements), and axial dystonia with an erect posture and difficulty bending or stooping. There is minimal tremor, and the dementia usually develops late in the syndrome and is relatively mild.

Corticobasal Ganglionic Degeneration

Corticobasal ganglionic degeneration is a degenerative movement disorder that occurs equally in men and women. The onset of symptoms typically occurs in the seventh decade of life, with the average patient surviving 5 to 10 years. The clinical features include unilateral extrapyramidal rigidity (difficulty moving, with rigidity and stiffness), tremor both at rest and during movement, apraxia (reduced higher mental function, which results in difficulty performing simple tasks), and "alien hand syndrome" of the involved upper extremity. Alien hand syndrome is an interesting phenomenon, where the affected hand or arm not only cannot be voluntarily controlled by the patient, but also appears to act in a fashion that actively opposes the goal the patient wishes to achieve. There can also be cortical sensory loss, clumsiness, and supranuclear gaze palsy (difficulty in making voluntary eye movements). The disorder is slowly progressive and eventually involves both sides of the body.

Sleep Disorders Associated with Movement Disorders

Parkinson disease is the most common of the movement disorders and has the most data regarding coexisting sleep disorders. There are virtually no data available for the more obscure degenerative diseases, and the incidence of sleep disorders remains largely unknown. Sleep-disordered breathing, which includes obstructive sleep apnea/hypopnea, central sleep apnea, Cheyne–Stokes breathing, and periodic breathing, is relatively common in Parkinson disease. Although it appears to occur at a frequency above that of the normal population, the exact epidemiology is not known. Many patients tolerate CPAP or bilevel PAP (BPAP) therapy, and experience significant functional improvement after the sleep apnea/hypopnea has been adequately treated. The spouse of a Parkinson disease patient with sleep apnea/hypopnea may also experience improved sleep efficiency and sleep architecture, with less daytime sleepiness when his or her bed partner with Parkinson disease and sleep apnea is effectively treated.

Insomnia can result from a primary sleep disorder such as RLS, psychophysiologic insomnia, poor sleep hygiene factors, side effects of medications, as well as the Parkinsonism resulting in the difficulty or inability to turn over in bed. Severe sleep maintenance insomnia is common in progressive supranuclear palsy. This may be related in part to immobility but appears to be more severe than in Parkinson disease (17).

RLS is one of the most common primary sleep disorders experienced by patients with Parkinson disease. Unfortunately, treatment of the neurologic symptoms with L-dopa commonly results in a worsening of the RLS by producing the daytime augmentation phenomenon in which RLS paradoxically worsens during the afternoons rather than evenings. Often, a change from L-dopa to a dopamine agonist such as pramipexole or ropinirole is needed, but this may result in less optimal control of the neurologic symptoms. Antiepileptic medications such as pregabalin or gabapentin enacarbil can be of benefit in the treatment of RLS. Alternatively, addition of an opioid such as hydrocodone or a benzodiazepine before bedtime may help improve RLS. Patients treated in this manner must be carefully monitored for worsening cognitive status and daytime sleepiness.

RBD is characterized by increased muscle tone during REM sleep and the "acting out of dreams." Limb movements and vocalization during REM sleep are frequently associated with violent behavior consistent with dream content. Injuries to the patient and/or the bed partner are common; however, directed violence is uncommon. The abnormal behavior does not occur with every REM period and may vary in frequency, duration, and the degree of violence. RBD may precede the onset of degenerative neurologic disorders by several years and then tends to reduce in severity as the specific neurologic disorder progresses (1). RBD is the initial manifestation in approximately half of patients with Parkinson disease (11). The frequency is even greater in patients with MSA. Interestingly, RBD in MSA occurs frequently in both males and females, whereas RBD in Parkinson disease occurs predominantly in male patients (18).

RBD has been reported but is rare in patients with progressive supranuclear palsy. Although most patients with MSA have RBD, REM sleep without atonia occurs in 95% of cases. REM sleep without atonia is also relatively common in corticobasal ganglionic degeneration but, unlike MSA, RBD is uncommon (19). Up to 80% of patients with RBD respond to clonazepam. Alternative treatments include carbamazepine, L-dopa, and dopamine agonists such as ropinirole and pramipexole.

Management of RBD in MSA is similar to that in the other degenerative neurologic disorders except that clonazepam should be avoided if possible because of its detrimental effect on respiratory stridor, autonomic respiratory instability, and significant gait instability. The use of this medication may, however, be necessary in some patients with MSA. When used, the patient should be monitored carefully for worsening of nocturnal stridor and periodic breathing. Fall precautions should be taken.

As in patients with dementia, excessive daytime sleepiness is very common in Parkinson disease. Potential causes include depression, sleep apnea, restless legs, and intrinsic hypersomnolence. Severe Parkinson disease is associated with excessive somnolence unrelated to any other sleep disorder. "Sleep attacks" or sudden, irresistible, and overwhelming episodes of sleepiness have been reported in a small number of patients with Parkinson disease, occurring more often in those receiving dopamine agonists (pramipexole, ropinirole, L-dopa, and bromocriptine) (20). The episodes of sleepiness improved following discontinuation of the dopamine agonist. Nocturnal stridor, a high-pitched inspiratory sound that is frequently unrecognized by the patient but commonly reported by the patient's bed partner, occurs in at least 10% to 15% of patients with MSA (21) and may be the presenting feature of the disorder (22). It probably has a central cause which produces abnormally enhanced vocal cord adduction. The stridor can lead to decreased oxygen saturation and severe respiratory compromise.

Tracheostomy has traditionally been the recommended treatment for nocturnal stridor, but the procedure has not been well received by patients. Treatment with CPAP has had mixed results. A number of other respiratory disorders have been associated with MSA, including central sleep apnea, obstructive sleep apnea, central hypoventilation, Cheyne–Stokes breathing, apneustic breathing, and irregular breathing. Brainstem degeneration is thought to be the common etiology for these disorders. Sleep-related breathing disorders are not common in corticobasal ganglionic degeneration but may occur as a concomitant disorder. The exact frequency of sleep-related breathing disorders is not known in the population of patients with corticobasal ganglionic degeneration. CPAP therapy can be problematic for such patients because their lack of motor control sometimes creates difficulty in wearing and adjusting the headgear.

Unilateral PLMs during sleep have been reported in patients with MSA (23) and progressive supranuclear palsy but are not as commonly seen as in Parkinson disease. PLMs can increase fragmented sleep if they cause EEG arousals and complicate the management of the sleep apnea/hypopnea syndrome.

Patient Management

When monitoring patients with known movement disorders, the sleep technologist should be prepared for parasomnias such as RBD, especially because the patient may demonstrate significantly better mobility during an episode of RBD than during wakefulness. Monitoring can be complicated by the patient's lack of motor control. Electrodes, monitors, and CPAP masks are frequently and repeatedly dislodged, and fall precautions should be employed at all times. The patient should be assisted to the restroom, and a bedside toilet should be made available if the patient wishes one. Patients may require assistance with turning during the night. The patient and the caregiver should be asked about these requirements before the sleep study is begun. It is also important to remember that mild dementia is a common component of many movement disorders, so possible cognitive impairment may also be present.

Technical Aspects of Recording

Abnormal sleep architecture may be seen in degenerative movement disorders and is prevalent in patients with progressive supranuclear palsy. Sleep spindles are typically decreased in both number and amplitude. One study in such patients revealed decreased total sleep time, reduced sleep efficiency, increased wake time after sleep onset, and increased stage N1 sleep. REM sleep was reduced with decreased REM period duration (20). Sleep-related breathing disorders are not common in progressive supranuclear palsy but may occur as a concomitant disorder.

OTHER DEGENERATIVE NEUROLOGIC DISORDERS

Amyotrophic Lateral Sclerosis (Lou Gehrig Disease)

ALS, or Lou Gehrig disease, causes relentlessly progressive weakness, which leads to death in 3 to 5 years after initial diagnosis. Death is usually secondary to respiratory failure and/or pneumonia. ALS occurs more frequently in men than in women and the onset of symptoms usually begins after age 50.

The clinical features of ALS include weakness, muscular atrophy, and fasciculations (involuntary muscle twitches). Hyperreflexia, spasticity, and upgoing toes also occur. Initial symptoms may be asymmetric, typically involving only the extremities (e.g., foot drop). As the weakness progresses, bulbar muscles of the throat and mouth become affected and result in dysphagia (difficulty swallowing) and dysarthria (difficulty speaking).

Associated Sleep Disorders

Central alveolar hypoventilation is a common component of ALS because of weakness of the respiratory muscles, including the diaphragm and intercostals. As bulbar weakness progresses, the muscle tone of the upper airway is decreased and obstructive sleep apnea/hypopnea may develop. Obstructive breathing events may be associated with hypoventilation, further complicating treatment. Patients may be intolerant of CPAP because they have difficulty exhaling against the pressure. BPAP or variable positive airway pressure may be more appropriate for such patients. Elevation of the head of the bed may alleviate this problem for several months or perhaps longer, and as the disease progresses, these patients typically require BPAP in the spontaneous or S mode. As the condition progresses, BPAP in the spontaneous-timed mode or noninvasive positive pressure ventilation may be necessary. As the disease progresses even further, tracheostomy with nocturnal ventilation may become the only effective treatment. Unfortunately, at this stage, many patients may elect to forgo further treatment because of end-of-life choices.

Patient Management Issues

Patients with ALS may require assistance with turning during the night and with other activities, including using the restroom. Because of bulbar weakness, aspiration is a constant hazard. Hypoventilation is also a concern. Because patients may have trouble exhaling, BPAP may be preferable over CPAP. Elevating the head of the bed, either with a wedge pillow or with a hospital bed, during sleep monitoring may reduce pressure requirement and improve patient comfort.

Technical Aspects of Recording

Patients with ALS are typically weak and may have difficulty cooperating with calibrations.

Fatal Familial Insomnia

Fatal familial insomnia is a rare familial autosomal dominant disorder caused by a mutation in a normal protein, the "prion protein," which causes it to transform into a prion, an infectious, self-reproducing protein structure. The prion subsequently damages the region in the thalamus, which regulates normal sleep patterns. There is severe disruption of the sleep–wake cycle, with extremely low sleep efficiency, reduced delta sleep, and reduced or absent REM sleep. Myoclonic jerks are frequent, and RBD or REM sleep without atonia may occur (24). Although insomnia is the most prominent feature of fatal familial insomnia, other features include cognitive decline, bradykinesia, ataxia, dysautonomia,

and hallucinations. Hypersomnolence may occur, but the affected patients, although sleepy, are unable to initiate restful sleep (25). The disease occurs equally in men and women, with a wide age of onset. The disorder progresses to death, usually within 4 years after onset. Death in fatal familial insomnia patients usually occurs secondary to pneumonia (25).

REFERENCES

1. Boeve, B., Silber, M., & Ferman, T. (2001). Current management of sleep disturbances in dementia. *Current Neurology and Neuroscience Reports, 2*, 169–177.
2. Engelman, H., Martin, S., Deary, J., et al. (1994). Effect of continuous positive airway pressure treatment on daytime function in sleep apnea/hypopnea syndrome. *Lancet, 343*, 572–575.
3. Engelman, H., Kingshott, R., Wraith, P., et al. (1999). Randomized placebo-controlled crossover trial of continuous positive airway pressure for mild sleep apnea/hypopnea syndrome. *American Journal of Respiratory and Critical Care Medicine, 159*, 461–467.
4. Borak, J., Cieslicki, J., Koziej, M., et al. (1996). Effect of CPAP treatment on psychological status in patients with severe obstructive sleep apnea. *Journal of Sleep Research, 5*, 123–127.
5. Bedard, M., Montplaisir, J., Malo, J., et al. (1993). Persistent neuropsychological deficits and vigilance impairment in sleep apnea syndrome after treatment with continuous positive airway pressure (CPAP). *Journal of Clinical Experience in Neuropsychology, 5*, 330–341.
6. Beninati, W., Harris, C., Herold, D., et al. (1999). The effect of snoring and obstructive sleep apnea on the sleep quality of bed partners. *Mayo Clinic Proceedings, 74*, 955–958.
7. Ferman, T., Boeve, B., Silber, M., et al. (1997). Hallucinations and delusions associated with the REM sleep behavior disorder/dementia syndrome. *Journal of Neuropsychology and Clinical Neuroscience, 9*, 692.
8. Ferman, T. J., Boeve, B. F., Smith, G. E., et al. (1998). The REM sleep behavior disorder/dementia syndrome: Neuropsychological differences when compared to Alzheimer's disease. *Neurology, 50*(Suppl. 4), A282.
9. Boeve, B., Silber, M., Ferman, T., et al. (2001). Association of REM sleep behavior disorder and neurodegenerative disease may reflect an underlying synucleinopathy. *Movement Disorders, 16*, 622–630.
10. McKeith, I. G., Perry, E. K., & Perry, R. H. (1999). Report of the second dementia with Lewy body International Workshop: Diagnosis and treatment. Consortium on dementia with Lewy bodies. *Neurology, 53*(5), 902–905.

11. Olson, E., Boeve, B., & Silber, M. (2000). Rapid eye movement sleep behavior disorder: Demographic, clinical, and laboratory findings in 93 cases. *Brain, 123,* 331–339.

12. Bamford, C. (1993). Carbamazepine in REM sleep behavior disorder. *Sleep, 16,* 33–34.

13. Ringman, J., & Simmons, J. (2000). Treatment of REM sleep behavior disorder with donepezil: A report of three cases. *Neurology, 55,* 870–871.

14. Ancoli-Israel, S., Kripke, D., Klauber, M., et al. (1991). Periodic limb movements in sleep in community-dwelling elderly. *Sleep, 14,* 496–500.

15. Vitiello, M., & Prinz, P. (1989). Alzheimer's disease: Sleep and sleep/wake patterns. *Clinics in Geriatric Medicine, 5*(2), 289–299.

16. Vitiello, M., Bliwise, D., & Prinz, P. (1992). Sleep in Alzheimer's disease and the sundown syndrome. *Neurology, 42*(Suppl. 6), 83–94.

17. Montplaisir, J., Petit, D., Decary, A., et al. (1997). Sleep and quantitative EEG in patients with progressive supranuclear palsy. *Neurology, 49,* 999–1003.

18. Plazzi, G., Corsini, R., Provini, F., et al. (1997). REM sleep behavior disorder in multiple system atrophy. *Neurology, 48,* 1094–1097.

19. Aldrich, M. S., Foster, N. L., White, R. F., et al. (1989). Sleep abnormalities in progressive supranuclear palsy. *Annals of Neurology, 25,* 577–581.

20. Frucht, S., Rogers, J. D., Greene, P. E., et al. (1999). Falling asleep at the wheel: Motor vehicle mishaps in persons taking pramipexole and ropinirole. *Neurology, 52*(9), 1908–1910.

21. Boeve, B., Silber, M., Ferman, T., et al. (2003). REM sleep behavior disorder in Parkinson's disease, dementia with Lewy bodies, and multiple system atrophy. In M. Bedard, Y. Agid, S. Chouinard, et al. (Eds.), *Mental and behavioral dysfunction in movement disorders* (pp. 383–397). Totowa, NJ: Humana Press.

22. Wenning, G., Shlomo, T., Magelhaes, M., et al. (1994). Clinical features and natural history of multiple system atrophy: An analysis of 100 cases. *Brain, 117,* 835–845

23. Iriarte, J., Alegre, M., Arbizu, J., et al. (2001). Unilateral periodic limb movements during sleep in corticobasal degeneration. *Movement Disorders, 16,* 1180–1183.

24. Scaravilli, F., Cordery, R. J., Kretzschmar, H., et al. (2000). Sporadic fatal insomnia: A case study. *Annals of Neurology, 48*(4), 665–668.

25. Kovacs, G. G., Trabattoni, G., Hainfellner, J. A., et al. (2002). Mutations of the prion protein gene phenotypic spectrum. *Journal of Neurology, 249*(11), 1567–1582.

chapter 26

Psychiatric Disorders That Affect Sleep

ROCHELLE ZOZULA   RITA BROOKS

LEARNING OBJECTIVES

On completion of this chapter, the reader should be able to:

1. Describe the characteristic changes in sleep architecture associated with specific psychiatric illnesses.
2. Appreciate changes in sleep structure caused by common psychotropic medications.
3. Anticipate problems in conducting sleep studies on various psychiatric patients.

KEY TERMS

Major depressive disorder
REM latency
Bipolar disorder
Seasonal affective disorder
Anxiety disorder
Alcoholism
Posttraumatic stress disorder
Antidepressant medication
Benzodiazepines
Schizophrenia

There is an intimate relationship between emotional functioning and sleep. Psychiatric disorders are common in our society, and as a result, patients with psychiatric disorders will be seen frequently in sleep disorder centers. Understanding the symptoms associated with these conditions is critical to evaluating the patient properly, creating the optimal sleep environment, and addressing the challenges that can arise during the polysomnographic (PSG) testing procedure. Psychiatric disorders are often treated with medications, and this usually occurs well before an overnight sleep study is performed. Some of the changes in sleep architecture observed during the study may reflect the effects of medications rather than primary illness. We will try to differentiate between the effects of the illness as opposed to medications.

This chapter will review the sleep characteristics of the major psychiatric disorders, including mood disorders, anxiety disorders, schizophrenia, and alcoholism. In this chapter, we will discuss the major disorders and their effects on sleep, including defining the disorder, discussing presenting symptoms, and determining what challenges the sleep technologist may face.

MOOD DISORDERS

It is normal for people to have changes in their mood or affect. However, when these mood changes are extreme, or when they shift from one extreme to the other, or when their mood is not consistent with their life events, they are said to have a mood disorder (1). The mood disorders include major depressive disorder (MDD), bipolar disorder, and seasonal affective disorder.

Major Depressive Disorder

MDD requires a minimum symptom duration of 2 weeks with no manic or hypomanic episodes. Symptoms include depressed mood; reduced level of interest in most or all activities; weight loss or gain; difficulty falling asleep or sleeping too much; feelings of inadequacy; feelings of extreme guilt; a reduced ability to think, concentrate, or make decisions; frequent thoughts of death or suicide; fatigue; and behavior that is agitated or slowed (2). MDD occurs some time in the lives of up to 20% of the North American population, and at any given time about 5% of the population is affected (3). Depression is most likely to begin in adolescence or in the early adult years, but the incidence seems to be increasing in younger populations (4). Between puberty and menopause, women are about two times as likely to develop major depression (5). The lifetime prevalence of MDD is 8% to 12% of men and 20% to 26% of women (6). Throughout a lifetime, an individual may experience several episodes of major depression, so it is a recurrent illness. Sleep disturbance is more pronounced during active illness, but sleep problems may persist during remission as well.

Sleep disturbance is so common in mood disorders that many individuals are given a diagnosis of depression on the basis of the symptom of insomnia. This may be due to a poor understanding in the general medical community of the variety of sleep disorders, or it may be because of an often erroneous assumption that antidepressant medications are good hypnotics. Although depression is perhaps overdiagnosed in patients with insomnia complaints, sleep disturbance is clearly a common feature of most psychiatric illnesses, including depression. For example, subjective sleep complaints are reported by more than 80% of MDD patients (7).

Although the specific cause of mood disorders has not been determined, there are several theories proposed that may elucidate the connection between mood disorders and sleep-related changes. First, a number of neurotransmitters have been implicated in mood disorders. Specifically, relative deficiencies of noradrenergic (NE) or serotonergic (5-HT) activity or increased cholinergic activity may be involved in depression (8). Notably, cholinergic activity is responsible for initiating rapid eye movement (REM) sleep, and norepinephrine and serotonin are responsible for terminating REM sleep and making the transition back to non-REM (NREM) sleep. Changes in these neurotransmitters would be expected to influence REM sleep, and in fact, REM sleep changes are among the most robust findings in depressive disorders. In addition, antidepressant medications typically enhance NE or 5-HT activity (by blocking the neurotransmitter uptake mechanisms), and patients taking these medications usually show characteristic changes in REM sleep (8, 9).

Another theory proposed for depression is that it may be caused by excessive amounts of REM sleep and a resulting decrease in REM sleep pressure (10). According to this theory, total or partial sleep deprivation can result in significant improvement in depression primarily through the mechanism of REM sleep suppression, and thereby, increasing the pressure to get into REM. Sleep deprivation studies have shown significant improvement in depressive symptoms in about 40% to 60% of patients, but the effect is only temporary and goes away after the REM sleep deprivation is stopped and that patient is allowed to have REM sleep again (11). Specifically, the improvement in mood is short-lived, because 50% to 80% of responders have partial or complete relapse after recovery of REM sleep.

A third theory regarding depression involves disruption of circadian and ultradian rhythms that control sleep–wake activity and REM–NREM cycles. It has been suggested that the circadian timing mechanism that controls REM sleep, core body temperature, and the hormone cortisol is phase-advanced (12). It has been hypothesized that REM sleep is phase-advanced relative to the sleep–wake cycle in depressive patients, and that depression occurs because of awakening at sensitive circadian phases. Other circadian models of depression have focused on the flattening (reduction) of the amplitude of circadian rhythms, including the core body temperature rhythm and rest–activity cycles (derived from actigraphy) (13). It has even been hypothesized that this circadian disruption may be linked to an increased susceptibility to having mood disorders across the life span.

Subjective Findings

Sleep disturbance can be assessed with subjective measures such as questionnaires, objectively with PSG, or inferentially with actigraphy. As previously noted, 80% of MDD patients complain about their sleep. These subjective complaints include difficulty falling asleep, frequent awakenings, early morning awakening with difficulty falling back to sleep, nonrestorative sleep, insufficient total sleep time (TST), and disturbing dreams. Some patients report increased daytime fatigue. The word *fatigue* is often used to reflect low energy or lethargy, as opposed to daytime sleepiness or drowsiness (difficulty remaining awake).

Subjective measures correlate well with some, but not all, objective measures. For example, patients are fairly good at reporting time in bed, TST, and sleep latency. They are less accurate when reporting the number of awakenings, sleep quality, sleep depth, and how rested they feel upon awakening (14).

Subjective reports on sleep quality may have clinical utility in managing MDD. Survey data have demonstrated that sleep disturbances can occur *before* the onset of other symptoms of MDD. For example, insomnia occurred as the first symptom in 41% of initial cases of MDD, and it was the first symptom in 56% of relapses. This association is so strong that some investigators can almost predict that a depressive episode will occur sometime in the future, perhaps even months or years, after insomnia first develops. Furthermore, improvement in sleep-related disturbances has been found to be positively correlated with the remission of depressive symptoms (15). This is in contrast to anxiety disorder, where the insomnia complaint typically begins with, or after, the onset of anxiety symptoms (16). The astute clinician should anticipate a relapse of depression in a "controlled" patient if such a patient starts complaining about a recurrence of his or her sleep disturbance (17).

Objective Findings

Many studies have objectively documented electroencephalographic (EEG) changes associated with MDD. Most studies show changes in the timing or distribution of sleep stages, particularly slow-wave sleep and REM sleep. A symptomatic but unmedicated adult with MDD typically shows a prolonged sleep-onset latency (SOL), bouts of intermittent wakefulness, increased N1 sleep, and reduced N3 sleep (5). The N3 deficits are greatest in the first NREM sleep period, whereas the amount of

N3 sleep is normal or even increased during the second NREM period. Even more profound and more consistent changes are seen in REM sleep parameters. Nonmedicated patients show a substantially shortened latency to the first REM period (REM latency). REM latency in depressed patients is often on the order of 30 to 50 minutes compared with the typical 90 to 100 minutes seen in nondepressed age- and sex-matched controls. There is also a significant increase in REM density (the number of eye movements per unit of time). Some studies show that the first REM period is longer and may have the highest REM density compared with later REM periods (18). This is just the opposite of normal sleepers, who have longer duration and more intense REM episodes later on in the sleep period. These sleep changes are not as robust in depressed children and adolescents (19, 20) as they are in nonmedicated adults with MDD. In fact, younger groups with depression are very similar to nondepressed individuals on most sleep variables.

The severity of the depression may or may not correlate with the severity of the sleep disturbance (21, 22). There is good evidence that disturbed sleep, particularly a shortened REM latency, may be a trait marker (show a propensity for) rather than a state marker (actively depressed). First-degree relatives of depressed individuals also commonly have short REM latencies (23). The abnormal REM changes may also be observed during remission of depression. These findings suggest that a shortened REM latency is associated with an increased risk of developing depression, as opposed to actively manifesting the disorder.

As previously noted, most antidepressant medication will influence REM sleep by lengthening the REM latency, decreasing REM density, and decreasing the REM percentage, particularly during the first third of the night. As stated previously, the mechanism for the antidepressant action was thought to be through REM suppression and increased REM sleep pressure. However, a number of effective antidepressant medications (e.g., bupropion, nefazodone, and trazodone) do not reduce REM sleep, which suggests another potential mechanism of action.

Cognitive behavioral therapy (CBT) has been shown to decrease REM density, but has no effect on REM latency (24). It is suggested that trait-dependent variables, such as shortened REM latency, decreased N3 sleep ratio, and decreased percentage of N3 sleep, remain stable over time; state-dependent measures, such as REM density and sleep efficiency, may improve with CBT treatment. However, a small percentage of subjects in remission have persistent sleep state–dependent abnormalities after CBT (25).

Bipolar Disorder

Bipolar disorder is characterized by the alternating pattern of two emotional extremes: depression and euphoria. The individual with bipolar illness cycles between periods of potentially severe depression and mania, an agitated and often elated emotional state. In addition to the aforementioned symptoms of depression, manic episodes may be characterized by irritable mood, thoughts of grandiosity, rapid or pressured speech, distractibility, and compulsive behavior (e.g., shopping sprees, drinking, sexual activity) (2).

Bipolar disorder is much less common than unipolar depression and has a lifetime prevalence rate of 2.8% to 6.5% (26). However, if the diagnostic criteria stipulate hypomania and not full mania (bipolar II), the incidence could include about one-half of currently diagnosed unipolar depression patients. There is no gender preference for bipolar disorder I, but bipolar II may affect more women than men (27). There may be a seasonal pattern for the occurrence of depressive and manic/hypomanic episodes. The onset of depression in bipolar disorder tends to be in the fall to winter, whereas mania tends to peak in the spring or fall (28).

Subjective Findings

The literature on sleep and bipolar disorder is not as complete as with unipolar depression. Subjective reports indicate that bipolar patients have concerns about their sleep much like unipolar depressives. In one study, 70% of a bipolar patient population had significant sleep concerns, including impaired sleep efficiency, higher levels of anxiety, fear about poor sleep quality, lowered daytime activity levels, and a tendency to misperceive sleep (29). One major difference between unipolar and bipolar disorder is a stronger tendency for bipolar patients to report symptoms of hypersomnia, with extended nocturnal sleep periods, difficulty awakening, and excessive daytime sleepiness, during the depressed phase (30). However, when the level of hypersomnia was objectively tested using the multiple sleep latency test, there was no increased physiologic sleep propensity demonstrated in the bipolar group. The authors stated that the reported hypersomnia might reflect lack of interest, social withdrawal, decreased energy, or psychomotor retardation, rather than a true increase in sleep propensity (31). Another notable subjective difference between bipolar disorder and MDD is that during the manic phase, although sleep may be severely curtailed, the patients have much less concern over their sleep. They feel that they do not need as much sleep (32). Prodromal episodes of insomnia tend to be more common in mania than depression and the shift to mania may be exacerbated by periods of sleeplessness (33).

Objective Findings

Objective data on sleep during mania indeed find decreased TST, increased time awake in the last 2 hours of the study, a short REM latency, and increased REM density. These findings were reported to be similar to the sleep changes seen in MDD (34, 35).

Manic episodes are often preceded by periods of sleeplessness, and case reports have suggested that mania can be triggered by sleep deprivation (36). It was speculated that the curtailed sleep time associated with mania may be potentially self-reinforcing for the clinical aspects of the disorder (37). However, it appears that sleep deprivation may have the same beneficial effects on bipolar disorder as it does on MDD patients (38). There is some concern that sleep deprivation can precipitate a manic episode. However, the rate of switching from depression to mania following sleep deprivation is no more pronounced than that observed using antidepressant medication (39).

Bipolar type II disorder is characterized by one or more depressive episodes accompanied by at least one hypomanic episode. In addition, there are no psychotic features such as delusions or hallucinations that can occur with bipolar I disorder. It should be noted that bipolar II is not a milder form of bipolar disorder. The depressive phase can be as severe in either disorder. As such, the increased sleep time seen in the depressive phase of either disorder can be similar. The manic phase is less pronounced in type II, but there is still a reduced need for sleep in over 80% of patients (40).

Seasonal Affective Disorder

Seasonal affective disorder (SAD) was first proposed in 1984 and is currently used as a specifier of either bipolar or recurrent MDD. The symptoms usually present during winter and remit during the spring. Symptoms also improve when the patient is exposed to daylight or bright light therapy. Although patients report depression, the other signs of SAD are quite different from those of MDD. SAD patients typically report increased appetite and increased need for sleep. The disorder is more common in young adults, particularly in women (41).

Disturbances of sleep are a primary component of SAD as they are of other mood disorders. However, SAD patients most often report hypersomnia. Among responses of 293 SAD patients on a symptom questionnaire, 95% acknowledged sleep concerns. The vast majority (80%) complained of winter hypersomnia, with only 10% reporting insomnia and 5% reporting insomnia and hypersomnia. TST increased by about 2.7 hours during the fall/winter months compared with the spring/summer months. Increasing sleep length by up to 2 hours during the winter months occurs in about one-half of a random sample of the general population. Thus, this symptom alone is not necessarily indicative of a disorder (42).

In contrast to the subjective impressions of increased sleep, actual sleep measurement of depressed SAD patients in winter showed reduced sleep efficiency, decreased N3 sleep percentage, and increased REM density, but normal REM latency. These findings were consistent when the patients were compared with themselves in the summer, compared with themselves following 9 days of bright light therapy, and compared with age- and gender-matched healthy controls. Although there may be a natural tendency to increase TST in the winter months, SAD patients show sleep architecture changes that are different from normal controls (42). Bright light therapy, especially morning light administration, appears to be an efficacious and safe treatment for this disorder (43). Bright light therapy is now being studied in more traditional forms of depression. There is some concern that light therapy can precipitate hypomanic or manic episodes, so caution is advised in using bright light therapy with bipolar patients (44).

Effect of Antidepressant Medications

A full review of medication and sleep appears elsewhere in this textbook. However, any discussion of psychiatric disorders and sleep must include some comments about the psychotropic medications. Generally, the antidepressant medications are REM-suppressing drugs. They tend to delay the onset of REM sleep and may decrease both the amount and the percentage of REM sleep. The REM suppression is most pronounced early in the treatment and tends to diminish with the long-term treatment (9). However, even in patients using these medications long term, a short REM latency is typically not seen. Although many of the older tricyclic antidepressants (e.g., amitriptyline, imipramine, clomipramine) are sedating, most of the selective serotonin reuptake inhibitor (SSRI) antidepressants (e.g., fluoxetine, paroxetine, sertraline) and other new agents (e.g., venlafaxine, bupropion) tend to be activating or alerting. As such, they may improve sleep by treating depression, but probably have little primary hypnotic efficacy, and they may actually worsen sleep (45). In addition, most antidepressants increase the incidence of periodic limb movements (PLMs) during sleep and may exacerbate restless legs syndrome (46). However, bupropion seems to be an exception, in that the drug does not exacerbate symptoms of restless legs syndrome (47, 48), nor does it suppress REM sleep like most of the other antidepressants (49). The SSRI fluoxetine can cause REMs in NREM sleep and scoring the record could be challenging if the scorer is unaware of this fact (50). Most antidepressants improve muscle tone in the upper airway and can slightly reduce snoring and the apnea–hypopnea index (AHI) in patients with obstructive sleep apnea syndrome (OSAS) (51, 52). This effect has been most studied with the antidepressants fluoxetine and protriptyline. In addition to increasing muscle tone, the REM-suppressing aspect of these drugs limits the time during sleep that is most conducive to having obstructive respiratory events.

Sleep Studies in Mood Disorders

In untreated depressed patients, the lengthened SOL, frequent awakenings, or early morning awakening may limit the amount of time available to allow for accurate assessment of other sleep disorders. A shortened REM latency is different from REM onset. Generally, individuals with depression show REM latencies in the 50- to 70-minute range as opposed to a "sleep-onset" REM period in which the REM latency is 15 minutes or less, sometimes being a true sleep-onset (0-minute latency) REM period.

If the depressed patient is being treated with antidepressant medication, a thorough understanding and documentation of the medications is helpful in completing an accurate interpretation of the results. Owing to the REM-suppressing characteristics of these medications, it may not be possible to diagnose narcolepsy in an individual taking an antidepressant medication if the patient's tendency to have a sleep-onset REM period is weak. The medication may also exacerbate leg movements during sleep and could slightly improve breathing during sleep. Fluoxetine can cause REMs in NREM sleep. All these changes can be misleading without good documentation. Moreover, the time of year that a study is conducted may be important if the patient has SAD. The phase of a bipolar illness that a patient is experiencing at the time of the study could produce drastically different results depending upon whether the patient is in the depressed or the manic phase of the disorder. Good technologist observations and documentation are important for all sleep studies, but particularly for the psychiatric/sleep disorder patient.

ANXIETY DISORDERS

Anxiety is a normal response to various situations that include threat. Dangerous or even important situations can elicit anxiety in almost anyone, and brief episodes of moderate anxiety are a normal part of life for most people. For some people, anxiety is so intense or long-standing that it becomes an anxiety disorder. There are several types of anxiety disorders:

1. Generalized anxiety disorder (GAD): Occurs when the anxiety is excessive and long-standing, but is not focused on any particular object or situation. Because the source of the anxiety cannot be specified, it is also called "free-floating" anxiety. This anxiety disorder affects about 5% of the U.S. population

at some time in their lives. Anxiety disorder is two times more common in women as compared to men (53).

2. Panic disorder (PD): Individuals experience recurrent extremely intense terrifying panic attacks that may come without warning or without an obvious cause. Symptoms may include heart palpitations, pressure in the chest, dizziness, nausea, sweating, and faintness. Many people with panic attacks feel they are having a heart attack. As many as 30% of the population may experience at least one panic attack within a given year (1).

3. Phobias: An intense, irrational fear of an object or situation that is not likely to be dangerous. There have been thousands of phobias described, but two of the most common are social phobia and agoraphobia. Social phobia is a fear of being negatively evaluated by others. Agoraphobia is a strong fear of being separated from a safe place like a home or from a safe person like a spouse or of being trapped in a place from which escape would be difficult or help would be unavailable (1).

4. Obsessive–compulsive disorder (OCD): Individuals with OCD experience persistent, upsetting, and unwanted thoughts (obsessions) that may motivate them to perform repetitive behaviors (compulsions) that the person believes will prevent the events associated with the obsession (1). Obsessions typically involve thoughts of contamination or harming one's self or others. Compulsions can take the form of incessant cleaning, checking behavior, or counting (1).

5. Posttraumatic stress disorder (PTSD): This is a stress reaction to a severe trauma. Among the characteristic reactions are anxiety, irritability, inability to concentrate, jumpiness, intense startle reactions, and hypervigilance. The most notable feature of PTSD is reexperiencing the trauma through nightmares or vivid memories. Occasionally, the individual will experience flashbacks in which the person behaves as if the trauma was happening again (1).

Anxiety is a state of increased cortical and peripheral arousal and, as such, is a state that makes sleep difficult. Sleep complaints are common in anxiety disorders and are among the diagnostic criteria for many of the anxiety disorders. Anxiety disorders clearly are among the most common causes of insomnia. In a study by the National Institute of Mental Health Epidemiologic Catchment Area, 7,954 respondents were questioned about their sleep complaints. Of these, 10.2% of the 811 respondents reported chronic insomnia. The single most common psychiatric diagnosis was anxiety disorder followed by depression and dysthymia (54).

According to a large European survey of over 14,000 individuals in the general population, insomnia was often a prodromal feature, or a coincident occurrence, in respondents with depression. When anxiety disorders were implicated, insomnia appeared concurrently or after the onset of the anxiety disorder (16).

Generalized Anxiety Disorder

Sleep difficulty is very common in GAD patients. Between 50% and 70% of these patients have difficulty sleeping (54). The principal cognitive feature associated with GAD is "excessive worry," which goes hand in hand with the development and maintenance of the insomnia complaint (55). Despite the high prevalence of sleep problems in these patients, there has been little research focusing specifically on this disorder. GAD patients report having difficulty both falling asleep and staying asleep and they feel that their sleep is unrefreshing. Objectively, PSG studies have shown that, relative to controls, GAD patients take longer to fall asleep, have lower sleep efficiency, have less N3 and more N1 sleep, and less TST. They have more frequent arousals during the first half of the sleep period and a lower REM density (56, 57). In contrast to depressed patients, GAD patients have a normal REM latency (of about 90 minutes). Sleep deprivation does not improve symptoms of anxiety as it does with depression (58).

Panic Disorder

As with GAD, most patients with PD have significant sleep complaints. Their subjective complaints are similar to those patients with GAD. They report difficulty falling asleep, difficulty remaining asleep, and decreased TST. The exceptional difference with PD patients is the presence of panic attacks. These attacks occur both during the day and during sleep. One study found 69% of PD patients had a lifetime occurrence of sleep panic attacks and 33% reported recurrent sleep panic attacks. Over one-half of the patients indicated that sleep deprivation and relaxation acted as a trigger for panic attacks (59). PD patients can differentiate REM sleep anxiety dreams from panic attacks. The panic attack has no dream content or vivid imagery. Patients have full awakenings from the event; they are not confused at the time of the event and are not amnestic for the events the following day, as is the case with night terrors. These findings help separate panic attacks from both REM-related nightmares and slow-wave sleep night terrors. Even PD patients without sleep panic attacks have disturbed sleep.

Objective studies show that sleep panic attacks occur from late N2 or early N3 sleep (60). If the attacks are frequent, some PD patients may develop a sleep phobia to avoid the panic symptoms. PD patients have longer sleep-onset latencies, reduced sleep efficiency, and decreased TST. However, N3 sleep is normal, REM latency is normal or increased, and REM density is normal (61, 62). In addition, increased motor activity during sleep has been reported in patients with PD, with evidence that they may move less on the nights when there is a sleep-related panic attack (63).

Phobia

Insomnia or other sleep complaints are rare in phobias unless the phobia is related to sleep itself. For example, individuals with sleep panic attacks may develop a fear of sleep as a way to avoid the panic attack. Other phobias such as fear of the dark can usually be dealt with by providing light or with cognitive therapy. Other than sleep-onset problems that are directly related to the phobia, sleep appears to be normal. However, some studies on social phobia have found subjective reports of poorer sleep quality, longer sleep latency, more frequent sleep disruption, and increased daytime dysfunction compared with control subjects (64). It is suggested that sleep problems in social phobia may be associated with comorbid depression in some individuals (55).

Obsessive–Compulsive Disorder

The core syndromal features of OCD do not include primary disturbances of sleep (55). Early studies have subjectively reported abnormal sleep patterns and objective changes in sleep characteristics (e.g., decreased TST, increased number of awakenings, shortened REM latency, reduced N3 sleep, and reduced sleep efficiency) (65). These findings are very similar to patients with MDD and they could suggest an overlap between OCD and MDD or they could indicate that many OCD patients also suffer from depression. In addition, the presence of the obsessions and compulsions may prevent individuals with OCD from going to bed because of the need to check their alarm clock or kitchen stove repeatedly. However, more recent studies on OCD patients failed to replicate these PSG findings and have concluded that sleep patterns in OCD are basically normal (66, 67).

The obsessions and compulsions of this disorder may lead to significant sleep disturbances. This can prove a challenge to performing a sleep study. A compulsion such as checking behavior may delay bedtime. Fears of contamination may keep patients from undergoing a sleep study owing to fears about the sleep environment or cleanliness of the electrodes. This may be particularly true with nasal continuous positive airway pressure (CPAP) and wearing a mask worn by previous patients (despite undergoing proper sterilization in-between patients).

Posttraumatic Stress Disorder

PTSD is characterized by the recurrent and intrusive distressing recollections of a traumatic event (e.g., violent attack with physical injury, sexual assault, death of a loved one), according to the *Diagnostic and Statistical*

Manual of Mental Disorders, 4th edition *(DSM-IV)* (55). Sleep complaints are varied and typically severe in patients with PTSD. Patients with PTSD may report poor sleep for decades, with corroborating evidence by their bed partners (68). In fact, insomnia (both sleep initiation and sleep maintenance subtypes) and nightmares (viewed as reexperiencing of the traumatic event) are part of the *DSM-IV* criteria for making the diagnosis (2). A survey conducted with male Vietnam War veterans with PTSD confirmed that insomnia complaints were very common, but the presence of recurrent nightmares was more specific for PTSD (69). In another community survey conducted in Canada, PTSD was frequently associated with violent behavior during sleep, sleep paralysis, sleep talking, and both hypnopompic and hypnagogic hallucinations (70). It is postulated that these sleep complaints are associated with features of heightened somatic arousal and hypervigilance, which are part of the diagnostic criteria for PTSD.

Some studies have objectively recorded increased awakenings and decreased N3 sleep in patients with PTSD (71, 72). Other studies have failed to find these changes (73, 74), and one study found no objective sleep differences at all, with the exception of an increase in brief arousals from REM sleep (75). The reason for these discrepancies is unknown. However, Kloss and Szuba (76) have speculated that a number of factors may be responsible. The amount of substance abuse, psychiatric comorbidities, degree or types of trauma, and patient demographics may substantially differ in study populations. They also propose that PTSD patients may be prone to sleep state misperception, or that they find the sleep laboratory a safe environment and, therefore, sleep better there than at home.

Although nightmares are commonly reported in PTSD, studies have also been inconsistent in REM-related changes associated with the disorder. Frequent nightmares occurred in 52% of combat veterans with PTSD compared with only 4.8% of combat veterans without PTSD (69). Some studies have found increases in REM density or shortened REM latencies (77, 78), whereas others have failed to detect these changes (74). It should be noted that the nightmare or "flashback" experienced during sleep may or may not be REM-related (79); this could account for some of the discrepancies in the findings.

Other studies have looked at sympathetic activation during REM and NREM sleep, using electrocardiographic data from early and late REM periods and the preceding NREM periods (80). By calculating the ratio of low- to high-frequency spectral densities in cardiac activity, the authors found that subjects who developed PTSD within a month of sustaining an acute injury had higher indices of sympathetic (NE) activation during REM sleep, when compared with subjects who did not develop PTSD postinjury. Moreover, these findings may lead to future pharmacologic interventions to prevent the development of PTSD in individuals who have experienced a traumatic life event.

One interesting line of investigation has found a high rate of obstructive sleep apnea (OSA) in both male and female PTSD patients. These investigators also reported improvement in insomnia, nightmares, and PTSD symptoms with treatment of the OSA with CPAP, independent of other psychiatric intervention (81). It is possible that once the REM sleep normalized with the continued use of CPAP, the intensity of the nightmares and sleep fragmentation diminished.

Treatment for sleep disturbances in PTSD has focused on both psychological and pharmacologic approaches. The use of evidence-based psychotherapy is essential as a primary or adjuvant therapy for PTSD (82). Pharmacologic therapy has focused on SSRI medications, mainly sertraline and paroxetine (83). More recent research has shown that prazosin, through the reduction of norepinephrine synthesis in the brain, may be effective in the reduction of nightmares in PTSD patients (84). This supports the hypothesis that NE stimulation may be contributing to the ongoing sleep disturbances and nightmares in PTSD.

Sleep Studies in the Anxious Patient

Stressors may exacerbate anxiety symptoms, and a sleep study can certainly be sufficiently stressful to cause a worsening of symptoms. Preparing the anxious patient for a sleep study is very important. Showing the room and fully explaining the procedure to the patient perhaps days before the actual study may be helpful. The interpersonal skills of the technologist are probably most important with the anxious patient. The ability to apply electrodes and to convey to the patient in a calm and reassuring manner that he or she will be able to complete the study will improve the likelihood of obtaining an accurate sleep study. In addition, anxious patients with sleep apnea may have particular problems with a CPAP mask, and spending time desensitizing the patient to CPAP therapy well before the study may allow for a more successful CPAP titration study. In particularly anxious patients, there may be a great deal of muscle tension artifact in the recording during wakefulness. This artifact may persist into stage N1 sleep and reappear with arousals during the study. This artifact can make determining sleep onset challenging and may cause wakefulness to be overscored.

The sleep-related panic attack might include symptoms of heart palpitations, shortness of breath, sweating, chest pain, and nausea (2). These symptoms are similar to the warning signs of a heart attack and many PD patients indeed feel that they are having a heart attack. It must be remembered that psychiatric patients also have medical problems, and it is important to take these symptoms seriously. If the patient experiences these symptoms during the sleep study, the technician should respond to the symptoms in a medically appropriate manner and not simply assume that they are a manifestation of a psychiatric illness.

Benzodiazepines (BZD) are often used to treat anxiety disorders. These medications will suppress N3 sleep and can slightly worsen the AHI in patients with OSAS, because of increased respiratory suppression. They can also reduce the arousal index related to leg movements, but may not actually decrease the number of leg movements. If the patient has an elevated PLM index, a low PLM arousal index, and is taking a benzodiazepine, it needs to be understood that the PLM arousal index would almost certainly be higher if the patient were not taking a BZD.

PSYCHOSES

Schizophrenia

Psychoses are defined as mental disorders characterized by the occurrence of delusions, hallucinations, incoherence, catatonic behavior, or inappropriate affect that cause impaired social or work functioning. Schizophrenia is a psychotic disorder and is considered one of the most severe and disabling of all mental disorders [1]. It is considered to be a neurodevelopmental disorder that manifests as a result of both hereditary and environmental factors.

The worldwide prevalence of schizophrenia is about 1% of the population; there are no gender differences. The severe symptoms of schizophrenia often dwarf sleep complaints. However, sleep can be severely disrupted in this disorder, and it was once hoped that understanding sleep would help explain the illness.

Severe insomnia is one of the prodromal features of the onset of schizophrenia, or psychotic relapse [85]. During episodes of intense psychotic agitation, schizophrenics may display insomnia or a total lack of sleep. Sleep–wake reversals, with daytime sleeping being the predominant pattern, are quite common. This sleep–wake pattern may also reinforce the social isolation that they desire during their psychotic break. Patients with schizophrenia who are considered "clinically stable" with the use of antipsychotic medication may still experience some sleep disturbance, such as early and middle of the night insomnia.

Dreaming associated with REM sleep can be thought of as a model for psychosis [86]. The discovery of REM sleep with its vivid hallucinations and perceptual distortions suggested that abnormalities of REM sleep might be related to the symptoms of schizophrenia. As early as 1955, attempts were made to establish a relationship between REM sleep and schizophrenia [87].

These investigations hoped to find intrusion of REM sleep into waking life or at least an unusual distribution or quality of REM sleep during the night. Unfortunately, PSG investigations have failed to find major changes in REM sleep in this group of patients.

Several studies have found a shortened REM latency in schizophrenic patients [88]. Studies also found that following REM sleep deprivation, schizophrenics do not show a "REM rebound" as would be expected [89]. This unusual finding led to speculation that REM phasic events could be intruding into wakefulness and causing, or at least contributing to, the thought and perceptual problems of the disorder. Studies have again failed to find much evidence supporting this hypothesis. The REM/NREM distribution of phasic events such as middle ear muscle activity does not differ in schizophrenics as the theory would predict [90]. Although a fascinating idea, there has not been any compelling evidence that REM sleep directly underlies the severe symptoms associated with schizophrenia.

One underlying theory for the possible REM findings has to do with the proposed model of a cholinergic–dopaminergic imbalance in schizophrenia [91]. According to this model, independent of sleep abnormalities, there seems to be a link between hyperactivity of the neurotransmitter system involving acetylcholine (which is also responsible for REM sleep regulation) and dopaminergic dysfunction (which controls the neurotransmitter dopamine). Studies of both depressed and schizophrenic patients have used drugs that enhance acetylcholine to induce REM sleep onset, called the cholinergic REM induction test [92]. Both psychiatric populations displayed shortened REM latencies during testing, implicating enhanced cholinergic sensitivity. Further research may, at last, find the long-sought-after connection between REM sleep and schizophrenia [93].

Subjective Findings

Subjectively, schizophrenic patients report that their sleep is frequently disrupted, and it is more fragmented during psychotic episodes. Although sleep quality may improve during remission, sleep problems can persist. Typically, the sleep complaint is difficulty falling asleep or remaining asleep during the night [76]. These patients are reported to have a higher incidence of nightmares, as do nonschizophrenic, highly creative individuals [94].

Objective Findings

The most reliable sleep changes found in schizophrenia occur in NREM sleep, particularly deficits of N3 sleep or delta wave (0.5 to 2 Hz) activity. Most studies have found a significant reduction in the total number of delta waves and an inverse correlation between delta activity and the severity of negative symptoms, such as affective flattening and impoverishment of speech.

In a review of the major studies on sleep in schizophrenia, Monti and Monti found that relative to controls, SOL was increased by about 36 minutes, wake time after sleep onset was increased, the number of awakenings was increased, TST was reduced by about 1 hour (54 minutes), sleep efficiency was reduced by about 15%, delta wave counts were decreased per minute of NREM sleep, and total delta wave counts were decreased. REM latency was found to be moderately decreased or normal (95). A longitudinal study of sleep in schizophrenia found that between baseline, 4 weeks, and 1 year, there were changes in the REM measures, but no significant changes in N3 parameters. The authors suggested that the stable N3 sleep changes reflect a trait of the schizophrenic patient, whereas the REM measures may reflect the state of the schizophrenic disorder (96).

Sleep Studies in the Psychotic Patient

Sleep studies in actively psychotic patients may have research interest, but probably have little clinical utility. Most patients obtaining a clinical sleep evaluation will do so either while in remission or while medicated. As with all patients, the interpersonal skills of the sleep technologist are very important with the psychotic patient. It may be difficult to explain the procedures, and there may be concerns that the equipment is doing more than is explained. For example, a schizophrenic patient may believe that the EEG is reading the mind or inserting thoughts.

Pharmacologic Treatment of Schizophrenia

Many of the antipsychotic medications can improve sleep quality, but may also be quite sedating. In addition, the older antipsychotics tend to have extrapyramidal side effects, and often are associated with movement disorders because of the effect of blockade of the dopaminergic postsynaptic receptors (e.g., parkinsonism and dystonia) (85). Some of the newer (atypical) antipsychotics (e.g., olanzapine and risperidone) are also sedating, because they increase slow-wave sleep, promote sleep maintenance, and enhance stage N2 sleep, but they have less effect on REM sleep than the older antipsychotic drugs (85). Flexible scheduling of studies to avoid psychotic exacerbations and approaching the patient in a calm, professional manner should allow for an accurate clinical study.

ALCOHOLISM

Ethyl alcohol (ethanol) is the second most commonly used psychoactive substance in the world, whereas caffeine is the first. It is similar to the sedative hypnotics and can have significant effects on both subjective sleep and the polysomnogram. The effects of alcohol use in normal subjects have been extensively studied. An adult can metabolize about 10 mL (1/3 oz) of 100% alcohol per hour regardless of the blood alcohol concentration. It takes an adult about 1 hour to metabolize a 1-oz glass (29.6 mL) of 80-proof whisky, a 4-oz glass (118.3 mL) of wine, or a 12-oz (354.9 mL) can of beer (97).

Although not all studies are consistent, generally it appears that acute alcohol use decreases SOL, suppresses REM sleep in a dose-dependent manner during the first half of the night, and may increase N3 sleep. However, the second half of the night shows increased N1 sleep and more awakenings. The sleep disruption observed in the second-half of the night is considered a rebound effect following the metabolism of ethanol. Metabolism may be completed in 4 to 5 hours after consumption, and the drug-induced sleep effects can rebound before the sleep cycle is completed. Studies that show REM suppression during the first half of the night may be followed by REM rebound during the second half of the night. With nightly dosing of alcohol, tolerance to these sleep changes can develop within 3 days, but a REM rebound may still be seen on discontinuation (98).

The effect of alcohol in alcoholics is different. When they are drinking, they may fall asleep rapidly, but their TST is decreased, and it is composed primarily of light NREM sleep because REM sleep and N3 are largely suppressed. The latter portion of the sleep cycle is fragmented with little REM sleep.

Patients often state that they cannot fall asleep without alcohol. With acute discontinuation of alcohol, there is decreased N3 and more frequent, although shorter, REM episodes. Total REM sleep time is not increased. Sober alcoholics often show very disturbed sleep. It takes them longer to fall asleep and they sleep for shorter periods of time. Their sleep can be fragmented with frequent brief arousals, and N3 sleep is decreased (98).

Insomnia occurs in 36% to 72% of alcoholic patients and may persist for months after beginning abstinence. Confounding factors with alcoholic patients and sleep are increased anxiety, depression, and tobacco use. Sober alcoholics may have more sleep-disordered breathing and more PLMs during sleep. Insomnia in alcoholism is important because it has been associated with relapse, possibly using alcohol to initiate sleep. It is not known if treatment of the insomnia can reduce relapse (99).

Ethanol also selectively decreases muscle tone in the upper airway (100) and can lead to the development or worsening of the degree of both snoring and obstructed breathing during sleep. This effect is more pronounced in men than in women, and older men are more vulnerable than younger men. Normal women are resistant to the development of sleep apnea after alcohol consumption regardless of menopausal status (101). In addition, ethanol may blunt the arousal response, so that obstructive apnea and hypopnea events become much longer in duration (102). The negative effects of alcohol on breathing are most pronounced during the first 1 to 2 hours following consumption, when alcohol concentrations are the highest. Therefore, proximity of alcohol consumption to bedtime is important. A single glass of wine several hours before bedtime would likely have little effect on sleep or breathing during sleep. An individual who routinely drinks alcohol in the evenings may not snore in the sleep center or may not have expected apnea if he or she happens to be studied without alcohol. Controlled use of alcohol in a sleep center or the use of a recording pulse oximeter at home may help clarify this issue. The use of alcohol may also bring into question the accuracy of a CPAP titration study if the pressure of a habitual drinker is set on an alcohol-free night. However, one study suggests that moderate alcohol consumption does not cause more apneas when the optimal pressure has been previously titrated (103).

CONCLUSION

Psychiatric patients often present a special challenge for the sleep technologist. Psychiatric illnesses generally have negative effects on sleep. The medications used to treat these illnesses also affect sleep architecture and may exacerbate other primary sleep disorders. This group of patients requires the utmost patience and interpersonal skills on the part of the sleep technologist, more than other patient groups. It is incumbent on the technologist to provide a calm, reassuring environment for conducting the sleep study. Explanation regarding the process of hooking up and conducting the study will help relax the patient before the study. Understanding the impact that psychiatric illnesses and medications have on sleep will allow an accurate interpretation of the sleep study and may provide some information on the patient's prognosis as well.

REFERENCES

1. Bernstein, D. A., Clarke-Stewart, A., Roy, E. J., et al. (1997). *Psychology* (4th ed.). Boston, MA: Houghton Mifflin Company.
2. American Psychiatric Association. (1995). *Diagnostic and statistical manual of mental disorders* (4th ed.). Washington, DC: Author.
3. Blazer, D. G., Kessler, R. C., McGonagle, K. A., et al. (1994). The prevalence and distribution of major depression in a national community sample: The national comorbidity survey. *American Journal of Psychiatry, 151,* 979–986.
4. Burke, K. C., Burke, J. K., Jr, Regier, D. A., et al. (1990). Age at onset of selected mental disorders in five community populations. *Archives of General Psychiatry, 47,* 511–518.
5. Armitage, R., & Hoffman, R. F. (2001). Sleep, EEG, depression and gender. *Sleep Medicine Reviews, 5*(3), 237–246.
6. Boyd, J. H. (1981). Epidemiology of affective disorders: A reexamination and future directions. *Archives of General Psychiatry, 38,* 1039–1046.
7. Reynolds, C. F., & Kupfer, D. J. (1987). Sleep research in affective illness: State of the art circa 1987. *Sleep, 10,* 199–215.
8. Janowsky, D. S., Davis, J. M., El-Yousef, M. K., et al. (1972). A cholinergic-adrenergic hypothesis of mania and depression. *Lancet, 2,* 632–635.
9. Wilson, S., & Argyropoulous, S. (2005). Antidepressants and sleep: A qualitative review of the literature. *Drugs, 65*(7), 927–947.
10. Vogel, G. W., Buffenstein, A., Minter, K., et al. (1990). Drug effects on REM sleep and on endogenous depression. *Neuroscience and Biobehavioral Reviews, 14,* 49–63.
11. Giedke, H., & Schwarzler, F. (2002). Therapeutic use of sleep deprivation in depression. *Sleep Medicine Reviews, 6*(5), 361–377.
12. Wehr, T. A., & Wirz-Justice, A. (1981). Internal coincidence model for sleep deprivation and depression. In W. P. Koella (Ed.), *Sleep 1980* (pp. 26–33). Basel, Switzerland: Karger.
13. Lyall, L. M., Wyse, C. A., Graham, N., et al. (2018). Association of disrupted circadian rhythmicity with mood disorders, subjective well-being, and cognitive function: A cross-sectional study of 91105 participants from the UK Biobank. *Lancet, 5*(6), 507–514.
14. Armitage, R., Trivedi, M., Hoffman, R., et al. (1991). Relationship between objective and subjective sleep measures in depressed patients and healthy controls. *American Journal of Psychiatry, 148*(9), 1177–1181.
15. Ford, D. E., & Kamerow, D. B. (1989). Epidemiologic study of sleep disturbance and psychiatric disorder: An opportunity for prevention? *Journal of the American Medical Association, 262,* 1479–1484.
16. Ohayon, M. M., & Roth, T. (2003). Place of chronic insomnia in the course of depressive and anxiety disorders. *Journal of Psychiatric Research, 37*(1), 9–15.
17. Gillin, J. C. (1998). Are sleep disturbances risk factors for anxiety, depressive and addictive disorders? *Acta Psychiatrica Scandinavica, 98*(S393), 39–43.
18. Riemann, D., Berger, M., & Voderholzer, U. (2001). Sleep and depression—Results from psychobiological studies: An overview. *Biological Psychology, 57*(1–3), 67–103.
19. Young, W., Knowles, J. B., & MacLean, A. W. (1982). The sleep of childhood depressives: Comparison with age-matched controls. *Biological Psychiatry, 17,* 1163–1168.

20. Emslie, G. H., Rush, A. J., Weinberg, W. A., et al. (1990). Children with major depression show reduced rapid eye movement latencies. *Archives of General Psychiatry, 47,* 119–124.

21. Stefos, G., Staner, L., Kerkhofs, M., et al. (1998). Shortened REM latency as a psychobiological marker for psychotic depression? An age-, gender-, and polarity-controlled study. *Biological Psychiatry, 44*(12), 1314–1320.

22. Kupfer, D. H., Ehlers, C. L., Frank, E., et al. (1991). EEG sleep profiles and recurrent depression. *Biological Psychiatry, 30*(7), 641–655.

23. Giles, D. E., Kupfer, D. J., Rush, A. J., et al. (1998). Controlled comparison of electrophysiological sleep in families of probands with unipolar depression. *American Journal of Psychiatry, 155*(2), 192–199.

24. Thase, M. E., Reynolds, C. F., Frank, E., et al. (1994). Polysomnographic studies of unmedicated depressed men before and after cognitive behavioral therapy. *American Journal of Psychiatry, 151*(11), 1615–1622.

25. Thase, M. E., Fasiczka, M. A., Berman, S. R., et al. (1998). Electroencephalographic sleep profiles before and after cognitive behavior therapy of depression. *Archives of General Psychiatry, 55,* 138–144.

26. Bauer, M., & Pfennig, A. (2005). Epidemiology of bipolar disorders. *Epilepsia, 46*(Suppl. 4), 8–13.

27. Barnes, C., & Mitchell, P. (2005). Considerations in the management of bipolar disorder in women. *Australian New Zealand Journal of Psychiatry, 39*(8), 662–673.

28. Benca, R. M. (2005). Mood disorders. In M. H. Kryger, T. Roth, & W. C. Dement (Eds.), *Principles and practice of sleep medicine* (4th ed., pp. 1311–1326). Philadelphia, PA: Elsevier Saunders.

29. Harvey, A. G., Schmidt, D. A., Scarna, A., et al. (2005). Sleep-related functioning in euthymic patients with bipolar disorder, patients with insomnia, and subjects without sleep problems. *American Journal of Psychiatry, 162*(1), 50–57.

30. Detre, T., Himmelhoch, J., Swartzburg, M., et al. (1972). Hypersomnia and manic-depressive disease. *American Journal of Psychiatry, 128,* 1303–1305.

31. Nofzinger, E. A., Thase, M. E., Reynolds, C. F., et al. (1991). Hypersomnia in bipolar depression: A comparison with narcolepsy using the multiple sleep latency test. *American Journal of Psychiatry, 148*(9), 1177–1181.

32. Riemann, D., Voderholzer, U., & Berger, M. (2002). Sleep and wake manipulations in bipolar depression. *Neuropsychobiology, 45*(Suppl. 1), 7–12.

33. Jackson, A., Cavanagh, J., & Scott, J. (2003). A systematic review of manic and depressive prodromes. *Journal of Affective Disorders, 74,* 209–217.

34. Hudson, J. I., Lipinski, J. F., Frankenburg, F. R., et al. (1988). Electroencephalographic sleep in mania. *Archives of General Psychiatry, 45*(3), 267–273.

35. Hudson, J. I., Lipinski, J. F., Keck, P. E., et al. (1992). Polysomnographic characteristics of young manic patients: Comparison with unipolar depressed patients and normal control subjects. *Archives of General Psychiatry, 49*(5), 378–383.

36. Wright, J. B. (1993). Mania following sleep deprivation. *British Journal of Psychiatry, 163,* 679–680.

37. Wehr, T. A., Sack, D. A., & Rosenthal, N. E. (1987). Sleep reduction as a final common pathway in the genesis of mania. *American Journal of Psychiatry, 144*(2), 201–204.

38. Colombo, C., Lucca, A., Bennedetti, F., et al. (2000). Total sleep deprivation combined with lithium and light therapy in the treatment of bipolar depression: Replication of main effects and interaction. *Psychiatry Research, 95*(1), 43–53.

39. Colombo, C., Bennedetti, F., Barbini, B., et al. (1999). Rate of switch from depression into mania after therapeutic sleep deprivation in bipolar depression. *Psychiatry Research, 86*(3), 267–270.

40. Wicki, W., & Angst, J. (1991). The Zurich study, X. Hypomania in a 28- to 30-year old cohort. *European Archives of Psychiatry and Clinical Neuroscience, 240,* 339–348.

41. Magnusson, A., & Partonen, T. (2005). The diagnosis, symptomatology, and epidemiology of seasonal affective disorder. *CNS Spectrums, 10*(8), 625–634.

42. Anderson, J. L., Rosen, L. N., Mendelson, W. B., et al. (1994). Sleep in fall/winter seasonal affective disorder: Effects of light and changing seasons. *Journal of Psychosomatic Research, 38*(4), 323–337.

43. Eastman, C. I., Young, M. A., Fogg, L. F., et al. (1998). Bright light treatment for winter depression: A placebo-controlled trial. *Archives of General Psychiatry, 55,* 883–889.

44. Terman, M., & Terman, J. S. (2005). Light therapy for seasonal and nonseasonal depression: Efficacy, protocol, safety, and side effects. *CNS Spectrums, 10*(8), 647–663.

45. Armitage, R., Emslie, G., & Rintelmann, J. (1997). The effect of fluoxetine on sleep EEG in childhood depression: A preliminary report. *Neuropsychopharmacology, 17,* 241–245.

46. Yang, C., White, D. P., & Winkleman, J. W. (2005). Antidepressants and periodic limb movements of sleep. *Biological Psychiatry, 58*(6), 510–514.

47. Kim, S. W., Shin, I. S., Kim, J. M., et al. (2005). Bupropion may improve restless legs syndrome: A report of 3 cases. *Clinical Neuropharmacology, 28*(6), 298–301.

48. Bayard, M., Bailey, B., Acharya, D., et al. (2011). Bupropion and restless legs syndrome: A randomized controlled trial. *Journal of the American Board of Family Medicine, 24*(4), 422–428.

49. Nofzinger, E. A., Reynolds, C. F., III, Thase, M. E., et al. (1995). REM sleep enhancement by bupropion in depressed men. *American Journal of Psychiatry, 152,* 274–276.

50. Schenck, C. H., Mahowald, M. W., Kim, S. W., et al. (1992). Prominent eye movements during NREM sleep and REM sleep behavior disorder associated with fluoxetine treatment of depression and obsessive-compulsive disorder. *Sleep, 15*(3), 226–235.

51. Hanzel, D. A., Proia, N. G., & Hudgel, D. W. (1991). Response of obstructive sleep apnea to fluoxetine and protriptyline. *Chest, 100*(2), 416–421.

52. Levy, P., Pepin, J. L., Mayer, P., et al. (1996). Management of simple snoring, upper airway resistance syndrome, and moderate sleep apnea syndrome. *Sleep, 19*(Suppl. 9), S101–S110.

53. Kessler, R. C., McGonagle, K. A., Zhao, S., et al. (1994). Lifetime and 12-month prevalence of DSM III-R psychiatric disorders in the United States. *Archives of General Psychiatry, 51*, 8–19.

54. Anderson, D. J., Noyes, R., & Crowe, R. R. (1984). A comparison of panic disorder and generalized anxiety disorder. *American Journal of Psychiatry, 141*, 572–575.

55. Benca, R. M. (2005). Anxiety disorders. In M. H. Kryger, T. Roth, & W. C. Dement (Eds.), *Principles and practice of sleep medicine* (4th ed., pp. 1311–1326). Philadelphia, PA: Elsevier Saunders.

56. Fuller, K. H., Waters, W. F., Binks, P. G., et al. (1997). Generalized anxiety and sleep architecture: A polysomnographic investigation. *Sleep, 20*(5), 370–376.

57. Saletu-Zhylarz, G., Saletu, B., Anderer, P., et al. (1997). Nonorganic insomnia in generalized anxiety disorder: 1. Controlled studies on sleep, awakening, and daytime vigilance utilizing polysomnography and EEG mapping. *Neuropsychobiology, 36*(3), 117–129.

58. Labbate, L. A., Johnson, M. R., Lydiard, R. B., et al. (1998). Sleep deprivation in social phobia and generalized anxiety disorder. *Biological Psychiatry, 43*(11), 840–842.

59. Mellman, T. A., & Uhde, T. (1989). Sleep panic attacks: New clinical findings and theoretical implications. *American Journal of Psychiatry, 146*, 1204–1207.

60. Hauri, P. J., Friedman, M., & Ravaris, C. L. (1989). Sleep in patients with spontaneous panic attacks. *Sleep, 12*(4), 323–337.

61. Uhde, T. W., Roy-Byrne, P., Gillin, J. C., et al. (1984). The sleep of patients with panic disorder: A preliminary report. *Psychiatry Research, 12*(3), 251–259.

62. Craske, M. G., & Tsao, J. C. (2005). Assessment and treatment of nocturnal panic attacks. *Sleep Medicine Reviews, 9*(3), 173–184.

63. Brown, T. M., & Uhde, T. W. (2003). Sleep panic attacks: A micromovement analysis. *Depression and Anxiety, 18*, 214–220.

64. Stein, M. B., Kroft, C. D. L., & Walker, J. R. (1993). Sleep impairment in patients with social phobia. *Psychiatry Research, 49*, 251–256.

65. Insel, T. R., Gillin, J. C., Moore, A., et al. (1982). The sleep of patients with obsessive–compulsive disorder. *Archives of General Psychiatry, 39*(12), 1372–1377.

66. Hohagen, E., Lis, S., Krieger, S., et al. (1994). Sleep EEG of patients with obsessive–compulsive disorder. *European Archives of Psychiatry and Clinical Neuroscience, 243*(5), 273–278.

67. Robinson, D., Walsleben, J., Pollack, S., et al. (1998). Nocturnal polysomnography in obsessive-compulsive disorder. *Psychiatry Research, 80*, 257–263.

68. Lavie, P. (2001). Sleep disturbances in the wake of traumatic events. *New England Journal of Medicine, 345*, 1825–1832.

69. Neylan, T. C., Marmar, C. R., Metzler, T. J., et al. (1998). Sleep disturbances in the Vietnam generation: Findings from a nationally representative sample of male Vietnam veterans. *American Journal of Psychiatry, 155*(7), 929–933.

70. Ohayon, M. M., & Shapiro, C. M. (2000). Sleep disturbances and psychiatric disorders associated with posttraumatic stress disorder in the general population. *Comprehensive Psychiatry, 41*, 469–478.

71. Schlosberg, A., & Benjamin, M. (1978). Sleep patterns in three acute combat fatigue cases. *Journal of Clinical Psychiatry, 39*(6), 546–549.

72. Mellman, T. A. (1997). Psychobiology of sleep disturbances in posttraumatic stress disorder. *Annals of the New York Academy of Sciences, 821*, 142–149.

73. Engdahl, B. E., Eberly, R. E., Hurwitz, T. D., et al. (2000). Sleep in a community sample of elderly war veterans with and without posttraumatic stress disorder. *Biological Psychiatry, 47*, 520–525.

74. Hurwitz, T. D., Mahowald, M. W., Kuskowski, M., et al. (1998). Polysomnographic sleep is not clinically impaired in Vietnam veterans with chronic posttraumatic stress disorder. *Biological Psychiatry, 44*, 1066–1073.

75. Breslau, N., Roth, T., Burduvali, E., et al. (2004). Sleep in lifetime posttraumatic stress disorder: A community based polysomnographic study. *Archives of General Psychiatry, 61*(5), 508–516.

76. Kloss, J. D., & Szuba, M. P. (2003). Insomnia in psychiatric disorders. In M. P. Szuba, J. D. Kloss, & D. Dingess (Eds.), *Insomnia—Principles and management* (pp. 43–70). Cambridge, UK: University Press.

77. Ross, B. J., Ball, W. A., Sanford, L. D., et al. (1999). Rapid eye movement sleep changes during the adaptation night in combat veterans with posttraumatic stress disorder. *Biological Psychiatry, 45*(7), 938–941.

78. Kauffman, C. D., Reist, C., Djenderedjian, A., et al. (1987). Biological markers of affective disorders and posttraumatic stress disorder: A pilot study with desipramine. *Journal of Clinical Psychiatry, 48*(9), 366–367.

79. van der Kolk, B., Blitz, R., Burr, W., et al. (1984). Nightmares and trauma: A comparison of nightmares after combat with lifelong nightmares in veterans. *American Journal of Psychiatry, 141*(2), 187–190.

80. Mellman, T. A., Knorr, B. R., & Pigeon, W. R. (2004). Heart rate variability during sleep and the early development of posttraumatic stress disorder. *Biological Psychiatry, 55,* 953–956.

81. Krakow, B., Melendrez, D., Warner, T. D., et al. (2002). To breathe, perchance to sleep: Sleep-disordered breathing and chronic insomnia among trauma survivors. *Sleep and Breathing, 6*(4), 189–202.

82. Ballenger, J. C., Davidson, J. R., Lecrubier, Y., et al. (2000). Consensus statement on posttraumatic stress disorder from the International Group on Depression and Anxiety. *Journal of Clinical Psychiatry, 61*(Suppl. 5), 60–66.

83. Sareen, J., & Stein, M. B. (2000). Pharmacotherapy for anxiety disorders in the new millennium. *Psychiatric Clinics of North America, 7,* 173–186.

84. Raskind, M. A., Peskind, E. R., & Kanter, E. D. (2003). Reduction of nightmares and other PTSD symptoms in combat veterans by prazosin: A placebo-controlled study. *American Journal of Psychiatry, 160,* 371–373.

85. Benson, K. L., & Zarcone, V. P., Jr. (2005). Schizophrenia. In M. H. Kryger, T. Roth, & W. C. Dement (Eds.), *Principles and practice of sleep medicine* (4th ed., pp. 1327–1336). Philadelphia, PA: Elsevier Saunders.

86. Hobson, J. A. (1997). Dreaming as delirium: A mental status analysis of our nightly madness. *Seminars in Neurology, 17*(2), 121–128.

87. Dement, W. C. (1955). Dream recall and eye movements in schizophrenics and normals. *Journal of Nervous and Mental Disease, 122*(3), 263–269.

88. Benca, R., Obermeyer, W., Thisted, R., et al. (1992). Sleep and psychiatric disorders: A meta-analysis. *Archives of General Psychiatry, 49*(8), 651–668.

89. Zarcone, V., Azumi, K., Dement, W., et al. (1975). REM phase deprivation and schizophrenia II. *Archives of General Psychiatry, 32*(11), 1431–1436.

90. Benson, K. L., & Zarcone, V. P. (1985). Testing the REM sleep phasic event intrusion hypothesis of schizophrenia. *Psychiatry Research, 15*(3), 163–173.

91. Tandon, R., & Greden, J. F. (1989). Cholinergic hyperactivity and negative schizophrenia symptoms. *Archives of General Psychiatry, 46,* 745–753.

92. Gillin, J. C., Sitaram, N., Nurnberger, J. I., et al. (1983). The cholinergic REM induction test. *Psychopharmacology Bulletin, 19,* 668–670.

93. Hobson, J. A. (2001). *The dream drugstore—Chemically altered states of consciousness* (pp. 238–241). Cambridge, MA: MIT Press.

94. Hartmann, E., Russ, D., van der Kolk, B., et al. (1981). A preliminary study of the personality of the nightmare sufferer: Relationship to schizophrenia and creativity? *American Journal of Psychiatry, 138*(6), 794–797.

95. Monti, J. M., & Monti, D. (2004). Sleep in schizophrenia patients and the effects of antipsychotic medications. *Sleep Medicine Reviews, 8,* 133–148.

96. Keshavan, M. S., Reynolds, C. F., Miewald, J. M., et al. (1996). A longitudinal study of EEG sleep in schizophrenia. *Psychiatry Research, 59*(3), 203–211.

97. Julien, R. M. (1995). *A primer of drug action* (7th ed., pp. 74–100). New York, NY: W.H. Freeman and Company.

98. Roehrs, T., & Roth, T. (2002). Sleep-wakefulness and drugs of abuse. In L. Lee-Chiong, M. Sateia, & M. Carskadon (Eds.), *Sleep medicine* (pp. 575–585). Philadelphia, PA: Hanley & Belfus.

99. Brower, K. J. (2003). Insomnia, alcoholism and relapse. *Sleep Medicine Reviews, 7*(6), 523–539.

100. Krol, R. C., Knuth, S. L., & Bartlett, D. (1984). Selective reduction of genioglossal muscle activity by alcohol in normal human subjects. *American Review of Respiratory Disease, 129*(2), 247–250.

101. Kryger, M. H. (1994). Sleep breathing disorders. In M. H. Kryger, T. Roth, & W. C. Dement (Eds.), *Principles and practice of sleep medicine* (2nd ed., pp. 603–620). Philadelphia, PA: W.B. Saunders.

102. Berry, R. B., Bonnett, M. H., & Light, R. W. (1992). Effect of ethanol on the arousal response to airway occlusion during sleep in normal subjects. *American Review of Respiratory Disease, 145*(2, Pt. 1), 445–452.

103. Berry, R. B., & Desa, M. M. (1991). Light RW: Effect of ethanol on the efficacy of nasal continuous positive airway pressure as a treatment for obstructive sleep apnea. *Chest, 99*(2), 339–343.

SECTION 4
Patient Care and Assessment

chapter 27

Patient Rights and the Provision of Sleep Medicine

JAYME R. MATCHINSKI

LEARNING OBJECTIVES

On completion of this chapter, the reader should be able to:

1. Describe various components of a Patient Bill of Rights.
2. Outline how to construct a Patient Bill of Rights for a sleep disorder center.
3. Identify risks and benefits of health care professionals ensuring patient privacy.
4. Discuss various health care regulations.
5. Describe how to maintain privacy of protected health information in the electronic health record.

KEY TERMS

Advance directives
Regulations
False Claims Act
Anti-Kickback Statute
Office of the Inspector General (OIG)
Safe harbor
Stark Law
HIPAA
HITECH Act
Breach notification
HIPAA Omnibus Rule
Covered entity
Business associate
Office for Civil Rights (OCR)
Protected health information (PHI)
Electronic health record (EHR)
Notice of privacy practices (NPP)

The provision of sleep medicine to patients by sleep disorder centers, sleep medicine professionals, and durable medical equipment (DME) companies requires compliance with applicable state and federal regulations. Patients have certain rights pursuant to state and federal regulations that govern the provision of patient care, maintenance and retention of the patient's medical records, and transfer of patient medical records to other entities and individuals.

Patient rights include the right to make decisions regarding medical care, the right to accept or refuse treatment, and the right to formulate advance directives, which may include written instructions, such as a living will or durable power of attorney for health care, as recognized by the state where the patient resides. This chapter focuses on patient rights and the provision of sleep medicine.

PATIENT BILL OF RIGHTS

Many states have promulgated a Patient Bill of Rights into state law to ensure the basic rights of patients for independence of expression, the patient's decision and action, concern for personal dignity, that human rights and relationships are preserved for all patients, and to define the responsibilities of patients who receive care from health care providers and facilities. Health care providers, including sleep disorder centers, sleep medicine professionals, and DME companies, must comply with the applicable state law related to Patient Bill of Rights. Sleep disorder centers, sleep medicine professionals, and DME suppliers should consider drafting a Patient Bill of Rights and posting the Patient Bill of Rights in the sleep disorder center and on its web sites. The Patient Bill of Rights should also be printed and included in the patient's orientation packet prior to the provision of a sleep study.

Outline of a Patient Bill of Rights for the Sleep Disorder Center

Sleep disorder centers will need to determine how to structure, draft, and implement a Patient Bill of Rights and related policies and procedures. State laws often require that certain provisions be included in a health care facility's Patient Bill of Rights. For example, the State of Illinois has promulgated a Medical Patient Rights Act, 410 ILCS 50/0.01, *et. seq.*, which sets forth certain rights that patients in Illinois have regarding the provision of health care by a health care provider, which is defined as any public or private facility that provides, on an inpatient or outpatient basis, preventative, diagnostic, therapeutic, convalescent, rehabilitation, mental health, or intellectual disability services, including general or special hospitals, skilled nursing homes, extended care facilities, intermediate care facilities, and mental health centers (410 ILCS 50/2.03).

The Illinois Medical Patient Rights Act requires that health care providers notify patients that they have the following rights regarding the provision of their health care:

- The right of each patient to care consistent with sound nursing and medical practices, to be informed of the name of the physician responsible for coordinating his or her care, to receive information concerning his or her condition and proposed treatment, to refuse any treatment to the extent permitted by law, and to privacy and confidentiality of records except as otherwise provided by law.
- The right of each patient, regardless of source of payment, to examine and receive a reasonable explanation of his or her total bill for services rendered by the physician or health care provider, including the itemized charges for specific services received.
- In the event an insurance company or health services corporation cancels or refuses to renew an individual policy or plan, the insured patient shall be entitled to timely, prior notice of the termination of such policy or plan.
- An insurance company or health services corporation that requires any insured patient or applicant for new or continued insurance or coverage to be tested for infection with human immunodeficiency virus or any other identified causative agent of acquired immunodeficiency syndrome shall (1) give the patient or applicant prior written notice of such requirement, (2) proceed with such testing only upon the written authorization of the applicant or patient, and (3) keep the results of such testing confidential. Notice of an adverse underwriting or coverage decision may be given to any appropriately interested party, but the insurer may disclose the test result itself only to a physician designated by the applicant or patient, and any such disclosure shall be in a manner that assures confidentiality.
- The right of each patient to privacy and confidentiality in health care. Each physician, health care provider, health services corporation, and insurance company shall refrain from disclosing the nature or details of services provided to patients, except that such information may be disclosed: (1) to the patient; (2) to the party making treatment decisions if the patient is incapable of making decisions regarding the health services provided; (3) for treatment

in accordance with state law; (4) for payment in accordance with state law; (5) to those parties responsible for peer review, utilization review, and quality assurance; (6) for health care operations in accordance with state law; (7) to those parties required to be notified under the Abused and Neglected Child Reporting Act or the Illinois Sexually Transmissible Disease Control Act; or (8) as otherwise permitted, authorized, or required by state or federal law. This right may be waived in writing by the patient or the patient's guardian or legal representative, but a physician or other health care provider may not condition the provision of services on the patient's, guardian's, or legal representative's agreement to sign such a waiver.
- Any patient who is the subject of a research program or an experimental procedure, as defined under the rules and regulations of the Hospital Licensing Act, shall have, at a minimum, the right to receive an explanation of the nature and possible consequences of such research or experiment before the research or experiment is conducted, and to consent to or reject it.
- Every health care facility in this state shall permit visitation by any person or persons designated by a patient who is 18 years of age or older and who is allowed rights of visitation unless (1) the facility does not allow any visitation for a patient or patients, or (2) the facility or the patient's physician determines that visitation would endanger the physical health or safety of a patient or visitor, or would interfere with the operations of the facility.

Most states have penalties and fines that will be assessed against a health care provider, including a sleep disorder center, that violates a patient's rights pursuant to the state's Patient Bill of Rights regulations. For example, in Illinois, if a health care provider violates a patient's rights pursuant to the state law, the health care provider will be found guilty of a petty offense and shall be fined $500.00, and if an insurance company or health care corporation violates a patient's rights pursuant to the regulatory requirements for a Patient Bill of Rights, the insurance company or health care corporation shall be found guilty of a petty offense and fined $1,000.00.

Sleep disorder centers and other health care providers are often required by state law to post a statement of the Patient Bill of Rights and provide a written statement of all the rights to the patient on admission to the facility. The statement shall also include the right not to be discriminated against by the sleep disorder center on the basis of the patient's race, color, or national origin, where such characteristics are not relevant to the patient's medical diagnosis and treatment. The statement shall further provide each admitted patient or the patient's representative or guardian with notice of how to initiate a grievance regarding improper discrimination with the facility and how the patient may lodge a grievance with the Illinois Department of Public Health and the Illinois Department of Human Rights regardless of whether the patient has first used the facility's grievance process.

A health care facility, including a sleep disorder center, that provides treatment or care to a patient in the State of Illinois shall require each employee of or volunteer for the facility, including a student, who examines or treats a patient to wear an identification badge that readily discloses the first name, licensure status, if any, and staff position of the person examining or treating the patient.

SAMPLE PATIENT BILL OF RIGHTS

Although sleep disorder centers will need to comply with the applicable state law regarding the regulatory requirements for Patient Bill of Rights, sleep disorder centers and sleep medicine professionals should also consider patient care issues and the delivery of patient care related to the screening, evaluation, testing, diagnosis, and treatment of sleep disorders when drafting a Patient Bill of Rights. The following is a sample Patient Bill of Rights Policy:

Patient Bill of Rights Policy

It is the policy of the sleep disorder center to respect the individual rights of all persons that come to this sleep disorder center for care. Patient rights include: the right to make decisions regarding medical care, the right to accept or refuse treatment, and the right to formulate advance directives, including: written instructions, such as a living will or durable power of attorney for health care as recognized under state law, relating to the provision of such, when an individual is incapacitated.

Patient responsibilities include those actions on the part of patients that are needed so that sleep disorder center and health care professionals can provide appropriate care, make accurate and responsible care decisions, address patient needs, and maintain a sound and viable health care sleep disorder center.

Access to Care

Patients shall be afforded impartial access to treatment that is available and medically indicated, regardless of race, creed, sex, national origin, religion, sexual orientation, disability, or source of payment. Free translation services are available if needed.

The patient has the right to considerate, respectful care at all times, under all circumstances, with recognition of his or her personal dignity and worth.

Privacy and Confidentiality

The patient has the right, pursuant to applicable state and federal law, to personal privacy and information privacy, as demonstrated by the right to the following:

- Be interviewed and examined in surroundings designed to assure reasonable audiovisual privacy.
- Expect that any discussion or consultation involving the patient's care will be conducted discreetly and that individuals not involved in direct care will not be present without permission of the patient.
- Have the patient's medical record read only by individuals directly involved in treatment or monitoring of quality, and by other individuals only on written authorization by the patient or his/her legally authorized representatives.
- Refuse to talk with or see anyone not officially connected with the sleep disorder center, including visitors and persons officially connected with the sleep disorder center but who are not directly involved in the patient's care.
- Wear appropriate personal clothing and religious or other symbolic items, as long as such clothing and religious or other symbolic items do not jeopardize safety or interfere with diagnostic procedures or treatment provided by the sleep disorder center and its professionals.
- Expect that all communications and other records pertaining to the patient's care, including the sleep study and source of payment for treatment, be treated as confidential.
- Expect that information provided to family members or significant other legally qualified person be delivered in privacy and with consideration of confidentiality.

Personal Safety and Security

The patient has the right to expect reasonable safety in the sleep disorder center including compliance with the sleep disorder center's policies and procedures, practices, and environment regarding patient safety and security. Other safety and security measures include: limited access to the sleep disorder center through the use of electronic access cards and readers on exterior entrances, video monitoring in numerous areas of the sleep disorder center, including the patient's treatment area, and the use of employee identification badges that are to be displayed by health care professionals providing services to the patient.

Identity

The patient has the right to know the identity and professional status of individuals providing service and which physician or other practitioner is primarily responsible for his or her care. This includes the patient's right to know of the existence of any professional relationship among individuals who are treating him or her, as well as the relationship to any health care or other institution, facility, or professional involved in his or her care. Participation by patients in research programs, or in the gathering of data for research purposes, shall be voluntary with a signed informed consent.

Communication

The patient has the right of access to people outside the sleep disorder center by means of oral and written communication. When the patient does not speak or understand the predominant language of the community, or is hearing impaired, the patient shall have access to an interpreter, if at all possible.

Information

The patient has the right to obtain from the health care professional responsible for coordinating his or her care complete and current information concerning his or her diagnosis, treatment, and any known prognosis. This information should be communicated in terms the patient can reasonably be expected to understand. When it is not medically advisable to give such information to the patient, the information shall be made available to a legally authorized representative.

The patient has the right to access his or her medical records. The patient shall complete the Authorization to Disclose Protected Health Information (PHI) form and submit it to the sleep disorder center.

The patient may access, request an amendment to, and/or receive an accounting of disclosures of his or her own PHI as permitted under applicable law, including the Health Insurance Portability and Accountability Act (HIPAA) regulations and standards.

Consent

The patient has the right to reasonably informed participation in decisions involving his or her health care. To the degree possible, this shall be based on a clear, concise explanation of his or her condition and of all proposed technical procedures, including the possibilities of any risk of mortality or serious side effects, issues related to the patient's diagnosis and treatment, and probability of success and outcomes. The patient shall not be subjected to any procedure without his or her voluntary, competent, and informed consent, or that of his or her legally authorized representative. Where medically significant alternatives for care or treatment exist, the patient shall be so informed.

The patient has the right to know who is responsible for authorizing and performing the diagnostic testing and/or treatment.

The patient shall be informed if the health care professional proposes to engage in or perform human experimentation or other research/educational projects affecting his or her care or treatment, and the patient shall sign an informed consent if participation is desired and maintains the right to refuse to participate or withdraw from any such activity at any time.

The patient may refuse treatment to the extent permitted by law. When refusal of treatment by the patient or his or her legally authorized representative prevents the provision of appropriate care in accordance with ethical and professional standards, the relationship with the patient may be terminated upon reasonable notice by the sleep disorder center.

If a patient is unconscious or is determined to be mentally incompetent and no consent can be obtained from an appropriate family member, legal action may be taken to obtain a court order for diagnostic testing procedures. In life-threatening emergencies, where the patient is incompetent or unconscious, appropriate treatment may be administered without consent.

Consultation

The patient, at his or her own request and expense, has the right to consult with a specialist.

Transfer and Continuity of Care

A patient may not be transferred to another facility unless he or she has received a complete explanation of the need for the transfer and the alternatives to such a transfer, and unless the transfer is acceptable to the other facility. The patient has the right to be informed by the responsible health care professional or his or her delegate of any continuing health care requirements following discharge from the sleep disorder center.

Regardless of the source of payment for his or her care, the patient has the right to request and receive an itemized and detailed explanation of his or her total finalized bill for services rendered in the sleep disorder center. The patient shall be informed of eligibility for reimbursement by any third-party coverage during the admission or preadmission financial investigation.

Sleep Disorder Center Rules and Regulations

The patient shall be informed of the sleep disorder center's rules and regulations applicable to his or her conduct as a patient. The sleep disorder center's notice of privacy practices (NPP) is available from the administrator and can be found on the sleep disorder center's web site.

Complaint Process

The patient has the right to file a complaint regarding services and is entitled to information regarding the sleep disorder center's mechanism for the initiation, review, and resolution of such complaints.

Patient Responsibilities

Patients have the responsibility for:

- Providing complete and accurate information about medical complaints and issues, past illnesses, hospitalizations, medications, pain, and other matters relating to the patient's health;
- Keeping appointments, arriving on time, and contacting the sleep disorder center if the appointment cannot be kept;
- Following the treatment plan recommended by those responsible for the patient's care;
- The patient's actions if they refuse treatment or do not follow the sleep disorder center's instructions;
- Providing complete and accurate information about the patient's health insurance coverage and promptly paying bills in a timely manner;
- Following the sleep disorder center's policies and procedures and applicable rules and regulations;
- Being considerate of the rights of other patients and the sleep disorder center's health care professionals; and
- Seeking information and, in the event the patient has any questions, asking such questions.

IDENTIFY RISKS AND BENEFITS OF HEALTH CARE PROFESSIONALS ENSURING PATIENT PRIVACY

Medicare and Medicaid

Payments by the federal Medicare program are currently made under a system whereby the secretary of the Department of Health and Human Services prospectively sets reimbursement amounts for medical services performed in sleep disorder centers and durable medical equipment supplied by DME companies. The Medicare Access and CHIP Reauthorization Act of 2015 ("MACRA") established new value-based payment models. The Department of Health and Human Services' Final Rule, published on October 14, 2016, replaced the Medicare sustainable growth rate methodology for updates to the physician fee schedule ("PFS") with a new payment approach called the Quality Payment Program that rewards the delivery of high-quality patient care through two methods. The first method is the Advanced Alternative Payment Model, and the second method is the Merit-based Incentive Payment System for eligible clinicians or groups under the PFS. Although MACRA went into effect on January 1, 2017, and requires the collection and submission of certain data, providers, including sleep disorder centers who provide services to Medicare patients, will not start getting paid under the new payment methods until January 1, 2019.

Under the Medicaid program, the federal government supplements funds provided by the state where the patient resides for medical assistance to indigent persons. At present, Medicaid payment to sleep disorder centers is based on a percentage of usual and customary charges. State Medicaid and other state health care programs are an important payor source to many health care providers and may become a proportionately larger source of revenue as federal health care reform continues to evolve, expanding Medicaid coverage, in those states that choose to expand Medicaid, to significant numbers of uninsured Americans. These programs often pay health care providers, including sleep disorder centers, at levels that may be below the actual cost of the care provided. As Medicaid and other state health care programs are partially funded by states, the often precarious financial condition of states may result in lower funding levels and/or payment delays in the future.

Health Care Reform

The Patient Protection and Affordable Care Act ("ACA") was enacted in March 2010. As a result of the ACA, substantial changes have occurred, and continued changes are anticipated in the U.S. health care system. The ACA is impacting the delivery of health care services, the financing of health care costs, reimbursement of health care providers, and the legal obligations of health insurers, providers, employers, and consumers, including regulatory compliance and enforcement activities. These provisions are slated to take effect at specified times over approximately the next decade from adoption, and therefore the full consequences of the ACA on the health care industry will not be immediately realized. The ramifications of the ACA may also become apparent only following implementation or through later regulatory and judicial interpretations. Thus, the health care industry is the subject of significant new statutory and regulatory requirements and consequently structural and operational changes and challenges for a substantial period of time. Portions of the ACA have already been limited and nullified as a result of legislative amendments and judicial interpretations, and future actions and amendments may further change its impact. In addition, the uncertainties regarding the implementation of the ACA create unpredictability for the strategic and business planning efforts of health care providers, and this in itself constitutes a risk.

The ACA addresses almost all aspects of health care delivery and has changed, and is changing, how health care services are covered, delivered, and reimbursed. These changes will result in new payment models with the risk of lower health care provider reimbursement from Medicare, utilization changes, increased government enforcement, and the necessity for health care providers to assess, and potentially alter, their business strategy and practices, among other consequences. Although many providers will receive reduced payments for care, millions of previously uninsured Americans may have coverage. Requirements for state "health insurance exchanges" could fundamentally alter the health insurance market and negatively impact health care providers, enabling insurers to aggressively negotiate rates. Federal deficit reduction efforts will likely curb federal Medicare and Medicaid spending further, to the detriment of health care providers, including ambulatory surgery centers. In June 2012, the Supreme Court upheld most provisions of the ACA, while limiting the power of the federal government to penalize states for refusing to expand Medicaid, and on June 25, 2015, the Supreme Court ruled that health insurance subsidies under the ACA would be available in all states, including those with a federally facilitated health insurance exchange. Efforts to repeal provisions of the ACA are, from time to time, pending in Congress. At this time, it is not possible to predict the outcomes of any legislative attempts to repeal or amend the ACA or any further judicial interpretations of the ACA.

The ACA makes changes to Medicaid funding and substantially increases the potential number of Medicaid beneficiaries. To fund this expansion, the ACA provides that the federal government will fund 100% of the costs of this expansion from 2014 to 2016, decreasing to 90% of the costs of this expansion by 2020 and thereafter. In June 2012, the U.S. Supreme Court held that the federal government cannot withhold existing federal funds for states that refuse to expand Medicaid as required by the ACA. Because Medicaid has historically reimbursed at rates below the cost of care, increases in the overall proportion of Medicaid patients pose a risk. The sleep disorder center cannot predict the effect of these legislative actions or proposals on the operations or results from operations.

HEALTH CARE REGULATION

Federal Issues

A wide array of regulatory issues impact sleep medicine and the provision of care to patients by sleep disorder centers and DME companies as related to the health care industry. Various levels of government agencies are involved with health care oversight, not only in the role of regulators but also as significant third-party payors.

Medicare, a federal health insurance program for the elderly and certain disabled persons, and Medicaid, a jointly administered federal and state program for certain indigent persons, are very important payors for most health care providers, including sleep disorder centers. There are numerous complex rules governing payments and methodology, documentation, claim forms, cost reporting forms, as well as certification processes for participation and conditions of participation in the Medicare and Medicaid programs.

The sleep disorder center must be approved for participation in the Medicare and Medicaid programs in order to become enrolled in the programs, receive provider numbers, and be permitted to bill Medicare and Medicaid for services rendered to patients who are Medicare and Medicaid beneficiaries. Failure to maintain certification by Medicare could have a materially adverse effect on the sleep disorder center's business. The sleep disorder center will also be required to revalidate its compliance with the Medicare regulations, including the conditions of participation, and such Medicare revalidation requirements have increased since the implementation of the ACA. Given the current regulatory environment, sleep disorder centers and DME companies will continue to be subject to intensive regulation, including increased audits and investigations to enforce regulatory compliance, at the state and federal levels.

"Fraud" and "False Claims"

Health care "fraud and abuse" laws have been enacted at the federal and state levels to broadly regulate the provision of services to government program beneficiaries and the methods and requirements for submitting claims for services rendered to the beneficiaries. Under these fraud and abuse laws, health care providers and suppliers who submit claims for services provided to government program beneficiaries can be penalized for a wide variety of conduct, including submitting claims for services that are not provided, billing in a manner that does not comply with government requirements or including inaccurate billing information, billing for services deemed to be medically unnecessary, and/or billings accompanied by an illegal inducement to utilize or refrain from utilizing a service or product.

Federal and state governments have a broad range of criminal, civil, and administrative sanctions available to penalize and remediate health care fraud, including the exclusion of the provider or supplier from participation in the Medicare or Medicaid programs, recoupment of previous payments, civil monetary penalties, suspension of Medicare or Medicaid payments, and criminal sanctions and imprisonment. Fraud and abuse cases may be prosecuted by one or more government entities and/or private individuals, and more than one of the available sanctions and penalties may be, and often is, imposed for each violation. The ACA authorizes the Secretary of the U.S. Department of Health and Human Services (DHHS) to exclude a provider's participation in Medicare and Medicaid, as well as suspend payments to a provider pending an investigation or prosecution of a credible allegation of fraud against the provider.

Laws governing fraud and abuse may apply to nearly all individuals and entities with which a health care provider does business. Fraud investigations, settlements, prosecutions, and related publicity can have a material adverse effect on health care providers. Major elements of these often highly technical laws and regulations are generally summarized below.

False Claims Act

The federal False Claims Act ("FCA") makes it illegal to knowingly submit or present a false, fictitious, or fraudulent claim to the federal government. Because the term "knowingly" is defined broadly under the law to include not only actual knowledge but also deliberate ignorance or reckless disregard of the facts, the FCA can be used to regulate and oversee a wide range of conduct. The ACA amends the FCA by expanding the numbers of activities that are subject to civil monetary penalties to include, among other things, failure to report and return known overpayments within statutory limits. FCA investigations and cases have become common in the health care industry and may cover a range of activity, from submission of incorrect billings, to highly technical billing infractions, to allegations of inadequate care. Penalties under the FCA are severe and can include damages equal to three times the amount of the alleged false claims, as well as substantial civil monetary penalties. Violation or alleged violation of the FCA frequently results in settlements that require multimillion-dollar payments and costly corporate integrity agreements. The FCA also permits individuals to initiate civil actions on behalf of the government in lawsuits called "qui tam" actions. Qui tam plaintiffs, or "whistle-blowers," can share in the damages recovered by the government or recover independently if the government does not participate. The FCA has become one of the government's primary tools against health care fraud and suspected fraud, and the government's enforcement activities related to the FCA have increased pursuant to the implementation of the ACA. FCA violations or alleged violations could lead to settlements, fines, exclusion, and/or reputation damage that could have a material adverse impact on a health care provider and the provider's future viability.

Under the ACA, the FCA has been expanded to include overpayments that are discovered by a health care provider and are not promptly refunded to the applicable federal health care program, even if the claims relating to the overpayment were initially submitted without any knowledge that they were false. The ACA requires that providers return identified overpayments within 60 days of identification, or the overpayment becomes an "obligation" under the FCA. There is great uncertainty in the industry as to when an overpayment is technically "identified" and the ability of a provider to determine the total amount of an overpayment and satisfy its repayment obligation within the 60-day time period. CMS, in its Final Rule published on February 12, 2016, provided some clarification as to the "identification" of overpayment. According to CMS, a facility has "identified" an overpayment when the facility has or should have, through the exercise of reasonable diligence, determined that the facility has received an overpayment and quantified the amount of the overpayment. This expansion of the FCA exposes hospitals and other health care providers to liability under the FCA for a considerably broader range of claims than in the past. Any violation of these laws could be financially devastating to the sleep disorder center.

Federal Anti-Kickback Statute

The federal "Anti-Kickback Statute" prohibits anyone from soliciting, receiving, offering, or paying any remuneration, directly or indirectly, overtly or covertly, in cash or in kind, in return for a referral (or to induce a referral) for any item or service that is paid by any federal or state health care program. The ACA amended the Anti-Kickback Statute to provide that a claim that includes items or services resulting from a violation of the Anti-Kickback Statute now constitutes a false or fraudulent claim for purposes of the FCA. Another amendment provides that an Anti-Kickback Statute violation may be established without showing that an individual knew of the statute's proscriptions or acted with specific intent to violate the Anti-Kickback Statute, but only that the conduct was generally unlawful. The new standards have significantly expanded criminal and civil fraud exposure for transactions and arrangements where there is no intent to violate the Anti-Kickback Statute, and these new standards have also led to increased enforcement activities by federal agencies, including audits and investigations of providers and suppliers.

Violation or alleged violation of the Anti-Kickback Statute often results in settlements that require significant dollar payments and the imposition of formal, government-monitored compliance programs. The Anti-Kickback Statute can be prosecuted criminally or civilly. Violation of the Anti-Kickback Statute is a felony, subject to potentially substantial fines for each act (which may be each item or each bill sent to a federal program), imprisonment, and/or exclusion from the Medicare and Medicaid programs, any of which would have a significant detrimental effect on the financial stability of most providers. In addition, significant civil monetary penalties may be imposed. Increasingly, the federal government and qui tam relators are prosecuting violations of the Anti-Kickback Statute under the FCA, on the basis of the argument that claims resulting from an illegal kickback arrangement are also the submission of false claims for FCA purposes.

The Anti-Kickback Statute applies to many common health care transactions between individuals and entities involved in the ownership and operation of a health care facility, including the ownership interests of physicians who refer patients to such health care facilities center, medical director agreements, and other related arrangements and agreements. Because the provisions of the Anti-Kickback Statute are so broad, the DHSS, Office of the Inspector General has published regulations, including "safe harbors," advisory opinions, and fraud alerts, outlining certain categories of activities that are deemed *not* to violate the Anti-Kickback Statute, provided all required elements of the safe harbor are met. The preambles to the safe harbor regulations state that the failure to comply with a safe harbor does not mean that the arrangement violates the Anti-Kickback Statute and that many legitimate ventures do not fall within one. If the statute is violated, the preambles state that the degree of the risk of prosecution depends on an evaluation of the many factors that are part of the decision-making process regarding case selection for investigation and prosecution.

Stark Law

The federal Stark Law and implementing regulation prohibits the referral of Medicare and Medicaid patients for certain designated health services ("DHS") (including inpatient and outpatient hospital services, clinical laboratory services, and radiation and other imaging services) to entities ("DHS Entities") with which the referring physician has a financial relationship unless the relationship fits within a stated exception. The Stark Law also prohibits a DHS Entity from furnishing the DHS and subsequently from billing Medicare for services performed pursuant to a prohibited referral. The government does not need to prove that the DHS Entity knew that the referral was prohibited to establish a Stark violation. Unless certain technical requirements are met, many ordinary business practices and economically desirable arrangements between hospitals and physicians arguably constitute improper "financial relationships" within the meaning of the Stark statute, thus implicating the prohibition on referrals and billing. Most providers of the DHS with physician relationships have some exposure to liability under the Stark Law.

Changes to the regulations issued under the Stark Law have rendered illegal a number of common arrangements under which physician-owned entities provide services and/or equipment to hospitals and may increase risk of violation because of lack of clarity of the technical requirements necessary to satisfy exceptions.

Medicare may deny payment for all services related to a prohibited referral, and a DHS Entity that has billed for prohibited services may be obligated to refund the amounts collected from the Medicare program. For example, if a medical director agreement between a DHS Entity and a physician is found to violate the Stark Law, the DHS Entity could be obligated to repay CMS for the payments received from Medicare for all of the Medicare-covered services performed by the physicians during the time the arrangement was out of compliance, a potentially significant amount, and the physician and DHS may be excluded from the Medicare program. The government may also seek substantial civil monetary penalties, and in some cases, a DHS Entity may be liable for fines up to three times the amount of any monetary penalty and/or be excluded from the Medicare and Medicaid programs. Potential repayments to CMS, settlements, fines, or exclusion for a Stark violation or alleged violation could have a material adverse impact on a health care provider. Increasingly, the federal government is prosecuting violations of the Stark Law under the FCA, on the basis of the government's position that claims resulting from an illegal referral arrangement are also false claims for FCA purposes. The federal government is also increasingly attempting to recover the federal portion of Medicaid claims referred to DHS Entities by physicians with whom they have a prohibited financial relationship.

State Issues

In addition to federal issues, compliance with state law by a sleep disorder center and a DME company is very important in the ongoing operation of the facilities and provision of sleep medicine. Most states regulate licensure, certificate of need, and other matters relative to medical practice and the operation of a health care facility, including sleep disorder centers and DME companies.

PRINCIPLES FOR EFFECTIVE AND PROFESSIONAL SOCIAL NETWORKING AND COMMUNICATION IN MAINTAINING PATIENT PRIVACY

HIPAA and Privacy Requirements
Health Insurance Portability and Accountability Act

HIPAA of 1996 adds additional civil penalties and criminal sanctions for health care fraud and applies to all health care benefit programs, whether public or private. HIPAA also provides for penalties and sanctions on a health care provider for knowingly and willfully embezzling, stealing, converting, or intentionally misapplying any money, funds, or other assets of a health care benefit program. A health care provider convicted of health care fraud could be subject to mandatory exclusion from Medicare.

HIPAA also addresses the confidentiality of individuals' health information, including privacy and security aspects of confidential health information. Disclosure of certain broadly defined PHI is prohibited unless expressly permitted under the provisions of the HIPAA statute and regulations, authorized by the patient, and meets exceptions related to the patient's treatment, payment, and health care operations. HIPAA's confidentiality provisions extend not only to patient medical records, but also to a wide variety of health care clinical and financial information. These patient privacy restrictions impose communication, operational, accounting, and billing restrictions that add costs and create potentially unanticipated sources of liability. HIPAA imposes civil monetary penalties for violations and criminal penalties for knowingly obtaining or using individually identifiable health information.

The HITECH Act

Provisions in the 2009 Health Information Technology for Economic and Clinical Health Act (the "HITECH Act"), enacted as part of the American Recovery and Reinvestment Act ("ARRA"), increase the minimum and maximum civil monetary penalties for violations of HIPAA and grant enforcement authority of HIPAA to state attorneys general. The HITECH Act also (1) extends the reach of HIPAA beyond "covered entities," (2) imposes a breach notification requirement on HIPAA-covered entities, (3) limits certain uses and disclosures of individually identifiable health information, (4) restricts covered entities' marketing communications, and (5) permits imposition of civil monetary penalties for a HIPAA violation even if an entity did not know and would not, by exercising reasonable diligence, have known of a violation.

The breach notification obligation, in particular, may expose covered entities such as sleep disorder centers and DME companies to heightened liability. Under the HITECH Act, in the event of a data privacy breach, covered entities are required to notify affected individuals and the federal government. If more than 500 individuals in any one state are affected by the breach, (1) the covered entity must also notify the media and (2) the federal government posts a description of the breach on its web site. Although HIPAA does not provide for a private right of action, these reporting obligations increase the risk of government enforcement as well as class action lawsuits filed under state privacy or consumer protection laws, especially if large numbers of individuals are affected by a breach.

On January 25, 2013, DHHS issued comprehensive modifications to the existing HIPAA regulations to implement the requirements of the HITECH Act, commonly known as the "HIPAA Omnibus Rule." The HIPAA Omnibus Rule became effective on March 26, 2013, and covered entities were required to be in compliance by September 23, 2013 (though certain requirements had a longer time frame). Key aspects of the HIPAA

Omnibus Rule include, but are not limited to: (1) a new standard for what constitutes a breach of private health information, (2) establishing four levels of culpability with respect to civil monetary penalties assessed for HIPAA violations, (3) direct liability of business associates for certain violations of HIPAA, (4) modifications to the rules governing research, (5) stricter requirements regarding nonexempt marketing practices, (6) modification and redistribution of notices of privacy practices, and (7) stricter requirements regarding the protection of genetic information. Although the effects of the HIPAA Omnibus Rule cannot be predicted at this time, the obligations imposed thereunder could have a material adverse effect on the financial condition of the Credit Group.

The HITECH Act revises the civil monetary penalties associated with violations of HIPAA as well as provides state attorneys general with authority to enforce the HIPAA privacy and security regulations in some cases through a damages assessment of $100 per violation or an injunction against the violator. The revised civil monetary penalty provisions establish a tiered system, ranging from a minimum of $100 per violation for an unknowing violation to $1,000 per violation for a violation due to reasonable cause, but not willful neglect. For a violation due to willful neglect, the penalty is a minimum of $10,000 or $50,000 per violation, depending on whether the violation was corrected within 30 days of the date the violator knew or should have known of the violation. Maximum penalties may reach $1,500,000 for identical violations. These levels of civil monetary penalties apply immediately for unknowing violations or violations due to reasonable cause.

Criminal penalties will be enforced against persons who obtain or disclose personal health information without authorization. DHHS is also beginning to perform periodic audits of health care providers and group health plans to ensure that required policies under the HITECH Act are in place. Finally, individuals harmed by violations will be able to recover a percentage of monetary penalties or a monetary settlement based on methods to be established by DHHS for this private recovery.

The Office for Civil Rights ("OCR") is the administrative office that is tasked with enforcing HIPAA. The OCR has stated that it has now moved from education to enforcement in its implementation of the law, and in March 2016, the OCR began its Phase 2 HIPAA Privacy, Security, and Breach Notification Audit Program, which requires providers to submit certain data to the OCR. Recent settlements of HIPAA violations for breaches involving lost data have reached millions of dollars. Any breach of HIPAA, regardless of intent or scope, may result in penalties or settlement amounts that are material to a covered health care provider or health plan.

Business Associates

Under existing HIPAA regulations, covered entities must include certain required provisions in their contractual relationships with organizations that perform functions on their behalf that involve use or disclosure of PHI. These organizations are called business associates and have been indirectly regulated by HIPAA through contractual obligations. The HITECH Act and the final rules promulgated thereunder provide that all of the HIPAA security administrative, physical, and technical safeguards, as well as security policies, procedures, and documentation requirements now apply directly to all business associates. In addition, the HITECH Act makes certain privacy provisions directly applicable to business associates. These changes are significant because business associates will now be directly regulated by DHHS for those requirements and, as a result, will be subject to penalties imposed by DHHS and/or state attorneys general. Likewise, to the extent a business associate is deemed to be an agent of the covered entity under the federal common law, the covered entity will be liable for the breaches of the business associate.

Security Breaches and Unauthorized Releases of Personal Information

State and local authorities are increasingly focused on the importance of protecting the confidentiality of individuals' personal information, including patient health information. Many states have enacted laws requiring businesses to notify individuals of security breaches that result in the unauthorized release of personal information. In some states, notification requirements may be triggered even where information has not been used or disclosed, but rather has been inappropriately accessed. State consumer protection laws may also provide the basis for legal action for privacy and security breaches and frequently, unlike HIPAA, authorize a private right of action. In particular, the public nature of security breaches exposes health organizations to increased risk of individual or class action lawsuits from patients or other affected persons, in addition to government enforcement. Failure to comply with restrictions on patient privacy or to maintain robust information security safeguards, including taking steps to ensure that contractors who have access to sensitive patient information maintain the confidentiality of such information, could consequently damage a health care provider's reputation and materially adversely affect business operations.

Sleep disorder centers qualify as a "covered entity" under the Administrative Simplification Provisions of HIPAA, and as a covered entity sleep disorder centers are required to comply with these regulations, including privacy and security standards. Failure to comply would expose the sleep disorder center to civil and criminal penalties. Also, failure to submit claims electronically in compliance with the EDI regulation may result in denial of claims and possible exclusion from participation in federal health care programs.

Understand How to Maintain Privacy of PHI in Electronic Health Records

The HIPAA regulations and security standards address how a patient's PHI must be protected from unauthorized disclosure to other entities and individuals. Many sleep disorder centers and DME companies utilize electronic health record (EHR) to document, retain, and transmit a patient's PHI. Given the utilization of EHR and potential for data breaches and unauthorized disclosure of patients' PHI, it is imperative that sleep disorder centers and DME companies comply with the HIPAA regulations and set up safeguards and security measures pursuant to the HIPAA security standards. The following is an overview of how a sleep disorder center and its sleep medicine professionals can maintain privacy of patients' PHI in an EHR pursuant to the HIPAA regulations and security standards.

Patients have the right to receive a notice explaining how a provider, including a sleep disorder center or health plan, uses and discloses their health information. Health care providers usually give patients this notice on their first visit to the sleep center and post it in the center where patients may see it. Health plans typically send their notices by mail after patient enrollment.

An NPP will often contain jargon that can be difficult for patients to understand.

The HIPAA regulations require that an NPP:

- include how the HIPAA Privacy Rule allows the covered entity to use and share PHI and state that it will obtain the patient's permission for any other reason;
- tell patients about their rights under the HIPAA Privacy Rule;
- tell patients how to file a complaint with the covered entity;
- tell patients how to file a complaint with the DHHS OCR;
- provide information about a patient's rights to restrict fund-raising solicitations; and
- explain the need to obtain a patient's written authorization for marketing or the sale of the patient's PHI.

For more information about notices of privacy practices, see the DHHS web site at: www.hhs.gov or 45 CFR §164.520.

Health care providers, including sleep disorder centers, should ask patients to sign a form saying that they received a copy of the NPP. The law does not require patients to sign this. However, signing does not waive a patient's rights under HIPAA and does not mean that the patient agrees with the privacy policy. If a patient refuses to sign, it does not prevent a health care provider from using or disclosing information in ways already permitted under HIPAA. A provider may not deny treatment if a patient refuses to sign an acknowledgment of having received an NPP.

The NPP will provide information about whom to contact with privacy questions and how to complain. If a patient does not have a copy of the notice, there may be one on the provider's or health plan's web site. If there is not an NPP on the health care provider's web site, a covered entity's administrative office will be able to provide the information and a copy of the notice.

HIPAA gives patients the right to see and receive a copy of their medical records but not the original medical records. To find out how to request access to a medical record, the patient should review the sleep disorder center's NPP. Patients can always request a copy of the notice, which should provide instructions for requesting records as well as contact information for asking questions or filing complaints.

Patients have the right to access both paper and electronic records. An individual may request information in a specific format, and the covered entity must comply with the request if the data are readily producible. If the data are not readily producible in the patient's specified format, the covered entity and the individual can agree on another format. If the sleep disorder center and the patient cannot reach an agreement, the covered entity will produce a hard copy.

For example, a patient might ask the sleep disorder center to provide his or her records on an external portable storage device such as a USB drive. If the sleep disorder center does not agree to use the USB drive because it believes it is a security risk, the sleep disorder center and the patient may reach agreement about another format. If they do not reach an agreement, the sleep disorder center may provide a hard copy to the patient.

Often, patients want providers to send their health information, including PHI, to third parties such as another doctor, a relative, or an attorney. To authorize this transfer and disclosure of PHI, the patient should sign a request that clearly identifies which medical records need to be sent, who has been designated to receive the medical records, and where the patient's medical records need to be sent. HIPAA allows covered entities, including sleep disorder centers, to charge a "reasonable, cost-based fee." The covered entity can charge for supplies, staff time for copying and processing, and mailing, if applicable.

The covered entity may charge for the time staff spends copying and processing the record. However, the sleep disorder center may not charge for the time a staff member spends searching for the record. In addition, the covered entity should not adopt a policy of charging a flat fee or charging a patient to view a record. Many states have laws that limit a covered entity's ability to charge for medical records. Sleep disorder centers should check the applicable state laws to ensure that its charges for patient medical records comply with the applicable state regulations.

A covered entity, including a sleep disorder center, must produce a patient's medical records 30 days from the date of request. HIPAA allows a covered entity one 30-day extension if the sleep disorder center provides written notice to the patient stating the reason for the delay and the expected date. This applies to both paper and electronic records.

A sleep disorder center, as the covered entity, may deny a patient's request for access under certain circumstances. Typically, the covered entity must issue a written denial letter, and in some cases, an individual may be able to appeal a denial. As a general rule, patients do not have the right to access their own psychotherapy notes or information a covered entity compiled for legal proceedings. Patients may be denied access to their PHI without the right to review the denial in the following situations:

- Correctional institutions may deny an inmate's request for a copy of PHI if it jeopardizes the health, safety, security, custody, or rehabilitation of the individual or other inmates. It may also deny a request that jeopardizes the safety of any person at the correctional institution or those responsible for transporting the inmate.
- If a covered health care provider obtains or creates PHI in the course of research, it may temporarily suspend access while the research is in process. This applies if the individual agreed to the denial when he or she decided to participate in a study and understands that the right will be reinstated when the research is complete.
- If a record that contains PHI is subject to the HIPAA privacy standards, there are certain circumstances where an individual may not be able to access the record.
- If the PHI was obtained from someone other than a health care provider under a promise of confidentiality and the access requested would likely reveal the source of the information, an individual may not be able to access the information.

Sometimes, patients have the right to have denials of access reviewed by a licensed health care professional. If so, the patient should receive instructions telling him or her how to appeal the denial. The covered entity will designate a reviewing official who did not participate in the original decision to deny access.

When patients access a medical record and find information they believe is inaccurate, they may file a written request that the record be corrected. The covered entity, including sleep disorder centers, must respond to the request within 60 days. The sleep disorder center may decide to take an additional 30 days but must provide the patient with a written explanation for the delay and a date by which it will complete the action.

If the covered entity denies the request, it must provide the patient with the following information in writing:

- The basis for the denial. For example, the covered entity did not create the medical record, the information is not part of the designated record set, the patient is not allowed to access the medical record under another HIPAA provision, or the medical record is accurate and complete;
- That the patient has a right to submit a written statement disagreeing with the denial;
- That the patient may request that the covered entity provide the request for amendment and the denial with any future disclosures that pertain to the request; and
- How the patient may complain.

Under the HIPAA regulations and privacy and security standards, covered entities, including sleep disorder centers, must allow a patient to make specific privacy requests. Although a patient has the right to make a request, in most situations the covered entity is not required to agree.

If a covered entity agrees to honor an individual's privacy request, it must comply unless the individual needs emergency treatment and the restricted PHI is necessary to provide the treatment. In an emergency situation where the covered entity must disclose information it agreed to restrict, it must request that the information not be further disclosed.

HIPAA enables patients to learn to whom the covered entity has disclosed their PHI. This is called an "accounting of disclosures." The accounting will cover up to 6 years prior to the patient's request date and will include disclosures to or by business associates of the covered entity. For each disclosure, the accounting must state:

- the date of the disclosure;
- the name of the entity or person who received the PHI, and, if known, the address;
- a brief description of the PHI disclosed; and
- a brief statement of the purpose of the disclosure.

The accounting does not include information about disclosures the covered entity made:

- to carry out treatment, payment, or health care operations;
- to the individual for information about him or her;
- incident to a use or disclosure that HIPAA permits or requires;
- that the patient authorized;

- for a sleep disorder center's directory or persons involved in the patient's care;
- for national security or intelligence purposes;
- to correctional institutions or law enforcement officials;
- as part of a limited data set that excludes a number of identifiers and is disclosed for research, public health, or health care operations; or
- that occurred prior to the date by which the covered entity had to comply.

Within 60 days of receiving a request for an accounting, a covered entity, including sleep disorder centers, must:

- provide the accounting; or
- extend the time by no more than 30 days as long as it provides the individual with a written statement of the reasons for the delay and date by which it will provide the accounting.

A covered entity must provide the first accounting, during any 12-month period, free of charge. If an individual requests more than one accounting during a year, the covered entity may impose a cost-based fee on subsequent requests. However, if it is going to charge, the covered entity must inform the individual of the fee in advance and give him or her an opportunity to withdraw or modify the request.

Under the HIPAA Privacy Rule, a covered entity can disclose a minor child's PHI to a parent acting as a child's "personal representative" as long as it is consistent with state and other law. DHHS provides the following examples of situations where a parent may not access a minor's medical record:

- a minor consents to care, and law does not require parental consent;
- a court or person appointed by the court directs a minor to obtain care; and
- a parent agrees that the minor and health care provider may have a confidential relationship.

Sleep disorder centers and DME companies should carefully review their policies and procedures and patient forms related to the provision of patient care, administration, and operational functions to ensure compliance with the applicable state and federal regulations, specifically regulations that address Patient Bill of Rights requirements, protection of patient's PHI, maintenance of privacy of patient's PHI in an EHR, and identify risks and benefits of health care professionals who provide sleep medicine services to patients to ensure patient privacy and protection of PHI.

chapter 28
Patient and Employee Safety

MARY KAY HOBBY

LEARNING OBJECTIVES

On completion of this chapter, the reader should be able to:

1. Recognize unsafe situations within the work environment.
2. Express that personal and patient safety involves each employee.
3. Participate in safe practices.
4. Describe how to prevent accidents or injury in the sleep center.
5. React appropriately to an unsafe environment or situation.
6. Describe the importance of infection control standards.

KEY TERMS

Proper lifting techniques
Chemical spills/waste
Performing cardiopulmonary resuscitation
Electrical grounding

The importance of effective workplace safety cannot be understated. The safety of employees affects morale, attendance, and workmen's compensation. Well-written policies and procedures play an imperative role in patient and employee safety. Policies help clarify and reinforce the standards expected of employees. Federal, state, and local organizations' and agencies' guidelines assure the occupational health and safety of the technologist and patients who visit the sleep center. The Occupational Safety and Health Administration (OSHA) is a division of the US Department of Labor. OSHA provides regulatory standards for workplace safety. These standards are intended to protect employers, employees, and patients in and around the work environment. Personal and environmental hazards that the sleep technologist may be subjected to should be addressed in the department policy and procedures manual. A Quality Improvement Plan is a formal documented action plan that targets areas of practice within an organization that will be the focus of safety and outcomes to obtain the highest quality of patient care. Quality assurance measures are then evaluated quarterly to track the effectiveness of the plan. The plan is adjusted appropriately to ensure that quality goals are being met. The American Academy of Sleep Medicine requires sleep centers to perform a safety risk analysis at a minimum every 5 years to identify and make a plan to lessen the risk of events such as falls, medical emergencies, or harassment allegations (1).

PERSONAL SAFETY/CHEMICALS

An aspect of personal safety in the sleep disorder clinic that may be neglected is a frequent exposure to fumes/odors from cleaning solutions and adhesive materials. Chemical exposure for health care workers is a possible threat at any sleep disorders center. Causes may include improperly used or maintained disinfectant solutions or sterilizing agents. OSHA requires manufacturers to provide safety information on chemical products in a uniform format to ensure safety and proper handling of the chemical products that are utilized in the workplace (2). Staff meetings discussing the hazards of chemicals and solutions used and, quick and easy access to safety data sheets (SDSs) are ways to educate workers about the potential dangers surrounding these compounds.

The SDS is not meant for consumers but is for employees who may be occupationally exposed to hazardous products or chemicals while in the working environment. The SDS is designed to provide workers with the proper procedures for handling, storing, and working with a particular substance. Basic supplies the sleep technologist uses during patient hookup procedures or cleaning equipment that require an SDS include the following:

- Electroencephalography (EEG) conductive paste or cream
- Disinfectant/cleaner concentrate
- Germicidal deodorizing cleaner
- Abrasive skin prep gel
- Adhesive to secure electrodes
- Alcohol prep pads
- Diaphoretic skin prep

The OSHA Quick Card identifies the required format for SDS (3).

Section 1, Identification includes product identifier; manufacturer or distributor name, address, phone number; emergency phone number; recommended use; restrictions on use.

Section 2, Hazard(s) identification includes all hazards regarding the chemical; required label elements.

Section 3, Composition/information on ingredients includes information on chemical ingredients; trade secret claims.

Section 4, First aid measures include important symptoms/effects, acute, delayed; required treatment.

Section 5, Firefighting measures list suitable extinguishing techniques, equipment; chemical hazards from fire.

Section 6, Accidental release measures list emergency procedures; protective equipment; proper methods of containment and cleanup.

Section 7, Handling and storage lists precautions for safe handling and storage, including incompatibilities.

Section 8, Exposure controls/personal protection lists OSHA's Permissible Exposure Limits; American Conference of Governmental Industrial Hygienists (ACGIH) Threshold Limit Values; and any other exposure limit used or recommended by the chemical manufacturer, importer, or employer preparing the SDS where available as well as appropriate engineering controls; personal protective equipment (PPE).

Section 9, Physical and chemical properties list the chemical's characteristics.

Section 10, Stability and reactivity lists chemical stability and the possibility of hazardous reactions.

Section 11, Toxicologic information includes routes of exposure; related symptoms, acute and chronic effects; numerical measures of toxicity.

Section 12, Ecologic information

Section 13, Disposal considerations

Section 14, Transport information

Section 15, Regulatory information

Section 16, Other information, includes the date of preparation or last revision.

It is crucial to the safety of sleep technologists to have access to a SDS manual containing information concerning each chemical used in the sleep center. This reference should be available for employees at all times.

INFECTION CONTROL

Infection control should be an integral part of the health care facility's objectives. It is the responsibility of each member of the health care team to ensure the use of proper techniques to eliminate the spread of infection (2). Cooperation from the organization's administration, medical staff, and other health care personnel is necessary to maintain infection control standards. The following elements are necessary to attain appropriate infection control:

- Coordination with other departments
- Medical evaluations
- Health and safety education
- Immunization programs
- Management of job-related illnesses and exposure to infectious diseases, including policies for work restrictions for infected or exposed personnel
- Counseling services for personnel on infection risks related to employment
- Maintenance and confidentiality of personnel health records (2)

According to the Centers for Disease Control and Prevention and OSHA, the use of "universal precautions" or "standard precautions" refers to an infection control system that assumes any direct contact with a patient, particularly with body fluids, has the potential for transmitting disease (4). Health care personnel are at risk for occupational exposure to blood-borne pathogens, including hepatitis B virus, hepatitis C virus, and HIV. Standard precautions are designed to reduce the risk of transmission of blood-borne pathogens and to reduce the risk of transmission of pathogens from moist body substances. Standard precautions apply to blood, secretions, excretions except sweat, and all other body fluids of patients receiving care in hospitals, regardless of their diagnosis or presumed infection status. It is important to note that bodily fluids can be considered contaminated whether or not they contain visible blood, nonintact skin, or mucous membranes (5). Exposures occur through needle sticks or abrasions caused by contaminated sharp objects. Infection may occur through contact with mucous membranes of the eyes and mouth, skin, or the patient's blood (6). Contact with any bodily fluid, regardless of quantity, is considered to be a potential source of infectious agents (5). Using appropriate barriers such as gloves, goggles, or gowns when contact with blood is expected can prevent many exposures. Remove gloves promptly after use and wash hands immediately to avoid the transfer of microorganisms (5). If exposure occurs, wash needlestick injuries and cuts with soap and water, flush splashes to the nose, mouth, or skin with water, and irrigate the eyes (6). Prompt reporting of exposures to the department that handles such situations is essential, so that proper treatment can be initiated.

Handwashing must occur after touching blood, body fluids, secretions, excretions, and contaminated items, whether or not gloves are worn. Wash hands immediately after gloves are removed, between patient contacts, and any time contamination has occurred, to avoid transfer of microorganisms to other patients or environments (5). Handwashing is also essential before eating and after using the bathroom.

It is important for technologists to handle used patient care equipment in a manner that prevents skin and mucous membrane exposure, contamination of clothing, and transfer of microorganisms to other patients and environments. Adequate procedures should be in place and followed for routine care, cleaning, and disinfection of environmental surfaces, beds, bedrails, bedside equipment, and other frequently touched surfaces (7).

Cleaning and disinfecting reusable equipment in the sleep center is a safety standard that cannot be compromised. It is the responsibility of *every* staff member to prevent the spread of infection with proper handwashing and effective cleaning of reusable equipment. Consider utilizing central processing for sterilizing reusable patient care equipment. Some facilities opt for disposable equipment to minimize the cost of disinfecting agents and staff time. Electrodes, masks, and even respiratory inductance plethysmography belts come in a disposable variety.

OSHA defines decontamination as the use of physical or chemical means to remove, inactivate, or destroy blood-borne pathogens on a surface or item to the point where they are no longer capable of transmitting infectious particles and the surface or item is rendered safe for handling, use, or disposal. Sterilization is the use of a physical or chemical procedure to destroy all microbial life, including highly resistant bacterial endospores (8).

In 1968, Spaulding (9) devised an approach to disinfect and sterilize patient care items or equipment that is still used today. This approach classifies medical equipment into categories according to a degree of risk of infection involved in the use of the items. Spaulding (9) describes these categories as critical, semicritical, and noncritical. Positive airway pressure (PAP) masks and airflow sensors fall into the category of semicritical, meaning that they come in contact with mucous membranes or skin that is not intact (9). Semicritical items require high-level disinfection, in a separate cleaning area, with wet pasteurization or a chemical disinfectant (9). Today most accrediting bodies recommend single-use PAP masks, tubing, humidifiers and headgear. If these items are cleaned there must be a method in place to track the number of times each item has been disinfected, and they must be discarded after they have been cleaned the maximum number of times indicated by the manufacturer. Reprocessing guidelines differ by manufacturer, by specific interface within manufacturers, and sometimes even for different parts of a CPAP mask–so this can be daunting to track and manage.

EEG electrodes and other sensors generally fall into the noncritical category (9). These items come in contact with skin but not with mucous membranes. Most noncritical reusable items may be disinfected where they are used and do not need to be transported to a central processing area. There is generally little risk of transmitting infectious agents to patients by means of noncritical items. A high-level disinfectant wipe should be used to clean most noncritical items (Table 28-1) (10).

PAP Mask Cleaning

According to the Spaulding criteria for medical device classification (9), PAP masks are considered semicritical medical equipment. Semicritical items contact mucous membranes or nonintact skin. Cleaning and disinfection requirements should adhere to those approved by the Food and Drug Administration (FDA) for each individual mask in order to ensure elimination of tuberculosis spores. Semicritical items minimally require high-level disinfection containing a tuberculocidal disinfectant. Glutaraldehyde, hydrogen peroxide, *ortho*-phthalaldehyde, and peracetic acid with hydrogen peroxide are FDA-approved semicritical method(s) of disinfection (i.e., Control III Elite, Cavicide, Sanizide Plus, and CIDEX OPA). Follow specific manufacturer's recommendations. Consider using a timer to remind you when the equipment can be removed from the disinfecting agent to avoid excessive wear.

Sleep centers have also found pasteurizing to be a cost-effective way to clean and disinfect equipment. Pasteurization is a form of cleaning/high-level disinfecting of health care equipment using water temperatures of 160° to 170° F (71° to 77° C). This eliminates or reduces the use of expensive toxic chemicals and saves labor costs of staff handwashing supplies. Guidelines on sterilization processes vary from state to state and, in some cases, from facility to facility.

The sleep center may have a maintenance agreement with a mask manufacturer that allows the patient to take home the mask that was used in the sleep center during the titration study. The manufacturer then replaces that mask for the sleep center. Small replacement fees may apply.

Patient Room, Electrode, and Sensor Cleaning

Work surfaces, bed rails, EEG electrodes, thermal airflow sensors, head straps, snore microphones, and belts are considered noncritical medical equipment. Noncritical items come in contact with intact skin but not mucous membranes. In addition, surfaces in patient rooms and work surfaces must be decontaminated to avoid

Table 28-1 Disinfecting Chart

	Noncritical Spaulding Category	Semicritical Spaulding Category	Cleaning
EEG electrodes	X		Rinse with warm water. Soak in general disinfectant according to manufacturer's directions after each patient use. Wipe lead wires using a cloth soaked in a solution of low-level disinfectant or wipe with a disinfectant towelette. Air dry prior to plugging into head box.
Snap electrodes	X		Wipe using a cloth soaked in a solution of low-level disinfectant or wipe with a disinfectant towelette.
Airflow sensors		X	Disposable airflow sensors are preferred. Wipe using a cloth with a high-level disinfecting agent or towelette that is not corrosive to metal or plastic. Air dry.
Belts	X		Disposable belts are preferred. Straps may be safely soaked in low-level disinfectant solution. Air dry.
			The wire-set may be wiped with disinfecting cloth or towelette. Do not immerse in liquid.
Body position sensor	X		Wipe using a cloth with a low-level disinfecting agent or towelette that is not corrosive to metal or plastic. Do not immerse in liquid. Air dry.
Snore microphone	X		Wipe using a cloth with a disinfecting agent or towelette that is not corrosive to metal or plastic. Do not immerse in liquid. Air dry.
SpO$_2$ sensor	X		Disposable sensors are preferred. Remove disposable adhesive from permanent sensors and discard; wipe with a low-level disinfecting agent or towelette that is not corrosive to metal or plastic. Do not immerse in liquid. Air dry.
Headgear	X		Should not be re-used. Single patient use headgear is preferred.
CPAP masks		X	Single-patient use CPAP masks are preferred. If re-used soak in a high-level disinfectant according to disinfectant manufacturer's guidelines or pasteurize. Rinse and dry thoroughly.
Linen	X		Blanket, sheets, and pillowcases must be washed between patients. Contaminated linens should be placed in impermeable bags.

Rutala, W. A., & Weber, D. J. (2008). MPH and the Healthcare Infection Control Practices Advisory Committee (HICPAC), *Guideline for Disinfection and Sterilization in Healthcare Facilities*. Centers for Disease Control, ©US Department of Health and Human Services. Retrieved from https://www.cdc.gov/infectioncontrol/pdf/guidelines/disinfection-guidelines.pdf

transmission of infection. A low-level disinfectant such as isopropyl alcohol (70% to 90%), sodium hypochlorite (5.25% to 6.15%) diluted with water at 1:500, or a germicidal (i.e., Control III, Sani-Cloth HB wipe, Super Sani-Cloth wipe, and Sani-Cloth Plus) wipe may be used to decontaminate noncritical items (10).

Proper handling and cleaning of sensors will prolong their durability and longevity. All equipment and sensors, masks, and belts coming into contact with the patient are considered contaminated. The sleep center must maintain a separation of "clean" and "dirty" equipment by keeping clean and dirty equipment in distinct areas designated as clean and dirty, respectively. All dirty equipment must be cleaned and disinfected after each use according to manufacturer guidelines. Single-use items must be discarded after each use.

Reusable equipment must be completely disassembled and thoroughly washed using an approved cleaning solution. OSHA requires staff to wear PPE such as gloves and goggles while cleaning equipment to reduce exposure to hazardous chemicals. Ensure that reusable equipment is not used for the care of another patient until it has been cleaned and processed appropriately (11). Personnel are more likely to comply with an infection control program if they understand the rules and the importance of such rules. Personnel education is the key element of an effective infection control program.

MEDICAL WASTE

Medical waste generated by health care providers can pose a risk of disease transmission if not managed properly. Hazardous waste and discarded chemicals that are toxic, flammable, or corrosive can cause fires, explosions, and pollution of air, water, and land. Knowing how to identify and properly dispose of medical and other hazardous waste is critical. Hazardous waste is a serious safety and health problem that continues to endanger human and animal life and environmental quality (12). Unless hazardous waste is properly treated, stored, or disposed, it will continue to do great harm to all living things that come into contact with it now or in the future.

Because of the seriousness of the safety and health hazards related to hazardous waste operations, OSHA has issued regulations to protect workers and help them handle hazardous wastes safely and effectively (13).

Medical "sharps" is the term used to describe any needle or sharp object including glass. If not cared for properly, sharps have the ability to cause puncture wounds and/or lacerations that may create a point of entry for infectious agents. Infectious agents are any organisms that cause disease or an adverse health impact to humans (2). Take care to prevent injuries when using needles and other sharp devices before, during, and after procedures, when cleaning used devices, and when disposing of used needles. Never recap used needles. Place used disposable syringes and needles and other sharp items in appropriate puncture-resistant containers and dispose of as regulated medical waste. Patient disposal of syringes, such as syringes used for insulin injection, should be monitored to prevent needles in the patient room. Sharps or products contaminated with blood or body fluids that are disposed of in the health care setting should be placed in properly identified and labeled containers to be sent to the waste treatment center for decontamination.

PROPER LIFTING TECHNIQUES

Back injuries account for nearly 25% of occupational injuries. Not only are these injuries costly to the Worker's Compensation program, but they also leave the worker prone to recurrent injury. Attention to posture, conditioning, and body mechanics are essential to maintaining a healthy back while on the job. Body mechanics refers to the way we use our body to accomplish a task (Table 28-2). Eighty percent of Americans will experience back pain

Table 28-2 Body Mechanics to Promote Back Injury Prevention

	Do	Do Not
Bending	Stoop with bent knees	Bend at the back
Reaching	Use step stool	Stretch overhead
Pulling or pushing	Use entire body	Use arms only
Lifting	Stand close to object	Reach
	Bend at knees and hips	Bend or twist at the waist

some time in their lives. Of these, 90% are due to strain of back muscles, ligaments, or soft tissue. These conditions generally heal completely, but often recur if prevention strategies are not used (14). The National Institute of Occupational Safety and Health (NIOSH) has researched and developed a lifting equation taking into account such things as weight of the object lifted, distance of the hands above the floor, angle of the distance of the object from the core of the body at the beginning or end of the lift, and twisting of the legs, shoulders, or torso in assessing physical stress with unassisted two-handed lifting.

Injury may occur when using poor posture, awkward positioning, or overreaching. When preparing to lift stand close to the object or individual being moved or lifted, position your feet a comfortable distance apart, bend at the knee, keep the back straight, and grip the item firmly. While lifting, slowly straighten your legs, keep the object close to your body, bring your back to a full upright position, and move your feet; never twist your shoulders or torso. Ask for help when necessary.

According to the NIOSH, back injuries cost American industry $10 to $14 billion in workers' compensation costs and about 100 million workdays annually (15). Lifting/pushing supplies and equipment; lifting, positioning, and/or transporting patients; and reaching, stooping, bending, kneeling, and crouching are physical abilities required of the sleep lab technologist to perform essential job functions. Care must be taken to maneuver correctly to avoid injury.

EMERGENCY PLAN

A workplace emergency is an unforeseen situation that threatens your employees or patients. It may even disrupt your business because of physical or environmental damage to your facility. Nobody expects an emergency or disaster. Yet, the simple truth is that emergencies and disasters can strike anyone, anytime, anywhere, and at any sleep center. The best way to protect yourself, your workers, and your patients is to expect the unexpected and develop a well-thought-out emergency action plan (EAP) to guide you when immediate action is necessary. An EAP is a written document required by OSHA standards and is often part of the sleep center's policy and procedure manual. Facilities must conduct and document emergency drills annually (1).

Emergencies may be natural or man-made and include the following:

- Floods
- Hurricanes
- Tornadoes
- Fires
- Toxic gas releases
- Chemical spills
- Radiologic accidents
- Explosions
- Civil disturbances
- Workplace violence resulting in bodily harm and trauma

It is best to prepare to respond to an emergency before it happens. A few people can think clearly and logically in a crisis, so it is important to do so in advance when you have time to be thorough.

An EAP covers designated actions that employers and employees must take to ensure employee safety from fire and other emergencies. Not all employers are required to establish an EAP. Even if you are not specifically required to do so, compiling an EAP is a good way to protect yourself, your employees, and your patients as well as your business during an emergency. An EAP should consist of the following:

- A preferred method for reporting fires and other emergencies
- An evacuation policy and procedure
- Emergency escape procedures and route assignments, such as floor plans, workplace maps, and safe or refuge areas
- Proper use of firefighting equipment such as extinguishers
- Contact list of names, titles, departments, and telephone numbers of individuals both within and outside your company to contact for additional information or explanation of duties and responsibilities under the emergency plan (16, 17)
- Procedures for employees who will perform critical tasks, such as shutting down critical plant operations, operating fire extinguishers, or carrying out other essential services before evacuating

- Rescue and medical duties for any workers designated to perform them. Designate an assembly location and procedures to account for all employees after an evacuation (1, 17).

When developing your EAP, it is important to determine the following:

- Conditions under which an evacuation would be necessary
- A clear chain of command and designation of the individual in your facility authorized to order an evacuation or shutdown. Consider designating an evacuation warden to assist others in an evacuation and to account for patients and personnel.
- Specific evacuation procedures including routes and exits. Post these procedures where they are easily accessible to all employees.
- Procedures for assisting people with disabilities or those who may have difficulty understanding verbal direction
- A designated group of people who will continue or shut down critical operations during an evacuation. These people must be capable of recognizing when to abandon the operation and evacuate themselves.
- A system for accounting for personnel and patients following an evacuation. Consider employees' transportation needs for community-wide evacuations.

Accounting for all employees and patients following an evacuation is critical. Confusion in the assembly areas can lead to delays in rescuing anyone trapped in the building, or unnecessary and dangerous search-and-rescue operations. To ensure the fastest, most accurate accountability of your employees and patients, you may want to consider including these steps in your EAP:

- Designate assembly areas where employees and patients should gather after evacuating.
- Take a head count after the evacuation. Identify the names and last-known locations of anyone not accounted for and pass them to the official in charge.
- Establish procedures for further evacuation in case the incident turns into a major one. This may consist of sending employees and patients home by normal means or providing them with transportation to an off-site location.

Protecting the health and safety of everyone in the facility should be the first priority. In the event of a fire, an immediate evacuation to a predetermined area away from the facility is the best way to protect employees and patients.

When preparing your EAP, designate primary and secondary evacuation routes and exits. To the extent possible, ensure that evacuation routes and emergency exits meet the following conditions:

- Clearly marked and well lit
- Wide enough to accommodate the number of evacuating personnel
- Unobstructed and clear of debris at all times
- Unlikely to expose evacuating personnel to additional hazards

If drawings are prepared to show evacuation routes and exits, post them prominently for all employees to see.

The best EAP includes employees in the planning process. Specify employee procedures during an emergency and ensure that employees receive proper training for emergencies. Encourage employees to offer suggestions about potential hazards, worst-case scenarios, and proper emergency responses. After developing the plan, allow employees to review procedures that take place before, during, and after the emergent event. Keep a copy of the EAP in a convenient location where employees can access it readily. With 10 or fewer employees, plans may be communicated orally (17, 18). A review of the EAP should be performed and documented annually.

SECURITY THREATS

Terrorist threats both inside and outside of hospitals and clinics have steadily grown over the years. But security has often remained unchanged. Facilities lack electronic lockdown capability, creating vulnerability of patient data and making it difficult to defend against cyberattacks. Insider threats against hospitals from fired or disgruntled employees, physicians, patients, or relatives of patients who may find reason for revenge are growing. Physician terrorist "suicide/homicide" bombers were and are a continuing threat. Intensive international background checks of physician groups found potential bombers (19). Extensive background checks revealed misrepresentation of certifications and education, which exposes trusting patient populations to unqualified practitioners or other dangers.

In the event of a bomb threat, it is imperative for employees to maintain a calm environment and gather as much information as possible from the caller. Ask the caller specific questions relating to the type, location, and time of detonation of the bomb. Listen carefully to assess voice quality of the caller. Are they calm? Excited? Angry? Do they speak fast? Slow? Loud? Slurred? With an accent? Note any background sounds such as traffic, airplanes, machinery, animals, music, or other details, which may assist in locating the caller. Once the call has been terminated, immediately call 911 and give the operator specific details. This should be done as confidentially as possible so as not to incite panic. Notify

management that a bomb threat has been received. Employees should awaken all patients and disconnect the head box from the amplifier. Evacuate and wait at a safe distance from the building for the authorities to arrive. During the evacuation, employees should make a visual sweep for any unusual or suspicious items. If such an item is found, make a mental note of its description and location and report it once the authorities are on the scene. Do not touch or attempt to move the item.

With many sleep facilities located off-site, physical separation of workers from patients or the general public through the use of bullet-resistant barriers or enclosures has been proposed. The height and depth of counters are important considerations in protecting workers because they introduce physical distance between employees and potential attackers. Consideration must be given to the continued ease of conducting business; a safety device that increases frustration for workers or patients may be self-defeating.

Sleep technologists often find themselves alone at night in an office complex awaiting patient arrival for sleep testing. Visibility and lighting of parking areas and entrances are environmental design considerations that can be implemented to discourage workplace assaults. There should be safeguards to prevent patients from entering the building through unlocked doors, particularly at night. Consider minimal use of landscaping near entrances where attackers could hide. Security devices such as entry buzzers, closed-circuit cameras, alarms, card key access, and an intercom system in the entryway may deter potential perpetrators and improve staff safety.

FIRE SAFETY

All employees should be trained about fire hazards in the workplace and on what to do in the case of fire (16). A popular acronym used to remember the best approach to fire safety is RACE (rescue, alarm, contain, and evacuate).

- **Rescue:** Assistance to the patient is priority. Remove all patients from immediate danger.
- **Alarm:** Alert coworkers to a fire emergency. This may be accomplished using an alarm system, voice communication, or sound signals such as bells, whistles, or horns (16). Alert emergency personnel using an alarm system such as a fire alarm pull box or by dialing 911.
- **Contain:** Close doors if possible to contain a fire. Attempts should be made to extinguish the flame by using an appropriate fire extinguisher for the classification of fire (Table 28-3). Many facilities have multipurpose extinguishers available. Multipurpose or "combination" extinguishers can be used for more than one classification of fire (16, 20).

Table 28-3 Fire Classifications

Class A Fires

Fires of this type consist of ordinary combustibles, such as wood, paper, or cloth, and can be put out with water. Approach the fire and aim the nozzle toward the base of the flames, sweeping the extinguisher nozzle from side to side across the base of the flame. Continue spraying until all smoldering material is saturated.

A multipurpose dry-chemical extinguisher can also be used on class A fires. Attack at the edge of the fire, directing the nozzle in a sweeping motion. The powdered chemical becomes sticky when heated, allowing it to form a film that clings to the heated material and smothers the fire.

Class B Fires

Fires that burn flammable liquids, such as oil, gasoline, solvents, and paints, as their primary fuel are class B.

Dry-chemical extinguishers are the type usually used—starting about 8 ft (2.1 m) away from the fire and slowly moving closer, applying the substance from side to side near the fire's base.

Carbon dioxide extinguishers are also effective on flammable liquid fires. You must use this type near the edge of the fire at close range in an enclosed area where no wind or draft exists. Fires can spread with the presence of oxygen, but carbon dioxide decreases the amount of oxygen surrounding the fire until the air can no longer support the combustion.

Class C Fires

These fires involve electrical equipment. Water cannot be safely used to extinguish this type of fire because of the electrical conduction properties of water, which may deliver a shock to the firefighter. If the equipment can be deenergized, extinguishers for class A or B fires may be safely used. Otherwise, carbon dioxide and dry-chemical extinguishers are the best. Carbon dioxide is nonconductive and noncorrosive and leaves no sticky film, making cleanup easy.

Class D Fires

Class D fires involve combustible metals, such as magnesium, titanium, zirconium, sodium, lithium, and potassium. Special dry-compound powders, such as powdered graphite and sodium chloride, powdered talc, soda ash, and limestone, are made to extinguish these fires. In case of emergency, dry sand can be used.

- **Evacuate:** Exit the building. The workplace must have exits suitably located and well-marked. Exits must be clearly visible and marked as an EXIT (17). Fire doors must not be blocked or locked. Exit routes must be kept clear of obstructions (17, 18). No materials or equipment may be placed, either permanently or temporarily, within the exit route (17, 18).

Emergency evacuation plans must also be implemented for other environmental disasters that may be common to your geographical area. All employees should understand evacuation plans, be familiar with how to alert emergency personnel, and always be prepared to respond to disasters, such as fire, or severe weather be it tornadoes, earthquakes, or hurricanes.

ELECTRICAL SAFETY

OSHA's electrical standards address electricity as a serious workplace hazard, exposing employees or patients to such dangers as electric shock, electrocution, burns, fires, and explosions. OSHA electrical standards help minimize these potential hazards by specifying safety aspects in the design and use of electrical equipment and systems. Almost every electrical accident is preventable. To avoid accidents and potential injuries, some basic precautions can be taken.

Computers, fans, PAP devices, home sleep apnea testing devices, televisions, and any other electrical equipment should be tracked, inspected, and monitored annually. Reports of failures of such equipment must be logged.

Volts, watts, and amps measure electricity. Volts measure the "pressure" under which electricity flows. Amps measure the amount of electric current. Watts measure the amount of work done by a certain amount of current at a certain pressure or voltage. To understand this relationship, think of water in a hose. Turning on the faucet supplies the force that is comparable with the voltage. The amount of water moving through the hose is like the amperage. A lot of water (more wattage) is needed to wash a muddy car. Less water (lower wattage) is needed to fill a glass.

Resistance to the flow of electricity is measured in ohms. Some substances, such as metals, offer very little resistance to the flow of electric current and are called conductors. Other substances, such as porcelain, pottery, and dry wood, offer such a high resistance that they can be used to prevent the flow of electric current and are called insulators. Dry wood has a high resistance, but when saturated with water, its resistance drops to the point where it will readily conduct electricity. This is also true of human skin. When it is dry, the skin has a fairly high resistance to electric current, but when it is moist, there is a radical drop in resistance. Pure water is a poor conductor, but small amounts of impurities, such as salt and acid (both of which are contained in perspiration), make it a ready conductor. When water is present either in the environment or on the skin, anyone working with electricity should exercise even more caution than they normally would.

Electricity travels in closed circuits, and its normal route is through a conductor. Ideally, current enters a device, flows through the electronics, and exits. Electric shock occurs when the body becomes a part of the electric circuit. The current must enter the body at one point and leave at another. If a person touches a bare conductor carrying current, this current will flow through the person to the ground (21). The effects of electric shock are variable depending upon the amount of voltage, current, and duration of the contact. Effects can range from a barely perceptible tingle to immediate cardiac arrest. A severe shock can cause considerably more damage to the body than is visible. One may suffer internal hemorrhages and destruction of tissues, nerves, and muscles. In addition, shock is often only the beginning in a chain of events. The final injury may be from a fall, cuts, burns, or broken bones associated with the shock (Table 28-4) (21).

Electrical accidents are typically caused by a combination of three possible factors:

- Unsafe equipment and/or installation
- Workplaces made unsafe by the environment
- Unsafe work practices

Ways of protecting people from the hazards caused by electricity include proper insulation, proper electrical grounding, and safe work practices. The power cord is a conductor that is insulated by the rubber cording. This prevents accidental exposure to electrical current (22). The integrity of all power cords must be checked routinely. Equipment with a damaged cord should be taken out of use (Table 28-5).

Grounding is another method for protecting employees from electric shock. The term "ground" refers to a connecting circuit from the equipment to the earth. By grounding a tool or electrical system, a low-resistance path to the earth is intentionally created. Electrical current will follow the path of least resistance. This does not guarantee that no one will receive a shock, be injured, or be killed. It will, however, substantially reduce the possibility of such accidents (23).

Equipment grounding for safety should not be confused with the patient–ground connection. A patient–ground connection is used to help prevent line-frequency interference (50 or 60 Hz) by providing a conductive pathway from the patient to ground through the recording system. In this case, the ground connection actually becomes a potential hazard because it may also become a pathway for a stray current. To prevent

Table 28-4	Effects of Electric Current in the Human Body

Current (mA)	Reaction
1	Perception level. Just a faint tingle.
5	Slight shock felt; not painful but disturbing. Average individual can let go. However, strong involuntary reactions to shocks in this range can lead to injuries.
6–25 (women)	Painful shock, muscular control is lost.
9–30 (men)	This is called the "freezing current" or "let-go" range.
50–150	Extreme pain, respiratory arrest, severe muscular contractions.ᵃ The individual cannot let go. Death is possible.
1,000–4,300	Ventricular fibrillation. (The rhythmic pumping action of the heart ceases.) Muscular contraction and nerve damage occur. Death is most likely.
10,000	Cardiac arrest, severe burns.

ᵃIf the extensor muscles are excited by the electric shock, the person may be thrown away from the circuit.

Table 28-5 Safety Tips for Power Cords
Replace, do not attempt to fix, cords that have been cut or damaged. Exposed strands of wire can cause shock or burns.
Never unplug a power cord by pulling the cord.
If a cord or plug is warm or hot to the touch, unplug it immediately.
Check wires, cords, and electrical equipment for signs of wear.
Never place electric cords across traffic areas or under a carpet.
Never bend or remove the ground (third prong on a plug). It is designed to help prevent shock.

this possibility, a patient–ground connection must be isolated and equipped with a circuit breaker. Technologists must also be aware that all wires connected to the patient pose a potential electrical hazard to the patient. Care must be taken to prevent the electrode leads from coming in contact with any electrical equipment or any conductive or wet surfaces.

Employees and others working with electric equipment need to use safe work practices. This includes unplugging electric equipment before inspecting or making repairs, using electric tools that are in good repair, and using appropriate protective equipment. To ensure that they use safe work practices, employees must be aware of the electrical hazards to which they will be exposed. Through cooperative efforts, employers and employees can learn to identify and eliminate or control electrical hazards (23).

PATIENT EMERGENCIES

Cardiovascular Events

Patients with comorbid conditions such as underlying cardiac or pulmonary disease, coupled with hypoxia due to sleep-disordered breathing, are susceptible to cardiac arrhythmias. Early detection of, and response to, cardiac arrhythmias can save lives. Each heartbeat is the result of an electrical impulse traveling through the heart, causing depolarization of the atria and ventricles (Fig. 28-1). Viewing the electrocardiogram (ECG) complex allows us to distinguish normal electrical conduction from cardiac ectopy, or abnormal electrical conduction. The P wave of the ECG complex represents atrial contraction. The P–R interval represents the hold time of the atrioventricular node. The QRS represents ventricular contraction. Knowing this helps us determine where in the electrical pathway the disruption occurs, thus better identifying the type of arrhythmia.

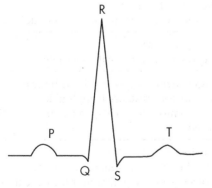

Figure 28-1 The electrocardiogram complex represents the electrical impulse traveling through the cardiac conductive pathway.

During sleep, heart rates of greater than 90 bpm indicate tachycardia, whereas a heart rate of less than 40 bpm indicates bradycardia (24). P waves of variable morphology indicate an atrial arrhythmia such as premature atrial contraction, atrial flutter, or atrial fibrillation. Atrial, or narrow complex, arrhythmias are generally not life-threatening. The technologist should document any occurrence in the technologist notes or study summary. The medical director must be notified if the patient becomes symptomatic, experiencing dizziness, light-headedness, syncope, cyanosis, or dyspnea.

A normal P–R interval has a duration of 0.12 to 0.20 seconds. An elongated P–R interval indicates a heart block. Varying degrees of heart blocks may be present. The normal duration of the QRS complex is 0.04 to 0.12 seconds. A longer, or wider, QRS segment indicates ventricular ectopy. Ventricular arrhythmias include premature ventricular contractions (PVCs), ventricular tachycardia, and ventricular fibrillation. Occasional PVCs are not uncommon and should be noted. Ventricular tachycardia and ventricular fibrillation are life-threatening. The technologist must activate the emergency medical system (EMS) and initiate cardiopulmonary resuscitation (CPR).

A pause of 3 seconds or greater between beats is considered an episode of asystole (24). In the event of a cardiac or respiratory arrest, the patient care staff is responsible for activating the EMS and administering CPR until the emergency medical personnel arrive (Table 28-6). Use mouthpieces, resuscitation bags, or other ventilation devices as an alternative to mouth-to-mouth resuscitation methods (4). Refer to Chapter 40 for more detail on arrhythmias.

The association between sleep apnea and systemic hypertension, stroke, congestive heart failure, and myocardial infarction has become more evident. Sudden cardiac arrest is the major complication of cardiovascular disease. The American Heart Association (AHA) has defined separate *chains of survival* for in-hospital and out-of-hospital events to summarize the present understanding of the best approach to the treatment of persons with sudden cardiac arrest (25). The chain of survival consists of five links:

1. *Surveillance and Prevention*
   - Recognize at-risk patients and have necessary equipment available to resuscitate if needed.
2. *Call for help*
   - Recognize the warning signs of heart attack or stroke and activate the EMS by calling 911 or code blue where available.
3. *Initiate CPR*
   - Immediate high-quality CPR increases positive outcomes. Compress the chest 2 in (5 cm) at a rate of 100 to 120 per minute. Allow for full recoil of the chest between compressions. Deliver 2 breaths after 30 compressions. Repeat as needed.

Table 28-6 **Medical Emergency Response**

Emergency Situation	Response
• Chest pain, neck, jaw, or arm pain	• Initiate 2 L/min O_2 through nasal cannula. • Call the medical director. • Monitor the patient.
• Mild-to-moderate difficulty breathing	• Call the medical director. • Monitor the patient.
• Severe difficulty breathing	• Activate EMS. • Monitor the patient.
• Seizures without cardiac arrest	• Turn the patient on the side in case of vomiting. • Call the medical director. • Remain at the bedside to monitor and protect the patient.
• Symptoms of stroke, that is, paralysis, weakness of limbs, difficulty speaking, difficulty comprehending	• Activate EMS. • Monitor the patient.
• Nausea/vomiting	• Provide emesis basin for patient. • Call the medical director.
• Fall/injury	• Call the lead technologist. • Complete the incident report.
• SpO_2 below 80% on 4 L/min of oxygen	• Awaken the patient. • Call the medical director. • Monitor the patient.
• Ventricular tachycardia for 10 s or more	• Awaken the patient. • Call the medical director. • Monitor the patient.
• Runs of premature ventricular contractions (six or more) occurring three or more times	• Awaken the patient. • Call the medical director. • Monitor the patient.
• Tachycardia 120 bpm or more over a minute or more or not associated with periods of apnea	• Awaken the patient. • Call the medical director. • Monitor the patient.
• Bradycardia <40 bpm over a minute or longer or not associated with periods of apnea	• Awaken the patient. • Call the medical director. • Monitor the patient.
• No electrocardiographic activity	• Assess the patient. • Activate EMS—first tech. • Begin cardiopulmonary resuscitation—additional staff.
• Parasomnia mobility (sleepwalking, active night terrors)	• Maintain patient safety. • Call security for assistance if applicable.
• Psychiatric emergency	• Maintain patient safety—remain with the patient. • Call security for assistance if applicable. • Visually monitor the suicidal patient until the situation is resolved.
• Grand mal seizures	• Activate EMS. • Go to the bedside to maintain patient safety. • Avoid placing anything in or near the patient's mouth. • Roll the patient on the side to prevent aspiration. • Document clinical observations.

EMS, emergency medical system.

4. *Provide defibrillation*
   - The interval between collapse and defibrillation is critical for successful conversion from ventricular fibrillation to a normal heart rhythm. Every minute that passes reduces the chance of survival. Without CPR and defibrillation, few attempts at resuscitation are successful. Automatic external defibrillators (AEDs) are easy to use and provide automatic recognition of a shockable cardiac arrhythmia. Voice commands warn before a shock is administered.
5. *Advanced life support and postarrest care*
   - Advanced cardiac life support provides equipment to support ventilation, establishes intravenous access, administers drugs, and controls arrhythmias.

These links are interdependent and must all be strong to increase the patient's chance of survival.

Warning signs of heart attack include lingering chest discomfort; discomfort in other areas of the upper body such as arms, back, neck, or stomach; sweating; nausea/vomiting; shortness of breath; and light-headedness. These signs may develop in persons of any age or sex, at any time or place. Signs and symptoms of acute stroke include alterations in consciousness (seizures, confusion, delirium, stupor, or coma), intense or unusually severe headache, incoherent speech, facial weakness, poor balance/clumsiness, visual loss, intense vertigo, double vision, unilateral hearing loss, and nausea or vomiting.

Sleep center personnel are first responders for medical emergencies. It is imperative that technologists are certified in CPR and are trained to recognize a change in a patient's condition that may be life-threatening (Table 28-7).

Table 28-7 | **American Heart Association 2016: Summary of Health Care Provider Basic Life Support Components for Adults, Adolescents, Children, and Infants**

	Adults/Adolescents	Children, Age 1 to Puberty	Infant, <1 y, Excluding Newborns
	Secure the scene, making it safe for victim and rescuers.		
Assessing patient	Check for responsiveness No breathing or gasping only No pulse (check for at least 5 s; no >10 s)		
Activate emergency response	Call for help Get AED Begin CPR		
Hand placement	Two hands on the lower half of the sternum	One or two hands on the lower half of the sternum	Two fingers in the center of the chest just below the nipple line
Compressions–ventilation ratio	30:2 (one rescuer)		
	30:2 (two rescuers)	15:2 (two rescuers)	
Compression rate	At least 100–120/min		
Compressions depth	2 in (5 cm)		1½ in (4 cm)
Chest recoil	Allow full recoil of the chest after each compression.		
AED—defibrillation	Use adult pads. Apply AED immediately for a witnessed arrest and CPR for an unwitnessed arrest.	Use AED after five cycles of CPR or as soon as AED is available. Use pediatric pads if available and adults pads if needed. Ensure pads do not touch one another. Use anterior/posterior pad placement as needed.	
Airway	Head tilt—chin lift		
Breathing, initial	Give 2 breaths • Each over 1 s • Visible chest rise with each breath • Resume compressions in <10 s		
Rescue breathing rate	1 every 5–6 s	1 every 3–5 s	

AED, automatic external defibrillator; CPR, cardiopulmonary resuscitation.

In 2010, the AHA changed the emphasis of CPR away from assessment and more toward action, changing the A-B-Cs (airway, breathing, and circulation) to C-A-Bs (circulation, airway, and breathing). The survivability rate is 40% to 70% when CPR is performed and an AED is utilized in the first 3 to 5 minutes postarrest (26). Compress the victim's chest at least 100 times per minute with enough force to circulate blood to the brain (see Table 28-6). Every interruption in chest compressions stops blood flow to the brain, which can lead to brain death. Cease compressions only long enough to allow the AED to analyze a cardiac rhythm or to deliver two breaths. Immediately resume compressions. It takes several compressions to get the blood moving again. Consider "hands-only CPR" if protective or airway equipment is not available. Reassess the victim every 2 minutes to evaluate the need for continued efforts.

Attach a defibrillator to the bare chest of anyone needing CPR, ensuring the pads do not touch. If the victim has an implantable pacemaker or port where the pads should reside, place the pad 1 in (2.5 cm) below the device. Dry-shave a hairy chest before placing the pads. Follow the AED voice prompts. The AED shocks for ventricular fibrillation only.

Pediatric adaptable AEDs are available. These use either pediatric pads or a dose attenuator adapter. If you are in a situation where a child requires CPR and no pediatric AED pads are available, use adult pads, but be sure that the pads do not touch. For a small child, place one pad on the sternum and the second pad on the victim's back between the shoulder blades.

Seizures

A seizure is a sudden discharge of electrical activity in the brain. There are two broad categories of seizures: generalized and partial (also called local or focal). Generalized seizures broadcast across the entire brain, whereas a small area of the brain produces partial seizures. Symptoms may include a brief loss of consciousness, lip smacking, chewing, muscle rigidity, spasms, or convulsions. The duration of a seizure may be several seconds to several minutes.

The technologist's response to patient seizure activity will vary according to the type of seizure occurring. The technologist's responsibility is to keep the patient safe. Knowing the patient history and the manifestation of the seizure will help with preparedness. Pad the headboard and use padded side rails as necessary. During grand mal seizures, also known as generalized tonic–clonic seizures, go to the patient bedside to keep the patient safe by turning him or her on the side to prevent aspiration. Never attempt to restrain a patient or to stop his or her movement, and never place any object in or near the patient's mouth.

Document clinical observations such as the duration of seizure, cyanosis, diaphoresis, movement type, and involvement. Speak calmly and reassuringly to the patient during and after the event. Give nothing by mouth until the patient is fully alert. Activate EMS if the seizure lasts 5 minutes or longer or if one seizure occurs right after another without the person regaining consciousness between seizures, seizures occur closer together than usual for that person, breathing becomes difficult, or the person appears to be choking.

VIOLENT PATIENTS

Although uncommon, the sleep technologist may encounter an aggressive or violent patient in the sleep center setting. The best way to reduce the chances of such an encounter is through careful screening of patients before a sleep study. However, to ensure the safety of the patient and the staff, it is important for sleep technologists to understand how to handle inappropriate behavior.

Aggression may take the form of angry shouting or accusing others of wrongdoing. Aggression may also involve physical violence such as breaking objects or harming others (27). When working with patients who have a history of mental illness or dementia, it is recommended that a familiar caregiver stays with the patient. Some individuals may be easily confused and suspicious that others are trying to do them harm. A recognizable caregiver may ward off such suspicions. Other causes of violence include delusions or hallucinations, reactions to drugs, and pain. Medication may reduce aggression and violence. On the contrary, medications that calm the patient may produce sleepiness or increase confusion (28).

Many patients who become violent are not violent from the moment they come through the door. A patient should be provided with alternatives to correct inappropriate behavior to enable him or her to maintain a good working relationship with the technologist and also dignity (27). There are a number of important things to keep in mind in order to avoid escalating a potentially violent situation. Some suggested methods of working with potentially violent patients include the following:

1. Avoid eye contact with the patient.
2. Do not block exits and leave the door to room open.
3. Maintain distance from a potentially violent patient; do not invade the patient's "space."
4. Adopt a passive, nonconfrontational posture and attitude, and allow the patient to ventilate feelings.
5. Develop a therapeutic alliance with the patient.
6. Treat the patient as you expect him or her to behave.
7. Offer food or drink.
8. Do not make challenging, provocative, or belligerent remarks.

9. If the patient acts out, tell him or her directly "your behavior is frightening others and we cannot allow such behavior."
10. Do not turn your back on a potentially violent patient.
11. Never underestimate the potential for violence.

If a situation arises in which the technologist feels uncomfortable with the patient, the former should call security and/or send the latter home.

Policies and procedures for training staff to recognize escalating behavior that might lead to violence and to assess and report threats allow employers to track and follow up on threats and violent incidents in the workplace. Training employees in nonviolent conflict resolution, cultural/ethical diversity training, and how to handle complaints will help alleviate behavior that could escalate to physical violence.

SUMMARY

Federal, state, and local agencies and accrediting bodies have developed guidelines to ensure the safety of all individuals visiting or working in the health care setting. A written emergency and safety plan will ensure that each employee understands the practices required to maintain the highest level of safety. It is the responsibility of each member of the health care team to understand and implement safety standards in order to prevent accident, injury, or illness from occurring.

REFERENCES

1. American Academy of Sleep Medicine. (2016). *Standards for accreditation of a sleep disorders center* (p. 20). Retrieved from http://www.aasmnet.org/Resources/PDF/AASMcenteraccredstandards.pdf
2. Centers for Disease Control and Prevention. (1998). Guidelines for infection control in health care personnel. *American Journal of Infection Control, 26*(3), 289–354.
3. United States Department of Labor. (2015). *OSHA QuickCard*. Retrieved February 10, 2018, from https://www.osha.gov/Publications/HazComm_QuickCard_SafetyData.html
4. OSHA Bloodborne Pathogen Standard. (n.d.). *Title 29 Code of Federal Regulation, Part 1910.1030*. Washington, DC: US Department of Labor.
5. Centers for Disease Control and Prevention. (1996). *Isolation precaution: Guideline for isolation precautions in hospitals*. Retrieved from http://www.cdc.gov/hicpac/2007IP/2007isolationPrecautions.html
6. Centers for Disease Control and Prevention. (2003). *Exposure to blood: What healthcare personnel need to know*. Washington, DC: Department of Health and Human Services, CDC. Retrieved July 2003, from https://www.cdc.gov/HAI/pdfs/bbp/Exp_to_Blood.pdf
7. Hobby, M. K. (2011). Requirements and techniques for cleaning equipment in the sleep lab. *A2Zzz, 20*(2), 24.
8. Centers for Disease Control and Prevention. (1987). Recommendations for prevention of HIV transmission in health-care settings. *Morbidity and Mortality Weekly Report, 36*(2S), 1S–18S.
9. Rutala, W. A., & Weber, D. J. (2008). MPH and the Healthcare Infection Control Practices Advisory Committee (HICPAC), *Guideline for Disinfection and Sterilization in Healthcare Facilities*. Centers for Disease Control, ©US Department of Health and Human Services. Retrieved from https://www.cdc.gov/infection-control/pdf/guidelines/disinfection-guidelines.pdf
10. Jones-Parker, M. (2005). Technical corner. *A2Zzz, 13*(4), 15.
11. Weber, D. J., & Rutala, W. A. (1993). Environmental issues and nosocomial infections. In R. P. Wenzel (Ed.), *Prevention and control of nosocomial infections* (2nd ed., pp. 420–449). Baltimore, MD: Williams and Wilkins.
12. United States Environmental Protection Agency. (1995). *The hazardous waste system* (p. ES-2). Washington, DC: Office of Solid Waste and Emergency Response.
13. Occupational Safety and Health Administration. (1997). *Hazardous waste operations and emergency response* (OSHA Publication No. 3114). Washington, DC: United States Department of Labor.
14. Apts, D. W. (1992). *Back injury prevention handbook*. Boca Raton, FL: Lewis Publishers.
15. National Institute on Occupational Safety and Health. (1996). *Back belts—Do they prevent injury?* (DHHS Publication No. 94-127). Retrieved from http://www.cdc.gov/niosh/docs/94-127/
16. OSHA Occupation Safety and Health Administration. (2002). *OSHA fact sheet*. Retrieved from http://www.osha.gov/OshDoc/data_General_Facts/FireSafetyN.pdf
17. Occupational Safety and Health Standards. (n.d.). *Exit routes, emergency action plans, and fire prevention plans. Title 29, Subpart E, Part 1910*. Retrieved from https://www.osha.gov/Publications/osha3088.html
18. Occupational Safety and Health Standards. (2001). *How to plan for workplace emergencies and evacuation* (OSHA 3088). Washington, DC: US Department of Labor.
19. *Time for healthcare reform: Hospital accreditation, blind spot, blinders or worse?* (2009). Washington, DC. Retrieved from https://www.osha.gov/laws-regs/federalregister/2016-12-07
20. Fire Extinguisher: 101. (n.d.). *Fire hazards (fire prevention tips)*. Retrieved from http://www.fire-extinguisher101.com/hazards.html

21. Seaba, P. J. (1984). Electrical safety. *American Journal of EEG Technology, 24*(1), 11–27.

22. Garneski, T. M. (1961). Electricity and electronics: Part I. *American Journal of EEG Technology, 1*(2), 51–56.

23. Occupational Safety and Health Administration. (1997). *Controlling electrical hazards* (OSHA Publication No. 3075). Washington, DC: United States Department of Labor.

24. Berry, R. B., Albertario, C. L., Harding, S. M, et al.; for the American Academy of Sleep Medicine. (2018). *The AASM manual for the scoring of sleep and associated events: Rules, terminology and technical specifications* [Version 2.5]. Darien, IL: American Academy of Sleep Medicine.

25. American Heart Association. (2010). *Basic life support for healthcare providers*. Dallas, TX: Author

26. American Heart Association. (2010). *CPR guidelines*. Dallas, TX: Author.

27. Hepburn, K. (1989). *Special care problems: Aggressive and violent behavior*. Minneapolis, MN: United States Department of Veterans Affairs, Veterans Health Services and Research Administration, Office of Geriatrics and Extended Care.

28. Allen, M. H., Currier, G. W., Hughes, D. H., et al.; Expert Consensus Panel for Behavioral Emergencies. (2001). The expert consensus guideline series: Treatment of behavioral emergencies. *Postgraduate Medical Specialties* (Spec No), 1–88.

chapter 29
Patient Interviewing and Assessment

KIMBERLY A. TROTTER

LEARNING OBJECTIVES

On completion of this chapter, the reader should be able to:

1. Review patient chart documentation including physician order, history, and physical examination.
2. Explain the principles of interviewing and observing the patient to assess special physical, cognitive, or emotional needs.
3. Orient the patient to the facility utilizing appropriate technologist–patient interaction.
4. Recognize patients with special needs (mental age, physical, or emotional discomfort) and assess patients' readiness to learn and their ability to cooperate.
5. Determine the need for any special precautions or special testing considerations (prosthetic devices, electromechanical devices, etc.).
6. Review protocols; analyze and respond to unclear, inappropriate, or contradictory orders.
7. Identify the patient's current sleep schedule, recent caffeine or alcohol intake, and current medications.
8. Orient the patient to the facility and testing procedure.
9. Interview the patient during the setup to clarify any gaps in history or symptoms identified during chart review.
10. Document any special needs identified or pertinent clinical information in the patient's chart.
11. Discuss positive airway pressure and other therapeutic modalities with the patient.
12. Assist with pre- and postprocedure questionnaires and follow-up processes.

KEY TERMS

Patient questionnaire
Patient orientation
Verbal interview
Readiness to learn
Patient assessment
Sleep pattern
Mental age

Prosthetic devices
Physical limitations
Emotional needs
Appropriateness of protocol
Universal precautions
Sundowning
Forensic patients

It is a new encounter every night when the sleep technologist comes to perform a polysomnography (PSG) and reviews a patient's chart for the first time. The technologist may not know anything about the patient he or she is about to see. Perhaps a sleep consultation was performed before the PSG; however, the needs of the patient have to be evaluated during the initial meeting in the sleep center by the technologist. Sometimes clinical notes are not as exact as we would like them to be. If the sleep consultation was completed by the referring physician, it may be vague and general. This is why patient interviewing and assessment is so important in making the most of the sleep study and, most importantly, making sure that the patient's accommodations are met.

CHART REVIEW

It is important for the daytime sleep technologists or chief technologist to review all charts before the night shift, because there may be special testing or equipment that needs to be set up before the night shift arrives. Once the nighttime sleep technologist arrives, he or she should thoroughly review the chart.

The chart should contain a recent history and physical (H&P). This is a report of the patient's general health status, regular medications, past surgeries, and family history. The H&P can come from the primary care physician or referring physician. Reviewing this information is helpful to understand the patient's general status. If the patient is a "direct referral," meaning he or she bypasses a sleep consultation and workup with the sleep specialist and is referred directly for a sleep study, then a comprehensive H&P, with sleep specific information, is very important and is required by the American Academy of Sleep Medicine standards of accreditation.

The sleep consultation is an integral part of the chart, and because it is sleep specific, it should be reviewed by the sleep technologist. Information such as sleep medications, sleep schedule, chief complaint, and family sleep history should all be addressed in the sleep consultation. During the consultation, a sleep questionnaire, sleepiness scale, and a sleep diary that usually consists of 2 weeks of data are usually obtained.

If the patient was referred directly to the sleep disorders center by the referring physician, the sleep questionnaire may be administered to the patient upon his or her arrival at the sleep center. The technologist will need to assess whether the patient is able to read, understand, and answer the questions. The technologist may need to assist the patient by asking the questions. Once the sleep questionnaire is filled out, then the technologist will have information he or she can use for determining what degree of special or accommodating treatment the patient may need. The technologist must make sure that the patient is able to fill out the pre- and postquestionnaires, as well, and assist if necessary.

The physician order form must be included in each PSG patient chart. It must be signed and must give clear instructions regarding what type of procedures are to be performed. It must also be clear if the patient has any special needs or considerations for his or her care. This documentation is very important to the technologist and, consequently, to the patient.

MEETING AND ASSESSING THE PATIENT

As mentioned, the sleep technologist is at a disadvantage before he or she first meets the patient, unless the former has prior information that he or she can review. Meeting and assessing the patient may be the only information he or she gets as far as special needs or considerations are concerned.

Visual Assessment

Visual assessment occurs when the sleep technologist first meets the patient. How is he or she dressed? Is the patient alert or sleeping in the chair? Does the patient seem nervous or relaxed? Are there any visible challenges?

Readiness to Learn

Once the formal introductions are made, and you escort the patient to the sleep room, it is time to check his or her readiness to learn. Readiness to learn is a phrase used to determine by casual interview of the patient if he or she is ready to learn. Obstacles to readiness to learn

include feeling nervous, being too sleepy to listen and participate in a conversation or presentation, not understanding the language, or not paying attention. Other reasons include diminished intellect and hearing loss.

Mental Age

Mental age is defined as the age level the patient functions at mentally or intellectually. Does he or she seem to understand simple words and phrases? Does the patient act like he or she is 13 years old, when he or she is really 35? This is important information, so the sleep technologist can simplify his or her presentation to the patient if necessary, assuring the patient will be able to understand the process and cooperate better.

Physical Limitations

Many times, physical limitations will be obvious when you first greet the patient. This valuable information may also be found in the patient's chart, the physician order form, sleep questionnaire, or consultation notes. If the patient was referred directly to the sleep center and the referring physician conducted the sleep consultation, this information may not be available because the referring physician is familiar with the patient and may not consider it an issue for the sleep technologist. This can result in a challenge for the technologist.

Emotional Needs

Emotional needs may be the most difficult to determine. If the patient seems withdrawn or distant, it will be a difficult night for both the sleep technologist and the patient, unless the technologist is able to break through and reach the patient, making him or her feel more comfortable and assured. Sometimes emotional needs are related to mental age; the patient may be immature and may need a lot of reassuring and attention. It is important to note that sometimes patients will act out in order to receive this added attention. In cases like this, the sleep technologist needs to set boundaries with the amount of attention and service he or she can give the patient. This is important when the sleep technologist is monitoring two patients because if he or she is overly busy with one patient, then the other patient suffers.

PATIENT ORIENTATION PROCESSES

Facility Orientation

When the patient arrives, escort him or her to the bedroom and show other pertinent areas of the facility that he or she may want to use, such as the bathroom, showers, and areas to store food. Show the patient how to operate the TV and fans. Allow them the opportunity to ask questions.

Patient Confidentiality and Patient Rights

The Health Insurance Portability and Accountability Act of 1996 regulations require each patient to sign an acknowledgment of receipt of patient confidentiality regulations. If this is the patient's first visit to the center and he or she has not previously signed this form, this must be collected by the technologist. Many facilities, particularly hospitals, also make a copy of information pertaining to patient rights and responsibilities available to the patient.

Procedure Consent

In many sleep centers, the technologist may have the patient review and sign a consent form, which describes the procedure. If the patient is to be videotaped, the technologist may obtain consent for this as well.

Recognizing and Accommodating Patients with Special Emotional Needs

Once the sleep technologist has had time to assess the patient's emotional needs, it is time to work with the patient to obtain the best PSG.

What Are Special Emotional Needs?

Special emotional needs are related to patients with disorders that include posttraumatic stress disorder (PTSD), depression, panic attacks, claustrophobia, and more serious mental illnesses. As stated previously, mental age can play a part in relation to special emotional needs.

The sleep technologist must develop strategies for dealing with these types of patients. For patients with PTSD, it is important to find out the best way to communicate with them during the night, and more importantly, the best way to wake them up should the technologist need to adjust sensors or apply positive airway pressure (PAP). Waking a patient with PTSD the wrong way can result in injury to the technologist! Ask the patient before lights out how he or she should be awakened. Some patients may prefer being awakened using the intercom, and others may need the light on and to be called from the doorway. A night light may also be appropriate.

PAP titration for these patients, as well as patients with claustrophobia, can be tricky, and these patients should be treated with caution and great care. Always allow the patient to be in control of the mask on the face. If the patient starts feeling panicky (a common

symptom of PTSD), then he or she can take the mask off the face and try again later. Always remind the patient to breathe slowly, focusing on breathing out. A full-face mask, which equalizes the positive pressure delivered between the nose and the mouth allowing the patient to breathe with the mouth open, may be helpful. Sometimes a nasal mask or nasal pillows can make the patient feel less claustrophobic. Nasal pillows or other types of small masks that do not touch the patient's face can be less restrictive and more comfortable. The technologist's impressions should always be documented in the patient's chart.

Depression is not evident in all patients, but in patients who seem down or disengaged, it is important to identify possible depression. It is important to note that the technologist is not licensed to diagnose the patient, but to merely document his or her impressions. Dealing with depressed patients is not easy, and the technologist should try to be sensitive to the patient's needs. Spending extra time with the depressed patient is important, especially if he or she seems withdrawn about the procedure.

Some patients may tell the technologist that they have panic attacks at night. These panic attacks may be related to obstructive sleep apnea (OSA) or PTSD. Assure such patients that you are nearby should they feel anxious.

The best way to handle the patient with a mental disorder is to be calm and not argumentative. Being argumentative with such patients can challenge their reality and can provoke them. Ideally, the medical director or sleep physician would have screened out unstable patients and you will not see them in the sleep center until they are stable. If the technologist feels threatened in any way, he or she should immediately leave the room and contact security if available, contact the medical director, or call 9-1-1. A technologist should never allow a patient to stand between him or her and the exit of the room. A sleep center policy for these types of situations should be available.

Recognizing and Accommodating Patients with Special Physical Needs

Patients who come to the sleep center with physical disabilities can be a challenge for the technologist. The referring physician should mention these disabilities in the H&P or consultation notes. If the patient is severely disabled, then it is important that a caregiver be present for the entire sleep study to assist with lifting and other personal needs.

If the patient has a prosthetic device or some other type of device necessary for mobility, the technologist must be aware of such devices and work around the device during the setup. If the patient has a prosthetic leg, the electromyographic electrodes must be placed on the leg above the prosthetic device or on the forearms for the detection of periodic limb movement disorder. If a patient has a prosthetic eye, it is important to document this information in the patient's chart, the technologist notes, and on the record, especially during patient calibrations when the patient moves the eyes to check the eye movement–monitoring electrodes.

If the patient has an unusually shaped head or has a plate or cover over a part of the skull, the technologist must modify the 10 to 20 electrode placement and document in the patient chart and in the technologist notes.

Infection control is another important area for using precautions with patients. If the patient is incontinent, then the technologist must know how to deal with body fluids properly. An in-service on infection control techniques by the hospital's infection control nurse is important, so that the technologist knows how to protect himself or herself and the patient. The same is true if the patient uses intravenous medications during the sleep study or even if the patient has a severe productive cough. Universal precautions (gloves and protective wear) must be strictly followed for all patients but are particularly important for patients requiring special precautions.

If the patient complains of pain, discomfort, or anxiety, immediate interventions are needed. The technologist must check on the patient, assess the situation, and determine a solution. The solution might be calling the ordering physician to get input or to have the physician talk to the patient over the phone to calm and reassure him or her. If the sleep center is in a hospital, it may involve paging the on-call physician, so he or she can evaluate the patient and determine if there is any risk in continuing the study. Some patients may need to end the study and be taken or sent to the emergency department for further evaluation and treatment.

OTHER CHALLENGES

Sundowning

Sometimes older patients can present as normal and fully functional during the daytime for the sleep consultation, but at night, they may exhibit "sundowning." Patients showing signs of sundowning become confused and agitated during the early evening. Patients with sundowning can be a challenge to work with. If a patient is known to have sundowning, then he or she should be required to bring a loved one or attendant for the sleep study. If the sundowning comes as a "surprise" to the technologist, then the technologist should calmly talk to the patient, with the lights on, so the patient can become accustomed to the surroundings and remember

that he or she is at the sleep center. If the patient continues to fight the testing procedure and becomes aggressive and agitated, then the technologist will have no other choice but to call a family member or caregiver to pick up the patient. This situation can be dangerous to the technologist who is not trained to deal with dementia or sundowning.

Violent/Inappropriate Behaviors

If a patient becomes violent or abusive to the technologist, be it verbal abuse, sexual innuendo, or physical movements or action, the technologist should immediately address the situation: Does the technologist feel physically threatened? If so, the technologist should leave the patient's room immediately and follow the sleep center policy, which may include calling security or the local police. If the technologist feels that the patient is being inappropriate, a technologist switch (if there is more than one technologist working) is usually the best first step and is usually successful in stopping such behavior. Simply have another technologist (same sex as patient) come in and assume care of the patient. If the patient is reminded that he or she is being videotaped, inappropriate behavior usually stops as well.

Forensic Patients

Another situation that appears to be dangerous, but is actually the safest of all patient interactions, is dealing with the forensic patient. Incarcerated patients, or forensic patients, are those who are brought in from prison for a sleep study. These patients are secured in shackles and are accompanied by two guards who remain in the sleep center for the entire night. Other than the shackles getting in the way of the hookup, and the space needed for two guards and a patient in one room, there is little threat. If the sleep center is in a hospital setting, then the hospital will have its own policy on forensic patients. Most policies involve contacting security on the day of the study and having the forensic patient and guards check in and out with security upon arrival and after the sleep study. It is important to be sensitive to the other patients by rooming the forensic patient, if possible, before others arrive.

Diabetes

Some medical disorders, such as diabetes, may involve the patient requiring medications and food during the night. Simply allow the patient to do what he or she needs to do, as if he or she were at home. It is, however, important that the patient be reminded to bring regular medication, supplies, and snacks for his or her sleep study because most sleep centers are outpatient based, with no readily available sources of food or medications. If the patient uses injections, the syringes will need to be disposed of properly.

Language Barriers

If the sleep center is in a geographic area with multicultural influences, the technologist is likely to see patients who do not speak English. If this is a recurring theme in the sleep center, the patient should bring an interpreter or family member who speaks English, and that person should remain with the patient for the entire sleep study to assure that the technologist can communicate with the patient. Another option is using a language line service. If the patient requires PAP during the night, the patient most likely will not understand the equipment or process being initiated without an interpreter present.

REVIEW PHYSICIAN ORDERS

When reviewing the chart, the physician orders need to make sense to the technologist. After assessing the patient, the technologist should ask himself or herself the question: Are the orders appropriate? If the orders are unclear or they are inappropriate or contradictory, it is important to contact the medical director to confirm the order or request a change in procedure. It is important to note that when a revised order is taken over the phone it must be documented, dated, and timed, and the sleep physician must sign the revised order the next day. This is easily completed, because most sleep centers use an electronic health record (EHR), which can be accessible securely and remotely.

ORIENT PATIENT TO TEST PROCEDURE

Explain PSG Protocol to Patient

Educating the patient about the setup and monitoring process will help the patient feel more at ease with the procedure. Explain that a PSG is a test that records various physiologic signals during sleep, and testing may vary on the basis of individual patient needs and physician's orders. Describe what the PSG measures, and the sensors as you apply them. A common concern voiced by patients is that they may be unable to sleep with all the monitoring leads attached. A reassuring response to this concern may be, "surprisingly, most people sleep very well. After a period of adjustment, you easily forget about the electrodes. All the attachments are made in such a way as to provide easy movement during sleep." Document how the patient feels about undergoing the PSG and his or her level of cooperation with the procedure.

Discuss Therapeutic Modalities

The most common therapeutic procedure technologists perform during PSG is PAP titration for sleep-related breathing disorders. The technologist has an important role in the orientation of the patient to the PAP device because the patient's first impression and experience with the device is likely to be very influential with his or her compliance. The patient should be shown and allowed to handle the equipment. Many centers utilize educational DVDs or YouTube videos, which are readily available through PAP equipment manufacturers. It is best to fit the patient and let the patient apply the PAP mask and experience PAP at a low level for a short trial period before the beginning of the study. This will avoid waking the patient to fit the mask or working with a sleepy, disoriented patient on becoming accustomed to the feel of the PAP therapy during the night.

The patient may display poor sleep hygiene, such as watching late night TV, or eating or drinking throughout the night. This should be documented in the chart, and good sleep hygiene education can be performed by the sleep technologist following the sleep study.

PATIENT–TECHNOLOGIST INTERVIEW

Patient Questionnaire

Most sleep centers require the patient to complete a sleep-focused questionnaire that is reviewed by the technologist. The technologist should discuss key notes in the questionnaire with the patient and clarify any incomplete or missing information. Ask for a brief history of medical illnesses and compare the patient's response with the physician consult notes. Patients often forget to discuss certain problems with their physician. A review of medications is also necessary, keeping in mind that many medications affect electroencephalographic patterns. The questionnaire has a section for additional technologist notes from this technologist–patient interview. The questionnaire may be your primary tool for understanding your patient and his or her needs, especially if he or she is a direct referral, with an abbreviated H&P.

Presleep Questionnaire

After you ask the patient to complete a presleep questionnaire (Fig. 29-1), review his or her responses and ask for missing information. This questionnaire generally reviews caffeine or alcohol intake, medications, physical complaints, sleep within the previous 24 hours, and unusual aspects of the day's activities. It may also include a sleepiness scale (Tables 29-1 and 29-2). For patients returning for a subsequent sleep study, further information

Name: _____   Date: _____

How many hours of sleep did you have last night? _____

How many hours do you normally have? _____

Did you take any naps today?   Yes   No

If yes, how long did you nap? _____ minutes

Did you get your normal amount of exercise today?   Yes   No

If no, why not? _____

Has today been an unusual day in any respect?   Yes   No

If yes, please explain: _____

_____

_____

Do you have any physical discomfort now?   Yes   No

If yes, what? _____

If you had alcohol, coffee, tea, or soft drinks today, specify amounts and times:

Type	Amount	Time
_____	_____	_____
_____	_____	_____
_____	_____	_____
_____	_____	_____

List all medications you took today:

Medications	Amount	Time
_____	_____	_____
_____	_____	_____
_____	_____	_____

Figure 29-1 Presleep questionnaire.

should be obtained regarding interim treatments, change in medications, or changes in sleep patterns.

Verbal Interview

In addition to the patient questionnaire, there are a number of verbal questions (Fig. 29-2) the technologist may ask the patient in order to get a clearer picture of his or her sleep habits and sleep problems. If the bed partner is present, obtain his or her input during the written or verbal interview. Many sleep problems, such as snoring or cessation of breathing, are not evident to the patient, and the bed partner is able to give a more objective assessment of these symptoms.

The best way for a technologist to begin the verbal interview is to discuss the patient's nighttime routine before bedtime. Assess whether the patient may have

special needs. Ask if there are any specific physical or psychological discomforts that may prevent a patient from achieving a normal night's sleep. If you are planning a PAP titration, ask if the patient has nasal congestion or blockage.

Patient Interaction/Interview during Testing

Reassure the patient that he or she can contact you at any time during the night using the intercom or call bell. If a patient is restless and not sleeping, check to see if he or she needs something to make him or her more comfortable and make sure that the patient's needs are met.

If the patient has difficulty tolerating initiation of PAP therapy, take the time to determine if there is a

Table **29-1** Stanford Sleepiness Scale

Degree of Sleepiness	Scale Rating
Feeling active, vital, alert, or wide awake	1
Functioning at high levels, but not at peak; able to concentrate	2
Awake, but relaxed; responsive, but not fully alert	3
Somewhat foggy, let down	4
Foggy; losing interest in remaining awake; slowed down	5
Sleepy, woozy, fighting sleep; prefer to lie down	6
No longer fighting sleep, sleep onset soon; having dream-like thoughts	7
Asleep	X

Table **29-2** Epworth Sleepiness Scale

0 = Would *never* doze or sleep

1 = *Slight* chance of dozing or sleeping

2 = *Moderate* chance of dozing or sleeping

3 = *High* chance of dozing or sleeping

Situation	Chance of Dozing or Sleeping
Sitting and reading	_____
Watching TV	_____
Sitting inactive in a public place	_____
Being a passenger in a motor vehicle for an hour or more	_____
Lying down in the afternoon	_____
Sitting and talking to someone	_____
Stopped for a few minutes in traffic while driving	_____
Total score	_____
Score results	
1–6	Within normal limits
4–8	Moderately sleepy
9 and over	Excessively sleepy

physical barrier such as nasal blockage or if the patient simply cannot or does not want to use the device.

If the technologist notices a significant physiologic event, such as a possible seizure or cardiac event, the technologist must immediately go to the patient and assess his or her vital signs and cognitive status through verbal questioning. All events and patient responses must be documented.

Medications

The technologist must also confirm the patient's general medications and document the medications taken on the day of the study, including over-the-counter medicines, vitamins, supplements, caffeine, and alcohol intake. In most states, medications cannot be administered by a sleep technologist. Medications can be brought in by the patient and self-administered. The technologist must document what medications were taken, dosage, and time. Medications, especially sleeping medications that the patient may take before the testing, must be closely monitored. If a patient takes a sleeping medication and then wants to discontinue the study, the sleep center and technologist would be liable if the patient drove home incapacitated from the medication. If a patient takes sleeping medication, then wakes up during the night and wants to discontinue the sleep study, the technologist must ensure that the patient is driven home or stays until morning and is evaluated for driving ability before being released. Patients who appear okay after sleep testing should

be evaluated before they are allowed to drive home if they have taken a hypnotic. It is important for the sleep technologist to understand the half-life (how long a medication stays in the patient's system) of the most common sleeping medications, so he or she can determine when it is safe for a patient to drive himself or herself home.

Sleep Schedule

The sleep questionnaire should have a section dedicated to documentation of the patient's normal sleep schedule. The technologist should make sure that all sections of sleep questionnaires and logs are filled out completely. If the patient normally goes to bed at 2 a.m. and the technologist's schedule has him or her ending his or her shift at 7 a.m., then this is a problem. The patient should not feel obligated to fall asleep unusually earlier or be awakened earlier than his or her normal time. Accommodations should always be made for the patient's sleep schedule.

What activities does the patient undergo before bedtime?

Does the patient bath, brush teeth, or perform other grooming activities before bedtime?

Does the patient watch TV in bed?

Does the patient perform rigorous mental work just before bedtime?

Does the patient perform rigorous physical exercise in the 3 to 4 hours before bedtime?

What time does the patient usually retire/begin sleeping?

How long does it take the patient to fall asleep?

What time does the patient usually awaken in the morning?

How does the patient feel after awakening? Is he or she still sleepy?

Is the patient a restless sleeper?

Does the patient snore, choke, gasp, or breathe noisily at night?

Is the snoring/noisy breathing intermittent or continuous?

Has the patient been told that he or she stops breathing at night?

Does the patient typically arise to use the bathroom during the night?

Does the patient typically awaken during the evening? Why? How often?

Does the bed partner have complaints about the patient's sleep symptoms?

How many pillows do you sleep with?

Can you lie on your back?

Do you keep the TV on at night?

Are you tired during the day?

Do you nap during the day? How much?

Is the bed partner complaining of abnormal movements or sounds at night?

Does the patient kick his or her legs at night?

Does the patient suffer from insomnia?

Does the patient have nasal congestion?

Does the patient frequently have headaches in the morning?

Does the patient have a dry mouth in the morning?

Does the patient fall asleep at inappropriate times?

What time of day is it the hardest to stay awake?

Does the patient smoke?

What time does he or she get home from work?

What does the patient do after dinner?

Does the patient fall asleep watching TV or reading?

Figure 29-2 Interview questions.

Postsleep Questionnaire and Follow-Up Process

A postsleep questionnaire (Fig. 29-3) will assess pertinent details of the patient's sleep period. Before the patient leaves the facility, answer any questions, remembering to be careful to avoid discussing detailed diagnostic results with the patient. Ensure the patient is aware of the follow-up process he or she is to undergo with the physician.

Chart Documentation

If special needs are not documented in the patient chart, then it is the technologist's duty to document these needs.

Postprocedure Documentation and Follow-Up Processes

After the procedure, the technologist will need to verify that all the PSG forms have been completed and signed,

Name: _____   Date: _____

How long did it take you to fall asleep last night? _____

How long does it usually take you to fall asleep? _____

How many times do you remember waking up last night? _____

How many times do you usually wake up?   _____

How long were you awake during the night?   _____

How long do you feel you slept last night?   _____

How long do you usually sleep every night?   _____

How would you say your sleep last night compares with your typical night?

Better _____   Same _____   Worse _____

Were you bothered by sleeping in the lab?   Yes   No

If yes, please explain _____

_____

Did you get enough sleep?   Too little   Just right   Too much

Do you have any physical discomfort at the present time?   Yes   No

If yes, please explain _____

_____

Please add any additional comments you might have: _____

_____

_____

_____

_____

Figure 29-3 Postsleep questionnaire.

including any consent forms. The technologist will want to administer a postsleep questionnaire in the morning to get a sense of how the patient felt when he or she slept. This is a subjective measure. A technologist's preliminary assessment is also completed in the morning which the sleep physician will review while interpreting the sleep study. Most sleep centers use an EHR; therefore, the technologist's documentation can be reviewed immediately by the medical director, which is helpful for patients. Also, remote access to sleep studies is common.

There is a fine line related to what the technologist should tell the patient after sleep testing. The patient wants to know if he or she has a sleep disorder or not. If the diagnosis was OSA and the patient tried PAP during a split-night study, it is most likely that he or she has OSA; however, it is important to leave the diagnosis to the sleep physician. It is inappropriate for the technologist to diagnose the patient. The technologist can simply tell the patient that the sleep physician will review the sleep study and discuss the diagnosis and treatment options with him or her.

After the study is over and the patient has left, it is important to make sure that the patient has a follow-up scheduled with the sleep physician to go over results, initiate treatment, and track his or her treatment success.

A follow-up visit and compliance documentation are required by the Medicare and many insurance providers. Follow-ups are usually scheduled through the sleep center office staff once the patient has completed testing.

SUMMARY

It is very beneficial to the sleep testing and treatment process for the sleep technologist to gather as much pertinent information about the patient as possible. This information gathering begins before the patient's arrival through chart review and continues until the patient has completed his or her sleep study and left the center. The process begins with a thorough review of the patient's chart, where the technologist will review the patient's H&P and physician orders for the sleep study. When the patient arrives, the technologist must orient the patient to the sleep facility and testing process. The patient questionnaire must be reviewed by the technologist and clarified with the patient. The technologist can ask additional clarifying questions pertaining to the patient's sleep complaints and document any additional information obtained.

POLICY:	All patients scheduled for sleep studies will either be seen in consultation by a sleep physician of the center and have a history and physical (H&P) placed in the patient chart, or the case will be discussed by the sleep physician and the referring physician, with the H&P in the chart. Patients with certain limitations will not be seen at the center for a polysomnography (PSG), until their condition changes.
PROCEDURE:	Any patients who need a PSG must first be either seen by the sleep physician or the sleep physician must discuss the case with the referring physician before the PSG is done. If the patient has certain limitations, then the PSG will not be done until his or her condition changes. These limitations include the following:
	24-hour nursing care, including catheters, intravenous medication, glucose checks, severe incontinence, or anything that requires a nurse or orderly (lifting, bed pan, and diaper changes).
	Mentally diminished capacity that could interfere with the PSG, such as dementia, severe developmental delay, or other disorders.
	Patients who may need additional care, and the sleep physician knows will benefit from a PSG, may be studied only if attended by a nurse or attendant, who will be able to perform nursing or patient care duties, and not interfere with the PSG testing, or the technologist performing the testing.
	Patients who require an attendant, but do not have one present will be sent home after the sleep physician has been notified. Sleep technologists are not licensed or trained in nursing care.

Figure 29-4 Acceptance policy and procedure.

The patient entrusts the sleep center, sleep physician, and the sleep technologist with his or her care. As a technologist, our duty is to screen patients and determine they are well enough to obtain a safe and valid sleep study. The first screening step rests with the physician. If the technologist has any doubt or discomfort related to testing a patient with special needs and there is no documentation in the patient's chart, a call to the ordering physician may be in order. If a patient's special needs are beyond the scope of practice of the technologist, such as requirements for lifting, personal care, or assisting the patient in the bathroom, then a decision needs to be made as to whether it is safe and in the best interest of the patient to continue the study. An acceptance policy that outlines the types of patients accepted for a sleep study should be upheld (Fig. 29-4). A well-trained, competent technologist is the expectation of every patient.

RECOMMENDED READING

1. Butkov, N. (2010). *Atlas of clinical polysomnography* (2nd ed.). Medford, OR: Synapse Media.
2. Chokroverty, S. (2009). Approach to the patient with sleep complaints. In *Sleep disorders medicine: Basic science, technical considerations, and clinical aspects* (3rd ed.). Philadelphia, PA: Saunders/Elsevier.
3. Kilkenny, T. M. (2002). *Fundamentals of polysomnography and sleep disorders.* New Hope, PA: Intellisleep Technology and Consulting LLC.
4. Kryger, M. H., Roth, T., & Dement, W. C. (2016). *Principles and practice of sleep medicine* (6th ed.). Philadelphia, PA: W.B. Saunders.
5. Mattice, C., Brooks, R., & Lee-Chiong, T. (2012). *Fundamentals of sleep technology* (2nd ed.). Philadelphia, PA: Lippincott Williams & Wilkins.

chapter 30

Preoperative Assessment and Perioperative Monitoring

DANIELIZA JUNIIS-JOHNSON   KRISTINA WEAVER

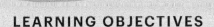

LEARNING OBJECTIVES

On completion of this chapter, the reader should be able to:

1. Define perioperative morbidity in patients with obstructive sleep apnea (OSA).
2. Describe comorbid conditions that may affect perioperative management.
3. Evaluate a known and suspected OSA patient preoperatively.
4. Describe perioperative risks associated with sleep-disordered breathing.
5. Minimize the risk posed by OSA intraoperatively.
6. Determine the postoperative disposition of a *suspected* and known OSA patient after general anesthesia.

KEY TERMS

Perioperative
Intraoperative
Hypertension
Diabetes
Multimodal analgesia
Opioids
Pain–sedation mismatch

Moderate obstructive sleep apnea (OSA) with an apnea–hypopnea index (AHI) greater than 15 is estimated to be present in 11.4% of men and 4.7% of women (1, 2). In the surgical population, a significant number of patients present for procedures that may have undiagnosed OSA. The use of the Berlin Questionnaire (BQ) found that 24% of patients were likely to have OSA when screened before surgery (3). Another screening questionnaire developed for perioperative use found a prevalence of 27.5% of patients who were likely to have OSA (4).

Identification of patients at risk for OSA is important to optimize perioperative outcomes. Patients with OSA may be more likely to have increased airway compromise with administration of sedative and anesthetic medications. These medications may decrease arousal responses that prevent collapse of the upper airway, leading to worsening of obstructive symptoms.

Because of concerns about perioperative morbidity in patients with OSA (diagnosed and undiagnosed), the American Academy of Sleep Medicine (AASM) provided recommendations regarding management (5). The Clinical Practice Review Committee found insufficient information from a review of the pertinent literature and thus provided a consensus statement. The statement included careful attention to identifying patients who may be at high risk for OSA, cautious use of sedating medications, and close monitoring postoperatively to note and address complications early. These comments, of course, were very general and did not offer very many specific processes for clinicians to implement.

The American Society of Anesthesiologists (ASA) also addressed the issue of perioperative management by creating a task force to develop guidelines regarding management of patients with OSA who may be at risk for perioperative morbidity (6). In October 2012, the ASA Committee on Standards and Practice Parameters elected to collect new evidence to determine if recommendations in the 2006 version of the ASA Practice Guidelines were supported by current evidence (7). The ASA Task Force made some more specific recommendations including the development of protocols to screen patients suspected of having OSA, the cautious administration of opioids postoperatively, and the use of telemetry or intensive care unit (ICU) monitoring for patients presumed at risk for events related to OSA in the postoperative period. The purpose of these guidelines is to improve the perioperative care and reduce the risk of adverse outcomes in patients with confirmed or suspected OSA who receive sedation, analgesia, or anesthesia for diagnostic or therapeutic procedures under the care of an anesthesiologist (7).

Perioperative risks associated with sleep-disordered breathing; preoperative assessment including screening tools, diagnostic testing, and intraoperative emergencies that may arise; and recommendations regarding management in the postoperative period will be reviewed. Sleep technologists involved in perioperative assessment of patients require an understanding of the problems encountered by OSA patients faced with upcoming surgical procedures.

PERIOPERATIVE RISKS ASSOCIATED WITH SLEEP-DISORDERED BREATHING

Sleep in the Hospitalized Patient

Sleep for the hospitalized patient leaves much to be desired, for it is often disrupted, fragmented, and/or minimally obtained. This disruption of sleep is often caused by environmental factors (noise, light, medical devices), patient characteristics (sex, age, pain intensity), or primary sleep disorders like OSA (8). Sleep deprivation or interruption decreases immune system function, slows healing, impairs cognitive function, and increases stress levels, stroke risk, and cardiovascular events, which can impact the overall health outcome of the patient, including length of stay (8) (Fig. 30-1). Medications also play a significant role in the disruption of sleep as well as increase in the incidence of OSA.

Perioperative Medications

Medications administered during the perioperative period can induce and exacerbate OSA. Drugs such as intravenous (IV) analgesics, opioids, pentothal, muscle relaxants, benzodiazepines, nitrous oxide, and propofol reduce the tone of the pharyngeal musculature, which maintains airway patency, thus increasing airway collapsibility (9). These medications cause loss

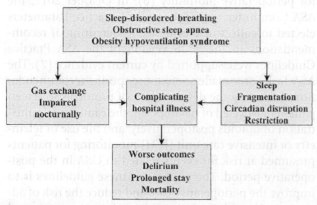

Figure 30-1 Effect of sleep-disordered breathing on the hospitalized patient. (Adapted with permission of Daedalus Enterprises Inc. from Gay, P. C. (2010). Sleep and sleep-disordered breathing in the hospitalized patient. *Respiratory Care*, 55(9), 1240–1254; permission conveyed through Copyright Clearance Center, Inc.)

of consciousness or deep sedation, which reduces the activity of the genioglossus and other extrinsic tongue muscles innervated by the hypoglossal nerve through central effects (9). Thus, perioperative patients with known or unknown OSA are at an even higher risk for complications. A cohort study reported that the risk of postoperative complications was 44% for subjects with OSA compared with 28% in those without OSA, in which most complications were due to respiratory events (10). The study also revealed that the patients with OSA who were not using continuous positive airway pressure (CPAP) and required CPAP after surgery had the highest rates of postoperative complications (10). An investigative report from the National Inpatient Sample found that patients with OSA had a higher incidence of postoperative pulmonary complications including pulmonary embolism, aspiration pneumonia, and respiratory failure (11).

Comorbid Conditions

It is imperative that health care providers involved in the care of the surgical patient be aware of comorbidities associated with OSA in order to provide the best possible health care outcome.

OSA is associated with multiple medical conditions that can affect management in the perioperative and postoperative period of surgical patients. Comorbidities associated with OSA include cardiovascular disease, arrhythmias, heart failure, hypertension, cerebrovascular disease, metabolic syndrome, and obesity (9).

Sleep Apnea and Its Link to Cardiac Disease

Sleep-disordered breathing is associated with significant cardiovascular disease (12). OSA contributes to cardiovascular risk by initiating or promoting heart failure, coronary artery disease, hypertension, atherosclerosis, cardiac arrhythmias, and stroke (13). There are an estimated 5.7 million Americans 20 years and older who have heart failure, with 870,000 new cases diagnosed every year (14). Heart failure patients have a high readmission rate into the hospital (15). Currently, 6.5 million hospital days every year are caused by heart failure, and by the year 2030, it is projected that the prevalence of heart failure will increase by 46%, resulting in 8 million diagnosed cases (14). However, heart failure patients diagnosed with OSA and treated with CPAP show a significantly reduced readmission rate into the hospital (16). Several studies have found that patients at risk for OSA who do not follow up with a physician evaluation to determine diagnosis increase their chance of exacerbating their current illness and increase the likelihood of being admitted and readmitted into the hospital in relation to a cardiac condition (16).

Sleep Apnea and Its Link to Obesity and Diabetes

Many Americans continue to maintain an unhealthy diet of fast food, and the increasing use of technology contributes to a reduction in physical activity and a more sedentary lifestyle. The prevalence of poor diet and increasing inactivity has led to rising rates of obesity (17). According to the Centers for Disease Control and Prevention, the prevalence of obesity was 39.8% and the disease affected about 93.3 million U.S. adults in 2015 to 2016. Many Americans fit into the category of obesity; a body mass index (BMI) greater than 30 is considered obese, and a BMI greater than 40 is viewed as morbidly obese (18). Those suffering from obesity, especially morbid obesity, are at a 77% increased risk for OSA (18). The cyclical respiratory obstructions of OSA cause fragmentation of sleep, which slows and impairs metabolism as a result of decreased oxygen levels (17). Obesity is also thought to cause OSA because of mechanical effects on airway size and lung volume due to excess adipose tissue and may also have neural effects that impair the neuromuscular response (12). According to the Sleep Heart Health Study, those individuals suffering from moderate-to-severe OSA were found to have BMI three times higher than individuals with the lowest BMI (12). Research conducted through the Wisconsin Sleep Cohort found that there is a 3% change of OSA severity for every 1% increase in weight over a 4-year period (12).

Those individuals suffering from OSA are more likely to be overweight, and they are also more likely to develop type 2 diabetes (T2D) (17). Glucose metabolism is the regulation of glucose and insulin via specific hormones (cortisol and growth hormone) (18). During sleep, these hormone levels rise, inducing insulin resistance that controls glucose tolerance (18). Glucose tolerance is lower in nonrapid eye movement (Stages 1 to 3) sleep, versus rapid eye movement (REM) sleep (18). OSA disrupts an individual's ability to transition into deeper stages of sleep as a result of apneas and arousals, which ultimately deteriorate glucose metabolism and impair glucose homeostasis (17). These factors contribute to the development of T2D in predisposed individuals (17).

Hospitalized inpatients and inpatients awaiting surgery who have OSA are at an increased risk for complications that can include longer hospitalization, higher reintubation rates, oxygen desaturations, hypercapnia, cardiac arrhythmias, myocardial injury, delirium, unplanned ICU transfers, and sudden unexpected death (19). Unfortunately, despite advances in sleep medicine and the role of sleep in regard to health and well-being, OSA still remains a highly undiagnosed disease (20). However, developing an inpatient assessment and monitoring program can assist when it comes to diagnosis, prognosis, patient care, interaction, and education for patients in the hospital setting.

INDICATIONS FOR PREOPERATIVE SLEEP ASSESSMENT

ASA guidelines highlight the importance of perioperative diagnosis and management of OSA, in which the "gold standard" screening tool continues to be the nocturnal polysomnogram (9). However, because of time constraints, cost, and personnel requirements, it can be an impractical screening tool for the perioperative patient (9). Thus, the use of other OSA screening tools that are less time-consuming and more cost-effective should be considered in perioperative management. Common screening tools include the Epworth Sleepiness Scale (ESS), STOP Questionnaire, STOP-BANG Questionnaire (SBQ), BQ, and the Wisconsin Sleep Questionnaire (21). These assessment tools are time efficient and have evidence-based reliability and validity (21). The user-friendly STOP-BANG screening tool was shown to have one of the lowest false-negative rates among screening tools for OSA (9).

METHODS FOR PREOPERATIVE SLEEP ASSESSMENT

The ASA guidelines were created by a task force to optimize care for patients with diagnosed or undiagnosed OSA who may have increased risk in the perioperative period (6). This group recommended the development of protocols to screen patients suspected of having OSA preoperatively for the identification of high-risk patients.

There are several screening tools that have been utilized in the preoperative assessment of patients suspected of having OSA. In addition, some physical findings may increase suspicion on initial physical examination. These include obesity and craniofacial abnormalities, such as retrognathia and macroglossia (22, 23). Questions regarding signs and symptoms of OSA should be asked, such as loud snoring, observed apnea, and daytime hypersomnolence. Several of the screening tools utilize these assessments as well.

The goal of administration of a screening tool is to identify high-risk patients and manage them as if they are likely to have OSA. Protocols have also been established at numerous medical centers on the basis of specific management of high-risk patients, and this will be discussed later.

One study identified 108 studies including a total of 47,989 participants. The summary estimates were calculated for the Berlin, STOP-BANG, STOP, and ESS questionnaires in detecting mild (AHI/respiratory distress index [RDI] ≥ 5 events per hour), moderate (AHI/RDI ≥ 15 events per hour), and severe OSA (AHI/RDI ≥ 30 events per hour). Compared with the BQ, STOP, and ESS, the SBQ is a more accurate tool for detecting mild, moderate, and severe OSA (24).

The BQ is a commonly utilized tool for screening for OSA. It asks patients to self-report on questions in three categories: snoring, daytime sleepiness, and hypertension history. This questionnaire has been utilized by primary care physicians, and in a study looking at 744 patients, half of those found to be at high risk were diagnosed with OSA by polysomnography (PSG) (25). In preoperative patients, the BQ was found to have moderately high sensitivity and specificity, with a sensitivity of 69% and a specificity of 54% (26).

The ASA checklist was one screening tool suggested by the ASA Task Force. It utilizes OSA severity, invasiveness of anesthesia and surgery, and postoperative opioid requirements to determine perioperative risk (6). This was found to have sensitivity and specificity similar to that of the BQ (4). Both the BQ and the ASA checklist may require more planning, time, and training of involved screeners than many centers are able to easily provide.

Another screening tool, the STOP-BANG (Snoring, Tiredness, Observed apneas, elevated blood Pressure–Body mass index, Age, Neck circumference, and male Gender) was developed and validated by Chung and colleagues specifically for surgical patients (4). In the initial study, 28% of 2,500 patients screened were at high risk of OSA. Of these, 10% underwent PSG, which found a sensitivity of 92.9% for OSA with AHI more than 15 events per hour.

Yet another screening tool developed specifically for preoperative screening is the perioperative sleep apnea prediction score (P-SAP). This was developed by a retrospective observational study to determine independent predictors of OSA by logistic regression. This involves demographic variables (age, male gender, and obesity), historical variables (snoring, diabetes mellitus, and hypertension), and airway measures (thick neck, reduced thyromental distance, and Mallampati class 3 or 4) (27). The Mallampati class is determined by the amount of the uvula visualized on airway inspection, with class 3 and 4 as the least optimal views. A P-SAP score of greater than or equal to 6 predicted OSA with excellent specificity (0.911), but poor sensitivity (0.239).

The sleep apnea clinical score (SACS) is a different screening tool that has been utilized in preoperative evaluation. The SACS was initially validated in outpatients and was found to have a high positive predictive value for OSA (28). In the perioperative setting, it was initially utilized to determine which patients were more likely to have oxygen desaturations postoperatively (29). The SACS was then evaluated in a prospective study and found to predict a much higher risk of postoperative oxygen desaturation (>4%), with an oxygen desaturation index (ODI) greater than 10 events per hour (30). In addition, these patients were significantly more likely to have postoperative respiratory and overall complications.

The use of a preoperative method to identify patients at high risk for undiagnosed OSA and perioperative complications is recommended by the ASA Task Force, and screening tools are being increasingly commonly utilized. Screening tools that are simple to teach and administer are likely to be most useful in this setting. Patients considered to be at high risk for OSA but without significant comorbidities can be identified preoperatively. These patients can then undergo their surgical procedure, with all care providers being aware of this increased risk. The STOP-BANG and SACS are simple tools that have been shown to identify high-risk patients, which may increase their utility in the perioperative setting.

Diagnostic Testing

PSG, as a preoperative diagnostic tool, is not feasible for all high-risk patients, because it is expensive, requires a significant time commitment for the study and preoperative initiation of therapy (if indicated), and would burden already busy sleep centers. PSG is typically limited to patients with severe comorbidities, such as decompensated heart failure, uncontrolled hypertension, or pulmonary hypertension. If the initiation of positive airway pressure (PAP) is indicated in those patients, the length of time of treatment before proceeding for surgery is not clear. This has not been studied, although it has been suggested that several weeks of PAP therapy may be necessary.

Overnight oximetry is an option in patients who are considered at risk for postoperative complications related to undiagnosed OSA. Figure 30-2 is an example of overnight oximetry in a patient with severe chronic obstructive pulmonary disease, obesity hypoventilation syndrome, and OSA. Review of this study indicates coexisting cardiopulmonary disease with reduced mean saturation. A prolonged time at low oxygen saturation may suggest that pulmonary hypertension is also present.

The utility of overnight oximetry routinely for patients suspected of undiagnosed OSA is not clear. In one study, patients with at least two clinical features of OSA during preoperative assessment were selected to undergo home oximetry before surgery (31). Using the desaturation index, overnight oximetry can be a sensitive and specific tool to detect sleep-disordered breathing in surgical patients (32). ODI has been used as an inexpensive marker for postoperative apnea-related events. It has been evaluated in the outpatient setting, and an ODI greater than 10 has been reported to have sensitivities of 71% to 85% with specificities of 90% to 95%. ODI, or RDI, has been shown to be a close estimate of AHI derived from PSG in patients suspected of having OSA and is a sensitive indicator to screen for mild-to-moderate OSA (33).

A total of 172 patients were evaluated, and the relationship between a 4% ODI and postoperative complications was investigated. The use of home overnight oximetry found that patients with 4% ODI greater than or equal to 5 events per hour had significantly more

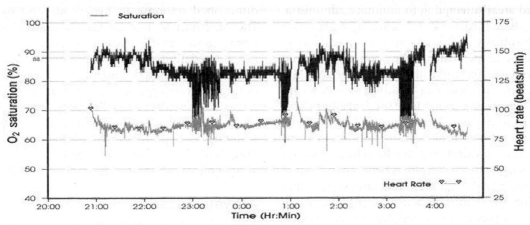

Figure 30-2 Oximetry result of a patient with severe obstructive sleep apnea (OSA) and chronic obstructive pulmonary disease with obesity hypoventilation. The reduced mean saturation is an indication that there is coexisting cardiopulmonary disease, and the prolonged time at low oxygen saturation suggests that pulmonary hypertension is also present. The frequency of 4% oxygen desaturations (4% oxygen desaturation index) per hour of 47 supports the diagnosis of severe OSA and corresponds with the patient's apnea–hypopnea index (AHI) from a polysomnogram showing an AHI of 40 per hour. Lastly, the clustered desaturations (icicles from the rooftop) to 59% identify the severe rapid eye movement desaturations typically occurring in this type of patient.

postoperative complications than patients with 4% ODI less than 5 events per hour (15.3% compared with 2.7%). In this study, many of the respiratory complications simply involved requiring more supplemental oxygen (33).

Thus, it is unclear if overnight oximetry to identify high-risk patients is beneficial. More work will be needed in this area.

Portable monitoring has recently become a useful diagnostic modality in the diagnosis of OSA (34). It is less expensive and much easier than PSG in sleep centers. Recently, certain portable monitors have become an acceptable alternative on the basis of the ruling of Centers for Medicare and Medicaid for the diagnosis of OSA and initiation of PAP. There is little information on the use of portable monitoring in the preoperative period. A recent abstract utilized portable monitoring with PSG in patients scheduled for elective surgery and found a high incidence of undiagnosed OSA that was not often recognized by the medical care team, with 47% severe OSA not suspected (35). Another abstract by the same group in Toronto utilized home-portable PSG in patients considered high risk by using the STOP-BANG tool (36). Patients at high risk by STOP-BANG and an ODI greater than 10 by nocturnal oximetry are very likely to have significant OSA. With more data, the use of a screening tool followed by portable monitoring with or without PSG in high-risk patients preoperatively may be found to be beneficial in the future.

With home sleep apnea testing (HSAT) on the rise and its ease of use, these devices potentially could be a possibility for utilization by presurgical teams in the perioperative and postoperative setting. HSAT can successfully identify OSA in 82% of adult surgical patients. HSAT provides a diagnosis of OSA accepted by most insurance carriers, enabling patients to obtain CPAP. Patients with significant cardiac, pulmonary, or neurologic conditions may require in-center sleep testing. In addition, in a patient highly suspected of having OSA, a negative HSAT usually requires in-center sleep testing (37).

Preoperative PAP

Patients with known OSA that are noncompliant with PAP therapy are a challenge in the perioperative period. Discussion with the patient regarding reinitiating PAP before surgery should be considered, but there are little data on this (38). Patients with OSA who have been utilizing PAP should continue this preoperatively (6). Documentation of this in the preoperative evaluation will allow all perioperative care providers, especially nurses and the anesthesia team, to have this information and plan for optimization in the perioperative period. Many patients cannot recall details of their PAP treatment, in which case an auto-titrating PAP device may be substituted while in hospital.

INTRAOPERATIVE MANAGEMENT

Because patients with diagnosed or suspected OSA are considered high risk, organizations including the ASA have developed specific guidelines with recommendations for intraoperative management (6). General principles of these guidelines include avoiding sedation in unsupervised areas, attempting to minimize administration of opioids and sedatives, and exercising vigilance for possible difficulties with intubation and airway management. There are limited data on the optimal intraoperative management of patients with OSA, or suspected OSA.

Ideally, general anesthesia could be provided with short-acting agents that do not have residual effects. This would limit the impact of prolonged sedation on the upper airway and obstructions in the immediate postoperative period. No ideal agent has been found, and no evidence to suggest that one agent is better than another has been proven, although ASA guidelines suggest that shorter-acting agents may be beneficial (6). The use of regional blocks (neuraxial or peripheral nerve blocks) as a sole anesthetic may be beneficial as another option to the OSA patient, because it circumvents the issue of upper airway patency in the perioperative period. Therefore, local and regional techniques may be preferred to general anesthesia (7). This may limit the amount of opioid and sedative agents required. Comparisons of the use of epidural local anesthetic to IV long-acting opioids found that opioid use led to more postoperative obstructive episodes and apneas, oxygen desaturations, and ventilatory compromise (31, 39).

It is known that general anesthesia leads to depression of upper airway muscle activity (40, 41). One commonly used IV agent, propofol, has been associated with increased collapsibility of the upper airway (41). This may be due to a combination of decreased central respiratory output to airway dilator muscles and upper airway reflexes (41).

Often, volatile inhaled anesthetics are utilized during general anesthesia (see Fig. 30-3). The residual effects of these volatile agents may affect respiration postoperatively. These agents could also worsen the respiratory depressant effects of opioids administered for analgesia. Choice of a volatile agent that is likely to lead to faster awakening may be useful. Morbidly obese patients undergoing abdominal surgery are found to have faster awakening after the use of desflurane than after sevoflurane, both commonly used volatile anesthetics (42, 43). Desflurane anesthesia is associated with higher oxygen saturation in the postanesthesia care unit (PACU). OSA patients receiving anesthetic care or regional anesthesia with sedation should have intraoperative capnography available to monitor for ventilation. If deep sedation is required, a secure airway is preferable to an unprotected airway (7, 30).

Monitored Anesthesia Care

Monitored anesthesia care (MAC) involves the use of IV sedation for a surgical procedure that does not require general anesthesia (44). Combinations of sedative medications are utilized, including benzodiazepines, opioids, and often propofol. These, individually and in combination, can lead to obstructive episodes and diminished response to hypoxemia and hypercarbia. The American Society for Gastrointestinal Endoscopy has suggested that patients with OSA are at increased risk for sedation-related complications (45). The ASA guidelines recommend careful monitoring for obstructions with capnography or other automated method because of increased risk in these patients (6). There are case reports regarding the use of PAP for patients with OSA or high risk of OSA during procedures under MAC (46). The use of PAP for MAC is a consideration, although there is limited information regarding its use.

Airway Management

Anatomic changes can be associated with OSA that may affect airway management intraoperatively. Patients may have increased neck circumference, macroglossia, retrognathia, and maxillary constriction. These anatomic features can be associated with difficult mask ventilation and intubation. High incidence of OSA has been reported in patients with difficult intubation (47). Difficult intubation has been found to occur eight times as often in patients with OSA (43, 48). Patients with severe OSA (AHI > 40) have been found to have a much higher incidence of difficult intubation (49). It has also been suggested that because of the association between OSA and difficult intubation, all patients who are found to be candidates for difficult intubation need referral for PSG (47).

Because of these issues, preparation for the induction of anesthesia and intubation should follow the ASA difficult airway guidelines (50). Preparations should be made for unanticipated difficulty in these patients. Sedatives should be administered slowly to avoid sudden loss of consciousness and resultant unanticipated obstructions. Obese patients should be placed in a ramped or sitting position. This involves elevation of the torso and head tilt with chin upward to optimize airway visualization and should be combined with approximately 30° head-up position (51, 52). Preoxygenation with 100% oxygen given by tight-fitting mask for 3 minutes should be performed. This can increase time of tolerance to apnea in case of intubation difficulties (53).

Alternate airway devices, such as laryngeal mask airway, video laryngoscope, or fiberoptic scope, should be readily available. If awake intubation is planned, topical anesthetics are utilized for the upper airway and oropharynx. If the surgical procedure is short in duration, care providers should be vigilant about residual topical anesthesia causing impaired upper airway reflexes at the end of the surgery (54).

Extubation following surgical procedure should be carefully planned, because residual anesthetics may increase the risk of obstruction. Often, nondepolarizing muscle relaxants are administered during surgery to optimize performance of the surgical procedure. It is important to ensure that the muscle relaxant is

Surgical Location	Management Strategies

Preoperative Evaluation
• Medical record review
  • Sleep apnea hx
  • Medical history of comorbids linked to sleep apnea
• Patient/family interview and screening
  • Evidence-based screening tool
  • Patient or family interview of symptoms
• Physical examination
  • Neck circumference, tongue size, BMI, cranial facial abnormalities
• Sleep study if undiagnosed and at risk to and allow for PAP therapy use if time permits
	Preoperative Management
	• Determination of inpatient vs. outpatient management
	• Sleep apnea status
	• Anatomic and physiologic abnormalities
	• Status of coexisting diseases
	• Nature of surgery
	• Type of anesthesia
	• Need for postoperative opioids
	• Patient age
	• Adequacy of postdischarge observation
	• Capabilities of the outpatient facility
	• Educate patient and family to bring PAP therapy if permitted
	• Educate patient and family of risk of apnea

Preoperative Preparation • PAP therapy should be considered if OSA is present • Patients with known or suspected OSA should be managed according to the "Practice Guidelines for Management of the Difficult Airway: An Updated Report"	**Intraoperative Management** • Consideration of general anesthesia vs. deep sedation • Use of local anesthesia or nerve blocks for superficial procedures • Ventilation should be continuously monitored by capnography. • Extubating while awake should be considered. Full reversal of neuromuscular block should be verified before extubating. • Extubating in the lateral, semi-upright, or other nonsupine positions when possible
Intraoperative • Choice of anesthesia technique • Airway management • Patient monitoring	**Postoperative (PACU) management** • Regional analgesic techniques should be considered to reduce or eliminate the requirements for systemic opioids. • To reduce opioid requirements, nonsteroidal anti-inflammatory agents and other modalities • Educate clinicians about the risk of respiratory depression and airway obstruction. • Supplemental oxygen should be administered to OSA risk patients to maintain their baseline oxygen saturation. • Caution on O_2—may increase apneic episodes and may hinder detection of atelectasis and hypoventilation. • When feasible, PAP therapy should be applied to patients who were using these modalities preoperatively unless contraindicated by the surgical procedure. • Avoid the supine position throughout the recovery process. • Hospitalized patients—continuous monitoring is ideal.
Postoperative (PACU) • Postoperative analgesia • Oxygenation • Patient positioning • Monitoring • Discharge to unmonitored settings	• Patient moved from recovery to a hospital-monitored critical care bed, step-down unit, and telemetry hospital bed or monitored by a dedicated appropriately trained observer in the patient's room. • Patients at increased risk should not be discharged from the recovery area to an unmonitored setting until no longer at risk of respiratory depression.

Figure 30-3 The intraoperative management of anesthetics. BMI, body mass index; OSA, obstructive sleep apnea; PACU, post anesthesia care unit; PAP, positive airway pressure. (Adapted from Gross, J. B., Bachenberg, K. L., Benumof, J. L., et al.; American Society of Anesthesiologists. (2014). Practice guidelines for the perioperative management of patients with obstructive sleep apnea: An updated report by the American Society of Anesthesiologists Task Force on Perioperative Management of Patients with Obstructive Sleep Apnea. *Anesthesiology, 120*(2), 268–286.)

fully reversed to avoid increased risk of upper airway obstruction. A nerve stimulation device should be utilized to assess appropriate reversal of muscle relaxant (55). Patients should be fully awake, breathing with adequate respiratory rate and tidal volume before extubation. Immediately after extubation, careful monitoring for evidence of obstruction and asynchrony of respiratory efforts should be performed.

MANAGEMENT OF SLEEP-DISORDERED BREATHING IN THE RECOVERY PERIOD

Postanesthesia Care Unit

Patients routinely go to a PACU following a surgical procedure. Cardiopulmonary monitoring is standard in the PACU. During this time, patients may have residual effects from anesthetic and analgesic agents administered. They are watched carefully by PACU nurses, who observe for any respiratory changes. Vigilant recovery care is provided by the nurses and includes assessment for pain and administration of IV opioids as needed. Patients who are at high risk for OSA on the screening questionnaires and have recurrent PACU respiratory events are more likely to have postoperative respiratory complications (56) (see Fig. 30-4).

Often, patients receive their highest doses of postoperative opioids in the PACU. Because of this combined with possible residual anesthetic effects, the PACU can be utilized to watch for respiratory events. A study utilizing the SACS preoperatively with a PACU respiratory assessment was able to identify patients at high risk for postoperative respiratory complications (30). PACU events documented were episodes of apnea, bradypnea, desaturations, and pain–sedation mismatch at three periods of 30 minutes each during the PACU stay. Patients then underwent recorded pulse oximetry on the nursing unit, with a calculation of 4% ODI of greater than 10 events per hour considered significant. A combination of both high SACS and PACU recurrent events identified the patients most likely to have ODI greater than 10 and respiratory complications

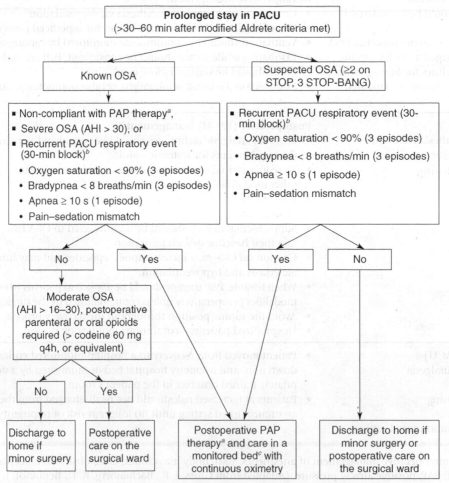

Figure 30-4 Postoperative management of the known or suspected obstructive sleep apnea patient after general anesthesia. [a]Recurrent postanesthesia care unit (PACU) respiratory event—any event occurring more than once in each 30-minute evaluation period (not necessary to be the same event). [b]Positive airway pressure (PAP) therapy—including continuous PAP, bilevel PAP, or auto-titrating PAP. [c]Monitored bed—environment with continuous oximetry and the possibility of early nursing intervention (e.g., intensive care unit, step-down unit, or remote pulse oximetry with telemetry in surgical ward). Pain–sedation mismatch, simultaneous occurrence of high pain scores and high sedation levels. (Reprinted with permission from Seet, E. & Chung, F. (2010). Management of sleep apnea in adults—Functional algorithms for the perioperative period: Continuing Professional Development, Figure 2. *Canadian Journal of Anesthesia, 57,* 849–865.)

with an odds ratio over 20. Thus, close observation in the PACU may assist in the determination of risks in the postoperative period.

Patients who are at risk should be placed in a sitting or lateral position in the PACU (57). A sitting position may also be useful. If patients have known OSA and utilize CPAP, this should be provided in the PACU. They can then be observed for any concerns while on preoperative PAP settings.

Patients with OSA who are noncompliant should be observed closely. If necessary, PAP can be initiated. These patients have been shown to have the highest risk of postoperative complications and need close monitoring after discharge from the PACU (10).

Patients who are at high risk for undiagnosed OSA can be challenging to manage. There are limited data on new initiation of PAP in suspected OSA postoperatively. If this appears to be indicated in the PACU, the patient should be placed in a monitored setting, which allows direct observation. It has been shown that patients with OSA not utilizing PAP in the postoperative period are at highest risk for complications (58).

Postoperative Analgesia

IV analgesics and opioids (common analgesic) not only increase airway collapsibility but suppress REM sleep (9). REM sleep allows the body to heal and restore itself for optimal function. The reduction of REM sleep has a higher occurrence after major surgery in which recovery REM (or REM rebound) is usually observed on the second or third postoperative day (9). During REM sleep, the neural drive to the pharyngeal muscles is minimized, causing hypotonia of the muscles, thus increasing severity of OSA during REM rebound (9). REM rebound can contribute to myocardial ischemia and infarction, stroke, hemodynamic instability, mental confusion, and wound breakdown (9). OSA patients are at higher risk for these affects.

Anesthetic and sedative drugs are central nervous system depressants that also inhibit respiration, causing oxygen desaturations, hypoxemia, and hypercapnia (59). In a case study of 23 patients with unrecognized sleep apnea, undergoing an outpatient procedure with conscious sedation, 17 (74%) patients developed OSA (59).

Postoperative Location

Patients with OSA or at high risk for OSA may require a higher level of care than that provided on a routine hospital unit after surgery. The ASA guidelines recommend high-risk patients may need a monitored setting or pulse oximetry that is continuously observed (6). Perioperative risk is dependent on the severity of OSA, whether PAP is being utilized, invasiveness of the surgery, and requirement for postoperative opioids.

The utilization of the SACS in combination with PACU respiratory events can assist in the determination of the level of care needed postoperatively (60). Recently, Seet and Chung (61) developed an algorithm to manage postoperative location (Fig. 30-4).

Using this algorithm, patients are at high risk if they have OSA (left) or high suspicion by preoperative screening. On the left-hand side of Figure 30-4, patients are at high risk when noncompliant with CPAP, AHI greater than 30, or recurrent PACU events. The PACU events are assessed at 30-minute intervals and are positive if they have events at two of the three periods. These events are as follows:

1. Apnea greater than or equal to 10 seconds
2. Bradypnea less than or equal to 8 breaths per minute (three episodes needed)
3. Desaturations less than 90% (three episodes needed)
4. Pain–sedation mismatch, high pain score with a high level of sedation. These patients may need a higher level of care, and possibly PAP.

The right-hand side of the algorithm guides the management of patients suspected of OSA, identified as high risk by screening tools. They are also considered high risk if they have recurrent PACU events in addition to high risk by screening and should be considered for a higher level of care postoperatively as well. If a patient requires initiation of PAP postoperatively, including someone with known OSA noncompliant with therapy, the patient should go to a step-down or monitored setting. Initiation of PAP on the unit without close observation will be difficult, and the acceptance of a new PAP is often difficult.

MONITORING

Oximetry

Pulse oximetry is a diagnostic tool that is used to indirectly measure the percentage of oxygenated hemoglobin in the blood capillaries (62). The pulse oximeter probe, which can be placed on the finger or earlobe, uses a red-infrared light source that measures the light absorption properties of hemoglobin (61). It is widely used in the perioperative and intensive care settings and in pediatric patients to identify hypoxemia or an indication of respiratory complication that may require clinical intervention (63). Pulse oximetry contributes to maintaining patient safety and reducing the risk of complications for the perioperative and postoperative patient, especially someone with a higher risk for OSA (63).

Capnograph

Capnography is used to assess alveolar hypoventilation and provides a measurement of carbon dioxide (CO_2)

that can assist with early detection of respiratory complications (63).

End-tidal CO_2 (EtCO$_2$) provides a noninvasive means of measuring CO_2 levels through a patient's exhaled breath (18) (see Fig. 30-5). Transcutaneous CO_2 (TcCO$_2$) provides a reading of CO_2 levels in the blood by a heated sensor placed on the skin (35 to 45 mm Hg—normal, >50 mm Hg—abnormal) (18).

A comprehensive meta-analysis of clinical trials shows clear and consistent evidence of reduced respiratory compromise when capnography monitoring is used during procedural sedation and analgesia (62). However, a mandate to include capnography in patient monitoring, as a means of early detection of alveolar hypoventilation, has remained a topic of debate (63).

Protocols

Continued use of sedative agents in the postoperative period can contribute to obstructions and apneas in OSA patients. Certain institutions have initiated protocols to limit sedative agents given to high-risk patients also receiving analgesic medications. This includes limitation of sleep-enhancing medications and benzodiazepines to minimize pharmacologic sedative effects that could worsen OSA symptoms. Often, these protocols include recommendations about

patient positioning. The ASA guidelines recommend the use of nonsupine positions, if possible, during the recovery period (6).

The role of protocols involving the initiation of PAP is unclear. There are several case reports regarding its use. One set of cases involved response to an adverse event that led to the development of an institutional protocol that included the initiation of PAP if needed (64).

A prospective study in patients undergoing orthopedic surgery involved the use of SACS (38). Patients were identified as high risk by SACS and randomized to receive routine postoperative care or initiation of auto-titrating PAP. The SACS was 85% sensitive in identifying patients with postoperative respiratory disturbance index greater than or equal to 15 by subsequent portable sleep studies. The use of preemptive PAP did not alter outcomes in patients at high risk for OSA. More than 50% of the high-risk group would not tolerate PAP use, and this may have affected ability to determine outcome difference. Of note, even low-risk patients desaturated on the first postoperative night but less severely than the high-risk group.

In a study looking at orthopedic patients with OSA, patients using CPAP postoperatively had significantly fewer complications postoperatively (58). Thus, it is important to continue postoperative CPAP in compliant patients.

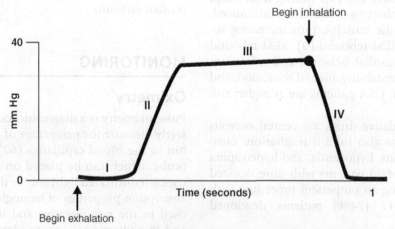

Figure 30-5 The "normal" capnogram is a waveform that represents the varying carbon dioxide level throughout the breath cycle. Phase I: Beginning of exhalation. Dead space is cleared from the upper airway. Phase II: Rapid rise in CO_2 concentration as alveolar CO_2 reaches the upper airway. Phase III: Plateau. Entire exhaled breath stream is alveolar gas. Maximum value for that tidal breath is the end-tidal CO_2. Phase IV: Beginning of inhalation. Atmospheric air replaces alveolar CO_2. (Reprinted with permission from Fleisher, G. R., & Ludwig, S. (2010). *Textbook of pediatric emergency medicine* (6th ed.). Philadelphia, PA: Wolters Kluwer; Figure 1 (Appendix). Copyright © LWW/Wolters Kluwer.)

PATIENTS AND METHODS

This retrospective, case-control study from a single academic medical institution included patients diagnosed as having OSAS between January 1995 and December 1998 and undergoing hip or knee replacement within 3 years before or anytime after their OSAS diagnosis. Patients with OSAS were subcategorized as having the diagnosis either before or after the surgery and also, regardless of time of diagnosis, by whether they were using continuous positive airway pressure (CPAP) prior to hospitalization. Matched controls were patients without OSAS undergoing the same operation. Interventions were defined specifically as administration of a particular treatment in the context of each complication, eg, supplemental oxygen, implementation of additional monitoring such as oximetry for hypoxemia, or transfer to the intensive care unit (ICU) for cardiac ischemia concerns. Postoperative complications were assessed for all patients in the different categories and included respiratory events such as hypoxemia, acute hypercapnia, and episodes of delirium. Serious complications were noted separately, including unplanned ICU days, reintubations, and cardiac events. The length of hospital stay was also tabulated.

SUMMARY

Patients with known and suspected OSA are at risk for complications in the perioperative period. Both the AASM and ASA have addressed this issue and provided recommendations to assist in management. Both intraoperative and postoperative management can be challenging. The ideal anesthetic management is not known, and difficult airway management is a concern for the intraoperative medical team. Postoperatively, OSA may be linked to multiple complications. Identification of patients with undiagnosed OSA may allow increased vigilance during their perioperative period. Careful history and physical examination and the use of clinical screening tools to identify patients at high risk for OSA should be utilized.

Patients with suspected OSA with comorbidities thought to be associated with OSA, such as heart failure and uncontrolled hypertension, should undergo further evaluation before proceeding with elective surgery. This will require evaluation by both sleep medicine and other subspecialists to optimize their medical condition. Patients with known OSA and those identified as high risk should be managed similarly in the perioperative period. Attention to the severity of OSA, invasiveness of the surgical procedure, postoperative opioid requirements, and positioning should be considered for the determination of requirements for postoperative monitoring.

Information regarding optimal management is limited. AASM and ASA guidelines should be reviewed in the development of institutional approaches to management of this high-risk group. Further work in this area is necessary to better understand the risks and optimal management strategies.

REFERENCES

1. Bixler, E. O., Vgontzas, A. N., Lin, H. M., et al. (2001). Prevalence of sleep-disordered breathing in women: Effects of gender. *American Journal of Respiratory and Critical Care Medicine, 163*, 608–613.
2. Bixler, E. O., Vgontzas, A. N., Ten Have, T., et al. (1998). Effects of age on sleep apnea in men: I. Prevalence and severity. *American Journal of Respiratory and Critical Care Medicine, 157*, 144–140.
3. Chung, F., Ward, B., Ho, J., et al. (2007). Preoperative identification of sleep apnea risk in elective surgical patients, using the Berlin questionnaire. *Journal of Clinical Anesthesia, 19*,130–134.
4. Chung, F., Yegneswaran, B., Liao, P., et al. (2008). STOP questionnaire: A tool to screen patients for obstructive sleep apnea. *Anesthesiology, 108*, 812–821.
5. Meoli, A. L., Rosen, C. L., Kristo, D., et al. (2003). Upper airway management of the adult patient with obstructive sleep apnea in the perioperative period–avoiding complications. *Sleep, 26*, 1060–1065.
6. Gross, J. B., Bachenberg, K. L., Benumof, J. L., et al.; American Society of Anesthesiologists. (2006). Practice guidelines for the perioperative management of patients with obstructive sleep apnea: A report by the American Society of Anesthesiologists Task Force on Perioperative Management of patients with obstructive sleep apnea. *Anesthesiology, 104*, 1081–1093.
7. Gross, J. B., Bachenberg, K. L., Benumof, J. L., et al.; American Society of Anesthesiologists. (2014). Practice guidelines for the perioperative management of patients with obstructive sleep apnea: An updated report by the American Society of Anesthesiologists Task Force on Perioperative Management of patients with obstructive sleep apnea. *Anesthesiology, 120*, 268–286.
8. Vincensi, B. (2016). Sleep in the hospitalized patient: Nurse and patient perceptions. *MEDSURG Nursing* [serial online], *25*(5), 351–356. Retrieved from CINAHL Complete.
9. Sundar, E., Chang, J., Smetana, G. W. (2011). Perioperative screening for and management of patients with obstructive sleep apnea. *Journal of Clinical Outcomes Management, 18*(9), 399–411.
10. Liao, P., Yegneswaran, B., Vairavanathan, S., et al. (2009). Postoperative complications in patients with obstructive sleep apnea: A retrospective matched cohort study. *Canadian Journal of Anaesthesiology, 56*, 819–828.

11. Memtsoudis, S., Liu, S. S., Ma, Y., et al. (2001). Perioperative pulmonary outcomes in patients with sleep apnea after noncardiac surgery. *Anesthesia & Analgesia, 112*, 113–121.

12. Kapur, V. K. (2010). Obstructive sleep apnea: Diagnosis, epidemiology, and economics. *Respiratory Care, 55*(9), 1155–1167.

13. Floras, J. S. (2014). Sleep apnea and cardiovascular risk. *Journal of Cardiology, 63*(1), 3–8. doi:10.1016/j.jjcc.2013.08.009

14. Mozaffarian, D., Benjamin, E., Go, A., et al. (2015). AHA statistical update: Heart disease and stroke statistics—2015 update. A report from the American Heart Association [Entire issue]. *Circulation, 131*, e29–e322. doi:10.1161/CIR.0000000000000152

15. Khayat, R., Abraham, W., Patt, B., et al. (2012). Central sleep apnea is a predictor of cardiac readmission in hospitalized patients with systolic heart failure. *Journal of Cardiac Failure, 18*(7), 534–540. doi:10.1016/j.cardfail.2012.05.003

16. Kauta, S. R., Keenan, B. T., Goldberg, L., et al. (2014). Diagnosis and treatment of sleep disordered breathing in hospitalized cardiac patients: A reduction in 30-day hospital readmission rates. *Journal of Clinical Sleep Medicine, 10*(10), 1051–1059.

17. Pallayova, M., & Taheri, S. (2013). Recognizing obstructive sleep apnea as a sign of developing diabetes. *Journal of Diabetes Nursing, 17*(8), 288–293.

18. Barkoukis, T. J., & Avidan, A. Y. (Eds.). (2007). *Review of sleep medicine* (2nd ed.). Philadelphia, PA: Butterworth Heinemann Elsevier.

19. Adesanya, A. O., Lee, W., Greilich. N. B., et al. (2010). Perioperative management of obstructive sleep apnea. *Chest, 138*(6), 1489–1498.

20. Adult Obstructive Sleep Apnea Task Force of the American Academy of Sleep Medicine. (2009). Clinical guideline for the evaluation, management and long-term care of obstructive sleep apnea in adults. *Journal of Clinical Sleep Medicine, 5*(3), 263–276.

21. Helvig, A. W., Minick, P., & Patrick, D. (2014). Post operative management of patients with obstructive sleep apnea: Implications for the medical surgical nurse. *Medsurg Nursing, 23*(3), 171–177.

22. Hillman, D. R., Platt, P. R., & Eastwood, P. R. (2010). Anesthesia, sleep, and upper airway collapsibility. *Anesthesiology Clinics, 28*, 443–455.

23. Young, T., Peppard, P. E., & Taheri, S. (2005). Excess weight and sleep-disordered breathing. *Journal of Applied Physiology, 99*, 1592–1599.

24. Chiu, H. Y., Chen, P. Y., Chuang, L. P., et al. (2017). Diagnostic accuracy of the Berlin questionnaire, STOP-BANG, STOP, and Epworth sleepiness scale in detecting obstructive sleep apnea: A bivariate meta-analysis. *Sleep Medicine Reviews, 36*, 57–70. doi:10.1016/j.smrv.2016.10.004

25. Netzer, N. C., Stoohs, R. A., Netzer, C. M., et al. (1999). Using the Berlin questionnaire to identify patients at risk for the sleep apnea syndrome. *Annals of Internal Medicine, 131*, 485–491.

26. Chung, F., Yegneswaran, B., Liao, P., et al. (2008). Validation of the Berlin questionnaire and American Society of Anesthesiologists checklist as screening tools for obstructive sleep apnea in surgical patients. *Anesthesiology, 108*, 822–830.

27. Ramachandran, S. K., Kheterpal, S., Consens, F., et al. (2010). Derivation and validation of a simple perioperative sleep apnea prediction score. *Anesthesiology and Analgesia, 110*, 1007–1015.

28. Flemons, W. W., Whitelaw, W. A., Brant, R., et al. (1994). Likelihood ratios for a sleep apnea clinical prediction rule. *American Journal of Respiratory and Critical Care Medicine, 150*, 1279–1285.

29. Gali, B., Whalen, F. X., Jr., Gay, P. C., et al. (2007). Management plan to reduce risks in perioperative care of patients with presumed obstructive sleep apnea syndrome. *Journal of Clinical Sleep Medicine, 3*, 582–588.

30. Gali, B., Whalen, F. X., Schroeder, D. R., et al. (2009). Identification of patients at risk for postoperative respiratory complications using a preoperative obstructive sleep apnea screening tool and postanesthesia care assessment. *Anesthesiology, 110*, 869–877.

31. Hwang, D., Shakir, N., Limann, B., et al. (2008). Association of sleep-disordered breathing with postoperative complications. *Chest, 133*, 1128–1134.

32. Rosenberg, J., & Kehlet, H. (1991). Postoperative episodic oxygen desaturation in the sleep apnoea syndrome. *Acta Anaesthesiologica Scandinavica, 35*, 368–369.

33. Kimoff, R. J., Morrison, D., Leblanc, M. H., et al. (2005). Prospective evaluation of nocturnal oximetry for detection of sleep-related breathing disturbances in patients with chronic heart failure. *Chest, 127*, 1507–1614.

34. Collop, N. A. (2008). Portable monitoring for the diagnosis of obstructive sleep apnea. *Current Opinions in Pulmonary Medicine, 14*, 525–529.

35. Chung, F., Liao, P., Singh, M., et al. (2010). *Undiagnosed obstructive sleep apnea in a surgical population, A770*. Retrieved from http://www.asaabstracts.com/strands/asaabstracts/abstract.htm?year=2010&index=18&absnum=927

36. Liao, P., Elsaid, H., Fazel, H., et al. (2010). *Perioperative strategy to identify OSA patients with STOP-Bang questionnaire and nocturnal oximeter, A771*. Retrieved from http://www.asaabstracts.com/strands/asaabstracts/abstract.htm?year=2010&index=18&absnum=1416

37. Finkel, K. J., Searleman, A. C., Tymkew, H., et al. (2009). Prevalence of undiagnosed obstructive sleep apnea among adult surgical patients in an academic medical center. *Sleep Medicine, 10*, 753–758.

38. Morgenthaler, T. I., & Gay, P. C. (2003). Identifying patients at high risk for postoperative sleep apnea [abstract]. *Sleep, 26* (Suppl.), A211.

39. Clyburn, P. A., Rosen, M., & Vickers, M. D. (1990). Comparison of the respiratory effects of i.v. infusions of morphine and regional analgesia by extradural block. *British Journal of Anaesthesia, 64,* 446–449.

40. Dahan, A., van den Elsen, M. J., Berkenbosch, A., et al. (1994). Effects of subanesthetic halothane on the ventilatory responses to hypercapnia and acute hypoxia in healthy volunteers. *Anesthesiology, 80,* 727–738.

41. Eastwood, P. R., Platt, P. R., Shepherd, K., et al. (2005). Collapsibility of the upper airway at different concentrations of propofol anesthesia. *Anesthesiology, 103,* 470–477.

42. Strum, E. M., Szenohradszki, J., Kaufman, W. A., et al. (2004). Emergence and recovery characteristics of desflurane versus sevoflurane in morbidly obese adult surgical patients: A prospective, randomized study. *Anesthesia and Analgesics, 99,* 1848–1853.

43. Gentil, B., de Larminat, J. M., Boucherez, C., et al. (1994). Difficult intubation and obstructive sleep apnoea syndrome. *British Journal of Anaesthesiology, 72,* 368.

44. Miller, R. D., Eriksson, L. I., Fleisher, L. A., et al. (2009). *Miller's anesthesia.* Cambridge, MA: Churchill Livingstone.

45. Lichtenstein, D. R., Jagannath, S., Baron, T. H., et al. Sedation and anesthesia in GI endoscopy. *Gastrointestinal Endoscopy, 68,* 815–826.

46. Huncke, T., Chan, J., Doyle, W., et al. (2008).The use of continuous positive airway pressure during an awake craniotomy in a patient with obstructive sleep apnea. *Journal of Clinical Anesthesia, 20,* 297–299.

47. Chung, F., Yegneswaran, B., Herrera, F., et al. (2008). Patients with difficult intubation may need referral to sleep clinics. *Anesthesiology and Analgesia, 107,* 915–920.

48. Cormack, R. S., & Lehane, J. (1984). Difficult tracheal intubation in obstetrics. *Anaesthesia, 39,* 1105–1111.

49. Kim, J. A., & Lee, J. J. (2006). Preoperative predictors of difficult intubation in patients with obstructive sleep apnea syndrome. *Canadian Journal of Anaesthesiology, 5,* 393–397.

50. Rosenblatt, W. H., & Whipple, J. (2003). The difficult airway algorithm of the American Society of Anesthesiologists. *Anesthesiology and Analgesics, 96,* 1233.

51. Dixon, B. J., Dixon, J. B., Carden, J. R., et al. (2005). Preoxygenation is more effective in the 25 degrees head-up position than in the supine position in severely obese patients: A randomized controlled study. *Anesthesiology, 102,* 1110–1115; discussion 5A.

52. Isono, S. (2007). Optimal combination of head, mandible and body positions for pharyngeal airway maintenance during perioperative period: Lesson from pharyngeal closing pressures. *Seminars in Anesthesia, Perioperative Medicine and Pain, 26,* 83–93.

53. Baraka, A. S., Taha, S. K., Aouad, M. T., et al. (1999). Preoxygenation: Comparison of maximal breathing and tidal volume breathing techniques. *Anesthesiology, 91,* 612–616.

54. Deegan, P. C., Mulloy, E., & McNicholas, W. T. (1995). Topical oropharyngeal anesthesia in patients with obstructive sleep apnea. *American Journal of Respiratory and Critical Care Medicine, 151,* 1108–1112.

55. Murphy, G. S., Szokol, J. W., Marymont, J. H., et al. (2008). Residual neuromuscular blockade and critical respiratory events in the postanesthesia care unit. *Anesthesiology and Analgesics, 107,* 130–137.

56. Seet, E., & Chung, F. (2010). Management of sleep apnea in adults - functional algorithms for the perioperative period. *Canadian Journal of Anesthesia, 57,* 849–864.

57. Isono, S., Tanaka, A., & Nishino, T. (2002). Lateral position decreases collapsibility of the passive pharynx in patients with obstructive sleep apnea. *Anesthesiology, 9,* 780–785.

58. Gupta, R. M., Parvizi, J., Hanssen, A. D., et al. (2001). Postoperative complications in patients with obstructive sleep apnea syndrome undergoing hip or knee replacement: A case-control study. *Mayo Clinic Proceedings, 76,* 897–905.

59. Sanjay, J. S., & Dhand, R. (2004). Perioperative treatment of patients with obstructive sleep apnea. *Current Opinion in Pulmonary Medicine, 10,* 482–488.

60. Gali, B., Whalen, F. X., Schroeder, D., et al. (2009). Identification of patients at risk for postoperative respiratory complications using a preoperative obstructive sleep apnea screening tool and postanesthesia care assessment. *Anesthesiology, 110,* 869–877.

61. Seet, E., & Chung, F. (2010). Obstructive sleep apnea: Preoperative assessment. *Anesthesiology Clinics, 28,* 199–215.

62. Ingram, G., & Munro, N. (2005). The use (or otherwise) of pulse oximetry in general practice. *The British Journal of General Practice, 55*(516), 501–502.

63. Saunders, R., Struys, M. M. R. F., Pollock, R. F., et al. (2017). Patient safety during procedural sedation using capnography monitoring: A systematic review and meta- analysis. *BMJ Open, 7,* e013402. doi:10.1136/bmjopen-2016-013402

64. Bolden, N., Smith, C. E., & Auckley, D. (2009). Avoiding adverse outcomes in patients with obstructive sleep apnea (OSA): Development and implementation of a perioperative OSA protocol. *Journal of Clinical Anesthesiology, 2,* 6–93.

chapter 31

Developing a Program for Identifying, Assessing, and Managing Hospitalized Patients for Sleep-Disordered Breathing

RENEA DAVIS

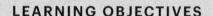

LEARNING OBJECTIVES

On completion of this chapter, the reader should be able to:

1. Identify hospitalized patients at risk for sleep-disordered breathing (SDB).
2. Develop an assessment appropriate to hospitalized patients with increased risk of SDB.
3. Discuss the primary comorbid disorders associated with multiple hospitalizations and readmissions.
4. Develop a program for hospitalized patients identified with SDB.

KEY TERMS

Sleep-disordered breathing (SDB)
Chronic obstructive pulmonary disease (COPD)
Congestive heart failure (CHF)
Obstructive sleep apnea (OSA)
Mallampati
Case management
Discharge planning
Outcomes measurement

INTRODUCTION

The purpose of this chapter is to provide sleep programs with a fundamental approach to developing a program for identifying, assessing, and managing hospitalized patients at increased risk for sleep-disordered breathing (SDB). The complex interactions between SDB and other common disorders such as treatment-resistant hypertension, chronic obstructive pulmonary disease (COPD), type 2 diabetes, atrial fibrillation, stroke, and congestive heart failure (CHF) have been associated with multiple

hospitalizations and readmissions in many patients as well as an increased risk of sedation complications and medication interactions.

RATIONALE

Despite widely available information about the clinical importance of screening for SDB, and the citation of SDB as a patient safety issue by the Joint Commission (1), the majority of patients with SDB remain unrecognized and undiagnosed. There may be a variety of reasons for this. The symptoms and risk factors for SDB are neither sensitive nor specific for SDB and overlap with many other important medical conditions, some of which may be the conditions driving admission to the hospital.

The recent declaration by the US Preventive Services Task Force that "the current evidence is insufficient to assess the balance of benefits and harms of screening for obstructive sleep apnea (OSA) in asymptomatic adults" has led to some unfortunate confusion (2). Health care professionals may mistakenly apply this recommendation to the acute care setting, where symptoms are often present, and where the balance of risk and benefit favors screening for SDB.

Adult and pediatric patients with SDB are at risk for complications during hospitalization or surgery. These patients may experience complications when receiving sedatives, opioid analgesics, or general anesthesia, increasing the risk of prolonged apnea and respiratory arrest. SDB can be worsened by the use of sedatives and narcotics.

Evidence suggests an association between SDB and COPD and CHF readmissions, conditions monitored closely by Medicare's Hospital Readmission Reduction Program. Untreated obesity hypoventilation syndrome increases the risk of acute and chronic hypercapnic episodes, as well as having a significant impact on long-term survival. SDB screening programs are an important way to identify these patient populations. Implementation of treatment in these patients has been shown to convey benefits. Studies have shown that patients hospitalized with CHF and/or COPD with SDB who are adherent to treatment have a lower 30-day readmission rate than untreated SDB patients.

Sleep technology professionals, especially sleep health educators with established core competencies, have an opportunity to participate in implementing procedures that help reduce readmission by establishing screening solutions. These strategies include building processes that identify, screen, and facilitate testing and initiate treatment of patients with SDB.

The Joint Commission issued an advisory on safety and quality issues relating to patients with OSA in June 2015 (2). The advisory cites sentinel events in which patients were diagnosed or suspected to have OSA, which may have been a contributing factor in some of the cases. In this advisory, staff in The Joint Commission's Division of Healthcare Improvement cite the following concerns regarding OSA:

- Lack of training for health care professionals to screen for and recognize OSA
- Failure to assess patients for OSA
- Lack of guidelines for the care and treatment of individuals at risk for, and those diagnosed with, OSA
- Failure to implement appropriate monitoring of patients with risk factors associated with OSA
- Lack of communication among health care providers regarding patients with OSA or potential risk factors associated with OSA
- Lack of postoperative evaluation and treatment for OSA

These concerns should be kept in mind as you develop your program to assure that they are addressed.

THE PURPOSE OF SCREENING

Screening of inpatients for SDB is intended to prevent SDB-related complications, protect patients from potential harm, reduce readmissions, and provide exceptional patient-centered care by improving patient wellness. The role of the sleep center technologist or clinical sleep health educator is to collect and summarize patient health information including vital signs and questionnaire results necessary for evaluation of risk for SDB. There should be set protocols in place to alert appropriate health care providers when patients meet criteria for an elevated risk of SDB. The clinical sleep health staff can manage the process of monitoring patients during hospitalization and work with the patient care team to coordinate an appropriate sleep care follow-up plan.

Building the Team

Development and implementation of a SDB screening program requires working with a variety of members of the patient care team and creation of policies and procedures to guide team members.

Composition of the team will vary from hospital to hospital and may require involvement of a variety of stakeholders to implement and manage the process. Some of the key players may be the following:

a. **Physician advocate:** One of the biggest assets to starting any hospital program is having a physician advocate. This physician should be well versed in the physician and hospital politics, know about the medical community, and understand the positive impact a program like this will have on patient care. This person does not necessarily have to be a sleep physician; a current referring physician such as a surgeon, cardiologist, or hospitalist may be a good option.

b. **Members of the sleep care team:** The medical director and other sleep physicians, practitioners, and staff need to be on board and well informed about the program. An inpatient program may require your sleep physicians and practitioners to see inpatients in consult, and order and interpret studies while the patient is in house. Adequate staff of registered polysomnographic technologists and certified clinical sleep health educators are essential to the program. These professionals will require sufficient time for chart review, patient education, and setting up, downloading, and scoring of the studies performed as part of the program.

c. **Administrators:** When a plan has been developed and you have a physician champion and staff on board, the next step is to present the plan to administration. Hospital administrators are responsible for the financial well-being of the hospital and a program that is focused on improving patient outcomes and reducing readmissions is one way of achieving that. Administrators are likely to be interested in the effect an inpatient screening program will have on the quality of patient care, meeting the Joint Commission's recommendations, achieving good outcomes, increasing referrals to the sleep center, and the risks of not identifying, testing, or educating these patients. The presentation should be short and factual, and include a financial analysis for the program.

d. **Hospital accountants:** The hospital finance department accountants can assist with the development of a cost analysis. A projection of the estimated number of patients based on patient population, current reimbursement, and payer mix will be needed to project possible revenue. They can typically pull numbers of patients by diagnosis (CHF or

COPD). This will help with the financial benefits of the program.

e. **Nursing administrators:** Determine if the nursing staff already use a STOP-Bang or modified sleep questionnaire about symptoms of OSA on admission. It will be important to develop an ongoing relationship with nursing as well as develop training for the nurses about the program and testing that will be performed on their patients.

f. **Risk management or patient safety officers:** Risk management involvement will guide you through the risks, safety precautions, and policies needed for the program.

g. **Surgical team members:** Preoperative screening can be beneficial in preemptively setting up appropriate monitoring during postoperative patient recovery and beyond for those at risk of OSA. Some of these teams include members from programs such as the following:
   • Bariatric surgery
   • Anesthesiology
   • General surgery
   • Cardiology

h. **Case managers and discharge planners:** It is important to educate this group because they are typically the last to see the patient before discharge. They can make a significant difference in assuring appropriate ongoing care for the patient after discharge.

Procedural Steps
Identify Hospitalized Patients with SDB

Identifying at-risk patients is the first step. Listed in the next paragraph are many different parameters used to identify these patients. It would be prudent to check to see if or how the admitting nurse is collecting sleep-related information and find out how to obtain access to it if it is being collected. If the hospital utilizes an electronic medical record (EMR), an established sleep screening tool like the Epworth Sleepiness Scale, Apnea Risk Evaluation System, the Berlin questionnaire, or the STOP-Bang should be implemented in the admitting process. One method to obtain referral to the program could be triggering the referral on the basis of a specific score on the screening questionnaire. If the admitting nursing staff administer the sleep questionnaire during admission, the application support team could develop a report to flag all new admissions that scored positive on the questionnaire. Additionally, or independently, further parameters collected such as diagnosis or a body mass index (BMI) of more than 35 could trigger a referral.

The following established risk factors can be used to identify populations at risk for SDB:

• Mallampati score
• BMI more than 35 kg per m^2
• Conditions that are often comorbid with SDB such as treatment-resistant hypertension, COPD, type 2 diabetes, atrial fibrillation, stroke, and CHF
• Symptoms of SDB such as complaints of witnessed apneas, snoring, gasping or choking at night, restless sleep
• Clinical manifestations such as nocturnal hypoxemia, nocturnal shortness of breath, waking with angina
• Previous diagnosis of sleep apnea and nonadherence to treatment
• Using medications such as opiates that may increase the risk of SDB.

Safeguard and Monitor At-Risk Patients

It is important to recognize that inpatients are acutely ill and, if suspected to have OSA or diagnosed but noncompliant with therapy, need to be monitored continuously upon admission. An automated alert system when a patient scores positive for OSA on admission to the following departments can help create a well-informed and active patient care team:

• The respiratory therapist initiates continuous telemetry, end-tidal or transcutaneous CO_2 and/or pulse oximetry monitoring, or even continuous positive airway pressure (CPAP) therapy.
• Pharmacy reviews the patient's medications and possible effects on SDB.
• Attending physicians and care extenders notified of patient risk
   • A sleep consult can be offered if appropriate, or referral to the sleep physician after discharge.
• Sleep center staff initiate patient education.
• Case managers/discharge planners informed to make appointments for the patient or arrange for home setup of CPAP.

Educate At-Risk Patients and Families

In some hospitals, it may be possible to automatically initiate a consult to the sleep physician who assesses the condition of the patients and the appropriateness for an inpatient home sleep apnea test (HSAT). Another option is an EMR alert for the attending physician who will discuss the risk with the patient and/or family and initiate a sleep physician consult if appropriate at that time. In all cases, the sleep center should provide an educational visit to the patient's room. Provide personalized patient information on sleep health and hygiene, sleep disorders, SDB and comorbidities, and therapeutic options. A discussion regarding possible OSA, screening and testing, and, if applicable, therapy adherence with the patient and family members may be appropriate. Always be respectful, because mostly patients will not be in a proper frame of mind to talk about snoring or how they are sleeping on account of their condition. In such a scenario, leave them with an educational sheet that includes a phone number to call when they feel better. Approach them later if an opportunity arises.

Tips to Remember

- Determine appropriate literacy level and educate the patient and family.
- Follow the American Association of Sleep Technologists (AAST) standardized Patient Education Curriculum guidelines.
- Document education provided in patients' medical record.
- Consider using the hospital patient education TV channel or videos of Expectation Management and Medical Information to provide accessible patient education.

Educate the Health Care Team

It is important to educate everyone on the health care team. Provide education on basic sleep hygiene, sleep disorders, and SDB, and the technology utilized to obtain sleep studies, especially HSAT if it will be utilized in hospitalized patients. The clinical staff need to be informed of the importance of monitoring pulse oximetry in at-risk patients and assuring that testing equipment remains on the patient during testing. It is important to acknowledge that patient care always comes first, and sleep study second.

The technologist applying the HSAT equipment is responsible for informing the attending nurse about the sleep study. Explain what the recording device is monitoring and that it will be retrieved and downloaded in the morning for review. The technologist educates the patient and nurse and verifies there is no impediment to testing that night.

In general, the education plan for the program should include the following:

- Outlining the program and educating hospitalists, nursing staff, cardiologists, pulmonologists, risk management, case management, and the respiratory therapy team (with special attention to night shift care teams) about the risk of SDB in hospitalized patients and available resources
- Referencing the AAST OSA Care Plan and the AAST Patient Education Curriculum
- Providing Continuing Education Credits (CEC)/ Continuing Education Units (CEU) in-service programs for staff
- Providing a method to contact the sleep health educator and other members of the sleep care team for support

Coordinate Diagnostic Testing

Work with the patient care team to assess patient risk and the benefits of immediate testing. Inpatients with chronically poor health may not return after discharge, and therefore, inpatient testing may be warranted.

- Triage patients on the basis of the risk assessment.
- Obtain an order for additional screening tests as needed (consider overnight oximetry or HSAT).
- Schedule postdischarge in-lab studies if appropriate.
- Report the outcome of testing to the attending physician and patient care team.
- Obtain an order for treatment from a sleep specialist or another physician if appropriate.

Assure Treatment Implementation

Identify any barriers to treatment and work with the health care team to resolve them. The hospital case manager and discharge planner will be assisting before discharge. There are many choices they must provide the patient to maintain compliance with state and federal regulations. Be sure to include them in the treatment planning process.

The sleep team should be prepared to do the following:

- Assist with implementation of positive airway pressure (PAP) therapy.
- Assure appropriate documentation to support the durable medical equipment (DME) order.
- Document the DME supplier, the interface type and size, and treatment settings.
- Coordinate with the DME supplier to assure appropriate equipment is in place upon discharge.

Monitor Patient Adherence and Outcomes

Implement a follow-up monitoring plan that includes the following:

- Frequent monitoring of adherence data, beginning with the first week and continuing until adherence to therapy is established.
- Technologist or educator telephone support for patients on PAP therapy as needed
  - Follow policies and procedures to determine and document the need for intervention.
- Assure timely and appropriate physician follow-up.
  - Provide clinical intervention when needed (further testing, evaluation, or support).
- Develop support of a DME liaison for home visits if necessary.
- Utilize digital patient engagement tools to support therapy adherence.
- Track and report patient outcomes.

- Establish metrics and reporting process (data collection tool or EMR).
  - Reporting should include previous history of readmission, adherence, and any readmission posttreatment.
- Collect data for American Academy of Sleep Medicine (AASM) outcome measures as indicated.
  - Track and report overall program outcomes.
- Maintain a database for outcomes tracking (readmission rates, adherence to therapy, improvement in quality of life, or other appropriate measures).

SUMMARY

Developing a program for identifying, assessing, and managing hospitalized patients at increased risk for SDB is a significant undertaking. In the inpatient arena, there are many overlapping priorities, and making the identification of hospitalized patients at risk for SDB that may extend or complicate their hospital stay, or result in readmissions, is no small undertaking.

An organized plan that includes all facets of the organization from administration and physicians to the nursing and ancillary staff is essential. Policies and procedures must be a part of the plan, and education for staff in all areas is key to the success of an inpatient program. Screening tools, diagnostic tools and processes, discharge and follow-up care, as well as measurement of outcomes and success of the program are each important pieces of the overall plan.

The success of an inpatient screening program depends on the cooperation and coordination of a multitude of people and services, but if done well, can result in improved care and better outcomes for hospitalized patients who are at risk for SDB. It is worth the effort!

REFERENCES

1. AAST Technical Guidelines. (February 2018). *Best practice for inpatient sleep disordered breathing screening and management.* American Association of Sleep Technologists. Retrieved July 2, 2018, from https://www.aastweb.org/hubfs/AAST%20Best%20Practice%20TG%202018%202-19-18%20FINAL%203-5-18.pdf?t=1530548876669

2. Quick Safety: An Advisory on Safety and Quality Issues. (June 2015). *At risk: Obstructive sleep apnea patients* (Issue 14). Oakbrook Terrace, IL: Joint Commission.

chapter 32

Medications and Their Effect on Sleep and Sleep Disorders

DEBBIE AKERS   JANET PRUETT   J. CATESBY WARE   ROBERT D. VORONA

LEARNING OBJECTIVES

On completion of this chapter, the reader should be able to:

1. Recognize major classes of drugs that may alter the polysomnogram.
2. Detect sleep disturbances that may occur because of specific medications.
3. Describe the relationship between sleep and medications.
4. Recognize when to intervene on behalf of patient safety.

KEY TERMS

Hypnotic
Antidepressant
Gamma-aminobutyric acid (GABA)
Sedative
Selective serotonin reuptake inhibitor (SSRI)
ACE inhibitor
Tricyclic antidepressant
Polysomnography (PSG)

The Center, for Disease Control and Prevention (CDC) reported in 2016 that 49% of the U.S. population used at least one prescription drug within the past 30 days; 23% used three or more prescription drugs, whereas 12% used five or more prescription drugs (1). Chances are that three out of four of the 84% using a prescription drug within the past 30 days are being seen in the sleep laboratory tonight. The purpose of this chapter is to assist the technologist to provide better patient care by understanding how daily medications can affect sleep and sleep disorders.

MEDICATIONS AND HOW THEY AFFECT SLEEP

About 89% of patients rely on some sort of prescribed medications. Most of these medications are for chronic conditions, whereas some are used for acute ailments. Medications for high blood pressure, heart disease, respiratory issues (asthma, chronic obstructive pulmonary disease), headaches, smoking cessation, colds and allergies, to name a few, can affect sleep by either depriving the patient of sleep or causing daytime sleepiness.

Some of the more commonly prescribed medications are antiarrhythmic drugs used to treat heart rhythm issues, which can cause difficulty initiating and maintaining sleep or insomnia. Beta-blockers are used to treat hypertension, arrhythmias, and angina. Beta-blockers increase the likelihood of awakenings during the night, nightmares, and/or insomnia. Cholesterol medications are associated with poor sleep. Asthma medications can cause insomnia because the chemicals in theophylline are related to caffeine and can make the patient feel fidgety. Thyroid conditions can cause tremendous sleepiness (specifically hypothyroidism), whereas the medication used to treat this disorder causes insomnia. These are a few of the common prescription medications often seen on the patient's medication list. This chapter will review medications that can affect a patient's sleep and the effects of medications on the polysomnography (PSG).

Hypnotics
Barbiturates

Barbiturates, sometimes called "downers," are medications that act on the central nervous system (CNS) by depressing or inhibiting nerve signals in the brain. They work by depressing the reticular formation, a comprehensive network of nerves found in the central area of the brainstem, thus promoting sleep. Other uses include, but are not limited to, anesthesia during surgery, an anticonvulsant, and for anxiety attacks. Barbiturates are derived from barbituric acid (2) that scientists have synthesized and are grouped according to how fast they produce an effect and how long that effect lasts, and are classified as sedative hypnotics that lead to the slowing down of the body's functions. This slowing down of the body's functions can include physical signs such as lethargy, slurred speech, shallow breathing, fatigue, drowsiness, and difficulty in concentrating.

Expected and possible effects on PSG (acute):

Decrease: Sleep latency (SL), wake after sleep onset (WASO), N1, rapid eye movement (REM), N3, arousals, and body movement.

Increase: Sleep efficiency (SE), total sleep time (TST), N2, spindles, N3, REM latency (RL), sleep apnea, and daytime sleepiness.

Withdrawal: Decrease TST and increase REM (REM rebound).

Barbiturates are now rarely used most likely because of the numerous adverse side effects and high incidence of tolerance and dependence. They used to be the "go-to drug" for insomnia but have lessened in popularity with the advent of benzodiazepines (BZDs).

Benzodiazepines

BZD is a psychoactive medication used as a sedative or muscle relaxant. When one suffers from anxiety or panic attacks, the brain becomes overactive and BZDs are chemicals that will help it to slow down. Although it is not clear how BZDs work, they are believed to affect the GABA receptors of the brain. GABA, or gamma-aminobutyric acid, is a major inhibitory brain chemical that blocks the transmission of a signal from one brain cell to another. Although GABA is an amino acid, it is classified as a neurotransmitter; it inhibits and relaxes, therefore inducing relaxation and sleep.

Expected and possible effects on PSG (acute):

Decrease: SL, WASO, REM, N3 (for most agents), periodic limb movements (PLMs), and arousals.

Increase: SE, TST, N1, N2, spindles, N3 (for some agents), RL, sleep apnea, and daytime sleepiness.

Withdrawal: Increase WASO, decrease TST, increase REM (REM rebound), increase SL, and arousals.

Although BZDs contain chemicals like those found in the body to induce calming, adding them to what is already in the body helps GABA receptors send out a greater number of these signals to the brain, resulting in sedation or relaxation. BZDs are also used for general anesthesia, sedation before medical procedures, alcohol withdrawal, nausea, and vomiting. Although BZDs are used for various reasons, some are more commonly prescribed for certain conditions (3):

Alcohol withdrawal: Chlordiazepoxide (Librium)

Anesthesia: Diazepam (Valium), lorazepam (Ativan), and midazolam (Versed)

Anxiety: Alprazolam (Xanax), chlordiazepoxide (Librium), clorazepate (Tranxene), diazepam (Valium), lorazepam (Ativan), and midazolam (Versed)

Insomnia: Estazolam (Prosom), flurazepam (Dalmane), quazepam (Doral), temazepam (Restoril), and triazolam (Halcion)

Irritable bowel syndrome: Chlordiazepoxide clidinium (Librax)

Muscle relaxant: Diazepam (Valium)

Seizure: Clonazepam (Klonopin), clorazepate (Tranxene), and diazepam (Valium)

Reduce PLMs: Clonazepam (Klonopin)

Keeping in mind that some BZDs have been used for a multitude of medical conditions, one should then not assume that a patient, who, for illustration purposes, takes diazepam, suffers from seizures. The sleep technologist should always take the time to read each patient's medical history (Table 32-1).

Nonbenzodiazepine (NBZD, Z-Drugs, and GABA Receptor Agonists)

NBZD, a relatively newer class of drugs, is also used for surgical anesthesia but is more widely advertised as a short-term treatment for insomnia. These drugs work in the same area of the brain as BZDs do but tend to be more specific for inducing sleep.

NBZDs are generally known to have a shorter half-life, so it is rare to wake up with a "hangover" feeling the following day. Newer controlled-release formulations may extend the half-life of the medication as in the case of zolpidem. Information released by the Food and Drug Administration (FDA), however, states that the termination half-life for controlled-release zolpidem (12.5 mg) is no different from that of the immediate release formula (10 mg).

The use of NBZDs is less likely to cause addiction but may cause amnesia and erratic behavior (as parasomnia). One should keep in mind, however, that these medications would not address any underlying medical problems that may cause insomnia and therefore should not be seen as a cure (Table 32-2).

Other Hypnotic Agents

Two examples of hypnotic agents are ramelteon and chloral hydrate. Ramelteon is considered a melatonin receptor agonist, thus inhibiting the wake-promoting activity of the suprachiasmatic nucleus. It also helps reduce SL and increase TST, while having no effect on sleep architecture. Chloral hydrate, an alcohol-type hypnotic,

Table 32-1 Benzodiazepines

Generic Name	Popularly Known as/Brand Name	Time to Peak (Onset of Action [h])	Elimination Half-life (h) (Active Metabolite)
Alprazolam	Xanax	1–2	6–12
Chlordiazepoxide	Librium	1.5–4	5–30 (36–200 h)
Clonazepam	Klonopin	1–4	18–50
Clorazepate	Tranxene	Varies	(36–100 h)
Diazepam	Valium	1–2	20–100 (36–200 h)
Estazolam	Prosom	0.5–5	10–24
Flunitrazepam	Rohypnol	0.5–3	18–26 (36–200 h)
Flurazepam	Dalmane	1–1.5	(40–250 h)
Halazepam	Paxipam	1–3	(30–100 h)
Lorazepam	Ativan	2–4	10–20
Midazolam	Versed	0.5–1	3 (1.8–6 h)
Oxazepam	Serax	3–4	4–15
Quazepam	Doral	1–5	25–120
Temazepam	Restoril	0.5–3	8–22
Triazolam	Halcion	0.5–2	2

Expected Effects of Benzodiazepines on Polysomnography

<	SL
>	SE
>	TST
<	WASO
>	NREM 1
>	NREM 2 > Spindles
<<	SWS
>	RL
<	REM
<	Arousals
<, >	PLMs
≥	Sleep apnea
>	Daytime sleepiness
	Withdrawal
<	TST
>	REM (REM rebound)
>	Arousals
>	SL

(*continued*)

Table 32-1 Benzodiazepines (continued)

Expected Effect on Polysomnography

<	SL
>	SE
>	TST
<	WASO
<	NwwwwREM 1
>	NREM 2 (spindles)
≤	SWS
>	RL
≤	REM
<, >	Arousals
=	PLMs
=	Sleep apnea
	Withdrawal
≥	WASO

NREM, nonrapid eye movement; PLM, periodic limb movement; REM, rapid eye movement; RL, REM latency; SE, sleep efficiency; SL, sleep latency; SWS, slow-wave sleep; TST, total sleep time; WASO, wake after sleep onset.

Table 32-2 Nonbenzodiazepines

Generic Name	Popularly Known as/Brand Name	Onset of Action (min)	Half-life (h)
Eszopiclone	Lunesta	60	4–6
Zaleplon	Sonata	15–30	1
Zolpidem	Ambien	15–30	2–3

Expected Effects of Nonbenzodiazepines on Polysomnography

<, >	SL
<, >	SE
>	TST
<	WASO
>	NREM 2 (spindles)
≥	SWS
>	RL
<<	REM
>	PLMs
≥	Daytime sleepiness
	Withdrawal
>	WASO
>	REM

NREM, nonrapid eye movement; PLM, periodic limb movement; REM, rapid eye movement; RL, REM latency; SE, sleep efficiency; SL, sleep latency; SWS, slow-wave sleep; TST, total sleep time; WASO, wake after sleep onset.

is occasionally used in the elderly. It has a short half life (4 to 6 hours) and will decrease SL and arousals. Slow-wave sleep (SWS) is also slightly depressed, but overall REM sleep is unchanged (4).

Antidepressants

There are occasions when doctors prescribe antidepressants to promote sleep despite none of these being specifically approved as sleep medications.

Antidepressants, the third most prescribed drug in this country, were first developed in the 1950s to help relieve the symptoms of depression. Tricyclic antidepressants (TCAs) and selective serotonin reuptake inhibitors (SSRIs) are the two most popular on the market today (5).

Tricyclic Antidepressants

TCAs are considered a first-generation antidepressant medication and are named for the molecular structure of most of the drugs in this class. They are one of the oldest classes of antidepressants and continue to be prescribed today. They are thought to act by blocking the reuptake or reabsorption of two critical brain hormones, the neurotransmitters serotonin and norepinephrine. Some block one, some the other, and some block both.

Neurotransmitters are different types of chemical messengers that the brain contains, which act as communication agents between various brain cells. Two of these transmitters are serotonin, also known as 5-hydroxytryptamine, and norepinephrine. Serotonin's effects are normally inhibitory. It diminishes appetite and sexual behavior and suppresses pain perception, and has also been correlated with eating and sleep disorders (6). Norepinephrine plays a significant role in how the body responds to stress. It is more involved in maintaining normal body functions such as heart rate, blood pressure, and blood sugar levels and in regulating attention, emotions, and sleep (7).

TCAs will also block the reuptake of histamine and acetylcholine (ACh) activity. Histamine helps control the sleep–wake cycle and promotes the release of epinephrine and norepinephrine, whereas ACh is a neurotransmitter with an important role in the enhancement of sensory perceptions when we are awake and in sustaining attention. ACh is known to be the most important inducer of REM sleep (8) (Table 32-3).

A low-dose doxepin formulation is approved by the FDA for the treatment of insomnia. Studies have shown that low-dose doxepin (3 and 6 mg) may be an alternative to hypnotics such as Ambien for primary insomnia. Doxepin decreases WASO and SL, increasing TST. These results were the same for chronic and transient insomnia patients.

Selective Serotonin Reuptake Inhibitors

SSRIs were developed in response to the need for better tolerated, if not safer, antidepressants than TCAs.

They were developed to inhibit the reuptake of only serotonin and not other neurotransmitters, which were also affected by TCAs. Because of this desired result, plus the benefit of improved tolerability and safety if taken in excess, SSRIs now replace TCAs as the drug of choice to treat depression. It should be noted, however, that there remain clinical situations where TCAs are still deemed more appropriate (e.g., severe depression).

SSRIs are stimulants and are more likely to produce insomnia. Several patients have reported sleeping better, and the remaining issues of insomnia are expected to improve with continued use. Although they may encourage better sleep, they have also been linked to REM behavior disorder (RBD). SSRIs' effect on sleep architecture includes a decrease in SL, SE, TST, and REM sleep and an increase in WASO, N1, and PLMs (Table 32-4).

Serotonin and Norepinephrine (Noradrenaline) Reuptake Inhibitors

Serotonin and norepinephrine (noradrenaline) reuptake inhibitors (SNRIs) are also known as "dual reuptake inhibitors" because they act on both serotonin and norepinephrine. The former regulates a variety of bodily functions and feelings, whereas the latter is a chemical messenger in the brain that influences sleep and alertness. Duloxetine (Cymbalta), venlafaxine (Effexor), and desvenlafaxine (Pristiq) are SNRIs. Aside from being antidepressants, duloxetine and venlafaxine are also indicated for the treatment of generalized anxiety and social anxiety disorders. Duloxetine may also be prescribed for painful diabetic neuropathy and may soon be used for stress urinary incontinence (9). Newly diagnosed with RBD? Effexor may be the culprit (Table 32-5).

Monoamine Oxidase Inhibitors

Monoamine oxidase inhibitors (MAOIs) are a class of antidepressants that affect serotonin, norepinephrine, and dopamine levels in the brain. Dopamine is responsible for motivation, interest, and drive and is also involved in muscle control and function. It is associated with positive stress states such as being in love, exercising, listening to music, and sex.

MAOIs are mostly effective in major depression and are typically prescribed for those who do not respond well to other antidepressants and as a last resort because of numerous side effects. They are effective for some forms of depression when other medications have failed (5).

Expected and possible effects on PSG:

Decrease: SE, TST, SWS, and REM.

Increase: SL, WASO, PLMs, and daytime sleepiness.

Table 32-3 Tricyclics

Generic Name	Popularly Known as/Brand Name	Half-life (h)
Amitriptyline	Elavil	10–50
Amoxapine	Asendin	8
Clomipramine	Anafranil	21
Doxepin	Silenor, Sinequan	8–24
Desipramine	Norpramin	12–24
Imipramine	Tofranil	11–25
Maprotiline	Ludiomil	8–16
Nortriptyline	Pamelor	18–44
Protriptyline	Vivactil	16–90
Trimipramine	Surmontil	14–46

Expected/Effects of Tricyclics on Polysomnography

<	SL
<	SE
<	TST
≥	WASO
</>	NREM 1
≤	SWS
>>	RL
<	REM
>	Arousals
≥	PLMs
≥	Daytime sleepiness
>	NREM eye movement
>	RBD

NREM, nonrapid eye movement; PLM, periodic limb movement; RBD, REM behavior disorder; REM, rapid eye movement; RL, REM latency; SE, sleep efficiency; SL, sleep latency; SWS, slow-wave sleep; TST, total sleep time; WASO, wake after sleep onset.

Atypical Antidepressants

There are some antidepressants that are both non-SSRI and non-TCA. An example of this is buspirone (Buspar). Because it lacks the anticonvulsant, sedative, and muscle relaxant properties associated with other anxiolytics, buspirone has been termed as "anxioselective" (10). It is nonsedating and shows no effect on SL, sleep continuity, SWS, or REM sleep and does not increase incidence of PLMs.

Cardiovascular Drugs

Antihypertensive Drugs

There are many different types of antihypertensive drugs, some of which affect how the heart pumps blood, whereas others cause vasodilation. The types that are most commonly used are beta-blocker drugs, angiotensin-converting enzyme (ACE) inhibitor drugs, angiotensin II blocker drugs, calcium-channel blocker drugs, and diuretic drugs.

Table 32-4 Selective Serotonin Reuptake Inhibitors

Generic Name	Popularly Known as/Brand Name	Half-life (h)
Citalopram	Celexa	35
Escitalopram	Lexapro	27–32
Fluoxetine	Prozac	48–96
Paroxetine	Paxil	20
Sertraline	Zoloft	26

Expected Effects of SSRIs on Polysomnography

>	SL
<	SE
<	TST
>	WASO
>	NREM 1
>	RL
<<	REM
>	PLMs
≥	Daytime sleepiness

NREM, nonrapid eye movement; PLM, periodic limb movement; REM, rapid eye movement; RL, REM latency; SE, sleep efficiency; SL, sleep latency; SWS, slow-wave sleep; TST, total sleep time; WASO, wake after sleep onset.

Table 32-5 Serotonin and Noradrenaline Reuptake Inhibitors

Generic Name	Popularly Known as/Brand Name	Duration of Effect/Elimination Half-life (h)
Desvenlafaxine	Pristiq	11
Duloxetine	Cymbalta	12
Venlafaxine	Effexor	5–7

Expected/Possible Effects of H1 Blockers on PSG

<	SL
>	TST
>	NREM 1
>	NREM 2
>	SWS
<	REM

Expected/Possible Effects of H2 Blockers on PSG

>	SWS (for cimetidine)
=	Usually have no effect on sleep stages or sleep continuity
+	Somnolence and lethargy for elder patients

NREM, nonrapid eye movement; PSG, polysomnography; REM, rapid eye movement; SL, sleep latency; SWS, slow-wave sleep; TST, total sleep time.

ACE Inhibitors

ACE inhibitors are drugs used to treat heart failure and high blood pressure and to treat diabetic kidney disease. ACE inhibitors help prevent, although not completely, the normal formation in the body of angiotensin II, which is a hormone that causes constriction (narrowing) of blood vessels. By reducing the amount of the hormone present in the blood, ACE inhibitors allow blood vessels to dilate. This dilation or widening of blood vessels throughout the body reduces blood pressure, making it easier for the heart to pump blood, and results in alleviating heart failure (11). Although these drugs help improve quality of life and cognitive performance, there is some question as to whether they may cause insomnia.

Angiotensin II Blockers

Like ACE inhibitors, angiotensin II drugs are used to treat heart failure, high blood pressure, and to prevent kidney failure. They are an alternative to ACE inhibitors and work by blocking the action of angiotensin II that is produced naturally by the body and causes blood vessels to constrict (12).

Beta-Blockers

Beta-blocker drugs, or beta-adrenergic blocking agents, are most often prescribed to treat high blood pressure. They work by blocking the action of epinephrine (adrenaline) and norepinephrine (noradrenaline), two chemicals produced by the body that increase heart rate and raise blood pressure (12).

Expected and possible effects on PSG:

Decrease: TST, SWS, and REM.
Increase: SL, WASO, N1, REM, total wake time, and daytime sleepiness (after daytime administration).

The effects on sleep quality and staging seem to be limited to lipophilic as opposed to hydrophilic beta-blockers (13). Lipophilic agents include propranolol, pindolol, and metoprolol, whereas hydrophilic agents include atenolol and sotalol. Beta-blockers have also been associated with complaints of insomnia, fatigue, hallucinations, and nightmares.

Calcium-Channel Blockers

Calcium-channel blockers reduce the amount of calcium entering the muscle cells in blood vessel walls. Muscle cells need calcium to contract, and reducing the amount of calcium induces the muscle cells to relax and the blood vessels to widen (12).

Calcium-channel blockers are not known to affect sleep, sleep continuity, or sleep stages. However, they are associated with insomnia and nightmares (14).

Diuretic Drugs

Diuretics work by reducing the amount of liquid and salts reabsorbed into the blood, thereby increasing the volume of urine that is produced. The reduced blood volume helps reduce blood pressure (12). Impact on sleep is secondary because of increased nocturia.

Centrally Acting Alpha-Adrenergic Agonists: Clonidine

Several studies have demonstrated that clonidine disrupted the quality of nighttime sleep by inducing more shifts to N1 or wakefulness (14, 15). Clonidine increases sedation and has also been known to suppress or reduce REM sleep.

Hypolipidemic Drugs

Cholesterol is a waxy, fat-like substance that is made by the liver. It forms part of every cell in the body, helps maintain healthy cell walls, and produces hormones, bile acids for the digestion of fat, and vitamin D. Excess cholesterol clogs blood vessels and increases the risk of heart disease and stroke.

Although cholesterol medications are often prescribed, there are no supporting data showing the relationship between the use of cholesterol medication and sleep architecture. Some reports, however, show that atorvastatin, lovastatin, and simvastatin may lead to insomnia or disrupt sleep, whereas Gemfibrozil and clofibrate are reported to cause sleepiness (16).

Stimulants

Stimulants are a class of drugs that work by increasing the dopamine levels in the brain. They include, among others, amphetamines, methylphenidate, modafinil, pemoline, and xanthene derivatives (namely caffeine and theophylline) (17). Xanthene derivatives, including caffeine, are also considered CNS stimulants. The exact mechanism of modafinil (Provigil) is not known. It is primarily used in the management of narcolepsy and is approved for persistent daytime sleepiness in patients on continuous positive airway pressure, circadian rhythm sleep disorder, and shift work. It is a wakefulness-promoting agent and decreases TST and REM sleep (18).

Stimulants, as a rule, affect wakefulness. They are known to increase SL and reduce both SE and SWS. Discontinuing their use may result in sleepiness as a rebound effect (except for modafinil) (17).

Caffeine users are more readily aroused by sudden noises and exhibit an increase in body movements during sleep and a reduction in the reported quality of sleep. When caffeine is used, REM sleep tends to occur earlier, but researchers have not yet determined whether the duration of REM sleep is increased or decreased (19).

Antihistamines

Histamine agonist or antihistamines are a class of medications used to treat millions who suffer from allergies and their symptoms. It is a pharmaceutical drug that inhibits the action of histamine by blocking it from attaching to histamine receptors. With the increase of allergy sufferers today, more and more people take antihistamines (Table 32-6).

Antihistamines are classified as either H1 receptor blockers (further grouped into first generation and second generation) or H2 receptor agonists. First-generation H1 blockers are sedating and the second generation, mild or nonsedating. The first-generation H1 blockers may decrease SL and REM and increase TST, N1, N2, and SWS. Cimetidine, an H2 receptor, is known to increase SWS. Other drugs in its class, including ranitidine and famotidine, have no documented effect on sleep stages or sleep continuity.

Anticonvulsants

Anticonvulsant or antiepileptic drugs can have either detrimental or beneficial effects on sleep. Most anticonvulsants appear to improve and stabilize sleep as a direct consequence of seizure suppression. Effect on sleep architecture is dependent on which anticonvulsant is prescribed (20).

> Gabapentin (Neurontin): Increase TST, SE, N1, SWS, REM, PLMs, and arousals.

> Clonazepam (Klonopin): Increase TST, N1, N2, and arousals while also decreasing SE, SWS, and REM.

Some anticonvulsants have been prescribed for other medical conditions. Gabapentin is also prescribed for neuropathic pain and hot flashes, and clonazepam for panic attacks.

Opioids/Opiates

Opiates are drugs derived from opium, whereas opioids refer to synthetic opiates, created to emulate opium; however, they are chemically different (21). Opioids refer to the entire family of opiates, including natural, synthetic, and semisynthetic.

An opioid is any agent that activates the opioid receptors, the protein molecules located on the membranes of some nerve cells. These receptors are found principally in the CNS and gastrointestinal tract. Opiates activate the receptors once they reach the brain, facilitate pain relief, and stimulate pleasure centers in the brain that then signal reward. They suppress perception of pain and calm an individual's emotional response to pain by reducing the number of pain signals sent by the nervous system. Drugs under this class include methadone, morphine, and oxycodone.

Opiates can cause sedation with acute use and insomnia with chronic use. They can increase wakefulness, thereby decreasing TST and SE. They are also known to increase N1 sleep. The limited data from sleep studies show a decrease in REM sleep and SWS. Subjective sleep has been reported as improved, possibly resulting from improved pain control (22). Withdrawal leads to sleep disturbances, affecting SL, SWS, and REM sleep (23).

Table 32-6 Antihistamines

Generic Name	Popularly Known as/Brand Name	Agent Type	Sedating	Nonsedating
Cetirizine[a]	Zyrtec	H1	☐	√
Chlorpheniramine	Chlor-Trimeton		√	☐
Cimetidine	Tagamet	H2	☐	☐
Cyproheptadine	Periactin	H1	√	☐
Desloratadine[a]	Clarinex	H1	☐	√
Diphenhydramine	Benadryl		√	☐
Fexofenadine[a]	Allegra	H1	☐	√
Levocetirizine	Xyzal		☐	√
Loratadine[a]	Claritin	H1	☐	√
Levocetirizine	Xyzal		☐	√
Montelukast	Singulair		☐	√

H1, effective in the symptomatic treatment of acute allergies.
H2, effective in the control of gastric secretions, often used in the treatment of gastroesophageal reflux.
[a]Second-generation H1 blockers considered less sedating. Cetirizine, however, may be (more sedating) in higher doses.

Antipsychotics

Antipsychotic drugs are a class of medications used to treat a serious mental disorder characterized by defective or lost contact with reality (psychosis) and other mental and emotional conditions. They are also known as tranquilizers used to treat conditions when a calming effect is desired.

Tranquilizers can be divided into different groups, called "major tranquilizers" and "minor tranquilizers." Although they are both groups of CNS depressants, their mechanisms of action, medical uses, and abuse potential are very different. Major tranquilizers (antipsychotics) are used to treat mental illnesses, whereas minor tranquilizers (BZDs) have therapeutic uses including the treatment of anxiety, insomnia, seizures, muscle spasms, and alcohol withdrawal. BZDs can be highly addictive, whereas antipsychotics are nonaddictive and have very little potential for abuse (24).

Reports on studies conducted on patients diagnosed with schizophrenia limit the drugs used to haloperidol, olanzapine, and clozapine. There is virtually no change in sleep architecture with haloperidol use except for an increase in RL. An increase or no change has been seen in N3, whereas a decrease, or no change, has been noted in REM density. The use of either olanzapine or clozapine shows an increase in N2 sleep. An increase in SWS is seen in the former, but a decrease is seen in the latter. The drug affects neither RL nor the duration of REM sleep (25).

Mood Stabilizers

Mood stabilizer drug types include antimania, anticonvulsant, antipsychotic, and antihypertensive medications. They are used to treat acute mania defined as an abnormally elevated mood state characterized by symptoms as inappropriate elation, increased irritability, severe insomnia, grandiose notions, increased speed and/or volume of speech, disconnected and racing thoughts, increased sexual desire, markedly increased energy and activity level, poor judgment, and inappropriate social behavior. They are also used to treat hypomania (a mild form of mania), depression, and mania + depression episodes. Regular use of mood stabilizers can help reduce the risk of suicide, prevent relapse, and improve the emotional well-being of any individual.

The use of an anticonvulsant, such as carbamazepine, has been an accepted treatment for mood disorders for some time. Studies in healthy volunteers have shown that carbamazepine and lithium carbonate, another mood-stabilizing drug, will increase SWS but will suppress REM sleep. Lithium carbonate also increases RL (26).

Other Sleep Aids

Over-the-counter (OTC) sleep aids and herbal supplements fall in this category. Most OTC products do contain antihistamines (diphenhydramine) and will cause drowsiness, so they can be effective for occasional use. Side effects include dry mouth, nausea, a hangover effect, blurred vision, and constipation.

Examples of herbal sleep aids include melatonin, valerian root, and chamomile tea. Melatonin is a natural hormone that regulates sleep cycles. It decreases SL and may help normalize irregular sleep–wake patterns, without affecting sleep architecture. It lost popularity, when the side effects became known: depression, weepiness, and headaches.

Some patients have found the use of valerian root calming and beneficial in treating mild cases of insomnia. It is somewhat like chamomile tea because it produces a soothing feeling of relaxation. Side effects for valerian root include headaches, indigestion, and restlessness, whereas chamomile tea can cause dermatitis or other allergic reactions. The use of chamomile tea with antiepileptic medications can increase their sedative effects. It can increase the risk of bleeding for individuals who are already taking aspirin or other blood-thinning medications (as in warfarin, etc.) (27).

This section will not be complete if two other popular OTC sleep aids are not mentioned: alcohol and nicotine (cigarettes).

The decision of when to consume alcohol appears to influence sleep. Taken too early (about 6 hours before bedtime), alcohol increases wakefulness by the second half of the night or taken at bedtime (about an hour before) causes fitful sleep by the second half of the night (28). Taken at bedtime, alcohol shortens SL, increases NREM, and reduces REM sleep. Whatever the timing, alcohol's depressant effects can increase the duration of periods of apnea or worsen any preexisting obstructive sleep apnea (29).

Nicotine can have a biphasic effect because it initially relaxes and then stimulates. It can raise blood pressure, speed up the heartbeat, stimulate brain wave activity, and can even make breathing shallower and faster (30). By stimulating the release of aminergic neurotransmitters (such as dopamine and serotonin), nicotine in cigarette smoke may disturb the normal regulation of NREM sleep and shift the distribution of sleep architecture toward lighter stages of sleep (31, 32). Use can decrease SL and increase frequency of arousals, resulting in reduced TST.

SUMMARY

The vast array of substances currently available to patients will always challenge the ability to interpret the PSG data. Many of these substances will alter sleep in some form. Sleep technologists need to be aware of the latest trends in the use and abuse of drugs, as well as the literature linking drugs to altered sleep. Technologists should ask themselves if and how each PSG might be affected by medications, whether taken on the day of the study or prior. Close attention to patients' medications will significantly aid in the interpretation of the PSG and increase the number of correct diagnoses (31, 32).

REFERENCES

1. National Center for Health Statistics. (2017). *Health, United States, 2016: With chartbook on long-term trends in health.* Hyattsville, MD. Accessed July 29, 2018, from https://www.cdc.gov/nchs/data/hus/hus16.pdf

2. Korsmeyer, P., & Kranzler, H. R. (Eds.). (2008). Barbiturates. In *Encyclopedia of drugs, alcohol, and addictive behavior* (3rd ed.). Farmington Hills, MI: Gale Cengage Learning.

3. Web MD, RXList. (n.d.). Benzodiazepine drug information. Retrieved from https://www.rxlist.com/benzodiazepines/drugs-condition.htm

4. Schatzberg, A. F., & Nemeroff, C. B. (2009). *Textbook of psychopharmacology.* Arlington, VA: American Psychiatric Publishing.

5. Mayo Foundation for Medical Education and Research. (1998–2011). *Antidepressants.* Rochester, MN: Author.

6. Carlson, N. (2001). *What is serotonin and what does it do?* Retrieved from https://www.macalester.edu/projects/UBNRP/placebo/serotonin2.html

7. New World Encyclopedia. (2007). *Norepinephrine.* Retrieved from http://www.newworldencyclopedia.org/entry/Norepinephrine

8. PediaView.com. (n.d.). *Acetylcholine.* Retrieved from http://pediaview.com/openpedia/Acetylcholine

9. Kaplan, H. I., & Saddock, B. J. (2007). *Synopsis of psychiatry: Behavioural sciences/clinical psychiatry.* Philadelphia, PA: Lippincott, Williams & Wilkins.

10. Taylor, D. P., Eison, M. S., Riblet, L. A., & Vandermaelen, C. P. (1985). Pharmacological and clinical effects of buspirone. *Pharmacology Biochemistry and Behavior, 23*(4), 687–694. Retrieved from https://www.sciencedirect.com/science/article/pii/0091305785904381

11. Patel, J., & Swierzewski, S. J. (2011). *High blood pressure medication.* Retrieved from http://www.healthcommunities.com/high-blood-pressure/pharm.shtml

12. Omudhome, O. (n.d.). *High blood pressure drugs: Side effects, types, uses, and names.* Retrieved from http://www.medicinenet.com/high_blood_pressure_medication/article.htm

13. Rosen, R. C., & Kostis, J. B. (1985). Biobehavioural sequelae associated with adrenergic-inhibiting antihypertensive agents: A critical review. *Health Psychology, 4*(6), 579–604.

14. Schweitzer, P. K. (2005). Drugs that disturb sleep and wakefulness. In M. Kryger, T. Roth, & W. Dement (Eds.), *Principles and practice of sleep medicine* (4th ed.). Philadelphia, PA: Elsevier Saunders.

15. Spiegel, R., & DeVos, J. E. (1980). Central effects of guanfacine and clonidine during wakefulness and sleep in healthy subjects. *British Journal of Clinical Pharmacology, 10*(Suppl. 1), 165S–168S.

16. Roman, F. (2008, May/June). Medication effects on sleep. *Focus Journal,* 52–53.

17. Qureshi, A., & Lee-Chiong, T. (2004). Therapeutic and adverse effects on sleep: Medications and their effect on sleep. *Medical Clinics of North America, 88,* 751–766.

18. Qureshi, A., & Lee-Chiong, T., Jr. (2004). Medications and their effect on sleep. *Medical Clinics of North America, 88*(33), 751–766, x.

19. Schneerson, J. M. (Ed.). (2000). Drugs and sleep. In *Handbook of sleep medicine* (pp. 33–58). Malden, MA: Blackwell Science.

20. Bazil, C. W., Malow, B. A., & Sammaritano, M. R. (2002). *Sleep and epilepsy: The clinical spectrum.* New York, NY: Elsevier Health Sciences.

21. National Alliance of Advocates for Buprenorphine Treatment. (n.d.). *Common buprenorphine side effects: Headache, constipation, dry mouth.* Retrieved from http://www.naabt.org/faq_answers.cfm?ID=3

22. Overeem, S., & Reading, P. (2010). *Sleep disorders in neurology: A practical approach.* Hoboken, NJ: Wiley-Blackwell.

23. Dimsdale, J. E., Norman, D., DeJardin, J., et al. (2007). The effect of opioids on sleep architecture. *Journal of Clinical Sleep Medicine, 3*(1), 33–36.

24. Addiction Technology Transfer Center. (n.d.). *Psychotherapeutic medications.* Retrieved from http://www.nattc.org/userfiles/file/MidAmerica/Psychmeds%202011_FINAL%20as%20of%203-1-11.pdf

25. Lader, M. H., Cardinali, D., & Pandi-Perumal, S. R. (2006). *Sleep and sleep disorders: A neuropsychopharmacological approach.* New York, NY: Springer.

26. Eisen, J., MacFarlane, J., & Shapiro, C. M. (1993). ABC of sleep disorders: Psychotropic drugs and sleep. *British Medical Journal, 306,* 1331–1334.

27. Hirshkowitz, M., & Smith, P. (Eds.). (2004). I can't sleep a wink: Examining insomnia. In *Sleep disorders for dummies.* Hoboken, NJ: Wiley Publishing, Inc.

28. Landolt, H. P., Roth, C., Dijk, D. J., et al. (1996). Late-afternoon ethanol intake affects nocturnal sleep and the sleep EEG in middle-aged men. *Journal of Clinical Psychopharmacology, 16*(6), 428–436.

29. Dawson, A., Lehr, P., Bigby, B. G., et al. (1993). Effect of bedtime ethanol on total inspiratory resistance and respiratory drive in normal non-snoring men. *Alcohol and Clinical Experience Research, 17*(2), 256–262.

30. Hirshkowitz, M., & Smith, P. (2004). Adopting a sleep-well lifestyle. In *Sleep disorders for dummies*. Hoboken, NJ: Wiley Publishing, Inc.

31. Zhang, L., Samet, J., Caffo, B., et al. (2006). Cigarette smoking and nocturnal sleep architecture. *American Journal of Epidemiology, 164*(6), 529–537.

32. Wettach, G. R., Ware, I. C., Vorona, R. D., et al. (2007). Pharmacologic effects on the polysomnogram. In N. Butkov & T. Lee-Chiong (Eds.), *Fundamentals of sleep technology* (pp. 393–412). Philadelphia, PA: Lippincott Williams & Wilkins.

chapter 33
Sleep Apps and Personal Tracking Devices

LAUREN TRIBOU

LEARNING OBJECTIVES

On completion of this chapter, the reader should be able to:

1. Compare currently available consumer technology for tracking sleep.
2. Describe potential uses, benefits, and limitations of personal sleep tracking devices for the public.
3. Describe potential uses, benefits, and limitations of personal sleep tracking devices for patients with sleep disorders.
4. Understand how sleep apps and personal sleep tracking devices could be utilized in sleep practice.

KEY TERMS

Accelerometer
Algorithm
Actigraph
Wearable sleep tracking device
Contact-free devices
Polysomnography (PSG)

As the consequences and adverse health effects associated with poor and limited sleep are becoming publicized and well known, personal sleep tracking products have risen in popularity. The purpose of this chapter is not to endorse or recommend any one specific sleep tracking product but rather to increase the understanding of available consumer sleep technology devices and to evaluate the potential uses for the tracking devices in both home and clinical settings. Sleep apps and personal tracking devices are nonprescription devices that monitor and record the user's sleep, and they are available for purchase through mobile app stores and in-store retailers (1).

Because devices must go through extensive testing and receive approval of the Food and Drug Administration (FDA) to be considered a mobile medical app, most consumer sleep technology devices are promoted as lifestyle enhancers instead of medical or diagnostic devices (2). As technology advances and sleep apps and personal tracking devices increase in popularity, it is necessary to recognize how personal sleep data can be utilized to monitor sleep health.

CONSUMER SLEEP TRACKING DEVICES

Many commercial sleep tracking devices are available to meet various consumer preferences. Consumers may choose wearable and contact-free accelerometers that sense and measure movements to predict sleep and wake periods (3). Although companies do not make device algorithms publicly available, many claim to be able to calculate light sleep, deep sleep, rapid eye movement (REM) sleep, and wake on the basis of movement alone (4).

WEARABLE SLEEP TRACKERS

Popular wearable sleep trackers include wrist-based devices such as Fitbit and finger-based devices like Thim. The wrist-based devices require a consumer to wear the device like a watch throughout the day and night and predict sleep time through the presence or absence of movement. According to its web site, Fitbit intends to improve sleep habits through tracking and recording sleep duration, light sleep/deep sleep/REM sleep, sleep schedule, heart rate, and movement. It also provides comparative "sleep insight" on the basis of consumer data, gender, and age (5). Consumers are then able to access and review nightly data through a mobile phone or tablet app and online software. Comparatively, the finger cup, Thim, is another wearable option and requires users to wear a "smart ring" at night to track movements and predict sleep. Instead of improving sleep habits through data monitoring, Thim claims to improve sleep quality through sleep training (6). During the first hour of sleep, the finger cup vibrates and interrupts sleep in 3-minute intervals in an attempt to condition the wearer to sleep better the remainder of the night. The cup then records finger movements and uses an algorithm to predict sleep stages (6). Like the wrist-based devices, recorded data can be viewed on a smartphone or tablet app to track sleep efficiency (SE).

CONTACT-FREE SLEEP TRACKERS

Consumers who do not wish to wear devices during the day or while in bed may opt to utilize contact-free devices to track their sleep. While also utilizing accelerometers to record movements and algorithms that estimate sleep stages and wake on the basis of the amount of movement, contact-free devices present a sleep tracking option on the basis of comfort. Several sleep tracking apps are available to download onto the user's smartphone or tablet from mobile app stores. Many sleep tracking apps offer a basic version for free with in-app optional purchases for more advanced versions with additional tracking features. Some contact-free devices may be used in conjunction with wearable devices but can function independently as well, offering consumers a low-cost option to monitor sleep.

Because sleep tracking apps rely on accelerometers to predict sleep, the recording device must be in close proximity to the user to sense and record movements. The Pillow app recommends that users position the device facedown on either the mattress or pillow about 15 to 25 cm from their bodies (7). In addition to an accelerometer, the Pillow app also utilizes audio input from nightly recordings in their algorithm to estimate sleep stages and quality (7). Users can access their nightly sleep report through the app and may opt to purchase app upgrades to access additional sleep statistics and tracking resources.

SLEEP TRACKING DEVICES FOR THE GENERAL PUBLIC

The wide accessibility and convenience of commercial sleep technology has increased the ease and popularity of monitoring personal sleep health. Apple watch *Sleep Watch* app and *Jawbone UP* app are both examples of commercial wearable devices that provide a daily sleep chart of the user. Information is displayed in easily interpreted charts and graphs (8). The data are recorded and can be viewed anytime through the associated app or web site. This method of collecting and monitoring personal health data can be fun and enlightening and gives users objective information about their personal rest and bedtime and wake patterns (3). Being personally involved in their own sleep health and analyzing their own sleep trends could motivate users to make changes and thus improve sleep hygiene and habits. They may further seek information on sleep disorders and/or medical treatment for consistently negative or concerning reports. Readily available sleep data empower the public to be engaged in, and knowledgeable about, their sleep health.

However, commercial sleep technology has limitations. Despite continuous technologic advances and product upgrades, technology is prone to inaccuracies and technical failures, which can result in misleading data. Polysomnography (PSG) is considered the gold standard in evaluating sleep quality because it measures brain activity, muscle tone, and eye movements, which are necessary to distinguish sleep stages (3). Movement and noise may be able to suggest periods of wake versus sleep, but they are not strong sleep stage indicators because there is little variation in the amount of movement between sleep stages (3). Additionally, the accelerometer and audio recorders in sleep tracking devices could detect and record sounds and movements from another person or pet sharing the bed and skew the user's sleep report: detecting outside movements could overestimate restlessness and periods of wake, or inversely, depending on the user's ability to lay still, misinterpret periods of motionless wake as sleep and overestimate sleep time (4). Misrepresenting sleep quality could lead to a false sense of security or concern, either of which could negatively impact health. Furthermore, multiple research studies evaluating commercial sleep technology accuracy have had to exclude participant data because of device malfunctions and user error in both wearable and contact-free devices (4, 8). Because of potential inaccuracies, data collected from commercial sleep trackers should be interpreted with caution.

Although sleep tracking devices provide insightful data about sleep trends, it is important to remember that commercial devices are unable to diagnose sleep disorders. "Consumer sleep technology must be cleared by the FDA and rigorously tested if it is intended to diagnose or treat sleep disorders" (9). In addition to the diagnostic and treatment criteria, the FDA requires regulation of any mobile platform that measures a physiologic property during sleep (2). In accordance with the FDA's regulation policy, Fitbit's web site explicitly states that its product is not as accurate as medical devices nor is it "intended to diagnose, treat, cure, or prevent any disease" (10). Thim and Pillow each have a similar disclaimer alerting users about their devices' medical limitations on their web sites (11, 12). Users concerned about their sleep health or the impact of sleep on their overall health should consult with a medical professional for possible evaluation and treatment.

SLEEP TRACKING DEVICES FOR PATIENTS WITH SLEEP DISORDERS

Individuals with a sleep disorder diagnosis may enjoy commercial sleep tracking devices in the same way as the general population does, with the understanding that the devices are unable to treat or monitor their condition. The tracking devices cannot measure specific sleep stages on the basis of accelerometer data but can indicate sleep trends that the user may wish to improve.

For example, seeing data that the user is typically in bed only 5 or 6 hours every night may encourage the user to go to bed earlier and increase sleep opportunity time.

Commercial sleep tracking devices do not have the means to monitor sleep-disordered breathing (SDB) because they do not measure airflow or respiratory effort. Meltzer et al. trialed a Fitbit Ultra using both the Normal mode and Sensitive mode, which the manufacturer recommended for individuals suspected of sleep disorders, in a pediatric population with varying levels of obstructive sleep apnea (OSA) (4). The study found that compared with a single-night PSG, the Fitbit Ultra Normal mode significantly overestimated total sleep time (TST) and SE, and the Sensitive mode significantly underestimated TST and SE in pediatric patients with no or mild OSA (4). In pediatric patients with moderate and severe OSA, the discrepancy in the Normal mode was not statistically significant; however, the Sensitive mode once again significantly underestimated TST and SE (4). Although the Fitbit web site claims that its devices are not intended for users under 13, the study results suggest that the Fitbit Ultra is not a reliable indicator of SDB, especially in modes specifically recommended for use in those with sleep disorders (4). The study further suggests that pediatric patients with moderate-to-severe OSA may move more in their sleep, which the accelerometer in the device detects and the algorithm calculates as wake (4). Depending on the mode and algorithm, users with sleep disorders could be receiving inaccurate data and have false conclusions about their nightly sleep.

Competing products and even different modes in the same product utilize unique algorithms with different equations and properties, so the sensitivity and accuracy between products vary (3). Toon et al. also compared commercial sleep devices with a single-night PSG in a pediatric population and found contradictory results compared with the Meltzer et al. study (8). Toon et al. examined a Jawbone UP wearable wrist device and a MotionX 24/7 contact-free sleep app and, unlike Meltzer et al., did not find any statistical differences in TST or SE across any OSA severity in the wearable device data (8). However, Toon et al. did note that the MotionX 24/7 "did not accurately measure any sleep parameter as measured by PSG" (8). Although additional research is necessary, the inconsistencies and conflicting study results indicated that commercial sleep tracking device users with sleep disorders should exercise caution when evaluating their sleep reports.

APPS FOR POSITIVE AIRWAY PRESSURE THERAPY

Even though commercial sleep tracking devices are unable to monitor breathing, individuals using positive airway pressure (PAP) machines to treat sleep apnea can access breathing data utilizing their PAP machine's complimentary app. The ResMed myAir and Philips Respironics DreamMapper apps, when linked to and used in conjunction with PAP therapy, track the user's therapy and provide data charts for a 30-day period (13, 14). In addition to documenting an apnea–hypopnea index (AHI) score, the devices record nightly therapy use time, mask leak value, and the treatment pressure or pressure range (13). The user may opt to set personal treatment goals and reminders, and the app can send tailored coaching messages to the user (14). Presenting data in an easy-to-understand format empowers users to be active in their treatment and to contact a health provider if frequent changes in AHI, mask leak, or pressure are observed (14). Patients should also be encouraged to contact a medical professional for any sleep concerns or excessive daytime sleepiness regardless of what the data indicate (9).

Utilizing the therapy tracking apps that record treatment progress and compliance encourages patient and clinician communication (9). Not only can PAP users view their therapy data through an app, durable medical equipment providers and health care providers can access the same data through the manufacturers' software. Clinicians and equipment providers can contact a patient if the data indicate that the therapy has not been used and the patient is in jeopardy of failing insurance compliance requirements. Further, clinicians also can adjust PAP settings if the current treatment does not appear to be optimal. Patients and clinicians have a convenient way to view the same data and contact each other with possible concerns. Adding to the convenience, telemedicine sleep apps are becoming increasingly popular as well and allow a sleep medicine provider to quickly assist a patient with treatment and sleep health questions when the patient's provider is unavailable or unable to do so (1).

SLEEP TRACKING DEVICES IN A SLEEP PRACTICE

Optimal treatment depends on accurate measurements and information, and personal sleep trackers may be beneficial when combined with clinical evaluations. Ibáñez et al. conducted a literature review investigating the uses and benefits of various sleep evaluation methods and determined that a combination of subjective and objective measures provided the most accurate insight into a patient's sleep habits and health (15). Although serving in a limited capacity, data obtained through a personal sleep app could help sleep providers identify a sleep disorder.

Even as PSG testing is considered the gold standard and the most accurate evaluation method, it still has flaws and should be supplemented with a questionnaire, sleep diary, or another method that provides sleep habit data (15). PSGs provide reliable data about a patient's sleep onset latency, sleep architecture, and sleep quality but may not be a true representation of a patient's typical night. PSGs are performed in a sleep center or hospital setting, which could be inconvenient and uncomfortable for a patient, and adding to the discomfort, the patient is attached to numerous electrodes and sensors before being monitored by a technologist throughout the night. Furthermore, because of the high cost, a patient is often monitored for a single night (8). A commercial sleep tracker could provide additional information about sleep trends over multiple nights while the patient sleeps in a natural environment. Unlike sleep diaries and questionnaires, which provide self-reported data, personal sleep tracking devices can serve as an objective and unbiased electronic diary and provide estimated data regarding bedtime, time asleep, number of awakenings, time out of bed, and sleep opportunity time (7, 15).

Because patients are increasingly bringing information from sleep apps and devices to clinicians for interpretation, clinicians should consider the data as supplemental sleep history information and not rely on this data for a diagnosis (15). Not only are the devices subjected to technical errors and user inconsistencies, Meltzer et al. found that the wearable device did not produce comparable results with either a PSG or an actigraph in a general pediatric population (4). Although Toon et al. found comparable results between the wearable device with a PSG and an actigraph in a general pediatric population, the contact-free device they tested significantly overestimated sleep (8). The differences in study results highlight device inconsistencies and unreliability in both wearable and contact-free devices. Although the devices may indicate general sleep habits and present an opportunity for sleep hygiene education, the algorithms in the devices do not provide the inter-device reliability or accuracy necessary to replace traditional diagnostic testing.

CONCLUSION

The benefits of good sleep are becoming increasingly known and accepted, and the interest in sleep health has grown in recent years. Commercial sleep tracking technology provides a fun and interactive way for individuals to monitor their sleep health and track their sleep trends. Because personal sleep tracking devices are not medical devices and are not intended to diagnose or treat medical conditions, users should still be advised to contact a medical professional for any sleep and health concerns.

As the data collected on commercial sleep trackers are currently inconsistent and unreliable, personal sleep trackers should be used only as supplemental information during a diagnostic evaluation. Especially as technology advances, further research is needed to determine if commercial sleep trackers could have a stronger role in sleep disorder evaluations and to examine the usefulness of sleep apps and tracking devices in patients with other sleep conditions like insomnia or periodic limb movement disorder. It will be exciting to see if any diagnostic materials will be integrated into personal sleep tracking devices in the future and if any of these devices will receive FDA approval as a mobile medical app.

REFERENCES

1. American Academy of Sleep Medicine. (2018, May). *Consumer sleep technology is no substitute for medical evaluation*. Retrieved May 16, 2018, from https://aasm .org/consumer-sleep-technology-position-statement/
2. U.S. Department of Health and Human Services, Food and Drug Administration, Center for Devices and Radiological Health, Center for Biologics Evaluation and Research. (2015, February). *Mobile medical apps: Subset of mobile apps that are the focus of FDA's regulatory oversight. Mobile medical applications. Guidance for Industry and Food and Drug Administration staff.* Retrieved May 16, 2018, from https://www.fda.gov/ downloads/MedicalDevices/UCM263366.pdf
3. Sleep Health Foundation. (2015, February). *Sleep tracker technology*. Retrieved January 30, 2018, from https://www.sleephealthfoundation.org.au/public-information/fact-sheets-a-z/sleeptracker.html
4. Meltzer, L. J., Hiruma, L. S., Avis, K., et al. (2015, August 1). Comparison of a commercial accelerometer with polysomnography and actigraphy in children and adolescents. *Sleep, 38*(8), 1323–1330.
5. Fitbit, Inc. (2018). *Fitbit*. Retrieved January 31, 2018, from https://www.fitbit.com/sleep-better
6. Re-Time Pty Ltd. (2017). *Thim*. Retrieved January 31, 2018, from https://thim.io/
7. Neybox. (2018). *Pillow on the iPhone basics*. Retrieved June 20, 2018, from https://pillow .uservoice.com/knowledgebase/ articles/755280-pillow-on-the-iphone-basics
8. Toon, E., Davey, M. J., Hollis, S. L., et al. (2016, March 15). Comparison of commercial wrist-based and smartphone accelerometers, actigraphy, and PSG in a clinical cohort of children and adolescents. *Journal of Clinical Sleep Medicine, 12*(3), 343–350.
9. Khosla, S., Deak, M. C., Gault, D., et al. (2018). Consumer sleep technology: An American Academy of Sleep Medicine Position Statement [Electronic version]. *Journal of Clinical Sleep Medicine, 14*(5), 877–880.

10. Fitbit, Inc. (2018). *Important safety and product information.* Retrieved June 16, 2018, from https://www.fitbit.com/legal/safety-instructions
11. Re-Time Pty Ltd. (2017). *Thim policies. Disclaimer.* Retrieved June 16, 2018, from https://thim.io/policies/
12. Neybox. (2018, May). *Pillow privacy policy. Disclaimer.* Retrieved June 16, 2018, from https://neybox.com/pillow-sleep-tracker-en/pillow-privacy-policy-en
13. ResMed. (2018). *myAir sleep apnea app.* Retrieved May 16, 2018, from https://www.resmed.com/us/en/consumer/airsolutions/personalized-support/myair.html
14. Philips Respironics. (2018). *DreamMapper.* Retrieved May 16, 2018, from https://www.sleepapnea.com/products/dreammapper/
15. Ibáñez, V., Silva, J., & Cauli, O. (2018, May 25). A survey on sleep assessment methods. *PeerJ, 6,* e4849.

10. Fitbit, Inc. (2018). Important safety and product information. Retrieved June 16, 2018, from https://www.fitbit.com/legal/safety-instructions

11. Re-Time Pty Ltd. (2017). Privacy policies. Disclaimer. Retrieved June 16, 2018, from https://fitbit.to/policies

12. Newbox. (2018, May). Pillow privacy policy. Disclaimer. Retrieved June 16, 2018, from https://neybox.com/pillow-sleep-tracker-en/pillow-privacy-policy-en

13. ResMed. (2018). An sleep apnea app. Retrieved May 16, 2018, from https://www.resmed.com/us/en/consumer/solutions/personalized-support/my-air.html

14. Philips Respironics. (2018). Dreammapper. Retrieved May 16, 2018, from https://www.sleepapnea.com/products/dreammapper/

15. Ibáñez, V., Silva, J., & Cauli, O. (2018, May 25). A survey on sleep assessment methods. PeerJ, 6, e4849.

SECTION 5
Adult Polysomnography

chapter 34
Digital Polysomnography

FRANK WALTHER

LEARNING OBJECTIVES

On completion of this chapter, the reader should be able to:

1. List the sources of all signals.
2. Describe how differential amplification effects signal voltage and polarity.
3. Discuss the source localization of electroencephalographic signals.
4. Apply Ohm's law and Nyquist's sampling theory to digital polysomnography (PSG).
5. Show the order in which signals are processed in PSG systems.
6. Discuss the filtering of PSG signals.
7. Outline the concepts of calibration.

KEY TERMS

Polysomnography
Biocalibrations
Bioelectric signals
Common mode rejection ratio
Conductivity
Polarity
Impedance
Sensitivity
Frequency
Amplitude
High-frequency filter
Low-frequency filter
Frequency response curve
Time constant
Rise time constant
Fall time constant
Notch filter
Analog-to-digital converter
Nyquist sampling theory
Ohm's law

The word *polysomnography* in its root derivation means many (*poly*) sleep (*somno*) writings (*graphy*). A polysomnogram is produced by a multiple-channel recording instrument comprised of a hardware device (often called an "amplifier") that interfaces with software to produce a digital record of multiple biophysical variables during the course of a sleep session.

Historically, polysomnographic (PSG) recordings were conducted with analog equipment that traced this physiologic activity by mechanical means to paper. Although these paper-based systems performed admirably, the machines were large and resource intensive. They required replenishment of paper and ink and ongoing maintenance of all the mechanical parts, not to mention extraordinary storage requirements. Because the activity was converted by mechanical means, each study required precise mechanical baseline calibrations. Scoring required page-by-page examination of each epoch, and event marking was done by hand. Present-day digital systems afford sleep professionals all the benefits of software programming and networking. Studies can be viewed on multiple screens, allowing for simultaneous acquisition and scoring. Montages can be adjusted across all parameters during and after the recording, video can be collected and synchronized with the recording, and indices can be estimated or tabulated in real time. Physicians are able to view studies remotely in real time and in review mode. Reports can be tailored to suit the needs of the health care provider.

The quality and validity of signal processing remains intact in modern digital PSG as long as adequate PSG system specifications and good PSG skills are observed. The American Academy of Sleep Medicine (AASM) Scoring Manual (1) has defined standards and best practices (i.e., sampling rates, bit rates, screen resolution, etc.) for the recording process to ensure that all studies accurately reflect the patient condition (see Table 34-1).

Table 34-1 Digital Specifications (1)

Maximum EEG and EOG electrode impedance	5 kΩ
Minimum digital resolution	12 bits per sample
Digital screen resolution	1,600 × 1,200
Notch filters 50/60 Hz	Per channel
Time scale range window view	5 s to entire recording

EEG, electroencephalography; EOG, electrooculogram.

PRINCIPLES OF ELECTRICAL CONDUCTION

Signal Sources

The basic function of a PSG system is to record signals associated with specific physiologic parameters and convert this activity into visible tracings that can be measured and analyzed. In PSG, there are three sources for these signals:

- Bioelectric potentials
- Transduced signals from sensors attached to the patient
- Signals derived from ancillary equipment

Bioelectric potentials are voltages generated by living tissue. Examples of bioelectric potential recordings include the electroencephalogram (EEG), electrooculogram, electromyogram, and electrocardiogram (ECG). Bioelectric signals are recorded using surface electrodes attached directly to the patient's skin over the area of interest. For the purposes of a discussion regarding the general pathway of these source signals, we concentrate on EEG recordings of the brain.

The brain's electrical charge is the result or summation of the electrical activity of billions of neurons. Neurons are electrically charged (or polarized) by transport proteins that pump ions across their cell membranes. When a neuron receives a signal from its neighbor, an action potential is triggered, it responds by releasing ions into the synaptic space outside the cell. Ions of like charge repel each other, and when many ions are pushed out of many neurons at the same time, they can push their neighbors, who push their neighbors, and so on, in a wave. When the wave of ions reaches the electrodes on the scalp, they can push electrons through the measuring circuit comprising the electrodes and a sensitive amplifier. Thus, the measuring circuit can measure the difference in this electron "push," or voltage, between any two electrodes. Recording these voltage differences over time gives us the EEG (2). Note that the EEG does not directly measure electrical impulses in the cells, but instead the EEG arises from changing ionic concentrations and the resulting charge in the extracellular space.

The electric potentials generated by a single neuron are far too small to be picked by the EEG (3), because the skull and skin act as capacitors and dampen the signal. EEG activity, therefore, always reflects the summation of the synchronous activity of thousands or millions of neurons that have similar spatial orientation (4).

Transduced signals are voltages usually supplied as DC voltages by sensors that are attached to the patient as opposed to voltages that are produced by the body. This can include position sensors, snore sensors, and respiratory sensors.

Ancillary equipment, such as continuous positive airway pressure devices, pulse oximeters, and end-tidal CO_2 ($EtCO_2$) monitors, can be interfaced with the PSG system by using one of many available DC inputs. The industry trend is to integrate pulse oximetry with the amplifier unit.

Electrodes

The first step of the signal pathway external to the body is the electrode. The electrodes, secured using a conductive paste, are the conduits for electron push and, as such, must have, as one of their properties, high electric conductivity. As seen in Table 34-2, the conductivities of copper, silver, and gold are all comparable.

These elements are all from group 12 of the periodic chart and are heavy, dense, malleable metals with high electric conductivity. This high conductivity is due to an atomic makeup of having free outer shell electrons in relation to a dense nucleus. The electrode cups commonly used in PSG are typically silver or gold plated. Those two metals have the additional desirable property of being resistant to the corrosive effects of oxygen, H_2O, and bodily fluids such as sweat. Gold is seen as superior because it optimizes contact impedance over the long duration of a sleep study. Silver–silver chloride and disposable electrodes made of these metals or plastic can also be used.

SIGNAL PATHWAY TO THE DIGITAL PSG

The signals previously discussed, whether they originate from the patient or are transduced or ascribed to the patient, follow a pathway that we shall refer to as a "channel." These input signals are amplified and processed, so that they are strong enough and clean enough to be converted into a digital signal that is ready for visual display, storage, and analysis.

Bioelectric signals are amplified with differential amplifiers, which reduce recording artifacts by subtracting

Table 34-2 Conductivity

Metal	Conductivity σ (1/Ωm) at 20° C
Silver	6.29×10^7
Copper	5.95×10^7
Gold	4.52×10^7

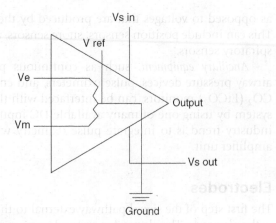

Figure 34-1 Differential amplifier.

voltages that are common to an electrode pair. The electrodes are usually routed to the amplifier through a small portable junction box, sometimes referred to as the "jackbox" or the "headbox." The industry trend is to integrate these functions even further by placing the jackbox, amplifier, and digitizer all in the same enclosure. A differential amplifier schematic is shown in Figure 34-1.

OHM'S LAW

The three electric properties that are the variables in the equation known as Ohm's law are voltage, current, and resistance. Ohm's law is commonly represented as

$$V = IR \text{ or voltage} = \text{current} \times \text{resistance.}$$

Ohm's law can be rearranged to show current as a function of voltage and resistance according to the formula $I = V/R$, and from this formula, one can deduce that under conditions of constant voltage, if resistance is increased, current or flow of electrons will be decreased. This concept has practical implications when we consider the fact that in our signal pathway, there are several factors that contribute to higher resistance. This means that the technologist must be vigilant in reducing these effects. Examples of things that could contribute to higher resistance are electrode cups inadequately filled with conductive paste, electrode damage, electrode wire damage, poor patient skin preparation, and incomplete removal of lotions and other skin products.

Notice that what is being measured is the difference in voltage of the two input electrodes as determined by their relation to the reference electrode (Fig. 34-1). The first input electrode is the exploring electrode. In PSG, we commonly refer to the mastoid electrodes as the reference electrodes because we have placed them on distant bony electrically neutral sites (M1 and M2). The M1 and M2 electrodes are considered the second input electrodes. The referential electrode is labeled "Vref."

Common ground is an additional connection (usually separate from the reference) and is necessary for equalizing electric potentials of the patient and the input circuits of the amplifier. Also, notice the power supply voltage, represented in the diagram by Vs in and Vs out. The power supply is necessary to carry out the function of amplifying the faint biopotential signals.

An essential function of the differential amplifier is that of common mode rejection, or in plain words, the cancelation of unwanted voltages that are common to both input electrodes. The ability of the differential amplifier to perform this vital function is expressed as the common mode rejection ratio (CMRR). This is the ratio of the differential voltage gain to the common mode voltage gain. If the differential amplifier were perfectly symmetrical, the common mode gain would be zero because both voltages would effectively cancel each other out, and the CMRR would be infinite. However, in reality, there is a slight amount of common voltage gain, resulting in industry standard CMRRs of 10,000 to 1 or even as high as 100,000 to 1.

SIGNAL PROCESSING

Signal Polarity and Summation

The processing of bioelectric signals includes conversion from analog to digital signal format. Electrodes on the surface of the scalp measure signals of constantly changing voltage, or amplitude, as a function of time. Differential amplifiers process the signals from two electrodes, an exploring electrode and a reference. Because the electrodes are positioned at various locations (according to the 10–20 system), the resulting tracing will vary according to the position of the electrodes and their distance and proximity to the source of voltage (see Fig. 34-2).

In EEG, it is conventional to represent negative voltage from a single input in relation to a reference as an upward deflection and, vice versa, a positive voltage is represented as a downward deflection. This relationship

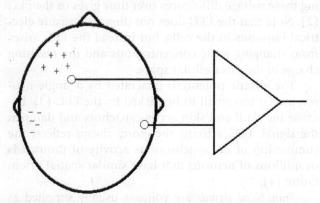

Figure 34-2 Differential amplification of exploring and reference electrodes.

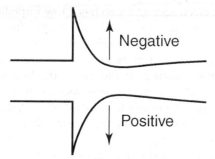

Figure 34-3 Polarity.

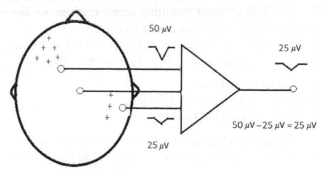

Figure 34-5 Two electrodes with equal polarity and different voltage inputs.

of the tracing to the electric zero above or below the baseline is referred to as "polarity," as illustrated in Figure 34-3.

With differential amplifiers, signal tracings shown on screen are the result of subtracting the voltage contributions from two input electrodes. This is accomplished by inverting the signal from the reference electrode. The formula for combining the signals is exploring electrode (V1) voltage minus reference electrode (V2) voltage (V1–V2), which we refer to as voltage drop.

In summation, under ideal conditions, the variables that determine bioelectric tracings are as follows:

1. Polarity
2. Voltage
3. Source
4. Electrode proximity
5. Time

Please examine the simple case of two electrodes detecting equal polarity and voltage (50 μV) at the same point in time, at the same distance from the source, in Figure 34-4. We apply the formula for voltage drop 50 – (50) = 0 and see by visual examination the result is no signal.

Now follow along with the case of simultaneous charges of equal polarity and equal proximity but differing voltages. 50 – (25) = 25. In this case, we see the resulting tracing having the same polarity (Fig. 34-5),

but if the reference electrode is higher in voltage than the input voltage, then the polarity flips. Now take the case of simultaneous charges of opposite polarity, equal proximity, and same voltages. 50 – (–50) = 100, as illustrated in Figure 34-6.

The number of possible combinations is infinite, but we will discuss one more example. That is the combination of two similar polarities, similar signal amplitudes but making their contributions at differing times. By using our formula, V1 – V2 as we go along the axis of time, we see the resulting (and recognizable) signal in Figure 34-7.

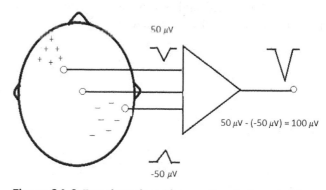

Figure 34-6 Two electrodes with opposite polarity and voltage.

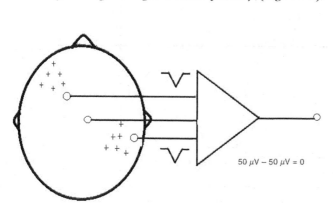

Figure 34-4 Two electrodes with equal polarity and voltage input.

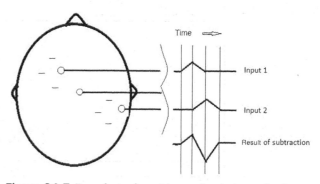

Figure 34-7 Two electrodes with equal polarity and voltage input at dissimilar times.

To a major extent, resulting signal tracings are dependent upon time, location of electrodes, source, and signal strength. Additional variables affect the resulting bioelectric tracings in practical applications. They are

1. Contact impedance
2. Common reference electrode(s)
3. Patient ground electrode

For optimal signal quality, it is necessary to match the input impedance of all electrode pairs as closely as possible. Impedance mismatching allows current to pass through to the amplifier and can lead to artifact (3). If two electrode sites produce a signal with the same amplitude and frequency, but one amplifier input receives less voltage because of a higher electrode impedance, then the signals are not perfectly canceling each other and the effect of common mode rejection is reduced. As a result, synchronized ambient signals can manifest as artifact in the record. The most common example of this is the noise from the 60 Hz (or 50 Hz) alternating current of the power grid. In order to avoid this kind of artifact, the technologist should strive for a uniform approach to site preparation and electrode application. By keeping impedances under 5 kΩ, the chances for wide variation in impedances are lessened.

Many amplifiers utilize a common referential electrode. This electrode allows for rereferencing after the recording has ended and is most effective when it is placed at a site on the skull that is equidistant to all exploring electrodes and also has a low impedance. For this reason, Cz is a good 10/20 site choice for this electrode as long as it is not required in a custom montage. Some systems have inputs for two common referential inputs, thus allowing for the use of the best signal. In addition to this, some modern systems also allow the user to assign a common reference electrode, thus alleviating dependence on referential signals that may go bad during the recording.

The patient ground electrode, as previously discussed, provides the electrical zero. Without a good stable ground electrode, the electrode pairs will not have a respective electric zero and will, therefore, wander with respect to equal inputs, thus picking up signals that would otherwise be canceled out. Even worse, this wandering common potential may cause amplifier saturation.

SIGNAL MEASUREMENT

Signal tracings are viewed on the display according to two variables, time and amplitude. Time is followed on the horizontal or *x* axis and is the basis for determining the frequency at which a signal intersects the *x* axis. The timescale used in sleep staging is 1 cm per second (see Fig. 34-8).

Frequency, expressed as cycles per second, is referred to in the unit of measurement known as Hertz (Hz). Frequency describes the period or width of the

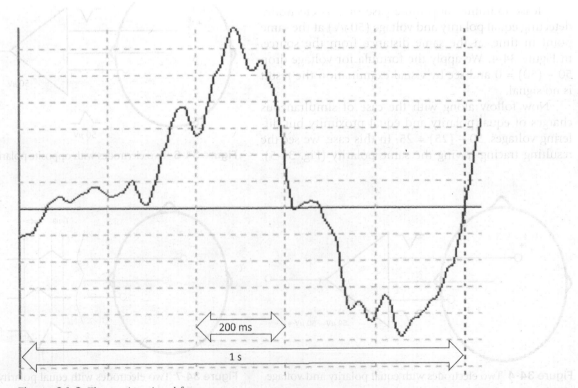

Figure 34-8 The *x* axis—signal frequency.

wave, whereas amplitude describes the height or voltage of the wave. In EEG, actual voltage from the electrodes is in microvolts, or millionth of a volt, and is represented as μV. This abbreviation is often spelled as uV on systems that cannot display Greek characters. Amplitude is followed on the vertical or y axis. The typical scale used in PSG to represent voltage amplitude is 50 μV per mm (see Fig. 34-9).

The two scales, frequency (time) and amplitude (voltage), can be combined into a useful waveform scale legend or key that can be displayed over the tracings and is available in many PSG systems (see Fig. 34-10). This is helpful when screens are resized to fit desktop workspaces and different monitor configurations, so that the observer will always be able to relate waveforms to a known scale. Another useful software tool commonly available allows the user to measure voltage and frequency by moving the mouse cursor over the tracing.

The ability to change the amplitude scale is referred to as "sensitivity setting." Sensitivity is determined by the formula

$$S = V/A$$

where S = sensitivity, V = voltage drop (expressed in μV), A = amplitude (expressed in mm or cm).

We see by our formula that increasing the sensitivity means that higher voltages are represented in the same amount of space, so increasing the sensitivity will decrease the size (amplitude) of the signal on screen.

According to the AASM recommended settings, sensitivities for EEG channels are 7 μV per mm.

LOW- AND HIGH-FREQUENCY FILTERS

In any practical setting, amplifier output contains not only the physiologic biopotential signals but also noise from various sources, both external (environmental) and internal (inherent in electronic circuit design). High-frequency muscle artifact and slow-frequency respiration or "sweat artifact" are examples of signals that are undesirable in PSG recording, even though they are physiologic in nature. Because there are so many competing signals of varying amplitude and frequency that can obscure the record, we need some way of filtering as much of this undesirable activity as possible. By the use of low-frequency filters (LFF) and high-frequency filters (HFF), we can limit a "window" of desirable frequency spectrum that is let through to the record. When we set an LFF, we are setting a lower limit of frequencies that are let into the recording. Only signals with frequencies above that limit, called the "cut-off frequency," are allowed to pass. For this reason, an LFF is also referred to as a "high-pass" filter.

Conversely, when we choose an HFF setting, we are setting an upper limit of allowed signal frequencies. This is also called the "low-pass" filter. By setting the LFF and the HFF cut-off frequencies, we choose the "window" or frequency band that we are interested in viewing.

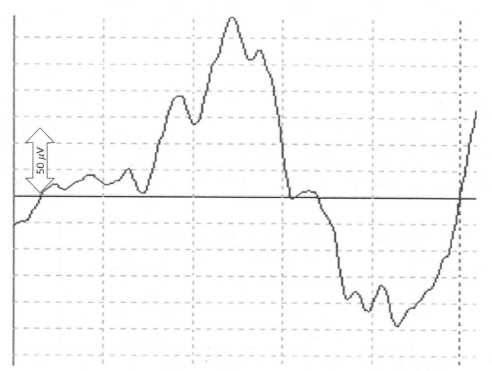

Figure 34-9 The y axis—signal amplitude.

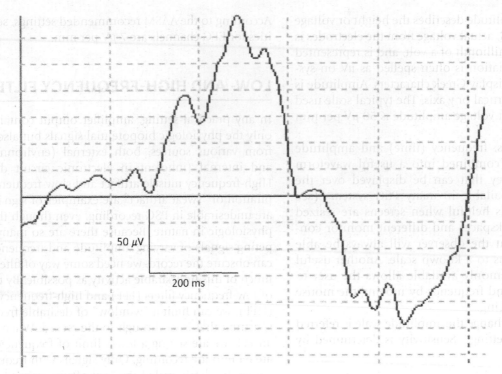

Figure 34-10 Waveform scale.

The extent to which the LFFs and HFFs are successful at filtering out unwanted frequencies is determined by the filter's frequency response. The amount of attenuation of a signal outside the pass band depends on the filter design. Digital filters do not affect the source data, and digital filters of high orders can be easily implemented in software. Digital filters used in PSG systems are usually limited to fourth or lower order to better preserve the signal shape (phase). Filter response can be visualized as a frequency response curve (see Fig. 34-11).

TIME CONSTANTS

In order to understand more fully what we see when we perform a digital machine calibration, it is necessary to understand the concept of time constants. A machine calibration is performed so that there is documentation of the validity of our filter settings. It should be understood that the term "calibrate" in this case is not strictly true because the calibration is actually done one time at the factory. The machine calibration shows the effect that amplification and filter settings have on a DC signal oscillating between +50 and −50 μV. This input signal is illustrated in Figure 34-12.

How quickly a signal falls back to the baseline (0 μV) as a function of the filters is known as the signal's time constant.

When a DC voltage is quickly turned on, the signal at the filter output is changing almost as quickly (but not immediately because the highest frequencies are filtered out by the HFF). After the signal reaches the peak, it immediately starts to decay back to the baseline (0) because the DC signal (0 Hz frequency) is filtered out by the LFF. As a result, the output after the effects of the filter settings will look as illustrated in Figure 34-13.

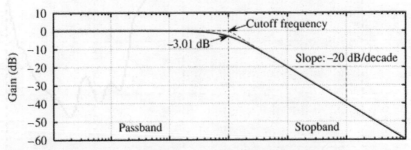

Figure 34-11 Frequency response curve. (Courtesy of Natus Medical Incorporated, Middleton WI.)

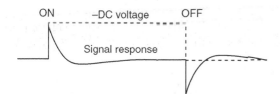

Figure 34-12 Square wave calibration signal.

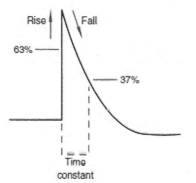

Figure 34-13 Effect of high-frequency filter and low-frequency filter settings on time constant.

Depending on the filter settings, we would see the signal decay at a faster or slower rate. The time it takes for the signal to decay to 37% of its original voltage is known as the "fall time constant." Conversely, the time it takes for the signal to reach 63% of its peak voltage is the "rise time constant." Now let us compare the effect of varying filter strengths on time constants as we look at Figure 34-14.

Notice that higher filter cut-off frequency settings result in lower fall time constants. This is important because it allows us to illustrate to all who would inspect our recorded studies that we were collecting data with verified correct filter settings as shown in Figure 34-15.

60-HZ (NOTCH) FILTERS

Otherwise known as the "notch filter," the purpose of the 60-Hz filter is to eliminate noise caused by power

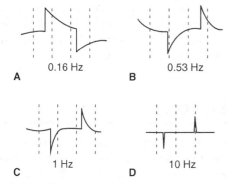

Figure 34-14 Effect of various filter settings on time constant.

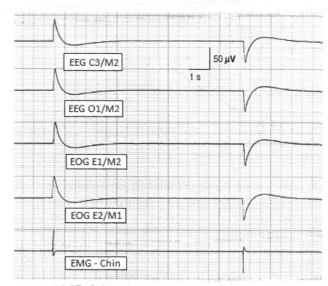

Figure 34-15 Calibration signals.

line interference from the record. Many countries use a 50-Hz power grid AC current; therefore, PSG systems often incorporate a 50-Hz notch filter as well. The notch filter allows strong suppression of unwanted electrical noise from the environment.

It is important to make sure that the record is as free of 60-Hz noise as possible without using a notch filter because very strong 60-Hz interference may result in artifacts or amplifier saturation that is not completely eliminated by a notch filter (see Fig. 34-16).

ANALOG-TO-DIGITAL CONVERTERS

The purpose of analog-to-digital conversion is to translate continuous (analog) bioelectric, transduced, and ancillary device signals into discrete numerical values (see Fig. 34-17). The analog-to-digital converter (ADC)

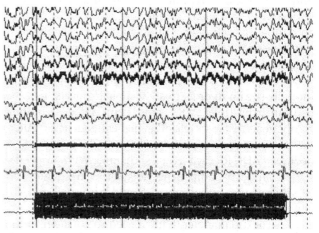

Figure 34-16 A 60 Hz artifact.

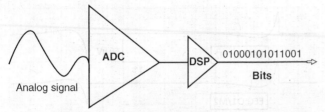

Figure 34-17 Analog-to-digital converter (ADC). DSP, digital signal processing.

captures analog signal periodically (at a sampling rate) and creates discrete numeric data points or samples. In order to properly reproduce the analog signal waveform, the sampling frequency needs to be sufficiently high. Specifically, it needs to be at least two times higher than the highest frequency that is being measured. This is known as "Nyquist theorem" (5). If this criterion is not followed, then incoming signals that are more than half the frequency of the sampling rate will be "aliased" or replaced with frequencies that are different from the original signal when the waveform is reconstructed for viewing.

This means that the incoming signal needs to be low-pass filtered in order to eliminate all frequencies higher than half the sampling rate before it gets to an ADC. This is accomplished by an antialiasing filter. In older systems, this type of filter had to be designed as a hardware circuit, making it potentially large, expensive, and suitable for only one fixed sampling frequency.

One of the most important advancements in system design is the shift in importance from hardware to software. The use of digital signal processing allows fewer circuitry components to accomplish the task. As a result, hardware can be miniaturized and costs reduced.

The sampling rate of a modern ADC can actually exceed 32,000 Hz, and by Nyquist sampling theory, this results in a reliable frequency spectrum of up to 16,000 Hz. This intermediate data stream can be then filtered in software before secondary sampling, which creates an output data stream typically at a sampling frequency of 200 to 512 Hz. This technique is called "oversampling" and allows a high degree of flexibility in selecting output data rate and aliasing elimination without the use of large and expensive electronic components for LFFs.

Multiplexing is the combination of multiple signals into one stream in order to allow digital conversion to be performed by fewer ADC components (albeit requiring components that work reliably at higher frequencies). Alternatively, multiple independent ADCs may be employed—a dedicated ADC for each recorded channel. With proper design and modern components, adequate signal quality can be achieved with either approach, and it is usually considerations such as size and cost that impact this choice.

The next parameter that we need to consider in the digitization process is voltage or amplitude resolution.

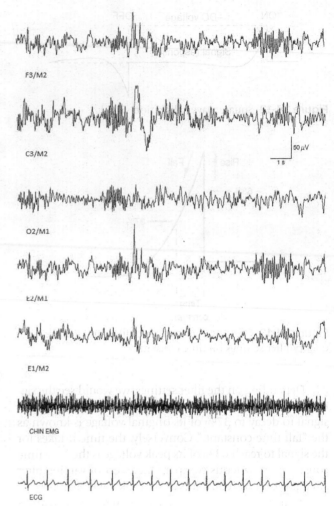

Figure 34-18 Accurate representation of the digitized signal.

In order to accurately display the EEG signal waveform, a minimum of 12 bits or $2^{12} = 4{,}096$ voltage points has been mandated by the AASM. In practice, most systems use at least 16 bit or higher ADCs, allowing larger dynamic range and smoother signals.

The number of data points may be further reduced by amplifier or software depending on relevant physiologic characteristics. This allows storage constraints to be met. The final result is accurate and noise-free representation of the original exceedingly weak signal at the desired electrode pairings, sensitivity, and filter settings, as exemplified in Figure 34-18.

CALIBRATIONS

In our discussion of calibrations, we must first be sure that we understand what the term "calibration" actually means. In its literal sense, calibration is the determination and documentation of the accuracy of a measurement or an observation. In PSG, there are several realms in which calibration comes into play.

Historically, machine calibration was necessary daily to ensure that the writing pens actually inked out tracings that accurately reflected recording parameters. This was due to the susceptibility of mechanical parts to gradually lose their position. In today's PSG systems, everything is digital, and true machine calibrations are no longer performed by the technologist. Rather, the conversion is innate to the amplifier circuitry, thus providing security in the knowledge that what you see is what you get. This does not mean that a well-run study does not attempt to document the scale used when viewing the recording. Therefore, at any time during a study, the technologist can usually initiate a software command that will produce several calibrations useful in the documentation process, including

1. Square wave—Many systems will produce a channel-by-channel scroll of a square wave that will trace a DC 50 μV per cm on/off signal.
2. Time constant—All PSG systems will record a channel-by-channel tracing that shows the aforementioned time constant as a function of time and filter settings.
3. Impedance check—Although not a true calibration, the impedance check will produce an electronic stamp that shows the contact impedance values of all electrodes. This varies among vendors in the way it is illustrated but usually documents the actual value in kΩ. While running the impedance check, it is possible to see whether the values are acceptable, and the technologist is alerted to any poor electrode connections. It is good practice to aim for similar values below 5 kΩ and to make sure that common and reference electrode impedance values are low.
4. Biocalibrations—These are physiologic maneuvers used to assess the integrity of the recording of various parameters. This is discussed in detail in other chapters, but we mention it here only to make sure that technologists do not confuse these patient calibrations with system calibrations.
5. External and integrated pulse oximetry calibrations—Most PSG systems have integrated pulse oximetry that conforms to AASM standards for accuracy and sampling rate. Because the readout of integrated oximetry is what the technologist views on the PSG monitor, the method for obtaining a calibration in this case would be to attach a separate clip from an independent oximeter to another finger and compare the readouts. In the case of using an ancillary oximeter that is plugged into a DC input, the technologist compares the readout on the bedside oximeter with what is being displayed on the PSG monitor and calibrates accordingly.

Table 34-3 Voltage Ranges for Direct Current Signals

Parameter	0 V	1 V
End-tidal CO_2 (mm Hg)	0	100
Transcutaneous CO_2 (mm Hg)	0	100

6. $EtCO_2$ and transcutaneous CO_2 involve the use of ancillary CO_2 monitoring devices that interface with the PSG system through one of the available DC inputs on the bedside amplifier. In either case, calibration involves the assigning of a voltage range to the minimum and maximum measurement values according to the example in Table 34-3.
7. Positive airway pressure (PAP) flow generators—Most manufacturers have developed flow generators capable of multiple measurements, including pressure, flow, leak rate, etc. Calibration of PAP to the PSG system involves the assigning of a voltage range to the desired minimum and maximum values according to the example in Table 34-4.

THE RECORDING MONTAGE

When the minimum criteria for channel recording as determined in the AASM scoring manual are met, a standard montage can be developed, as shown in Table 34-5.

Digital PSG allows the technologist to rereference during and after the recording as necessary to maintain signal clarity. This includes the ability to choose an arithmetic average of the left and right mastoid references when ECG artifact contaminates the recording. This has been referred to as "linked ears," and the digital benefit is that because the rereferencing is done using software, the technologist no longer needs to enter the room and combine M1 and M2 with jumper cables. The technologist is able to change many additional recording

Table 34-4 Calibration Ranges for Positive Airway Pressure Outputs

Parameter	0 V	1 V
Pressure (cm H_2O)	0	30
Flow (L/min)	−60	60
Leak (L/min)	0	60

Table 34-5 Sample Montage

Channel	Derivation	Sensitivity (μV/mm)	High Filter (Hz)	Low Filter (Hz)	Sample Rate (Hz)
L outer canthus	E1–M2	5–7	35	0.3	256
R outer canthus	E2–M1	5–7	35	0.3	256
Chin EMG	EMG1–EMG2–EMG3	10	100	10	256
Central EEG	C3–M2 or C4–M1	5–7	35	0.3	256
Occipital EEG	O1–M2 or O2–M1	5–7	35	0.3	256
Frontal EEG	F3–M2 or F4–M1	5–7	35	0.3	256
Left anterior tibialis	LAT1 LAT2	10	100	10	256
Right anterior tibialis	RAT1 RAT2	10	100	10	256
ECG	ECG1 ECG2	20	70	0.3	256
Snore		20	100	10	256
P flow AC*		20	15	0.1	100
P flow DC*	DCx	20	15	N/A	100
Thermo flow*		20	15	0.1	100
Thoracic effort belt		10–100	15	0.1	100
Abdominal effort belt		10–100	15	0.1	100
CPAP*	DCx	–	5	–	100
SpO₂	DCx	–	5	–	25

*flow channel options. CPAP, continuous positive airway pressure; ECG, electrocardiogram; EEG, electroencephalogram; EMG, electromyogram; SpO_2, pulse oximetry.

variables in order to examine more closely those aspects of the recording that warrant documentation. For example, any number of montages can be selected in order to satisfy the requirements of the ordering physician and aid in diagnosis.

VIDEO AND AUDIO RECORDING IN PSG SYSTEMS

The ability to synchronize digital video to the PSG recording introduces an additional valuable diagnostic tool to digital PSG. By converting the analog signal from a high-resolution camera into a digital format, such as MPEG4, video can be streamed into the collection computer, and using various software programs, the video can be time-synchronized with the raw PSG data stream. Modern systems no longer require cumbersome add-on

hardware to process the video stream but utilize conversion algorithms such as software compression and available USB ports. On most systems, the video capture bit rate can be adjusted in order to decrease the video file size. Reviewing physicians can quickly navigate to desired epochs to view video synchronized with the recording. Large video files can also be deleted or clipped to desired epoch ranges or be copied to separate data storage locations to suit the facilities' retention requirements. During the collection process, technologists can pan, tilt, and even zoom to capture the most articulate and fine aspects of patient movement and behavior during the recording.

In the same regard, refined directional and omnidirectional microphone configurations also make it possible to capture even the faintest sounds emanating from the recording bedroom. The end result is a true detailed composite of all recording parameters of the patient's sleep experience.

PRESENT AND FUTURE CONSIDERATIONS FOR DIGITAL PSG

The needs of health care providers and testing facilities demand that present-day diagnostic and treatment platforms are cost-efficient. Owing to software developments and hardware miniaturization, sleep facilities are now able to incorporate improvements in such areas as database customization, storage, networking, portability/mobility, and interfacing with other facility information platforms. Digital PSG has also become more reliable with the inclusion of such technologies as automatic disaster recovery, which, in the case of interruptions to the recording such as power outages, automatically restarts and appends to the existing record.

In the area of patient data and information, there is the issue of ever-expanding storage requirements. Smaller facilities can archive studies to various media. Larger networked facilities can leverage existing infrastructure to make use of more elegant solutions. Study data can be backed up over networks to storage servers that automate periodic redundant backups. Depending on regulatory requirements, data can be archived for the requisite period before they are deleted if they are deleted at all. Some facilities may also print study reports and interpretations for inclusion in paper files.

With the advent of sophisticated database programming, it is now possible to keep track of patient records using any number of variables, including demographic data and information clinically specific to the patient. Physicians and other users can easily sort patients they are interested in viewing, and management and retrieval of salient information is now as quick as a click of the pointing device.

There is also concurrent application or "multitasking" technology, allowing technologists to simultaneously acquire and review patient data, making it possible to view live recording on one monitor while scoring the same record on a different monitor, or by splitting the screen. Virtualization technology makes it possible to serve multiple instances of the application. Larger facilities may find this technology prudent and actually dedicate servers of this type, so that all stakeholders can access patient information regardless of time or place.

Users can also make use of autoscoring algorithms, although these outcomes require review for clinical confirmation. Another valuable addition is the capability of multiuser comparison scoring. This is known as "Interscorer reliability." All of these advancements necessitate increased vigilance and protection of sensitive personal health information. This is accomplished using encryption protocols, password-protected user logins, and other administrative forms of data protection.

In other areas of data exchange, most PSG systems now integrate with the facility's electronic medical record. This initiative is known as HL7. Integration of the PSG system with the facility information system means that patient demographics and personal health care information can be imported from existing databases, so that valuable clinical history is not overlooked by the sleep specialists. This is important in view of the fact that sleep medicine is particularly concerned with differential diagnosis and comorbid conditions. Along those same lines, most modern PSG systems will also export study files in European Data Format and other standard file formats, so that patient records can be viewed across varying platforms. Modern PSG systems also integrate with spreadsheets and word processing programs, so that reports can be tailored to show data in every way imaginable.

Portable or remote PSG occurs when the technologist is not in the same physical location as the patient is. Digital PSG has also made possible portable monitoring or home sleep apnea testing (HSAT). Most PSG vendors now offer portable amplifiers that do not sacrifice any channels typically included in normal facility–based PSG. These devices can be set up in the facility and taken home with the patient. The technology is quite similar to full PSG with the option of audio and video capture. These devices usually record information to flash storage on the order of 2 GB to as high as 10 GB. This technology is categorized as a type II device. Type III and type IV devices are simpler devices that record fewer channels and they comprise the devices that are used for HSAT. The next area of improvement in portable diagnostics may well be streaming data from the home to the facility for remote viewing and "real-time" observation and processing. All of these improvements will be governed by data integrity, data security, and Health Insurance Portability and Accountability Act (HIPAA) concerns. With the ever-changing landscape of sleep medicine, one thing is certain, PSG will forever be inextricably linked to digital technology.

Special thanks to Valery Arkhangorodsky from Natus Medical Incorporated and currently with Google, and to Michael Tamayo of Natus Medical Incorporated, whose technical consulting and assistance was invaluable.

REFERENCES

1. Berry, R. B., Albertario, C. L., Harding, S. M., et al.; for the American Academy of Sleep Medicine. (2018). *The AASM manual for the scoring of sleep and associated events: Rules, terminology and technical specifications* [Version 2.5]. Darien, IL: American Academy of Sleep Medicine.

2. Tatum, W. O., Husain, A. M., & Benbadis, S. R. (2008). *Handbook of EEG interpretation*. New York, NY: Demos Medical Publishing.

3. Nunez, P. L., & Srinivasan, R. (1981). *Electric fields of the brain: The neurophysics of EEG*. New York, NY: Oxford University Press.

4. Klein, S., & Thorne, B. M. (2006). *Biological psychology*. New York, NY: Worth.

5. Forouzan, B. A., & Fegan, S. C. (2001). *Data communications and networking* (2nd ed., p. 105). Boston, MA: McGraw-Hill.

chapter 35
Recording the Biopotentials of Sleep

REGINA PATRICK

LEARNING OBJECTIVES

On completion of this chapter, the reader should be able to:

1. Explain the frequency and voltage characteristics of the primary biopotentials recorded during polysomnography.
2. Recognize and correct problems with biopotential signals.
3. Explain the purpose and procedures for pre- and postphysiologic calibrations.
4. Recognize common artifacts and determine the appropriate action or monitoring required.
5. Identify and respond to physiologic data, clinical events, patient needs, and medical emergencies.

KEY TERMS

Artifact
Biopotential
Clinical event
Electrocardiogram
Electroencephalogram
Electromyogram
Electrooculogram
High-frequency filter
Low-frequency filter
Medical emergency
Physiologic calibration
Respiratory airflow
Respiratory effort

The desired signals of brainwaves on an electroencephalogram (EEG), eye movements on an electrooculogram (EOG), heartbeats on an electrocardiogram (ECG), and thoracic and abdominal movements on the respiration channels occur in association with signals that are stronger. The stronger signals may obscure the desired signals. On a polysomnograph (PSG), low-frequency filters and high-frequency filters make it possible to record desired signals while excluding undesired signals. The low-frequency filter setting will not allow any frequency less than that setting to be recorded, and the high-frequency filter setting will not allow any frequency above the setting to be recorded. Thus, any frequency falling between the high- and low-frequency filters will be detected and recorded.

The low- and high-frequency filters are set just below and above, respectively, the desired signal frequency. The American Academy of Sleep Medicine (AASM) (Darien, IL) recommends the following high- and low-frequency filter settings for EEG, EOG, electromyogram (EMG), ECG, and respiratory channels.

RECORDING THE BIOPOTENTIALS OF SLEEP

Electroencephalogram

The EEG frequencies of interest range from less than 1 cycle per second (i.e., <1 Hz) to 14 Hz. Therefore, a low-frequency filter setting of 0.3 Hz (which allows the detection of slow waves) and a high-frequency filter setting of 35 Hz (which allows the detection of alpha waves) are typically used for the EEG channels.

Electrooculogram

A low-frequency filter setting of 0.3 Hz allows the detection of the slow-rolling eye movements that occur with sleep onset, and a high-frequency filter setting of 35 Hz allows the detection of rapid eye movements (REMs) and the fast, low-amplitude EOG activity occurring throughout sleep.

Electromyogram

A low-frequency filter setting of 10 Hz and a high-frequency filter setting of 100 Hz are used to detect EMG frequencies of the skeletal muscles (e.g., legs and chin). This range is sufficient to record the faster firing rate of the muscles (i.e., increased muscle tone) during arousals, wake, or nonrapid eye movement (NREM) sleep and the decreased firing rate of the muscles (i.e., atonia [lack of muscle tone]) during REM sleep.

Electrocardiogram

A low-frequency filter setting of 0.3 Hz and a high-frequency filter setting of 70 Hz are used to detect ECG frequencies. The low-frequency filter setting of 0.3 Hz (i.e., 0.3 cycles per second = 1 cycle per 3.33 seconds) allows the recording of each heartbeat (which normally takes about 0.8 seconds) and a high-frequency filter setting of 70 Hz (i.e., 70 cycles per second = 1 cycle per 0.014 second) allows the recording of a heartbeat's individual waves (i.e., P, QRS complex, and T wave, the duration of these waves ranges from <0.10 to 0.25 seconds).

Respiratory Effort

The low-frequency filter setting is 0.1 Hz and the high-frequency filter setting is 15 Hz for the respiratory effort sensors, usually, respiratory inductance plethysmography belts. (Some centers may use piezoelectric belts for recording respiratory effort; however, the AASM no longer considers these belts acceptable for recording respiratory effort.) The low setting allows the slower sinusoidal waves of inhalation and exhalation to be recorded, whereas the high setting excludes frequencies that would obscure these waves.

Respiratory Airflow

For the airflow sensors (thermistor or thermocouple, pressure transducer), the low-frequency filter setting is 0.1 Hz and the high-frequency filter setting is 15 Hz. As with the respiratory effort channel, these settings allow the sinusoidal waves of inhalation and exhalation to be recorded while excluding frequencies that would obscure these waves.

PROBLEMS RECORDING BIOPOTENTIAL SIGNALS

Even with the correct filter settings, undesired signals (i.e., artifacts) can appear in a channel and interfere with the recording of a desired signal. The following are some common problems that can lead to artifact in a channel.

Skin/Electrode Issues

Some skin problems (e.g., rash) can affect the electrical properties of the skin by altering normal cellular interactions. This alteration may result in a high impedance reading. If the skin problem is localized, a technologist may need to place the electrode in a slightly different position to avoid the problem area. If the problem is more widespread, a technologist may need to forgo placing an electrode on that area of the skin. In this case, the technologist should thoroughly notate in the patient's chart why the electrode was not placed on the patient.

Problems Recording EEG Signals
Sweat Artifact

Sweat may cause low-frequency artifact to appear in the EEG, resulting in rolling in the EEG channels. Cooling the patient by increasing air circulation (turning on a fan or air conditioner, opening the door) may eliminate rolling by ameliorating sweating. However, sweat contains salt and the salt that remains on the skin after the skin cools can cause chemical changes in the electrolyte gel used in the electrode. This factor can cause continued problems with a poor signal. If a poor signal continues, the poorly recording electrode(s) should be replaced.

Movement Artifact

Muscle activity during movement can obscure underlying EOG and EEG signals. During movement, it may be necessary for the technologist to describe exactly what is happening—especially if a patient is being monitored for nocturnal seizures or REM sleep behavior disorder (RBD) (i.e., a sleep disorder in which muscle atonia does not occur during REM sleep, thereby allowing the person to act out dreams).

Problems Recording EOG Signals

The retina has a negative charge (reflected by an upward deflection on the EOG channel) and the cornea has a positive charge (reflected by a downward deflection on an EOG channel). The difference between the two, called the "corneoretinal potential," is approximately -60 mV. The corneoretinal potential makes it possible to record eye movements from sensors placed on the outer canthus of each eye. When the eyes move in the same direction, one electrode will be close to the retina and record a negative charge, whereas the other electrode will be close to the cornea and record a positive charge.

To ensure equal amplitude of conjugate eye movements, the AASM recommends placing one EOG electrode 1 cm above and 1 cm lateral to the midline of the outer canthus of one eye (typically the right eye) and one EOG electrode below and 1 cm lateral to the midline of the outer canthus of the other eye (typically the left eye). In general, both EOG electrodes are referenced

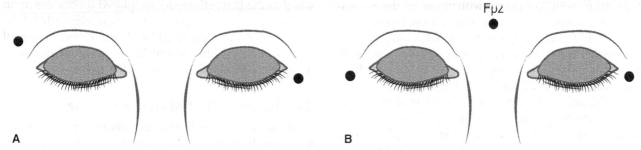

Figure 35-1 The recommended (**A**) and alternate (**B**) electrode placement for the electrooculogram channels.

to the same mastoid site (M2); however, it is acceptable for each EOG electrode to be referenced to the contralateral ear mastoid reference (i.e., E1-M2 and E2-M1). If both electrodes are placed above or below the midline of the outer canthus, the EOG signals will deflect in phase (i.e., in the same direction) rather than out of phase (i.e., in opposite directions). When using the recommended placement, the out-of-phase deflections of the EOG signals are greater for horizontal eye movements than for vertical eye movements.

An alternate placement allowed by the AASM for the EOG electrodes is to place each electrode 1 cm below and lateral to the midline of the outer canthus of its respective eye. Both electrodes are referenced to Fpz. In this configuration, vertical eye movements are in phase and horizontal eye movements are out of phase (Figs. 35-1 and 35-2).

An advantage of using the AASM's recommended eye placement is that all conjugate eye movements produce out-of-phase deflections. However, the deflections of vertical eye movements are greater than those of horizontal eye movements and eye blinks. As a result, it can be difficult to determine the direction of all eye movements, and eye movements with low amplitude may be missed. Using the alternate AASM eye placement, the vertical and horizontal eye movement deflections are

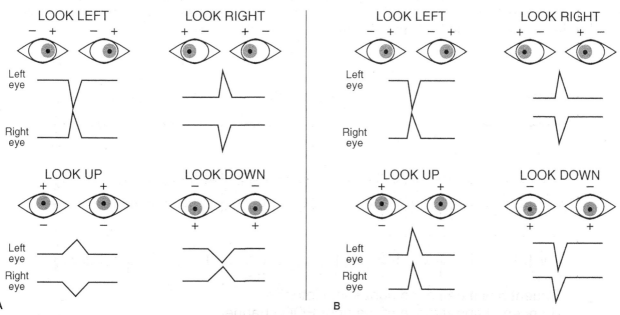

Figure 35-2 Eye deflections with the American Academy of Sleep Medicine (AASM)-recommended electrode placement (**A**) and the AASM alternate electrode placement (**B**). The deflections with alternate placement are larger for the vertical movements, compared with those of the recommended placement.

more prominent, compared with those of the recommended placement, and the signals for eye blinking are more readily detected (as in-phase deflections). However, with the alternate placement, the Fpz electrode may allow some EEG activity in the EOG recording, which can make it difficult to distinguish EEG activity from EOG activity, particularly during vertical eye movements. Even if electrodes are correctly placed using the recommended or alternate EOG electrode placement, several physiologic conditions can affect the recording of biopotential changes in an EOG channel.

An Artificial Eye

An artificial eye does not generate the electrical potential changes as would a natural eye. Therefore, an electrode placed by the artificial eye does not reflect eye movements of the affected eye. However, recording eye movements during REM sleep is still possible. Rather than placing an electrode on the outer canthus of each eye, the technologist can place both electrodes on the unaffected eye. The first electrode should be placed 1 cm from the edge and 1 cm above the midline of the outer canthus and the second electrode (which would have been used on the channel of the affected eye) should be placed 1 cm below the midline of the outer canthus of the same eye. Thus, the electrodes will still pick up the deflections needed to record REMs.

If a technologist were to place an electrode by the outer canthus of the affected eye, the EOG signals on that channel would appear dampened or distorted because the electrode continues to record frontal EEG activity. The technologist should make a note in the patient's chart that the patient has an artificial eye and indicate whether the EOG electrodes are placed on one eye or on both eyes. If the technologist places an electrode by the affected eye, he or she needs to describe how the signal is affected (e.g., "the patient has an artificial right eye; the right EOG signal is dampened").

Eye Diseases That Affect the Retina

Damage to or destruction of the rods or cones in the retina alters these cells' ability to undergo a photochemical reaction. The retina's electrical potential consequently decreases, and this factor can affect the corneoretinal potential. A diminished corneoretinal potential may dampen the EOG signal of one or both eyes in people who have diseases that affect the retina, such as Best disease (i.e., congenital macular dystrophy) (Fig. 35-3). The technologist may need to increase the sensitivity of the channels to record the EOG signal. The technologist should make a note in the patient's chart if sensitivity was increased for the affected eye.

Eye Muscle Problems

Six muscles in the eye, which are arranged as three sets of opposing muscles, allow a person to move the eyes in all four directions (up, down, left, and right) and obliquely. If a problem such as a stroke affects how these muscles move, one or both eyes will not move correctly. As a result of impaired muscle movement, EOG signals may be altered (nonexistent or dampened). The technologist may need to increase the sensitivity of the EOG channels to record the signal. The technologist should make a note in the patient's chart if sensitivity was increased for the affected eye.

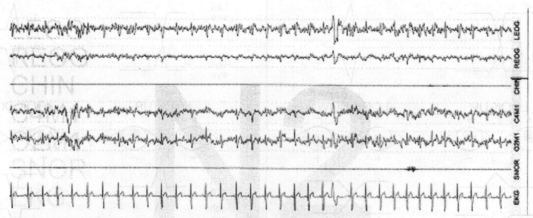

Patient has a damaged right eye. Note the dampened appearance of the right EOG channel.

Figure 35-3 Electrooculogram (EOG) recording of a patient who suffered a right eye injury. (Image used with permission of Regina Patrick, RPSGT, RST, and obtained on the SomnoStar system, version 9 [2008; Cardinal Health Respiratory Technologies, Palm Springs, CA].)

Problems Recording EMG Signals

Problems recording biopotential changes on the chin or leg EMG channels usually result from improper electrode placement, from high impedances (e.g., the skin is insufficiently cleaned), or from electrodes becoming dislodged during sleep. To reduce the likelihood of poor signal quality in the EMG channels, the technologist must show the same care in preparing the electrode sites as when applying EEG and EOG electrodes, and he or she should obtain a low-impedance reading (<10 Ohms [Ω]). The electrodes must also be securely attached to the chin or legs to prevent their being easily dislodged during the night. For example, an extra piece of tape may be placed on the leg sensors to ensure that they remain on the patient during the night. However, vigorous movement by a patient may dislodge an electrode, no matter how well secured. If the PSG recording system provides re-referencing capabilities, the EMG channel can be re-referenced to a backup electrode. If necessary, electrodes may need to be reapplied.

Problems Recording ECG Signals

Problems with the ECG recording are generally caused by poorly attached or dislodged ECG electrodes. If an ECG electrode becomes dislodged during the study (Fig. 35-4), an ECG tracing may be temporarily obtained from alternate electrode derivations, provided that the PSG recording system offers re-referencing capabilities.

If re-referencing is not possible, the electrode will need to be reapplied.

Problems Recording Respiratory Effort

People with certain neurologic problems that affect the abdominal and thoracic muscles or who have chest deformities such as kyphosis (commonly called "hunchback") may be unable to fully expand and contract the chest wall. This insufficient movement may result in reduced respiratory signals, even if the abdominal and thoracic sensors are properly placed on the patient. The technologist may, therefore, need to increase the sensitivity of a respiratory channel to record respiratory signals.

Problems Recording Respiratory Airflow

A common problem with recording airflow pressure changes is that the pressure transducer sensor may become plugged by excessive mucus, especially in a person with an upper respiratory infection or sinus infection. This obstruction will interfere with the proper recording of the signal. The technologist may need to clean or replace the sensor during the study to obtain a clear airflow signal. Another common problem with the airflow transducer sensor is that the air tube becomes kinked or the patient lies on the air tube. The technologist may need to enter the patient's room to unkink the air tube or dislodge it from under the patient.

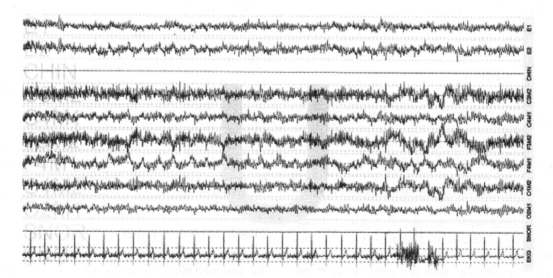

Patient movement dislodged EKG electrode slightly, resulting in interference in the signal.

Figure 35-4 Poor electrocardiogram (ECG) signal. (Image used with permission of Regina Patrick, RPSGT, RST, and obtained on the SomnoStar system, version 9 [2008; Cardinal Health Respiratory Technologies, Palm Springs, CA].)

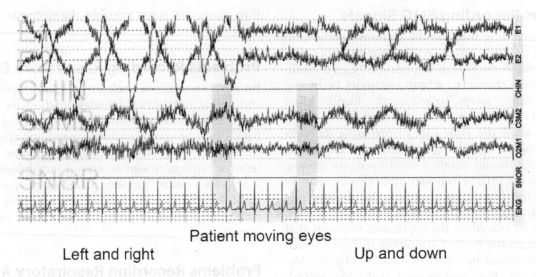

Patient moving eyes

Left and right   Up and down

Figure 35-5 Eye deflections with the AASM-recommended electrode placement. (Image used with permission of Regina Patrick, RPSGT, RST, and obtained on the SomnoStar system, version 9 [2008; Cardinal Health Respiratory Technologies, Palm Springs, CA].)

PROCEDURES FOR PRE- AND POSTPHYSIOLOGIC CALIBRATIONS

Physiologic calibrations (sometimes called "biocalibrations" or "patient calibrations") are performed before and after a sleep study. The physiologic calibrations are a series of instructions that are designed to determine that the sensors are correctly recording signals from a patient, the polarity of the signals is correct, the strength of the signal is sufficient for recording, and no unwanted interference exists. The following are features that should appear for each channel during the physiologic calibration procedure.

The EOG Channels

For these channels, it is important that the eye signals of each channel deflect in opposite directions when the person's eyes move conjunctively (i.e., in the same direction). To mimic the conjunctive eye movements of REM sleep, ask the patient to look left and right five times, then up and down five times (Fig. 35-5). As a result of the corneoretinal potential, the signal on one eye channel should deflect upward and the signal on the other eye channel should deflect downward with each movement. (However, if one uses the alternate EOG electrode placement, horizontal eye movements produce deflections in the opposite direction and vertical eye movements produce deflections in the same direction.)

The next physiologic calibration that involves the eyes elicits alpha waves. To do this, ask the patient to close the eyes for 30 seconds and then open the eyes for 30 seconds. In most people, when the eyes are closed, alpha waves become prominent in the EEG, especially

in the occipital channels. When the eyes are opened, the EEG resumes its original waking activity, which consists of a mixture of fast, low-frequency waves, primarily alpha and beta waves (the latter of which have a frequency of 18 to 30 Hz) (Fig. 35-6).

The third physiologic calibration involving the eyes involves having the patient blink the eyes five times rapidly (Fig. 35-7). During wake, a patient may blink at a rate of 0.5 to 2.0 Hz. As drowsiness develops, the blinking rate begins to slow and may be replaced by slow oscillating eye movements.

The Chin EMG Channel

For this channel, it is important to sufficiently detect muscle tone when the person is in NREM sleep. To ensure muscle tone is being recorded appropriately, ask the patient to grit the teeth together or chew (for 5 seconds), and then relax (Fig. 35-8). There should be greater than or equal to 0.5 cm increase in the amplitude of the signal, which reflects the increase in muscle tone. For patients who have no teeth, ask them to open the mouth or yawn instead.

The Snore Channel

For this channel, it is important that the sensor detects the increased vibration of the upper airway muscles that occurs with snoring. Ask the patient to make a snoring noise or hum for 5 seconds (Fig. 35-9). If the patient is unable to make a sufficient snoring noise, an alternative is to ask the patient to make a vocalization such as counting "1, 2, 3," or saying "A, B, C." The signal should increase briefly with each vocalization.

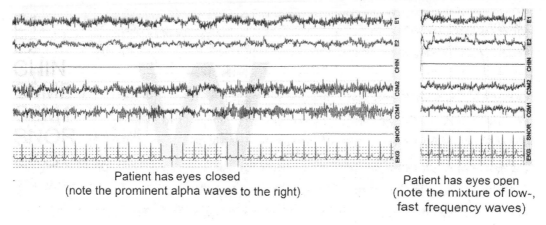

Patient has eyes closed
(note the prominent alpha waves to the right)

Patient has eyes open
(note the mixture of low-,
fast frequency waves)

Figure 35-6 Electroencephalogram changes with eyes closed **(left)** and open **(right)** (Image used with permission of Regina Patrick, RPSGT, RST, and obtained on the SomnoStar system, version 9 [2008; Cardinal Health Respiratory Technologies, Palm Springs, CA].)

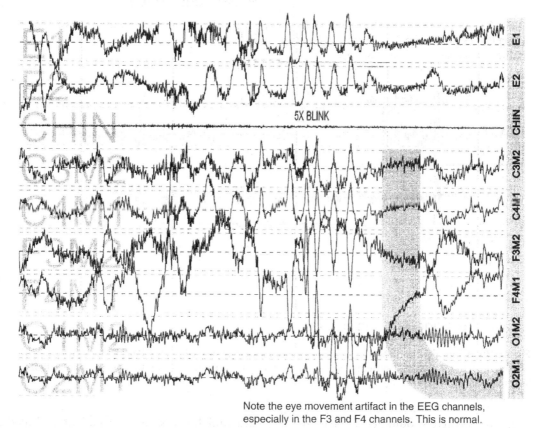

5X BLINK

Note the eye movement artifact in the EEG channels,
especially in the F3 and F4 channels. This is normal.

Figure 35-7 The appearance of the electrooculogram channels with eye blinking. EEG, electroenceph-alogram. (Image used with permission of Regina Patrick, RPSGT, RST, and obtained on the SomnoStar system, version 9 [2008; Cardinal Health Respiratory Technologies, Palm Springs, CA].)

The Leg EMG Channels

For these channels, it is important to detect the leg movements that occur with periodic leg movement (PLM) disorder or restless legs syndrome. Some patients with PLM disorder may bend the legs at the knee or hip level; however, more often, a person with PLM disorder may flex the ankle or toes. Therefore, it is important that the leg sensors are able to detect the smallest leg movements (e.g., flexing of the toes) occurring during a sleep study. To mimic PLMs, ask the patient to flex the foot/raise the toes of the right (or left) foot five times and then to flex the foot/raise the toes of the opposite foot

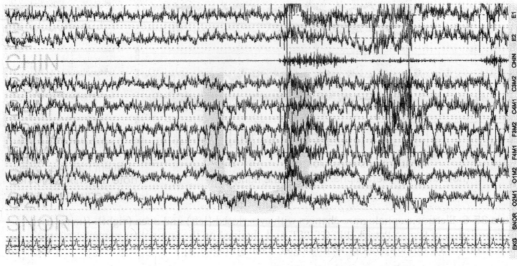

Patient gritting teeth

Figure 35-8 Change in chin electromyogram activity with gritting. (Image used with permission of Regina Patrick, RPSGT, RST, and obtained on the SomnoStar system, version 9 [2008; Cardinal Health Respiratory Technologies, Palm Springs, CA].)

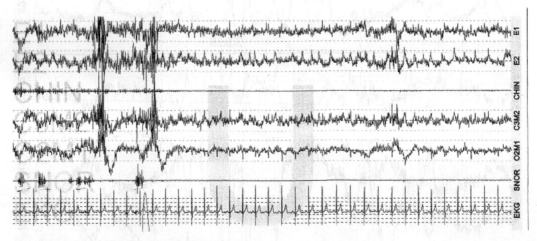

Patient making snoring noises

Figure 35-9 Simulation of snoring. (Image used with permission of Regina Patrick, RPSGT, RST, and obtained on the SomnoStar system, version 9 [2008; Cardinal Health Respiratory Technologies, Palm Springs, CA].)

five times (Fig. 35-10). There should be a burst of activity with each flex.

The Airflow Channels

For these channels, it is important that the airflow sensor (i.e., thermistor or thermocouple) and pressure transducer sensor are detecting airflow and air pressure changes, respectively, occurring with inhalation and exhalation. It is also important that these sensors detect the lack of airflow during an apnea episode. To ensure that the airflow sensors are detecting nasal breaths and oral breaths, ask the patient to breathe through the nose only for 10 seconds and then to breathe for 10 seconds through the mouth only (Fig. 35-11). As the person inhales and exhales, the thermistor or thermocouple should generate sinusoidal signals on the airflow channel. Nasal pressure transducers typically only measure nasal airflow; therefore, the signal in this channel should be flat during oral breathing maneuvers.

To mimic apnea, ask the patient to take a deep breath in and hold it for 10 seconds. The airflow and air pressure signals should be flat because no air is passing through the nose or mouth (Fig. 35-12).

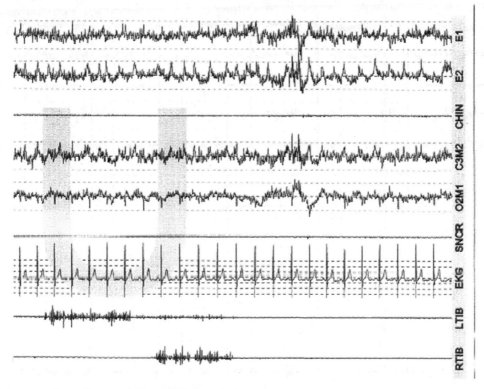

Patient flexing left and right toes

Figure 35-10 Change in leg electromyogram activity with toe flexes. (Image used with permission of Regina Patrick, RPSGT, RST, and obtained on the SomnoStar system, version 9 [2008; Cardinal Health Respiratory Technologies, Palm Springs, CA].)

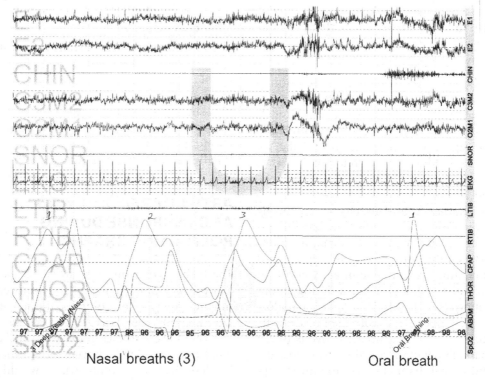

Nasal breaths (3)   Oral breath

Figure 35-11 Oral/nasal airflow tests. (Image used with permission of Regina Patrick, RPSGT, RST, and obtained on the SomnoStar system, version 9 [2008; Cardinal Health Respiratory Technologies, Palm Springs, CA].)

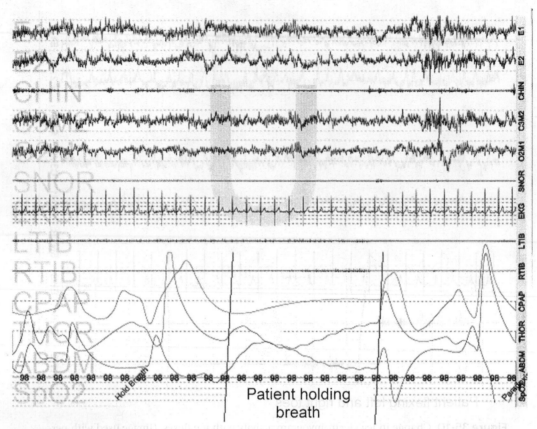

Figure 35-12 Simulation of apnea. (Image used with permission of Regina Patrick, RPSGT, RST, and obtained on the SomnoStar system, version 9 [2008; Cardinal Health Respiratory Technologies, Palm Springs, CA].)

The Abdominal and Thoracic Effort Channels

For these channels, it is important that the sensors detect the movements of the abdomen and chest during normal respiration and during an apnea. During the airflow tests, the abdominal and thoracic effort channels should have a sinusoidal signal moving in correlation with the airflow signal for inhalation and exhalation. When the patient is holding the breath to mimic apnea, the abdominal and thoracic channel signals should be flat (see Fig. 35-12).

Another respiratory feature usually tested during physiologic calibrations is paradoxical breathing—the movement of the abdomen and thorax in opposite directions—when the upper airway is fully blocked but the person continues to make respiratory efforts to breathe. Paradoxical breathing can occur during an obstructive sleep apnea (OSA) episode. To mimic paradoxical breathing, ask the person to hold the breath while making breathing movements. An alternative is to ask the person to pant. Either of these actions will cause the thoracic and abdominal channel signals to move in opposite directions (Fig. 35-13).

The ECG Signal

The ECG signal is not tested as part of the physiologic calibrations procedure. However, the technologist should note that the ECG signal has the correct polarity. The P wave should deflect upward, the QRS complex should have a down-up-down deflection, and the T wave should deflect upward. If the waves are in the wrong directions, the polarity should be corrected before lights out (Figs. 35-14 and 35-15).

ARTIFACT RECOGNITION AND RESPONSE DURING POLYSOMNOGRAPHY

The biggest contributor to artifact on a PSG during a study is patient movement. Patient movement increases muscle activity to the point that the activity obscures the EEG and EOG signals as artifact (Fig. 35-16).

The muscle artifact in these channels cannot be filtered out. A patient's movement is usually short, lasting less than 30 seconds, which would normally not interfere with the scoring of the record. However, if the

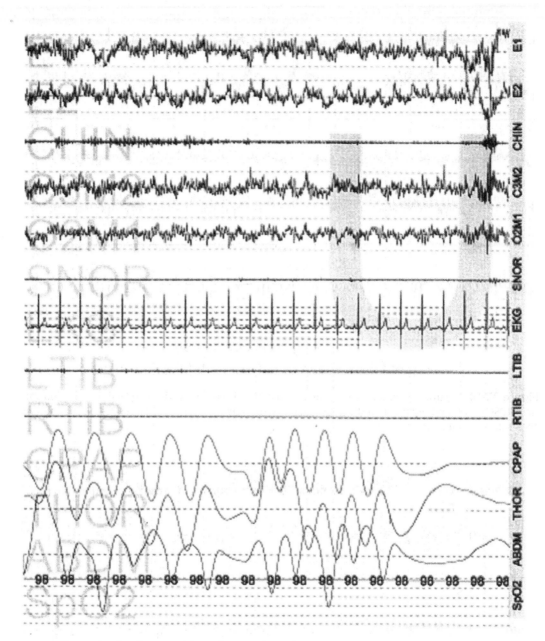

Paradoxical breathing (note that the thoracic and abdominal channels deflect in opposite directiions)

Figure 35-13 Simulation of paradoxical breathing. (Image used with permission of Regina Patrick, RPSGT, RST, and obtained on the SomnoStar system, version 9 [2008; Cardinal Health Respiratory Technologies, Palm Springs, CA].)

movement is prolonged (e.g., patient is tossing and turning in bed), the technologist needs to make a notation of this on the PSG.

Muscle artifact can also result from fast rhythmic muscle contractions induced by a seizure. During a seizure, a technologist needs to record on the PSG and in the patient's chart what activity occurred (e.g., patient flailed arms; patient jerking leg) and in what order. This description may later help a physician determine the origin and progression of the seizure in the patient's brain.

Patient movement may also dislodge electrodes. If a ground electrode, system electrode, or reference electrode (e.g., M_1 or M_2) becomes dislodged, all channels referenced to that electrode will contain artifact. The

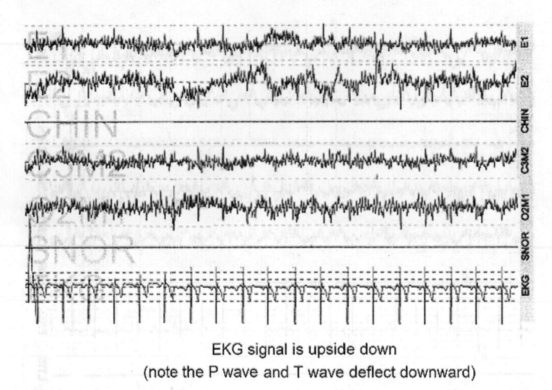

EKG signal is upside down
(note the P wave and T wave deflect downward)

Figure 35-14 Electrocardiogram (ECG) before correction. (Image used with permission of Regina Patrick, RPSGT, RST, and obtained on the SomnoStar system, version 9 [2008; Cardinal Health Respiratory Technologies, Palm Springs, CA].)

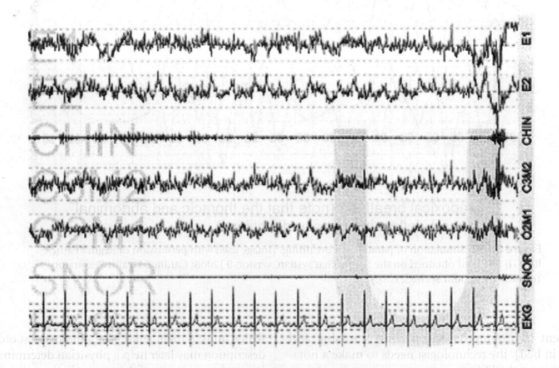

Same patient with the ECG corrected

Figure 35-15 Electrocardiogram (ECG) after correction. (Image used with permission of Regina Patrick, RPSGT, RST, and obtained on the SomnoStar system, version 9 [2008; Cardinal Health Respiratory Technologies, Palm Springs, CA].)

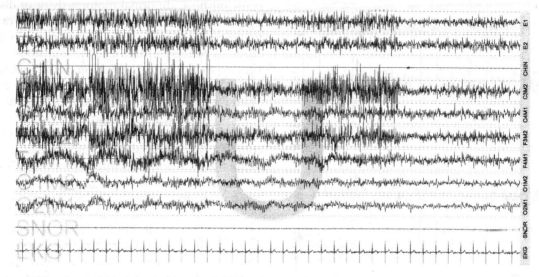

Muscle artifact (note it obscures the underlying EEG and EOG signals)

Figure 35-16 Patient movement resulting in muscle artifact. EEG, electroencephalogram; EOG, electrooculogram. (Image used with permission of Regina Patrick, RPSGT, RST, and were obtained on the SomnoStar system, version 9 [2008; Cardinal Health Respiratory Technologies, Palm Springs, CA].)

solution is to switch to the other reference or to a second ground or system reference electrode, if it is available, or to replace the electrode.

Another source of artifact is 60-Hz interference from external sources such as electronic equipment, television, and radios. This artifact appears as a somewhat thick line that may overlay the EEG, ECG, or EOG signals (Figs. 35-17 and 35-18). If the patient has any electronic devices operating near the electrode headbox, turning off the device should clear up the signal. At times, accessory equipment (such as a continuous positive airway pressure machine) near the electrode headbox may emit 60-Hz interference. If possible, moving the equipment away from the headbox may reduce the interference. If the interference remains, the technologist may need to look for other sources of 60-Hz interference or, as a last resort, apply the 60-Hz notch filter.

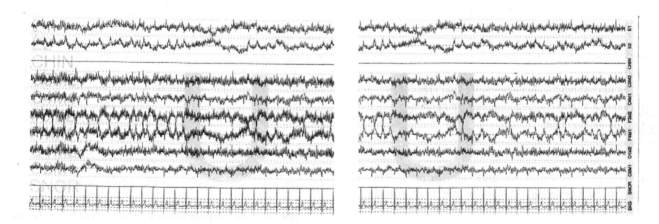

60-Hz interference in EEG and EOG channels

EEG and EOG channels after filtering out the interference

Figure 35-17 Sixty-hertz interference in the EEG and EOG channels. EEG, electroencephalogram; EOG, electrooculogram. (Image used with permission of Regina Patrick, RPSGT, RST, and obtained on the SomnoStar system, version 9 [2008; Cardinal Health Respiratory Technologies, Palm Springs, CA].)

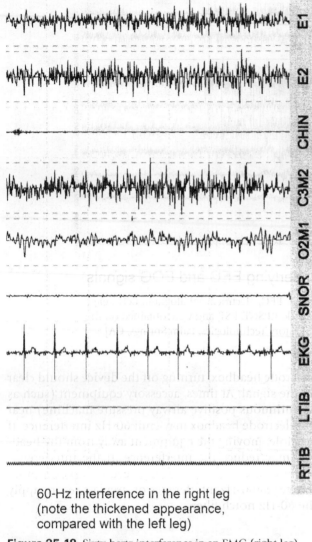

60-Hz interference in the right leg
(note the thickened appearance,
compared with the left leg)

Figure 35-18 Sixty-hertz interference in an EMG (right leg) channel. (Image used with permission of Regina Patrick, RPSGT, RST, and obtained on the SomnoStar system, version 9 [2008; Cardinal Health Respiratory Technologies, Palm Springs, CA].)

IDENTIFYING AND RESPONDING TO CLINICAL EVENTS AND MEDICAL EMERGENCIES

Some clinical events that can occur during a study are seizures, ECG arrhythmias, and parasomnias. The advent of these events during a study may require technologist and/or clinical intervention.

CLINICAL EVENTS

Seizures

A seizure is the sudden transient disturbance of brain activity that may result in sensory disturbances, loss of consciousness, abnormal motor activity, or disturbance of the autonomic nervous system. A seizure can be partial or generalized. A partial seizure occurs if the origin of the dysfunctional activity is limited to a discrete area (i.e., the focus) in the brain. A generalized seizure occurs if the dysfunctional activity involves a large area of the brain (e.g., one hemisphere) or if the dysfunctional activity involves the whole brain.

There are two types of partial seizures: simple and complex. During a simple partial seizure, a person maintains consciousness throughout the episode; however, impaired neuronal firing may manifest in a variety of ways, depending on the location of the focus and the pathway the dysfunctional signals travel. The person may have uncontrolled motor phenomenon (e.g., muscle twitching); sensory dysfunction (e.g., olfactory hallucination such as smelling rotten meat); autonomic symptoms (e.g., urinary urgency); or psychic signs (e.g., sense of *déjà vu* [i.e., the sense of having experienced something before]). During a complex partial seizure, an episode may begin with an "aura"—a preliminary sign of an impending seizure. (An aura is in actuality the manifestation of a simple partial seizure.) For example, an aura may involve muscular twitching in one arm. As the complex seizure continues, the person may exhibit altered consciousness or may lose consciousness. For example, during a complex partial seizure the person may have automatisms (i.e., involuntary aimless behavior such as lip smacking or picking at clothing) but later have no memory of the activity.

Simple and complex partial seizures can progress to a generalized seizure. A generalized seizure involves a loss of consciousness. At its simplest, a generalized seizure may involve a 1- to 10-second lapse of awareness (i.e., absence seizure), after which the person may continue the preseizure activity, unaware of the passage of time. However, during the seizure, onlookers may note the person staring unresponsively or blinking or rolling the eyes.

A tonic–clonic seizure is a generalized seizure at its worst. This type of generalized seizure begins with a sudden rigid extension of muscles (i.e., tonic phase), which is soon followed by violent shaking—the result of extremely fast, rhythmic muscular contractions (i.e., clonic phase). A tonic–clonic seizure may last from 2 to 5 minutes. Afterward, a person may be confused, be extremely sleepy, or may complain of headache, muscle aches, or muscle weakness.

The violent muscle contractions occurring during a tonic–clonic seizure obscure the signals in all of the channels on the PSG. The technologist needs to go into the patient's room to ensure that the patient does not harm himself or herself as a result of the violent jerking. The patient should be turned to the side to prevent aspiration of fluids (e.g., saliva), and the sleep center's emergency protocol should be followed.

Other types of generalized seizures are tonic seizures, which involve muscle rigidity but are not followed by a clonic phase; clonic seizures, which involve violent rhythmic contractions but are not preceded by a tonic phase; myoclonic seizures in which a person has brief involuntary jerking of the torso or extremities; and atonic seizures in which the skeletal muscles lose all tone, causing the person to suddenly drop to the floor.

A person with epilepsy (i.e., recurrent episodes of seizures) may have spikes or spike-and-slow wave complexes in the EEG channels on a PSG. On observing this activity in the EEG, a technologist should make a notation of it in the patient's chart.

Cardiac Arrhythmias

Cardiac arrhythmias may appear on the ECG channel during a sleep study, even in a person who does not have a diagnosed heart problem. Some common arrhythmias that may be seen on the ECG channel during a sleep study are sinus tachycardia (i.e., a fast heart rhythm), atrial tachycardia, sinus bradycardia (i.e., a slow heart rhythm), bradytachycardia (i.e., slowing of the heart rhythm, followed by a sudden increase in the heart rhythm), premature atrial contraction (PAC), premature ventricular contraction (PVC), atrioventricular branch block (AV block), premature junctional contraction (PJC), junctional tachycardia, and bundle branch block (BBB). Some arrhythmias require immediate emergency intervention.

Sinus tachycardia is a heart rhythm of greater than or equal to 100 bpm in adults. This rate is initiated by the sinoatrial (SA) node. Sinus tachycardia can occur in association with other illnesses such as hyperthyroidism, chronic obstructive pulmonary disease, and congestive heart failure.

Atrial tachycardia is a heart rhythm of 150 to 250 bpm. This rate is initiated by an atrial focus outside the SA node. Atrial tachycardia usually occurs in association with heart problems such as Wolff–Parkinson–White syndrome, but can occur with excessive use of stimulants (e.g., caffeine), use of certain drugs (e.g., marijuana), electrolyte imbalances, hypoxia, and psychological or physical stress.

Sinus bradycardia is a heart rhythm of less than or equal to 60 bpm. This rate is initiated by the SA node. Sinus bradycardia can occur as a result of a drug effect (e.g., beta-blocker drugs) or occur in association with other disorders such as hypothyroidism. However, bradycardia can be a normal finding in athletes.

Bradytachycardia most often occurs during an OSA episode, although it can occur in association with heart problems (e.g., sick sinus syndrome in which SA node dysfunction causes episodes of tachycardia, bradycardia, sinus arrest or pause, or bradytachycardia). In an OSA episode, the heart rhythm progressively slows to less than or equal to 60 bpm during the cessation in breathing (i.e., apnea). With an apnea-induced arousal, the heart rate suddenly speeds up to greater than or equal to 100 bpm as a person resumes breathing. The heart rate soon returns to normal as the blood oxygen level is restored.

A PAC is an atrial contraction that occurs too soon after the preceding beat because a focus in an atrium but outside of the SA node (which would normally induce an atrial contraction) instead triggers the contraction of the atria. A PAC may or may not be followed by a ventricular contraction. The P wave appears different from one that originates in the SA node. If the premature signal travels the normal pathway through the SA node, through the atrioventricular (AV) node, and down the bundle of His, the heartbeat will appear normal. PACs can occur in association with heart disease (e.g., heart failure), respiratory failure, hypoxia, electrolyte imbalances (i.e., improper levels of minerals such as calcium and potassium or molecules such as phosphate [HPO_4^-] and bicarbonate [HCO_3^-]), as in adverse drug effect (e.g., digitalis toxicity), or with the use of certain substances (e.g., alcohol, cigarettes). An occasional PAC in some people may be normal and present no danger. However, in people with heart disease, the presence of PACs can lead to more serious arrhythmias (e.g., atrial flutter, atrial fibrillation).

A PVC occurs when a focus in the ventricle triggers a ventricular contraction before the atria contract. The result is a deformed and wide QRS complex because the signal has not passed through the normal route (i.e., SA node to AV node, and through the bundle of His). PVCs can occur in people without heart problems; however, they often occur in association with heart disease and can be a prelude to a lethal ventricular arrhythmia (e.g., ventricular tachycardia, ventricular fibrillation). PVCs can occur because of metabolic acidosis (i.e., acidic state in the body resulting from an improper acid–base balance), hypoxia, a drug effect (e.g., tricyclic antidepressants, amphetamines), a heart defect, or damage to the ventricles.

An AV block occurs when the conduction of a signal from the atria to the ventricles is impeded (i.e., blocked). A problem at the level of the AV node, bundle of His, or the right or left branches of the bundle of His can result in an AV block. An AV block can be first degree (i.e., delayed conduction of signals from the atria to the ventricles), second degree (i.e., partial disconnection between atrial contractions and ventricular contractions so that not every atrial contraction results in a ventricular contraction), or third degree (i.e., complete disconnection between atrial contractions and ventricular contractions so that the atria and ventricles contract independently). An AV block can occur because of ischemia (i.e., low blood flow) or infarction (i.e., dead tissue caused by blocked blood flow) of the heart muscle, an adverse drug effect, structural defect in the ventricles, or damage to the AV node.

In a first-degree block, each P wave is followed by a QRS complex, and the P wave and the QRS complex appear normal. However, after the P wave, there is a delay lasting greater than 0.2 seconds before the QRS complex appears. (The normal interval between the end of the P wave and the beginning of the QRS complex is 0.12 to 0.20 seconds.) The delay occurs because the signal from the SA node cannot be conducted quickly through the AV node because of a problem at the level of the AV node (Fig. 35-19—first-degree block).

A second-degree block consists of two types: type I block (also called Mobitz I block or Wenckebach phenomenon) and type II block (also called Mobitz II block). In a type I block, P waves appear rhythmically. However, the interval between each P wave and the following QRS complex progressively lengthens until a QRS complex does not appear after a P wave. Therefore, the ventricular contractions are irregular, but the atrial contractions are regular (Fig. 35-19—second-degree block: type I and type II).

In a type II block, a signal is occasionally not conducted from the AV node. The type II block can result from a problem at the level of the bundle of His or bundle of His branches. Atrial contractions are regular, whereas ventricular contractions may or may not be regular in a type II block.

In a third-degree block, the atria and the ventricles contract regularly but independently of each other. The atrial contractions do not induce ventricular contractions. For example, the atria may contract at a rate of 90 bpm, whereas the ventricles contract at a rate of 30 bpm (Fig. 35-19—third-degree block).

A PJC occurs before a normal sinus contraction can occur. The origin of the junctional signal is the area around the AV node and bundle of His (collectively called the "AV junction"). A junctional signal travels simultaneously toward the atria and through the bundle of His. The result is an inverted P wave but normal QRS and T waves. PJCs can occur with excessive use of caffeine, digoxin toxicity, and heart problems affecting the heart wall (e.g., inferior wall infarction, swelling of the AV junction after heart surgery).

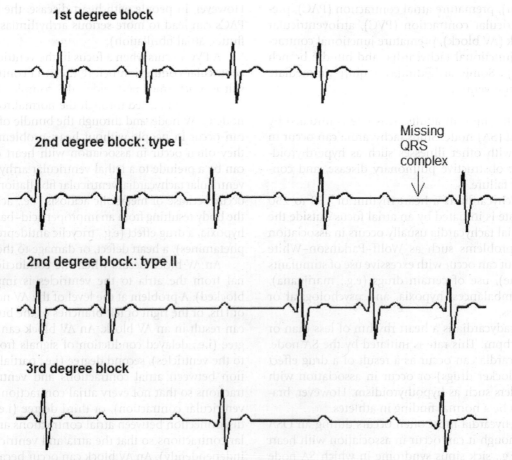

Figure 35-19 Schematic of first-degree, second-degree (type I [Mobitz I] and type II (Mobitz II]), and third-degree atrioventricular block.

Junctional tachycardia is when three or more successive PJCs occur. The rate of the contractions is 100 to 200 bpm.

Atrial arrhythmias, ventricular arrhythmias, and BBBs may require emergency intervention. When to intervene will be discussed later in the Medical Emergencies section.

Parasomnias

RBD, night terrors (i.e., sleep terrors), nightmares, sleepwalking, and enuresis are parasomnias for which a technologist may need to intervene to protect a patient from hurting himself or herself. RBD typically occurs in elderly men, although it can occur in women. The other parasomnias typically occur in children. However, they can also occur in adults. Each of these parasomnias is associated with a specific sleep stage. Therefore, a technologist needs to be vigilant when a patient enters the stage during which a particular parasomnia is likely to occur.

REM Sleep Behavior Disorder

RBD is often a prodrome (i.e., an early symptom indicating the onset of a disease or illness) of Parkinson disease. Symptoms of RBD manifest during REM sleep. In a person with RBD, REM sleep muscle atonia does not occur, which leaves the person free to act out dreams. Dreams reported by people with RBD are usually violent with themes of being chased or attacked. As a result, people with RBD may strike out against an attacker, unaware that they are in actuality striking a bed partner or a wall or other hard object. During REM sleep, the technologist monitoring a patient with RBD needs to record exactly what the patient does. If the patient is hurt during an episode, the technologist may need to initiate the sleep center's emergency protocol.

Night Terrors (Pavor Nocturnus)

Night terrors (also called pavor nocturnus) occur most commonly in children during slow-wave sleep in the early part of the night. Night terrors are more common in boys but can occur in girls. A child with night terrors awakens screaming and apparently in distress. Parents often note the child looks dazed. Attempts to calm the child agitate the child more, and a child is unable to respond or explain what scared him or her. After a few minutes, the episode is usually over and the child goes back to sleep as if nothing has happened. In the morning, the child has no awareness of having awakened with a night terror. During a sleep study, the technologist needs to be vigilant to note the onset of slow-wave sleep (night terrors tend to occur during this sleep stage), to anticipate the occurrence of a night terror, and to note everything a child does during an episode.

Sleepwalking (Somnambulism)

Sleepwalking (also called "somnambulism") occurs most often during slow-wave sleep in children. A child who sleepwalks gets out of bed and begins to walk in a somewhat haphazard fashion. The child appears dazed and may or may not respond to questions put to him or her by onlookers. The child may settle back in bed or settle in another setting. During a sleep study, the technologist needs to be vigilant to note the onset of slow-wave sleep and to note everything a child does during an episode of sleepwalking. If the child gets out of bed and appears to be in danger of hurting himself or herself, the technologist may need to enter the room to intervene.

Enuresis

Enuresis is bed-wetting. It occurs in children who are beyond the age by which urinary control is normally accomplished. It generally occurs during slow-wave sleep. During a sleep study, the technologist needs to be vigilant to note the onset and the end of slow-wave sleep. Enuresis alarms can be used to signal an episode of bed-wetting. If an alarm is unavailable, then at the end of the slow-wave sleep episode, the technologist needs to enter the child's room to assess whether the child has urinated. If so, the bedding should be changed. Afterward, the child can return to bed.

MEDICAL EMERGENCIES

A medical emergency is an acute injury or illness that results in an immediate risk to a person's life or long-term health. Medical emergencies in a sleep center are rare, but can occur. To effectively manage a medical emergency and potentially reduce the risk of injury or death to a patient, a technologist should be aware of the medical emergency protocols of his or her sleep center and when to implement them. Cardiorespiratory arrest and falls are the most common events that occur in a sleep center and would require a technologist to initiate the center's medical emergency protocol. Other events that would require a technologist to initiate a center's medical emergency protocol are certain cardiac arrhythmias, stroke, asthma attack, and diabetic ketoacidosis. A technologist's awareness of the impending signs of an adverse event or implementing steps to prevent an adverse event from occurring could potentially save a patient's life or mitigate injury to a patient. Patients experiencing a medical emergency may need to be transported to an emergency room. Depending on the severity of the emergency, the patient may then be admitted to a hospital.

Cardiorespiratory Arrest

Cardiorespiratory arrest is a cessation in the heartbeat and in breathing. A patient who goes into cardiac arrest, respiratory arrest, or both (i.e., cardiorespiratory arrest) during a sleep study can die within minutes and, therefore, requires immediate medical attention. Delayed response by a technologist could jeopardize the patient's life and health. For a patient in cardiac and/or respiratory arrest, a technologist should utilize an automated external defibrillator (AED), initiate cardiorespiratory resuscitation, alert the emergency medical service (EMS), and follow the emergency protocol of the sleep center.

Heart Attack

A heart attack (i.e., myocardial infarction) is a sudden episode in which blood flow in one or more vessels supplying the heart becomes blocked and thereby damages or results in the death of a part of the heart muscle. As a heart attack progresses, the heart rhythm may become unstable and ultimately stop, which may result in a person's death. Some warning signs of a heart attack are the patient has shortness of breath; complains of squeezing or crushing chest pain originating below the breast bone, which may radiate to the left arm, jaw, neck, or shoulder blades; has cool extremities (a sign that the heart is not pumping efficiently); has sweating; or complains of indigestion (individuals often mistake a heart attack for indigestion). If a technologist suspects a heart attack in a patient who is alert but manifesting these symptoms, the technologist should initiate the center's emergency protocol.

Cardiac Arrhythmias

A normal heartbeat will contain a P wave that represents atrial contraction, a QRS complex that represents ventricular contraction, and T wave that represents repolarization of the ventricles (Fig. 35-20). Atrial repolarization occurs during ventricular contraction; however, the much stronger signals produced by a ventricular contraction obscure the atrial repolarization signal. The normal heart rhythm is typically 60 to 100 bpm. Cardiac arrhythmia is a change from the normal rhythm and results from changes in the heart rate, regularity of signals, pathway of signals, or sequence in the activation of the heart. Cardiac arrhythmias may arise from the atria, ventricles, AV junction, and bundle of His branches.

Atrial Arrhythmias

Atrial arrhythmias that may be of concern during a sleep study are sinus tachycardia and atrial tachycardia, sinus bradycardia, PACs, atrial flutter, and atrial fibrillation. Atrial tachycardia, atrial bradycardia, and PACs may not be problematic in healthy people without heart disease. However, in people with an underlying heart condition, these atrial arrhythmias can lead to serious life-threatening arrhythmias. Atrial fibrillation is a serious life-threatening rhythm that requires implementing a center's emergency protocol.

Sinus Tachycardia and Atrial Tachycardia

Sinus tachycardia is a heart rhythm greater than 100 bpm. The origin of the signals is the SA node. Sinus tachycardia can be nonclinical (e.g., a person's heart rate can rise to more than 100 bpm with exercise), an adverse drug effect (e.g., amphetamine use), or the effect of using stimulants (e.g., caffeine, nicotine, alcohol). In a healthy person with no known heart problems, a technologist should make a notation of the rhythm in the patient's chart and follow the center's protocol regarding arrhythmias (e.g., contacting the center's medical director to make the person aware of the situation; ending a study, if necessary). However, if a patient with sinus tachycardia but no known heart problems complains of symptoms such as heart pain and palpitations, or faints, the technologist should implement the center's emergency protocol (e.g., initiating the AED and cardiopulmonary resuscitation, contacting EMS, transferring the

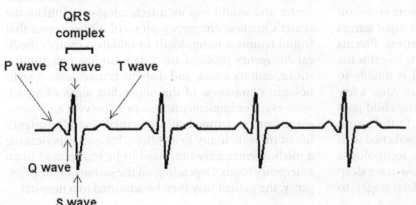

Figure 35-20 Schematic of a normal heart rhythm.

patient to an emergency room, and calling a staff physician [if the center is located in a hospital]).

Sinus tachycardia can be problematic in people with heart problems. The increased rate of contractions increases the heart's requirement for oxygen. If the heart muscle cannot meet this demand, a person with heart trouble and tachycardia may complain of chest pain, palpitations, a pounding chest, or skipped beats. The patient may also have blurred vision and hypotension, or may faint. The center's emergency protocol should be implemented for a patient with heart problems and tachycardia who is experiencing these symptoms. Sinus tachycardia can progress to heart failure (i.e., inability of the heart to pump blood efficiently throughout the body), stroke, sudden cardiac arrest, and death. Features of sinus tachycardia are (1) a regular but fast rhythm, (2) normal P wave, QRS complex, and T wave, and (3) the P wave is close to the T wave (Fig. 35-21).

Atrial tachycardia is the abrupt appearance of three or more atrial contractions that originate from a focus other than the SA node. The sinus rhythm resumes after the episode. These atrial contractions have a rate of 150 to 250 bpm. At this rate, the ventricles cannot properly fill with blood. Therefore, the amount of blood the heart pumps in a minute (i.e., cardiac output) throughout the circulatory system is reduced. In a healthy person without heart disease, episodes of atrial tachycardia may be benign. It can occur in people who ingest excessive amounts of stimulants such as caffeine, who use marijuana, who have electrolyte imbalances, or who are undergoing psychological or physical stress. Atrial tachycardia can also occur with hypoxia or as an adverse effect of digitalis toxicity. A technologist should make a notation of atrial tachycardia in the patient's chart and follow the center's protocol regarding cardiac arrhythmias. If the person complains of palpitations, angina, blurred vision, dizziness, trouble breathing (i.e., dyspnea); has syncope (i.e., faints); or has hypotension, a technologist should implement the center's emergency protocol.

In a person with a heart problem, atrial tachycardia can precede serious ventricular arrhythmias. Therefore, on noting this rhythm, a technologist should follow the center's protocol regarding cardiac arrhythmias and carefully monitor the person. If the ECG pattern changes to a life-threatening rhythm (e.g., atrial fibrillation) or

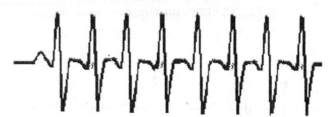

Figure 35-22 Schematic of atrial tachycardia.

a patient complains of palpitations or angina, faints, or has hypotension, the center's emergency protocol should be initiated. Features of atrial tachycardia: (1) each P wave induces a QRS complex; however, the P wave may be indiscernible because of the rapid rate of 150 to 250 bpm and (2) the QRS complex appears normal (Fig. 35-22).

Sinus Bradycardia

Bradycardia is a heart rhythm initiated by the SA node at a rate of less than or equal to 60 bpm. Bradycardia is problematic when the rhythm falls to less than 45 bpm. In a healthy person without heart disease, sinus bradycardia may be benign. For example, a slow heart rhythm can be a normal finding in athletes. It can also be a drug effect (e.g., beta-blocker drugs such as propranolol). A technologist should make a notation of bradycardia in the patient's chart and follow the center's protocol regarding cardiac arrhythmias.

Patients with known heart problems and bradycardia should be monitored carefully because bradycardia can lead to more serious arrhythmias such as ventricular tachycardia and ventricular fibrillation. A patient who is experiencing symptoms of bradycardia may complain of dizziness, may faint, or may have hypotension. If a patient has these complaints, the technologist should implement the center's emergency protocol. Features of sinus bradycardia are (1) the P waves and QRS complex are normal and (2) each P wave is followed by a QRS complex (Fig. 35-23).

Premature Atrial Contraction

A PAC occurs because a focus outside the SA node initiates one or more beats independently of the SA node. A PAC may or may not trigger a ventricular contraction.

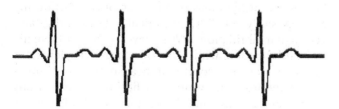

Figure 35-21 Schematic of sinus tachycardia.

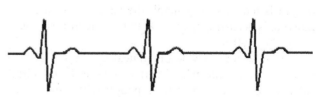

Figure 35-23 Schematic of sinus bradycardia.

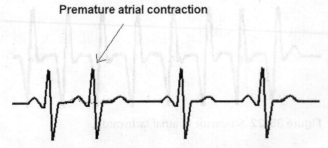

Figure 35-24 Schematic of premature atrial contraction.

In a person without heart problems, a PAC is rarely dangerous. PACs can be associated with pain, anxiety, use of alcohol or cigarettes, fever, and infectious diseases. A patient may experience them as palpitations or as a skipped beat. However, if PACs are frequent, a technologist should follow the center's protocol regarding cardiac arrhythmias.

PACs are problematic in people with coronary heart disease, hypoxia, respiratory failure, pulmonary disease, electrolyte imbalances, or digitalis toxicity because they can lead to more serious arrhythmias such as atrial flutter and atrial fibrillation. If a patient with PACs complains of heart palpitations, skipped beats, or a fluttering sensation, a technologist should initiate the center's emergency protocol. Features of a PAC are (1) the P wave occurs prematurely and may or may not be followed by a QRS complex, (2) the P wave may appear abnormal because the signal does not arise from the SA node, and (3) PACs may occur every other beat (i.e., bigeminy), every third beat (i.e., trigeminy), or in couplets (i.e., two sequential PACs) (Fig. 35-24).

Atrial Flutter

Atrial flutter is a form of atrial tachycardia in which atrial contractions occur at a rate of 250 to 400 bpm (typically 300 beats). At this rate, not every atrial contraction will induce a ventricular contraction. Instead, every second, third, or fourth atrial signal may be conducted through the ventricles because the AV node can only respond to signals up to 180 bpm. The number of atrial contractions that occur with each ventricular contraction is called the "conduction ratio" (e.g., four atrial contractions per one ventricular contraction is a 4:1 conduction ratio; the normal conduction ratio is 1:1). If the ventricular rate that occurs with atrial flutter is too slow (<40 bpm) or too fast (>150 bpm), the cardiac output is reduced. In general, the faster the ventricular rate that is occurring with atrial flutter, the more dangerous is the rhythm.

Atrial flutter rarely occurs in healthy people. It tends to occur in people with heart problems (e.g., mitral valve disease) and can occur in people with chronic obstructive pulmonary disease or systemic arterial hypoxia.

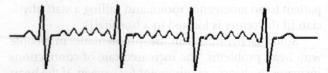

Figure 35-25 Schematic of atrial flutter.

People with atrial flutter may experience symptoms of low cardiac output, complain of dizziness and light-headedness, or faint. Technologists should implement the center's emergency protocol for patients complaining of these symptoms. Atrial flutter can lead to the life-threatening arrhythmia, atrial fibrillation. Features of atrial flutter are (1) not every P wave is followed by a ventricular contraction, (2) the P waves that appear between ventricular contractions occur so rapidly that they have a sawtooth appearance, and (3) the QRS complex appears normal (Fig. 35-25).

Atrial Fibrillation

In atrial fibrillation, many foci in the atria fire rapidly at a rate of 400 to 600 times per minute. This phenomenon may occur in association with heart problems such as severe mitral valve stenosis and coronary artery disease, with hyperthyroidism, with the use of stimulants (e.g., coffee, alcohol, nicotine), or with the use of medications (e.g., digitalis, aminophylline). The result of signals from multiple foci in the atria is that the atria cannot contract but instead quiver. Some atrial signals are conducted from the atria to the AV node, which allows the ventricles to contract. However, because of the lack of coordinated contractions from the atria, the ventricles consequently cannot properly fill with blood and the cardiac output is reduced. A patient with atrial fibrillation may complain of symptoms such as light-headedness, dizziness, mild shortness of breath, pain, and blurred vision, or the patient may faint or be unresponsive. Atrial fibrillation is a dire emergency because it can lead to sudden death. On noting this rhythm, a technologist should immediately implement the center's emergency protocol. Features of atrial fibrillation are (1) P waves are lost and appear as a thin narrow wavy line and (2) QRS complexes typically occur at a rate of 100 to 150 bpm (but can be lower) (Fig. 35-26).

Ventricular Arrhythmias

Ventricular arrhythmias that may be of concern during a sleep study are PVCs, ventricular tachycardia, and ventricular fibrillation. PVCs may not be problematic in healthy people with no known heart problems but may be serious in people with heart problems. Ventricular tachycardia and ventricular fibrillation are serious life-threatening rhythms in people with and without heart problems and require medical intervention.

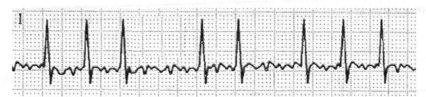

Figure 35-26 Electrocardiograph of atrial fibrillation.

Premature Ventricular Contraction

A PVC occurs when a focus located below the level of the bundle of His fires a signal before a P wave can be conducted. The subsequent QRS complex has a widened appearance because the ventricular signal is not conducted through the normal path. In addition, because the ventricles contract before the atria contract, cardiac output is decreased. Patients with PVCs may complain of symptoms associated with low cardiac output such as hypotension, angina, syncope, and respiratory distress.

PVCs can be benign in healthy people with no heart problems. However, if PVCs are frequent (i.e., six or more PVCs per minute), a technologist should make a notation of the arrhythmia in the patient's chart, follow the center's protocol regarding cardiac arrhythmias, and monitor the patient.

A technologist should carefully monitor a person with heart problems who has PVCs because such a person is at greater risk of PVCs progressing to ventricular tachycardia or ventricular fibrillation. If a patient with a heart problem is known to have PVCs, a technologist should carefully monitor the patient for an increase in frequency or a change from the baseline pattern. On noting an increase in the number of PVCs from the baseline or on noting a change from the baseline pattern such as the appearance of paired PVCs, bigeminy or trigeminy, or PVCs that look different from each other (i.e., multifocal PVCs, which indicates they have different foci), a technologist should immediately implement the emergency protocol of the sleep center. Paired PVCs, bigeminy or trigeminy, and multifocal PVCs are dangerous patterns that can induce ventricular tachycardia or ventricular fibrillation, either of which can lead to death. Features of a PVC are (1) it is not preceded by a P wave, (2) the QRS complex is wide and distorted, (3) it can regularly alternate with normal beats (e.g., bigeminy [Fig. 35-27] or trigeminy [Fig. 35-28]), (4) two PVCs can occur in succession (i.e., PVC couplet [Fig. 35-29]), and (5) PVCs may have multiple foci (Fig. 35-30).

Ventricular Tachycardia

Ventricular tachycardia is when three or more PVCs occur successively and the ventricular rate is greater than or equal to 100 bpm. The rapid ventricular contractions

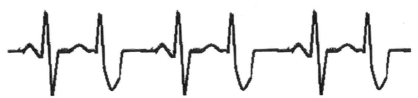

Figure 35-27 Schematic of bigeminy (every second beat is irregular).

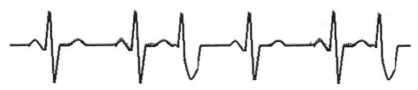

Figure 35-28 Schematic of trigeminy (every third beat is irregular).

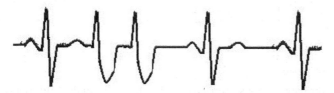

Figure 35-29 Schematic of a premature ventricular contraction couplet.

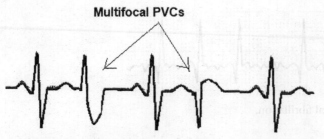

Multifocal PVCs

Figure 35-30 Schematic of multifocal premature ventricular contraction (PVC).

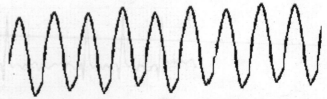

Figure 35-31 Electrocardiograph of ventricular tachycardia.

prevent the ventricles from properly filling with blood, which can quickly lead to ventricular fibrillation, followed by cardiac arrest and death. Ventricular tachycardia can be associated with the use of certain drugs (e.g., digitalis, cocaine, procainamide), heart disease (e.g., myocardial infarction, coronary heart disease), and electrolyte imbalances. A patient experiencing ventricular tachycardia may complain of angina, will have hypotension, and may have a decreased level of consciousness that may progress to unresponsiveness.

Ventricular tachycardia can occur in short bursts lasting less than 30 seconds and cause few to no problems. However, sustained ventricular tachycardia is a serious rhythm that requires the immediate implementation of a center's emergency protocol, which may include the use of an AED. Ventricular tachycardia appears as a somewhat sinuous pattern, which represents successive and uniformly distorted QRS complexes (Fig. 35-31).

Ventricular Fibrillation

As with atrial fibrillation, ventricular fibrillation occurs because many foci in the ventricles but outside the AV node fire rapidly, which results in the ventricles quivering rather than contracting. There is no cardiac output during ventricular fibrillation. As ventricular fibrillation progresses, the ventricles ultimately come to a standstill and death occurs. On noting this pattern, a technologist should immediately initiate a center's emergency protocol, which may include the use of an AED device. Features of ventricular fibrillation are (1) there are no discernible P waves, (2) there are no QRS complexes, and (3) there are no T waves. On an ECG, ventricular fibrillation appears as a fine squiggly line (i.e., fine ventricular fibrillation) or a coarse line (i.e., coarse ventricular fibrillation); on a PSG, because of its slower recording speed, ventricular fibrillation appears as a low thick somewhat flat line or as a compact angular zig-zag line, respectively (Fig. 35-32).

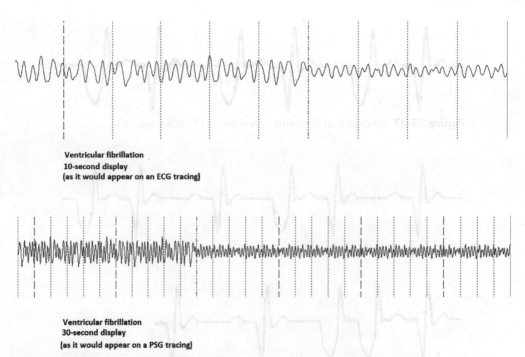

Ventricular fibrillation
10-second display
(as it would appear on an ECG tracing)

Ventricular fibrillation
30-second display
(as it would appear on a PSG tracing)

Figure 35-32 Ventricular fibrillation (coarse, seconds 1–6 [left]; fine, seconds 7–10 [right]) as it would appear on an ECG (top) and on a PSG (bottom). ECG, electrocardiogram; PSG, polysomnograph. (Courtesy of Jon Atkinson.)

Junctional Arrhythmias

Junctional arrhythmias arise from improper signals from the AV junction. Junctional arrhythmias that may be of concern during a sleep study are PJC and junctional tachycardia.

Premature Junctional Contraction

A PJC occurs when a focus in the area of the AV node and bundle of His (collectively called the "AV junction") initiates a heart contraction before the SA node can initiate an atrial contraction. When a signal originates from the AV junction, a wave of depolarization simultaneously travels upward toward the SA node and downward through the bundle of His branches. A PJC is usually not dangerous, although patients should be monitored for symptoms (e.g., light-headedness). PJCs can occur in people with certain heart conditions (e.g., Wolf Parkinson–White syndrome, rheumatic heart disease, myocardial infarction), with the use of certain drugs (e.g., digitalis), and with excessive use of caffeine.

A technologist should make a notation of this arrhythmia in a patient's chart and follow the center's protocol regarding cardiac arrhythmias. If a patient complains of palpitations or feeling a "quickening" in the chest, a technologist should implement the sleep center's emergency protocol. Features of a PJC are (1) an upside-down P wave (the result of retrograde depolarization) and (2) a normal QRS complex; however, the P wave may precede the QRS complex, come after the QRS complex, or be embedded within the QRS complex (Fig. 35-33).

Junctional Tachycardia

In junctional tachycardia, three or more successive junctional contractions occur. This phenomenon occurs because a focus in the AV junction takes over as the heart's pacemaker at a rate of approximately 100 to 200 bpm. Junctional tachycardia typically occurs in people who have heart problems that affect the heart's wall such as congenital heart disease, infarction in the inferior or posterior wall, or trauma-induced swelling of the AV junction after heart surgery. It can also occur with digitalis

toxicity. The rapid ventricular contractions can reduce cardiac output and decrease blood flow into the ventricles. As a result, a patient may complain of palpitations or feeling a "quickening" in the chest, or may show signs of low cardiac output (e.g., light-headedness, fainting, dizziness). For a patient experiencing symptoms, a technologist should implement the center's emergency protocol. Features of junctional tachycardia are (1) a regular but fast ventricular rhythm (100 to 200 bpm), (2) an inverted P wave, which may appear just before, within, or after the QRS complex, (3) a normal QRS complex, and (4) a normal T wave (unless the rate is so rapid the T wave cannot be detected) (Fig. 35-34).

Branch Bundle Block

In the upper portion of the interventricular septum, the bundle of His fibers divide into two branches, the left bundle branch and the right bundle branch. Each branch travels down its respective side of the interventricular septum and then spreads throughout its respective ventricle. When stimulated, the bundle branch fibers allow the simultaneous contraction of ventricles. Injury to the heart (e.g., heart attack) can impede the conduction of a signal through the left bundle branch or right bundle branch; this impedance is called a "left bundle branch block" (LBBB) or "right bundle branch block" (RBBB), respectively. Both types of blocks can occur with heart disease or injury. However, an RBBB can occur in people without heart disease, whereas an LBBB never occurs in a healthy person. If a signal is impeded in one branch, the P wave and T wave will be normal because the SA node and AV node are functioning correctly, but the QRS complex is wider than normal and may appear doubled (reflecting the slower contraction of the ventricle affected by the BBB).

Many people do not experience symptoms with a BBB. However, some people with a BBB may have a slow heart rate, which may cause fainting. In addition, people with a BBB are at greater risk of sudden cardiac

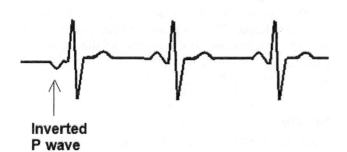

**Inverted
P wave**

Figure 35-33 Schematic of premature junctional contraction.

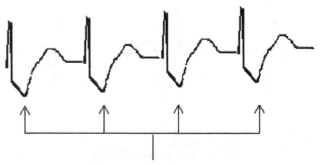

**Inverted P wave occurs after
the QRS complex**

Figure 35-34 Schematic of junctional tachycardia.

death because of faulty conduction in the heart. On noting a BBB, a technologist should make a notation of the arrhythmia and follow the center's protocol for cardiac arrhythmias. If the ECG pattern changes to a life-threatening rhythm (e.g., severe bradycardia) or a patient with a BBB faints or complains of feeling as if he or she will faint, the technologist should implement the center's emergency protocol. Features of a branch bundle block are (1) the QRS complex will be wider than normal (i.e., >0.12 seconds), (2) the QRS complex is wider than normal and may appear doubled, (3) the QRS complex has an M pattern in LBBB and a "rabbit ear" pattern in RBBB, and (4) the heart rhythm may be normal (~60 to 100 bpm) but can be slower or faster (Fig. 35-35).

Falls

A fall is a sudden unexpected descent to the floor from standing, sitting, or other positions (e.g., rolling out of a bed) with or without injury to the patient. Neurologic conditions such as Alzheimer disease and Parkinson disease, stroke, cerebral palsy; musculoskeletal disorders such as scoliosis; and the use of ambulatory devices such as wheelchairs and walkers can increase a patient's risk of falling. Fall precautions involve practices with the goal of preventing a patient from falling. Examples of precautions that a technologist may need to take to reduce the likelihood of a fall in patients with a fall risk

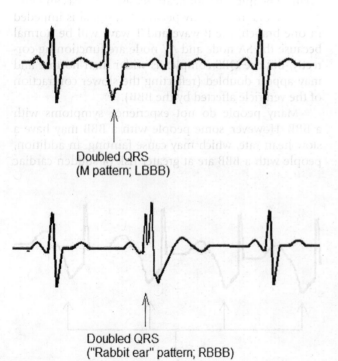

Doubled QRS
(M pattern; LBBB)

Doubled QRS
("Rabbit ear" pattern; RBBB)

Figure 35-35 Schematic of bundle branch block: left bundle branch block (LBBB) **(top)** and right bundle branch block (RBBB) **(bottom)**.

are assisting the patient with ambulation to and from the toilet or during walks to various areas in the sleep center (e.g., to and from the hookup room, lounge, office); allowing the patient to use a bedpan, portable toilet placed by the bedside, or urinal (male patients); and removing items from the floor such as area rugs that could become caught on a patient's foot or in an ambulatory device and cause a fall.

In elderly patients in particular, the risk of falls can be increased by the use of certain types of medications, such as hypnosedatives (e.g., zolpidem, ramelteon) and benzodiazepines (e.g., lorazepam, diazepam), antidepressants (e.g., tricyclic drugs such as amitriptyline and imipramine; serotonin reuptake inhibitors [SSRIs] such as fluoxetine and paroxetine; non-SSRIs such as mirtazapine), neuroleptics (e.g., risperidone), and antipsychotics (e.g., thioridazine), or by the use of four or more medications that are known to increase the risk of falls. Knowledge of the medications a patient is taking can allow a technologist to be more diligent in following the fall prevention protocols of a sleep center.

Once a patient is in the center, some methods that can help prevent falls include the following:

- Increase the lighting level. In some patients, reduced vision can increase the risk of falls. Increasing lighting in an area could allow patients to see objects more readily and thereby help reduce the risk of fall.
- Keep floors free of clutter and remove area rugs or other objects that can become entangled on a patient's feet or in walking assistance devices.
- Provide a nonskid bath mat in a shower or tub.
- Administer a questionnaire to assess a patient's fall risk. Examples of questions are "Have you fallen in the last year?"; "Are you taking four or more medications?"; "Do you have any vision problems?" (peripheral vision loss [i.e., "tunnel vision"] may prevent a person from seeing objects on the floor and consequently tripping over the object); "Have you had a stroke or been diagnosed with Parkinson disease?"; "Have you had any problems with balance or walking?"; "Do you have difficulty getting up from a chair?" (difficulty arising from a chair can be related to leg weakness or poor balance, which increases fall risk).

If a patient falls despite these efforts and is injured, the technologist should initiate the center's emergency protocol. Depending on the severity of the injury, the patient may need to be transported to a hospital for assessment and treatment.

Stroke

It is important for a technologist to recognize the warning signs of a stroke in a patient. As with a heart attack, a delayed response could jeopardize the patient's life and health. Some warning signs of a stroke are slurred speech or incoherent speech (e.g., a person may speak in "gibberish" or use the wrong words for an object); uncoordinated gait; weakness or numbness in part of the body such as the face; altered consciousness; drowsiness; and patient complaints of dizziness, headache, and double vision or unilateral blindness (i.e., blindness in only one eye). If a technologist suspects a stroke in a patient who is alert but manifesting these symptoms, the former should initiate the center's emergency protocol and record symptoms in the patient's record.

Asthma Attack

Asthma is an overactive immune response to an allergen. After exposure to the allergen, the air passages in the lungs contract, thereby causing difficulty in breathing, which is manifested by wheezing, coughing, and a sense of chest tightness. The sudden appearance of these symptoms is called an "asthma attack." An asthma attack can be a life-threatening condition. During such an attack, the bronchial airway passages suddenly narrow after exposure to an allergen. As the narrowing in the air passages worsens, wheezing may become louder, the person may begin to use neck muscles (i.e., accessory muscles) to raise the ribcage in an effort to get air into the lungs, or the person may begin to breathe fast (i.e., "pant"). As an asthma attack continues, airway inflammation and narrowing prevent oxygenation and a person may become cyanotic (i.e., has a blue tinge to the skin, especially the lips, face, and fingers). Continued reduction in oxygenation can result in unconsciousness and death.

For some asthmatic patients, positive airway pressure (PAP) treatment can trigger an asthma attack. The force of the air into the lungs or the plastic particles from the PAP mask or both may induce an asthma attack. Depending on the severity of the symptoms, a patient may be able to continue PAP treatment by using an inhaler to open the airway. However, if symptoms worsen (e.g., wheezing becomes significantly worse, the person begins using accessory muscles to breathe, the person becomes cyanotic), the technologist should immediately stop PAP treatment and implement the center's emergency protocol.

Diabetic Ketoacidosis

Diabetic ketoacidosis is a complication of diabetes, a disease involving improper blood glucose levels. Diabetic ketoacidosis occurs when insulin insufficiency (i.e., lower-than-normal insulin production) or insulin resistance (i.e., inability to use insulin correctly) causes the body to sense a "starvation" state. (Insulin is a hormone that removes glucose from the blood, so that body tissues can utilize glucose.) Typically, in a starvation state, stores of carbohydrates (i.e., sugars, starches) from which glucose could be synthesized have been depleted. To restore glucose levels, the body forms glucose from noncarbohydrate sources such as fat; this process is called "gluconeogenesis." However, a by-product of gluconeogenesis is ketone bodies (i.e., acetone, acetoacetic acid, and beta-hydroxybutyric acid). These molecules are acidic and raise the acidity of the blood, which can result in altered consciousness, coma, and ultimately death, if left untreated.

Ketoacidosis can result from insulin insufficiency, having a severe infection or other illness, not eating for a prolonged time, being severely dehydrated, or a combination of these factors. Ketoacidosis typically occurs in people with type 1 (i.e., insulin-dependent) diabetes. People with this type of diabetes produce little or no insulin. However, ketoacidosis can occur in people with type 2 (i.e., noninsulin-dependent) diabetes when blood sugar levels are high because of poor blood sugar control or poor treatment compliance. In people with type 2 diabetes, insulin resistance allows excessive amounts of glucose to remain in the blood and not enter the body's tissues; thus, the body erroneously senses a starvation state and initiates gluconeogenesis.

Signs and symptoms of diabetic ketoacidosis develop quickly—sometimes within 24 hours—as the levels of ketone bodies increase. At its onset, a person with ketoacidosis may have excessive thirst, dry mouth, frequent urination, and dry or flushed skin. As ketoacidosis progresses, the patient may experience nausea and vomiting, abdominal pain, weakness or fatigue, and shortness of breath. In the later stages of ketoacidosis, the person develops a fruity or nail polish remover–like smell to the breath because of the excessive production of acetone and other ketone bodies; rapid deep breathing; confusion; coma; and, at worse, death.

The treatment for ketoacidosis involves correcting a person's blood glucose and insulin levels. Some patients may recognize early symptoms of improper blood glucose or insulin levels and attempt to take precautions. For example, a patient may state "My blood sugar feels like its high, I better take my insulin" or "My sugar feels like its low, I better eat something." To confirm whether blood glucose levels need to be decreased (i.e., taking insulin) or raised (ingesting a meal or candy), a patient may use test strips to test the blood for high glucose level or test the urine for high ketone level and act accordingly. The sleep technologist should record this information in the patient's record. If a patient does not improve or appears to be getting worse within 20 to 30 minutes after attempting to correct blood glucose or insulin levels, a sleep technologist should initiate the sleep center's emergency protocol or contact EMS.

SUMMARY

Recording biopotentials accurately during a sleep study and recording factors or events that affect the recording of biopotentials are very important aspects of a sleep technologist's job. The quality of a record produced by a technologist can affect the quality of care a patient receives. If a sleep physician is unable to read a record because of uncorrected artifacts or improper signals (e.g., low-amplitude respiratory signals), the physician may be unable to accurately diagnose a patient's sleep problem and effectively treat it. Factors (e.g., blindness) and events (e.g., the onset of a seizure, parasomnias) that affect a recording need to be recognized, addressed (if necessary), and recorded in a patient's chart by the technologist. Recording these factors and events gives a sleep physician a clearer picture of what is occurring with a patient during sleep. This information may then impact how a physician diagnoses and treats a sleep disorder in a patient.

In addition to recording a PSG, it is important that technologists recognize when a patient may be in danger of injury or experiencing a life-threatening event during the sleep center visit. A technologist's quick and appropriate actions in managing medical emergencies could lessen injury to a patient, avoid the long-term consequences of an injury to a patient, or avoid the death of a patient in a sleep center.

SUGGESTED READINGS

Ambrose, M. L., Mauro, E., Nash, J., et al. (Eds.). (1997). *ECG interpretation made incredibly easy*. Springhouse, PA: Springhouse Corporation.

American Heart Association. (2016). *Basic life support*. Dallas, TX: Author.

Berry, R. B., Albertario, C. L., Harding, S. M., et al.; for the American Academy of Sleep Medicine. (2018). *AASM manual for the scoring of sleep and associated events: Rule, terminology and technical specifications* [Version 2.5]. Darien, IL: American Academy of Sleep Medicine.

Bromfield, E. B., Cavazos, J. E., & Sirven, J. I. (Eds.). (2006). Chapter 2: Clinical epilepsy. In *An introduction to epilepsy* [Internet]. West Hartford, CT: American Epilepsy Society. Retrieved February 26, 2018, from https://www.ncbi.nlm.nih.gov/books/NBK2511/?report=classic

de Jong, M. R., Van der Elst, M., & Hartholt, K. A. (2013). Drug-related falls in older patients: Implicated drugs, consequences, and possible prevention strategies. *Therapeutic Advances in Drug Safety, 4*, 147–154.

Duce, B., Rego, C., Milosavljevic, J., et al. (2014). The AASM recommended and acceptable EEG montages are comparable for the staging of sleep and scoring of EEG arousals. *Journal of Clinical Sleep Medicine, 10*, 803–809.

Food and Drug Administration. (2008). *Drug approved labeling: Ambien (zolpidem tartrate); NDA 19908 S027 FDA*. Silver Spring, MD: Author. Retrieved February 26, 2018, from https://www.accessdata.fda.gov/drugsatfda_docs/label/2008/019908s027lbl.pdf

Hammond, T., & Wilson, A. (2013). Polypharmacy and falls in the elderly: A literature review. *Nursing and Midwifery Studies, 2*, 171–175.

Iber, C., Ancoli-Isreal, S., Chesson, A. L., et al. (2007). *AASM manual for the scoring of sleep and associated events: Rules, terminology and technical specifications*. Westchester, IL: American Academy of Sleep Medicine.

Kolla, B. P., Lam, E., Olson, E., et al. (2013). Patient safety incidents during overnight polysomnography: A five-year observational cohort study. *Journal of Clinical Sleep Medicine, 9*, 1201–1205.

Kolla, B. P., Lovely, J. K., Mansukhani, M. P., et al. (2013). Zolpidem is independently associated with increased risk of inpatient falls. *Journal of Hospital Medicine, 8*, 1–6.

Kothare, S. V., Vendrame, M., Sant, J. L., et al. (2011). Fall-prevention policies in pediatric sleep laboratories. *Journal of Clinical Sleep Medicine, 7*, 9–10.

Leach, J. P., & O'Dwyer, R. (2011). *Epilepsy simplified*. Shrewsbury, UK: TFM Publishing, Ltd.

Mehra, R., & Strohl, K. P. (2004). Incidence of serious adverse events during nocturnal polysomnography. *Sleep, 27*, 1379–1383.

National Health Service. (2014). Bulletin 87. Care homes—Medication and falls. *PrescQIPP*. London, UK: Author. Retrieved February 26, 2018, from https://www.gov.im/media/1347552/care-homes-medication-and-falls-december-2014.pdf

Richardson, K., Bennett, K., & Kenny, R. A. (2015). Polypharmacy including falls risk-increasing medications and subsequent falls in community-dwelling middle-aged and older adults. *Age and Ageing, 44*, 90–96.

U.S. National Library of Medicine. (2018). Diabetic ketoacidosis. *Medline Plus*. Bethesda, MD: Author. Retrieved February 26, 2018, from https://medlineplus.gov/ency/article/000320.htm

chapter 36
Preparing the Patient for Polysomnography

EILEEN B. LEARY

LEARNING OBJECTIVES

On completion of this chapter, the reader should be able to:

1. Apply the standard electrodes and sensors used in polysomnography.
2. Perform measurements for electroencephalogram using the International 10/20 System of Electrode Placement.
3. Troubleshoot if a signal has poor quality.
4. Develop personal techniques for electrode and sensor application.

KEY TERMS

Biocalibration
Calibration
Diode
Electroencephalogram
Electromyogram
Electrooculogram
Impedance
Inion
Nasion
Piezo-sensor
Preauricular points
Respiratory inductance plethysmography
Thermistor
Thermocouple

The application of electrodes and sensors to the patient is one of the most important parts of a sleep study. If done poorly, the quality of the data will be compromised and a significant part of the night will be spent troubleshooting and problem-solving. Filters should not be used to compensate for poor-quality electrode application. Excessive use of filtration can significantly alter the integrity of the data and impact how the study is analyzed.

There are many different approaches to preparing a patient for a sleep study. This chapter will focus on the standard or classic method. In addition to the varied techniques utilized by different sleep centers, each sleep technologist will develop his or her own method of performing the application. Exchanging ideas with other technologists is an excellent way to continue to improve and refine one's technique.

BASIC SUPPLIES AND EQUIPMENT

To expedite the hookup process, it is helpful to have all your supplies close at hand while preparing the patient (Table 36-1). Applying electrodes takes dexterity and care, so being well organized is essential.

BEFORE THE PATIENT ARRIVES

It is critical to allow time at the beginning of the shift before the patient arrives to prepare for the night ahead. The technologist should use this time to review the practitioner's orders, set up and calibrate the recording equipment, prepare the necessary supplies, and assess and respond to any special needs the patient may have.

Undergoing a sleep study can be stressful for a patient. An informed and knowledgeable technologist helps reduce that anxiety and creates a positive patient experience. Become familiar with the patient's medical history by reviewing the chart before the patient arrives. Be sure to label any questionnaires or forms that require completion and check the physician's order to determine which type of study has been prescribed (positive airway pressure [PAP] titration, diagnostic study, split-night study, or extended channel montage). If an order is unclear, contact the sleep center manager, on-call physician, or the practitioner who made the order for clarification.

The hookup procedure will be faster and more efficient if the supplies are prepared and organized in advance. For example, you can precut the tape and gauze, lay out gold cup electrodes, check for broken or damaged sensors, and stock the supply tray before the patient arrives. Ensure all items that will come into contact with a patient have been cleaned and disinfected according to infection control standards before use.

Table 36-1 Basic Supplies

General supplies

- Nonlatex gloves
- Scissors
- Towels
- Various types of medical tape (Transpore, Hypafix, or Medipore, and Scanpor)
- Impedance meter

For applying scalp and face electrodes (to record EEG, EOG, and chin EMG)

- Air compressor (if using collodion)
- Tape measure
- Grease pencil
- Hair pins/clips
- Hair comb
- Electrodes (gold cup with center hole)
- Alcohol swabs
- Abrasive skin preparation (NuPrep or Lemon Prep)
- Cotton-tip applicators
- EEG conductive paste
- Electrolyte gel or cream
- Collodion/EC2 paste
- Collodion remover/acetone
- Gauze (4 × 4 squares and/or roll of single-ply gauze)
- Medical tape (Micropore, Transpore, and fabric tape)
- Double-sided electrode collars

For applying ECG electrodes (to record the ECG)

- Disposable ECG snap pads
- ECG electrodes

For applying leg EMG electrodes (to record leg movements)

- Gold cup electrodes with extra long leads (72 in [182.9 cm])
- Small ECG patches (optional)

For applying respiratory belts (to record respiratory effort)

- Thoracic/abdominal belts in various sizes
- Inductive plethysmography belts

For applying airflow sensor (to record respiratory airflow)

- Nasal cannula with pressure transducer and thermocouple, or thermistor

For applying snore sensor

- Snore sensor

For applying oximeter probe (to record SpO$_2$)

- Oximeter probe (disposable or reusable)
- Oximeter calibration tool (may have autocalibration)

ECG, electrocardiogram; EEG, electroencephalogram; EMG, electromyogram; EOG, electrooculogram.

APPLYING THE ELECTRODES AND SENSORS

Proper electrode and sensor placement is essential for recording a quality polysomnogram. Every technologist should be familiar with all electrodes and sensors, what they measure, where they are placed, and how they plug into the headbox (also called a jackbox). All electrodes and sensor leads should be easily identifiable to avoid confusion when connecting them to the headbox. Some technologists prefer to use labeled gold cup electrodes, whereas others plug each electrode into the headbox immediately after it is attached.

Suggested Routine for Electrode and Sensor Application

This chapter provides a suggested sequence for applying electrodes and sensors, but all technologists develop their own routine. Don't be afraid to experiment and develop a system that suits your individual style.

1. Scalp and face electrodes
2. Snore sensor
3. Electrocardiogram (ECG) electrodes
4. Leg electrodes
5. Respiratory bands
6. Airflow sensor(s)
7. Oximeter probe

The airflow sensor and oximeter probe are typically applied shortly before bedtime as these sensors are more cumbersome to the patient. However, for some patients, it may be helpful to have a longer assessment of the individual's waking oxygen levels. In those cases, the oximeter should be attached upon arrival to allow oxygen levels to be monitored throughout the hookup procedure.

General Suggestions to Optimize Electrode Application

- During the application procedure, the technologist should explain the procedure to the patient. This is an ideal time to provide education on sleep hygiene, obstructive sleep apnea, and/or whatever sleep topic seems appropriate for the patient.
- The patient's skin and hair should be clean and dry. Electrodes applied to oily skin or hair will likely have high impedance levels, resulting in poor signal quality, and are more susceptible to becoming detached during the night. Patients should be instructed by the daytime staff to shower or bathe before arriving. If necessary and if shower facilities are available, ask the patient to shower at the sleep center before beginning the hookup. If the patient has very dirty or oily hair and a shower is not

possible, use alcohol or acetone wipes to remove the excess oil. Alcohol dries quickly, so the site can be prepped and the electrode attached almost immediately.

- When using tape or gauze to adhere an electrode, scrub only the small area where the electrode will be placed. If excess prep material remains in the vicinity of the electrode, gently cleanse the area with rubbing alcohol because tape will not stick to the gritty prep.
- Facilitate tape removal in the morning by using small pieces of tape and making tabs by folding down one end. The tape should be just large enough to secure the sensor and wire throughout the study (Fig. 36-1).
- Point the wires toward the crown of the head or nape of the neck to make them more manageable. Consider where the headbox will be placed during the night when selecting how to bundle the wires.
- Provide extra slack in the wires to avoid putting stress on the electrodes.

Attaching Gold Cup Electrodes

Before starting the application process, all electroencephalogram (EEG) electrode sites should be measured and marked using the International 10/20 System (1) described later in the chapter. Scalp electrodes can be attached using paste or collodion. When deciding which method to use, signal quality, stability of sensor, convenience of application, and removal as well as cleanup should be considered. Collodion requires an air compressor to dry the glue, has a strong odor, is highly combustible, and requires storage in fireproof safe and a solvent to remove in the morning. Paste is removed with water, but electrodes may move slightly or loosen during the night, particularly if the patient sweats. Although collodion is more secure, most labs use paste because it is more convenient and less caustic.

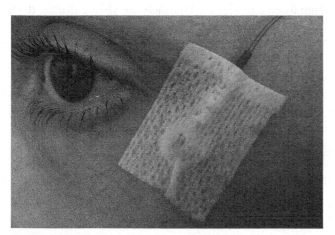

Figure 36-1 Suggested approach to tabbing tape. Note the small crease at the bottom center of the tape.

Preparing the Electrode Sites

Preparing the skin before attaching the electrode is essential for reducing impedance levels and ensuring signal quality. Be sure to discuss the procedure with the patient so that he or she is not surprised by the process. First, clean the area with an alcohol swab to remove any makeup or oil on the skin. Then, using a small cotton-tipped applicator, gently scrub the area where the sensor will be placed with an abrasive skin preparation, such as NuPrep or Lemon Prep, for 5 to 10 seconds, applying moderate pressure. The skin may redden slightly from the procedure.

To prevent signal contamination and possible bridging with other electrode sites, be sure to only scrub the area covered by the electrode cup. Likewise, avoid using excessive amounts of prep material because it has conductive properties and electrodes attached with tape will not stick to the prep. If there is excess prep material, the area can be cleaned again with rubbing alcohol. Be sure to wipe away from the electrode site to avoid transferring skin oils from the surrounding area.

Attaching Gold Cup Electrodes with Electrode Paste

Fill the electrode disk with conductive paste, so the surface is slightly rounded, making sure that there are no air pockets. Using the wooden side of the cotton-tipped applicator or a comb, part the hair in the same direction in which the lead wire will be positioned. Hair clips can be used to keep the site clear. Spread a small amount of electrode paste evenly on one side of a 3-cm square of gauze. Position the electrode in the center of the prepped site so the paste is against the skin. Cover the electrode with the gauze square, paste side down. Distribute the electrode paste around the head of the electrode, keeping it firmly in place until the paste begins to set. Check for a secure application by gently tugging on the electrode wire.

Attaching Gold Cup Electrodes with Collodion

When using collodion, the hookup process should be performed in a well-ventilated area as the glue is very pungent and flammable. If there is limited space available, an air filtration or exhaust system can be used to reduce the fumes. For safety purposes, collodion and acetone should always be handled carefully and stored in a fireproof safe. Collodion and acetone spills pose a safety risk; consequently, all sleep centers should have a protocol for handling and properly disposing of these materials.

A towel should be placed around the patient's shoulders to protect his or her clothing from the glue. Separate the hair using a comb or the wooden side of the cotton-tipped applicator so that the skin is visible. Hair clips can be used to help hold the hair in place and keep the electrode site in view. Once the site is prepped, position a clean gold-cupped electrode on the scalp and place a small square of single-ply gauze on top (~2 to 3 cm). Insert the air compressor stylus through the gauze into the hole at the top of the electrode to hold it in place against the scalp. Using a syringe or another disposable applicator, apply just enough glue to saturate the gauze. If the electrode is moved after the glue is applied, the collodion may seep between the scalp and the electrode, which will raise the impedance level and compromise signal quality. Smooth the gauze tightly over the scalp while the glue is dried with the air compressor, taking care not to adhere your gloves to the electrode. If long enough, the patient's hair can be used to help anchor the electrode to the scalp. Before removing the stylus, twist the end to break any seal that may have formed from the glue. The collodion bottle should be kept tightly closed when not in use to avoid spills and maintain the liquid nature of the glue. When collodion is exposed to air for an extended time, it becomes viscous and difficult to apply in moderation.

When all electrodes are glued in place, use a blunt-tipped needle syringe to fill the electrodes with electrolyte gel or cream. Be careful not to overfill the electrode cup, or the gel may leak out the side and break the collodion seal, causing electrode popping artifact during the recording.

Attaching Gold Cup Electrodes with Tape

Fill the electrode cup with conductive paste or electrolyte gel so it is slightly rounded, making sure there are no air pockets. To help ensure a solid connection with the skin, center a double-sided electrode collar over the cup and remove the paper backing. Place the electrode onto the prepped site, paste side down, with the wire pointed toward the crown of the head, and cover with a piece of tape. Press firmly around the rim of the cup to obtain a good seal. To facilitate removal in the morning, fold one end of the tape, creating a small tab; this makes it easier to pull the tape off at the end of the study (Fig. 36-1):

Managing the Electrode Leads

Organizing and securing the wires during the electrode application procedure will reduce the likelihood of electrodes being inadvertently pulled off during the night. After attaching the electrodes to the face and scalp, gather all the wires together into a ponytail at the crown of the head or nape of neck, making sure no wire is pulled taut. Bundle the wires together with pieces of tape or Velcro strips. If tape is used, both ends should be folded over for easy removal. The wires should be secured every 4 to 6 in (10.2 to 15.2 cm) to reduce tangling. The leads

from the other sensors can also be grouped separately and taped together to make the wires more manageable.

If using tape to bundle the electrodes becomes problematic because of the sticky tape residue, try using Coban tape. This tape sticks to itself, comes in many colors, and is disposable. Posey straps, or even the ends of old PAP headgears, can also be used, although they have a tendency to slide and the added weight may put extra strain on the sensors.

Experienced sleep technologists usually develop their own approach for arranging and managing the wires, which helps facilitate easy removal in the morning. A neatly organized application also makes it easier to troubleshoot recording problems and replace sensors when necessary.

EEG Scalp Electrodes

According to the standard practice, EEG electrodes are applied using the International 10/20 System of Electrode Placement (1). When applying the electrodes, there are three key elements that are vital to collecting quality data:

1. Electrodes must be placed in the correct location.
2. Electrode sites must be properly prepared.
3. Electrodes must be securely attached.

The current AASM Scoring Manual (2) recommends six EEG scalp electrodes for polysomnography (PSG): two frontal electrodes (F3 and F4), two central electrodes (C3 and C4), and two occipital electrodes (O1 and O2). In addition, two mastoid electrodes M1 and M2 are placed on the mastoid processes, the bony protrusion located behind each ear.

The primary recording derivations are F4-M1, C4-M1, and O2-M1. Backup electrodes should be placed in order to record the backup derivations F3-M2, C3-M2, and O1-M2 in the event an electrode signal becomes compromised during the study. Most sleep centers include both the recommended and the backup electrode derivations in a standard PSG recording montage to ensure all EEG channels are visible during data collection and allow for troubleshooting.

Determining the EEG Electrode Placements: The International 10/20 System

The International 10/20 System of Electrode Placement (1) is a standardized method for identifying equally spaced electrode positions on the scalp on the basis of four identifiable skull landmarks. This method was developed in 1958 to provide a consistent procedure for collecting EEG data and to develop common terminology. The system is termed 10/20 because the measurements are spaced either 10% or 20% of the distance between a given pair of skull landmarks. Percentages are used rather than absolute distances to allow for normal variations in head shape and size.

Each location is named with a letter indicating the corresponding lobe of the brain and a number or letter identifying the exact site. The locations on the left side of the head are odd numbered, the right side are even numbered, and the midline is represented by the letter 'z'. From front to back, the lobes are: pre-frontal (Fp), frontal (F), temporal (T), central (C), parietal (P) and occipital (O).

Before starting the measuring process, have the patient sit in a chair that is low enough to allow you to see the top of the head. Ensure that all reusable equipment (grease pencil, hair clips, measuring tape) has been cleaned and disinfected according to facility protocols for infection control. When using a paper measuring tape, be sure to fold the end down at the zero line to avoid computation errors.

Identifying the Landmarks

The four standard landmarks used in the 10/20 system are the nasion, inion, and left and right preauricular points (Fig. 36-2). If the landmarks are not correctly identified, electrode placement will not be accurate.

Each site should be marked to facilitate the measuring process keeping in mind that these sites are used as landmarks only and are not electrode positions.

Preauricular Points

The opening of the ear canal is protected by a small piece of cartilage called the "tragus." The preauricular points are the indentations just above this cartilage. If you are unsure of the location, place a finger on the patient's cheek, touching the tragus, and ask the patient to open and close his or her jaw. The indentation will become more pronounced with this movement.

Nasion

The nasion is the indentation between the forehead and the nose formed by the intersection of the frontal bone and two nasal bones of the skull. While facing the patient, find the small dip at the bridge of the nose between the eyes and lightly mark the point with a grease pencil.

Inion

The inion is the ridge or knob at the back of the head. When running your finger up the back of the neck to the skull, you should feel a depression with the ridge of the protruding inion just above it. This landmark may

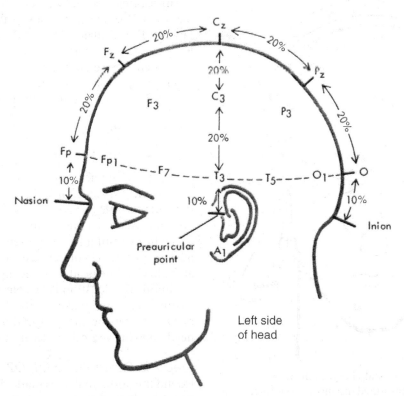

Figure 36-2 Identifying the landmarks. (From Harner, P. F., & Sannit, T. (1974). *A review of the International Ten–Twenty System of Electrode Placement.* Quincy, MA: Grass Instrument Co. Courtesy of Natus Medical Incorporated, Middleton, WI.)

be difficult to find on some individuals, so ask the patient to tilt his or her head all the way back, or forward, while you try to feel the ridge. If you are unable to locate the inion, mark it at the same level as the preauricular points. A common mistake is to use the underside of the protrusion instead of the tip, which will impact the accuracy of electrode placement.

Measuring the Scalp Electrode Sites

Each electrode site is determined by the intersection of two lines created by calculating distances, measured in centimeters, stemming from the four main landmarks (Fig. 36-3). Start the measuring process by marking each of these landmarks with the grease pencil.

Step 1 in Determining Cz

Many PSG software systems use Cz for the system reference electrode, which is not the same as the patient ground. Even if an electrode is not attached at Cz, it should be marked as a reference point for identifying other electrode sites.

While standing to one side of the patient, place the zero line of the measuring tape on the marked inion. Stretch the tape measure upward, over the crown of the

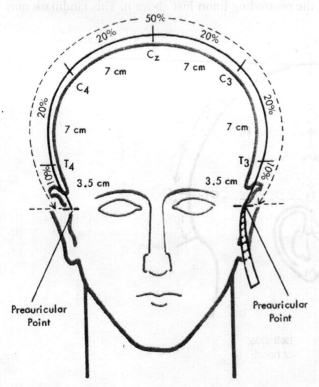

Figure 36-3 Measuring the scalp between the two preauricular points. The measured distances in centimeters are provided as an example; actual distances will vary depending on the size and shape of the scalp. (From Harner, P. F., & Sannit, T. (1974). *A review of the International Ten–Twenty System of Electrode Placement*. Quincy, MA: Grass Instrument Co. Courtesy of Natus Medical Incorporated, Middleton, WI.)

head, until it reaches the marked nasion. Determine the total distance between the inion and the nasion in centimeters. Using your grease pencil, mark the values for 10%, 50%, and 90% of that total distance. The marks at 10% and 90% will be used for identifying other electrode sites. Next, measure the distance between the marks made at 10% (will become Fpz) and 50% (will become Cz) and draw a line halfway between the two for Fz. Be sure to mark these sites with straight horizontal lines that are prominent enough to be easily located later.

Step 2 in Determining Cz

Standing behind the subject, reposition the zero end of the tape measure on one of the preauricular marks. Stretch the measuring tape over the top of the head through the 50% mark that was made during step 1, until it reaches the opposite preauricular mark. Determine the total distance from preauricular to preauricular point. Calculate 10%, 50%, and 90% of the total distance and mark each location. The point where the 50% mark intersects with the line drawn indicating 50% of the distance between nasion and inion is the site for Cz.

Step 1 in Determining C3 and C4

Standing to one side of the patient, place the zero line of the measuring tape on Cz and measure the distance to the mark made at 10% above one of the preauricular points (T3 or T4). Calculate 50% of this distance and mark the location. Repeat the process standing on the other side of the patient. These are the first set of marks necessary in determining C3 and C4. The second set of marks will be established after O1 and O2 have been identified.

Step 1 in Determining O1, O2, Fp1, and Fp2

Standing in front of the patient, draw a vertical line in the middle of the forehead (lining up with the bridge of the nose), intersecting the line drawn 10% up from the nasion. This location is Fpz. Standing to the side of the patient, place the zero end of the measuring tape at Fpz and wrap the tape around the entire circumference of the head, until it meets the zero end at Fpz. Calculate 50% of the head circumference and make a vertical mark at the back of the head, intersecting the 10% mark above the inion. This location is Oz. Next, calculate 5% of the circumference and make a vertical mark 5% to each side of Oz. Repeat the same procedure at the front of the head, drawing vertical marks 5% to each side of Fpz.

Step 2 in Determining O1, O2, Fp1, and Fp2

Extend the horizontal lines marked at Oz and Fpz during step 1 in determining Cz until they intersect with these new lines. At the back of the head, the points at which the lines intersect are O1 and O2, with O1 being on the patient's left side and O2 on the right. At the front of the head, the intersecting lines identify Fp1 and Fp2.

To double-check these locations, measure the distance between the two new vertical lines drawn on the back of the head. This distance should equal 10% of the total head circumference, with the original 50% line (Oz) in the center. Fp1 and Fp2 should be verified in the same manner on the forehead.

Step 1 in Determining F3 and F4

Place the zero line of the measuring tape on the newly marked Fp1 and stretch the tape to the line you made 10% up from the left preauricular point (T3) and mark 10% of the total head circumference to create F7, which will be used later to calculate F3. Repeat the process on the right side to identify F8. The total distance between F7 and F8, passing through Fpz, should be 30% of the total head circumference, and all measurements should be in the same plane.

Step 2 in Determining C3 and C4 and F3 and F4

Standing to the left of the patient, place the zero end of the measuring tape at O1 and extend the tape over the left side of the head to Fp1. Calculate 50% of the distance between O1 and Fp1 and make a vertical mark, intersecting the line drawn during step 1 in determining C3 and C4. The intersection of these two lines determines the location for C3.

Once C3 has been identified, measure the distance between Fp1 on the forehead and C3 and mark the halfway point. This will be the first line for F3.

Repeat the process standing on the right side of the patient, measuring the distance between O2 and Fp2 to determine the location for C4 (Fig. 36-4). Then mark 50% between Fp2 and C4 to identify the first mark for F4.

Step 3 in Determining F3 and F4

To complete the process of locating F3 and F4, measure the distance between F7 and F8, passing through the line marked earlier for Fz. Determine 50% of this distance to identify the second mark for Fz. Locate the final mark for F3 halfway between Fz and F7. Repeat the process to identify the second mark for F4 between Fz and F8.

Preparing the Electrode Site

The EEG electrode sites must be prepared using the procedure described earlier. Perform a visual check as the sites are prepped to ensure that the sites are correctly aligned. If the pattern does not match Figure 36-4, the measurements should be checked before attaching electrodes.

Attaching the Electrode

The EEG electrodes are generally attached using paste, although collodion or taping using double-sided electrode collars and paper tape may also be used.

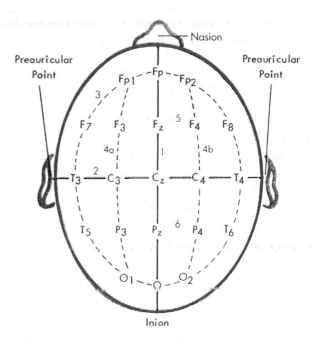

Figure 36-4 Overview of electrode locations. (From Harner, P. F., & Sannit, T. (1974). *A review of the International Ten–Twenty System of Electrode Placement*. Quincy, MA: Grass Instrument Co. Courtesy of Natus Medical Incorporated, Middleton, WI.)

Reference Electrodes

Determining the Reference Electrode Placement (M1 and M2)

The reference electrodes M1 and M2 are placed over the mastoid process (bone behind the earlobe). The electrodes should be placed on the skin between the crease of the earlobe and where the hairline begins. To reduce artifacts, the sensors should be placed over the flattest and boniest area. M1 is placed behind the left ear and M2 behind the right ear.

Preparing the Electrode Site

The reference electrode sites should be prepared using the same procedure described earlier for attaching gold cup electrodes.

Attaching the Electrode

The reference electrodes can be attached with tape if there is enough space between the ear and the hairline to secure the tape. Paste or collodion application can also be used.

Ground Electrode

Determining the Ground Electrode Placement

The ground electrode is typically placed in the middle of the forehead between the nasion and the start of the hairline at the site that was identified as Fpz during the measurement process. However, the exact location for the ground electrode is not critical. It is more important to ensure a good connection, so avoid areas with deep creases or wrinkles. A flat area just below the hairline also works well for this application.

Preparing the Electrode Site and Attaching the Electrode

The ground electrode site should be prepared using the procedure described earlier. The ground electrode may be attached with either conductive paste and tape or electrolyte gel, a double-sided electrode collar, and tape.

Electrooculogram Electrodes

Two electrodes, E1 and E2, are used to measure eye movements. Both electrooculogram (EOG) electrodes are referenced to the M2 electrode. In keeping with the International 10/20 System's naming convention, E1 is near the patient's left eye and E2 is near the right eye.

Determining EOG Electrode Placements (E1 and E2)

The standard placement for EOG electrodes (2) is designed to record both vertical and horizontal eye movements. To accomplish this, the left eye electrode (E1) is attached 1 cm below and 1 cm lateral to the left outer canthus (outside corner of the eye), whereas the right eye electrode (E2) is secured 1 cm above and 1 cm lateral to the outer canthus of the right eye. Use caution when prepping and placing these electrodes because the skin near the eye tends to be very thin and sensitive.

The AASM alternate placement is to position both electrodes 1 cm lateral and 1 cm below the outer canthus of each eye (2). When using the alternate derivation, both electrodes are referenced to Fpz.

Preparing the Electrode Sites and Attaching the Electrodes

The sites should be prepared using the procedure described earlier. Use caution with prepping and attaching electrodes close to the eye to prevent discomfort and skin irritation. The EOG electrodes are attached using paste and tape or a combination of double-sided electrode collars and tape. It is important to remember that the skin around the eye is very sensitive, particularly in elderly patients, so use tape sparingly. There are specialty tapes and skin barrier products commercially available to make removal of tape more comfortable for sensitive patients.

Chin Electromyogram Electrodes

The AASM recommends using three electrodes: two primary electrodes referenced to each other to create a bipolar signal and one backup electrode in the event

that one of the primary sensors fails. Obtaining an adequate signal can be challenging with obese subjects, so a third electrode can be particularly helpful in this population. The muscle tone information relayed through this channel is essential for determining rapid eye movement (REM) onset and bruxism. It can also help identify sleep onset and arousals. For an extended bruxism montage, two additional electrodes can be placed on the masseter muscles when clinically indicated. The masseter muscles are located just below the cheekbone and can be easily felt by having the patient grit his or her teeth.

Determining the Chin Electromyogram Electrode Placements

Three electrodes are placed for recording chin electromyogram (EMG) (2). The third chin EMG electrode is useful as a backup, in case one of the EMG electrodes becomes loose or detached during the night. The first electrode, ChinZ, is placed at the midline of the chin, 1 cm above the inferior edge of the mandible.

The other two electrodes, Chin1 (lower left lateral) and Chin2 (lower right lateral), are placed on the submentalis, which is the large muscle located below the chin. It is important to place the electrodes over the muscle. The submental electrodes are placed 2 cm below the inferior edge of the mandible and 2 cm to the right and left of the midline so they are 4 cm apart. As with any pair of electrodes, it is imperative that they are far enough apart to avoid electrode bridging; not even the tape should touch.

Preparing the Electrode Sites and Attaching the Electrodes

The sites should be prepared using the procedure described earlier. Chin EMG electrodes typically need extra security to guarantee they will stay in place through the night. Using a paste and tape or a double-sided electrode collar and gauze tape reduces the chance of these electrodes coming off during the study. For patients with facial hair, collodion or EC2 paste is recommended.

Electrocardiogram Electrodes

The ECG data collected during a polysomnogram is an abbreviated ECG generally using only one ECG channel instead of twelve. Therefore, the ECG is not typically used as a definitive test to diagnose subtle arrhythmias. However, signal quality must be sufficiently clear to allow recognition of significant arrhythmias, which should be reported to the clinician. Standard ECG electrodes should be used to record the ECG to minimize artifact and assure signal quality. Additional ECG leads can be ordered by the physician and added to the montage if clinically indicated.

Locating the ECG Sites

To record a modified lead II ECG using the recommended torso electrode placement (2), one ECG electrode is placed approximately 3 to 5 cm (two finger widths) below the right clavicle. The other ECG electrode is placed on the left lower ribcage. The electrodes should be aligned in parallel to the right shoulder and left hip.

An alternate (modified lead I) placement is sometimes used on very obese patients, whereby the second electrode is positioned below the left clavicle.

Preparing the Electrode Sites and Attaching the Electrodes

Standard ECG electrodes with snap leads should be used to record the ECG. The electrode sites should be cleaned with rubbing alcohol to remove skin oils. The area should be lightly scrubbed with a prep material to reduce impedance before the electrode is attached. For male patients, it may be necessary to shave the area before applying the electrodes. This will reduce artifact and make it easier to remove the sensors in the morning.

Snap the electrode to the lead wire before applying it to the patient's skin. Remove the backing from the electrode and place the gel side down. Feed the connector end of the wire up through the patient's bedclothes.

Be sensitive to the patient's modesty when attaching ECG electrodes; lift only as much of the garment as necessary. It is important to put your patients at ease and make them as comfortable as possible during the electrode application process. Communication is key; understanding what to expect will make patients feel more relaxed.

If the polarity of the ECG derivation is reversed, the ECG recording will be inverted, so be sure the leads are plugged into the headbox correctly to avoid confusion. Polarity can also be corrected using the PSG software to invert the signal.

Anterior Tibialis (Leg) EMG Electrodes

Movement activity from both legs should be monitored during a PSG on two separate channels. The recommended approach for collecting this data is to use surface electrodes. Gold cup electrodes are the most sensitive for recording EMG activity. Because the leg electrodes have the longest wires, they are more likely to have 50/60-Hz interference and can be difficult to manage. Taking time during the application to ensure that the electrodes and lead wires are securely in place and protected will improve the signal and reduce the likelihood that an electrode will be pulled off during the night. An extended EMG montage (2) can be used to monitor arm movements or another specific EMG activity if clinically indicated.

Locating the Electrode Sites

To monitor lower limb movements, two electrodes are attached to the anterior tibialis muscle that runs along the edge of the tibia (shin bone). The electrodes should be placed vertically along the muscle ridge 2 to 3 cm apart or one-third of the length of the anterior tibialis muscle, whichever is shorter.

It is essential to position the sensors on the muscle rather than the tibia bone. To ensure you have the correct placement, ask the patient to flex the foot back and forth to see the muscle move. Once you have correctly identified the location, mark the sites with a pencil. Figure 36-5 illustrates the correct electrode placement.

To monitor upper limb movements, two electrodes should be placed 2 cm apart on the anterior of the forearm along the flexor digitorum superficialis muscle and/or the extensor digitorum communis muscle that is located on the posterior of the forearm. To ensure correct placement on the flexor digitorum superficialis muscle, ask the patient to flex the hand at the base of the fingers (where fingers attach to the hand, not at the finger joints) to see the muscle move and mark the site. To identify extensor digitorum communis muscle electrode placement, ask the patient to extend the fingers back without moving the wrist and mark the site.

Preparing the Electrode Sites and Attaching the Electrodes

Standard prepping procedure should be used. In male patients, it may be necessary to shave the area where tape will be applied. This will improve impedance and reduce discomfort when the tape is removed after the study.

Each electrode is attached to the leg, arm, or other EMG recording site with paste and tape or double-sided electrode collars and about 2 in (5.1 cm) of tape to ensure that the sensor will remain in place throughout the night. A stress loop should be used after both electrodes are attached to reduce the likelihood of the electrodes

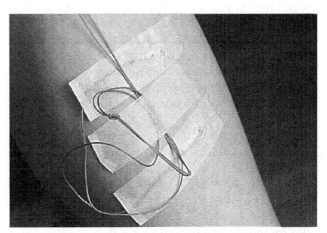

Figure 36-5 Stress loop used to avoid tension on leg electrodes.

being pulled off during the study (Fig. 36-5). Using a 2-in (5.1-cm) piece of tape, secure the loop between or above the two electrodes. With this method, if the wires are inadvertently tugged, the tape from the stress loop will be pulled off rather than the electrodes.

Managing the Electrode Leads

The limb EMG lead wires should be threaded up through the patient's night clothes to keep them from becoming tangled and unmanageable. Ask the patient to reach down from the waist and pull the sensors up through the pajamas. You can help by passing the ends up from the bottom of the bedclothes. Be sure that the leads are not pulled too tightly; there should be enough slack in the lines so the patient can stand up and move around comfortably. If the patient is wearing shorts or a nightgown, tape the wires to the thigh, again making sure to leave enough slack for movement. Use similar techniques to secure upper limb electrode lead wires.

Respiratory Effort Sensors

Accurately assessing ventilatory effort and the differentiation between abdominal and thoracic movement is critical for distinguishing between obstructive, central, and mixed breathing events. The 2018 AASM Scoring Manual Version 2.5 (2) specifies that either esophageal manometry or inductance plethysmography (calibrated or uncalibrated) may be used to classify abnormal breathing events.

Esophageal manometry is considered the gold standard because it is a calibrated signal that can measure subtle changes in breathing effort. However, it is an invasive measure and therefore is employed judiciously. Although esophageal pressure manometry is recommended for scoring respiratory effort–related arousals, nasal pressure and inductance plethysmography are acceptable alternatives.

Most sleep centers use respiratory inductance plethysmography (RIP) bands to meet the AASM criteria for monitoring respiratory effort. The bands are placed around the chest and abdomen and generate a respiratory effort signal on the basis of changes in body circumference associated with breathing. The RIP bands are embedded with wires, woven in a sinusoidal pattern, that encircle the body. An electrical current is applied to the wires, generating an oscillating signal in response to variations in resistance associated with changes in body circumference.

Dual thoracoabdominal polyvinylidene fluoride (PVDF) belts are an acceptable alternate method to detect breathing effort. PVDF belts produce an electrical signal when subjected to force, sound, acceleration, pressure, or heat and do not require an external battery. Piezo-sensor bands do not meet AASM recommendations for monitoring respiratory effort.

Selecting the Band Size

Selecting the correct RIP band or PVDF belt size will simplify the process of fitting the effort sensors and reduce the need to make adjustments during the night. Bands and belts are available in both pediatric and adult sizes and should be chosen according to the size of the subject. If the bands are too small, they will cause patient discomfort and the band will be stretched too tight, distorting the signal. If the bands are too long, they may be loose and difficult to adjust properly.

Determining the Position of the Bands

The bands are placed around the thorax and abdomen. The thoracic band is positioned just below the armpits. The abdominal band is secured around the waist, below the lower edge of the rib cage. For obese patients, find the location that will provide a snug fit and allow the bands to stay in place throughout the night. Have the subject stand and move around to ascertain whether the bands are likely to shift during the night.

Fitting the Bands

A buckle may be used to fasten the bands, or they may be self-adhering where the ends of the bands overlap. Fit the bands so they are snug, but not too tight or too loose, with the lead wires pointing upward toward the headbox. Bands may need to be taped in place to assure that they will stay in place for the entire night. Incorrect placement can cause poor signals and restrict the patient's comfort.

Snore Sensor

There are multiple AASM-approved devices to detect snoring, including an acoustic sensor, a piezoelectric sensor, and a nasal pressure transducer (cannula). The acoustic sensor is thought to detect snore events with lower volume and higher fundamental frequency than both the nasal pressure transducer and the piezoelectric sensor (3). However, the piezoelectric sensor is more commonly used and works by measuring vibration at the skin surface. The cannula measures snoring by pressure vibration in the nares.

Locating the Appropriate Site

To locate the ideal position, place two fingers on the anterior side of the patient's neck above the larynx and ask him or her to hum. The sensor should be secured over the area with the strongest vibration.

Preparing the Site and Attaching the Sensor

Clean the area with rubbing alcohol to remove any oil from the skin, because tape will adhere better to clean skin; no site preparation is required.

Attach the sensor using tape. The tape should be applied in such a way as to ensure a solid connection between the sensor and the skin, as well as to secure the wire. To be sure that the tape will not restrict movement, ask the patient to hold the head naturally, looking straight ahead while attaching the sensor. Avoid placing the sensor or tape along the slope of the jaw or on the jawbone.

Airflow Sensors

Airflow is monitored using an oronasal thermal sensor and nasal cannula pressure transducer. AASM standards require both types of sensors for scoring breathing events (2). The thermal sensor is used to identify apneas, and a thermistor, thermocouple, PVDF sum signal can be used. Many sleep centers use oronasal PVDF sensors in place of a thermal sensor; however, these are not currently AASM approved (2).

Thermistors generate their signal by changes in temperature. When a patient breathes out, the heat that is applied to the thermistor produces a signal. An oronasal thermocouple measures change in temperature and does not require a power source. The oronasal thermistor creates a signal by passing a constant current through the thermistor junction of two dissimilar metals and requires a voltage source. The PVDF sum signal is a derived flow signal from the PVDF belts. PVDF airflow sensors use a specially treated plastic film that is flexible and lightweight to generate a voltage when exposed to temperature changes, pressure changes, force changes, vibration, and sound; so it is responsive to changes in both air temperature and pressure and does not require an external voltage source.

The nasal air pressure transducer (with or without square root transformation of the signal) is used to identify hypopneas. It measures qualitative change in air pressure with inspiration and expiration but does not measure oral breathing. Although each system uses a different technology, the sensor placement at the nares and in front of the oral airway is similar.

Securing the Sensors

Thermal sensors are typically designed to monitor both nasal and oral airflow. A three-pronged sensor is placed under the patient's nose, with the two nasal prongs positioned directly in the flow of nasal air, whereas the third prong is situated in front of the mouth. Most oronasal sensors are secured by looping the wires around the ears and connecting them under the chin. Additionally, small pieces of tape can be used to fasten the wires to the cheeks to prevent the sensor from becoming dislodged. The tips of the sensors should not touch the lips, skin, or nasal membranes.

Pressure transducers use nasal cannula–type sensors that fit into the nares to record nasal pressure. These cannulas also loop around the patient's ears and can be taped to the cheeks if necessary. When both a pressure transducer and a thermal sensor are used, the thermal transducer is generally placed over the nasal cannula.

Oximeter Probe

The finger oximeter indirectly records pulse and blood oxygen levels using a small light that shines through the finger to a photodetector on the other side. The maximum acceptable signal averaging time for pulse oximetry during PSG is 3 seconds.

Determining the Appropriate Recording Site

If possible, the sensor should be placed on the index finger of the hand closest in proximity to the oximeter. If the index finger does not yield an accurate reading, the ring or pinkie finger can be used as an alternate placement. There are alternate sensors available for most pulse oximeters that can record from the bridge of the nose and pediatric sensors that can be used to record from the base of the foot in infants.

Preparing the Recording Site

The fingernail should be free of nail polish and cleaned with rubbing alcohol before the sensor is attached. Artificial fingernails may prevent the probe from accurately measuring the oxygen saturation. Ideally, nail polish and artificial nails should be removed before the study, but in reality, that is not always possible. If the patient has artificial fingernails, try applying the sensor to one of the patient's toes.

Applying a Disposable Oximeter Probe

To gauge accurate placement of a disposable probe and to ensure that the light-emitting diode (LED) aligns with the receptor diode, bend the probe in half before removing the tape so the two diodes line up and place it over the patient's finger. Once the correct fit is assured, peel off the paper backing, place the LED above the nail, fold the sensor over the top of the finger so that the receptor diode is positioned opposite the LED against the pad of the fingertip. Wrap the tape around the finger, making sure the two sides are vertically aligned and the diodes face each other directly. Then to secure the finger sensor, tape the sensor wire to the wrist.

Take care to assure that the probe is not taped too tightly around the finger. After securing the sensor, ask the patient if any discomfort is felt. If the finger throbs, loosen and reapply the sensor.

Applying a Reusable Oximeter Probe

Place a flexible fingertip sensor over the tip of the finger with the LED positioned above the nail and the receptor diode opposite the LED against the pad of the fingertip.

Secure the sensor with tape and tape the sensor wire to the wrist. After securing the sensor, check to be sure that the tape is not too tight. Ask the patient if any discomfort is felt. If there is throbbing, loosen the tape and re-apply the sensor.

A clip-type finger sensor fits over the tip of the finger. This type of sensor is typically placed on an index finger, but in some patients may be placed on another finger. Check for an acceptable signal and then tape the wire to secure it to the wrist.

Position Sensor

The AASM recommends a position sensor to monitor the patient's sleeping position (2). However, some sleep centers still require the technologist to document any changes in body position in technologist notes to ensure that accurate information is available to the physician reviewing the study. Most position sensors are attached to one of the respiratory effort bands and recognize five different patient positions (standing/sitting, supine, prone, left side, and right side).

SETTING UP AND CALIBRATING THE EQUIPMENT

Enter the patient information into the computer, select the correct montage, test the equipment, and document the performance of the equipment. Equipment calibrations are essential for accurate signal measurement and data interpretation, so a 30-second machine calibration must be performed and stored as part of the record before and after every sleep study. More detailed information about technical settings can be found in other chapters in this textbook.

The mechanism to perform the calibration process will vary depending on the type of equipment and software used. The industry standard is to apply a negative 50-μV DC voltage to all channels to evaluate individual channel signal responses. This will document the correct signal polarity, amplitude, and time constant for each channel. During the calibration, the following features should be assessed:

- Correct signal polarity (confirm that there is an upward deflection in response to the negative voltage)
- Appropriate sensitivity settings for each channel (gauge the amplitude or height of the calibration wave in relation to the applied voltage)
- Correct filter settings for each channel (inspect the time constant or duration of the calibration wave)

If one of the channels does not give the expected response to the 50-μV DC voltage input, check the filter settings to be sure they are correct. For all channels, sensitivity (also called gain) should be adjusted

at the beginning of the recording. Although in digital PSG changes made during the acquisition process are not permanent alterations to the incoming signal, the technologist should avoid unnecessary changes unless an adjustment is required to preserve the quality of the signals. Any changes to settings should be documented in the technologist notes.

CHECKING ELECTRODE IMPEDANCES AND SIGNAL QUALITY

After the machine calibrations are completed, the impedance levels of each electrode, including the ground and reference electrodes, must be checked. The impedance readings should be stored as part of the recording to document the quality and accuracy of the recorded signals. This is followed by a series of patient calibrations, also called "biocalibrations." AASM standards require repeat impedance checks and biocalibrations in the morning to document that signals did not deteriorate during the night (2).

Low-individual impedance levels ensure accurate signal transmission from each electrode and minimize the possibility of external signal interference by providing a clean pathway for the signal. High impedances defeat the passage of signals between the subject and the electrode, resulting in a poor signal. Most PSG recording systems use an internal impedance meter, although older software packages may still require the use of an external meter.

It is critical to understand the system you are using because some of the internal meters do not read individual impedance levels; instead, they measure the imbalance between selected pairs of electrodes. Therefore, to achieve accurate impedance readings, it is necessary to identify problematic electrodes or use an external meter such as a handheld AC impedance meter to check electrode impedances.

Ideally, the *individual* impedance level of all electrodes on the face and scalp should not exceed 5 kΩ. The impedance *differences* between paired EEG electrodes are also critical for preventing undesirable artifacts. Maintaining low-individual impedance readings (below 5 kΩ) assures that the difference in impedance levels between paired electrodes will be minimal. On some systems, the ground electrode connection may yield an artificially elevated reading because of the safety circuit breaker in the headbox, sometimes reporting as much as 5 kΩ more than the true impedance. Move this electrode to another position in the headbox or use a handheld meter to evaluate the true impedance level.

It is not always possible to obtain ideal impedance readings, particularly for the leg EMG channels. If the electrode impedance at a particular site remains high despite troubleshooting, the efforts to resolve the problem should be documented in the technologist notes.

TROUBLESHOOTING TECHNIQUES

Troubleshooting equipment issues begins with the basics; always start by checking that the system is plugged in properly, turned on, and that all cables and wires are securely connected.

- If an electrode has a high impedance level (>5 kΩ), it should be removed and the site reprepped before the electrode is reattached. Care should be taken not to overscrub an area, because patient discomfort, bruising, or, in extreme situations, skin injury can result from too much scrubbing.
- If electrical noise is seen in all channels, check the patient ground and/or system reference connection.
- If the impedance reading is still high after reprepping and reattaching an electrode, there are two possible problems. The lead wire or electrode may be damaged or the area of skin has unusually high impedance. A faulty electrode should be removed and replaced. If necessary, the electrode may be reattached immediately adjacent to the previous site.

BIOCALIBRATIONS

Biocalibrations are a series of exercises performed before initiating a study to verify correct input derivations, signal quality, and accurate signal response. It is essential to record the AASM-recommended biocalibrations at the beginning and end of each study to facilitate scoring and interpretation of the study (2). Additional calibrations must be performed if additional signals, such as upper limb EMG, are recorded. During biocalibrations, be sure to allow enough time between each set of instructions to make the corresponding signal response distinct and easily identifiable. Record each step of the process in the technologist notes.

If a signal does not respond in the expected fashion, always repeat the instruction and watch the video monitor to ensure that the patient correctly carried out the procedure. It may be helpful to explain the exercise in a different way or go into the bedroom to demonstrate the action. See Table 36-2 for an example set of biocalibrations.

ECG Channel

Take a moment to verify that the polarity of the ECG signal is correct. If it is reversed, the ECG leads should be switched in the headbox. If changing the leads in the headbox is not possible or does not correct the problem, the ECG signal can be inverted using the PSG software and the alteration should be documented.

EEG Channels

Ask the patient to relax with his or her eyes open for at least 30 seconds and then with the eyes closed for 30 seconds. Alpha waves are typically prominent and should be seen in the occipital channels when the eyes are closed.

If no alpha waves are present and the patient definitely has his or her eyes closed, check the electrode placement of O1 and O2 to be sure that the electrodes are in the correct location. If the measurements are confirmed, it is possible that the individual is not an alpha producer, which should be documented in the technologist's notes along with all troubleshooting efforts.

EOG Channels

Instruct the patient to keep the head still and move just the eyes left and right several times. Then instruct him or her to look up and down several times. Next, ask the patient to blink the eyes slowly and distinctly five times. The tracings should show prominent deflections in the EOG channels, with a significant difference between the three types of movements.

If no movement is detected on the EOG channels, it may be necessary to demonstrate the exercise to the patient to confirm whether he or she understood the instructions. If the patient is following the instructions correctly but the waveforms are still not responding, the derivations and filter settings should be confirmed. Finally, the placement of the two eye electrodes (E1 and E2) should be verified.

Chin EMG Channel

Ask the patient to grit the teeth or chew for 5 seconds. The EMG tracing should show a burst of activity when the teeth are clenched or the patient is chewing. Next, instruct the patient to relax, to be sure the EMG tracing shows an adequate level of baseline muscle tone (at least 0.5 cm in amplitude).

If the chin EMG does not pick up the muscle activity and you are sure the patient is gritting their teeth, confirm whether the derivation and filter settings are correct and whether the EMG electrodes are correctly placed. Try rereferencing the EMG channel to the backup electrode in an effort to improve the signal and identify which electrode is the source of the problem.

Snore Channel

Ask the patient to simulate a snore or hum for 5 seconds. The snore channel tracing should show a high degree of deflection during this maneuver. If the snore channel does not show a response, the filter settings should be checked and, if necessary, the sensor should

Table 36-2 Example Set of Biocalibrations

Instruction	Channel	Expected Response	Possible Fixes
None	ECG	Correct signal polarity, R wave should deflect upward.	Change headbox or invert signal.
None	EEG, EOG, EMG	Impedances within acceptable range	Check electrode, reattach if necessary.
Eyes open (30 s)	EEG	Mixed-frequency EEG	Check electrode placements.
Eyes closed (30 s)	EEG	EEG should change from mixed frequency to alpha rhythm.	Check electrode placements.
Look left and right (5 times each direction)	EOG	Distinct, opposite deflections that are somewhat blunt or squared. Looking left should bring the signals together; looking right should take the signals apart.	Check derivations, filter settings, and electrode placements.
Look up and down (5 times each direction)	EOG	Distinct, opposite deflections that come together in a peak. Looking down should bring the signals together; looking up should take the signals apart.	Check derivations, filter settings, and electrode placements.
Blink (5 times)	EOG	Distinct, opposite deflections going first apart and then coming together before returning to baseline	Check derivations, filter settings, and electrode placements.
Grit teeth or chew (5 s)	Chin EMG	Bursts of activity on chin EMG channel	Check derivations, filter settings, and electrode placements or try rereferencing to backup electrode.
Simulate a snore or hum (5 s)	Snore	Bursts of activity on snore channel, which may bleed over to the chin EMG	Check filter settings and position of sensor or replace sensor.
Breathe normally (10 s)	Respiratory	Clean sine wave, without spikes or electrical noise with all respiratory channels in phase (move together). Check polarity and note IN vs. OUT.	Adjust sensitivity or gain levels or invert signal if appropriate.
Hold breath (10 s)	Respiratory	Simulates a central apnea. Respiratory effort and flow channels should be flat.	Reposition or replace bands or flow sensors.
Breathe through nose only (10 s)		Clean sine wave, without spikes or electrical noise on nasal cannula.	Reposition or replace bands or flow sensors.
Breathe through mouth only (10 s)		Clean sine wave, without spikes or electrical noise on oral thermal sensor.	Reposition or replace bands or flow sensors.
Transfer breath	Respiratory	Simulates paradoxical breathing. Respiratory effort deflections should be out of phase (opposite movements) and flow channels should be flat.	Reposition or replace bands or flow sensors.
Flex right foot (5 times)	Leg EMG	Bursts of activity on right leg EMG channel	Check electrode placements.
Flex left foot (5 times)	Leg EMG	Bursts of activity on left leg EMG channel	Check electrode placements.

This table includes an example of instructions to give the patient at both the beginning and the end of the study, which electrode should be impacted, how the recording should change during the task, and suggested corrections. If a signal does not show the anticipated response, always confirm if the patient correctly performed the exercise before making any adjustments.
ECG, electrocardiogram; EEG, electroencephalogram; EMG, electromyogram; EOG, electrooculogram.

be repositioned. If moving the sensor does not rectify the problem, replace the sensor.

Respiratory Channels

With normal breathing, the airflow and respiratory effort channels should show a clean sine wave, without spikes or electrical noise. All channels should be in phase. The sensitivity or gain levels of the respiratory channels should be adjusted to obtain adequate deflections and to avoid signal blocking.

During the night, as the subject moves or changes body positions, the respiratory bands may shift and cause changes in signal amplitude, requiring channel sensitivity adjustments. If the bands become too loose, or the airflow sensor becomes displaced, manual readjustment of the sensors may be necessary to maintain a quality signal. Any changes to the bands or to the settings made after lights out should be well documented in the technologist notes.

To test the signals, instruct the patient to lie still and breathe normally for 15 to 20 seconds and then hold his or her breath for 10 seconds. During the breath hold, the respiratory channels should show a flat line. Next, ask the patient to breathe through the nose for only 10 seconds and then through the mouth again for only 10 seconds. To simulate paradoxical breathing effort, you may ask the patient to make breathing efforts during a breath hold. This instruction can be relayed as trying to sip a very thick milkshake through a clogged straw. This should result in out-of-phase (opposite) deflections in the respiratory effort channels while the airflow channels remain flat.

Leg EMG

Ask the patient to flex or extend the big toe of each foot several times to see a burst of activity in the recording. Each leg should be tested separately. If there is no change in recorded muscle activity, it may be necessary to demonstrate the exercise to the patient to confirm if he or she understood the instructions. If the patient is correctly performing the task and there is still no change in signal, the derivation and filter settings should be checked. If the problem persists, verify that the leg EMG electrodes are in the proper position over the anterior tibialis muscle. If upper limb EMG is recorded, the appropriate maneuvers to verify correct operation of these sensors must also be completed.

CONCLUDING A PSG STUDY

Overnight polysomnograms are typically run for at least 6 hours to ensure sufficient data are collected to adequately assess the patient's sleep. PAP titrations should continue for at least 3 hours after initiating treatment in order to allow adequate time for the patient to progress through all the sleep stages and body positions at the optimal PAP level.

Because of the higher percentage of REM sleep in the last third of the night, it is not unusual for a patient to be in REM when it is time to end the study. If time permits, allow patients to complete the REM period before calling lights on and waking the patient up.

After the patient is awake but before being disconnected, check and document impedance levels, and repeat biocalibrations and machine calibrations before stopping the recording. If a polysomnogram is terminated early at the specific request of the patient, the technologist may need to complete an against medical advice form and the technologist must document the circumstances.

Procedure for Waking a Patient

1. Enter "lights on" in the technologist notes and record the time in the study log.
2. Enter the patient's room and explain that the test is over and that calibrations will be performed. If conducting a PAP study, remove the mask and turn off the PAP machine.
3. Repeat the impedance check and biocalibrations performed at the beginning of the night. Note any equipment that is malfunctioning in the technical summary.
4. End the acquisition according to system software instructions.
5. Ask if the patient needs to use the bathroom. When the patient is comfortable, remove all the electrodes and sensors from the patient.
   a. Remove electrode paste from the scalp and face with warm water.
   b. Remove electrodes attached with collodion using acetone or collodion remover, taking care to avoid the patient's eyes. A syringe with collodion remover or small cotton balls or pieces of gauze is best used for this procedure. Carefully soak each electrode site until the electrode loosens and then wipe away any excess collodion residue. Ask the patient to tilt the head backward, to prevent any acetone or remover from dripping toward the face.
   c. Loosen tape by moistening with water, alcohol, or adhesive remover as needed for patient comfort.

Documentation

Documentation protocols vary by sleep center; however, the key information to be relayed is usually fairly standard. It is standard in most sleep centers to include the following information in the technical summary report at the end of a shift:

- "Lights off" and "lights on" times
- Patient's overall sleep quality
- Degree of snoring, if any
- Positions in which the patient slept, positional effects on respiratory events, oxygen saturation levels, and sleep quality
- Presence, frequency, and severity of respiratory disturbances
- Presence, frequency, and severity of ECG abnormalities
- Presence, frequency, and severity of periodic limb movements
- Lowest oxygen saturation recorded
- Any cardiac, respiratory, seizure, or other medical conditions that may require follow-up or medical attention
- Any other pertinent patient observations (unusual sleep patterns or unusual behaviors)
- Optimal PAP setting(s), if used
- Equipment problems or persistent recording artifacts, if any

Before signing off on a patient chart, confirm whether all the necessary patient and technologist paperwork has been completed and then place all patient records in locked storage, following standard procedures of the Health Insurance Portability and Accountability Act. In case of medical conditions that require immediate attention, contact the attending or on-call physician before allowing the patient to leave the sleep center.

Discharging the Patient

Be sure to allow adequate time in the morning for the patient to complete any morning paperwork required by the sleep center protocol and get ready for the patient's day. It may be helpful to ask the patient the night before how long he or she will need to shower and get dressed once disconnected from the electrodes. After a long, overnight shift it may be tempting to rush the patient out in the morning, but customer service is an important part of the job. Taking a few extra minutes to attend to the patient's needs will significantly improve his or her experience. After the patient has been

discharged from the sleep center or while he or she is getting ready to leave, clean all the equipment and the work area.

SUGGESTED READINGS

A review of the international ten–twenty system of electrode placement. (1974). Quincy, MA: Grass Instrument.

American Association of Sleep Technologists. (2012). *Standard polysomnography: Technical guideline*. Retrieved January 13, 2018, from https://www .aastweb.org/hubfs/Technical%20Guidelines/ StandardPSG.pdf?t=1510785704439

Harner, P. F., & Sannit, T. (1974). *A review of the International Ten–Twenty System of Electrode Placement*. Quincy, MA: Grass Instrument.

Kapur, V. K., Auckley, D. H., Chowdhuri, S., et al. (2017). Clinical practice guideline for diagnostic testing for adult obstructive sleep apnea: An American Academy of Sleep Medicine clinical practice guideline. *Journal of Clinical Sleep Medicine, 13*(3), 479–504.

Kushida, C. A., Littner, M. R., Morgenthaler, T., et al. (2005). Practice parameters for the indications for polysomnography and related procedures: An update for 2005. *Sleep, 28*, 499–521.

REFERENCES

1. Harner, P. F., & Sannit, T. (1974). *A review of the International Ten–Twenty System of Electrode Placement*. Quincy, MA: Grass Instrument.
2. Berry, R. B., Albertario, C. L., Harding, S. M., et al.; for the American Academy of Sleep Medicine. (2018). *The AASM manual for the scoring of sleep and associated events: Rules, terminology and technical specifications* [Version 2.5]. Darien, IL: American Academy of Sleep Medicine.
3. Arnardottir, E. S., Isleifsson, B., Agustsson, J. S., et al. (2016). How to measure snoring? A comparison of the microphone, cannula and piezoelectric sensor. *Journal of Sleep Research, 25*(2), 158–168.

chapter 37
Polysomnographic Recording Procedures

EILEEN B. LEARY

LEARNING OBJECTIVES

On completion of this chapter, the reader should be able to:

1. Identify the key prerequisites for obtaining quality artifact-free data.
2. Describe appropriate patient monitoring and documentation procedures.
3. Recognize clinical and technical issues that require a technologist response.
4. Recognize common causes of recording artifacts.
5. Identify and correct common artifacts in various recording parameters.
6. Utilize the principles of system referencing, rereferencing techniques, and other strategies to maintain recording quality.
7. Describe the processes related to ending the study and discharging the patient.

KEY TERMS

50/60-Hz artifact
Artifacts
Montage
Signal derivations
System referencing
Rereferencing

The basic concepts of obtaining high-quality, artifact-free recordings have not changed despite considerable technologic advancements over the years that have impacted how we collect, process, and view polysomnographic (PSG) data. The three major factors include the following:

- Proper electrode and sensor application
- Accurate signal processing
- Conscientious maintenance of the recording

This chapter touches on the patient element, but really focuses on how to utilize the available tools offered by today's digital sleep recording systems to obtain a high-quality, artifact-free sleep study.

ELECTRODE APPLICATION

The first step toward obtaining an artifact-free polysomnogram is the proper application and correct placement of the electrodes and sensors. Although all data collection systems have mechanisms to filter data, they are meant to fine-tune the signal being collected, not disguise or repair a nonexistent or bad signal related to poor electrode application. Poor electrode application cannot be fixed through aggressive filtration and signal manipulation because excessive signal filtering will obscure or alter the data.

Careful attention should be paid to each of the following steps during the hookup process to attain a quality recording:

- Precise head measurements for the electroencephalogram (EEG) electrodes
- Careful site preparation, scrubbing an area no larger than the size of the electrode cup
- Utilization of high-quality electrodes (typically, gold cup electrodes)
- Secure adhesion of the electrodes to the skin
- Low and relatively equal electrode impedances (<5 kΩ as measured by an AC impedance meter)
- Proper management of the electrode wires

For a more detailed explanation of electrode application techniques, see Chapter 36, *Preparing the Patient for Polysomnography*.

SIGNAL PROCESSING

Once the electrodes and sensors are in place, the resulting signal must be processed in a standardized manner to ensure consistent output across individuals as well as sleep centers. Signal processing includes amplification of the signal, filtration, analog-to-digital conversion, and signal display.

Basic considerations for proper signal processing include the following:

- The use of high-quality amplifiers
- Sturdy electrical connections
- Adequate electrical shielding
- Proper electrical grounding of equipment
- Appropriate filter settings for each recorded parameter

- Adequate sampling rates for each recorded parameter
- Correct signal polarity
- Adequate computer screen resolution (digital screen and video card must be at least 1,600 × 1,200)
- Documentation of all signal manipulations

The American Academy of Sleep Medicine (AASM) updates their guidelines (1) regularly. Every technologist is responsible for reviewing the current standards, including requirements for digital PSG recording, because they represent the essential requirements for performing and scoring polysomnograms.

Today, it is recommended that a digital PSG system include the following features:

- A mechanism to perform visual (on-screen) electrical calibrations for all channels by applying a negative 50 μV DC voltage to document correct signal polarity, amplitude, and time constant
- A separate 50/60-Hz notch filter for every channel
- The ability to program sampling rates for each channel
- The capacity to measure individual impedance levels for each electrode against a common reference (may be the sum of all other applied electrodes)
- The capability to retain and display all settings used by the attending technologist, including adjustments to derivations, sensitivity, filters, and temporal resolution
- A filter design that mimics conventional, analog-style frequency response curves

The AASM also suggests as an optional feature that all systems have the flexibility to choose and/or change the electrode input signal derivations without relying on a common reference electrode.

SELECTING THE APPROPRIATE MONTAGE

Today, virtually all digital sleep systems allow you to select which channels to monitor during a study by allowing customizable settings for the electrode derivation, sensitivity, filter settings, label, color, and analysis properties for each channel. The arrangement of the recording channel selections and their settings is called a montage. Multiple montages can be developed and saved for use on multiple patients. An example of a sleep apnea diagnostic montage using the AASM-recommended specifications is shown in Table 37-1 (1, 2). The technologist must ensure that the correct montage is chosen during the setup process because the montage cannot be changed once the recording is initiated.

Examples of common montages include the following:
- Sleep apnea diagnostic evaluation
- Positive airway pressure (PAP) titration

- Seizure
- Multiple sleep latency test/maintenance of wakefulness test
- Specialty equipment (transcutaneous CO_2, end-tidal CO_2)

Before choosing a montage, carefully review the physician's order to be sure you select the montage that will record the appropriate physiologic data. A quality hookup is a wasted effort if the appropriate information is not recorded and the study has to be repeated.

INITIATING THE RECORDING

It is time to initiate the recording when the montage has been selected, patient demographics have been entered in the system, and the patient is properly hooked up. Once the study is recording, system calibrations are performed for at least 30 seconds to document that the equipment is functioning properly and the correct filter settings and sampling rates have been selected.

The next step is to test the impedance levels of each electrode to confirm a secure attachment. Most sleep systems have an impedance meter built into the software, but an external AC impedance meter can be used if necessary. Ideally, all electrodes should have relatively equal and low (<5 kΩ) impedance readings. If any channel reports a high level of interference, the electrode should be reapplied or replaced before starting the recording.

After verifying that each electrode is providing an optimal signal, perform biocalibrations to assess whether the sensors are in the correct location and recording appropriate physiologic information. The patient should be walked through a series of exercises designed to provide a baseline signal for each channel. It is important to document each of these instructions in the technologist notes and allow several seconds between each exercise to allow time for the signals to return to baseline.

Once all these items have been completed, the patient is ready for bed. Turn the lights off in the bedroom and document the "lights out" information in the technologist's notes. It is common to record details such as the bedtime, body position, and oxygen saturation at the beginning of a study.

MONITORING THE PATIENT AND DOCUMENTING DURING THE RECORDING

Once the patient is in bed for the night, the pace of the night usually changes significantly, but that does not mean the work is done. Every patient must be carefully monitored over the course of the night to ensure the patient is safe, the necessary information is collected, and there are no disruptions to data collection.

Table 37-1 Example of a Sleep Apnea Diagnostic Montage Using the AASM-Recommended Technical Specifications[a]

Channel	Derivation	Type	Sampling Rates		LFF (Hz)	HFF (Hz)
			Minimal (Hz)	Desirable (Hz)		
1	F3-M2	EEG	200	500	0.3	35
2	F4-M1	EEG	200	500	0.3	35
3	C3-M2	EEG	200	500	0.3	35
4	C4-M1	EEG	200	500	0.3	35
5	O1-M2	EEG	200	500	0.3	35
6	O2-M	EEG	200	500	0.3	35
7	E1-M2 (LOC)	EOG	200	500	0.3	35
8	E2-M2 (ROC)	EOG	200	500	0.3	35
9	EMG-chin	EMG	200	500	10	100
10	ECG	ECG	200	500	0.3	70
11	Snore	Snore	200	500	10	100
12	Nasal	Nasal pressure	25	100	≤0.03	100
13	Oronasal	Airflow	25	100	0.1	15
14	Chest (thoracic)	Respiration	25	100	0.1	15
15	Abdominal	Respiration	25	100	0.1	15
16	Limb	EMG	500	200	10	100
17	SaO$_2$	Oximetry	10	25	N/A	N/A
18	Position	Body position	1	1	N/A	N/A

[a]Channel selections and settings may vary based on sleep center policy and the sleep acquisition system utilized (1).
ECG, electrocardiogram; EEG, electroencephalogram; EMG, electromyogram; EOG, electrooculogram; HFF, high-frequency filter; LFF, low-frequency filter; LOC, left outer canthus; ROC, right outer canthus.

Q30 Documentation

One element of cohesive data collection is the detailed and professional documentation, throughout the night. Some sleep centers require Q30 documentation, which is a structured technologist note entered every 30 minutes. It is possible to program some of the digital systems to prompt for a technologist note at preselected intervals with a pop-up dialog box. The content of these notes varies depending on sleep center policy. Standard comments include information such as body position, PAP setting (if appropriate), heart rate, SaO$_2$, CO$_2$ levels (if available), and any other relevant patient updates like sleep stage, snoring, or unresolved artifact. Keep in mind that the technologist notes are part of the official medical record, so they should contain facts rather than opinions or speculations about a diagnosis.

Waveform Recognition

A sleep technologist must be able to read and interpret the data being collected to effectively run a sleep study. A basic knowledge of sleep stages is necessary to differentiate wake from sleep and assess the quality of sleep throughout the night. However, monitoring a patient is more than just identifying sleep spindles or rapid eye movements. A sleep technologist must also be able to understand how the various channels of data impact one another to truly understand whether the data being viewed are a true physiologic event or artifact requiring correction.

Sleep apnea in particular is a complex phenomenon that impacts multiple biologic systems. Abnormal breathing events not only impact respiration and oxygen saturation but also affect cardiac function, muscle tone, and, of course, sleep consolidation. Therefore, the data should be interpreted as a whole in addition to assessing each channel independently.

Assessment of Sleep Disorders

The most common reason patients undergo overnight PSG is for evaluation of sleep-related breathing disorders (SRBDs), which is an umbrella term for disorders related to abnormal breathing during sleep where breathing is repeatedly interrupted. There are several different types of sleep-disordered breathing including obstructive sleep apnea (OSA), central sleep apnea (CSA), mixed sleep apnea (MSA), and upper airway resistance syndrome. During sleep, apneas can be caused by a physical obstruction, such as is seen in OSA, the most common type of SRBD. Breathing pauses can also be caused by a disruption of the central nervous system, as is seen in CSA. Each disorder has a spectrum of severity levels ranging from mild to severe.

Each type of sleep apnea has a different approach to treatment; therefore, it is imperative that every sleep technologist understands the differences between the disorders and be able to correctly identify which type of event is being witnessed. The technologist must also be able to differentiate between different obstructive events (respiratory effort–related arousal [RERA], hypopnea, and apnea).

Although sleep apnea is the most prevalent disorder seen in the sleep center, other disorders should not be overlooked. Understanding the physiologic data that are seen during the recording is key to obtaining relevant data. Most sleep centers have a copy of the *International Classification of Sleep Disorders*, third edition (*ICSD-3*), which can be consulted when necessary.

RESPONDING TO PATIENT NEEDS

For many patients, a night in the sleep center is uneventful. However, the technologist must be vigilant throughout the night to ensure the patient is safe and comfortable at all times.

Responding to Physiologic Data

There are a number of factors that require the technologist to intervene during a sleep study ranging from a medical emergency to a restroom break. The technologist must be alert and attentive to identify a potential issue, assess the situation, and, if appropriate, take action.

Signal Issues

There are numerous opportunities for signal failure during a sleep study. The key is to identify a compromised signal as soon as possible and take the appropriate corrective action based on the situation.

Medical Emergencies

Medical emergencies are fairly uncommon; however, the unexpected can occur at any time, so it is imperative that every sleep technologist is certified in cardiopulmonary resuscitation and basic life support, is able to use an automated external defibrillator, and is familiar with the sleep center's emergency protocol.

Cardiac issues are the most likely to be encountered in patients with sleep-disordered breathing, so a base knowledge of cardiac arrhythmias is essential to distinguish life-threatening issues such as ventricular tachycardia from benign irregularities.

Medication Needs

Today, many sleep centers are not located in a hospital, so there is no convenient way to distribute medications. Therefore, patients are typically instructed by the daytime staff to bring with them any medications they need to take while at the sleep center on the night of the sleep study. Even if the sleep center is situated in a hospital with access to medications, most sleep centers avoid dispensing medications because sleep technologists are not generally authorized to administer medications. In most sleep centers, the patient will bring and self-administer the medication. If a patient arrives for the sleep study without the necessary medications, the on-call physician or medical director should be contacted.

Treatment Interventions

When a split-night study is indicated, it is imperative to clearly understand when the study should transition from diagnostic to PAP titration. Criteria for starting PAP are typically based on Medicare guidelines, although the exact policy may vary from one sleep center to another. The key is to obtain sufficient diagnostic data to document the presence of sleep apnea to both the clinician and the insurance company while leaving enough time to identify a therapeutic PAP.

Early Termination of the Study

On occasion, a patient may ask to end the study early and leave the sleep center in the middle of the night. In this situation, the technologist should make a reasonable effort to convince the patient to stay and complete the study. However, if the patient insists on leaving, the technologist should document the situation and terminate the study. Early termination may result in patient safety and possible billing issues. Depending on the sleep center protocol, it may be necessary to have the patient complete an against medical advice form.

MAINTAINING THE RECORDING

A quality sleep recording requires vigilance to ensure the data recorded at the end of a study is just as accurate as the data collected at the beginning. Patients, especially children, often move, perspire, change body position, and pull at the electrode wires in their sleep. The sleep technologist is responsible for monitoring the data as it is recorded and making appropriate adjustments and corrections to the signals or replacing electrodes that have been inadvertently dislodged during the study. See Figure 37-1 for an example of a high-quality, artifact-free sleep tracing.

Selecting Display Features

The viewing resolution of each signal is dependent on the size and resolution of the computer monitor as well as the number of channels being displayed. When too many channels are viewed simultaneously, the subtle nuances of the waveform become lost due to their small size. Therefore, an overcrowded display can alter the recording technologist's perception as well as the scorer's or interpreter's perception of the data. In essence, viewing a limited number of flawlessly acquired channels may be more clinically relevant than viewing a large number of poorly recorded ones.

The 2018 AASM criteria (1) for scoring and review of sleep study data must meet or exceed the following standards:

- A 15-in screen size with a minimum of 1,600 pixels horizontal and 1,050 pixels vertical
- A minimum digital resolution of 12 bits per sample
- Histograms with stage, respiratory events, leg movement events, O_2 saturation, and arousals to be displayed
- Ability to position the cursor on the histogram and jump to the page selected
- Ability to view a screen on a timescale ranging from .5 seconds to the entire night
- Ability to synchronize the recorded video data with the PSG data and have an accuracy of at least one video frame per second
- Ability to display whether sleep staging scoring was performed visually or computed automatically by the software

The AASM also suggests the following optional criteria:

- Ability to turn pages automatically or scroll through the study
- Control key or toggle to turn off or invert a channel
- Ability to click and drag a channel to change display order
- Display setup profiles (including colors) that may be activated at any time
- Analysis options such as fast Fourier transformation or spectral analysis on specifiable intervals including omission of data tagged as artifact
- Ability to turn on and off highlighting of EEG patterns used to make sleep stage decisions (e.g., sleep spindles, K complexes, alpha activity)
- Ability to turn on and off highlighting of respiratory patterns used to make sleep stage decisions

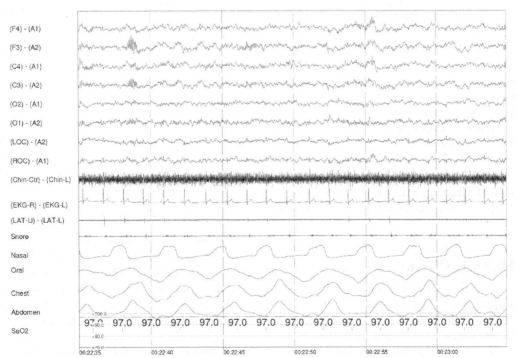

Figure 37-1 Artifact-free tracing. Example of a high-quality, artifact-free sleep tracing using the 2018 AASM-recommended derivations.

Utilizing System References

The original analog amplifiers that processed sleep study data included an electrode selector panel used to specify the electrode derivations for each channel. During the night, the technologist could easily rereference the signal by changing the selector panel to avoid waking the patient if an electrode became dislodged during the night. Although this technique was very convenient, all changes to the data were permanent and, therefore, impossible to reverse once recorded. Today, digital recording systems are designed to collect and store each signal separately. The most common method references all EEG signals to a common electrode, typically placed on the midline of the scalp (Cz). This approach is known as system referencing. It has the advantage of allowing the viewer to change the electrode derivations at any time through software functions without permanently altering the raw data. Any desired derivation can then be viewed by digitally subtracting the common reference from any pair of EEG electrodes. For example, the signal for C3-M2 is created by simultaneously subtracting Cz from C3 and M2.

Despite the advantages of this technique, such as preserving data integrity, system referencing does create opportunities for error because any electrode, including the system reference, may potentially become the source of artifact. If the system reference signal becomes degraded, the entire recording is affected and no amount of rereferencing will resolve the issue. Therefore, sleep technologists as operators of digital recording equipment featuring system referencing must be especially aware of the possibility of reference-generated artifacts and be cognizant of how signals should be combined to produce reliable, accurate waveforms.

Most software systems use a common reference to record and store data. The AASM suggestion that all systems include the flexibility to choose and/or change the electrode input signal derivations without relying on a common reference electrode is currently an optional feature on most digital systems. It is essential that the recording software allows the capability of storing all derivation changes or any other signal manipulations performed by the technologist during the study, so that the scorer/interpreter does not have to duplicate this process.

Utilizing Multiple Channel Recordings

An alternative solution to using a common system reference is to program the montage to include multiple derivations for each parameter. For example, both C3/M2 and C4/M1 can be recorded, which gives the viewer the option to change from C3/M2 to C4/M1 if the M2 channel should fail. The rationale is that if an electrode becomes dislodged, another derivation will be able to produce a readable alternative signal. The drawback to this approach is that preselecting the derivations limits the options for rereferencing during the night. This is especially important if multiple electrodes go bad and creativity is needed to correct the issue. For example, if the C3 and M1 signals are both degraded, neither the C3-M2 nor the C4-M1 derivation will be acceptable. With rereferencing capabilities, a derivation of C4-M2 may be selected, at least temporarily, until the problem can be corrected without unduly disturbing the patient.

Utilizing Filters and Filtering

Filters are used in PSG to isolate and record specific frequency bandwidths relevant to each recording parameter while eliminating surplus signal information. The AASM has set standard filter configurations for each channel to minimize the presence of unwanted signal frequencies while preserving the signals of interest (1, 2) (see Table 37-1). As a general rule, the filter settings should only be changed when all other efforts to eliminate unwanted artifact have failed. There are three different types of filters that can be employed to correct artifact: low-frequency filter (LFF), high-frequency filter (HFF), and 50/60-Hz notch filter.

Low-Frequency Filter

The LFF (high-pass filter) allows high-frequency signals through while reducing signals with frequencies lower than the cutoff value, which is determined by the time constant. The LFF can be increased to diminish or eliminate the presence of slow-wave artifact resulting from sweat or respiratory artifact (see section Common Recording Artifacts). The standard LFF setting for EEG and electrooculogram (EOG) is 0.3 Hz.

High-Frequency Filter

The HFF (low-pass filter) does the exact opposite of the LFF by attenuating high-frequency signals while preserving low-frequency signals. It is unusual to alter the HFF during the night. The HFF is generally set at 35 Hz for EEG and EOG channels.

50/60-Hz Notch Filter

The 50/60-Hz notch filter reduces interference caused by outside electrical interference from outlets, power cords, and electrical ancillary equipment. Common mode rejection should eliminate most 50/60-Hz artifact if the electrodes have been properly attached and the surrounding equipment is functioning correctly; therefore, additional filtration should not be needed. However, the 50/60-Hz notch filter can be used to temporarily resolve artifact until the problem can be identified and corrected.

Overfiltering affects the integrity of the recording by hiding problems that should be corrected at the source rather than filtered. Care must be taken, therefore, not to overprocess the input signals. Using filters to reduce artifacts is only appropriate when the underlying physiologic signals are intact, which means the electrode impedances are in an acceptable range and the connections are sound. Filters can be used to temporarily correct an artifact that is caused by body movements, sweat, or direct pressure against one of the electrodes. If the underlying physiologic signals from the patient are lost or distorted, filtering the signal will not solve the problem.

RECORDING ARTIFACTS

Even when careful attention is devoted to the hookup process, some degree of artifact can be expected to occur in virtually every sleep study. By definition, artifacts are extraneous signals appearing within any of the recorded parameters of the polysomnogram. These signals can originate from the patient's body, from recording instruments and devices used on the patient, or from the surrounding environment. The task of the sleep technologist includes recognizing the artifact, determining its origin, and deciding on the most appropriate way to address the problem.

It is important to keep in mind that not all artifacts are considered undesirable. For example, "snoring artifact," often seen in the chin electromyogram (EMG) channel, is useful for confirming the accuracy of the snore channel (see Fig. 37-2). Muscle-generated artifacts seen during patient movement help identify arousals. These and certain other physiologic artifacts can be quite useful in the interpretation of the polysomnogram and should not be removed from the recording.

However, many types of artifacts are undesirable and can severely impede the scoring and interpretation process. These include 50- or 60-Hz power line frequencies, slow-frequency artifacts caused by sweat, electrode "popping" artifacts, electrocardiogram (ECG) artifacts recorded in the EEG, EOG, or EMG channels, and various other interfering signals recorded within any of the channels.

Artifact Recognition

Most recording artifacts can be recognized by their exaggerated appearance. However, in some cases, it may be difficult to discern between artifacts and physiologic signals of interest. For example, sweat artifact in the EEG is usually identified by its excessively slow frequency, but sometimes the intruding waves may appear similar to high-amplitude delta waves. An advantage offered by multichannel PSG is the ability to cross-examine the recording to see whether the signals in question correlate with other recorded parameters. For example, if questionable slow waves are seen in the central EEG channel, but are not appropriately reflected in the occipital or eye movement channels, they are likely artifact. For this reason, EEG frequencies are not filtered from the eye channels. In addition to detecting eye movements, EOG

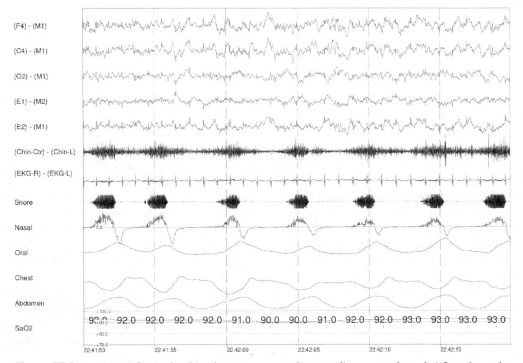

Figure 37-2 Snoring artifact in the chin electromyogram, electrocardiogram, and nasal airflow channels. Notice that the respiratory effort bands are out of phase, which may suggest paradoxical breathing.

channels record frontal EEG activity. The combined tracings from the central, occipital, and eye movement channels allow for cross-examination of these signals to confirm normal voltage distribution (higher voltages in the frontal region and lower voltages in the occipital region) and identify exaggerated, stray voltages that do not correlate with adjoining channels.

Cross-examining channels can also help identify the source of the artifact by comparing adjacent channel tracings. For example, if an identical artifact is seen in two or more channels sharing the same reference (e.g., C3-M2 and O1-M2), it can be assumed that the artifact originates from the reference electrode. Alternatively, if an artifact appears in only one channel (sharing a common reference with other channels), the problem can be attributed to the exploring electrode.

Artifact Correction

When unwanted artifact is detected, whether environmental or biologic in nature, it should be documented and corrected as soon as possible. As a general rule, when an artifact is localized to just one channel, it typically indicates that the problem lies with just one electrode. Unfortunately, there is no hard and fast rule for how to correct artifact, because there are many different causes of signal interference and often multiple solutions. In some scenarios, like muscle artifact, no corrective action is required because the situation will resolve itself. Other circumstances require immediate intervention to correct the problem, such as a displaced airflow sensor or an oximeter.

If a problem is detected during the impedance check or biocalibrations, every effort should be made to resolve the issue before starting the study, even if it requires re-attaching electrodes or replacing sensors. However, if an artifact develops after the patient has fallen asleep, replacing the electrode may not be the best course of action. Often, it is possible to eliminate undesirable artifacts by rereferencing the input signal derivation to an alternate exploring or reference site, with proper documentation. For example, if an artifact contaminates the C4 channel, the signal input can be changed to C3. If the artifact originates from a reference site, such as M2, then the reference input may be changed to the opposite side (M1). However, if the patient awakens to use the restroom, the problematic electrode should always be fixed at the source and the system returned to the standard derivations.

Artifacts often originate from the side of the head or face on which the patient is lying, usually due to sweat or direct pressure against the electrode. It may be necessary to make several derivation changes during the course of a sleep study, because the patient changes body position. To perform signal derivation changes, the recording equipment must provide a method for making these

changes. Essentially all digital systems have this functionality through either system referencing or the ability to simultaneously record multiple electrode derivations.

Although a sleep center may have a policy regarding rereferencing or artifact tolerance, often the sleep technologist must use judgment to assess whether the problem warrants waking the patient. For instance, if the recording is compromised to the point where the sleep stage cannot be determined, the patient should be disturbed to correct the issue. However, if there is still sufficient readable data being recorded to adequately monitor the patient, the best course of action may be to wait until the patient awakens naturally to repair the problem.

COMMON RECORDING ARTIFACTS

50/60-Hz Artifact

The most pervasive interfering signal is the 50- or 60-Hz power line frequency (60 Hz in the United States and 50 Hz in many other countries). Artifact caused by 50/60-Hz interference appears as a regular, sinusoidal wave, which completely obscures the physiologic signal, turning it into a thick, dark tracing. To qualify as 50/60-Hz interference, there must be exactly 60 oscillations (if recorded in the United States) per second. The oscillations should be counted on a 1-second display. If there are not exactly 60 oscillations, there is another cause for the artifact such as increased muscle tone. Figure 37-3A shows how 50/60-Hz artifact can obscure an EEG channel, and Figure 37-3B presents the same channel at a slower speed to demonstrate the regular appearance of the 60-Hz artifact. With the signal expanded from 30 seconds to 1 second, the 60-Hz artifact on the O1/M2 channel is easily distinguished from muscle artifact by the uniformed sinusoidal pattern (Fig. 37-3C).

Normal levels of 50/60-Hz interference are minimized or eliminated with common mode rejection, provided the impedance levels among the electrodes are low (<5 kΩ) and relatively equal. The patient–ground electrode, which is not the same as the electrical ground, also helps dissipate 50/60-Hz interference. Despite these routine measures to combat 50/60-Hz interference, abnormally high levels of interference may still impact a recording. Excessive 50/60-Hz artifact is usually caused by high-electrode impedance levels or a poor electrical connection.

Another cause for 50/60-Hz artifact is an excessive amount of current leakage, originating from electrical ancillary equipment, extension cords, lamps, televisions, electric beds, fans, and so on. When the artifact originates from poorly shielded electrical equipment, it will impact all channels that include the 50/60-Hz frequency bandwidth.

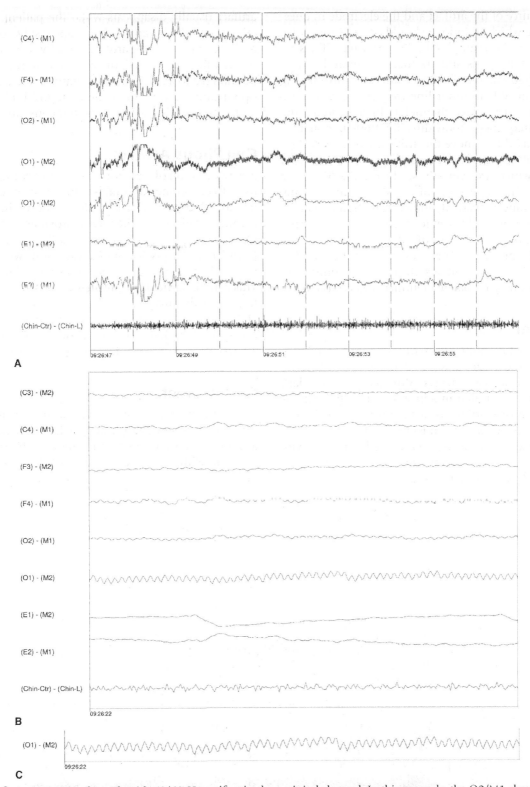

Figure 37-3 A: A 30-second epoch with 50/60-Hz artifact in the occipital channel. In this example, the O2/M1 channel appears twice. The top display shows the channel with the 60-Hz interference. The second instance uses the 60-Hz notch filter to correct the display and confirm the cause of the problem. In this scenario, the electrode should be reattached at the next available opportunity. **B:** 50/60-Hz artifact in occipital channel with a 1-second epoch. **C:** With the signal expanded from 30 seconds to 1 second, the 60-Hz artifact on the O1/M2 channel is easily distinguished from muscle artifact by the uniformed sinusoidal pattern.

The source of the artifact and the electrode in question dictate which technique should be used to resolve the problem. For example, the leg EMG recordings require extra-long leads and are therefore more likely to absorb 50/60-Hz interference from the surrounding environment. When minor line frequency interference appears in a leg EMG channel (which includes the 50/60-Hz frequency bandwidth), a 50/60-Hz notch filter can be used to remove the artifact. However, 50/60-Hz notch filters should not be used in the EEG or EOG channels, which are typically set below the 50/60-Hz bandwidth. The appearance of 50/60-Hz artifact in any of these channels invariably indicates high impedances, a poor connection, a broken lead wire, or an unplugged lead. In these cases, the use of 50/60-Hz filters merely conceals the problem. To eliminate 50/60-Hz interference in EEG or EOG channels, the electrode connection causing the artifact must be identified and corrected.

Muscle Artifact

Muscle artifact is another form of fast or high-frequency artifact routinely encountered in the EEG, EOG, and, occasionally, the ECG tracings. Although the thick, dark tracing can look similar in appearance to 50/60-Hz interference, muscle artifact is distinguished by its irregular high frequency, as seen in Figure 37-4.

Muscle artifact is caused by localized muscle activity in the vicinity of an exploring or reference electrode and is commonly seen in tense or anxious patients. Muscle artifact usually disappears when the patient relaxes or falls asleep. If the artifact does not resolve on its own and the source of the artifact (usually a reference electrode) can be identified, the electrode derivation should be changed to a back-up configuration. Then, at the next opportunity, correct the issue by repositioning the M1 and M2 electrodes to decrease extraneous muscle signals.

Cell Phone Artifact

A new variation of electrical interference comes from the use of cell phones and tablets in the sleep center. If a patient places a device near the headbox, intermittent communication with the service provider and incoming messages or alerts may result in 100-μV low-frequency (5 to 9 Hz) sharply contoured waveforms with intermittent high-frequency (20 to 50 Hz) sinusoidal waves (2). This can be particularly problematic because EEG interference at this frequency can mimic spindles (11 to 16 Hz) and cause confusion with sleep staging. To mitigate this type of interference, mobile devices should be kept at least 32 in away from recording equipment.

ECG Artifact

ECG artifact consists of a visible intrusion of the ECG signal on the EEG, EOG, and/or EMG channels. ECG artifact is easily recognizable by the spike-like waves that coincide with each QRS complex of the ECG channel. Refer to Figure 37-5 for an example of ECG artifact.

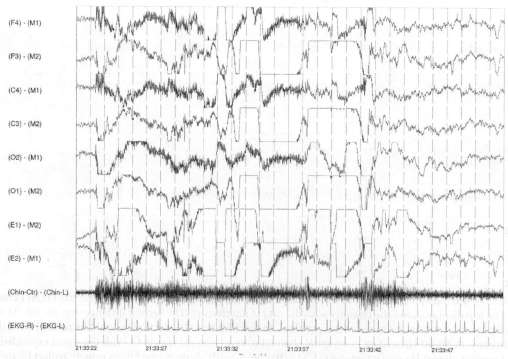

Figure 37-4 Muscle artifact in the electroencephalogram and electrooculogram channels. In this example, note how the artifact coincides with the increase in muscle activity measured by the chin electromyogram at the start of the epoch. As the muscle tone decreases, the artifact disappears and the waveforms are once again readable.

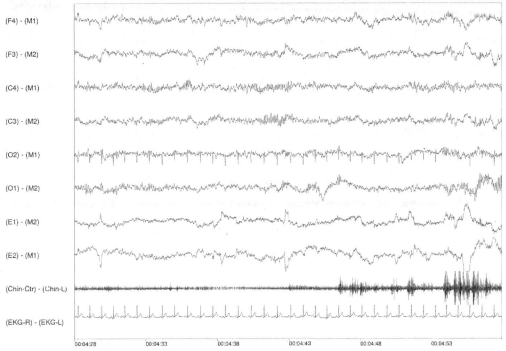

Figure 37-5 Electrocardiogram (ECG) artifact in the O2 channel. In this example, a prominent ECG signal can be clearly detected in the O2/M1 channel, but not in the other electroencephalogram or electrooculogram channels. Because the artifact is localized to just one channel, double referencing M1 and M2 is unlikely to resolve the problem.

Extraneous ECG signals are normally canceled by common mode rejection. However, due to the relatively long interelectrode distances used in standard PSG derivations (such as C3 referenced to M2), sometimes it is impossible to eliminate a small amount of ECG artifact in the EEG and EOG channels. This is particularly true when studying obese patients.

When ECG artifact is found in just one channel, it is usually caused by impedance imbalances between the exploring and the reference electrodes. As with any form of undesirable artifact, utilizing proper electrode application techniques minimizes ECG interference. If excessive ECG artifact originates in one of the reference electrodes, multiple channels will be affected. The electrodes should be reattached slightly above the mastoid process, over the firm bony area behind the ear (taking care not to place them too high). As a general rule, to reduce the possibility of ECG artifacts, avoid soft, fatty tissue behind the ears when applying the reference EEG electrodes M1 and M2 during the initial hookup procedure. If altering the placement of the reference electrodes does not correct the problem, the interference can be minimized or eliminated by linking the two reference electrodes M1 and M2. Double referencing an EEG or EOG channel essentially creates three divergent ECG signals that cancel each other out, thereby reducing the artifact. Using analog equipment, this was accomplished by double referencing the EEG and EOG channels through the electrode selector panel. Digital systems

have provisions for double referencing using the system reference approach described earlier.

There are drawbacks to double referencing electrodes, so this technique should not be used routinely. Once the channels are double referenced, any other signal interference (such as sweat or muscle artifact) originating from either of the cross-linked reference electrodes will contaminate all the linked channels. In addition, if the artifact is originating from one of the reference electrodes, cross-linking the reference electrodes will increase the artifact rather than reduce it. Furthermore, the use of additional reference electrodes in any channel may attenuate the signal of interest.

Slow-Frequency Artifacts

There are three main categories of slow-wave frequency artifacts routinely seen in PSG: sweat artifact, respiratory artifact, and electrode popping. These artifacts are occasionally confused with slow-wave sleep because of their slow frequency.

Sweat Artifact

Perspiration induces chemical changes in the electrolyte interface between the electrode and the patient's skin, causing the slow-oscillating wave patterns commonly referred to as "sweat artifact." The huge, slow sways and wandering baseline differentiate sweat artifact from slow-wave sleep. See Figure 37-6 for an example of sweat artifact in the EEG and EOG channels.

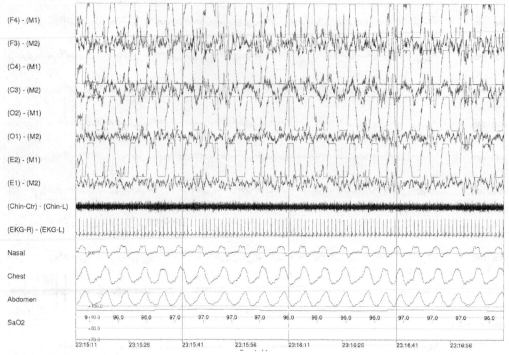

Figure 37-6 Slow-frequency artifact. The slow-frequency artifact originating in the M2 lead has caused multiple channels to block. Notice how the sway of the electroencephalogram (EEG) coincides with the respiration. In this situation, the technologist should rereference the EEG and electrooculogram to M1 until the room cools.

If a patient perspires enough to cause sweat artifact in multiple channels, the technologist should attempt to cool the room with a fan or air-conditioning. If the artifact is affecting one side of the head, changing the derivation or rereferencing the electrodes is appropriate while waiting for the temperature in the room to decrease. As a last resort, the LFF in the EEG and/or EOG channel(s) can be raised from 0.3 to 1 Hz to reduce the amount of slow-wave activity in that channel. Any changes to the electrode derivation or filters must be properly documented.

Respiratory Artifact

Slow-frequency artifact often appears synchronous with the patient's breathing patterns, as shown in Figure 37-6. However, "respiratory artifact" is a misleading term because it is unlikely that respiration alone is responsible for the problem. Although the slight movement of the head associated with breathing is often a contributing factor to slow artifacts, the underlying cause of these artifacts can usually be attributed to either a chemical or a mechanical instability of the electrode/patient interface. Body movements associated with respiration may further aggravate slow-frequency artifacts, but again are rarely the direct cause of the problem.

It is very difficult to eliminate artifact caused solely by the slight head or body movements associated with respiration. If the artifact is excessive, the LFF in the EEG and/or EOG channel(s) can be raised from 0.3 to 1 Hz to decrease the slow-wave artifact. Modifications to the filter settings must be documented in the technologist

notes. If another type of slow-frequency artifact is being exacerbated by respiration, the primary cause of the artifact should be addressed.

Electrode Popping

The difference between sweat and popping artifact may not always be readily apparent. In general, electrode popping produces sharper, higher amplitude waves, causing a signal blocking effect in the EEG or EOG channels, which is illustrated in Figure 37-7. Popping artifacts in the EMG channels will produce a sharper, spiky wave due to the higher filter settings of these channels.

Electrode popping can be generated by applying pressure against an electrode or by creating tension on an electrode wire. Dirty or faulty electrodes can also cause electrode popping. Maintaining a tight seal between the electrodes and the patient's skin will minimize electrode popping artifact. When direct pressure against one of the electrodes causes artifact, a solution (other than repositioning the patient) is to temporarily raise the channel's LFF. This strategy is only effective if the electrode is well attached and the underlying physiologic signal remains intact. An alternative technique when the artifact is limited to the side of the head on which the patient is lying is to change the input derivation to the opposite side of the head.

In many cases, a combination of all three scenarios described (sweat, pressure against an electrode, and slight body movements associated with breathing) contributes

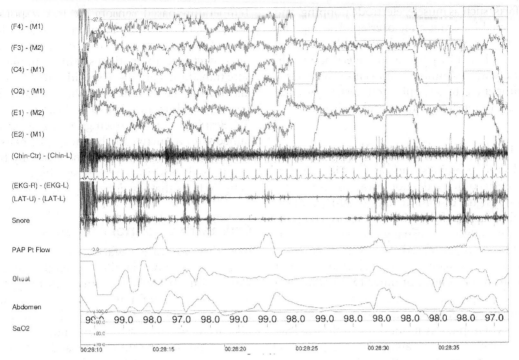

Figure 37-7 Electrode popping artifact in the electroencephalogram and electrooculogram channels. This sample shows popping in the M1 lead, which has caused a significant disruption to multiple signals, causing them to block out of range.

to slow-frequency artifacts. As with most signal interference, slow-frequency artifacts can be minimized by paying close attention to the quality of the electrode application. This prevents the electrode from "floating" over the electrode site, which can cause a disruption of the input signal with even the slightest movement.

Movement Artifacts

The term "movement artifact" is a general expression that describes a mixture of artifacts caused by body movement, which obscure multiple channels. When major body movements occur, as seen in Figure 37-8, different

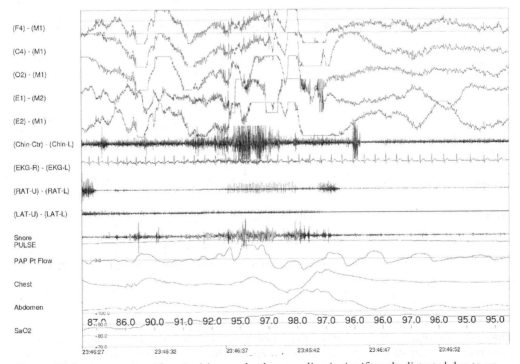

Figure 37-8 Movement artifact. In this sample, the recording is significantly distorted due to patient movement. Note the electrode popping in the electroencephalogram and the artifact on the channel monitoring the right leg (RAT).

types of artifacts, such as muscle, electrode popping, and generalized signal blocking, may overlap. Although artifacts related to movement are unavoidable, they can be further exacerbated by poor-quality electrode application. The only way to minimize movement artifacts is to practice proper electrode application techniques and to reduce strain or tension on the electrode leads.

Artifacts in the Respiratory Channels

Unlike bioelectric recordings, such as the EEG, inaccurate respiratory recordings do not always demonstrate obvious signs of signal distortion, like 50/60-Hz artifact. Instead, artifacts appearing in the respiratory channels tend to be more subtle and usually consist of conflicting information being displayed. Therefore, it is essential to examine all available respiratory channels and view them within the context of other PSG parameters to avoid treating signal inaccuracies caused by patient movement or transducer displacements as factual data.

Most forms of respiratory monitoring in clinical PSG are based on external, noncalibrated, indirect representations of the patient's breathing patterns. These representations are generally imprecise and susceptible to signal distortion. For example, respiratory airflow sensors are typically either temperature based or pressure based. Both types of sensors are susceptible to signal loss or distortion due to sensor displacement. In addition, each type of sensor has its own peculiarities and limitations.

Temperature-based sensors are less responsive to minor changes in airflow than pressure transducers. They are also more susceptible to drift caused by air currents or contact with the patient's skin. Cannula-based pressure transducers are more sensitive to minor changes in airflow, but are more susceptible to signal loss due to mouth breathing or cannula occlusion.

Respiratory effort tracings are most commonly obtained with inductive plethysmography belts, which are susceptible to signal distortion caused by body movements, body position changes, shifting or twisting of the belts, or belts that are either too loose or overtightened.

Oximetry Channel Artifacts

As with respiratory artifact, inaccuracies of the oximetry channel can be identified when the oximetry output varies with no apparent correlation to respiratory pattern (see Fig. 37-9 for an illustration). Oximetry artifact may be caused by improper probe attachment, probe displacement, poor perfusion, motion artifact, or imprecise equipment calibrations, and/or faulty oximeter/computer interface. All these factors must be considered when evaluating the oximetry tracing. To ensure signal accuracy, sleep technologists must know how to recognize a potentially false signal and be adequately trained in the proper use and calibration of the oximeter. Typically replacing the probe or recalibrating the system will correct the issue.

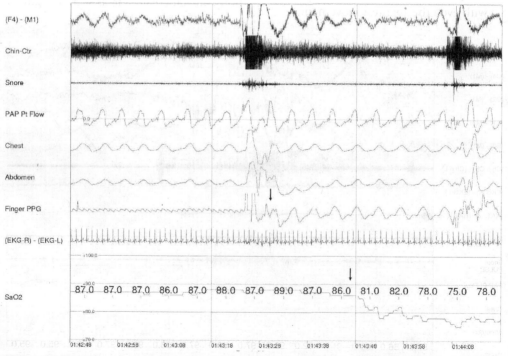

Figure 37-9 Oximetry channel artifact. The oximetry signal in the second half of this epoch is erroneous. The sharp drop in SaO_2 does not correspond with the breathing pattern, and the finger photoplethysmography (PPG) signal confirms the tracing is invalid.

Most present-day recording systems provide some form of oximetry signal verification and/or method of deleting "bad" data. However, no signal detection system is foolproof; therefore, a visual inspection of the entire oximetry channel tracing should be conducted for every study. False oximetry readings may significantly alter the interpretation of the recording; therefore, any false readings must be tagged or deleted, so they do not appear as factual data in the sleep study report.

Artifacts Specific to Digital Recording Systems

There are numerous digital recording systems and each one uses a different technology; as a result, the appearance of recording artifacts may vary across systems. Some systems may overprocess signals, minimizing the appearance of artifacts, at the cost of losing essential detail. Other systems generate tracings that resemble conventional paper recordings, preserving all the necessary detail and allowing the presence of artifacts to alert the technologist of a potential problem.

Using an analog recording system, when a connection to the patient deteriorates or is lost, the technologist is immediately alerted by the obvious presence of artifact, usually in the form of 60-Hz artifact. Some digital systems generate a flat line when a signal is lost. This is equally problematic because a brief or intermittent loss of signal could be misinterpreted as a physiologic event, such as an asystole in the ECG channel.

Miscellaneous Artifacts

In addition to the commonly recognized recording artifacts, many other atypical or unique artifacts may be encountered during PSG. Some may have physiologic origins, whereas others may be related to the equipment or to external signal interference. The task of the sleep technologist involves a careful evaluation of any unusual patterns that do not seem to be related to the signal of interest. As noted previously, care must be exercised not to remove all suspicious patterns arbitrarily. Instead, the technologist should develop strategies to identify the cause of the pattern, decide whether its presence is useful or detrimental to the evaluation of the sleep study, and then proceed accordingly.

ENDING THE STUDY

When morning arrives and it is time to wake your patient(s), do your best to put whatever technical issues you may have struggled with during the night behind you to ensure you are polite, cheerful, and courteous to your patient. This is a key time to exercise good customer service. For additional details about ending a sleep study, see Chapter 36.

Morning Calibrations

After marking "lights on" and waking the patient, perform and record an impedance check and repeat biocalibrations to confirm that all the electrodes are still collecting relevant data. When the calibrations have been completed, the patient can be disconnected from the equipment and allowed to get out of bed.

Removing and Cleaning Sensors, Electrodes, and Equipment

Unhooking a patient is much faster and easier than applying the electrodes, but it should still be performed with care. Acetone or collodion remover should be used if the EEG electrodes were attached with collodion. If paste was used, warm water can be used to soften the paste for removal. If it is difficult to remove tape, moisten it with alcohol or adhesive remover to avoid causing the patient discomfort.

Documentation

At the end of your shift, review the documentation completed during the night to ensure all relevant information has been relayed according to sleep center policy. Typically, in addition to technologist notes, most sleep centers have the patient complete a morning questionnaire to gather subjective information about the night.

Patient Discharge Procedures

Once the patient has completed all the necessary paperwork and is ready to leave the sleep center, be sure to explain what he or she can expect to happen next. Typically, that will include a follow-up phone call or appointment with the clinician to discuss the test results. Providing a time frame for when that contact is likely to happen will facilitate the process and keep the individual's expectations in line with what the sleep center can provide. Be careful not to predict what the doctor may say about the sleep study results. Conflicting information will complicate the process and undermine the reputation of the facility.

SUMMARY

The sleep technologist has a very complex role that requires a unique range of skills in addition to a strong understanding of sleep and sleep disorders. A good technologist must be able to interact well with patients, be dexterous enough to apply the electrodes and sensors, and be adept at troubleshooting equipment and software issues. The technologist must be able to identify medical emergencies and know when to intervene as well as identify and correct different types of artifact quickly and effectively. By properly maintaining the sleep recording, the attending sleep technologist assures the safety of the patient and records a polysomnogram with minimal signal distortion caused by artifacts.

SUGGESTED READINGS

Barkoukis, T. J., & Avidan, A. Y. (2007). *Review of sleep medicine* (2nd ed.). Philadelphia, PA: Butterworth-Heinemann.

Butkov, N. (1994). *The all-night sleep recording manual.* Medford, OR: Synapse Media.

Butkov, N. (1996). *Atlas of clinical polysomnography* (Vols. I & II). Medford, OR: Synapse Media.

REFERENCES

1. Berry, R. B., Albertario, C. L., Harding, S. M., et al.; for the American Academy of Sleep Medicine. (2018). *The AASM manual for the scoring of sleep and associated events: Rules, terminology and technical specifications* [Version 2.5]. Darien, IL: American Academy of Sleep Medicine.
2. Rasquinha, R. J., Moszczynski, A. J., & Murray, B. J. (2012). A modern artifact in the sleep laboratory. *Journal of Clinical Sleep Medicine, 8*(2), 225–226.

chapter 38
Adult Sleep Scoring

HARRY WHITMORE   RITA BROOKS

LEARNING OBJECTIVES

On completion of this chapter, the reader should be able to:

1. Recognize the electroencephalogram waveforms of wakefulness and sleep.
2. Define and implement the rules for staging sleep in adults.
3. Define and implement the rules for scoring events in adults.

KEY TERMS

Alpha rhythm
Low-amplitude mixed-frequency activity
Vertex sharp waves
K complexes
Sleep spindles
Slow-wave activity
Rapid eye movements
Obstructive apnea
Central apnea
Mixed apnea
Hypopnea
Respiratory effort–related arousals

The scoring of sleep and its events represents at least half of what the technologist must do on a nightly basis, whether the technologist is doing hookups at night, running multiple sleep latency tests (MSLTs) during the day, or scoring records as a scoring technologist. Although the scoring technologist might spend most of the day scoring polysomnograms (PSGs), the technologist working at night must understand and implement the scoring rules to run a PSG well. Similarly, the technologist working during the day running MSLTs and maintenance of wakefulness tests must also understand and implement the scoring rules to execute the respective procedure properly. In short, all technologists should understand the scoring rules.

Scoring is usually performed using a two-pass method, meaning that the entire recording is looked through at least twice. In the first pass, the recording is viewed in 30-second epochs and a sleep stage is assigned to each epoch between lights out and lights on. Arousals are also generally scored during sleep staging. In the second pass, the resolution of the display is changed to 60 seconds, 120 seconds, or even 5 minutes and events are marked. The summary data that result from this process are then tabulated and reported according to the current version of the *AASM Manual for the Scoring of Sleep and Associated Events* (1).

HISTORICAL PERSPECTIVE

The history of how we describe and quantify sleep is the story of how technology has helped us observe the rhythms of the human in a relatively nonintrusive manner. The first person to report recording the electrical biopotentials of the brain in mammals was Richard Caton, who recorded brain waves from the exposed brains of dogs and rabbits in 1875 (2). It was not until brain waves could be recorded through the skin and scalp that the field of electroencephalogram (EEG) was born. Hans Berger reported the presence of what he called the *alpha rhythm* using electrodes attached to the scalp of himself and his son in 1929 (Figs. 38-1 and 38-2).

Loomis and others at Harvard adopted this technology and were the first to describe sleep stages using features of the EEG in 1937. They classified five different stages of what we would now call nonrapid eye movement (NREM) sleep (stages A through E). Several other investigators added to this early work in EEG, but it was not until the landmark paper in 1953 by Eugene Aserinsky and Nathaniel Kleitman that described regularly occurring bouts of rapid eye movements (REMs) during sleep that the standard of the recording montage including more than simply the EEG was recognized.

Eugene Aserinsky adopted Jacobson's technique of monitoring eye movements using EEG electrodes to study infants. It should be noted that he spent many hours collecting the data himself, much like the sleep technologist does today. He noticed regularly occurring periods of "jerky eye movements" in more than 50

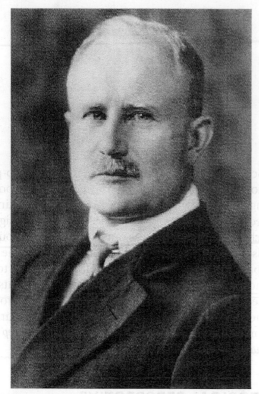

Figure 38-1 German psychiatrist Hans Berger (1873 to 1942) is best known as the inventor of electroencephalography and is the discoverer of the alpha wave rhythm.

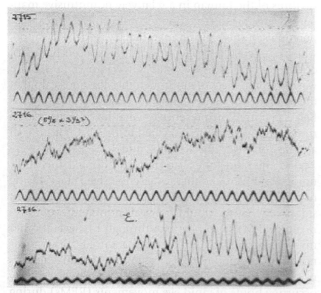

Figure 38-2 Hans Berger reported the presence of what he called the *alpha rhythm* using electrodes attached to the scalp of himself and his son in 1929.

recordings by 1952. This added the electrooculogram (EOG) to what we now know as the PSG.

A few years later, a young medical doctor named William Dement joined the Kleitman group at the University of Chicago. In 1957, Dement and Kleitman

published a landmark article entitled *Cyclic Variations in EEG During and Their Relation to Eye Movements, Body Motility, and Dreaming.* This article outlined four stages of what we now call NREM sleep as well as REM sleep.

In 1968, *A Manual of Standardized Terminology, Techniques and Scoring for Sleep Stages of Human Subjects* was published (2). This manual was the result of the efforts of a committee led by Allan Rechtschaffen and Anthony Kales and represents the first consensus-based set of rules for the scoring of sleep in humans. Its intended application was for the sleep research community to aid in the standardization and compatibility of research data in adults. This R&K manual, as it has become known, was the most widely used set of rules in scoring sleep until 2007, when the American Academy of Sleep Medicine (AASM) put together a task force to compose a new set of rules that would address its shortcomings.

Although the R&K manual was the most widely used scoring system for 39 years, it was not the only scoring system in use. Several years later, in 1971, a similar set of scoring rules was published by a committee led by Anders, Emde, and Parmelee. *A Manual for Standardized Terminology, Techniques, and Criteria for Scoring of States of Sleep and Wakefulness in Newborn Infants* was intended to serve much the same purpose as the R&K manual: a set of rules by which increased comparability of research results might be achieved, but for PSG data from newborns and infants instead of adults.

A group from the University of Florida also published a scoring system at about the same time as the R&K manual was being developed. The scoring rules put forth by Williams, Karacan, and Hursch used 1-minute epochs instead of the 20- or 30-second epochs suggested in the R&K manual, as well as slightly different frequency bands and amplitude requirements. Although not widely used, the group did publish an impressive summary of normative PSG data using their guidelines in 1974 (3).

The R&K manual has several significant drawbacks that have been described in detail elsewhere (4, 5). Many of these drawbacks stem from the fact that the manual ended up being used for purposes other than its intended original purpose: to aid in the standardization of sleep research data between laboratories. The clarity and economy of its rules made it easy to use and thus, with no other clear alternative in existence, clinicians began to use the scoring rules for sleep studies in the clinical setting. In the clinical setting, several additional channels were added: channels to monitor respiratory airflow and effort, an electrocardiogram (ECG) channel, and electromyogram (EMG) channels to monitor limb movements (LMs). There are no definitions for respiratory events, arousals, or rules for the scoring of limb movements in the R&K manual. To address these other features of sleep, additional guidelines were developed (6–8).

A second drawback of the R&K manual is the fact that it was intended only for adults and thus does not address the effect of age on sleep. Although a separate manual was developed for the scoring of sleep in newborns and infants (9), the changes in sleep due to advancing age are not addressed in the R&K manual. For example, the 75 μV criteria for the scoring of slow-wave sleep has been questioned (5).

A third issue not addressed in the R&K manual is the absence of digital specifications for the acquisition and scoring of PSG data. The R&K manual was developed in the late 1960s before the use of computers became the norm for recording sleep. Thus, R&K only provides guidelines for the use of paper machines and many of the choices for the number of channels to be recorded were determined by the use of eight-channel recorders. As such, only one central EEG signal was required as a minimum EEG channel because all of the waveforms of sleep can be seen from this derivation. Two EOG leads were suggested, as well as a single chin EMG channel. This allowed two participants to be recorded on a single machine. The advancement of digital technologies now allows for as many as 256 channels to be recorded and analyzed with relative ease.

Taken together, these many drawbacks led to the re-evaluation of the R&K manual. To this end, the board of the AASM approved the development of a new scoring manual. Over the course of 2 years, a steering committee and eight task forces were brought together with members of the board of the AASM and content experts in various aspects of sleep. Six of the eight task forces were developed to investigate and report on major content areas of the new manual: visual scoring, digital scoring, arousal, movement, respiratory issues, and cardiac issues. The issue of age effects was addressed by the two remaining task forces, one for pediatrics and one for geriatrics.

Each task force followed the same process for the development of the new manual. They performed a literature search and review, from which they produced evidence tables and a review paper, which served to provide transparency about the decisions made in the new manual. Each of these papers was published in a single issue of the *Journal of Clinical Sleep Medicine* in 2007 and provides a thorough review for the curious reader.

Since 2007, there have been eight versions of the *AASM Manual for the Scoring of Sleep and Associated Events*, with the most recent ninth version 2.5 being released in early 2018. The reader is encouraged to read page 75 of version 2.5 for a brief review of the committee-recommended changes made since the 2007 manual was written. Some of the changes introduced in these eight updates to the manual have been minor to the terms to be used, while other changes were more substantive, including the addition of home sleep apnea testing (HSAT) and infant rules for scoring sleep and associated events. These substantive changes have been examined in detail in other chapters.

TECHNICAL SPECIFICATIONS

The AASM Manual for the Scoring of Sleep and Associated Events contains important technical specifications for the collection of PSG data. These rules represent the first consensus-based set of rules for the use of digital technology in polysomnography.

The maximum impedance allowed for EEG and EOG is 5 kΩ. The minimum digital resolution is 12 bits per sample. The sampling rates and filter settings for each channel are detailed in Table 38-1 (1).

The minimal sampling rate for the EEG, EOG, EMG, and ECG channels is 200 samples per second, the preferred sampling rate is 500 samples per second for these parameters. The sampling rate is chosen on the basis of what the frequency of interest is in the signal being viewed. The AASM Scoring Manual suggests that the sampling rate and high filter settings may be increased if needed to more accurately display EEG spikes. In this case, the sampling rate should be "at least three times the high frequency of interest" (1).

Usually, a sleep study is scored in two passes. The scorer will first view the sleep study in 30-second epochs to determine the appropriate sleep stage. After determining sleep and wakefulness, the scorer will do a second pass in a more compressed view, usually a 60- to 120-second epoch, to determine sleep-related events.

RECOGNIZING WAVEFORMS

There are four features of the EEG signal that are informative to the categorization of the signal as a distinct waveform (Table 38-2). They are the *amplitude*, *frequency*, *morphology*, and *distribution* of the waveform. We use these four features of the EEG signal to identify the waveforms that are a part of the definition of sleep stages. The *amplitude* of the signal refers to its vertical distance from the isoelectric baseline, measured in microvolts (μV). The *frequency* refers to the number of waves per second, measured in Hertz (Hz) or the number of cycles per second. The *morphology* of the waveform refers to its shape. The *distribution* of the waveform is the source of the signal, or the region in which the amplitude is the highest.

Alpha Rhythm

The first waveform that we must recognize is the *alpha rhythm* or Berger's rhythm. As with several waveforms, the alpha rhythm is defined by its frequency, which is

Table 38-1 Recommended Digital Specifications and Filter Settings from the *AASM Manual for the Scoring of Sleep and Associated Events*

Channel	Desirable Sampling Rate in Hz	Minimal Sampling Rate in Hz	Low-Frequency Rate in Hz	High-Frequency Rate in Hz
Electroencephalogram	500	200	0.3	35
Electrooculogram	500	200	0.3	35
Electromyogram	500	200	10	100
Electrocardiogram	500	200	0.3	70
Airflow	100	25	0.1	15
Oximetry	25	10	(not filtered)	(not filtered)
Nasal pressure	100	25	Direct current (DC) or ≤0.03	15
Esophageal pressure	100	25	0.1	15
Body position	1	1	(not filtered)	(not filtered)
Snoring sounds	500	200	10	100
Rib cage and abdominal movements	100	25	0.1	15
Positive airway pressure device flow	100	25	DC	DC

Reprinted with permission from Berry, R. B., Albertario, C. L., & Harding, S. M. (2018). *The AASM manual for the scoring of sleep and associated events: Rules, terminology and technical specifications* (Version 2.5). Darien, IL: American Academy of Sleep Medicine.

between 8 and 13 Hz (Fig. 38-3). Different people have slightly different alpha frequencies and some people have no alpha frequency at all. Some people display alpha that cycles at about 11 Hz, whereas others may have an alpha rhythm that cycles at around 9 Hz. Although they are different frequencies, both are considered alpha since they fall between 8 and 13 Hz.

Another helpful feature of alpha is its occipital distribution (Fig. 38-4). Although alpha can usually be seen in each of the three EEG channels, its amplitude is the highest in the occipital channel.

Low-Amplitude Mixed-Frequency Activity (Theta)

The second waveform to recognize is theta activity, also known as *low-amplitude mixed-frequency (LAMF) activity* (Fig. 38-5). The frequency of LAMF activity is 4 to 7 Hz.

Table 38-2 Summary of Waveforms Used in Scoring Sleep and Wakefulness

	Alpha Activity	Low-Amplitude Mixed Frequency	Vertex Sharp Wave	Spindle	K Complex	Slow Wave
Amplitude	Not defined	"Low"	Not defined	Not defined	Not defined	75 μV
Frequency	8–13 Hz	4–7 Hz	≥2 Hz	11–16 Hz	<2 Hz	0.5–2 Hz
Waveform	Sinusoidal	Mixed	Sharp	"Distinct"	Negative followed by positive	Not defined
Distribution	Occipital	Not defined	Central	Central	Frontal	Frontal

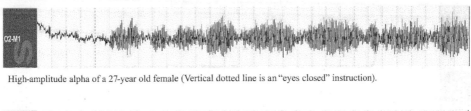

High-amplitude alpha of a 27-year old female (Vertical dotted line is an "eyes closed" instruction).

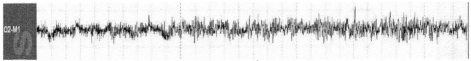

Moderate-amplitude alpha of a 20-year old male (Vertical dotted line is an "eyes closed" instruction).

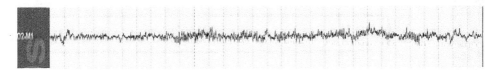

Low-amplitude alpha of a 20-year old male (Vertical dotted line is an "eyes closed" instruction).

Figure 38-3 Varying amplitudes of the alpha rhythm.

The amplitude is quite loosely defined as "low." In the R&K manual, the term "low-voltage mixed frequency" was used and the frequency range was from 2 to 7 Hz, a slightly larger frequency range. This overlapped with what is referred to as *theta* activity by the International Federation of Clinical Neurophysiology (10). The amplitude is quite loosely defined as "low." The distribution of the activity is diffuse, meaning it occurs in all channels.

Vertex Sharp Waves

The third waveform to recognize is the *vertex sharp wave* (Fig. 38-6). The AASM Scoring Manual defines vertex sharp waves as "sharply contoured waves with duration <0.5 seconds maximal over the central region and distinguished from the background activity" (1). There is no amplitude criterion for a vertex sharp wave. The distribution is central, meaning that the vertex sharp wave

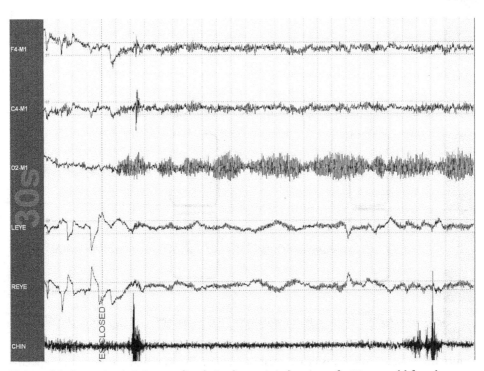

Figure 38-4 Maximal alpha amplitude in the occipital region of a 27-year-old female (horizontal dotted line is an "eyes closed" instruction).

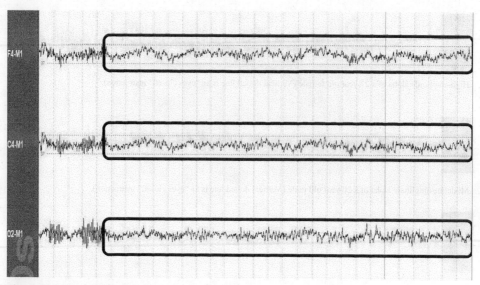

Figure 38-5 Alpha in the first 4½ seconds is replaced by low-amplitude mixed-frequency electroencephalography activity in a 27-year-old female.

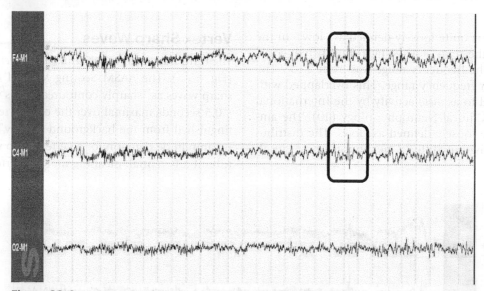

Figure 38-6 An example of a vertex sharp wave in a 26-year-old male.

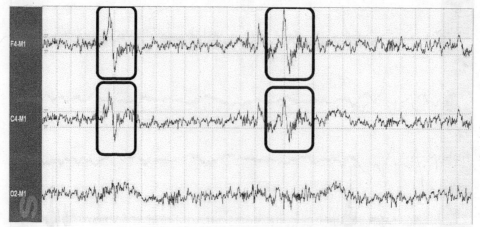

Figure 38-7 Two K complexes in a 27-year-old female. The first at 4th second of the epoch has no spindle associated with it, while the second at the 16th second does. Both are considered K complexes. Note also the higher amplitude in the frontal derivations.

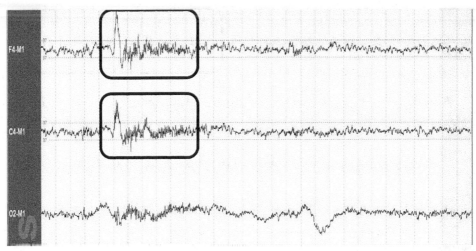

Figure 38-8 A K complex associated with an arousal. Although a K complex, we would not use it to score N2 sleep in this example.

will usually have its highest amplitude in the central channels. The most recognizable feature of the vertex sharp wave is its characteristic morphology.

K Complex

The fourth waveform to recognize is the K complex (Fig. 38-7). The AASM Scoring Manual defines a K complex as "a well delineated negative sharp wave immediately followed by a positive component standing out from the background EEG, with a total duration ≥0.5 seconds, usually maximal in amplitude when recorded using the frontal derivations" (1). K complexes may or may not be associated with arousals. When a K complex

is part of an arousal (Fig. 38-8), it is not used as evidence of stage N2 sleep. A common misconception of K complexes is that they must have a spindle immediately following them, thus making them a complex. This is not the case.

Sleep Spindle

The fifth waveform to recognize is the sleep spindle (Fig. 38-9). The AASM Scoring Manual defines a sleep spindle as "a train of distinctive waves with a frequency 11 to 16 Hz (most commonly 12 to 14 Hz) with a duration ≥0.5 seconds, usually maximal in amplitude in the central regions" (1).

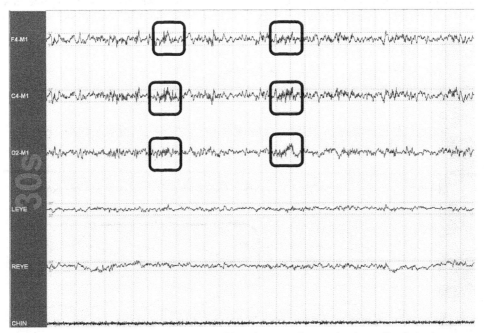

Figure 38-9 Sleep spindles in a 25-year-old male; note the maximal amplitude in the central derivation.

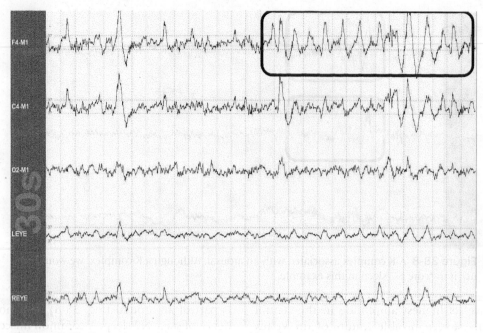

Figure 38-10 Slow-wave activity in a 19-year-old male; note the maximal amplitude in the frontal derivation.

Slow-Wave Activity

The sixth waveform to recognize is slow-wave activity (Fig. 38-10). Slow-wave activity consists of waves with a frequency of 0.5 to 2 Hz and a peak-to-peak amplitude greater than 75 μV. This wave activity is measured over the frontal region. This definition can be difficult to apply to the EEG signal in practice. Although we know we are to measure the "peak-to-peak" amplitude, the current definition does not tell us whether to begin counting at the most negative part of the wave or the most positive part. In addition, some K complexes may fit the definition of slow-wave activity. Although several automated algorithms have been developed, none have replaced the human as the gold standard for detecting slow waves. The AASM Inter-Scorer Reliability (ISR) Committee has proposed a "zero-cross" method for measuring slow-wave activity.

Slow Eye Movements

The seventh waveform to recognize is slow eye movements (Fig. 38-11). The AASM Scoring Manual defines

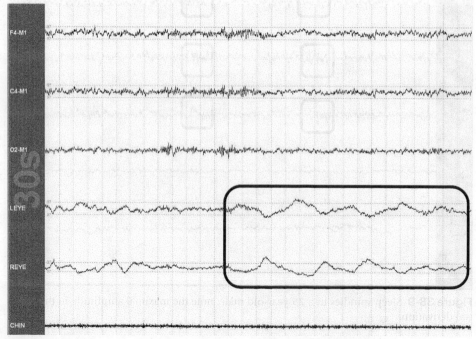

Figure 38-11 Slow-rolling eye movements in a 19-year-old male.

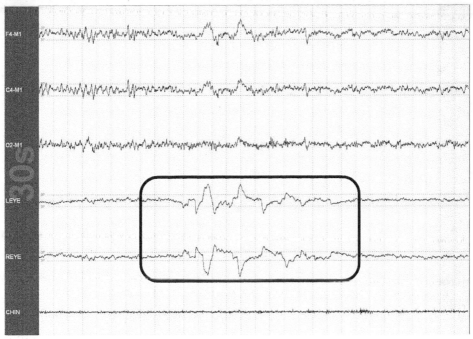

Figure 38-12 Rapid eye movements in a 27-year-old female.

slow eye movements as "conjugate, reasonably regular, sinusoidal eye movements with an initial deflection usually lasting >500 ms" (1).

Rapid Eye Movements

The eighth waveform to recognize is REMs (Fig. 38-12). The AASM Scoring Manual defines REMs as "conjugate, irregular, sharply peaked eye movements with an initial deflection usually lasting <500 ms" (1).

SCORING SLEEP STAGES

Sleep staging is usually done on the first pass of the two-pass approach to sleep scoring. In the first pass, the scorer views the recording in 30-second epochs, using an epoch-by-epoch approach. One sleep stage (Stage wake [W], N1, N2, N3, R) is assigned to each 30-second epoch between lights out and lights on. In the event that two or more stages occur in a single 30-second epoch, the stage making up the greatest portion of the epoch is assigned to that epoch. In the event that three or more stages appear in a single 30-second epoch, observe the following:

I. Score the epoch as sleep if the majority of the epoch meets criteria for stage N1, N2, N3, or R.

II. Assign the sleep stage that occurs for the majority of sleep within the epoch (1).

Stage Wake

Stage W is scored when 50% or more of the epoch has alpha rhythm over the occipital region in people who produce the alpha rhythm (Fig. 38-13). In people who do not produce alpha rhythm, stage W is scored when any of the following is present; eye blinks at a frequency of 0.5 to 2 Hz, reading eye movements, or REMs associated with high muscle tone (1).

Scoring Arousals

There is one rule for scoring arousals, but understanding it is important because arousals have implications for stage scoring (Fig. 38-14). "Score an arousal during sleep stages N1, N2, N3, or R if there is an abrupt shift of EEG frequency including alpha, theta and/or frequencies greater than 16 Hz (but not spindles) that lasts at least 3 seconds, with at least 10 seconds of stable sleep preceding the change" (1). This is true for arousals scored in stages N1, N2, and N3 sleep. When scoring arousals in R, there must also be a simultaneous increase in submental EMG for at least 1 second (1).

Identifying Major Body Movements

The AASM Scoring Manual defines a major body movement as "movement and muscle artifact obscuring the EEG for more than half an epoch to the extent that the sleep stage cannot be determined" (1). There are three rules for what to do with epochs that contain major body movements:

1. If alpha rhythm is present for part of the epoch (even <15 seconds duration), score the epoch as stage W.
2. If no alpha rhythm is discernible, but an epoch scored as stage W either precedes or follows the epoch with a major body movement, score the epoch as stage W.
3. Otherwise, score the epoch as the same stage as the epoch that follows it (1).

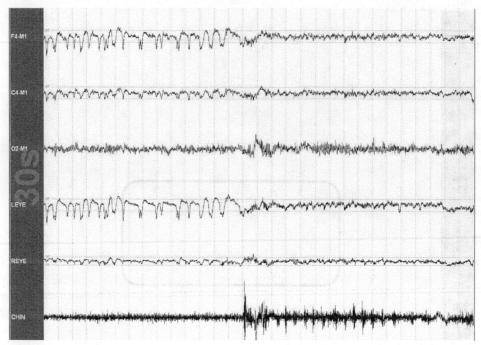

Figure 38-13 Wakefulness in a 31-year-old male. Note the eye blinks in the first 14 seconds and the alpha throughout.

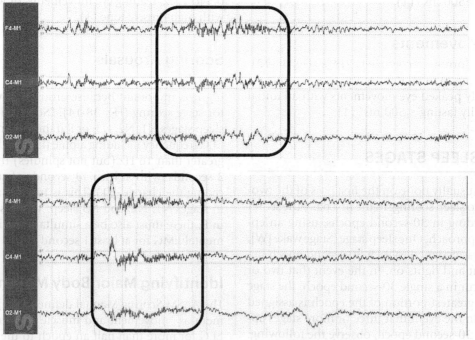

Figure 38-14 An example of an arousal without a K complex in a 22-year-old male at the top and an arousal with a K complex at the bottom in a 33-year-old male.

Major body movements are thus not scored as events themselves, but they are used to help the scorer decide how to score epochs with very little or no readable EEG activity due to movement or muscle artifact.

Stage N1 (NREM 1)

Stage N1 sleep (Fig. 38-15) is scored when alpha rhythm drops out and 50% of the epoch comprises LAMF EEG in people who produce the alpha rhythm. In people who

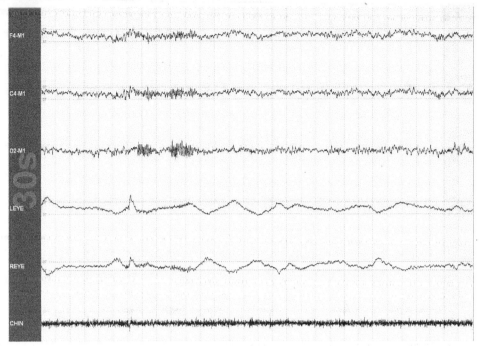

Figure 38-15 An N1 sleep in a 27-year-old female. Alpha activity is replaced by low-amplitude mixed-frequency electroencephalography activity. There are also slow-rolling eye movements present.

do not produce the alpha rhythm, stage N1 is scored at the earliest appearance of any of the following: slowing of the background frequency by greater than or equal to 1 Hz and in the range of 4 to 7 Hz, the presence of vertex sharp waves, or the presence of slow eye movements. Further, an epoch is scored as stage N1 if the *majority* of the epoch meets the criteria for stage N1 and there is no evidence of another sleep stage. Continue to score stage N1 until there is evidence of another sleep stage (1).

There are two other situations when a score of stage N1 is recommended. When stage N2 is interrupted by an arousal, the following epochs are scored as stage N1 if LAMF EEG is present and K complexes and sleep spindles are absent, until there is evidence of another stage of sleep. When an arousal interrupts stage R and is followed by LAMF EEG and slow eye movements, score as stage N1, even with continued low chin EMG activity, until there is evidence of another stage of sleep (1).

Stage N2 (NREM 2)

Stage N2 sleep makes up the majority of total sleep time in most individuals (Fig. 38-16). Stage N2 sleep is scored when there is a K complex or spindle in the first half of the epoch or the second half of the epoch that precedes it, with a background of LAMF activity. In the event that stage N2 sleep is interrupted by an arousal, score N1 sleep until the next K complex or sleep spindle appears (1). There are specific rules for

the continuation and termination of stage N2 sleep, as well as a special set of rules for the transitions between N2 and REM sleep.

Continue to score stage N2 unless an arousal or stage change interrupts the EEG activity, even in epochs without K complexes or sleep spindles if preceding epochs contain either K complexes or sleep spindles. Transition from stage N3 to stage N2 when the EEG no longer meets criteria for scoring stage N3 as long as there is no arousal and criteria for stage W or stage R are not present.

Stage N2 ends when there is a transition to another stage (including stage W), an arousal results in a stage change, or a major body movement occurs. If a major body movement interrupts stage N2, score the epoch following the movement as stage N2 if there are no slow eye movements and as stage N1 if there are slow eye movements present (1). See the major body movement scoring rules for additional information.

Stage N3

Stage N3 (Fig. 38-17) is scored when 20% or more of a 30-second epoch contains slow-wave activity. Thus, 6 seconds of activity in the frequency range of 0.5 to 2 Hz with an amplitude of greater than 75 μV measured in the frontal channels in a single epoch is sufficient to score N3 sleep. K complexes are scored as slow waves if they meet the definition of slow-wave activity. Pathologic slow-wave activity and artifact are not scored as stage N3 activity.

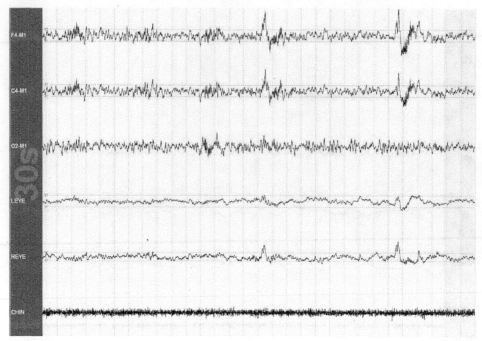

Figure 38-16 An N2 sleep in a 27-year-old female.

Stage R

Stage R (Fig. 38-18) is scored when all of the following are present in the epoch: LAMF EEG, low chin EMG tone, and REMs. Sawtooth waves are a distinctive waveform observed during stage R, but are not required to score the epoch as stage R. REMs are transient during stage R and are not required to be on each epoch to sustain scoring stage R. The continuation and termination rules address this. Stage R usually transitions from stage N2 or another NREM stage.

Definite stage R includes LAMF EEG activity without K complexes or sleep spindles, low EMG tone, and REMs. Score epochs that do not demonstrate REMs but precede or follow an epoch of definite stage R as stage R if chin EMG remains low, if EEG does not demonstrate K complexes or sleep spindles, and if there are no arousals

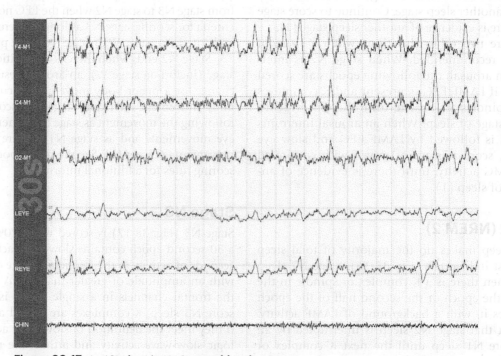

Figure 38-17 An N3 sleep in a 19-year-old male.

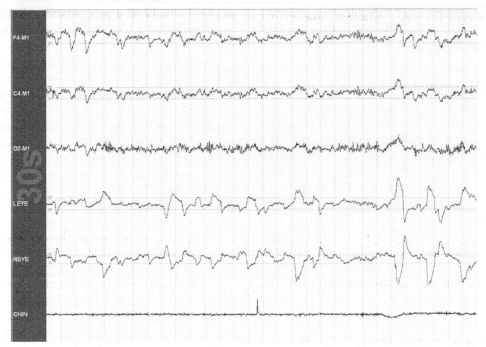

Figure 38-18 REM sleep in a 27-year-old female.

or slow eye movements present. This is essentially the R&K lookback rule.

Note that stage R takes precedence over stage N2 rules. If the majority of an epoch meets stage R criteria, the epoch should be scored as stage R. Specific rules are outlined in the AASM Scoring Manual to address epochs that have a mixture of stage R and stage N2 features. In this instance, we need to determine which stage comprises the majority of the epoch. In an epoch that exhibits low chin EMG tone and a mixture of REMs, sleep spindles, and K complexes, score as follows:

- Segments of the epoch with no REMs that are between two K complexes, two sleep spindles, or between a K complex and a sleep spindle (regardless of which comes first) are stage N2.
- Segments with REMs and no intervening K complexes or sleep spindles are stage R.
- Score the epoch stage R or stage N2 on the basis of the segment that represents the majority of the epoch (1).

Stage R ends when there is a transition to another sleep stage or an awakening. Following an arousal or major body movement, score the following epoch on the basis of the features of the epoch. If increased chin EMG tone and slow eye movements are present, score the epoch as stage N1. If chin EMG tone remains low and no slow eye movements are seen, score the epoch as stage R. If K complexes and/or sleep spindles are present, even with low chin tone, score the epoch as stage N2 (1).

SCORING RESPIRATORY EVENTS

The AASM Scoring Manual provides technical considerations for scoring respiratory events. More specifically, it specifies channels to focus on for the scoring of different types of events as well as backup channels for times when the primary channels may fail or are not used due to the type of sleep study being done (positive airway pressure [PAP] titrations).

Identifying Apnea

During a diagnostic study, the recommended sensors for identification of apnea are the oronasal thermal airflow sensor for monitoring airflow and dual respiratory inductance plethysmography (RIP) belts (calibrated or uncalibrated) for monitoring respiratory effort. During a PAP titration study, the PAP device flow signal and dual RIP belts are recommended. Esophageal manometry is also a recommended technique for monitoring respiratory effort; however, it is rarely used today because it is an invasive measure.

Several alternate sensors are either recommended or acceptable if the primary sensors are not functioning properly. Recommended alternative flow measures for identification of apnea include a nasal pressure transducer (with or without square root transformation) or the RIP sum or RIP flow signal derived from calibrated or uncalibrated RIP belts. The polyvinylidene fluoride (PVDF) sum signal derived from PVDF belts is considered an acceptable alternative flow measure. An acceptable alternative respiratory effort measure is dual thoracoabdominal PVDF belts.

Identifying Hypopnea

During a diagnostic study, the nasal pressure transducer (with or without square root transformation of the signal) is the recommended sensor for monitoring airflow. Dual RIP belts (calibrated or uncalibrated) are recommended for monitoring respiratory effort. During a PAP titration study, the PAP device flow signal and dual RIP belts are recommended (1). The recommended alternative measures, if the nasal pressure transducer fails, are the oronasal thermal airflow sensor and the RIP sum or RIP flow signal from dual thoracoabdominal belts (calibrated or uncalibrated). An acceptable alternative for respiratory effort measurement is dual thoracoabdominal PVDF belts, and for monitoring airflow the PVDF sum (1).

Additional Respiratory Event Monitors

Oxygen saturation is an essential measure for determining oxygenation during sleep as well as for scoring hypopnea. Pulse oximetry with a signal averaging time of less than or equal to 3 seconds at a heart rate of 80 bpm is recommended. Monitoring snoring assists in the determination of respiratory event type and should be accomplished using an acoustic sensor (microphone), a piezoelectric sensor, or a nasal pressure transducer. A measure of carbon dioxide levels is essential for the detection of hypoventilation. During a diagnostic study end-tidal or transcutaneous PCO_2 may be used for this purpose. During a PAP titration, transcutaneous PCO_2 is recommended (1). Arterial PCO_2 measurement is a recommended alternative for use during a PAP titration study, but is rarely used because this is an invasive measure.

There are four primary parameters to consider for scoring respiratory events, usually performed during the second pass of the diagnostic portion of a sleep study: the thermal channel, the nasal pressure transducer, the two respiratory effort channels (chest and abdomen), and the oximetry channel. There is a fifth channel that may be useful for scoring hypopneas and respiratory event–related arousals (RERAs): the EEG channel used for scoring arousals. The thermal channel and pressure transducer channel are replaced by the PAP machine–generated flow channel during PAP titrations. If hypoventilation is scored, a measure of PCO_2 must also be recorded. Of note, with subsequent versions of the scoring manual there has been an addition of PVDF belts as an acceptable alternative to esophageal manometry and RIP belts.

Any respiratory event requires the event to meet certain duration criterion to be scored. The 2007 version of the manual had a problematic rule for determining the duration of a respiratory event that was updated in version 2 (11).

Currently, the AASM Scoring Manual indicates that event duration should be measured from the nadir preceding the first breath that is clearly reduced to the beginning of the first breath that approximates the baseline breathing amplitude (1). The question of what we consider baseline breathing and what is considered clearly reduced is one that may pose problems in the actual practice of scoring respiratory events. The AASM Scoring Manual indicates when baseline breathing amplitude is difficult to determine, events can be determined to have ended when either there is a sustained increase in breathing amplitude or, with events associated with oxygen desaturation, the oximetry channel indicates a resaturation of at least 2% (1).

The recommended or alternate sensors for monitoring apnea must be used to determine event duration: preferably the oronasal thermal sensor signal for a diagnostic study or the PAP device flow signal for a PAP titration study. For hypopnea, the nasal pressure signal (diagnostic study) or PAP device flow signal (PAP titration study) should be used to determine event duration (1).

In adults, duration must be 10 seconds at minimum to score a respiratory event.

Scoring an Apnea

An apnea is scored when an almost complete absence of airflow (at least a 90% drop in amplitude) is seen on the thermal or PAP flow sensor. If the period of decreased amplitude lasts at least 10 seconds, then an apnea should be scored (1). Although a physiologic consequence such as a desaturation or arousal is often seen after an apnea, no such consequence is needed to score an apnea.

An apnea must be categorized in one of three ways: obstructive (Figs. 38-19 and 38-20), mixed (Fig. 38-21), or central (Fig. 38-22). The AASM Scoring Manual describes the categories as given here:

Obstructive—"meets apnea criteria and is associated with continued or increased inspiratory effort throughout the entire period of absent airflow" (1). Most apneas that we score are of the obstructive type.

Central—"meets apnea criteria and is associated with absent inspiratory effort throughout the entire period of absent airflow" (1). Central apneas are seen less frequently than obstructive events.

Mixed—"meets the apnea criteria and is associated with absent inspiratory effort in the initial portion of the event, followed by resumption of inspiratory effort in the second portion of the event" (1). Mixed apneas are generally considered to be obstructive events in terms of treatment decisions.

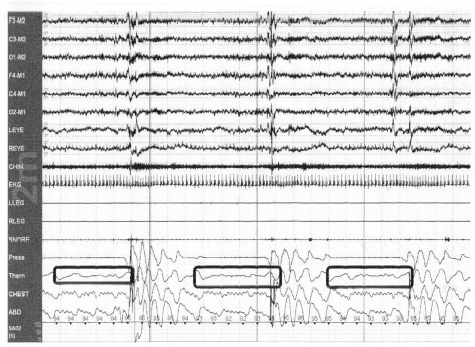

Figure 38-19 Three obstructive apneas in a 58-year-old female. Note the paradoxical breathing during the obstructive events.

The apnea requires an almost complete cessation of airflow to be scoring. Events that have a smaller decrease in airflow are scored as hypopneas. The definition of hypopnea has undergone several changes from the 2007 version of the manual. These changes primarily were related to the definitions of the recommended and alternative hypopnea rules. Today, the recommended rule allows scoring a hypopnea on the basis of a *greater than 30% reduction in the flow signal lasting at least 10 seconds accompanied by either a 3% oxygen desaturation or an arousal. The alternative rule (required by Medicare and some insurers) requires a 4% oxygen desaturation and does not allow scoring a hypopnea on the basis of an arousal.* An additional change allows the clinician or investigator to

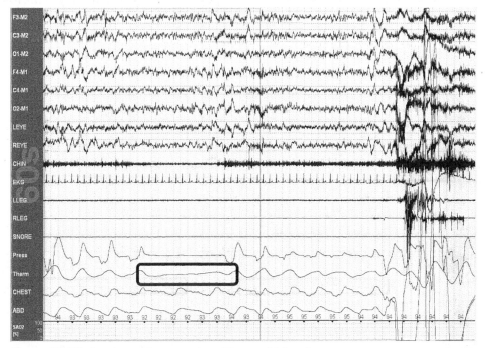

Figure 38-20 An obstructive apnea in a 59-year-old female.

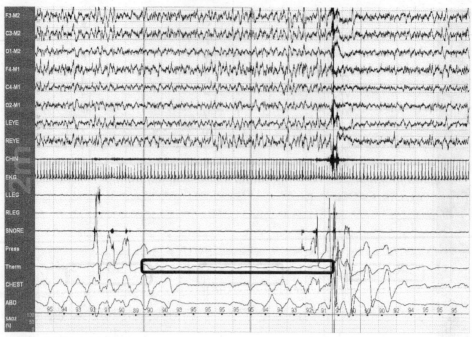

Figure 38-21 A mixed apnea in a 67-year-old male.

further define hypopneas as either obstructive or central. The reader is encouraged to review the article by Berry and colleagues that explains these changes in detail (11).

Scoring a Hypopnea

Hypopneas are scored when at least a 30% reduction of airflow is seen in the nasal pressure signal (or PAP flow for a PAP titration) with a duration of at least 10 seconds. Unlike apnea, the scoring of hypopneas requires

a physiologic consequence. Thus, scoring hypopneas requires a 3% desaturation or an arousal (Fig. 38-23) or a 4% desaturation using the alternate scoring rule (Fig. 38-24) (1).

Hypopneas may be further differentiated as either *obstructive* or *central* at the discretion of the medical director of the sleep center. If electing to categorize hypopneas as *obstructive* or *central*, the presence or absence of three features determines this categorization. *Obstructive* hypopneas may be scored if any of the following features

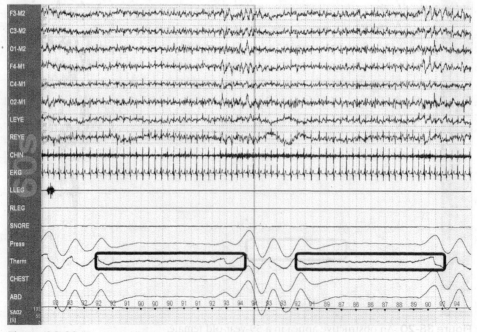

Figure 38-22 Two central apneas in a 60-second epoch in a 45-year-old male.

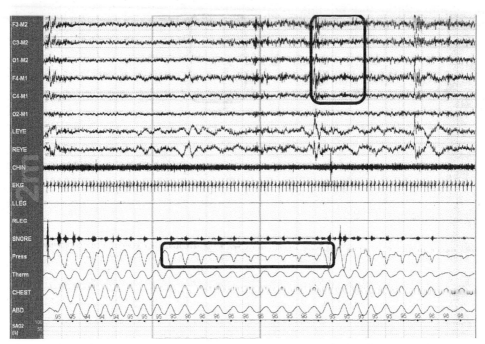

Figure 38-23 A 2-minute epoch displaying a hypopnea associated with an arousal in a 29-year-old male.

are seen: snoring during the event, increased inspiratory flattening during the event, or thoracoabdominal paradoxic respiratory motion during the event. If one or more of these features are seen, then the event should be scored as *obstructive*. Only if *none* of these three features are seen may a *central* hypopnea be scored (1).

Scoring Respiratory Effort–Related Arousal

There are events that do not meet the criteria for either of the hypopnea rules or criteria to be scored as an apnea. These events are known as RERAs (Fig. 38-25).

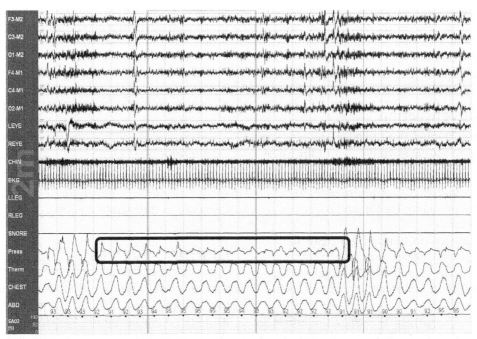

Figure 38-24 A 2-minute epoch displaying a hypopnea with 4% desaturation.

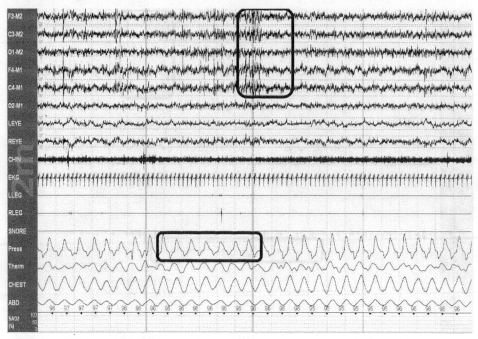

Figure 38-25 A 2-minute epoch displaying a respiratory event–related arousal in a 24-year-old male.

The RERA always causes an arousal. The AASM Scoring Manual criteria for scoring a RERA requires a sequence of breaths showing increasing respiratory effort or flattening of the inspiratory portion of the nasal pressure (diagnostic study) or PAP flow (PAP titration) waveform that leads to an arousal (1).

Earlier versions of the manual specifically indicated the preferred method for monitoring respiratory effort when scoring RERAs was esophageal pressure monitoring; however, RERAs are commonly scored on the basis of pressure transducer signal in clinical practice and thus the current version of the manual mentions nasal pressure and PAP flow as adequate for scoring RERAs.

Scoring Hypoventilation

The AASM Scoring Manual also provides a rule for scoring hypoventilation during sleep if either of the following occurs:

a. Increase in the arterial PCO_2 (or surrogate) to a value greater than 55 mm Hg for greater than or equal to 10 minutes
b. Greater than or equal to 10 mm Hg increase in arterial PCO_2 (or surrogate) during sleep (in comparison to an awake supine value) to a value exceeding 50 mm Hg for greater than or equal to 10 minutes (1).

The reader is encouraged to review the article by Berry and colleagues that discusses monitoring hypoventilation in more detail (11).

Scoring Cheyne–Stokes Breathing

Scoring Cheyne–Stokes breathing requires meeting two specific criteria. This breathing pattern includes changes in breathing amplitude that follow a crescendo/decrescendo pattern and repetitive central apneas or hypopneas. Both of the following criteria are required to score Cheyne–Stokes breathing:

a. There are episodes of greater than or equal to three consecutive central apneas and/or central hypopneas separated by a crescendo and decrescendo change in breathing amplitude with a cycle length of greater than or equal to 40 seconds.
b. There are greater than or equal to five central apneas and/or central hypopneas per hour of sleep associated with the crescendo/decrescendo breathing pattern recorded over greater than or equal to 2 hours of monitoring (1).

Note that central apneas that meet duration criteria and occur during Cheyne–Stokes breathing must also be scored as independent events.

CARDIAC EVENTS

Scoring cardiac events is done on the basis of a single two-lead ECG signal. This signal is derived using a modified lead II placement of ECG electrodes, meaning that one electrode is placed on the right side of the patient's chest between the nipple and the clavicle bone and the second electrode on the left side of the patient near the bottom of the rib cage.

The AASM Scoring Manual outlines six rules of cardiac events that must be scored during sleep in adults:

1. Score sinus tachycardia with a sustained sinus heart rate of greater than 90 bpm.
2. Score bradycardia with a sustained heart rate of less than 40 bpm.
3. Score asystole for cardiac pauses greater than 3 seconds.
4. Score wide complex tachycardia for a rhythm lasting a minimum of three consecutive beats at a rate greater than 100 per minute with QRS duration of greater than or equal to 120 ms.
5. Score narrow complex tachycardia for a rhythm lasting a minimum of three consecutive beats at a rate greater than 100 per minute with a QRS duration of less than 120 ms.
6. Score atrial fibrillation if there are irregularly irregular QRS complexes associated with replacement of consistent P waves by rapid oscillations that vary in size, shape, and timing (1).

SCORING MOVEMENTS

The movements most commonly scored in sleep are limb movements (LMs) (Fig. 38-26). Limb movement EMG is monitored using surface electrodes on specific muscles. The technical guidelines for the recording of limb movements outlined in the AASM Scoring Manual must be utilized to accurately score LMs. For limb movements, the anterior tibialis muscle on both legs is always monitored. Additional upper extremity monitoring for limb movement activity is optional.

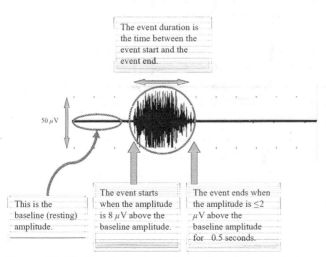

Figure 38-26 Duration criteria for the LMs from the *AASM Manual for the Scoring of Sleep and Associated Events.*

The AASM Scoring Manual has defined a significant LM event as an 8 μV increase in EMG voltage above resting EMG with a duration of 0.5 to 10 seconds. The onset of an LM is defined as the point at which there is an 8 μV increase in EMG voltage above the resting EMG, and the end of the LM event is defined as the start of a period lasting at least 0.5 seconds during which the EMG does not exceed 2 μV above resting EMG (1).

Limb movements are scored either as isolated (in which case they are simply marked) or as a part of a series. The rules that define a periodic limb movement (PLM; Fig. 38-27) series indicate there must be at least four consecutive LM events with at least 5 seconds no more than 90 seconds between onset of the events. LMs on different limbs separated by less than 5 seconds between onsets are counted as a single LM (1). Note that PLMs that occur during an epoch of wake (stage W) are not counted as part of the series. However, it is important to also note that if the onset of the next scorable LM in the series occurs in an epoch staged as sleep and onset of the two events in sleep epochs on either side of the wake epoch is less than 90 seconds, the PLM series continues uninterrupted.

Arousals may be associated with LMs. When an arousal occurs simultaneously with or overlaps with the LM, or there is less than 0.5 seconds between the LM and the arousal, they are considered to be associated (1). LMs are typically scored with and without arousals. Scoring of LMs is also affected by the presence of respiratory events. For this reason, respiratory events should be scored before LM scoring.

An LM should not be scored if it occurs within 0.5 seconds preceding or following an apnea, hypopnea, or RERA.

There are several additional movement events that can be scored and reported. Alternating leg muscle activation (ALMA), hypnagogic foot tremor (HFT), and excessive fragmentary myoclonus are optionally reported. Both ALMA and HFT are benign postarousal occurrences, and thus are considered to be polysomnographic findings.

Bruxism

Bruxism is monitored using chin EMG and, if suspected, additional masseter muscle EMG. Bruxism in sleep (Fig. 38-28) is scored when brief (phasic) or sustained (tonic) elevations of chin EMG activity at least twice the amplitude of background EMG are seen. Phasic chin EMG activity of 0.25 to 2 seconds in duration is scored as bruxism when at least three episodes occur in a regular sequence. Tonic (sustained) chin EMG activity of greater than 2 seconds is also scored. To score a new episode of bruxism, either tonic or sustained, there must be at least 3 seconds of steady baseline chin EMG before scoring a new episode. It is important to note that bruxism can

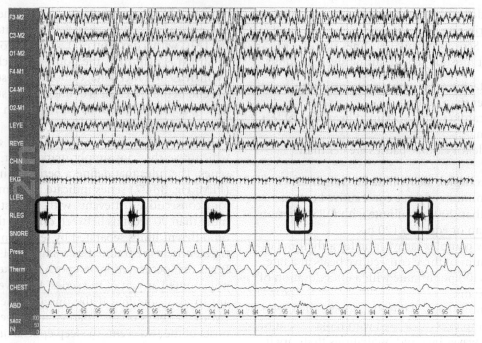

Figure 38-27 A periodic limb movement series in a 43-year-old female.

also be scored on the basis of audible tooth-grinding episodes. Specifically, there must be a minimum of two audible tooth-grinding episodes in the absence of epilepsy to audibly score bruxism (1).

REM Sleep Behavior Disorder

To score REM sleep behavior disorder (RBD), a time-locked video with recorded sound is essential to record dream enactment episodes occurring during REM

sleep. Absent the occurrence of an episode during the polysomnography, demonstration of REM sleep without atonia is required. Scoring rules for RBD require identification of sustained tonic muscle activity and/or excessive transient muscle activity (phasic muscle activity) in REM sleep. To score tonic activity in REM sleep, 50% of the REM epoch must have chin EMG activity of an amplitude greater than that seen during NREM sleep. To score transient muscle activity, 30-second epochs of REM sleep are divided into 10 sequential 3-second mini

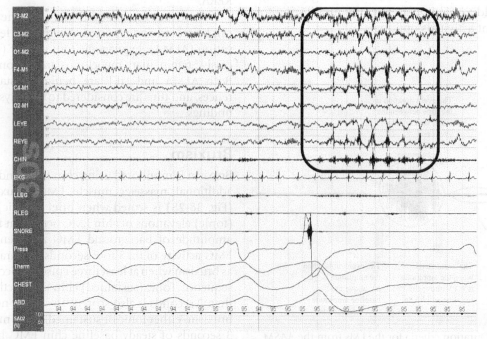

Figure 38-28 A 30-second epoch that displays bruxism.

epochs. To score RBD in an epoch of REM thus divided, at least five of the mini epochs (50% of the 30-second epoch) must contain transient muscle activity bursts 0.1 to 5 seconds in duration and at least four times as high in amplitude as the background EMG activity (1).

Rhythmic Movement Disorder

To record the movements associated with rhythmic movement disorder, a pair of electrodes are placed on the neck paraspinal muscles and referenced to each other in a bipolar montage. Scoring is based on evaluating movements recorded in this montage as follows:

Movements must have a minimum frequency of 0.5 Hz and a maximum frequency of 2 Hz. A cluster of rhythmic movements is identified as a minimum of four movements. The amplitude of the individual rhythmic bursts must be at least two times the background EMG activity to score rhythmic movements (1).

CONCLUSION

Scoring a PSG involves learning the rules outlined in the current version of the AASM Scoring Manual and reviewing as many PSGs as possible with an experienced scorer. It takes most people new to scoring about 2 weeks to become minimally proficient at scoring sleep stages and events. It takes frequent scoring practice to become an expert. The first time we score a record, we are tempted to try and get everything right, and this is a good instinct. There is an old saying in sleep though, "don't take as much time to score a record as it did to record it." So, make a decision about each epoch and move on, making a note of questionable epochs to be reviewed later with a more experienced scorer.

The AASM's ISR program is an online resource that allows scorers to score a common sample of PSG recording and compare their scores to a gold standard panel as well as other scorers who participate in the ISR program. In addition to participation in an ISR program being an AASM accreditation requirement, it is a convenient way to receive expert feedback on one's scoring. This is a valuable resource to the novice and expert scorer alike.

SUGGESTED READING

American Academy of Sleep Medicine. (2009). *A technologist's handbook for understanding and implementing the AASM manual for the scoring of sleep and associated events: Rules, terminology, and technical specifications.* Westchester, IL: Author.

REFERENCES

1. Berry, R. B., Albertario, C. L., & Harding, S. M. (2018). *The AASM manual for the scoring of sleep and associated events: Rules, terminology and technical specifications* [Version 2.5]. Darien, IL: American Academy of Sleep Medicine.
2. Silber, M. H., Ancoli-Israel, S., Bonnet, M. H., et al. (2007). The visual scoring of sleep in adults. *Journal of Clinical Sleep Medicine, 3*(2), 121–131.
3. Williams, R. L., Karacan, I., & Hirsch, C. J. (Eds.). (1974). *Electroencephalography (EEG) of human sleep: Clinical applications.* New York, NY: John Wiley & Sons.
4. Himanen, S. L., & Hasan, J. (2000). Limitations of Rechtschaffen and Kales. *Sleep Medicine Review, 4*(2), 149–167.
5. Webb, W. B. (1986). Recording methods and visual scoring criteria of sleep records: Comments and recommendations. *Perception and Motor Skills, 62,* 664–666.
6. American Sleep Disorders Association. (1992). EEG arousals: Scoring rules and examples: A preliminary report from the Sleep Disorders Atlas Task Force of the American Sleep Disorders Association. *Sleep, 15*(2), 173–184.
7. American Academy of Sleep Medicine Task Force. (1999). Sleep-related breathing disorders in adults: Recommendations for syndrome definition and measurement techniques in clinical research. *Sleep, 22*(5), 667–689.
8. Atlas Task Force. (1993). Recording and scoring leg movements. *Sleep, 16*(8), 748–759.
9. Anders, T., Emde, R., & Parmelee, A. (1971). *A manual of standardization terminology, techniques and criteria for scoring states of sleep and wakefulness in newborn infants.* Los Angeles, CA: UCLA Brain Information Service, NINDS Neurological information Network.
10. A glossary of terms most commonly used by clinical electroencephalographers. (1974). *Electroencephalography and Clinical Neurophysiology, 37*(5), 538–548.
11. Berry, R. B., Budhiraja, R., Gottlieb, D. J., et al. (2012). Rules for scoring respiratory events in sleep update of the 2007 *AASM manual for the scoring of sleep and associated events.* Deliberations of the Sleep Apnea Definitions Task Force of the American Academy of Sleep Medicine. *Journal of Clinical Sleep Medicine, 8*(5), 597–619.

chapter 39

Scoring Respiratory Events

LAREE J. FORDYCE

LEARNING OBJECTIVES

On completion of this chapter, the reader should be able to:

1. Identify sleep-related breathing events according to the American Academy of Sleep Medicine adult respiratory scoring rules.
2. Define the various types of sleep-related breathing events.
3. Identify common artifacts that occur in the respiratory channels.

KEY TERMS

Obstructive apnea
Mixed apnea
Central apnea
Hypopnea
Respiratory artifact
Respiratory event–related arousal (RERA)
Hypoventilation

Scoring respiratory events is an important part of our jobs as sleep technologists. The *AASM Manual for the Scoring of Sleep and Associated Events* has outlined the respiratory scoring rules for both adults and pediatrics. In this chapter, we review the respiratory scoring rules in adults as well as show examples to illustrate respiratory events and how these events should be scored.

The current Parameters to Be Recorded as well as the Technical Specifications for Respiratory Rules for both adults and pediatrics are outlined in the *AASM Manual for the Scoring of Sleep and Associated Events* and should be reviewed to ensure collection of data meets these standards (1).

When scoring respiratory events, it is important to record the proper signals using the appropriate sensors (1). We should be recording airflow using an oronasal thermal sensor (this includes thermistors, thermocouples, or polyvinylidene fluoride airflow sensors) or a nasal pressure transducer. For respiratory effort channels, thoracic and abdominal respiratory inductance plethysmography (RIP) belts are recommended. The RIPsum and RIPflow channels can be a helpful tool for scoring respiratory events. See Figure 39-1 for an example of a normal respiratory pattern.

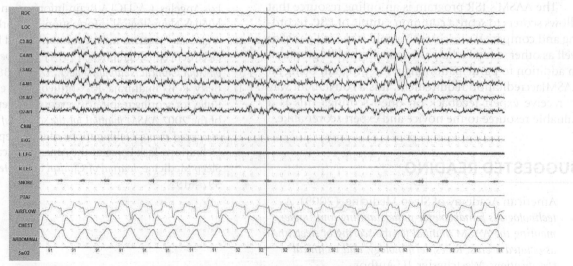

Figure 39-1 Normal respiratory pattern.

APNEA

An apnea should be scored using the oronasal thermal airflow sensor; however, alternatives such as a nasal transducer, RIPsum, or RIPflow may be used if this sensor is not functioning. When performing a positive airway pressure (PAP) titration study, use the PAP device flow signal to score apneas. There are three types of apneas: obstructive, central, and mixed.

Obstructive Apnea

1. An obstructive apnea (see Fig. 39-2A, B) is defined as cessation of airflow (drop in signal by ≥90% of the preevent baseline using an oronasal thermal airflow sensor) with continued respiratory effort throughout the event.
2. The duration of the event is greater than or equal to 10 seconds.

Central Apnea

1. A central apnea (see Fig. 39-3A, B) is defined as cessation of airflow (drop in signal by ≥90% of the preevent baseline using an oronasal thermal airflow sensor) with absent respiratory effort throughout the entire event.
2. The duration of the event is greater than or equal to 10 seconds.

Mixed Apnea

1. A mixed apnea (see Fig. 39-4A, B) is defined as cessation of airflow (drop in signal by ≥90% of the preevent baseline using an oronasal thermal airflow sensor) for at least 10 seconds, with resumption of respiratory effort in the second part of the event.
2. The duration of the event is greater than or equal to 10 seconds.

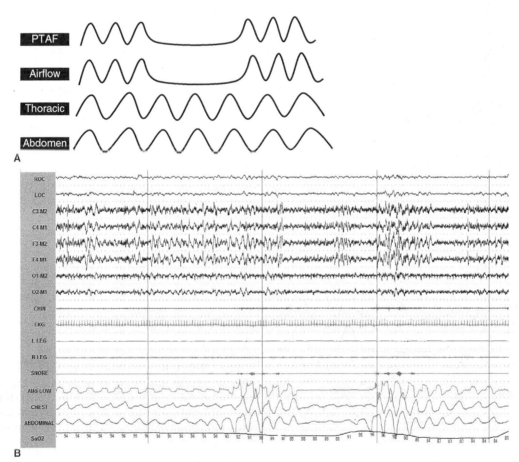

Figure 39-2 A, B: Obstructive apnea. PTAF, pressure transducer airflow.

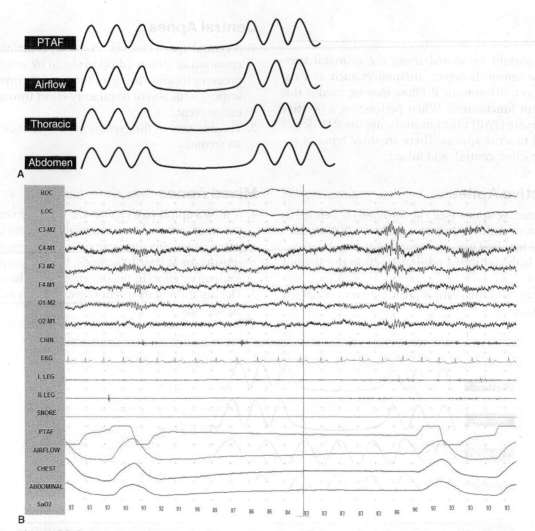

Figure 39-3 A, B: Central apnea. In this example, the airflow as well as the respiratory effort is completely absent. PTAF, pressure transducer airflow.

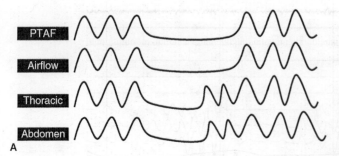

Figure 39-4 A, B: Mixed apnea. The airflow stops completely and does not resume until the end of the event. At the beginning of the event, there is no effort; then effort resumes before the end of the event. Most often, a snore event is seen with resumption of airflow. PTAF, pressure transducer airflow.

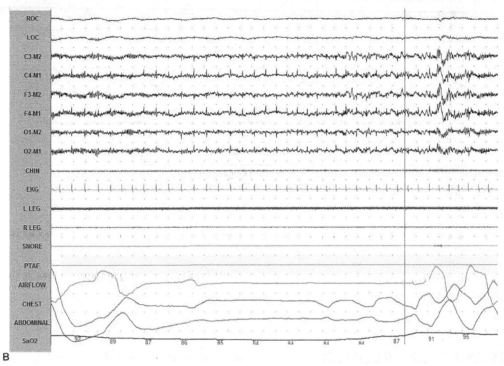

B

Figure 39-4 (*Continued*)

HYPOPNEA

A hypopnea (see Fig. 39-5A, B) should be scored using a nasal pressure transducer; however, alternatives such as an oronasal thermal airflow sensor, RIPsum, or RIPflow may be used if this sensor is not functioning. When performing a PAP titration study, use the PAP device flow signal to score a hypopnea.

There are two rules that can be used to score hypopnea. It is important that your report specifies which scoring rule you have used to score hypopnea.

Hypopnea Rule 1A

1. A hypopnea is defined as a decrease in airflow (drop in signal by ≥30% of the preevent baseline using a nasal pressure transducer) with continued respiratory effort throughout the event.

2. The duration of the event is greater than or equal to 10 seconds.

3. The event is associated with either a greater than or equal to 3% oxygen desaturation (from preevent baseline) or an arousal. See Figure 39-6 for an example of a hypopnea with an arousal.

Hypopnea Rule 1B

1. A hypopnea is defined as a decrease in airflow (drop in signal by ≥30% of the preevent baseline using a nasal pressure transducer) with continued respiratory effort throughout the event.

2. The duration of the event is greater than or equal to 10 seconds.

3. The event is associated with a greater than or equal to 4% oxygen desaturation (from preevent baseline). An example of a hypopnea scored on the basis of an arousal is seen in Figure 39-7.

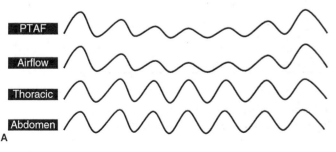

A

Figure 39-5 A: Hypopnea. B: A hypopnea scored using rule 1A with greater than 3% desaturation. There is at least a 30% reduction in the flow channel. The event lasts a minimum of 10 seconds and is accompanied by at least a 3% decrease in oxygen saturation. PTAF, pressure transducer airflow.

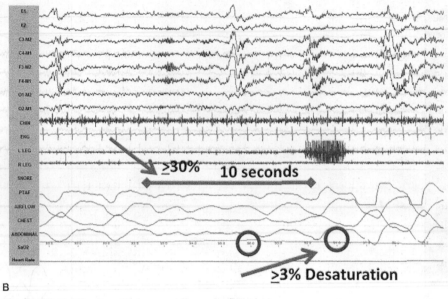

B

Figure 39-5 (*Continued*)

RESPIRATORY EFFORT–RELATED AROUSAL

Scoring respiratory effort–related arousals (RERAs) is optional, as noted in the AASM scoring manual, Parameters to Be Reported.

A RERA is scored when an event that does not meet the criteria to be scored as an apnea or hypopnea occurs, and yet leads to an arousal from sleep. A RERA should be scored if the event is greater than or equal to 10 seconds in duration. The event is characterized by increasing respiratory effort or by flattening of the inspiratory portion of the nasal pressure (diagnostic study) or PAP device flow (titration study) waveform followed by an arousal. An example of a RERA is seen in Figure 39-8.

HYPOVENTILATION

Monitoring hypoventilation in adults is optional, as noted in the AASM scoring manual, Parameters to Be Reported. To score hypoventilation in sleep requires monitoring a measure of CO_2 (see Fig. 39-9).

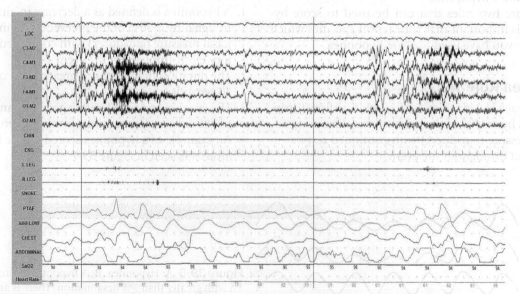

Figure 39-6 A hypopnea with arousal scored using rule 1A. There is at least a 30% reduction in the flow channel. The event lasts a minimum of 10 seconds. There is no oxygen desaturation, but there is an arousal associated with the event.

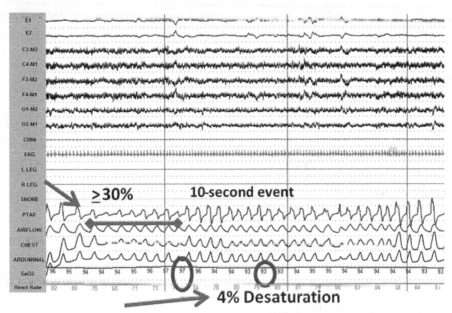

Figure 39-7 A hypopnea scored using rule 1B. There is at least a greater than or equal to 30% decrease in airflow using PTAF. The event lasts at least 10 seconds and there is an associated 4% oxygen desaturation.

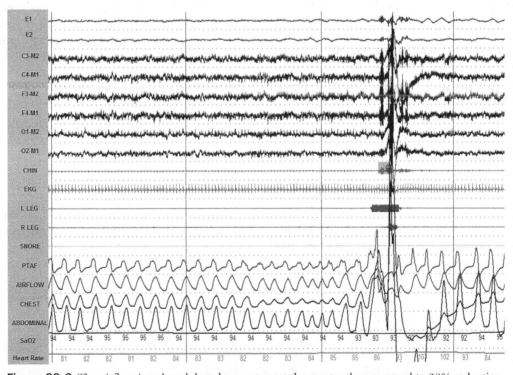

Figure 39-8 The airflow is reduced, but does not meet the greater than or equal to 30% reduction required to score a hypopnea. There is no desaturation. The event does, however, lead to an arousal and can be scored as a respiratory event–related arousal.

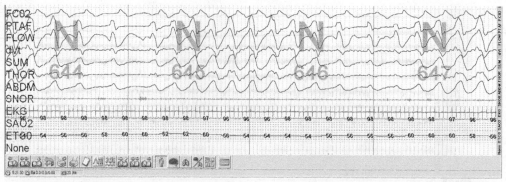

Figure 39-9 Hypoventilation identified in this recording by consistent high levels of CO_2 in the end-tidal CO_2 channel and the absence of discrete scorable events.

Hypoventilation is scored when either of the following occurs:

1. There is an increase in the arterial PCO_2 (or surrogate) to a value greater than 55 mm Hg for more than or equal to 10 minutes.
2. There is greater than or equal to 10 mm Hg increase in arterial PCO_2 (or surrogate) during sleep (in comparison to an awake value) to a value exceeding 50 mm Hg for greater than or equal to 10 minutes (1).

CHEYNE–STOKES RESPIRATION

We often see patients with Cheyne–Stokes respiration (CSR) who have other medical conditions such as heart failure, atrial fibrillation, or stroke. The pattern of CSR can be easily identified (see Fig. 39-10 for a classic example). Cheyne–Stokes breathing can be scored when there are episodes of greater than or equal to three consecutive central apneas and/or central hypopneas separated by a crescendo and decrescendo change in breathing amplitude with a cycle length of greater than or equal to 40 seconds. This looks like pearls on a string. Cheyne–Stokes breathing can also be scored when there are greater than or equal to five central apneas and/or central hypopneas per hour of sleep associated with

a crescendo and decrescendo breathing pattern over greater than or equal to 2 hours of monitoring (1).

RESPIRATORY ARTIFACTS

When recording and scoring respiratory events, it is important to ensure that the signals recorded are accurate and appropriate for scoring the type of event occurring in the recording. As mentioned earlier, thermal sensors, pressure transducer cannulas, and effort sensors are used to differentiate between apneas and hypopneas. If any of these signals are not working properly, other channels can be substituted to identify respiratory events. However, if there are few working signals or if there is artifact in the respiratory channels, it can be difficult to identify and score the correct respiratory events. See Figures 39-11 and 39-12 for examples of common respiratory artifacts.

SUMMARY

Scoring respiratory events can be challenging. Clinical examples of challenging events are not as clean as textbook examples. Figure 39-13 is another example of an obstructive apnea. Figure 39-14 shows a mixed apnea, and Figure 39-15 a hypopnea. It is essential to record

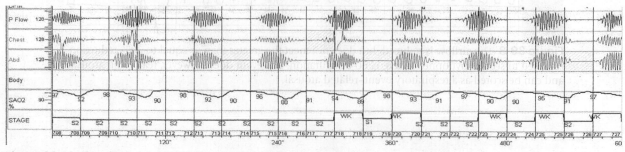

Figure 39-10 A sample of classic Cheyne–Stokes respiration over a period of 10 minutes.

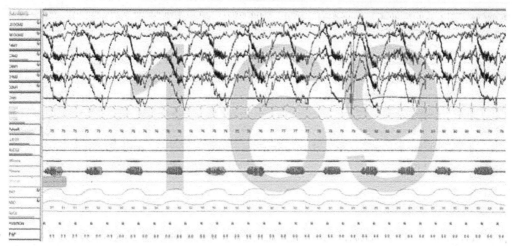

Figure 39-11 Respiratory artifact in the electroencephalogram can be mistaken for sweat artifact or a poor reference or ground electrode. Identifying the correct cause of artifact enables the technologist to fix the problem.

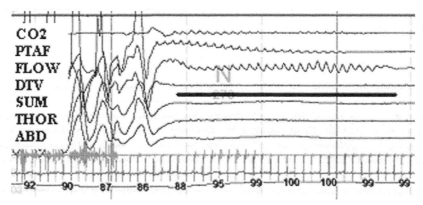

Figure 39-12 Cardioballistic artifact in the respiratory channels can be mistaken for respiratory effort or airflow. The ability to identify artifact in the respiratory channels enables correct scoring of the respiratory event—in this case, a central apnea.

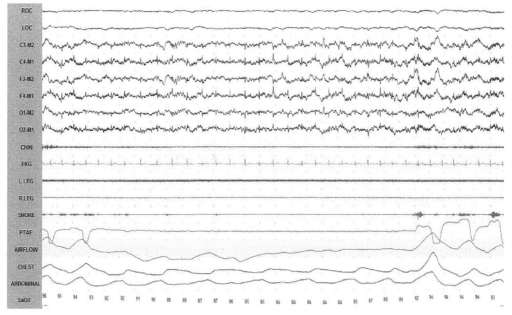

Figure 39-13 Obstructive apnea.

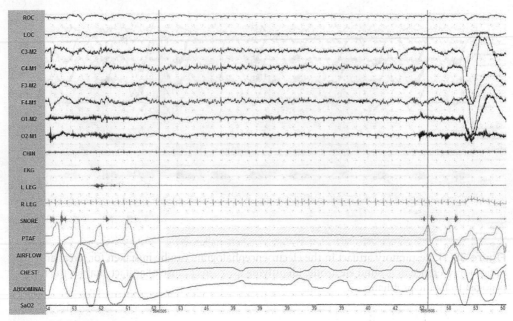

Figure 39-14 Mixed apnea.

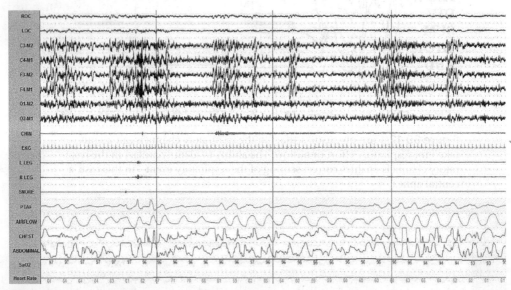

Figure 39-15 Hypopnea.

the appropriate signals to identify the various defined respiratory events and score them according to accepted AASM scoring rules. The *AASM Manual for the Scoring of Sleep and Associated Events* outlines the appropriate parameters and sensors to utilize for collection of data as well as respiratory event scoring rules and examples that can assist in the scoring process (1). The wise technologist will keep a scoring manual handy!

REFERENCE

1. Berry, R. B., Albertario, C. L., Harding, S. M., et al.; for the American Academy of Sleep Medicine. (2018). *The AASM manual for the scoring of sleep and associated events: Rules, terminology and technical specifications* [Version 2.5]. Darien, IL: American Academy of Sleep Medicine.

chapter 40
Understanding Cardiac Arrhythmias

JON W. ATKINSON

LEARNING OBJECTIVES

On completion of this chapter, the reader should be able to:

1. State the reporting guidelines of the American Academy of Sleep Medicine (AASM).
2. Describe normal electrocardiogram parameters.
3. Understand systematic arrhythmia analysis steps.
4. Explain the rule of differing morphology.
5. Use the algorithm for the AASM reporting of cardiac arrhythmias.
6. Understand polysomnographic monitoring and recording techniques.

KEY TERMS

Normal sinus rhythm
Sinus bradycardia
Accelerated junctional and ventricular rhythms
Atrial, junctional, and ventricular tachycardias
First-, second-, and third-degree AV block
Atrial and ventricular fibrillation
Atrial and ventricular flutter

THE AMERICAN ACADEMY OF SLEEP MEDICINE MONITORING AND REPORTING GUIDELINES

In 2007, shortly after the first edition of *Fundamentals of Sleep Technology* was published, the American Academy of Sleep Medicine (AASM) published *The AASM Manual for the Scoring of Sleep and Associated Events: Rules, Terminology and Technical Specifications* (1). This manual contains information about the technical aspects of recording the electrocardiogram (ECG) as well as recommendations for reporting abnormal cardiac events. Little change in the cardiac section of the scoring manual has occurred through the different versions, including the latest version 2.5 (2) except a slight revision of the definition of atrial fibrillation.

Technical Considerations

The AASM manual provides the following technical specifications for the recording of ECG during polysomnography:

1. The sampling rate should be 500 Hz desirable, 200 Hz minimum, with a digital resolution of 12 bits per sample.
2. The maximum electrode impedance for ECG is not specifically stated; however, 5 kΩ is appropriate.
3. Recommended low-frequency filter is 0.3 Hz and high-frequency filter 70 Hz.
4. The recommended recording derivation is a modified lead II with the right shoulder negative and the left lower torso positive.

Notes provided suggest that the recommended filters may be prone to various artifacts such as movement, perspiration, and muscle. Employing standard ECG electrodes instead of electroencephalogram (EEG) electrodes may make these problems less likely to occur. Additional ECG electrodes may be placed at the discretion of the practitioner.

Scoring Rules

The AASM manual recommends indicating the presence of the arrhythmias listed in the next paragraph, which should be acknowledged by responding "yes" if they occur and providing the heart rate (HR) or the duration of the pause.

1. Sinus tachycardia (ST) during sleep for sustained (>30 seconds duration) sinus HR greater than 90 bpm for adults
   - Report (yes/no); report highest HR observed
2. Bradycardia during sleep for sustained HR of less than 40, ages 6 through adult
   - Report (yes/no); report lowest HR observed (defined as HR <40 bpm)
3. Asystole for pauses greater than 3 seconds duration for ages 6 through adult
   - Report (yes/no); report longest event
4. Wide complex tachycardia for a rhythm of 3 or more consecutive beats at a rate greater than 100 bpm with a QRS duration of more than or equal to 0.12 seconds
   - Report (yes/no); report highest HR observed

5. Narrow complex tachycardia for a rhythm of 3 or more consecutive beats at a rate greater than 100 bpm with a QRS duration of less than 0.12 seconds

   • Report (yes/no); report highest HR observed

6. Atrial fibrillation for an irregularly irregular ventricular rhythm where the normal, consistent P waves have been replaced by rapid oscillations of varying timing, size, and shape

   • Report (yes/no)

The notes in the cardiac scoring section of the manual state that significant arrhythmias should be reported if the single lead recorded is sufficient for accurate scoring. This would include type II and type III atrioventricular (AV) blocks, escape rhythms, atrial flutter, and so on. Ectopic beats should also be reported if deemed clinically significant. Included in this group are frequent premature ventricular contractions (PVCs), patterned PVCs, ventricular couplets, and frequent atrial or junctional extrasystoles. These events may be reported similar to the aforementioned:

7. Other arrhythmias (yes/no); report the arrhythmia (such as heart block or significant ectopy)

ANATOMY AND PATHWAYS

This portion of the chapter is reproduced with modification from Atkinson JW, with permission (3). There are numerous other excellent resources for arrhythmia interpretation (4–6).

Arrhythmia recognition and identification is a fairly logical process that is based on a good working knowledge of the anatomy and pathways of the conduction system of the heart. Within the myocardium, there are areas of specialized tissue that have the primary function of generating electrical impulses or transmitting these impulses to other areas of the conduction system and finally to the cardiac muscle mass. The main areas of interest are the sinoatrial (SA) node, the AV node, the AV bundle or bundle of His, the left and right bundle branches, and the Purkinje system (fibers).

The normal sequence of events is as follows:

1. The cycle begins with a discharge of the SA node, which causes the atria to depolarize.
2. The AV node receives input through the internodal pathways and holds the signal for a brief period (a brief pause between atrial and ventricular depolarization that facilitates ventricular filling).
3. The impulse is passed from the AV node to the AV bundle.
4. The signal is then sent down the right and left bundles (the left bundle divides into an anterior and a posterior fascicle).

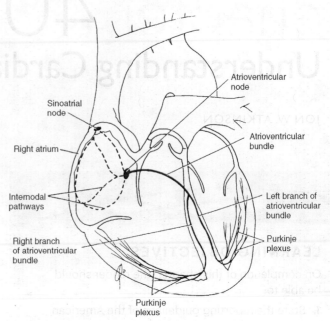

Figure 40-1 The conducting system.

5. The left and right bundles distribute the impulse through the Purkinje system to the ventricular myocardium such that all the cardiac muscles contract simultaneously as a unit.

See Figure 40-1 for a graphic illustration of the conducting system.

CARDIAC CYCLE

The cardiac cycle is the repetitive sequence of atrial depolarization, atrial repolarization, ventricular depolarization, and ventricular repolarization. The corresponding electrophysiologic events appear as the main components of the ECG. These are identified as the P wave, the QRS complex, and the T wave. Furthermore, there is a relationship between the physiology of the cardiac cycle and the waveforms and intervals of the ECG. Table 40-1 shows the physiologic event and related ECG component. Figure 40-2 shows a graphic representation of the events in Table 40-1.

NORMAL PARAMETERS

Any presentation of arrhythmias requires an understanding of the ECG in its normal state. The normal ranges for key parameters needed to diagnose arrhythmias are shown in Table 40-2.

The basis for observing and identifying arrhythmias is the normal sinus rhythm (NSR). The following samples are presented in both a 30-second window and a 10-second window for comparison.

Table 40-1	Physiologic Event and Related Electrocardiogram Component
Physiologic Event	**Electrocardiogram Waveform**
Atrial depolarization	P wave
Atrial repolarization	None seen (hidden by the timing and magnitude of the QRS complex)
Pause between atrial depolarization and ventricular depolarization	PR interval (the last portion following the P wave, PR segment)
Ventricular depolarization	QRS complex
Ventricular repolarization	T wave

Table 40-2	The Normal Adult Ranges for Key Electrocardiogram Parameters Needed to Diagnose Arrhythmias
Key Parameter	**Value Range**
Heart rate	60–100 bpm, awake 40–90 bpm, during sleep
Rhythm	Regular
PR interval	0.12–0.20 s
QRS interval	0.04–0.11 s
Sinoatrial node discharge rate	60–100/min
Atrioventricular node discharge rate	40–60/min
Ventricular discharge rate	20–40/min

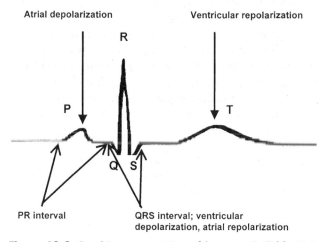

Figure 40-2 Graphic representation of the events in Table 40-1.

One of the better features of digital recordings is the ability to change time scales without changing how the recording is saved to the hard drive. For the purpose of arrhythmia analysis, it is frequently beneficial to view the ECG utilizing a 10-second screen (Fig. 40-3[1]) rather than the usual 30-second window (epoch; Fig. 40-4) used for sleep staging. This functionality demonstrates a basic concept: If you want to view rapidly occurring activities (ECG, EEG, etc.), spread the display out; if you want to view slowly occurring events (apneas, hypopneas, limb movements, etc.), compress the display.

---

[1]Record samples have been reduced to fit the format of this book. The actual appearance of the ECG on a computer screen or printout will vary according to the selected time scale, as well as the size of the active screen display.

Features of the NSR

P wave: Present, each appears the same

QRS complex: Present, each appears the same

PR interval (start of P wave to start of QRS complex). See Figure 40-2: 0.12 to 0.20 seconds

QRS interval (start of Q wave to end of S wave). See Figure 40-2: 0.04 to 0.11 seconds

P to QRS ratio: 1:1

Rhythm: Regular

Rate: 60 to 100

ARRHYTHMIA BASICS

An ECG arrhythmia occurs if there is a difference from NSR in impulse formation, impulse conduction, or both. Heart beats that originate outside of the SA node, such as other areas in the atrium, the AV node, or the ventricle, are some examples of impulse formation abnormalities. These abnormal beats will not have a sinus P wave. Abnormal beats with only conduction abnormalities will exhibit a sinus P wave but then show prolonged conduction across the AV node or through the ventricular conduction pathway. The AV blocks and bundle branch blocks are good examples of impulse conduction abnormalities. When both impulse formation and impulse conduction are affected, neither a normal sinus P wave nor a normal QRS complex is present. Any of the ventricular arrhythmias demonstrate both impulse formation and impulse conduction abnormalities. Essentially, an arrhythmia is present if the rate is too fast or too slow, the rhythm is irregular, the site of origin

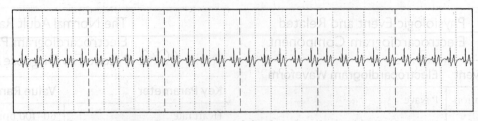

Figure 40-3 Normal sinus rhythm, 30-second display.

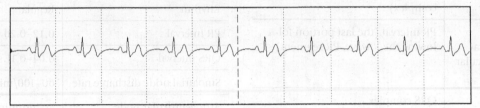

Figure 40-4 Normal sinus rhythm, 10-second display.

is abnormal, or the movement of the impulse through the conductive system is abnormal.

ARRHYTHMIA ANALYSIS

Far too often, there is the temptation to "guess" the type of arrhythmia that is presented on the polysomnogram. This section presents a systematic method to accurately analyze cardiac rhythm disturbances. If possible, a second ECG derivation should be added to the montage. This is easily accomplished unless the equipment manufacturer has only a dedicated, two-input amplifier for recording the ECG. Utilizing a second ECG channel may reveal changes in P wave or QRS complex configuration that are difficult to ascertain with a single-channel recording. When examining the ECG for detail, use a 10- or 6-second window to examine the intervals or subtle changes in morphology.

Routine use of the following methodical evaluation system will improve the accuracy of identifying arrhythmias.

Step 1. Examine the P wave.

Is the P wave absent or present? Absence of a distinct P wave would indicate that the arrhythmia is not of atrial origin (except atrial fibrillation or atrial flutter). Do the P waves all look the same (have the same morphology)? A basic concept that should be remembered is as follows: If an ECG complex starts from the same location and takes the same pathway, it will always look the same. This is the *rule of identical morphology*. The corollary to the rule of identical morphology is as follows: If the complex originates from a different location or takes a different pathway, the appearance will be different. This is the *rule of differing morphology*.

Step 2. Examine the QRS complex.

Check for absence or presence and similar appearance of the QRS complex. Absence of the QRS indicates some type of second- or third-degree AV block, or severe ventricular disturbance such as ventricular fibrillation or asystole. Differing morphologies of the QRS indicate a shift from a supraventricular origin of the abnormal beat(s) or a different pathway in the ventricle, such as bundle branch block or multifocal ventricular origin.

Step 3. Examine the P and QRS relationship.

Ask the following questions. Is there a P wave for every QRS complex? Is there a QRS complex for every P wave? Is there a 1:1 P to QRS ratio? A P to QRS ratio of more than 1 (more P waves than QRS complexes) indicates some sort of AV block. A P to QRS ratio of less than 1 (more QRS complexes than P waves) indicates a junctional or ventricular arrhythmia.

Step 4. Measure the intervals.

Is the PR interval normal, or is it too long or too short? An abbreviated PR interval may indicate a junctional beat (retrograde P wave) or an accessory pathway (such as in Wolff–Parkinson–White syndrome). A prolonged PR interval indicates that some type of AV block is occurring. Is the QRS interval normal or too long? (Seldom, if ever, will it be too short.) A widened QRS complex likely indicates bundle branch block, a beat of ventricular origin, or, in some cases, an aberrantly conducted beat of supraventricular origin (the beat originates before the ventricular conductive pathway is repolarized during the relative refractory period).

Step 5. Regular or irregular rhythm.

Examine the P–P and the R–R intervals. If the intervals are constant, the rhythm is regular. If they vary, the rhythm is irregular. Using calipers on a computer monitor is not advised, so either print the screen image and measure the intervals with calipers on paper or use something like a 3 × 5 index card. Make pencil marks corresponding to a succession of two or more P waves, while holding the card against a stationary screen display. Move the card from one set of P–P intervals to the next and see if they fall on the marks. Do the same for the R waves.

Step 6. Determine the rate.

An accurate determination of HR is obtained from the ECG. Do not rely on the readout from a pulse oximeter. Using the ECG display, HR can be determined in a variety of fashions:

Times two method: Count the number of beats in a 30-second screen display and multiply by two. This can be a bit cumbersome but is quite accurate. Make sure you do this in a frozen screen view.

Times four method: Count the number of beats in a 15-second display and multiply by four. Again, use a stationary screen.

Times six method: Count the number of beats in a 10-second display and multiply by six.

Interval method: Measure the active screen width in millimeters. If you have a 30-second window, multiply this number by two to get the number of millimeters in 60 seconds. If you are using a 10-second window, multiply the active screen width by six to obtain the number of millimeters in 60 seconds. Measure the R–R interval with a ruler and divide into the number of millimeters in 60 seconds.

COMMON ATRIAL ARRHYTHMIAS

- Premature atrial contractions (PACs)
- Sinus bradycardia (SB)
- Atrial tachycardia (AT); ST; supraventricular tachycardia (SVT)
- Sinus arrhythmia
- Sinus pause
- Paroxysmal atrial tachycardia
- Atrial fibrillation
- Atrial flutter

PREMATURE ATRIAL CONTRACTION

Features of PACs

P wave: Present, appearance of the P wave of the abnormal beat will be different (it arises from a different location)

QRS complex: Present, each appears the same

PR interval: 0.12 to 0.20 seconds, may vary slightly with the abnormal beat

QRS interval: 0.04 to 0.11 seconds

P to QRS ratio: 1:1

Rhythm: Irregular because of the premature beat; P–P will be different, so will be the R–R

Rate: 60 to 100

Comments: Note the different appearance of the P wave (origin is from a different source and travels a different pathway) at the arrows in Figures 40-5 and 40-6. There may also be subtle PR interval changes. The QRS and the T wave are normal in appearance, unless the ectopic atrial focus fires so early that it captures the ventricle, whereas the bundle branches or the Purkinje system is still relatively refractory to conduction (PAC with aberrancy).

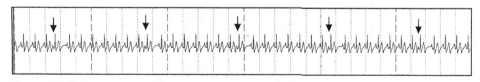

Figure 40-5 Premature atrial contraction, 30-second display.

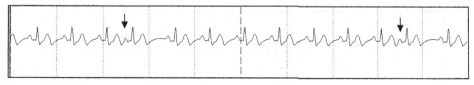

Figure 40-6 Premature atrial contraction, 10-second display.

SINUS BRADYCARDIA

Features of SB

P wave: Present, each appears the same

QRS complex: Present, each appears the same

PR interval: 0.12 to 0.20 seconds

QRS interval: 0.04 to 0.11 seconds

P to QRS ratio: 1:1

Rhythm: Regular

Rate: Less than 50, some authors say less than 60 awake. Bradycardia during sleep is regarded as a sustained HR of less than 40 bpm (1).

Comments: Sinus bradycardia (Figs. 40-7 and 40-8) looks like NSR except the rate is slower. This is not uncommon in athletic individuals and patients on beta-blockers.

ATRIAL TACHYCARDIA; SINUS TACHYCARDIA; SUPRAVENTRICULAR TACHYCARDIA

Features of Supraventricular Tachyarrhythmias

P wave: Present, each appears the same, may not be well defined in SVT

QRS complex: Present, each appears the same

PR interval: 0.12 to 0.20 seconds

QRS interval: 0.04 to 0.11 seconds

P to QRS ratio: 1:1

Rhythm: Regular

Rate: Greater than 100 bpm. ST during sleep is regarded as a sustained sinus rhythm of more than 90 bpm (1).

Comments: Supraventricular tachyarrhythmias are rapid, regular rhythms with normal-appearing QRS complexes. ST will have a normal sinus P wave. In AT, the P wave will have a morphology different from that of the sinus P wave (Figs. 40-9 and 40-10). SVT will not have a clearly defined P wave. It is difficult to distinguish one from the other on the surface ECG. Electrophysiologic studies may be necessary to determine the precise focus. *Sustained tachyarrhythmias will decrease cardiac output. The patient should be assessed for the level of consciousness, chest pain, and blood pressure and the physician notified.* The AASM recommends reporting ST during sleep if sustained. Otherwise, brief runs of these arrhythmias are reported as narrow complex tachycardia.

SINUS ARRHYTHMIA

Features of Sinus Arrhythmia

P wave: Present, each appears the same

QRS complex: Present, each appears the same

PR interval: 0.12 to 0.20 seconds

QRS interval: 0.04 to 0.11 seconds

P to QRS ratio: 1:1

Rhythm: Irregular

Rate: 60 to 100

Comments: Sinus arrhythmia (Figs. 40-11 and 40-12) is frequently seen in infants and children. It is often seen in obstructive sleep apnea as a result of the vagal effect of intrathoracic pressure fluctuations. Minor fluctuations of HR associated with inspiration and expiration are quite normal and indicate a "healthy" autonomic control of HR. Lack of HR fluctuation may indicate an underlying pathologic condition such as diabetes mellitus.

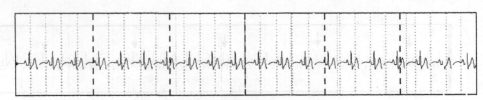

Figure 40-7 Sinus bradycardia, 30-second display.

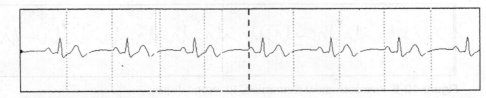

Figure 40-8 Sinus bradycardia, 10-second display.

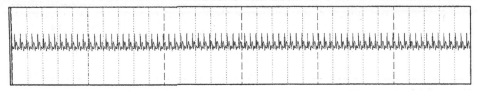

Figure 40-9 Atrial tachycardia, 30-second display.

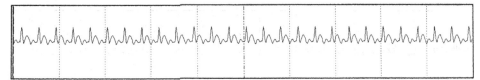

Figure 40-10 Atrial tachycardia, 10-second display.

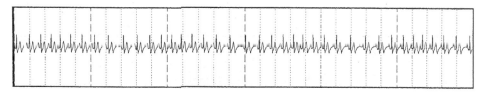

Figure 40-11 Sinus arrhythmia, 30-second display.

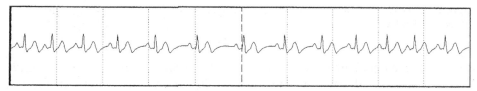

Figure 40-12 Sinus arrhythmia, 10-second display.

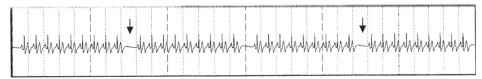

Figure 40-13 Sinus pause, 30-second display.

SINUS PAUSE

Features of Sinus Pause

P wave: Absent during pause

QRS complex: Absent during pause

PR interval: Absent during pause

QRS interval: Absent during pause

P to QRS ratio: 1:1

Rhythm: Irregular

Rate: 60 to 100, but can occur at any rate

Comments: One cannot distinguish arrest from block on surface ECG. This requires electrophysiologic studies of the heart. *If a sinus pause is prolonged, notify appropriate medical personnel according to protocol.* The arrows in Figs. 40-13 and 40-14 indicate the areas of absence of the P waves. The AASM recommendation is to report heart rate pauses of more than 3 seconds duration as asystole.

PAROXYSMAL ATRIAL TACHYCARDIA, PAROXYSMAL SUPRAVENTRICULAR TACHYCARDIA

Features of Paroxysmal Supraventricular Tachyarrhythmias

P wave: Present, aberrant, often hidden

QRS complex: Present, appearance is the same, may be aberrant

PR interval: Not measurable

QRS interval: 0.04 to 0.11 seconds

P to QRS ratio: 1:1

Rhythm: Regular during paroxysm

Rate: 150 to 250

Comments: Supraventricular tachyarrhythmias often occur with reentry phenomena from an accessory pathway.

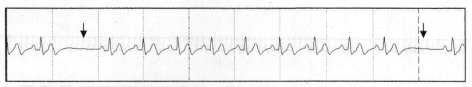

Figure 40-14 Sinus pause, 10-second display.

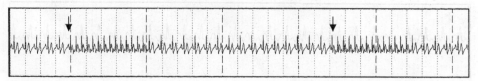

Figure 40-15 Paroxysmal atrial tachycardia, paroxysmal supraventricular tachycardia, 30-second display.

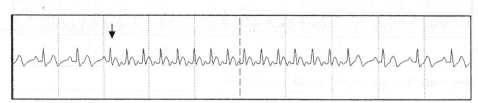

Figure 40-16 Paroxysmal atrial tachycardia, paroxysmal supraventricular tachycardia, 10-second display.

The term *paroxysmal* describes a phenomenon that arises abruptly from the background and abruptly returns to that background. Generally, these arrhythmias are self-limiting, but *if sustained, assess patient and notify appropriate medical personnel according to protocol.* Report these arrhythmias as narrow complex tachycardia. The arrows in Figures 40-15 and 40-16 indicate the onset of the paroxysm.

ATRIAL FIBRILLATION

Features of Atrial Fibrillation

P wave: None, per se; chaotic deflections called "fibrillatory waves"

QRS complex: Present, appearance is the same

PR interval: Not measurable

QRS interval: 0.04 to 0.11 seconds

P to QRS ratio: Not applicable

Rhythm: Irregularly irregular

Rate: Ventricular rate is highly variable.

Comments: Central sleep apnea, Cheyne–Stokes respirations, and mixed apneas (often with a long central component) are frequently seen with atrial fibrillation. This is likely due to decreased cardiac output and a prolonged circulation time rendering the breathing control centers ineffective. *If sustained or previously*

undocumented, notify appropriate medical personnel according to protocol. Indicate in the polysomnographic report as atrial fibrillation. Note the absence of true P waves and the replacement by chaotic fibrillatory waves in the preceding examples (Figs. 40-17 and 40-18).

ATRIAL FLUTTER

Features of Atrial Flutter

P wave: None, per se; sawtooth deflections called "flutter waves"

QRS complex: Present, appearance is the same

PR interval: Not measurable

QRS interval: 0.04 to 0.11 seconds

P to QRS ratio: Variable 2:1, 3:1, 4:1, and so on.

Rhythm: Regular or irregular depending on the variability of the block

Rate: Atrial: 250 to 400; ventricular rate depends on the degree of the block and atrial rate

Comments: Atrial flutter often occurs with reentry phenomena from accessory pathway. *If sustained or previously undocumented, notify appropriate medical personnel according to protocol.* Note under Other Arrhythmias on the polysomnographic report. Note the "sawtooth" flutter wave indicated by the arrows in Figures 40-19 and 40-20.

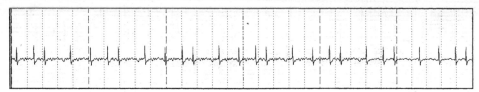

Figure 40-17 Atrial fibrillation, 30-second display.

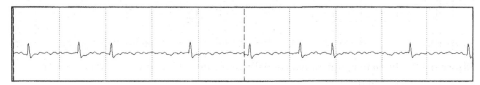

Figure 40-18 Atrial fibrillation, 10-second display.

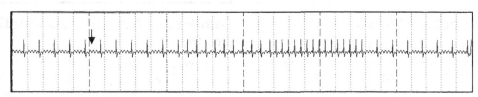

Figure 40-19 Atrial flutter, variable block, 30-second display.

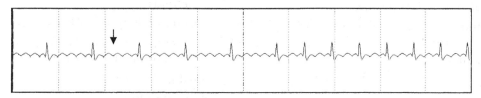

Figure 40-20 Atrial flutter, variable block, 10-second display.

JUNCTIONAL ARRHYTHMIAS

- Premature junctional contraction (PJC)
- Junctional rhythm
- Accelerated junctional rhythm
- Junctional tachycardia

Junctional arrhythmias can occur if the AV nodal tissue fires prematurely or if the atrial mechanism for initiating the cardiac cycle fails. Key features of the junctional arrhythmias are normal-appearing QRS complexes (the pathway distally from the AV bundle is intact). P waves may or may not be seen. If the P waves are seen, they will be inverted (a reverse from the normal P wave vector) and can occur before or after the QRS complex. If they occur before the QRS, the PR interval will be shorter than normal in contrast to the preceding ECG samples.

PREMATURE JUNCTIONAL CONTRACTION

Features of PJCs

P wave: Premature and abnormal configuration, will be inverted; can be before (with shortened PR interval), after, or hidden in the QRS

QRS complex: Present, appearance is the same

PR interval: Shorter than normal

QRS interval: 0.04 to 0.11 seconds

P to QRS ratio: Less than 1:1 if hidden; 1:1 if inverted P is seen

Rhythm: Irregular

Rate: Usually normal, but can occur in ST or SB

Comments: The premature beats with normal-appearing QRS complexes and absent or hidden P waves are seen at the arrows in Figures 40-21 and 40-22.

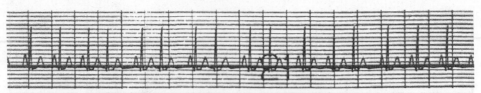

Figure 40-21 Premature junctional (nodal) contraction, 30-second timescale; uncompressed, partial epoch display.

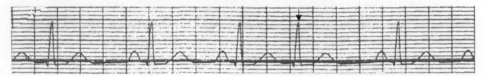

Figure 40-22 Premature junctional (nodal) contraction, 10-second timescale; uncompressed, partial epoch display.

JUNCTIONAL RHYTHM

Features of Junctional Rhythms

P wave: Premature and abnormal configuration, will be inverted; can be before (with shortened PR interval), after, or hidden in the QRS

QRS complex: Present, appearance is the same

PR interval: Shorter than normal; less than 0.12 seconds

QRS interval: 0.04 to 0.11 seconds

P to QRS ratio: Less than 1:1 if hidden; 1:1 if inverted P is seen

Rhythm: Regular

Rate: 40 to 60

Comments: Junctional rhythms are often seen as an escape rhythm with sinus node dysfunction. This type of rhythm should be listed under Other Arrhythmias in the report. Note the inverted P wave and short PR interval in Figures 40-23 and 40-24 at the arrows.

ACCELERATED JUNCTIONAL RHYTHM

Features of Accelerated Junctional Rhythm

P wave: Premature and abnormal configuration, will be inverted; can be before (with shortened PR interval), after, or hidden in the QRS

QRS complex: Present, appearance is the same

PR interval: Shorter than normal; less than 0.12 seconds

QRS interval: 0.04 to 0.11 seconds

P to QRS ratio: Either less than 1:1 if hidden; or 1:1 if inverted P is seen

Rhythm: Regular

Rate: 60 to 100

Comments: Accelerated junctional rhythm is often seen as escape rhythm with sinus node dysfunction. This type of rhythm should be listed under Other Arrhythmias in the report (Figs. 40-25 and 40-26).

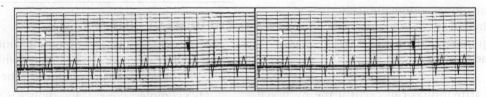

Figure 40-23 Junctional rhythm, 30-second display.

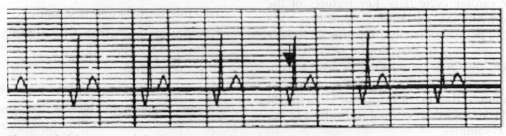

Figure 40-24 Junctional rhythm, 10-second window.

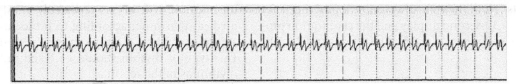

Figure 40-25 Accelerated junctional rhythm, 30-second window.

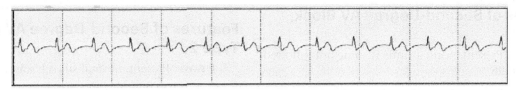

Figure 40-26 Accelerated junctional rhythm, 10-second window.

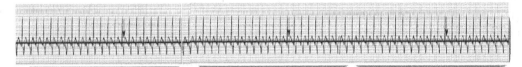

Figure 40-27 Junctional tachycardia, 30-second window.

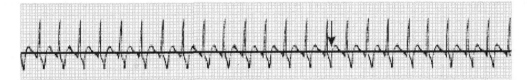

Figure 40-28 Junctional tachycardia, 10-second window.

JUNCTIONAL TACHYCARDIA

Features of Junctional Tachycardia

P wave: Premature and abnormal configuration, will be inverted; can be before (with shortened PR interval), after, or hidden in the QRS

QRS complex: Present, appearance is the same

PR interval: Shorter than normal; less than 0.12 seconds

QRS interval: 0.04 to 0.11 seconds

P to QRS ratio: Less than 1:1 if hidden; 1:1 if inverted P is seen

Rhythm: Regular

Rate: Greater than 100

Comments: Note the inverted P wave following the QRS at the arrows in Figures 40-27 and 40-28. Assess the patient if sustained and notify appropriate medical personnel according to protocol. This type of rhythm should be listed under Narrow Complex Tachycardia in the report.

BLOCKS

- First-degree AV block
- Second-degree AV block, type 1
- Second-degree AV block, type 2
- Third-degree AV block
- Left bundle branch block (LBBB)
- Right bundle branch block (RBBB)

FIRST-DEGREE AV BLOCK

Features of First-Degree AV Block

P wave: Present, appearance is the same

QRS complex: Present, appearance is the same

PR interval: Longer than normal; more than 0.20 seconds

QRS interval: 0.04 to 0.11 seconds

P to QRS ratio: 1:1

Rhythm: Regular

Rate: Usually normal

Comments: Note the difficulty seeing a prolonged PR interval on a 30-second display and the clarification provided with a 10-second display (Figs. 40-29 and 40-30).

SECOND-DEGREE AV BLOCK, TYPE 1 (WENCKEBACH)

Features of Second-Degree AV Block, Type 1

P wave: Present, normal sinus P, some not followed by QRS

QRS complex: Present, appearance is the same

PR interval: Progressively lengthening

QRS interval: 0.04 to 0.11 seconds

P to QRS ratio: More than 1:1, may be 1:1 if the nonconducted P wave is hidden

Rhythm: Irregular

Rate: Usually slow, but can be normal

Comments: As in Figures 30-29 and 30-30, the progressively lengthening PR intervals are better appreciated on a 10-second display. This type of block is not uncommon. If it occurs repeatedly, notify appropriate medical personnel according to protocol. The P waves are indicated by the arrows in Figures 40-31 and 40-32. This type of rhythm should be listed under Other Arrhythmias in the report.

SECOND-DEGREE AV BLOCK, TYPE 2

Features of Second-Degree AV Block, Type 2

P wave: Present, normal sinus P wave, 2, 3, or more P waves before QRS

QRS complex: Present, appearance is the same

PR interval: Constant PR interval before dropped QRS, PR interval may be normal or prolonged.

QRS interval: 0.04 to 0.11 seconds

P to QRS ratio: More than 1:1

Rhythm: Irregular

Rate: Usually slow, but can be normal

Comments: If second-degree AV block is prolonged, escape beat may occur. Note the constant PR interval

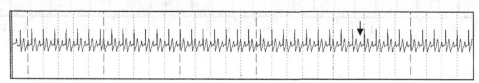

Figure 40-29 First-degree atrioventricular block, 30-second display.

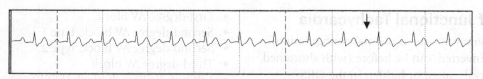

Figure 40-30 First-degree atrioventricular block, 10-second display.

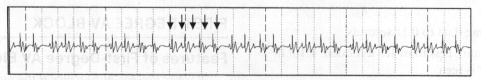

Figure 40-31 Second-degree atrioventricular block, type 1, 30-second display.

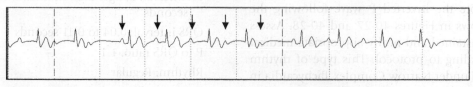

Figure 40-32 Second-degree atrioventricular block, type 1, 10-second display.

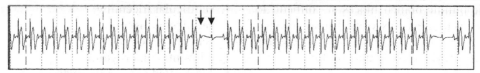

Figure 40-33 Second-degree atrioventricular block, type 2, 30-second display.

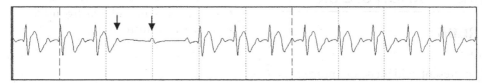

Figure 40-34 Second-degree atrioventricular block, type 2, 10-second display.

before dropped QRS in Figures 40-33 and 40-34. This may lead to a string of P waves without QRS complexes. This arrhythmia is worthy of a call to medical personnel according to protocol. Nonconducted P waves are indicated by the arrows in the preceding examples. This type of rhythm should be listed under Other Arrhythmias in the report.

THIRD-DEGREE AV BLOCK, A–V DISSOCIATION

Features of Third-Degree AV Block

P wave: Present, but has no relationship with QRS; often hidden in QRS and T waves

QRS complex: Present, appearance is the same

PR interval: Varies greatly

QRS interval: Less than 0.12 seconds if block is in a bundle of His; more than 0.12 seconds if block is in bundle branches.

P to QRS ratio: More than 1:1

Rhythm: Regular P–P and regular R–R but not the same rate

Rate: 40 to 60 if bundle of His is blocked; 30 to 40 if bundle branches are involved.

Comments: Note the constant P–P interval and the constant R–R interval in Figures 40-35 and 40-36. That is, there is a regular atrial rhythm and a regular ventricular rhythm, just not at the same rate. P waves are noted at the arrows and are sometimes difficult to see when simultaneously occurring with other waveforms such as the T wave and QRS complex. This type of rhythm should be listed under Other Arrhythmias in the report.

LEFT BUNDLE BRANCH BLOCK

Features of LBBB

P wave: Normal

QRS complex: Present, widened, and notched (M-shaped pattern), best seen in V6, lead I, or AVL

PR interval: Normal, can be prolonged with first-degree block

QRS interval: More than 0.12 seconds

P to QRS ratio: 1:1

Rhythm: Regular

Rate: Usually 60 to 100, but can occur with slower or faster rates

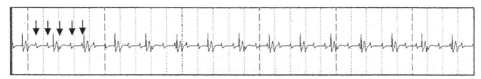

Figure 40-35 Third-degree atrioventricular block, 30-second display.

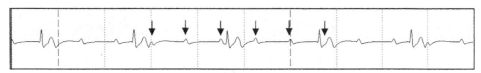

Figure 40-36 Third-degree atrioventricular block, 10-second display.

Comments: The bundle branch blocks are difficult to visualize. The key is to use a 10-second display (or less) and look for the increased QRS interval and notching (may be quite subtle) (Figs. 40-37 and 40-38).

RIGHT BUNDLE BRANCH BLOCK

Features of RBBB

P wave: Normal

QRS complex: Present, widened, and notched (rabbit-eared appearance), best seen in V_1 or MCL_1, hence not well seen in most sleep studies

PR interval: Normal, can be prolonged with first-degree block

QRS interval: More than 0.12 seconds

P to QRS ratio: 1:1

Rhythm: Regular

Rate: Usually 60 to 100, but can occur with slower or faster rates

Comments: RBBB is often difficult to visualize during polysomnography. Use a 10-second screen and look for widened QRS. You might see W-shaped waves in lead I (Figs. 40-39 and 40-40).

VENTRICULAR ARRHYTHMIAS

- PVCs
- Unifocal PVCs
- Multifocal PVCs

- Ventricular trigeminy
- Ventricular bigeminy
- Ventricular couplets
- Idioventricular rhythm
- Accelerated ventricular rhythm
- Ventricular tachycardia
- Runs of ventricular tachycardia
- Sustained ventricular tachycardia
- Ventricular fibrillation

PREMATURE VENTRICULAR CONTRACTIONS, UNIFOCAL PVCS

Features of PVCs and Variants

P wave: Not present with abnormal beat

QRS complex: Occurs earlier than expected, widened and bizarre appearing in abnormal beat

PR interval: None

QRS interval: More than 0.12 seconds with abnormal beat

P to QRS ratio: Less than 1:1

Rhythm: Irregular

Rate: Usually 60 to 100, but can occur with slower or faster rates

Comments: The arrows in Figures 40-41 to 40-50 indicate areas of ventricular ectopy (not all are annotated). Note that Figures 40-41 and 40-42 have different-appearing PVCs. This sample was taken from the same recording

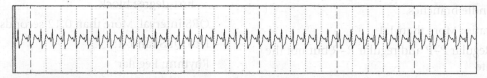

Figure 40-37 Left bundle branch block, 30-second display.

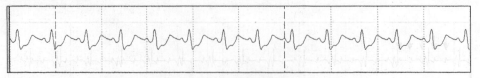

Figure 40-38 Left bundle branch block, 10-second display.

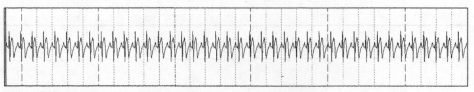

Figure 40-39 Right bundle branch block, 30-second display.

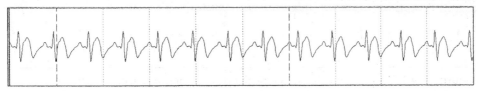

Figure 40-40 Right bundle branch block, 10-second display.

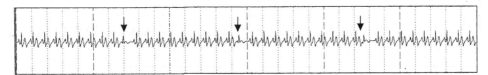

Figure 40-41 Unifocal premature ventricular contractions, 30-second display.

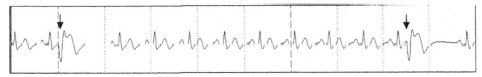

Figure 40-42 Unifocal premature ventricular contractions, 10-second display.

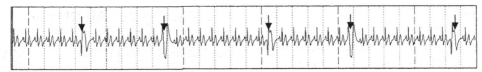

Figure 40-43 Multifocal premature ventricular contractions, 30-second display.

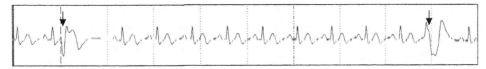

Figure 40-44 Multifocal premature ventricular contractions, 10-second display.

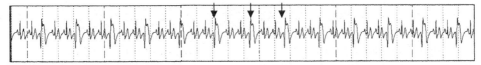

Figure 40-45 Trigeminal premature ventricular contractions, ventricular trigeminy, 30-second display.

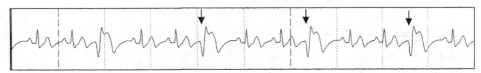

Figure 40-46 Trigeminal premature ventricular contractions, ventricular trigeminy, 10-second display.

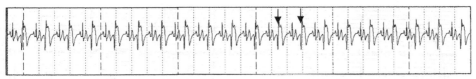

Figure 40-47 Bigeminal premature ventricular contractions, ventricular bigeminy, 30-second display.

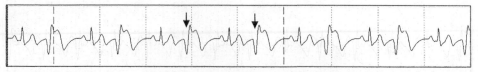

Figure 40-48 Bigeminal premature ventricular contractions, ventricular bigeminy, 10-second display.

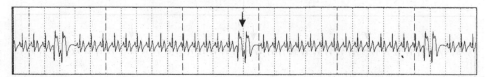

Figure 40-49 Ventricular couplets, 30-second display.

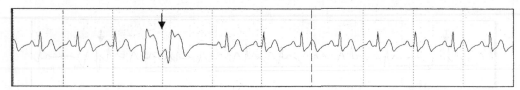

Figure 40-50 Ventricular couplets, 10-second display.

but using a different lead combination. Figure 40-41 is lead I and Figure 40-42 is lead II. Changing lead combinations may make the abnormality more apparent. In Figures 40-43 and 40-44, note the different appearance of the PVCs. Apply the *rule of differing morphology.* These beats originate from different areas of the ventricle (separate foci) and are therefore called "multifocal PVCs." Figures 40-45 and 40-46 display PVCs every third beat (ventricular trigeminy) and Figures 40-47 and 40-48 present PVCs every other beat (ventricular bigeminy). Note that the terms trigeminy and bigeminy can also refer to atrial and junctional extrasystoles bearing similar patterns. Figures 40-49 and 40-50 show paired PVCs (ventricular couplets). The aberrant waves have the same appearance; hence, they originate from the same location. Multifocal couplets are paired ventricular beats arising from different locations. These arrhythmias should be listed under Other Arrhythmias in the report if frequent or are of clinical significance.

IDIOVENTRICULAR RHYTHM

Features of Idioventricular Rhythm

P wave: No P waves associated with abnormal

QRS complex: Wide and bizarre

PR interval: None

QRS interval: More than 0.12 seconds

P to QRS ratio: Less than 1:1

Rhythm: Regular

Rate: Less than 40 bpm

Comments: Idioventricular rhythm (Figs. 40-51 and 40-52) is often seen as escape rhythm with sinus node and AV node dysfunction. If sustained, assess the patient and notify appropriate medical personnel according to protocol. Indicate as Bradycardia on the polysomnographic report, although it may also be indicated under Other Arrhythmias.

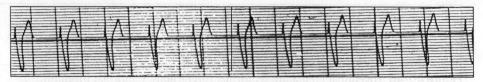

Figure 40-51 Idioventricular rhythm, 30-second timescale.

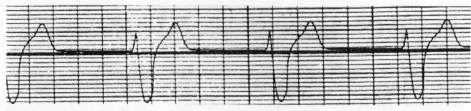

Figure 40-52 Idioventricular rhythm, 10-second timescale.

ACCELERATED VENTRICULAR RHYTHM

Features of Accelerated Ventricular Rhythm

P wave: No P waves associated with abnormal

QRS complex: Wide and bizarre

PR interval: None

QRS interval: More than 0.12 seconds

P to QRS ratio: Less than 1:1

Rhythm: Regular

Rate: 40 to 100 bpm

Comments: Accelerated ventricular rhythm (Figs. 40-53 and 40-54) is often seen as escape rhythm with sinus node and AV node dysfunction. Cardiac output is generally adequate. If sustained, assess the patient and notify medical personnel according to protocol. This type of rhythm should be listed under Other Arrhythmias in the report.

VENTRICULAR TACHYCARDIA

Features of Ventricular Tachycardia

P wave: No P waves associated with abnormal

QRS complex: Wide and bizarre

PR interval: None

QRS interval: More than 0.12 seconds

P to QRS ratio: Less than 1:1

Rhythm: Regular

Rate: 100 to 250

Comments: If ventricular tachycardia is not sustained, notify medical personnel according to protocol. If it is sustained, assess the patient and activate emergency medical system according to protocol (see Figs. 40-55 to 40-58). This type of rhythm should be listed under Wide Complex Tachycardia in the report.

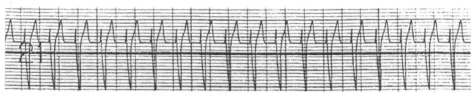

Figure 40-53 Accelerated ventricular rhythm, 30-second timescale.

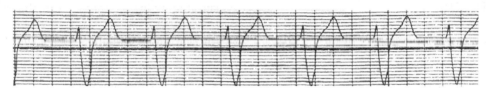

Figure 40-54 Accelerated ventricular rhythm, 10-second timescale.

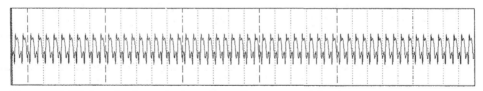

Figure 40-55 Sustained ventricular tachycardia, 30-second display.

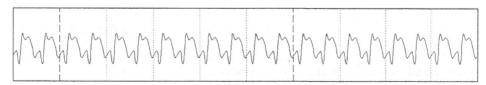

Figure 40-56 Sustained ventricular tachycardia, 10-second display.

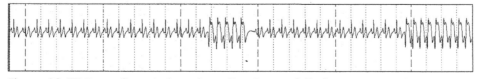

Figure 40-57 Runs of ventricular tachycardia, 30-second display.

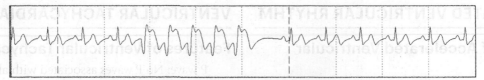

Figure 40-58 Runs of ventricular tachycardia, 10-second display.

VENTRICULAR FIBRILLATION

Features of Ventricular Fibrillation

P wave: No P waves seen

QRS complex: None; wave deflections are disorganized, chaotic, varying in size and shape.

PR interval: None

QRS interval: Not measurable

P to QRS ratio: Not measurable

Rhythm: Chaotic

Rate: Not measurable

Comments: Ventricular fibrillation (Figs. 40-59 and 40-60) is a medical emergency. Assess the patient and activate EMS. When the ECG looks like the EEG, take immediate action. This type of rhythm should be listed under Other Arrhythmias in the report.

INTERVENTIONS

Each facility should have a policy for dealing with significant arrhythmias. Sustained tachyarrhythmias (atrial or junctional tachycardias and ventricular tachycardias), atrial fibrillation and flutter with rapid ventricular response, and sustained ventricular arrhythmias (idioventricular or accelerated ventricular rhythm) require immediate assessment of the patient. Assessment should include the level of consciousness; dizziness or light-headedness; the presence of chest, arm, or neck pain; oxygen saturation; and blood pressure. Of course,

emergency protocol for Code Blue or activating the emergency medical system should be initiated in the case of unresponsiveness. Other arrhythmias such as nonsustained runs of ventricular tachycardia, asystoles, second- and third-degree blocks, and previously undocumented atrial fibrillation or flutter warrant a call to the medical director, referring the physician or house officer for direction, according to protocol.

RECORDING AND MONITORING TECHNIQUES

Many sleep centers have a prescribed electrode placement for recording the ECG. This usually involves recording from the right and left subclavicular areas (essentially lead I) or the right subclavicular area and the lower left thorax (essentially lead II, the AASM-recommended derivation). However, the chosen ECG derivation may not always demonstrate a good P wave and a QRS complex of adequate amplitude necessary for arrhythmia identification. The ECG quality should be observed before or during the physiologic calibration procedure. Different lead combinations should be sampled to provide the best ECG display before "lights out." Some recording systems have a dedicated paired input for the ECG. In this case, one must physically move the electrodes to another location. Other systems will allow the user to reference any recording electrode to any other using the system input selection panel. In this case, it is fairly simple to reference an ECG electrode to another recording electrode (such as a left leg electrode) and obtain a different view of the ECG.

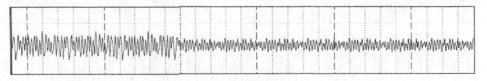

Figure 40-59 Ventricular fibrillation, 30-second display.

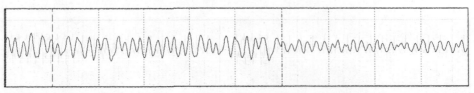

Figure 40-60 Ventricular fibrillation, 10-second display.

A more advanced tactic is to routinely monitor two separate ECG leads (a lead I and a lead II, or a lead I and a lead III simultaneously). There are recording systems that have the capability of averaging recording signals. It is possible in these systems to provide a semblance of the precordial leads by averaging left arm, left leg, and right arm signals as a reference for any of the V leads. In addition, a reasonable facsimile of the augmented limb leads (aVR, aVL, and aVF) may be obtained by recording the right arm versus the average of the left arm and left leg (aVR), etc.

To ensure a quality recording, ECG electrodes should be applied with the same care and proper skin preparation as with any other electrodes used in the sleep study. The AASM guidelines recommend the use of standard ECG electrodes rather than EEG electrodes (1). High electrode impedances or sloppy application techniques will result in artifacts, which in some cases may resemble ectopic beats. To avoid misinterpretation of the ECG, any questionable patterns should be confirmed by examining alternate derivations (as described earlier).

Viewing the ECG for arrhythmia recognition is facilitated by "spreading the recording out," utilizing a 10-second display or less (the author has used a 6-second display to try to find evidence of "hidden" P waves). Intervals are nearly impossible to assess using a standard 30-second screen width. Measurement of the PR and QRS intervals can be accomplished by printing the 10-second screen and then measuring the intervals with a millimeter ruler and dividing this measurement by the number of millimeters per second on the print out. Standard calipers can be used to determine regularity on these printouts. If the system is incapable of printing during recording, it is possible to measure the intervals and test regularity by using a stationary 10-second window and an index card. Make tick marks at the beginning and end of the interval of interest, measure this distance in millimeters, and divide by the number of millimeters per second provided by your display. Regularity can be checked by making tick marks at three successive R waves (or P waves) and then moving the card from R wave to R wave (or P wave to P wave). If the tick marks fall in line, the rhythm is regular.

At the end of the numbered references are a few web references that were recently accessed. The author has found them an interesting "challenge" and learning experience and would recommend them to the student or technologist as an additional learning resource after studying arrhythmias and developing a degree of confidence in arrhythmia identification.

REFERENCES

1. Iber, C., Ancoli-Israel, S., Chesson, A., et al. (2007). *The AASM manual for the scoring of sleep and associated events: Rules terminology and technical specifications* (1st ed.). Westchester, IL: American Academy of Sleep Medicine.

2. Berry, R. B., Albertario, C. L., Harding, S. M., et al.; for the American Academy of Sleep Medicine. (2018). *The AASM manual for the scoring of sleep and associated events: Rules, terminology and technical specifications.* Version 2.5. Darien, IL: American Academy of Sleep Medicine.

3. Atkinson, J. (2005). Cardiac arrhythmias. In T. Lee-Chiong & W. Brown (Eds.), *Respiratory clinics of North America* (Vol. 11, p. 4). Philadelphia, PA: W.B. Saunders.

4. Dubin, D. (2000). *Rapid interpretation of EKGs* (6th ed.). Tampa, FL: Cover Publishing.

5. Huff, J. (2011). *ECG workout: Exercises in arrhythmia interpretation* (6th ed.). Philadelphia, PA: Lippincott Williams & Wilkins.

6. Thaler, M. S. (2007). *The only EKG book you'll ever need* (5th ed.). Philadelphia, PA: Lippincott Williams & Wilkins.

Web References

Arrhythmia recognition: The art of interpretation. Retrieved March 23, 2018, from http://www.12leadecg.com/arrhythmias

EKG Academy. *EKG interpretation practice.* Retrieved March 26, 2018, from https://ekg.academy/ekg-interpretation-practice

Medical Intensive Care Nursing. *Cardiology in critical care: EKG and arrhythmia recognition.* Retrieved March 23, 2018, from http://www.micunursing.com/#Section_3_Cardiology_in_Critical_Care

Practical Clinical Skills. *EKG arrhythmia practice drill.* Retrieved March 26, 2018, from https://www.practicalclinicalskills.com/ekg-practice-drill

chapter 41

Scoring Movement Rules

LAREE J. FORDYCE

LEARNING OBJECTIVES

On completion of this chapter, the reader should be able to:

1. Describe movement events and movement event scoring rules according to the standards of the American Academy of Sleep Medicine.
2. Identify the common artifact that occurs in leg movement channels.

KEY TERMS

Periodic limb movements in sleep (PLMS)
Rhythmic movement disorder (RMD)
Bruxism
REM sleep behavior disorder (RBD)
Hypnagogic foot tremor (HFT)
Excessive fragmentary myoclonus (EFM)

In polysomnography (PSG), scoring movements is necessary but can be tricky. The *AASM Manual for the Scoring of Sleep and Associated Events* has outlined the scoring rules for scoring movements in both adults and pediatrics. Review the current sections Parameters to Be Recorded as well as the Technical Specifications for Movement Rules in the *AASM Manual for the Scoring of Sleep and Associated Events* to verify you are using the most updated recording parameters for collection of data. In this chapter, we will review the movement scoring rules as well as provide examples to illustrate how these events should be scored.

When scoring movements, it is important that we are recording the proper channels and using appropriate sensors. To assess movement activity in the lower limbs, both legs should be monitored. Surface electrodes are placed on the belly of the tibialis anterior muscle of each

leg, about 2 to 3 cm apart (1). If upper limb movements are being assessed, both arms should be monitored. Surface electrodes should be placed on either the extensor digitorum communis or flexor digitorum superficialis muscles, or both (1).

Surface electrodes are placed on the neck over the paraspinal muscles (1) to record movement activity typical of rhythmic movement disorder (RMD). To record the electromyographic (EMG) activity seen with bruxism, surface electrodes are placed on the masseter muscle (1). For exact placements of the electrodes used for these EMG recordings, see the chapter on Movement Rules in the current version of the *AASM Manual for the Scoring of Sleep and Associated Events*.

PERIODIC LIMB MOVEMENTS IN SLEEP

1. Periodic limb movements in sleep (PLMS) are defined as leg movements with a duration between 0.5 and 10 seconds.
2. The maximum amplitude of the event must be an 8 μV increase from the baseline limb EMG signal.
3. PLMS events may cause arousals. Arousals are scored as long as they occur within 0.5 seconds of the movement.

See Figure 41-1 for an example of a periodic limb movement that resulted in an arousal.

PERIODIC LIMB MOVEMENT SERIES

1. A periodic limb movement series is defined as four leg movements (see Fig. 41-2) with a duration between 5 and 90 seconds.
2. The maximum amplitude of the event must be at minimum an 8 μV increase from the baseline limb EMG signal.
3. Events may cause arousals. Arousals are scored as long as they occur within 0.5 seconds of the movement.

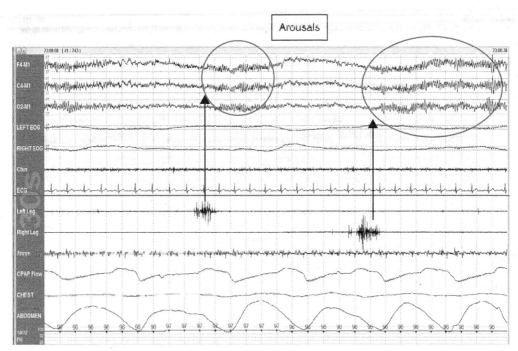

Figure 41-1 There is a greater than 8 μV increase in the leg electromyogram channels from baseline. The event duration is between 0.5 and 10 seconds. At the end of the movement event, there is an arousal.

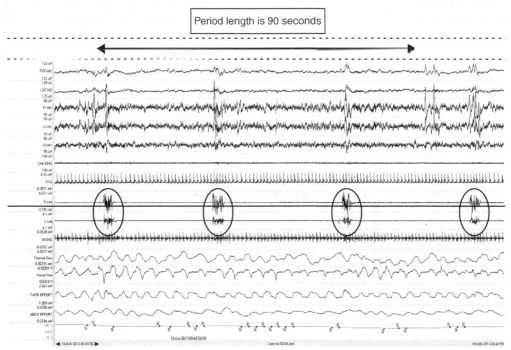

Figure 41-2 There is a greater than 8 μV increase from baseline. There are four leg movements. The period length is between 5 and 90 seconds. At the end of each movement event, there is an arousal.

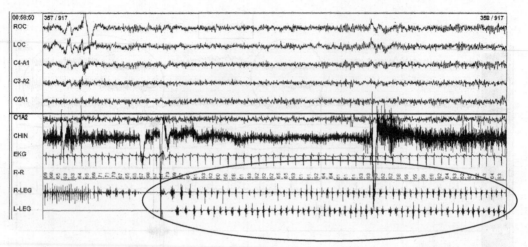

Figure 41-3 This epoch shows movements consistent with rhythmic movement disorder. There are more than four clustered movements. The activity is twice the amplitude of the baseline electromyogram activity.

RHYTHMIC MOVEMENT DISORDER

1. RMD will show a minimum of four individual clustered movements.
2. The amplitude of the activity will be twice that of the background EMG activity.
3. The frequency of RMD activity is 0.5 to 2.0 Hz.

   See Figure 41-3 for an example of rhythmic movement activity.

LEG MOVEMENTS WITH RESPIRATORY EVENTS

1. Leg movements may occur in conjunction with respiratory events. It is important to know whether the leg movement or the respiratory event came first. Only one type of event is scored: either the limb movement or the respiratory event (see Fig. 41-4).
2. Leg movements should not be scored if they occur within 0.5 seconds of a respiratory event.

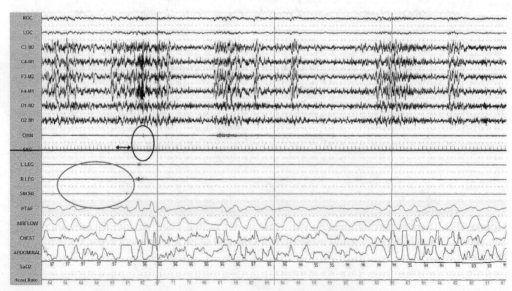

Figure 41-4 If a leg movement occurs within 0.5 seconds of a respiratory event, it is not scored. The respiratory event caused a leg movement at the end of this event.

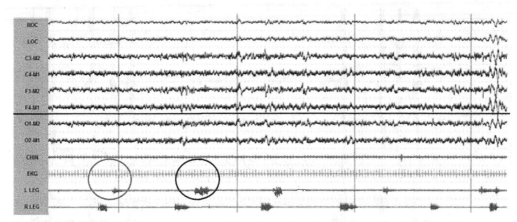

Figure 41-5 Alternating leg movement with a greater than 8 μV increase from baseline. There are four alternative leg muscle activations (ALMAs) circled in this figure. Each ALMA lasts between 100 and 500 ms.

ALTERNATIVE LEG MUSCLE ACTIVATION

1. Alternative leg muscle activation (ALMA) is defined as small bursts of muscle activity that alternate from one leg channel to the other.
2. For the activity to be considered ALMA, there must be a series of at least four alternating limb movements (see Fig. 41-5).
3. The frequency between ALMA events is 0.5 to 3.0 Hz, with a duration of 100 to 500 ms.
4. ALMA may also be a form of hypnagogic foot tremor (HFT).

HYPNAGOGIC FOOT TREMOR

1. HFT will show a series of at least four EMG bursts (see Fig. 41-6).
2. The frequency will be between 0.3 and 4.0 Hz.

BRUXISM

1. Bruxism is characterized by grinding or clenching of the teeth during sleep, usually associated with arousals from sleep.
2. The events consist of sustained (tonic) and phasic (brief) contractions of the jaw, usually 0.25 to 2 seconds in duration.
3. On the PSG, audio should be recorded to score bruxism more reliably.
4. A series of repetitive bruxism movements is called "rhythmic masticatory muscle activity."

See Figure 41-7 for an example of bruxism that was audible to the technologist and is reflected on the electroencephalogram (EEG) tracing as muscle activity in the EEG.

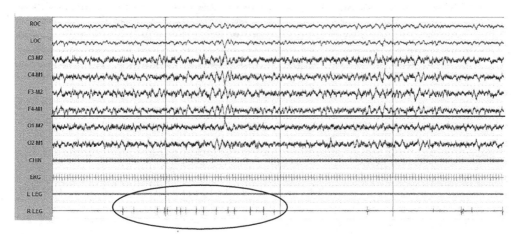

Figure 41-6 In this 120-second epoch, note the movements in the right leg channel. They meet the criteria to be scored as hypnagogic foot tremor.

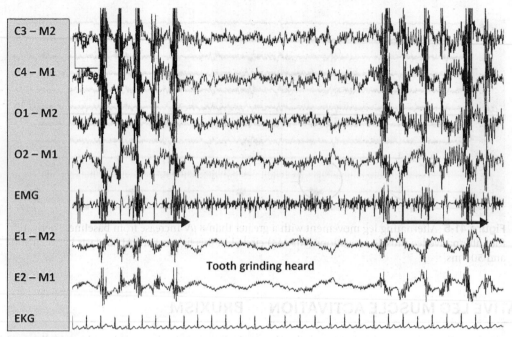

Figure 41-7 This is an example of bruxism reflected in the electroencephalogram channels. The technologist notes that audible tooth grinding was heard. EKG, electrocardiography; EMG, electromyograph.

EXCESSIVE FRAGMENTARY MYOCLONUS

1. Excessive fragmentary myoclonus (EMF) is described as a benign movement. It is reported to not have any clinical consequences. See Figure 41-8 for an example of EMF activity.
2. The EMG burst duration is 150 ms.
3. A minimum of five EMG potentials per minute must be recorded.

4. During the PSG recording, 20 minutes of EMF activity must be seen during nonrapid eye movement (NREM) sleep in order to score EMF.

REM SLEEP BEHAVIOR DISORDER

REM sleep behavior disorder (RBD) is parasomnia that occurs in REM sleep where normal paralysis in REM is

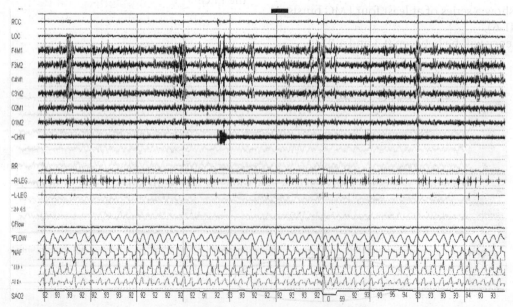

Figure 41-8 This is an example of excessive fragmentary myoclonus in the right leg electromyogram channel.

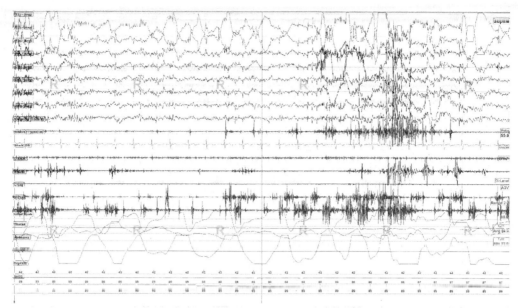

Figure 41-9 A 60-second sample of excessive chin and limb electromyogram activity during rapid eye movement (REM) sleep consistent with scorable transient muscle activity seen in REM behavior disorder.

absent or incomplete. During REM sleep, RBD can be scored when the following criteria are present:

1. Sustained chin EMG muscle activity in REM sleep. The epoch will show at least 50% duration of chin EMG activity greater than the minimum amplitude seen in NREM sleep.

2. Excessive transient muscle activity occurring during REM sleep in the chin or limb EMG channels. The

epoch will show bursts of EMG activity lasting 0.1 to 5.0 seconds with an amplitude that is four times greater than the background EMG activity.

Figures 41-9 and 41-10 are examples of scorable transient and sustained excessive EMG activity during REM sleep, respectively.

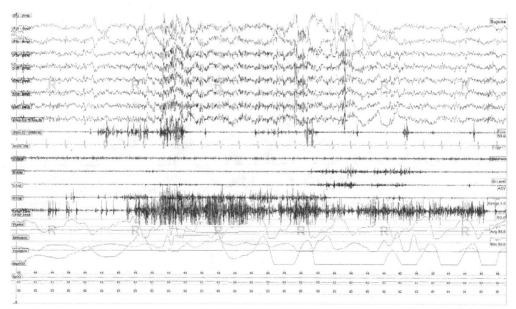

Figure 41-10 A 30-second epoch showing excessive chin and limb electromyogram activity during rapid eye movement (REM) sleep consistent with a scorable epoch of sustained muscle activity consistent with REM behavior disorder.

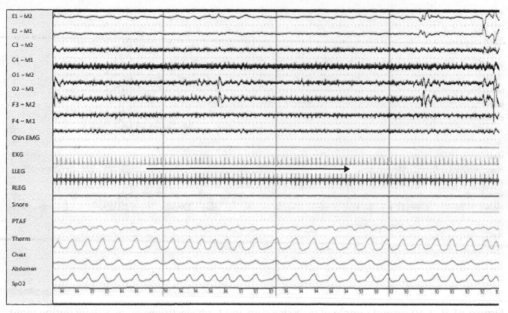

Figure 41-11 In this 120-second epoch, there is electrocardiogram artifact in the left leg channel. This artifact may mask any leg movements that might be occurring, such as REM sleep motor disorder. REM, rapid eye movement.

MOVEMENT ARTIFACTS

When recording and scoring movement events, it is important to evaluate the proper signals to determine what type of event is occurring. Physiologic signals such as electrocardiogram can obscure the desired activity and make it difficult or impossible to score limb movements (see Fig. 41-11). Patient movement itself can obscure activity in all of the channels, as seen in Figure 41-12.

If there are few working signals, poor signals, or artifact in the channels, this will prevent identifying or scoring significant movements occurring during sleep.

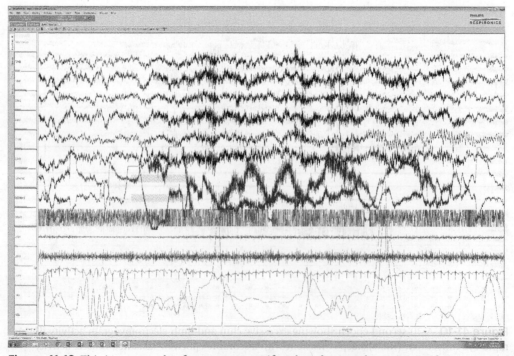

Figure 41-12 This is an example of a movement artifact that obscures the entire epoch.

SUMMARY

Scoring movements in sleep can be challenging, even when the primary events being scored routinely are simple PLMS. Most importantly, the EMG signals recorded to assess movement disorders must be obtained using appropriate electrodes and accurate placements. The scorer must be well versed in general sleep and arousal scoring as well as respiratory event scoring to accurately score PLMS. Scoring RBD, bruxism, and other unusual movements that are not so commonly seen may require a review of the scoring rules. Both the recording and scoring technologist should always be aware of the patient history and the indication for the PSG in order to ensure that unusual events are not missed and the patient receives an appropriate diagnosis.

REFERENCE

1. Berry, R. B., Albertario, C. L., Harding, S. M., et al.; for the American Academy of Sleep Medicine. (2018). *The AASM manual for the scoring of sleep and associated events: Rules, terminology and technical specifications* [Version 2.5]. Darien, IL: American Academy of Sleep Medicine.

chapter 42
Generating the Polysomnography Report

JON W. ATKINSON

LEARNING OBJECTIVES

On completion of this chapter, the reader should be able to:

1. Describe the purpose of the sleep study report.
2. Define the parameters to be reported according to the American Academy of Sleep Medicine (AASM) guidelines set forth in *The AASM manual for the scoring of sleep and associated events: Rules, terminology and technical specifications version 2.5*.
   a. Cite the definitions and use formulae to calculate common sleep architectural parameters.
   b. Cite the definitions and use formulae to calculate common event parameters.
3. Derive and utilize histograms.
4. Develop derivations of unique/detailed event parameters and tables.
5. Validate the use of summary reports.
6. Describe archiving and data storage procedures.
7. Describe the AASM reporting guidelines for Home Sleep Apnea Testing set forth in *The AASM manual for the scoring of sleep and associated events: Rules, terminology and technical specifications version 2.5*.

KEY TERMS

Polysomnography
Reporting
Data analysis
Home Sleep Apnea Testing (HSAT)

In the early days of sleep medicine, polysomnographic studies were recorded on paper. Utilizing a paper speed of 10 mm per second, these records usually contained 800 to 1,000 pages of data. The purpose of the polysomnographic report was to summarize these data, presenting an overview of the patient's sleep architecture and allowing for comparisons among sleep studies (1). In the late 1960s, a standard scoring system was developed to provide guidelines for staging human sleep, and this scoring system was the gold standard for decades (2). This document was based on data from normal, young adult subjects. As the practice of clinical sleep medicine evolved and a variety of sleep-related pathologies were recognized, it became clear that additional descriptive statistics were necessary to convey adequately the various aspects of normal and abnormal sleep. Guidelines for identifying and scoring arousals (3), periodic limb movements (PLMs) (4), and respiratory events (5) were then developed in an effort to standardize the tabulation of these data.

Manual scoring and data tabulation was a daunting task, even for a very experienced technologist, often consuming hours of time per recording. Before the advent of personal computers to assist with "number crunching," the tabulation of data and generation of the report summary sometimes involved more time than the identification of sleep stages and abnormal events. Today, a polished report representing the visual scoring of sleep and events, replete with graphics and charts, can typically be produced within 1 to 2 hours (depending on the complexity of the recording and the severity of the patient's condition). This type of report would have been virtually impossible to produce in the formative years of polysomnographic technology.

The advent of digital polysomnography recording systems with intrinsic scoring and data tabulation has rendered the report generation task much less cumbersome. Although this represents a significant advance in technology, it has also given rise to several problems:

1. The digitization of polysomnographic data allows use of various automated functions, including computer-assisted or automated scoring. To date, most of these functions have not been validated for clinical use.
2. Automated scoring is generally not accurate for sleep staging and abnormal event recognition. This is particularly true in light of the high incidence of mechanical, physiologic, and medication-induced artifacts that can occur in unison or in combination. Computer-scored recordings must always be reviewed and edited by a competent technologist. In essence, the technologist must manually corroborate the sleep stage scoring and review/edit computer-scored abnormal events, such as apneas, hypopneas, oxygen desaturations, and limb movements. This editing process is generally more time-consuming and cumbersome than scoring the record manually.
3. Reliance on automated data tabulation and report generation built into these programs allows the

technologist to be uninformed about the theory, concepts, and formulae involved in the generation of these reports.

a. The knowledge base related to the theory, concepts, and formulae used to generate reports becomes very important when installing new systems and developing report templates or developing specialized reports or data points. The data points in a report must be checked for accuracy and appropriateness before the report is used to present patient data. It is not uncommon to find inaccurate numbers in the initial reports developed following a new installation.

b. Back in the days of analog paper–based recordings, the manual data tabulation theories, concepts, and formulae presented in this chapter were utilized many times daily. There was continuous reinforcement of this knowledge and a practical reason for learning and maintaining this information. Currently, many technologists have little exposure to this knowledge and do not spend time exploring its intricacies. Consequently, reports may be of lesser quality or relevance than those designed and maintained by knowledgeable users.

PURPOSE OF A SLEEP STUDY REPORT

The purpose of the polysomnographic report is dependent on the needs of the end user. This may be the interpreting physician, the referring physician, the homecare company or durable medical equipment (DME) supplier, or the third-party payer. With the advent of digital recordings, there is an ability to overanalyze and therefore produce reports with overwhelming, often superfluous amounts of data. Fortunately, it is also easy to develop multiple reports using the same data to meet the needs of multiple users.

For in-depth data analysis or research purposes, a report can contain multiple tables, statistics, graphs, and customized charts to meet the needs of the interpreter or research project. Histographic summaries can correlate events with sleep staging, body position, and treatment settings. Event tabulations, percentages, and indices can be provided for every conceivable condition encountered during the study. A report of this nature can be quite lengthy, but not necessarily practical. Figure 42-1 is an example of a Split-Night Study—Long Report for Sleep Center Use.

Split-Night Study (Long Report for Sleep Center Use)

Patient Name: Walker, Ima			
Gender	Female	Study date	September 13, 2011
D.O.B.	December 6, 1946	Subject code	98765
Age	64	Referring physician	Frequent referral, MD
Height	66.0 in	Sleep specialist	Sleep doctor, MD
Weight	190.0 lbs	Recording tech	IM Sleepy, RPSGT
BMI	30.7	Scoring tech	JW Atkinson, RPSGT

Study Indications:
Daytime complaints of EDS (ESS=9), loud snoring, nonrestorative sleep. Sleep complaints of breathing/snoring stops in sleep, wakes for unknown reasons, restless sleep, somniloquy, occasional heartburn, and bruxism.

Recording/Collection Notes:
Insert recording/collection technician notes here.

Scoring/Analysis Notes:
Insert scoring/analysis technician notes here.

Hypopnea Rule:	VIII.4.A
Stage Scored by:	TECH
Hypoventilation:	NO
Cheyne–Stokes Breathing:	NO
Arrythmias:	NO

Figure 42-1 Split-night study. CPAP, continuous positive airway pressure; PLM, periodic limb movement; REM, rapid eye movement; TIB, time in bed; TST, total sleep time; WASO, wake after sleep onset (long report for Sleep Center use and third-party payer).

Channel information Chart

Channel Input Label	Channel Name	Channel Type	Frequency
Snore (Amp 1)	Snore	Snore	256
Chest (Amp 1)	Chest	Chest	32
Abd (Amp 1)	Abdomen	Abdomen	32
C3 (Amp 1)	C3	EEG,C3,CZ	256
C4 (Amp 1)	C4	EEG,C4,CZ	256
O1 (Amp 1)	O1	EEG,O1,CZ	256
L Eye (Amp 1)	E1	Ocular, Left	256
R Eye (Amp 1)	E2	Ocular, Right	256
O2 (Amp 1)	O2	EEG,O2,CZ	256
A1 (Amp 1)	M1	EEG,A1,CZ	256
A2 (Amp 1)	M2	EEG,A2,CZ	256
L EMG (Amp 1)	EMG1	EMG, Left	256
R EMG (Amp 1)	EMG2	EMG, Right	256
L EKG (Amp 1)	ECG1	EKG,1	256
R EKG (Amp 1)	ECG2	EKG,2	256
L Leg+ (Amp 1)	L-Leg1	Legs, Left,1	256
L Leg– (Amp 1)	L-Leg2	Legs, Left,2	256
R Leg+ (Amp 1)	R-Leg1	Legs, Right,1	256
R Leg– (Amp 1)	R-Leg2	Legs, Right,2	256
Thermistor (Amp 1)	Airflow	AirFlow	32
Pressure (Amp 1)	Nasal pressure	Nasal canula	32
Body position (Amp 1)	Body position	Body position	1
OP. 1+ (Amp 1)	F3	EEG,F3,CZ	256
OP. 2+ (Amp 1)	F4	EEG,F4,CZ	256
OP. 3+ (Amp 1)	EMG3	EMG, Submental	256
SpO₂ (Amp 1)	SaO2	SaO2	16
Pulse (Amp 1)	Pulse	Pulse	16
Pleth (Amp 1)	Pleth	Pleth	16
DC X1 (Box 1)	CPAP flow	CPAP (flow)	16
DC X2 (Box 1)	CPAP	CPAP (pressure)	16
DC X3 (Box 1)	CPAP leak	CPAP (leak)	16

Figure 42-1 (*continued*)

Sleep Architecture

Lights out clock time (h:min)	9:47:00 p.m.
Lights on clock time (h:min)	12:50:56 a.m.
Total recording time (TRT; in min)	183.9
Sleep period time (SPT)*	3:03:03
Total sleep time (TST; in min)	161.0
Sleep efficiency (SE)	87.5%
Sleep latency (SL)	0:00:54
Total stage changes (after sleep onset [SO])	84
Awakenings (after SO)	19
WASO	22.0
REM periods	2
REM latency*	1:35:00
REM latency (less wake time)*	1:32:30

*Time formats are in h:min:s

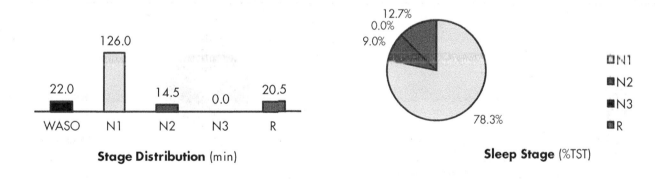

Stage Distribution (min)   **Sleep Stage** (%TST)

Sleep Stage	Latency (min)
N1	0.0
N2	30.5
N3	N/A
R	95.0

Stage latency = 0.0 denotes start of sleep.

Figure 42-1 (*continued*)

Respiratory Events	Cen. Apneas	Obs. Apneas	Mxd. Apneas	Hypopneas	Total Apneas	Apnea+ Hypopnea	RERA	All Resp. Events*
Count:	0	52	0	155	52	207	0	207
Index (events/h)	0.0	19.4	0.0	57.8	19.4	77.1	0.0	77.1
Mean duration (s)	N/A	29.4	N/A	24.0	29.4	25.3	N/A	25.3
Longest event (s)	N/A	66.1	N/A	81.9	66.1	81.9	N/A	81.9
REM count	0	10	0	7	10	17	0	17
Non-REM count	0	42	0	148	42	190	0	190
REM index	0.0	29.3	0.0	20.5	29.3	49.8	0.0	49.8
Non-REM index	0.0	17.9	0.0	63.2	17.9	81.1	0.0	81.1

*Note: Does not contain Cheyne–Stokes breathing, hypoventilation, or periodic breathing.

Respiratory Events (by body position)	Supine Sleep Count	Supine Sleep Index	Prone Sleep Count	Prone Sleep Index	Left-Side Sleep Count	Left-Side Sleep Index	Right-Side Sleep Count	Right-Side Sleep Index	Upright Sleep Count	Upright Sleep Index
Duration (h:min:s)	2:40:50		0:00:00		0:00:00		0:00:00		0:00:00	
Obstructive apneas (OA)	52	19.4	N/A	N/A	N/A	N/A	N/A	N/A	N/A	N/A
Central apneas (CA)	0	0.0	N/A	N/A	N/A	N/A	N/A	N/A	N/A	N/A
Mixed apneas (MA)	0	0.0	N/A	N/A	N/A	N/A	N/A	N/A	N/A	N/A
Hypopneas	155	57.8	N/A	N/A	N/A	N/A	N/A	N/A	N/A	N/A
RERAs	0	0.0	N/A	N/A	N/A	N/A	N/A	N/A	N/A	N/A
Total	207	77.2	N/A	N/A	N/A	N/A	N/A	N/A	N/A	N/A

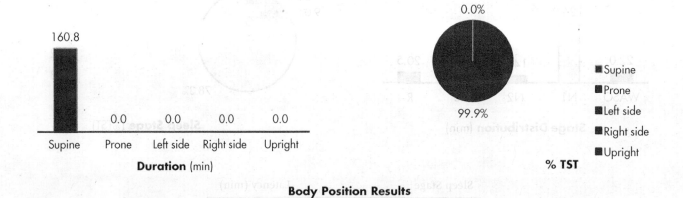

Body Position Results

Arousals	Resp. Count	Resp. Index	Spontaneous Count*	Spontaneous Index*	Total Count	Total Index
TST	153	57.0	25	9.3	178	66.3
Non-REM	141	60.2	25	10.7	166	70.9
REM	12	35.1	0	0.0	12	35.1

*EEG arousal activity *not* associated with *respiratory* or *PLM* events.

Figure 42-1 (*continued*)

Limb Movements	LM w Arousals		LM w/o Arousals		Total LMs		PLM Series	
(by sleep stage)	Count	Index	Count	Index	Count	Index	Count	Index
TST	0	0.0	0	0.0	0	0.0	0	0.0
N1	0	0.0	0	0.0	0	0.0	0	0.0
N2	0	0.0	0	0.0	0	0.0	0	0.0
N3	N/A	N/A	N/A	N/A	N/A	N/A	N/A	N/A
R	0	0.0	0	0.0	0	0.0	0	0.0

Oxygen Desaturation Events	Count	Index
TST	200	74.5
Wake (after SO)	5	13.6
Non-REM	181	77.3
REM	19	55.6

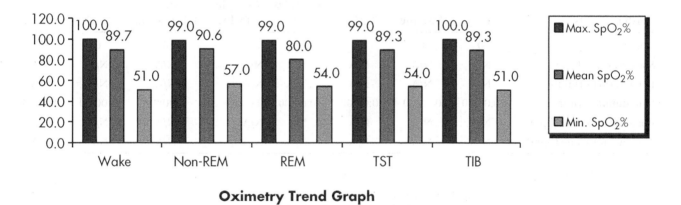

Oximetry Trend Graph

Oxygen Saturation	Wake	Non-REM	REM	TST	TIB
Max. SpO_2%	100.0	99.0	99.0	99.0	100.0
Mean SpO_2%	89.7	90.6	80.0	89.3	89.3
Min. SpO_2%	51.0	57.0	54.0	54.0	51.0
SpO_2% ≤ 89% (min)	0.1	49.3`	14.5	63.8	67.7
% Time in range					
90–100%	36.7%	59.6%	26.6%	55.4%	53.0%
80–89%	12.7%	35.3%	23.3%	33.7%	31.1%
70–79%	1.0%	3.9%	23.9%	6.4%	5.7%
60–69%	3.2%	0.8%	21.5%	3.4%	3.4%
50–59%	1.0%	0.1%	4.7%	0.7%	0.8%
<50%	0.0%	0.0%	0.0%	0.0%	0.0%
% Artifact/bad data	45.4%	0.4%	0.0%	0.3%	6.0%

Figure 42-1 (*continued*)

Heart Rate (HR) Results	Wake	Non-REM	REM	TST	TIB
Max. HR (bpm)	79.0	79.0	81.0	81.0	81.0
Mean HR (bpm)	64.6	61.7	60.7	61.4	61.6
Min. HR (bpm)	9.0	54.0	49.0	49.0	9.0
			% Time in range		
>100 (bpm)	0.0%	0.0%	0.0%	0.0%	0.0%
90–100 (bpm)	0.0%	0.0%	0.0%	0.0%	0.0%
80–89 (bpm)	0.0%	0.0%	0.1%	0.0%	0.0%
70–79 (bpm)	7.4%	1.7%	0.9%	1.5%	1.9%
60–69 (bpm)	48.1%	55.0%	51.4%	54.0%	53.6%
50–59 (bpm)	10.9%	43.2%	47.6%	44.3%	42.1%
<50 (bpm)	2.1%	0.0%	0.0%	0.0%	0.1%
% Artifact/bad data	31.4%	0.2%	0.0%	0.1%	2.2%

Cardiac Events	Brady.	Asystole	Tachy.	Narrow Complex Tachy.	Wide Complex Tachy.	Atrial Fibrillation	Accel.	Decel.
Count	0	0	0	0	0	0	0	0
Shortest event (min:s)	N/A	N/A	N/A	N/A	N/A	N/A	N/A	N/A
Longest event (min:s)	N/A	N/A	N/A	N/A	N/A	N/A	N/A	N/A
Sum duration (min:s)	0:00:00	0:00:00	0:00:00	0:00:00	0:00:00	0:00:00	0:00:00	0:00:00
Absolute max. rate (bpm)	N/A	N/A	N/A	N/A	N/A	N/A	N/A	N/A
Absolute min. rate (bpm)	N/A	N/A	N/A	N/A	N/A	N/A	N/A	N/A

Sleep Architecture

Lights out clock time (h:min)	12:52:00 a.m.
Lights on clock time (h:min)	5:36:59 a.m.
TRT (in min)	285.0
SPT*	4:44:36
TST (in min)	278.0
SE	97.5%
SL	0:00:24
Total stage changes (after SO)	64
Awakenings (after SO)	10
WASO	6.6
REM periods	3
REM latency*	0:15:30
REM latency (less wake time)*	0:15:30

*Time formats are in h:min:sec

Figure 42-1 (*continued*)

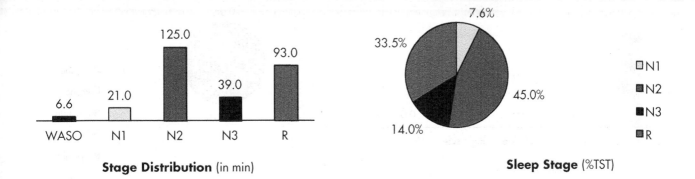

Stage Distribution (in min)   **Sleep Stage** (%TST)

Sleep Stage	Latency (min)
N1	0.0
N2	2.0
N3	13.0
R	15.5

Stage latency = 0.0 denotes start of sleep.

Respiratory Events	CA	OA	MA	Hypopneas	Total Apneas	Apnea+ Hypopnea	RERA	All Resp. Events *
Count	3	0	0	19	3	22	0	22
Index (events/h)	0.6	0.0	0.0	4.1	0.6	4.7	0.0	4.7
Mean duration (s)	13.5	N/A	N/A	28.5	13.5	26.4	N/A	26.4
Longest event (s)	18.4	N/A	N/A	56.3	18.4	56.3	N/A	56.3
REM count	0	0	0	14	0	14	0	14
Non-REM count	3	0	0	5	3	8	0	8
REM index	0.0	0.0	0.0	9.0	0.0	9.0	0.0	9.0
Non-REM index	1.0	0.0	0.0	1.6	1.0	2.6	0.0	2.6

*Note: Does not contain Cheyne–Stokes breathing, hypoventilation, or periodic breathing.

Respiratory Events (by body position)	Supine Sleep		Prone Sleep		Left-Side Sleep		Right-Side Sleep		Upright Sleep	
	Count	Index	Count	Index	Count	Index	Count	Index	Count	Index
Duration (h:min:s)	4:38:00		0:00:00		0:00:00		0:00:00		0:00:00	
OA	0	0.0	N/A	N/A	N/A	N/A	N/A	N/A	N/A	N/A
CA	3	0.6	N/A	N/A	N/A	N/A	N/A	N/A	N/A	N/A
MA	0	0.0	N/A	N/A	N/A	N/A	N/A	N/A	N/A	N/A
Hypopneas	19	4.1	N/A	N/A	N/A	N/A	N/A	N/A	N/A	N/A
RERAs	0	0.0	N/A	N/A	N/A	N/A	N/A	N/A	N/A	N/A
Total	22	4.7	N/A	N/A	N/A	N/A	N/A	N/A	N/A	N/A

Figure 42-1 (*continued*)

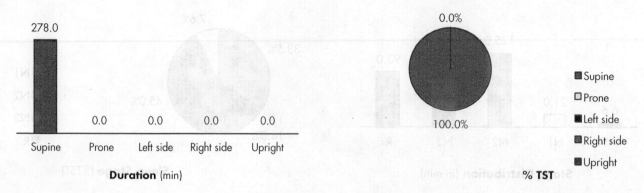

Body Position Results

Arousals	Resp. Count	Resp. Index	Spontaneous Count*	Spontaneous Index*	Total Count	Total Index
TST	1	0.2	27	5.8	28	6.0
Non-REM	1	0.3	21	6.8	22	7.1
REM	0	0.0	6	3.9	6	3.9

*EEG arousal activity *not* associated with *respiratory* or *PLM* events.

Limb Movements (by sleep stage)	LM w Arousals Count	LM w Arousals Index	LM w/o Arousals Count	LM w/o Arousals Index	Total LMs Count	Total LMs Index	PLM Series Count	PLM Series Index
TST	0	0.0	2	0.4	2	0.4	0	0.0
N1	0	0.0	1	2.9	1	2.9	0	0.0
N2	0	0.0	1	0.5	1	0.5	0	0.0
N3	0	0.0	0	0.0	0	0.0	0	0.0
R	0	0.0	0	0.0	0	0.0	0	0.0

Oxygen Desaturation Events	Count	Index
TST	28	6.0
Wake (after SO)	0	0.0
Non-REM	12	3.9
REM	16	10.3

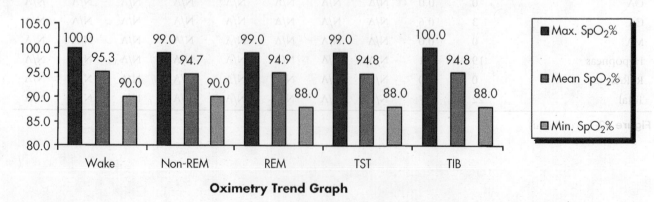

Oximetry Trend Graph

Figure 42-1 (*continued*)

OXYGEN SATURATION	Wake	Non-REM	REM	TST	TIB
Max. SpO$_2$%	100.0	99.0	99.0	99.0	100.0
Mean SpO$_2$%	95.3	94.7	94.9	94.8	94.8
Min. SpO$_2$%	90.0	90.0	88.0	88.0	88.0
SpO$_2$% ≤ 89% (min)	0.0	0.0	0.6	0.6	0.6
% Time in range					
90–100%	99.0%	100.0%	99.0%	99.6%	99.6%
80–89%	1.0%	0.0%	1.0%	0.4%	0.4%
70–79%	0.0%	0.0%	0.0%	0.0%	0.0%
60–69%	0.0%	0.0%	0.0%	0.0%	0.0%
50–59%	0.0%	0.0%	0.0%	0.0%	0.0%
<50%	0.0%	0.0%	0.0%	0.0%	0.0%
% Artifact/bad data	0.0%	0.0%	0.0%	0.0%	0.0%

HR Results	Wake	Non-REM	REM	TST	TIB
Max. HR (bpm)	79.0	79.0	81.0	81.0	81.0
Mean HR (bpm)	64.6	61.7	60.7	61.4	61.6
Min. HR (bpm)	9.0	54.0	49.0	49.0	9.0
% Time in range					
>100 (bpm)	0.0%	0.0%	0.0%	0.0%	0.0%
90–100 (bpm)	0.0%	0.0%	0.0%	0.0%	0.0%
80–89 (bpm)	0.0%	0.0%	0.1%	0.0%	0.0%
70–79 (bpm)	7.4%	1.7%	0.9%	1.5%	1.9%
60–69 (bpm)	48.1%	55.0%	51.4%	54.0%	53.6%
50–59 (bpm)	10.9%	43.2%	47.6%	44.3%	42.1%
<50 (bpm)	2.1%	0.0%	0.0%	0.0%	0.1%
% Artifact/bad data	31.4%	0.2%	0.0%	0.1%	2.2%

Cardiac Events	Brady.	Asystole	Tachy.	Narrow Complex Tachy.	Wide Complex Tachy.	Atrial Fibrillation	Accel.	Decel.
Count	0	0	0	0	0	0	0	0
Shortest event (min:s)	N/A	N/A	N/A	N/A	N/A	N/A	N/A	N/A
Longest event (min:s)	N/A	N/A	N/A	N/A	N/A	N/A	N/A	N/A
Sum duration (min:s)	0:00:00	0:00:00	0:00:00	0:00:00	0:00:00	0:00:00	0:00:00	0:00:00
Absolute max. rate (bpm)	N/A	N/A	N/A	N/A	N/A	N/A	N/A	N/A
Absolute min. rate (bpm)	N/A	N/A	N/A	N/A	N/A	N/A	N/A	N/A

Figure 42-1 (*continued*)

CPAP/Bilevel Titration Chart

Treatment Level (cm H₂O)	TIB	Time		Respiratory									Oximetry		
		REM (h:min:s)	Non-REM	OA	CA	MA	All Hypn's	A + H TOTAL	AHI	RERA	All Resp	RDI	Max. SpO₂%	Min. SpO₂%	Mean SpO₂%
CPAP 8	0:21:54	0:05:30	0:15:30	0	1	0	3	4	11.4	0	4	11.4	98.0	88.0	93.8
CPAP 9	0:11:52	0:11:52	0:00:00	0	0	0	3	3	15.2	0	3	15.2	98.0	90.0	94.3
CPAP 10	1:36:40	0:19:10	1:16:30	0	1	0	6	7	4.4	0	7	4.4	98.0	90.0	94.6
CPAP 11	1:07:10	0:45:58	0:18:12	0	1	0	4	5	4.7	0	5	4.7	98.0	91.0	95.2
CPAP 12	1:27:54	0:10:30	1:14:48	0	0	0	3	3	2.1	0	3	2.1	99.0	90.0	95.1

CPAP / BiLevel (IPAP / EPAP)

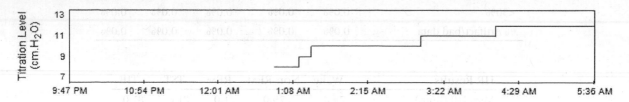

Hypnogram

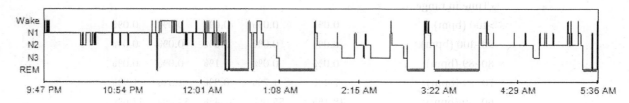

Respiratory Events

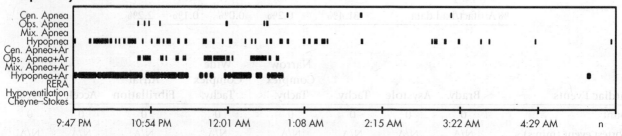

SpO₂%

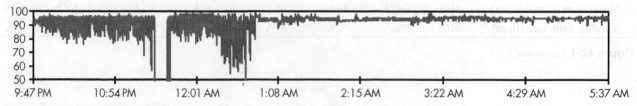

Figure 42-1 *(continued)*

Body Position

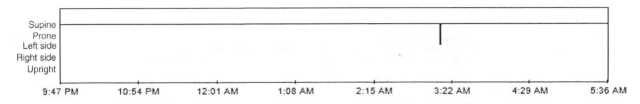

Limb Movement Events

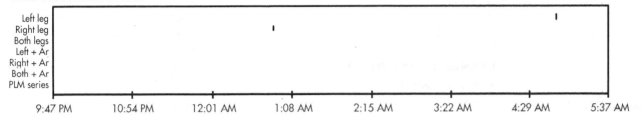

Figure 42-1 (*continued*)

A report generated for clinical use should be relevant, concise, and easily understood by the referring physician (6). This type of report generally serves the needs of the third-party payer as well. It typically includes a summary of sleep architecture, respiratory events, oxygen saturation levels, limb movements, arousals, and heart rate (HR) in a tabular form. A graphic summary is usually also presented. This report should not exceed two or three pages at the most. Figure 42-2 is an example of a Split-Night Study—Referring Physician Report.

Split Night Report (Referring Physician Report)

Patient Name: Walker, Ima			
Gender	Female	Study date	September 13, 2011
D.O.B.	December 6, 1946	Subject code	98765
Age	64	Referring physician	Frequent referral, MD
Height	66.0 in	Sleep specialist	Sleep doctor, MD
Weight	190.0 lbs	Recording tech	IM Sleepy, RPSGT
BMI	30.7	Scoring tech	JW Atkinson, RPSGT

Study Indications:
Daytime complaints of EDS (ESS=9), loud snoring, nonrestorative sleep. Sleep complaints of breathing/snoring stops in sleep, wakes for unknown reasons, restless sleep, somniloquy, occasional heartburn, and bruxism.

Figure 42-2 Split-night report. CPAP, continuous positive airway pressure; PLM, periodic limb movement; REM, rapid eye movement; RERA, respiratory effort–related arousal; TIB, time in bed; TST, total sleep time; WASO, wake after sleep onset (referring physician report).

Diagnostic Analysis

Sleep Architecture	
Lights out clock time (h:min)	9:47:00 p.m.
Lights on clock time (h:min)	12:50:56 a.m.
TRT (in min)	183.9
SPT*	3:03:03
TST (in min)	161.0
SE	87.5%
SL	0:00:54
Total stage changes (after SO)	84
Awakenings (after SO)	19
WASO	22.0
REM periods	2
REM latency*	1:35:00
REM latency (less wake time)*	1:32:30

*Time formats are in h:min:s

Respiratory Events	CA	OA	MA	Hypopneas	Total Apneas	Apnea+ Hypopnea	RERA	All Resp. Events*
Count	0	52	0	155	52	207	0	207
Index (events/h)	0.0	19.4	0.0	57.8	19.4	77.1	0.0	77.1
Mean duration (s)	N/A	29.4	N/A	24.0	29.4	25.3	N/A	25.3
Longest event (s)	N/A	66.1	N/A	81.9	66.1	81.9	N/A	81.9
REM count	0	10	0	7	10	17	0	17
Non-REM count	0	42	0	148	42	190	0	190
REM index	0.0	29.3	0.0	20.5	29.3	49.8	0.0	49.8
Non-REM index	0.0	17.9	0.0	63.2	17.9	81.1	0.0	81.1

*Note: Does not contain Cheyne–Stokes breathing, hypoventilation, or periodic breathing.

Arousals	Resp. Count	Resp. Index	Spontaneous Count*	Spontaneous Index*	Total Count	Total Index
TST	153	57.0	25	9.3	178	66.3
Non-REM	141	60.2	25	10.7	166	70.9
REM	12	35.1	0	0.0	12	35.1

*EEG arousal activity not associated with respiratory or PLM events.

Figure 42-2 (*continued*)

Limb Movements (by sleep stage)	LM w Arousals Count	LM w Arousals Index	LM w/o Arousals Count	LM w/o Arousals Index	Total LMs Count	Total LMs Index	PLM Series Count	PLM Series Index
TST	0	0.0	0	0.0	0	0.0	0	0.0
N1	0	0.0	0	0.0	0	0.0	0	0.0
N2	0	0.0	0	0.0	0	0.0	0	0.0
N3	N/A	N/A	N/A	N/A	N/A	N/A	N/A	N/A
R	0	0.0	0	0.0	0	0.0	0	0.0

Oxygen Desaturation Events	Count	Index
TST	200	74.5
Wake (after SO)	5	13.6
Non-REM	181	77.3
REM	19	55.6

Oxygen Saturation	Wake	Non-REM	REM	TST	TIB
Max. SpO$_2$%	100.0	99.0	99.0	99.0	100.0
Mean SpO$_2$%	89.7	90.6	80.0	89.3	89.3
Min. SpO$_2$%	51.0	57.0	54.0	.0	51.0
SpO$_2$% ≤ 89% (min)	0.1	49.3	14.5	63.8	67.7
% Time in range					
90–100%	36.7%	59.6%	26.6%	55.4%	53.0%
80–89%	12.7%	35.3%	23.3%	33.7%	31.1%
70–79%	1.0%	3.9%	23.9%	6.4%	5.7%
60–69%	3.2%	0.8%	21.5%	3.4%	3.4%
50–59%	1.0%	0.1%	4.7%	0.7%	0.8%
<50%	0.0%	0.0%	0.0%	0.0%	0.0%
% Artifact/bad data	45.4%	0.4%	0.0%	0.3%	6.0%

HR Results	Wake	Non-REM	REM	TST	TIB
Max. HR (bpm)	79.0	79.0	81.0	81.0	81.0
Mean HR (bpm)	64.6	61.7	60.7	61.4	61.6
Min. HR (bpm)	9.0	54.0	49.0	49.0	9.0
% Time in range					
>100 (bpm)	0.0%	0.0%	0.0%	0.0%	0.0%
90–100 (bpm)	0.0%	0.0%	0.0%	0.0%	0.0%
80–89 (bpm)	0.0%	0.0%	0.1%	0.0%	0.0%
70–79 (bpm)	7.4%	1.7%	0.9%	1.5%	1.9%
60–69 (bpm)	48.1%	55.0%	51.4%	54.0%	53.6%
50–59 (bpm)	10.9%	43.2%	47.6%	44.3%	42.1%
<50 (bpm)	2.1%	0.0%	0.0%	0.0%	0.1%
% Artifact/bad data	31.4%	0.2%	0.0%	0.1%	2.2%

Figure 42-2 (*continued*)

Cardiac Events	Brady.	Asystole	Tachy.	Narrow Complex Tachy.	Wide Complex Tachy.	Atrial Fibrillation	Accel.	Decel.
Count	0	0	0	0	0	0	0	0
Shortest event (min:s)	N/A	N/A	N/A	N/A	N/A	N/A	N/A	N/A
Longest event (min:s)	N/A	N/A	N/A	N/A	N/A	N/A	N/A	N/A
Sum duration (min:s)	0:00:00	0:00:00	0:00:00	0:00:00	0:00:00	0:00:00	0:00:00	0:00:00
Absolute max. rate (bpm)	N/A	N/A	N/A	N/A	N/A	N/A	N/A	N/A
Absolute min. rate (bpm)	N/A	N/A	N/A	N/A	N/A	N/A	N/A	N/A

Treatment Analysis

Sleep Architecture

Lights out clock time (h:min)	12:52:00 a.m.
Lights on clock time (h:min)	5:36:59 a.m.
TRT (in min)	285.0
SPT*	4:44:36
TST (in min)	278.0
SE	97.5%
SL	0:00:24
Total stage changes (after SO)	64
Awakenings (after SO)	10
WASO	6.6
REM periods	3
REM latency*	0:15:30
REM latency (less wake time)*	0:15:30

*Time formats are in h:min:s

Respiratory Events	CA	OA	MA	Hypopneas	Total Apneas	Apnea+ Hypopnea	RERA	All Resp. Events*
Count	3	0	0	19	3	22	0	22
Index (events/h)	0.6	0.0	0.0	4.1	0.6	4.7	0.0	4.7
Mean duration (s)	13.5	N/A	N/A	28.5	13.5	26.4	N/A	26.4
Longest event (s)	18.4	N/A	N/A	56.3	18.4	56.3	N/A	56.3
REM count	0	0	0	14	0	14	0	14
Non-REM count	3	0	0	5	3	8	0	8
REM index	0.0	0.0	0.0	9.0	0.0	9.0	0.0	9.0
Non-REM index	1.0	0.0	0.0	1.6	1.0	2.6	0.0	2.6

*Note: Does not contain Cheyne–Stokes breathing, hypoventilation, or periodic breathing.

Figure 42-2 (*continued*)

Respiratory Events (by body-position)	Supine Sleep Count	Index	Prone Sleep Count	Index	Left-Side Sleep Count	Index	Right-Side Sleep Count	Index	Upright Sleep Count	Index
Duration (h:min:s)	4:38:00		0:00:00		0:00:00		0:00:00		0:00:00	
OA	0	0.0	N/A	N/A	N/A	N/A	N/A	N/A	N/A	N/A
CA	3	0.6	N/A	N/A	N/A	N/A	N/A	N/A	N/A	N/A
MA	0	0.0	N/A	N/A	N/A	N/A	N/A	N/A	N/A	N/A
Hypopneas	19	4.1	N/A	N/A	N/A	N/A	N/A	N/A	N/A	N/A
RERAs	0	0.0	N/A	N/A	N/A	N/A	N/A	N/A	N/A	N/A
Total	22	4.7	N/A	N/A	N/A	N/A	N/A	N/A	N/A	N/A

Arousals	Resp. Count	Resp. Index	Spontaneous Count*	Spontaneous Index*	Total Count	Total Index
TST	1	0.2	27	5.8	28	6.0
Non-REM	1	0.3	21	6.8	22	7.1
REM	0	0.0	6	3.9	6	3.9

*EEG arousal activity not associated with respiratory or PLM events.

Limb Movements (by sleep stage)	LM w Arousals Count	Index	LM w/o Arousals Count	Index	Total LMs Count	Index	PLM Series Count	Index
TST	0	0.0	2	0.4	2	0.4	0	0.0
N1	0	0.0	1	2.9	1	2.9	0	0.0
N2	0	0.0	1	0.5	1	0.5	0	0.0
N3	0	0.0	0	0.0	0	0.0	0	0.0
R	0	0.0	0	0.0	0	0.0	0	0.0

Oxygen Desaturation Events	Count	Index
TST	28	6.0
Wake (after SO)	0	0.0
Non-REM	12	3.9
REM	16	10.3

Oxygen Saturation	Wake	Non-REM	REM	TST	TIB
Max. SpO_2%	100.0	99.0	99.0	99.0	100.0
Mean SpO_2%	95.3	94.7	94.9	94.8	94.8
Min. SpO_2%	90.0	90.0	88.0	88.0	88.0
SpO_2% ≤ 89% (min)	0.0	0.0	0.6	0.6	0.6
% Time in range					
90–100%	99.0%	100.0%	99.0%	99.6%	99.6%
80–89%	1.0%	0.0%	1.0%	0.4%	0.4%
70–79%	0.0%	0.0%	0.0%	0.0%	0.0%
60–69%	0.0%	0.0%	0.0%	0.0%	0.0%
50–59%	0.0%	0.0%	0.0%	0.0%	0.0%
<50%	0.0%	0.0%	0.0%	0.0%	0.0%
% Artifact/bad data	0.0%	0.0%	0.0%	0.0%	0.0%

Figure 42-2 (*continued*)

HR Results	Wake	Non-REM	REM	TST	TIB
Max. HR (bpm)	79.0	79.0	81.0	81.0	81.0
Mean HR (bpm)	64.6	61.7	60.7	61.4	61.6
Min. HR (bpm)	9.0	54.0	49.0	49.0	9.0
% Time in range					
>100 (bpm)	0.0%	0.0%	0.0%	0.0%	0.0%
90–100 (bpm)	0.0%	0.0%	0.0%	0.0%	0.0%
80–89 (bpm)	0.0%	0.0%	0.1%	0.0%	0.0%
70–79 (bpm)	7.4%	1.7%	0.9%	1.5%	1.9%
60–69 (bpm)	48.1%	55.0%	51.4%	54.0%	53.6%
50–59 (bpm)	10.9%	43.2%	47.6%	44.3%	42.1%
<50 (bpm)	2.1%	0.0%	0.0%	0.0%	0.1%
% Artifact/bad data	31.4%	0.2%	0.0%	0.1%	2.2%

Cardiac Events	Brady.	Asystole	Tachy.	Narrow Complex Tachy.	Wide Complex Tachy.	Atrial Fibrillation	Accel.	Decel.
Count	0	0	0	0	0	0	0	0
Shortest event (min:s)	N/A	N/A	N/A	N/A	N/A	N/A	N/A	N/A
Longest event (min:s)	N/A	N/A	N/A	N/A	N/A	N/A	N/A	N/A
Sum duration (min:s)	0:00:00	0:00:00	0:00:00	0:00:00	0:00:00	0:00:00	0:00:00	0:00:00
Absolute max. rate (bpm)	N/A	N/A	N/A	N/A	N/A	N/A	N/A	N/A
Absolute min. rate (bpm)	N/A	N/A	N/A	N/A	N/A	N/A	N/A	N/A

CPAP/Bilevel Titration Chart

Treatment Level (cm H$_2$O)	Time			Respiratory										Oximetry		
	TIB	REM (h:min:s)	Non-REM	OA	CA	MA	All Hypn's	A + H Total	AHI	RERA	All Resp	RDI	Max. SpO$_2$%	Min. SpO$_2$%	Mean SpO$_2$%
CPAP 8	0:21:54	0:05:30	0:15:30	0	1	0	3	4	11.4	0	4	11.4	98.0	88.0	93.8
CPAP 9	0:11:52	0:11:52	0:00:00	0	0	0	3	3	15.2	0	3	15.2	98.0	90.0	94.3
CPAP 10	1:36:40	0:19:10	1:16:30	0	1	0	6	7	4.4	0	7	4.4	98.0	90.0	94.6
CPAP 11	1:07:10	0:45:58	0:18:12	0	1	0	4	5	4.7	0	5	4.7	98.0	91.0	95.2
CPAP 12	1:27:54	0:10:30	1:14:48	0	0	0	3	3	2.1	0	3	2.1	99.0	90.0	95.1

Figure 42-2 (*continued*)

Hypnogram

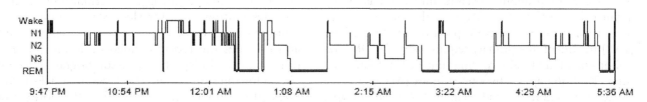

Respiratory Events

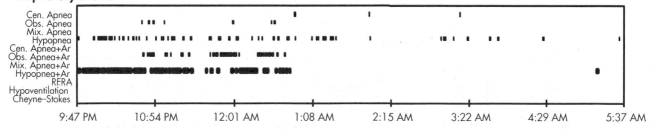

CPAP / BiLevel (IPAP / EPAP)

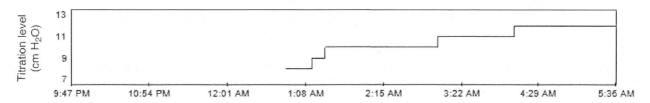

Body Position

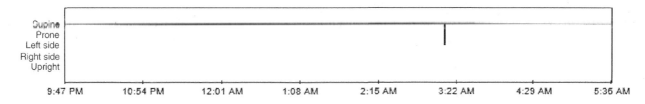

SpO$_2$%

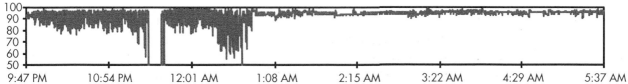

Limb Movement Events

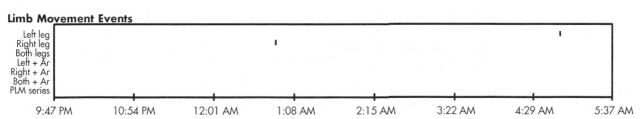

Figure 42-2 (*continued*)

A report to the homecare company or DME provider may be even more abbreviated and limited to basic sleep architecture, respiratory events, arousals, and oxygen saturation summaries. For basic positive airway pressure (PAP) treatment, the primary requirements for DME reimbursement are total recording time (TRT), total sleep time (TST), the apnea–hypopnea index (AHI), and the oxygen (O$_2$) saturation nadir. Figure 42-3 is an example of a Split-Night Report—DME/Insurance Co. Report.

The AASM manual for the scoring of sleep and associated events: Rules, terminology and technical specifications includes scoring rules for sleep stages, arousals, respiratory events, cardiac events, and movement events and provides the recommended minimum information to be included in a polysomnographic report. The following summarizes the AASM manual's recommended parameters for inclusion in the polysomnographic report (7).

Split-Night Report (DME/Insurance Co. Report)

Patient Name: Walker, Ima			
Gender	Female	Study date	September 13, 2011
D.O.B.	December 6, 1946	Subject code	98765
Age	64	Referring physician	Frequent referral, MD
Height	66.0 in	Sleep specialist	Sleep doctor, MD
Weight	190.0 lbs	Recording tech	IM Sleepy, RPSGT
BMI	30.7	Scoring tech	JW Atkinson, RPSGT

Study Indications:
Daytime complaints of EDS (ESS=9), loud snoring, nonrestorative sleep. Sleep complaints of breathing/snoring stops in sleep, wakes for unknown reasons, restless sleep, somniloquy, occasional heartburn, and bruxism.

Diagnostic Section

Sleep Architecture

Lights out clock time (h:min)	9:47:00 p.m.
Lights on clock time (h:min)	12:50:56 a.m.
TRT (in min)	183.9
SPT*	3:03:03
TST (in min)	161.0
SE	87.5%
SL	0:00:54
Total stage changes (after SO)	84
Awakenings (after SO)	19
WASO	22.0
REM periods	2
REM latency*	1:35:00
REM latency (less wake time)*	1:32:30

*Time formats are in h:min:s

Figure 42-3 Split-night report (durable medical equipment/Insurance Co. report). CPAP, continuous positive airway pressure; PLM, periodic limb movement; REM, rapid eye movement; TIB, time in bed; TST, total sleep time; WASO, wake after sleep onset.

Respiratory Events	CA	OA	MA	Hypopneas	Total Apneas	Apnea+ Hypopnea	RERA	All Resp. Events *
Count	0	52	0	155	52	207	0	207
Index (events/h)	0.0	19.4	0.0	57.8	19.4	**77.1**	0.0	77.1
Mean duration (s)	N/A	29.4	N/A	24.0	29.4	25.3	N/A	25.3
Longest event (s)	N/A	66.1	N/A	81.9	66.1	81.9	N/A	81.9
REM count	0	10	0	7	10	17	0	17
Non-REM count	0	42	0	148	42	190	0	190
REM index	0.0	29.3	0.0	20.5	29.3	49.8	0.0	49.8
Non-REM index	0.0	17.9	0.0	63.2	17.9	81.1	0.0	81.1

*Note: Does not contain Cheyne–Stokes breathing, hypoventilation, or periodic breathing.

Oxygen Desaturation Events	Count	Index
TST	200	74.5
Wake (after SO)	5	13.6
Non-REM	181	77.3
REM	19	55.6

Oxygen Saturation	Wake	Non-REM	REM	TST	TIB
Max. SpO_2%	100.0	99.0	99.0	99.0	100.0
Mean SpO_2%	89.7	90.6	80.0	89.3	89.3
Min. SpO_2%	51.0	57.0	54.0	54.0	51.0
SpO_2% ≤ 89% (min)	0.1	49.3	14.5	63.8	67.7
% Time in range					
90–100%	36.7%	59.6%	26.6%	55.4%	53.0%
80–89%	12.7%	35.3%	23.3%	33.7%	31.1%
70–79%	1.0%	3.9%	23.9%	6.4%	5.7%
60–69%	3.2%	0.8%	21.5%	3.4%	3.4%
50–59%	1.0%	0.1%	4.7%	0.7%	0.8%
<50%	0.0%	0.0%	0.0%	0.0%	0.0%
% Artifact/bad data	45.4%	0.4%	0.0%	0.3%	6.0%

Figure 42-3 (*continued*)

TREATMENT SECTION

Sleep Architecture

Lights out clock time (h:min)	12:52:00 a.m.
Lights on clock time (h:min)	5:36:59 a.m.
TRT (in min)	285.0
SPT*	4:44:36
TST (in min)	278.0
SE	97.5%
SL	0:00:24
Total stage changes (after SO)	64
Awakenings (after SO)	10
WASO	6.6
REM periods	3
REM latency*	0:15:30
REM latency (less wake time)*	0:15:30

*Time formats are in h:min:s

Oxygen Desaturation Events	Count	Index
TST	28	6.0
Wake (after SO)	0	0.0
Non-REM	12	3.9
REM	16	10.3

Respiratory Events	CA	OA	MA	Hypopneas	Total Apneas	Apnea+ Hypopnea	RERA	All Resp. Events*
Count	3	0	0	19	3	22	0	22
Index (events/h)	0.6	0.0	0.0	4.1	0.6	4.7	0.0	4.7
Mean duration (s)	13.5	N/A	N/A	28.5	13.5	26.4	N/A	26.4
Longest event (s)	18.4	N/A	N/A	56.3	18.4	56.3	N/A	56.3
REM count	0	0	0	14	0	14	0	14
Non-REM count	3	0	0	5	3	8	0	8
REM index	0.0	0.0	0.0	9.0	0.0	9.0	0.0	9.0
Non-REM index	1.0	0.0	0.0	1.6	1.0	2.6	0.0	2.6

*Note: Does not contain Cheyne–Stokes breathing, hypoventilation, or periodic breathing.

Figure 42-3 (*continued*)

Oxygen Saturation	Wake	Non-REM	REM	TST	TIB
Max. SpO$_2$%	100.0	99.0	99.0	99.0	100.0
Mean SpO$_2$%	95.3	94.7	94.9	94.8	94.8
Min. SpO$_2$%	90.0	90.0	88.0	88.0	88.0
SpO$_2$% ≤ 89% (min)	0.0	0.0	0.6	0.6	0.6
% Time in range					
90–100%	99.0%	100.0%	99.0%	99.6%	99.6%
80–89%	1.0%	0.0%	1.0%	0.4%	0.4%
70–79%	0.0%	0.0%	0.0%	0.0%	0.0%
60–69%	0.0%	0.0%	0.0%	0.0%	0.0%
50–59%	0.0%	0.0%	0.0%	0.0%	0.0%
<50%	0.0%	0.0%	0.0%	0.0%	0.0%
% Artifact/bad data	0.0%	0.0%	0.0%	0.0%	0.0%

Figure 42-3 (*continued*)

Recording Parameters

The AASM manual recommends listing the recording parameters employed during the sleep study in the report. These include the following:

a. Electroencephalogram (EEG) derivations
b. Electrooculogram (EOG) derivations
c. Chin electromyogram (EMG)
d. Leg EMG derivations
e. Airflow parameters
f. Effort parameters
g. Oxygen saturation
h. Body position
i. Electrocardiogram (ECG)

These are the typical parameters recorded. Although not specifically addressed, additional parameters such as carbon dioxide (CO_2) monitoring (end-tidal or transcutaneous) and esophageal pH monitoring should also be included in the list of recording parameters if they are utilized.

I. Sleep scoring data
   a. Lights out (off) time in hour:minute format
   b. Lights on time in hour:minute format
   c. TRT; lights off time to lights on time given in minutes
   d. TST; summation of all epochs of sleep given in minutes
   e. Sleep latency (SL); the time in minutes from lights out to the first epoch of sleep given in minutes (calculated by subtracting the lights out epoch number from the epoch number of the first epoch of sleep and dividing by 2)
   f. Stage R latency, RL; the time in minutes between the first epoch of sleep and the first epoch of stage R in minutes (calculated by subtracting the first epoch of sleep from the first epoch of stage R and dividing by 2)
   g. Wake after sleep onset (WASO); stage W in TRT minus the SL in minutes
   h. Percent sleep efficiency (SE); 100 × TST/TRT
   i. Time in each stage in minutes
   j. Percent of TST for each stage, %N1, %N2, and so on; 100 × time in each stage/TST

II. Arousal events
   a. The number of arousals
   b. Arousal index (ArI); 60 × # of arousals/TST

III. Respiratory events
   a. Number of obstructive apneas (OA)
   b. Number of mixed apneas (MA)
   c. Number of central apneas (CA)
   d. Number of hypopneas (H)
   e. Number of apneas and hypopneas
   f. Apnea index (AI); 60 × (OA + MA + CA)/TST
   g. Hypopnea index (HI); 60 × (H/TST)
   h. AHI; 60 × (OA + MA + CA + H)/TST
   i. Number of respiratory effort–related arousals* (RERA)
   j. Respiratory effort–related arousal index* (RERAI); 60 × (RERA)/TST
   k. Number of oxygen desaturations ≥3% or ≥4%**
   l. Oxygen desaturation index (ODI) ≥3% or ≥4%**; 60 × (O_2 desats/TST)
   m. Mean continuous oxygen saturation
   n. Minimum oxygen saturation in sleep (nadir)
   o. Occurrence of hypoventilation (a "yes/no" response)*
   p. Occurrence of Cheyne–Stokes breathing (a "yes/no" response)

---

*These are optional statistics.
**These are also optional and depend on the hypopnea rule employed; 3% desaturation or arousal (AASM alternate rule), or 4% desaturation (AASM-recommended rule).

IV. Cardiac events
    a. Average HR during sleep
    b. Highest HR during sleep
    c. Highest HR during the recording
        The presence of the arrhythmias listed in the following paragraph should be acknowledged by responding "yes" if they occur and providing the HR or the duration of the pause.
    d. Bradycardia (yes/no); report lowest HR observed (defined as HR <40 bpm, asleep)
    e. Asystole (yes/no); report longest event observed (defined as pause >3 seconds)
    f. Sinus tachycardia during sleep (yes/no); report highest HR observed (defined as sinus HR >90 bpm, asleep)
    g. Narrow complex tachycardia (yes/no); report highest HR observed
    h. Wide complex tachycardia (yes/no); report highest HR observed
    i. Atrial fibrillation (yes/no)
    j. Other arrhythmias (yes/no); report the arrhythmia such as heart block or significant ectopy

V. Movement events
    a. Number of PLMS
    b. Number of PLMS with arousals
    c. PLMS index (PLMSI); $60 \times$ (PLMS/TST)
    d. PLMS arousal index (PLMSArI); $60 \times$ (PLMS w arousal/TST)

VI. Summary statements
    a. Findings related to the diagnosis
    b. EEG abnormalities
    c. ECG abnormalities

    d. Behavioral observations
    e. Sleep hypnogram (this is optional)

The minimum recommended parameters will be expanded upon in the following sections.

COMMON SLEEP ARCHITECTURAL DEFINITIONS AND FORMULAE

Sleep architecture parameters generally include latencies, summation of time spent in each sleep stage and body position, and the percent of TST spent in each sleep stage. Latencies are defined as the time periods from one hallmark event, such as "lights out" or sleep onset (SO), to another hallmark event, such as REM onset or SO. The classic reporting parameters are TRT, TST, WASO, time spent in each sleep stage, and time spent in each body position. Computers can now subclassify these time frames to a much more stratified level. For example, a continuous positive airway pressure (CPAP) titration report may include a time value for each pressure setting, relative to every combination of sleep stage and body position (back/REM/CPAP $\times$ time). If you can define a parameter, it can be tabulated and reported!

Another reported parameter is the percentage of time spent in each sleep stage, relative to TST. In addition, the percent of TST relative to TRT establishes the SE. Variations from established normative data are often reported to help identify pathology and provide insight into the patient's clinical condition.

Table 42-1 presents common sleep architectural terms with definitions and formulae where indicated.

Table 42-1 Common Sleep Architectural Terms with Definitions and Formulae

Term	Definition/Formula
%Stage N1	The percentage of TST spent in stage N1 sleep $$(\text{Minutes of N1/TST}) \times 100$$ May also be presented as the percentage of TRT spent in N1, in which case the formula is $$(\text{Minutes of N1/TRT}) \times 100$$ Because TRT almost always includes some WASO, these presentations will always give a lower value than that of TST. Tables should clearly define the denominator for the statistic.
%Stage N2	The percentage of TST spent in N2 sleep $$(\text{Minutes of N2/TST}) \times 100$$ May also be presented as the percentage of TRT spent in N2, in which case the formula is $$(\text{Minutes of N2/TRT}) \times 100$$

Table 42-1 (continued)

Term	Definition/Formula
%Stage N3	The percentage of TST spent in N3 sleep $$(\text{Minutes of N3/TST}) \times 100$$ May also be presented as the percentage of TRT spent in N3, in which case the formula is $$(\text{Minutes of N3/TRT}) \times 100$$
%Stage R	The percentage of TST spent in REM sleep $$(\text{Minutes of R/TST}) \times 100$$ May also be presented as the percentage of TRT spent in REM, in which case the formula is $$(\text{Minutes of R/TRT}) \times 100$$
%Wake time, stage W	The percentage of time spent awake. This statistic can be based only on TRT $$(\text{Minutes of W/TRT}) \times 100$$ Tables including this statistic should clearly define the denominator
SO	The first epoch of sleep
Latency to stage R	The period of time from SO to the first epoch of stage R sleep. This could be 0.0 min if the first epoch of sleep is REM. To calculate in minutes, count the number of epochs and divide by two $$\frac{(\text{Criterion epoch} - \text{SO epoch})}{2}$$
Latency to N2	The period of time from SO to the first epoch of N2 sleep. This could indeed be 0.0 min if the first epoch of sleep is N2. To calculate in minutes, count the number of epochs and divide by two $$\frac{(\text{Criterion epoch} - \text{SO epoch})}{2}$$
Latency to N3	The period of time from SO to the first epoch of N3 sleep $$\frac{(\text{Criterion epoch} - \text{SO epoch})}{2}$$
SE	The portion of the TRT spent asleep. Usually expressed as a percentage $$(\text{TST/TRT}) \times 100$$
SL	The time from lights out to SO (first of any epoch of sleep) $$\frac{(\text{SO epoch} - \text{lights out epoch})}{2}$$
TRT	The time from "lights out" to "lights on." To calculate in minutes, count the number of epochs and divide by two $$\frac{(\text{"Lights on" epoch} - \text{"lights out" epoch})}{2}$$
TST	The total amount of sleep recorded during the TRT. The basis for many of the additional statistics and indices. Derived by summing the total of all the minutes of N1, N2, N3, and R sleep $$\text{Sleep time}_{Total} = N1_{Total} + N2_{Total} + N3_{Total} + R_{Total}$$

(continued)

Table 42-1 *(continued)*

Term	Definition/Formula
TWT	Total time spent awake during the TRT. It is the sum of SL, WASO, and WASP $$TWT = SL + WASO + WASP$$
Unequivocal sleep	Primarily used to determine the end point of a maintenance of wakefulness test. Unequivocal sleep is defined as follows: 1. The first of three consecutive epochs of N1 sleep 2. The first epoch of N2, N3, or R (e.g., unequivocal sleep occurs at the underscored stage R in the following sequence: W W W 1 W W R) 3. The first epoch of N1 that is contiguous with a non-N1 stage of sleep (e.g., unequivocal sleep is at the underscored stage N1 in the following sequence: W W W 1 W W 1 2)
WASO	Wakefulness occurring between the SO and the last epoch of sleep
TIB or TRT	The time from "lights out" to "lights on." To calculate in minutes, count the number of epochs and divide by two $$\frac{(\text{"Lights on" epoch} - \text{"lights out" epoch})}{2}$$

REM, rapid eye movement; SE, sleep efficiency; SL, sleep latency; SO, sleep onset; TIB, time in bed; TRT, total recording time; TST, total sleep time; TWT, total wake time; WASO, wake after sleep onset; WASP, wake after the sleep period.

ABNORMAL EVENT DEFINITIONS AND FORMULAE

In addition to the above-mentioned information, a reporting of abnormal events (apneas/hypopneas, limb movements, arousals, and indicated cardiac events) occurring during the polysomnogram provides the data to support the absence or presence and severity of sleep pathology. The number of event types and the data analysis statistics available to describe these events are practically limitless, depending only on one's needs and imagination. Traditionally, events commonly included in the sleep report are apneas and hypopneas, arousals, limb movements, and O_2 desaturations. The statistics reported can include any or all of the following:

- Number of events
- Maximum duration of events
- Average (mean) duration of events
- %TST occupied by a given event type
- Number of events of a given type per unit time, that is, TST (index)
- The lowest value of a given event type (nadir)

The number of events is self-explanatory; once the events have been described, simply count the number of events meeting the definition criteria.

The maximum duration is the longest event matching the definition criteria.

The mean duration of the event is determined by adding the durations of all the events and dividing by the total number of events.

The percentage of the TST occupied by a given event is the total of the durations of all the events divided by TST × 100.

The calculation of an *index* represents the average number of a specific event per hour of sleep time. Utilizing a standard epoch length of 30 seconds per epoch, the total number of epochs scored as sleep is counted and divided by two. This provides the total number of minutes of sleep. The events of interest are then counted, multiplied by 60, and divided by the total minutes of sleep.

The *nadir* is the lowest value recorded of an event type.

Table 42-2 presents common event parameters and formulae where indicated.

HISTOGRAPHIC PRESENTATION

The old adage "A picture is worth a thousand words" holds true for polysomnographic reports. Graphic representation of the sleep histogram aligned with the graphic representation of oxygen saturation levels, body position, abnormal respiratory events, PLMs, arousals, and CPAP treatment levels provides a wealth of valuable information even to the inexperienced viewer. Most polysomnographic recording systems provide this reporting capability.

The graph (or histogram) included with the reports shown in Figures 42-1 and 42-2 shows repetitive apneas and hypopnea with severe desaturations and limited sleep other than N1 in the baseline portion of the recording. The treatment condition shows scattered

Table 42 2 Common Event Parameters and Formulae

Term	Definition/Formula
Total apneas	The total of all apneas recorded $$\text{Apneas}_{\text{Total}} = \text{obstructive apneas}_{\text{Total}} + \text{mixed apneas}_{\text{Total}} + \text{central apneas}_{\text{Total}}$$
Total hypopneas	The total of all hypopneas recorded $$\text{Hypopneas}_{\text{Total}} = \text{obstructive hypopneas}_{\text{total}}$$ $$+ \text{mixed hypopneas}_{\text{total}} + \text{central hypopneas}_{\text{total}}$$
AI	The number of apneas per hour of sleep $$AI = \text{\# apneas/hour of sleep}$$ or $$AI = (\text{\# apneas/minutes of sleep}) \times 60$$
Hypopnea index	The number of hypopneas per hour of sleep $$AI = \text{\# hypopneas/hour of sleep}$$ or $$AI = (\text{\# hypopneas/minutes of sleep}) \times 60$$
AHI	The number of apneas and hypopneas per hour of sleep. This statistic is useful to compare baseline with treatment conditions and one treatment condition to another because the time base is the same or $$AHI = \text{\# apneas} + \text{\# hypopneas/hour of sleep}$$ or $$AHI = (\text{\# apneas} + \text{\# hypopneas}) \times (60)/\text{minutes of sleep}$$
Polysomnography RDI	Formerly synonymous with AHI, more recently it has come to mean number of apneas and number of hypopneas and number of RERAs per hour of sleep $$RDI = (\text{apneas}) + (\text{\# hypopneas}) + (\text{RERAs})/\text{hours of sleep}$$ or $$RDI = (\text{\# apneas} + \text{\# hypopneas} + \text{RERAs}) \times (60)/\text{minutes of sleep}$$
Home sleep apnea testing RDI	Ever since the recognition of type III home sleep testing, RDI has been defined by the Centers for Medicare & Medicaid Services as the number of apneas and hypopneas per hour of recording time because sleep staging parameters are not recorded. $$RDI = \text{\# apneas} + \text{\# hypopneas} /\text{hours of recording time}$$ or $$RDI = (\text{\# apneas} + \text{\# hypopneas}) \times (60)/\text{minutes of recording time}$$
Mean duration apnea	The sum of all apnea durations (Σ apnea duration) per number of apnea events $$\text{Mean duration apnea} = \frac{\Sigma \text{ apnea duration}}{\text{No. apnea}}$$
Mean duration hypopnea	The sum of all hypopnea durations (Σ hypopnea duration) per number of hypopneic events. $$\text{Mean duration hypopnea} = \frac{\Sigma \text{ hypopnea duration}}{\text{No. hypopneas}}$$
Maximum duration apnea	The longest apneic event recorded

Table 42-2 *(continued)*

Term	Definition/Formula
Maximum duration hypopnea	The longest hypopneic event recorded
DI	The number of desaturation events per hour of sleep or DI = # desaturation events/hours of sleep or DI = (# desaturation events/minutes of sleep) × 60
Saturation nadir	The lowest saturation recording during the recording
PLMI	The number of PLMs per hour of sleep or PLMSI = #PLMS/hours of sleep or PLMSI = (#PLMS/minutes of sleep) × 60
Total PLM	The number of period limb movement events scored
Total PLM with arousal	The number of PLMs with corresponding arousals
PLMArI	The number of PLMs with arousal per hour of sleep or PLMArI = #PLMS with arousal/hours of sleep or PLMArI = (#PLMS with arousal/minutes of sleep) × 60
Desaturation events	The number of desaturation events meeting the criterion

AHI, apnea + hypopnea index; AI, apnea index; DI, desaturation index; PLMArI, PLM with arousal index; PLMI, periodic limb movement index; PLMS, periodic limb movements of sleep; PLMSI, PLMS index; RDI, respiratory disturbance index; RERA, respiratory effort–related arousal.

respiratory events, mostly in stage R and marked improvement in oxygen saturation. Significant amounts of N2 and N3 sleep are also present compared with the baseline condition.

DEVELOPING OTHER RELEVANT STATISTICS

Digital recording systems and their data manipulation abilities make it possible to develop statistics and reports that can provide significant amounts of data for the end user. As an example, it is common to report the AHI in both the baseline and the treatment segments of a split-night protocol recording. Understanding the concept of indices (the number of events per unit of time for a given condition) makes the derivation of the requisite formulae a relatively simple task. The key is to define the condition(s), calculate the time spent in that condition, and then tabulate the events occurring in that condition. To obtain the relevant index, the

number of events is multiplied by 60 and then divided by the minutes of time. For example, to calculate the AHI before and after CPAP initiation, the following formulae would be used:

$$\text{AHI}_{\text{baseline}} = (\text{\# apneas}_{\text{baseline}} + \text{\# hypopneas}_{\text{baseline}})/\text{TST (hours)}_{\text{baseline}}$$

or

$$\text{AHI}_{\text{baseline}} = (\text{\# apneas}_{\text{baseline}} + \text{\# hypopneas}_{\text{baseline}}) \times 60/\text{TST (minutes)}_{\text{baseline}}$$

and

$$\text{AHI}_{\text{treatment}} = (\text{\# apneas}_{\text{treatment}} + \text{\# hypopneas}_{\text{treatment}})/\text{TST (hours)}_{\text{treatment}}$$

or

$$\text{AHI}_{\text{treatment}} = (\text{\# apneas}_{\text{treatment}} + \text{\# hypopneas}_{\text{treatment}}) \times 60/\text{TST (minutes)}_{\text{treatment}}$$

To take this concept a bit further, suppose you are interested in finding the AHI for a given treatment condition such as a CPAP level of 10 cm H_2O in the supine position. Again, define the condition and tabulate the number of events and sleep time spent in that condition.

$$AHI_{CPAP\ of\ 10/SUPINE} = (\#apneas_{CPAP\ of\ 10/S} + \\ \#hypopneas_{CPAP\ of\ 10/S})/ \\ TST\ (hours)_{CPAP\ of\ 10/S}$$

or

$$AHI_{CPAP\ of\ 10/SUPINE} = (\#apneas_{CPAP\ of\ 10/S} + \\ \#hypopneas_{CPAP\ of\ 10/S}) \\ \times 60/TST\ (minutes)_{CPAP\ of\ 10/S}$$

It may be that you would like to see the AHI for each CPAP or bilevel treatment level. As aforementioned, define the treatment condition, calculate the number of events for each level of treatment, and divide by the sleep time spent in that condition.

As another example, if you are interested in determining the percentage of apnea relative to the total AHI, the following formula is applied:

$$\%apnea = (\#apneas \times 100)/(\#\ apneas + \#\ hypopneas)$$

As can be seen from these few examples, the number of statistical data points is limited only by the imagination and the need of the user. Most equipment manufacturers provide the capability of tailoring reports to the specific requirements of the customer and have prescribed fields that may be used to generate customized statistics and reports. It is interesting to consider the number of hours that would be necessary to calculate something such as the AHI for each CPAP treatment level in the days before digital recordings.

THE DICTATED SUMMARY

The dictated summary of the recording should be presented in an orderly manner. The following outline is generally accepted:

I. Findings related to sleep diagnosis include the following:
   a. Patient history and indications for the study
   b. A description of the monitoring parameters and recording montage
   c. A description of the sleep architecture
   d. Respiratory events and O_2 saturation levels
   e. PLMs
   f. Arousals

II. Cardiac events

III. Other events (EEG abnormalities and parasomnias/behavioral observations)

IV. Impression

V. Comments

VI. Recommendations

Note that much of the report can be obtained from the information derived directly from the demographics and the recording data from the sleep study. See Figure 42-4 as a good example of a Split-Night Report—Dictated Final Report.

Split-Night Report (Dictated Final Report)

Patient's Name: Ima Walker

Date of Study: September 13, 2011
Referring Clinician: Frequent Referral, MD
Date of Interpretation: September 15, 2011

Demographics:
The patient is a 64-year-old, 66.0 tall, 190.0 pound female with a BMI of 30.7, who completed a split-night study. The patient presents to the sleep lab with complaints of excessive daytime sleepiness (ESS=9), loud snoring, non-restorative sleep. Sleep complaints of breathing/snoring stops in sleep, wakes for unknown reasons, restless sleep, somniloquy, occasional heartburn, and bruxism. Patient previously smoked for 15 years, she quit Dec. 1984. She drinks two alcoholic drinks per week and 2 to 4 diet sodas daily. She is being treated for HTN, Heart Cath in June '06, Neck circumference=16".

Current Medications:
Lipitor, Tricor, Ramipril, Triamterene/HCTZ, Levocetirizine, Buspirone HCl, Metoprolol Tartrate, Nabumetone, Aspirin, Fish Oil, Niacin, Centrum Silver MVI.

Study Methods:
The polysomnography study included recording and monitoring of EEG, EMG, ECG, pulse oximetry, respiratory effort and flow, body position, and snoring. Video recordings were obtained as needed. A qualified sleep technologist continuously monitored the patient throughout the night. Sleep staging and respiratory events were scored manually using the AASM standards. The data were digitally collected using XXX software.

Figure 42-4 Split-night report (dictated final report) Sample report D.

Diagnostic Period:

The diagnostic period took place from 9:47:00 p.m. to 12:50:56 a.m. The patient took 0.9 minutes to fall asleep, and slept for a total of 161.0 minutes out of 183.9 minutes of TRT, which resulted in a SE of 87.5%. REM latency is recorded at 92.5 minutes.

The patient's sleep architecture consisted of

Stage N1 (NREM 1):	78.3%	(126.0 minutes)
Stage N2 (NREM 2):	9.0%	(14.5 minutes)
Stage N3 (NREM 3):	0.0%	(0.0 minutes)
Stage R (REM)	: 12.7%	(20.5 minutes)

The patient had an average AHI of 77.1, with oxygen saturation falling to a low of 51.0%. The patient had a mean oxygen saturation of 89.3% throughout the diagnostic period of the study. The patient experienced 0 PLM events, resulting in a PLM index of 0.0 (events per hour).

Treatment Period:

The treatment period took place from 12:52:00 a.m. to 5:36:59 a.m. The patient took 0.4 minutes to fall asleep, and slept for a total of 278.0 minutes out of 285.0 minutes of TRT, which resulted in a SE of 97.5%. REM latency is recorded at 15.5 minutes.

The patient's sleep architecture consisted of

Stage N1 (NREM 1):	7.6%	(21.0 minutes)
Stage N2 (NREM 2):	45.0%	(125.0 minutes)
Stage N3 (NREM 3):	14.0%	(39.0 minutes)
Stage R (REM)	: 33.5%	(93.0 minutes)

With PAP therapy, the overall AHI was recorded as 4.7, with oxygen saturation falling to a low of 88.0%. The patient had a mean oxygen saturation of 94.8% throughout the treatment period of the study. With PAP therapy of 12 cm H_2O, the AHI was reduced to 2.1. The patient experienced two PLM events, resulting in a PLM index of 0.4 (events per hour).

Interpretation:

Severe sleep apnea was treated with PAP therapy of 12 cm H_2O. The Periodic Limb Movement Index of 0.3 is considered to be insignificant.

Recommendations:

1. Sleep hygiene information.
2. Avoid the use of depressant medication and alcohol in the evenings.
3. The patient may benefit from upper airway evaluation if clinically indicated.
4. Avoid sleeping in the supine position.
5. The patient may benefit from weight loss.
6. Begin CPAP therapy of 12 cm H_2O using heated humidification and optional use of pressure relief.

Sleepy Doctor, MD

Figure 42-4 (*continued*)

TECHNOLOGIST COMMENTS

A key component of the polysomnographic report is the attending and scoring of the technologist's comments. These key individuals, who have spent the most time with the patient and the data, respectively, can add further insight into the study. Examples may include an account of the patient's physical and emotional status, a description of audible breathing or snoring sounds, and any atypical findings that are not evident in the routine tabulation of sleep stages and events, such as alpha intrusion, medication effects on the EEG, atypical motor activity during REM sleep, or any other pertinent observations of parasomnia-like activity. This type of information is generally intended for the reading physician only and should not be distributed to insurers, referral sources, or DME/homecare vendors.

DATA ARCHIVING AND STORAGE

Once record scoring and report generation are completed, the data must be archived and stored for a period of time. This period may vary, but typically this is regulated by state statute. A typical period required to keep records is 7 years or 7 years beyond the age of majority for unemancipated minors. Check the statutes in your state as they may vary.

The archiving process usually involves removing the data and video/audio recording to a remote server for access by the interpreter and then long-term archiving on a large file server with off-site backup. This type of system can be expensive but is usually fairly low in labor intensity. Other alternatives involve archiving to external hard drives or CD/DVD media.

When archiving the recording, one should always *copy* rather than move the record from the recording device to the storage device. Copying provides a safety net to prevent loss of data due to corruption during the transfer. The *move* process deletes the data from the original device as the transfer is being completed and hence risks data loss if the data become corrupt during the transfer process. *Check the integrity* of the data on the archival medium before *deleting* the recording from the original device.

Home Sleep Apnea Testing

The following rules for scoring and reporting Home Sleep Apnea Testing (HSAT) have been developed and are included in *The AASM manual for the scoring of sleep and associated events: Rules, terminology and technical specifications, version 2.5*, for recording devices that utilize respiratory flow and effort parameters or peripheral arterial tonometry (PAT).

Reporting HSAT Using Respiratory Flow and/or Effort Parameters

I. General reporting parameters
  a. Type of device
  b. Type of airflow sensor(s)
  c. Type of respiratory effort sensor(s)—could be single or dual
  d. Oxygen saturation
  e. HR (from ECG or from pulse oximetry)
  f. Body position—optional
  g. Sleep/wake or monitoring time (MT) (if sleep/wake is reported, EEG, EOG, and chin EMG must be recorded; if MT is used, the method of determining the recording time should be specified)—optional
  h. Snoring (from nasal pressure cannula, piezo, or acoustic sensor)—optional

II. Recording data required to be reported
  a. Start time of the recording (hour:minute)
  b. End time of the recording (hour:minute)
  c. Total recording time (TRT) in minutes including wake and artifact
  d. MT in minutes (the divisor used to calculate the respiratory event index [REI])
  e. TST in minutes if EEG, EOG, and chin EMG are recorded (the divisor for calculating AHI if sleep is recorded and scored)
  f. HR (maximum, minimum, average)

  g. Number of respiratory events (REs)
    i. Number of apneas
      1. Number of central mixed and obstructive events (phenotyping of apneic events is optional)
    ii. Number of hypopneas
  h. REI 60 × (apneas + hypopneas/MT)
  i. Apnea–hypopnea index (AHI) 60 × (apneas + hypopneas/TST) if sleep is recorded
  j. REI and AHI, supine and nonsupine—optional
  k. Central apnea index (CAI = 60 × # CA/MT)—optional
  l. A measure of oxygen desaturation using at least one of the following three parameters:
    i. ODI >3% or ≥4%; ODI − 60 × # of desaturation events ≥3% or ≥4% per MT in minutes. The employed threshold level ≥3% or ≥4% must be specified.
    ii. SpO_2 saturation (maximum, minimum, and mean values)
    iii. SpO_2 saturation (% time at or below 88% or other designated thresholds
  m. Presence of snoring (if recorded)—optional

III. Summary statements
  a. Testing date/interpretation date
  b. Study technical adequacy (as defined in sleep center policies and procedures)
    i. Document repeat studies caused by technical failure
    ii. Limitations of the study
  c. Interpretation of REI (based on MT) or AHI (if sleep recorded)
  d. Occurrence of snoring, if recorded
  e. Interpretation
    i. Whether or not the study supports the diagnosis of obstructive sleep apnea
    ii. Statement of diagnostic severity, if applicable
    iii. If study is nondiagnostic, recommendation of in-laboratory polysomnogram, if indicated by clinical history
  f. Printed name and signature of interpreting physician (verification of raw data review)
  g. Recommendation for management of patient meeting AASM clinical practice guidelines and practice parameters
  h. Chain of custody, if applicable—optional

Reporting HSAT Using PAT

I. General reporting parameters
  a. Type of device
  b. Sleep, wake, REM times derived from actigraphy

c. Airflow/effort surrogate signals (based on peripheral arterial tone)

d. Oxygen saturation

e. HR

f. Body position—optional

g. Snoring, if recorded—optional

II. Recording data required to be reported

a. Start time of the recording (hour:minute)

b. End time of the recording (hour:minute)

c. TRT in hours:minutes

d. Estimated sleep time (in minutes)

   i. Estimated % REM, light sleep, deep sleep—optional

e. HR (maximum, minimum, average)

f. Number of RE

g. REI (use PAT AHI [pAHI] as a surrogate for REI)

h. ODI ≥4%, ODI = 60 × # of desaturation events ≥4% per MT in minutes

III. Summary statements

a. Testing date/interpretation date

b. Study technical adequacy (as defined in sleep center policies and procedures)

   i. Document repeat studies caused by technical failure

   ii. Limitations of the study

c. Interpretation of estimated sleep time

d. Occurrence of snoring, if recorded—optional

e. Interpretation

   i. Whether or not the study supports the diagnosis of OSAS

   ii. Statement of diagnostic severity, if applicable

   iii. If study is nondiagnostic, recommendation of in-laboratory polysomnogram, if indicated by clinical history

f. Printed name and signature of interpreting physician (verification of raw data review)

g. Recommendation for management of patient meeting AASM clinical practice guidelines and practice parameters

h. Chain of custody, if applicable—optional

REFERENCES

1. Aldrich, M. (1999). Approach to the patient. In M. Aldrich (Ed.), *Sleep medicine* (pp. 95–110). New York, NY: Oxford University Press.

2. Rechtschaffen, A., & Kales, A. (1968). *A manual of standardized terminology, techniques, and scoring system for the sleep stages of human subjects.* Los Angeles, CA: UCLA BIS/BRI Publications.

3. Bonnet, M., Carley, D., Carskadon, M., et al. (1992). ASDA report: Atlas and scoring rules: EEG arousals; scoring rules and examples. *Sleep, 15*(2), 174–184.

4. Bonnet, M., Carley, D., Carskadon, M., et al. (1993). ASDA report: Atlas and scoring rules: Recording and scoring leg movements. *Sleep, 16*(8), 749–759.

5. American Academy of Sleep Medicine. (1999). Sleep related breathing disorders in adults: Recommendations for syndrome definition and measurement techniques in clinical research: The report of the American Academy of Sleep Medicine Task Force. *Sleep, 22,* 667–789.

6. Butkov, N. (2002). Polysomnography. In T. Lee-Chiong, M. Sateia, & M. Carskadon (Eds.), *Sleep medicine* (p. 636). Philadelphia, PA: Hanley and Belfus.

7. Berry, R. B., Albertario, C. L., Harding, S. M., et al.; for the American Academy of Sleep Medicine. (2018). *The AASM manual for the scoring of sleep and associated events: Rules, terminology and technical specifications* [Version 2.5]. Darien, IL: American Academy of Sleep Medicine.

chapter 43

Multiple Sleep Latency Test and Maintenance of Wakefulness Test

DAVID MOORE   S. JUSTIN THOMAS

LEARNING OBJECTIVES

On completion of this chapter, the reader should be able to:

1. Recognize the potential consequences of excessive sleepiness.
2. Identify the difference between subjective and objective evaluation of sleepiness.
3. Discuss the indications for performing the multiple sleep latency test (MSLT) and the maintenance of wakefulness test (MWT).
4. Describe the general considerations regarding the MSLT and MWT.
5. Describe the specific protocols for performing and interpreting the MSLT and MWT.

KEY TERMS

Excessive daytime sleepiness (EDS)
Narcolepsy
Idiopathic hypersomnia
Sleep latency
Sleep-onset rapid eye movement period (SOREMP)

The American Academy of Sleep Medicine (AASM) has defined excessive daytime sleepiness (EDS) as sleepiness occurring in a situation when an individual would be expected to be awake and alert (1). Excessive sleepiness is a complex issue that has had a profound impact on society. The cost of accidents due to excessive sleepiness has been estimated at approximately $43.15 to $56.02 billion during 1988 alone (2). Although these figures were criticized as overestimated (3), even a fraction of this amount would be a costly figure. Furthermore, it is important to recognize that when these accidents include the loss of life, the cost is incalculable.

Sleepiness on the job may cause accidents in the workplace. It is estimated that 42% to 49% of commercial vehicle accidents are caused by sleepiness or inattention.

Twenty-five percent of Americans perform shift work (most of these in the transportation industry) and 4% work nights (2). Considering that humans are not biologically wired to be nocturnal, attempting to work during one's biologically natural sleep time produces a tendency to be sleepy while at work. Additionally, shift workers often have to take extreme measures to sleep efficiently during the day. This leads to a generally sleepy working population at risk for accidents. Ironically, most sleep technologists have worked or currently work nights. It is not unusual to hear stories of fellow sleep technologists who have had trouble with sleepiness, including falling asleep while driving home.

The total number of motor vehicle accidents and ensuing fatalities due to sleepiness reported in the literature varies greatly from 1% to 41.6% (2, 4). The variation in these reports may be due to several factors. Until recently, the issue of sleepiness in relation to accidents has not been routinely assessed, and in many cases, the individuals involved are unaware of falling asleep or will not admit to falling asleep at the wheel at the risk of assuming responsibility for an accident. Unlike alcohol-related accidents, there is no blood test to determine one's level of sleepiness when an accident occurs, and therefore, sleepiness is often merely speculation. However, the association between sleepiness and motor vehicle accidents is undeniable. In clinical situations, large numbers of patients with diagnosed sleep disorders report having had motor vehicle accidents (2). Furthermore, when polled, nine out of ten police officers had pulled over at least one motorist under the suspicion of driving under the influence when the person was actually sleepy. The National Highway Traffic Safety Administration reported that between 2009 and 2013, drowsy driving resulted in an average of 72,000 crashes, 44,000 injuries, and 800 deaths per year (5).

As sleepiness becomes a recognized problem in society, the role of the sleep center in documenting pathologic sleepiness has increased in importance. However, measuring sleepiness is a difficult and often an elusive task. Several scales, such as the Epworth Sleepiness Scale and the Stanford Sleepiness Scale, have been developed to subjectively measure sleepiness. Because of their subjective nature, these scales are used in conjunction with the sleep history and more objective measures to aid in the diagnosis of sleep disorders. Objective measures of sleepiness are the multiple sleep latency test (MSLT) and the maintenance of wakefulness test (MWT).

The MSLT measures one's tendency to fall asleep. It is used as part of the evaluation of patients with suspected narcolepsy and may be used in evaluating patients with suspected idiopathic hypersomnia (1). The MSLT consists of five nap opportunities, each separated by 2 hours. A shorter four-nap test may be performed; however, this test is not reliable for the diagnosis of narcolepsy unless at least two sleep-onset rapid eye movement (REM) periods (SOREMPs) have been recorded (1). The MWT measures one's ability to resist the urge to fall asleep. The MWT may be used to evaluate treatment response or to assess patients whose inability to remain awake may constitute a public or personal safety issue (1). The MWT consists of four 40-minute trials, each separated by 2 hours. Currently, the MSLT and MWT are the only objective measures available to the clinician to quantify sleepiness in a patient. They should be used in conjunction with other clinical information to determine the correct diagnosis and best course of treatment. The importance of quantifying sleepiness lies in the impact that sleepiness has on the patient and society as a whole. In this regard, technologists play an important role in the diagnosis of the disorders of excessive sleepiness.

INDICATIONS

The MSLT is indicated in the diagnosis of narcolepsy and *may be* indicated in the diagnosis of idiopathic hypersomnia. The mean sleep latency (MSL), calculated as the arithmetic mean of the individual sleep latencies for the total number of naps or trials, is used as a component in the diagnosis of the disorders of excessive sleepiness. The difference in the MSL between controls and narcoleptics is statistically significant, with 84% of narcoleptics having an MSL less than 5 minutes (6). REM latency is defined as the time from sleep onset to the first epoch of REM sleep. SOREMPs are defined as a REM onset during an MSLT, with two or more SOREMPs being highly indicative of narcolepsy (6). However, other sleep disorders may produce similar results in an MSLT and, therefore, must be ruled out in the previous night's polysomnogram. Complications arise when attempting to use the MSLT to diagnose idiopathic hypersomnia. The MSL for idiopathic hypersomnia falls between that of narcoleptics and normal controls and is similar to that of sleepier normal controls (1).

The MWT may be indicated in two instances: determining treatment success, whether it is with medication or continuous positive airway pressure (CPAP), or with one's ability to remain awake as a measure of safety. However, in both of these cases, normative data

are sparse. Because both the MSLT and the MWT assess sleepiness but from two different angles, it has been suggested that they may be performed during the same day to assess more accurately the individual's level of sleepiness than if they were performed independently (7). This is an interesting proposition that warrants more investigation.

GENERAL CONSIDERATIONS AND PROCEDURES

Before the start of the MSLT or the MWT, several factors must be taken into account. A 2-week sleep diary is helpful in assessing the patient's sleep schedule before the study. Furthermore, actigraphy is a powerful tool in verifying the sleep diary. Used appropriately, actigraphy in coordination with a sleep diary will validate the patient's reported sleep, ensure adequate sleep is achieved, and rule out other disorders such as delayed phase syndrome. Once a history of adequate sleep has been obtained and circadian sleep disorders are ruled out as a possible differential diagnosis, an overnight polysomnogram must be performed before the MSLT to rule out other sleep disorders that would affect sleep architecture and produce excessive sleepiness. The prerequisites for the MWT are less stringent, and the need for a sleep diary or a prior polysomnogram is based on the clinician's judgment (1).

For both tests, a patient's normal sleep schedule should be considered. Shift workers may need a daytime polysomnogram before a nocturnal MSLT or MWT. Of course, one issue with such a schedule is that competition with the circadian rhythm may be affecting the MSLT or MWT. It may be quite normal, even after sleeping during the day, to experience sleepiness at 4 a.m. (8) and have a lower than normal sleep latency on a nocturnal MSLT.

Medication should also be considered before the performance of the MSLT or MWT. Numerous medications affect levels of sleepiness, including alcohol, caffeine, antihistamines, stimulants, barbiturates and other anticonvulsants, benzodiazepines, and narcotics (9–16). Furthermore, some medications may need to be stopped for a period so that a valid test could be conducted. Stimulants should be stopped 2 weeks before the performance of the MSLT. REM suppressants should also be stopped if narcolepsy is suspected so that the suppression of possible SOREMPs is prevented (1).

Selective serotonin reuptake inhibitors (SSRIs) suppress REM sleep, and therefore, discontinuation of this medication should be considered before the performance of an MSLT. From a technical standpoint, SSRIs may produce atypical eye movements throughout sleep. Every attempt should be made, in consultation with the patient's prescribing primary care physician or psychiatrist, to discontinue these drugs if feasible, practical, and safe in order to fully interpret the data obtained.

These considerations may not be necessary for the MWT, particularly if the purpose is to document the effectiveness of the stimulant. Although not required, a urine drug screen may be performed for any substance that might not have been reported. These general procedures should be followed before any MSLT or MWT. Omission of any of these preliminary considerations may lead to questions regarding the validity of the test and final diagnosis.

The recording montage for both the MSLT and the MWT is generally less complicated than a standard polysomnographic (PSG) montage, and in fact, it is more comfortable for the patient and also common practice to remove the unnecessary leads following the overnight polysomnogram. However, there are essential elements to each montage (Table 43-1). They include a frontal electroencephalogram (EEG [F3-M2 and/or F4-M1]), a central EEG (C3-M2 and/or C4-M1), an occipital EEG (O1-M2 and/or O2-M1), a left and right electrooculogram (EOG), a mental/submental electromyogram (chin EMG), and an electrocardiogram (8, 17). For the MSLT, extra EOG leads may also be added to provide a clearer picture of lateral and vertical eye movements (a total of four EOG leads, including one above and one below the outer canthus of each eye). Although not routine, a snoring microphone and/or respiratory channels may be added if indicated (8).

MULTIPLE SLEEP LATENCY TEST

Beyond the general procedures that encompass both the MSLT and the MWT, specific criteria must be met to complete a valid MSLT. The previous night polysomnogram should mimic the patient's normal sleep schedule as much as possible and record a total sleep time (TST) of at least 6 hours (1). Performing an MSLT following a polysomnogram that is shorter than normal, is longer than normal, or at a time differs from the patient's routine sleep time may affect the overall results. Specifically, the MSLT should not be performed if the patient had insufficient sleep the night before the test.

The MSLT protocol consists of five nap opportunities, each separated by 2 hours. A shorter four-nap test may be performed; however, it is not reliable for the diagnosis of narcolepsy unless at least two SOREMPs have been recorded (1). The first nap should be started 1.5 to 3 hours after the completion of the polysomnogram. Each successive nap should be started 2 hours after the commencement of the previous nap (8, 17). At the termination of the polysomnogram, it is imperative—because it is between naps—to keep the patient awake and out of the bed. The patient should be continuously monitored to ensure that sleep between naps does not occur. This can be a difficult task with a severely sleepy patient.

Original reports by Mitler et al. (8) recommended having the patient wear street clothing during the MSLT. However, the current practice parameters submitted by the AASM do not mention this requirement (1). Allowing the patient to wear sleepwear all day may be psychologically associated with bedtime or sleep activity, potentially reducing the sleep latency, and this issue should be considered when drafting policy and procedures. However, it is unclear whether this difference is clinically significant. A breakfast and lunch are typically provided; however, it is important to note that caffeine should not be consumed at any point during the day of study. Just before each nap, it is a good idea to make sure that the patient has used the bathroom recently, has turned off his or her cellular phone, and is generally ready for the nap. Any interruption in the nap has serious consequences for the entire study. Also, the time just before the first nap, or after breakfast, provides an ideal opportunity to obtain a urine specimen for drug screening if one has been ordered by the physician.

Table 43-1	Multiple Sleep Latency Test and Maintenance of Wakefulness Test Montages

Minimally Required Channels

Frontal EEG (F3-M2 or F4-M1)
Central EEG (C3-M2 or C4-M1)
Occipital EEG (O1-M2 or O2-M1)
Left EOG (E1)
Right EOG (E2)
Chin EMG
ECG

Optional Channels

Vertical EOG
Additional frontal EEG
Additional central EEG
Additional occipital EEG
Snore microphone
Respiratory channels

ECG, electrocardiogram; EEG, electroencephalogram; EMG, electromyogram; EOG, electrooculogram.

Current guidelines allow the physician to determine whether a urine drug screen is needed and the conditions under which the sample is collected (1).

Additional considerations for the MSLT include the following: no vigorous physical activity during the day of the study, cessation of smoking at least 30 minutes before each nap, and cessation of any stimulating activity 15 minutes before lights out (1). It is important to note that different forms of nicotine delivery have different pharmacodynamics. Nicotine ingestion through inhalation is eliminated significantly faster than through other means of delivery (Fig. 43-1). Therefore, although it is acceptable for the patient to stop smoking 30 minutes before the nap, the use of items such as chewing tobacco, nicotine patches, and nicotine gum should not be allowed during the day of the study.

A recommended routine just before initiating each nap includes performing electrode impedance checks 10 minutes before lights out, performing biocalibrations 5 minutes before lights out obtaining a subjective sleepiness assessment 45 seconds before lights out requesting the patient to lie down in a comfortable position 30 seconds before lights out, and instructing the patient to "please lie quietly, keep your eyes closed, and try to fall asleep" at lights out (8, 17, 18).

Scoring and Ending Each Nap

Sleep onset for the MSLT is defined as the first 30-second epoch scored as any stage of sleep (1). Sleep latency is the elapsed time in minutes from lights out to sleep onset. If no sleep is achieved after 20 minutes, then the nap is ended, and the sleep latency for that nap is reported as

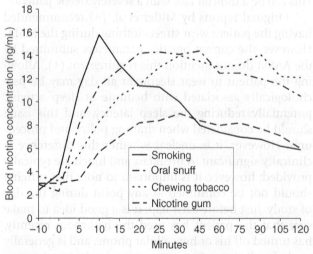

Figure 43-1 Blood nicotine levels using various forms of delivery. (Data from U.S. Department of Health and Human Services. [1988]. *The health consequences of smoking: Nicotine addiction: A report of the Surgeon General.* Rockville, MD: Centers for Disease Control, Office on Smoking and Health.)

20 minutes. The MSL is calculated as the sum of the individual sleep latencies for each nap divided by the total number of naps. REM latency is defined as the elapsed time in minutes from the first 30-second epoch of sleep to the first 30-second epoch of REM sleep.

In order to assess for the occurrence of REM sleep, the clinical MSLT test is continued for 15 minutes after the first epoch of any stage of sleep (8). If any REM sleep occurs during this 15-minute window, it is considered a SOREMP (1). This differs from research-based MSLT protocols, where the nap is terminated after the onset of unequivocal sleep, which is defined as the first of three consecutive 30-second epochs of stage 1 sleep or the first 30-second epoch of any other stage of sleep. The research protocol ensures that sleep has been achieved but does not allow for accumulated sleep. The clinical protocol serves two purposes: it establishes a level of sleepiness by measuring sleep latency and allows time for SOREMPs to occur, which allows the diagnosis of narcolepsy.

Ending the Test and Interpretations

The MSLT can be ended after four or five naps have been completed. The literature is varied regarding the use of four or five naps (19–24). However, the most current report recommends running a five-nap MSLT, particularly when diagnosing narcolepsy (1). A four-nap MSLT is unreliable in the diagnosis of narcolepsy unless two SOREMPs have already occurred during the first four naps. In addition, there is a statistically significant difference in the MSL between a four-nap MSLT and a five-nap MSLT, with the latter generally producing a longer MSL. The number of naps was found to be one of four factors that significantly impact the MSL. The other factors were age, definition of sleep latency, and prior TST (6). MSL increases with age in adults. In fact, one analysis suggests that MSL will increase by 0.6 minutes per decade (6). In general, an MSL less than 5 minutes is consistent with pathologic sleepiness. However, an isolated MSL value should not be used for diagnostic purposes outside of the clinical context (1, 17, 25). Normative MSL data may be found in Table 43-2.

MSL alone is generally not a good indicator of pathologic sleepiness in individuals suspected of idiopathic hypersomnia. This is due to the large overlap in MSL between individuals with idiopathic hypersomnia and controls in the normative data (1). Once the MSL is calculated, it is used in conjunction with other symptoms to determine the final diagnosis.

Special Considerations

Pediatric PSG presents unique issues that must be considered. This is especially true when conducting a pediatric MSLT. Disorders of excessive sleepiness, particularly

Table 43-2 **Multiple Sleep Latency Test Mean Sleep Latency Based on Age**

Age Range (y)	Mean Sleep Latency (SD)
10–19	10.0 (4.5)
20–29	10.4 (5.4)
30–39	10.8 (3.9)
40–49	11.7 (4.4)
50–59	12.1 (1.1)
60–69	11.2 (5.2)
70–79	No data
80–89	15.2 (6.0)

Data from Arand, D., Bonnet, M., Hurwitz, T., et al. (2005). Review by the MSLT and MWT Task Force of the Standards of Practice Committee of the American Academy of Sleep Medicine. *Sleep, 28,* 123–144.

narcolepsy, often go unnoticed or undiagnosed until early adulthood. Children may simply be considered long sleepers or lazy. There is a paucity of normative data for pediatric MSLT, and MSLT has not been validated for use in children less than 8 years of age.

The testing environment may be particularly unsettling for a child and could potentially produce a prolonged MSL, even in the most hypersomnolent child. For this reason, associated symptoms in a child may play a stronger role in diagnosis and treatment than in an adult. For example, an MSL of 12 to 14 minutes may be more pathologic in a child than in an adult. In general, prepubescent patients will have the longest MSL, whereas young adults will have the shortest MSL (6). Another consideration with pediatric patients is that narcolepsy tends to be an evolving disorder in childhood. Therefore, although SOREMPs may not be present, a child may still have narcolepsy with other classical symptoms such as cataplexy. For this reason, MSLTs may need to be repeated throughout childhood to account for developmental changes (26, 27). Under these conditions, other symptoms are just as important as the MSLT in making a diagnosis in a pediatric patient.

Because of the possible comorbidity of obstructive sleep apnea (OSA) and narcolepsy, it may be necessary to perform an MSLT on a patient wearing CPAP. In fact, if a patient presents with a chief complaint of excessive sleepiness or any other narcolepsy symptoms and OSA is present on the polysomnogram, it is necessary to treat the OSA first, before attempting to perform the MSLT (6, 18). However, if excessive sleepiness or any other narcolepsy symptoms persist after a history of compliant CPAP use, performing the MSLT with CPAP in place

is advised. It is important that the patient wear CPAP during the preceding overnight polysomnogram at the optimal pressure setting and during the MSLT naps. If the MSLT is performed without CPAP, the patient's 15 minutes of sleep may be disrupted because of sleep-disordered breathing.

MAINTENANCE OF WAKEFULNESS TEST

In contrast to the MSLT, the MWT measures the ability to resist the urge to fall asleep. Instead of being used as a tool in diagnosing sleep disorders, MWTs are more commonly used to evaluate treatment response or assess one's ability to remain awake for safety purposes. Increasingly, the transportation industry is recognizing the value of the MWT in assessing sleepiness (28). Unfortunately, there are fewer data available concerning standardized practices and normals for the MWT than for the MSLT. However, the practice parameters provided by the AASM make recommendations regarding the MWT collection and interpretation (1).

On the basis of clinical circumstances, the clinician should determine the necessity of a polysomnogram before the MWT. At present, no consensus has been reached regarding the use of a sleep diary; however, it is important to note that chronic sleep deprivation, or even a poor night's sleep before the test, may affect the outcome of the MWT. The AASM standards advise that if the patient reports having inadequate sleep before the MWT, if the patient does not feel normally alert, or if reliable information is unavailable, the MWT should not be performed (1).

Overall, the general procedures for the MSLT and the MWT are similar. The need to perform a preceding overnight polysomnogram is determined by the clinician (1). The first trial should be started 1.5 to 3 hours after the individual wakes up, with no sleep occurring between the time when the individual wakes up and the start of the first trial. The MWT is performed in a dimly lit room with the patient in bed in the seated position with the head and limbs fully supported. Subsequent trials are performed at 2-hour intervals (1, 29). Breakfast is generally provided an hour before the first trial, and lunch should be provided immediately following the second trial. A urine drug screen may be collected, similar to the MSLT protocol, just before the first trial.

There has been disagreement concerning the duration of each trial, with a 20-minute trial (similar to the MSLT) being used in some studies and a 40-minute trial being used in others. However, it has been shown that the use of a 40-minute trial avoids the "ceiling effect" produced by the 20-minute trial. For example, an individual who might fall asleep at minute 23 would show a sleep onset using the 40-minute protocol, whereas the same individual would show no sleep if the 20-minute protocol were used. For this reason, a four-trial, 40-minute protocol is recommended for maximizing sensitivity. One substantial difference between the MSLT and the MWT protocols is the test environment. Instead of a completely dark room, there should be a light of 0.10 to 0.13 lux positioned behind the patient's head, out of direct or peripheral vision at the level of the cornea. The patient should be sitting comfortably in bed with the back and head supported (29, 30).

Before each trial, the general routine should be performed as in the MSLT. However, at the conclusion of the biocalibrations, the instructions differ significantly, whereby the individual should be instructed to "Please sit still and remain awake for as long as possible. Look directly ahead of you, and do not look directly at the light." Furthermore, it is usually necessary to ensure that the individual does not employ extreme measures to maintain wakefulness during the trials (30, 31).

Scoring and Ending Each Trial

As in the MSLT, sleep onset for the MWT is defined as the first epoch of any stage of sleep as defined by the AASM practice parameters (1). However, other definitions for sleep onset have been used. Different protocols, including differing sleep-onset definitions, have been indicated for different clinical purposes as determined by the clinician (31). The trial is terminated if no sleep is achieved during the 40 minutes on the basis of the 40-minute MWT protocol recommended by the AASM, or if the patient exhibits three consecutive epochs of stage N1 sleep or one epoch of any other stage of sleep.

Ending the Test and Interpretations

The MWT is terminated after four trials (1). Following the AASM-recommended 40-minute trial protocol, an MSL of less than 8 minutes is considered abnormal. As stated earlier, there are fewer normative data for the MWT than for the MSLT (Table 43-3) (31). The paucity of normative data, combined with the fact that the predictive value of the MSL in regard to safety issues has not been established, indicates the need to combine other clinical factors in making a determination of safety and occupational risk (1).

SUMMARY

The guidelines for the MSLT and MWT were published by the AASM in 2005 and a revised set of guidelines are expected to be published in 2019. However, it is not expected that the revisions will be substantial and many of the proposed revisions are addressed in this

Table 43-3 Maintenance of Wakefulness Test Mean Sleep Latency Based on Age

Age Range (y)	Mean Sleep Latency (SD)
30–39	30.86 (2.04)
40–49	36.52 (1.88)
50–59	36.73 (1.59)
60–69	38.03 (1.06)

Data from Arand, D., Bonnet, M., Hurwitz, T., et al. (2005). Review by the MSLT and MWT Task Force of the Standards of Practice Committee of the American Academy of Sleep Medicine. *Sleep, 28,* 123–144.

chapter. In summary, both the MSLT and the MWT are invaluable tools in diagnosing and evaluating disorders of excessive sleepiness when they are combined with a thorough sleep history and subjective measures of sleepiness. However, for all their merit, they are not without their weaknesses. Consequently, they should be part of the diagnostic process, and not the process in its entirety. The impact of excessive sleepiness has become a societal issue, as evidenced by legislation aimed at drowsy driving. The diagnosis of idiopathic hypersomnia or narcolepsy has a far greater impact on the patient than ever before. To avoid false positives or negatives, strict guidelines must be followed not only by the clinician but also by the technologist performing these tests. For this reason, the MSLT and MWT guidelines outlined in the most recent AASM practice parameters dictate, "sleep technologists who perform MSLTs (and MWTs) should be experienced in conducting the test (1)." Therefore, the role of the sleep technologist is crucial in the diagnosis of disorders of excessive sleepiness, and a thorough understanding of the test, its indications, procedures, and interpretation is essential in performing a valid test.

REFERENCES

1. Littner, M. R., Kushida, C., Wise, M., et al. (2005). Practice parameters for clinical use of multiple sleep latency test and the maintenance of wakefulness test. *Sleep, 28*(1), 113–121.
2. Leger, H. (1994). The cost of sleep related accidents: A report for the National Commission on Sleep Disorders Research. *Sleep, 17,* 84–93.
3. Webb, W. B. (1985). The cost of sleep-related accidents: A reanalysis. *Sleep, 18*(4), 276–280.
4. U.S. Department of Transportation. (1985). *Report to the Senate Committee on Appropriations and the House Committee on Appropriations. Transportation-related research: CARfile study.* Washington, DC: Author.

5. National Highway Traffic Safety Administration (NHTSA). *NHTSA Drowsy Driving Research and Program Plan*. Retrieved from https://www.nhtsa.gov/sites/nhtsa.dot.gov/files/drowsydriving_strategicplan_030316.pdf

6. Arand, D., Bonnet, M., Hurwitz, T., et al. (2005). The clinical use of the MSLT and MWT. *Sleep, 28*(1), 123–144.

7. Cresswell, P., Kenny-Foy, T., & Hart, I. K. (2005). The MWT and MSLT can be performed on the same day in normal controls and patients with narcolepsy/cataplexy without confounding the MWT [Abstract]. *Sleep, 28*(Suppl.), A325.

8. Mitler, M. M., Carskadon, M. A., & Hirshkowitz, M. (2000). Evaluating sleepiness. In M. H. Kryger, T. Roth, & W. C. Dement (Eds.), *Principles and practice of sleep medicine* (3rd ed., pp. 1251–1257). Philadelphia, PA: W.B. Saunders

9. Roehrs, T., Lumley, M., Asker, D., et al. (1986). Ethanol and caffeine effects on daytime sleepiness. *Sleep Research, 15*, 41.

10. Roth, T., Roehrs, T., Koshorek, G., et al. (1986). Central effects of antihistamine. *Sleep Research, 15*, 43.

11. Roehrs, T., Papineau, K., Rosenthal, L., et al. (1999). Sleepiness and the reinforcing and subjective effects of methylphenidate. *Experimental and Clinical Psychopharmacology, 7*(2), 145–150.

12. Bishop, C., Roehrs, T., Rosenthal, L., et al. (1997). Alerting effects of methylphenidate under basal and sleep-deprived conditions. *Experimental and Clinical Psychopharmacology, 5*(4), 344–352.

13. Manni, R., Ratti, M. T., Perucca, E., et al. (1993). A multi-parametric investigation of daytime sleepiness and psychomotor functions in epileptic patients treated with phenobarbital and sodium valproate: A comparative controlled study. *Electroencephalography and Clinical Neurophysiology, 86*(5), 322–328.

14. Dement, W., Seidel, W., & Carskadon, M. A. (1982). Daytime alertness, insomnia and benzodiazepines. *Sleep, 5*(Suppl. 1), S28–S45.

15. Carskadon, M. A., Seidel, W. F., Greenblatt, D. J., et al. (1982). Daytime carryover of triazolam and flurazepam in elderly insomniacs. *Sleep, 5*(4), 361–371.

16. Roehrs, T., Kribbs, N., Zorick, F., et al. (1986). Hypnotic residual effects of benzodiazepines with repeated administration. *Sleep, 9*(2), 309–316.

17. Roth, T., Roehrs, T. A., & Rosenthal, L. (1999). Measurement of sleepiness and alertness: Multiple sleep latency test. In S. Chokroverty (Ed.), *Sleep disorders medicine: Basic science, technical considerations, and clinical aspects* (2nd ed., pp. 223–229). Boston, MA: Butterworth Heinemann.

18. Carskadon, M. A., Dement, W. C., Mitler, M., et al. (1986). Guidelines for the multiple sleep latency test (MSLT): A standard measure of sleepiness. *Sleep, 9*, 519.

19. Levine, B., Roehrs, T., Zorick, F., et al. (1988). Daytime sleepiness in young adults. *Sleep, 11*(1), 39–46.

20. Zwyghuizen-Doorenbos, A., Roehrs, T., Schaefer, M., et al. (1988). Test-retest reliability of the MSLT. *Sleep, 11*(6), 562–565.

21. Hartse, K. M., Roth, T., & Zorick, F. J. (1982). Daytime sleepiness and daytime wakefulness: The effect of instruction. *Sleep, 5*(Suppl. 2), S107–S118.

22. Carskadon, M. A., & Dement, W. C. (1979). Effects of total sleep loss on sleep tendency. *Perception and Motor Skills, 48*(2), 495–506.

23. Richardson, G. S., Carskadon, M. A., Flagg, W., et al. (1978). Excessive daytime sleepiness in man: Multiple sleep latency measurement in narcoleptic and control subjects. *Electroencephalography and Clinical Neurophysiology, 45*(5), 621–627.

24. Alloway, C. E., Ogilvie, R. D., & Shapiro, C. M. (1997). The alpha attenuation test: Assessing excessive daytime sleepiness in narcolepsy-cataplexy. *Sleep, 20*(4), 258–266.

25. Carskadon, M. A., & Dement, W. C. (1981). Cumulative effects of sleep restriction on daytime sleepiness. *Psychophysiology, 18*, 107–113.

26. Sheldon, S. H. (1996). *Evaluating sleep in infants and children*. Philadelphia, PA: Lippincott-Raven.

27. Guilleminault, C. (1987). Narcolepsy and its differential diagnosis. In C. Guilleminault (Ed.), *Sleep and its disorders in children*. New York, NY: Raven Press.

28. National Sleep Foundation. *Sleep news*. Retrieved from http://www.sleepfoundation.org/hottopics/index.php

29. Doghramji, K. (1999). Maintenance of wakefulness test. In S. Chokroverty (Ed.), *Sleep disorders medicine: Basic science, technical considerations, and clinical aspects* (2nd ed., pp. 231–236). Boston, MA: Butterworth Heinemann.

30. Mitler, M. M., Doghramji, K., & Shapiro, C. (2000). The maintenance of wakefulness test: Normative data by age. *Journal of Psychosomatic Research, 49*, 363–365.

31. Doghramji, K., Mitler, M. M., Sangal, R. B., et al. (1997). A normative study of the maintenance of wakefulness test (MWT). *Electroencephalography and Clinical Neurophysiology, 103*, 554–562.

chapter 44
Home Sleep Apnea Testing

SUSAN PURDY   RICHARD B. BERRY

LEARNING OBJECTIVES

On completion of this chapter, the reader should be able to:

1. Compare the use of polysomnography and home sleep apnea testing (HSAT) in the diagnosis of obstructive sleep apnea.
2. Determine the accuracy of HSAT.
3. Describe the clinical use of HSAT.
4. Integrate the use of HSAT into overall patient care.

KEY TERMS

American Academy of Sleep Medicine (AASM)
Peripheral arterial tonometry (PAT)
G-Codes
Common Procedural Terminology (CPT)
Local Coverage Determination (LCD)
Type 3 HSAT Device
Respiratory event index (REI)
Oxygen desaturation index (ODI)

INTRODUCTION

Obstructive sleep apnea (OSA) is a common disorder associated with significant morbidity and mortality and requires accurate assessment and proper management. Polysomnography (PSG) is the standard test for the diagnosis of suspected sleep-related breathing disorders and for positive airway pressure (PAP) titration to determine an effective level of PAP for treatment (1–4). Attended PSG requires highly trained personnel for adequate study performance and interpretation and can be costly. Access to PSG in a timely manner may be limited or delayed in some locales, and this has prompted the use of limited channel monitoring outside the sleep center for the diagnosis of OSA. This type of testing has been called "portable monitoring" (PM), out-of-center sleep testing (OCST or OOCST), or home sleep testing (HST) (5–9). The term HST is used by the Centers for Medicare and Medicaid Services (CMS) to describe unattended home testing (10–12). The American Academy of Sleep Medicine (AASM) currently recommends the terminology "Home Sleep Apnea Testing" (HSAT) (4, 13). Unattended limited channel testing can be performed in the sleep center or hospital. Additionally, this testing does not usually determine the amount of sleep (no electroencephalogram [EEG] recorded). Therefore, the names PM, HST, OCST, or HSAT are not ideal but are used in much of the literature on this subject. For the sake of simplicity, unattended limited channel sleep monitoring will be termed HSAT in this chapter, except when discussing Medicare coverage, where the term HST will be used.

Although PSG is the standard test to diagnose OSA in the United States (1–4), in other locales, more limited studies are routinely used. For example, Flemons et al. (14) stated in 2004 that in the United Kingdom PSG comprised approximately 10% of all sleep studies. Approximately two-thirds of the studies used oximetry alone, with the rest being limited channel studies. In the Veterans Administration (VA) Health Care System, where demand exceeds in-lab testing capacity, HSAT is commonly used in place of PSG for uncomplicated patients. However, despite the widespread use of HSAT worldwide, such testing was only approved in the United States by the CMS to qualify patients for continuous positive airway pressure (CPAP) treatment in 2008 (10, 11). Reimbursement for HSAT was subsequently approved in 2009 (12). Since that time, the number of HSAT studies has continued to increase every year. In 2014, 845,569 sleep studies were completed by 1.4% of Medicare beneficiaries for a total cost of $189 million. Since 2010, annual expenditures for sleep studies have declined, whereas the number of studies performed has increased by 9.1%. In 2014, PSG, split-night PSG, and unattended home sleep studies accounted for 40%, 48%, and 12%, respectively, of the total sleep studies. This represents a dramatic growth in the number of unattended sleep studies performed since 2000, when they represented only 0.9% of the total studies (15). Today, some insurance providers mandate the use of HSAT for the diagnosis of OSA in all uncomplicated patients.

Table 44-1 Classification of Sleep Testing

	Level I (Type 1)	Level II (Type 2)	Level III (Type 3)	Level IV (Type 4)
	Attended PSG	Unattended PSG	Cardiorespiratory monitoring	Continuous single or dual bioparameter recording
Parameters	Minimum of 7 parameters: EEG, EOG, chin EMG, ECG, airflow, respiratory effort, and oxygen saturation	Minimum of 7 parameters: EEG, EOG, chin EMG, ECG, airflow, respiratory effort, and oxygen saturation	Minimum of 4: ventilation (at least 2 parameters of respiratory movement or respiratory movement and airflow), heart rate or ECG, and oxygen saturation	Minimum of 1 oxygen saturation: flow or chest movement
Body position	Documented or objectively measured	Possible	Possible	No
Leg movement	EMG or motion sensor desirable but optional	Optional	Optional	No
Personnel interventions	Possible	No	No	No

The terminology of Level I to IV was used, but recent terminology is Type I to IV or Type 1 to 4.
ECG, electrocardiogram; EEG, electroencephalogram; EMG, electromyogram; EOG, electrooculogram; PSG, polysomnography.
From Ferber, R., Millman, R., Coppola, M., et al. (1994). Portable recording in the assessment of obstructive sleep apnea. ASDA standards of practice. *Sleep*, 17(4), 378–392. Adapted by permission of American Sleep Disorders Association and Sleep Research Society.

TYPES OF HSAT

The commonly used classification of sleep testing was proposed by Ferber et al. (16) in a 1994 American Sleep Disorders Association review (Table 44-1). This classification used the terminology Level I, II, III, and IV. This terminology was later modified to Type 1, 2, 3, and 4 (or Type I, II, III, and IV) (17). In 2008, the CMS issued a decision to allow HST to qualify a patient for CPAP (10, 11). CMS defined HST types slightly differently and created G-codes (G0398, G0399, and G0400) to describe HST services (Table 44-2) (11, 12). The G-codes are found in the Healthcare Common Procedure Coding System Level II codebook and are maintained and valued by the CMS. G-codes are procedure codes developed by the CMS to identify products, supplies, and services that do not have an assigned Common Procedural Terminology (CPT) code for

Table 44-2 Centers for Medicaid and Medicare Classification of Sleep Testing

Code	Type	Setting	Monitoring
	I	Attended in facility	Minimum of 7 channels including EEG, EOG, EMG, ECG/heart rate, and oxygen saturation
G0398	II	Unattended in or out of a sleep lab facility or attended in a sleep lab facility	Minimum of 7 channels including EEG, EOG, EMG, ECG/heart rate, and oxygen saturation
G0399	III	Unattended in or out of a sleep lab facility or attended in a sleep lab facility	Minimum of 4 channels and must record ventilation, oximetry, and ECG or heart rate
G0400	IV	Unattended in or out of a sleep lab facility or attended in a sleep lab facility	Minimum of 3 channels, *one of which is airflow*
–		Unattended in or out of a sleep lab facility or attended in a sleep lab facility	PAT, minimum of 3 channels: PAT, actigraphy, and oximetry

ECG, electrocardiogram; EEG, electroencephalogram; EMG, electromyogram; EOG, electrooculogram; PAT, peripheral arterial tonometry.
Based on Centers for Medicare and Medicaid Services. (2009, March 3). *Decision memo for sleep testing for obstructive sleep apnea* (CAG-00405N). Baltimore, MD: Author; Berry, R. B., Albertario, C. M., Harding, S. M., et al.; for the American Academy of Sleep Medicine. (2018). *The AASM manual for the scoring of sleep and associated events: Rules, terminology and technical specifications* [Version 2.5]. Darien, IL: American Academy of Sleep Medicine.

Table 44-3 Common Procedural Terminology (CPT) Codes* for Home Sleep Apnea Testing

95800	Sleep study, unattended, simultaneous recording; heart rate, oxygen saturation, respiratory analysis (e.g., by airflow or peripheral arterial tone), and sleep time.
95801	Sleep study, unattended, simultaneous recording; minimum of heart rate, oxygen saturation, and respiratory analysis (e.g., by airflow or peripheral arterial tone).
95806	Sleep study, unattended, simultaneous recording of heart rate, oxygen saturation, respiratory airflow, and respiratory effort (e.g., thoracoabdominal movement).

which there is a programmatic operating need to separately identify them on a national level. Reimbursement is determined regionally by the specific local coverage determination (LCD). Later HSATs were assigned CPT codes: 95800, 95801, and 95806 (Table 44-3). The method of determination of sleep time (95800) is not specified. CPT codes are copyrighted and maintained by the American Medical Association. Although CPT codes exist for HSAT studies, many insurance providers require the use of G-codes for billing. The AASM uses the HSAT CPT codes in their recommended standards for such testing (7, 13). The CPT classification of HSAT differs somewhat from the G-code classification. However, 95806 describes most Type 3 devices. Sleep testing using peripheral arterial tonometry (PAT), actigraphy, and oximetry was also approved for HST by the CMS, but a G-code was not assigned to this type of testing (11). This type of testing would fall under the CPT classifications 95801 or 95802. An estimate of total sleep time (TST) is determined by PAT devices on the basis of actigraphy, heart rate, and characteristics of the sympathetic tone (PAT signal) in different sleep stages (18). However, unless EEG and electrooculogram (EOG) are recorded, the AASM standards (10) require that monitoring time (MT) rather than TST be reported. In the original classification, Type 4 testing required one or two bioparameter recording (Table 44-1). However, in 2009 when the CMS issued a memo approving reimbursement for HST (Table 44-2), Type IV devices were mandated to record three or more channels, one of which was airflow (10–12). Most Type 4 devices monitor oximetry (oxygen saturation, SaO_2) as one of the channels being recorded.

Type 1 testing is an attended PSG in a facility. Type 2 testing (unattended or ambulatory PSG) records similar parameters, although often a reduced number of parameters are recorded. Both Type 1 and 2 testing allow the scoring of arousals and sleep staging. Type 2 studies allow recording of either heart rate (usually from oximetry) or electrocardiogram (ECG). Most Type 2 devices have the capability of recording ECG. Type 2 studies have been used in the Sleep Heart Health Study, testing a large population for the effect of sleep apnea

on cardiovascular morbidity (19, 20). However, Type 2 studies are rarely used outside the research setting because of the expertise required and limited reimbursement when compared with Type 1 studies.

A Type 3 study, also called "cardiorespiratory testing," consists of at least two channels of respiratory monitoring, oximetry, and ECG or heart rate. The G0399 classification requires a minimum of four channels and must record ventilation, ECG/heart rate, and SaO_2. Typically, airflow and respiratory effort (e.g., chest and abdominal respiratory inductance plethysmography [RIP]) are used for respiratory monitoring. The CPT 95806 classification specifies monitoring of airflow and respiratory effort. Some of the simpler HSAT devices use only one respiratory effort belt. In most Type 3 devices, the heart rate is derived from the oximetry data. An example of a Type 3 study from a comprehensive HSAT device is shown in Figure 44-1. When reading CMS documents, it is important to note that *the respiratory disturbance index (RDI) is the number of apneas and hypopneas per hour of MT.* This RDI definition differs from the one used in the AASM scoring manual that specifies the RDI to equal the number of apneas, hypopneas, and respiratory effort–related arousals *per hour of TST* (10). The AASM also recommends that the term "respiratory event index" (REI) be used to describe the number of apneas and hypopneas per hour of MT in HSAT reports (9, 13).

HISTORY OF HSAT IN THE UNITED STATES

The history of HSAT in the United States has been characterized by a slow acceptance of this type of testing as data supporting the use of the devices accumulated. CMS considered HSAT several times before finally approving the method for the diagnosis of sleep apnea. A detailed step-by-step description of the developments in evaluation and subsequent approval of HSAT for the diagnosis of OSA is provided in two of the references (21, 22). An editorial discussing the rationale for the CMS decision to approve HSAT describes the final stages of the process (23). Early studies of the utility of HSAT for

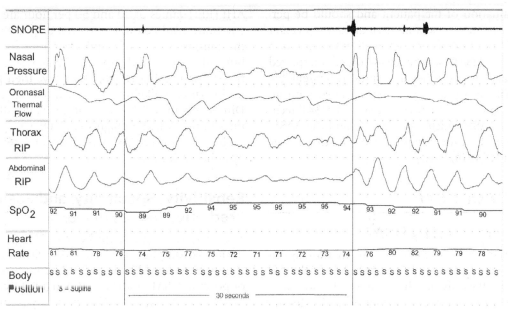

Figure 44-1 Tracings (120-second window) from a Type 3 home sleep apnea testing device (PDX, Philips Respironics) showing a hypopnea. In this study, the signal from the oronasal device was suboptimal. RIP, respiratory inductance plethysmography.

the diagnosis of OSA focused on a comparison of the ability of devices to rule in or rule out sleep apnea with that of PSG (17, 24–30), and AASM practice parameters recommended narrow indications for HSAT (31, 32). However, in 2007 before the approval of HSAT by the CMS, the AASM did publish important clinical guidelines for the use of HSAT in a wider spectrum of indications (8) if certain evaluation and testing procedures were followed. The guidelines influenced the requirements for reimbursement of HSAT studies by insurance providers. The ultimate decision of CMS to allow HSAT for the diagnosis of OSA in patients to be treated with CPAP was heavily influenced by studies showing that clinical pathways using HSAT devices resulted in equivalent outcomes from CPAP treatment, including improvement in daytime sleepiness and the amount of

adherence to treatment (33, 34). These and later studies documenting the effective use of HSAT (35–40) will be discussed in another section.

The AASM clinical guidelines for the use of unattended portable monitors in the diagnosis of OSA in adults (8) provide important recommendations on how HSAT is to be performed and used. The guidelines provided a recommendation that HSAT be performed under the auspices of AASM-accredited sleep centers. Subsequent to the national carrier determination of CMS, a number of LCDs by regional durable medical equipment Medicare administrative contractors or private insurance providers were published, further defining requirements for the performance of HST (HSAT) (Table 44-4). The requirements vary by region and funding entity but in general require HSAT following

Table 44-4 Typical Requirements for Reimbursement for Home Sleep Apnea Testing

- Treating physician who orders the study must perform a face-to-face evaluation. Evaluation must include the following:
  1. Sleep history and symptoms including, but not limited to, snoring, daytime sleepiness, observed apneas, choking or gasping during sleep, morning headaches
  2. Epworth Sleepiness Scale
  3. Physical examination documents body mass index, neck circumference, and a focused cardiopulmonary and upper airway evaluation
- Sleep center performing home sleep apnea testing study must be accredited by the American Academy of Sleep Medicine (AASM), The Joint commission (TJC), or Accreditation Commission for Health Care (ACHC).
- Raw data must be reviewed by a sleep physician who is a board-certified, Diplomate in Sleep Medicine by a member board of the American Board of Medical Specialities (ABMS), or an active physician staff of sleep center AASM, TJC, or ACHC accredited.

a clinical evaluation of the patient and should be performed under the auspices of an accredited sleep center (AASM, Joint Commission, or Accreditation Commission for Health Care). HSAT must be reviewed and interpreted by a physician who is either a board-certified/eligible sleep physician or a staff physician associated with an accredited sleep center. An AASM review of HSAT technology, recent AASM practice guidelines, and the AASM scoring manual also provide guidance on the technology to be used for HSAT (4, 9, 13).

ACCURACY OF HSAT

AHI PSG versus REI by HSAT

There are a number of potential reasons that the apnea + hypopnea index (AHI) by HSAT and PSG might differ. The AHI by PSG divides the number of respiratory events by the TST in hours. The AHI by HSAT divides the number of events by the hours of monitoring. The TST is always less than or equal to the MT and is often shorter than the MT by an hour or more. Thus, even if the same number of events is detected by PSG and HSAT devices, the AHI will be greater by PSG as the TST is less than the total MT. For example, if 100 events are recorded and the TST is 5 hours and the MT is 6 hours, the AHI for PSG is 20 per hour, but the AHI by HSAT will be 16.6 per hour.

The AHI values may vary from HSAT and PSG studies if the respiratory sensors used in the studies are not the same. For example, a study by Dingli et al. used a thermal sensor to detect apnea and hypopneas during PSG and nasal pressure during HSAT (25). If PSG and HSAT studies are done on different nights, night-to-night variability may also contribute to differences in AHI. Many patients have a much higher AHI in the supine position or during rapid eye movement (REM) sleep. In these patients, the relative amounts of supine and REM sleep contribute to night-to-night variability in the AHI. Of interest, a study by Levendowski et al. (41) found greater night-to-night variability with PSG compared with HSAT. Another study by Smith et al. comparing HSAT with PSG found that patients had less supine sleep at home compared with the sleep center (42). Having less supine sleep at home would often result in a lower HSAT AHI compared with a PSG AHI. In addition, if some events are missed by HSAT because of sensor dislodgement for a portion of the night, this will also reduce the AHI. On the contrary, patients may sleep better at home and have a greater amount of REM sleep. Individuals may consume more alcohol at home, therefore changing the HSAT REI (AHI).

Exact agreement between AHI values by PSG and REI by HSAT is less important than correct classification of a patient as having OSA or not having OSA. Although AHI (REI) values of 30 and 50 per hour are quite different, both would clearly support a diagnosis of OSA. On the contrary, values of 3 and 8 per hour are very similar, but only one would support a diagnosis of OSA. It is not surprising that HSATs often have their greatest utility in patients likely to have a moderate-to-high AHI. Differences in AHI by HSAT and PSG usually have minimal impact on the diagnosis of OSA in patients with moderate-to-severe OSA who have a relatively high AHI by either technique.

Sensitivity, Specificity, and Positive Predictive Values of HSAT

The analysis of agreement between different diagnostic devices is complex (43). The sensitivity of HSAT for detecting OSA using PSG as the gold standard is the number of positive HSAT studies × 100 divided by the number of positive PSG studies. The specificity is the number of negative HSAT studies × 100 divided by the number of negative PSG studies. A high number of false-negative studies reduce the sensitivity, whereas a high number of false-positive studies will reduce the specificity of HSAT compared with PSG. The positive predictive value is the number of true positives by HSAT × 100 divided by the total number of positive HSAT studies. For example, if the positive predictive value is 80%, then there is an 80% chance that a positive HSAT study is correct. The negative predictive value is the number of true negative tests divided by the total number of negative studies. The positive predictive value and negative predictive values depend on the *prevalence* of the disorder being diagnosed as well as the sensitivity and specificity of the diagnostic test (43). If one assumes a sensitivity of 80% and specificity of 89%, then the positive predictive value is only 47% with a 10% prevalence of a disorder, but 89% when the prevalence of the disorder is 50%. Using the same sensitivity and specificity assumptions, the negative predictive value when there is a 10% prevalence is 98.9%, but only 89.8% when the prevalence is 50%. Thus, a HSAT study with a given sensitivity and specificity will result in a higher positive predictive value when used in a high prevalence population (high pretest probability of OSA). On the contrary, if the prevalence is high, the negative predictive value of a negative HSAT study is typically lower. If HSAT is negative and there is a high clinical suspicion of sleep apnea, PSG should be ordered (4, 8).

Comparison of HSAT with PSG (Accuracy)

The AHI by PSG can be compared with HSAT using a number of study designs. Some studies have compared AHI values from a simultaneous recording of PSG and

HSAT in a sleep center (42, 44). This approach eliminates night-to-night variability issues, but this is not the way HSAT devices are typically used. Other studies evaluating the accuracy of HSAT have compared the AHI by PSG in the sleep center with the AHI by HSAT at home (on different nights). A few studies recorded HSAT both simultaneously with PSG in the sleep center and at home on a different night (44). In general, the AHI by HSAT and PSG tends to have better agreement when both HSAT and PSG are recorded the same night of sleep. For example, Santos-Silva and coworkers compared AHI values determined by a Type III device (Philips Respironics Stardust) at home with those determined by PSG (44), as well as AHI values determined by simultaneous PSG and HSAT recording. As expected, the best sensitivity and specificity were found when studies were performed simultaneously.

The trisociety systematic evidence review of the use of HSAT for the diagnosis of OSA analyzed a total of 51 studies, published between 1990 and 2001. The studies analyzed included 35 Type 4 monitors, 12 Type 3 monitors, and 4 Type 2 monitors (17, 27). Most of the studies excluded patients with comorbid sleep disorders or medical disorders, such as heart failure. The PSG AHI results were considered the gold standard, and the ability of HSAT to rule in or rule out OSA was determined. Finding a single HSAT AHI cutoff that was both sensitive and specific was problematic. The best evidence was for Type 3 devices in the attended setting; however, Type 3 devices are rarely used for attended studies. A number of studies comparing unattended HSAT and PSG have been published since the trisociety evidence review (42, 44). In general, they have shown reasonable sensitivity and specificity. The findings vary with the population studied and the methodology. The use of a higher HSAT AHI cutoff value for diagnosis results in a lower sensitivity and a higher specificity for the test.

OUTCOME STUDIES USING HSAT

The ultimate decision of the CMS (10) in 2008 to allow HSAT for the diagnosis of OSA in patients to be treated with CPAP was heavily influenced by studies showing that clinical pathways using HSAT devices resulted in equivalent outcomes from CPAP treatment, including improvement in daytime sleepiness and the amount of adherence to treatment (32, 33). One of the Agency for Healthcare Research and Quality (AHRQ) evidence reviews published in 2007 focused on outcomes rather than agreement in AHI (30). Studies by Whitelaw et al. (33) and Mulgrew et al. (34) were two important evaluations that influenced the CMS decision. Ever since those outcome studies were published, others have also been published showing similar findings (35–40). Whitelaw et al. (33) randomized 288 patients referred by a family physician

to either standard PSG or a SnoreSat home monitor (only oximetry data were actually utilized). A randomly selected subset of eligible patients referred to the sleep center was studied. Inclusion criteria contained a history suggestive of OSA in association with somnolence or significant physiologic consequences of OSA. Only 44% of patients were considered eligible and, of those, only 11% actually completed the trial. All patients underwent treatment with an auto-titrating PAP (APAP). The patients were followed after a 4-week period to determine their improvement with treatment. There was no difference in the ability of the AHI by PSG and the RDI by HSAT (desaturations per hour) to predict the response to APAP treatment in terms of adherence to treatment or improvement in the quality of life. Mulgrew et al. (34) compared a pathway using PSG (Dx PSG, CPAP PSG separate nights) with a pathway using auto-titration followed by CPAP treatment (95% pressure determined during autotitration). CPAP was further adjusted on the basis of oximetry in this group. Patients were chosen on the basis of the Epworth Sleepiness Scale (ESS), Sleep Apnea Clinical Score, and desaturations per hour greater than 15. Thus, patients in both treatment pathways had a high probability of having moderate-to-severe OSA. Once patients met inclusion and exclusion criteria, they were randomized to the PSG pathway or to the APAP pathway (oximetry → auto-titration → CPAP). At 3 months, the improvement in ESS and quality of life was similar between the two pathways. CPAP adherence was actually better with the pathway not using PSG (e.g., oximetry → auto-titration → CPAP). At the end of the study, PSG was performed on CPAP at the final pressure chosen for each patient. The two pathways had similar AHI values (similar treatment effectiveness).

Berry and coworkers (35) compared a pathway using HSAT, APAP titration, and CPAP treatment with a pathway utilizing PSG for diagnosis and titration (most PSGs were split studies) and CPAP treatment. Patients were required to have daytime sleepiness and a moderate-to-high probability of OSA on the basis of history. An AHI greater than 5 per hour was used to diagnose OSA (either by HSAT or PSG), and all patients diagnosed with OSA were offered CPAP. After 6 weeks of CPAP treatment, the percentage of patients using CPAP, the mean CPAP adherence, and the improvements in ESS and quality of life did not differ between clinical pathways. The study used a HSAT device on the basis of peripheral aterial tonometry (PAT).

Antic and coworkers (36) identified a high-risk patient group for OSA with ESS greater than 8 and an oxygen desaturation index (ODI) (2% dips) greater than or equal to 27 per hour. Patients were randomized to a pathway using auto-titration, CPAP at the 95th percentile pressure determined during auto-titration, and treatment directed by a specialist nurse (visits at 1 and 3 months) OR a pathway consisting of diagnostic

PSG, CPAP PSG, CPAP treatment, nurse visits, and MD visits if needed. At 3 months, the groups did not differ in ESS improvement or CPAP adherence.

Skomro and coworkers (37) randomized patients to a PSG arm or home monitoring (HM) arm. The patients in both arms had a PSG performed (usually split night in PSG arm, and diagnostic PSG in HM arm). The HSAT device was the Embletta (Embla, Denver CO). The HM arm underwent APAP for 1 week and then CPAP for 3 weeks on the basis of the APAP data. Patients in the PSG arm underwent CPAP treatment for 4 weeks. The pathways were equivalent in CPAP adherence, improvement in ESS, and quality of life. A large study in VA patients found a pathway using HSAT to not be inferior to one using PSG for diagnosis and PAP titration (38). Rosen and coworkers found a higher PAP adherence in patients diagnosed by HSAT (39) who underwent auto-titration at home to determine an effective level of CPAP rather than PSG for diagnosis and PAP titration. Of note, in all the above-mentioned studies, patients with significant comorbidities were excluded. The studies do suggest that diagnosis by HSAT in a group with moderate-to-high probability of having OSA (without comorbidity), followed by CPAP treatment based on APAP titration, results in equivalent outcomes compared with pathways using PSG. However, because auto-titration is not reimbursed, this is not a viable clinical pathway in most circumstances. A more recent study found that a clinical pathway using the diagnosis of OSA by HSAT and *treatment with AutoCPAP* (no auto-titration) resulted in equivalent outcomes to one using PSG (40). This approach is the one commonly used for treatment after diagnosis by HSAT (unless a PSG titration study is performed).

CLINICAL USE OF HSAT

Advantages and Limitations of Type 3 HSAT

HSAT has a number of potential advantages (Table 44-5), including sleep in the normal home environment with fewer sensors (patients may sleep better), and ease of study for patients with immobility, those with special needs (claustrophobia), or unstable medical conditions requiring intensive care. HSAT may also be useful in verifying an adequate CPAP before discharge from the hospital, until a follow-up by PSG titration can be obtained. HSAT monitoring is less complex and requires less expertise than PSG devices. The number of diagnostic studies is not limited by the number of rooms in the sleep center. In locales with limited PSG capacity,

Table 44-5 Potential Advantages and Limitations for Unattended Type 3 Home Sleep Apnea Testing

Advantages	Limitations
• Sleep in normal home environment (patients may sleep better)	• Some patients very anxious about becoming disconnected without someone available for reconnection
• Some patients may find HSAT more comfortable than PSG (fewer monitoring leads)	• Unattended—so potential for monitoring leads becoming unhooked or technically inadequate study
• Good for patients who are immobile or who might find PSG challenging (claustrophobia)	• 10%–15% technically inadequate studies (up 30% in some studies if patient places the sensors)
• Flexible setting: home, hospital room, hotel	• TST and amounts of different sleep stages are not documented (Type III and IV HSAT). Were the TST and amount of REM sleep adequate?
• HSAT monitoring less technically complex than PSG	• Apnea + hypopnea index underestimated because of division by monitoring time, which is greater than total sleep time
• Each device less costly than PSG equipment	• May not determine amount of supine monitoring time (some HSAT devices)
• Less expertise needed to set up HSAT device and sensors	• HSAT device loss or damage can be a significant problem
• Less expertise needed to score and interpret HSAT studies than PSG	• Good-quality HSAT studies require trained personnel and have substantial costs (education, setup, download, cleaning units, analysis, report generation)
• Virtual sleep center—number of patients who can be studied is not limited by the size of a sleep center	• Less cost to perform HSAT but much less reimbursement
• Some locales may decrease wait time for diagnosis and treatment (depends on availability of PSG)	• Need to perform PSG for negative studies in most sleepy patients
	• If diagnosis of significant obstructive sleep apnea is made—still need to perform PSG CPAP titration in most patients unless alternate approach used (APAP titration, APAP treatment, empiric CPAP level)
	• Cannot detect arrhythmias if pulse rate by oximetry rather than electrocardiogram recorded

APAP, auto-titration positive airway pressure; CPAP, continuous positive airway pressure; HSAT, home sleep apnea testing; PSG, polysomnography; TST, total sleep time; REM, rapid eye movement.

the use of HSAT may reduce the wait time to study and treatment. On the contrary, there has been a dramatic increase in the number of sleep centers (23), so access to PSG may not be limited in many locales.

There are also a number of disadvantages to HSAT. Some patients are quite anxious about sensors becoming disconnected and would actually prefer an attended study. If sensors do become dislodged during an unattended study, it may be technically inadequate. In fact, a significant proportion of HSAT studies are technically inadequate (from 5% to 30%) (45). HSAT is less cost-effective if a high proportion of studies must be repeated. HSAT devices are less expensive than PSG equipment but may not be returned or may be damaged in the patients' home. Type 3 (95806) HSAT studies do not determine the amount of sleep, or the amount of REM sleep. It may be difficult to determine if a study underestimates the severity of OSA caused by limited amounts of sleep or REM sleep. Some HSAT devices determine body position. This is important if the patient has much more severe apnea in the supine position. Good-quality HSAT studies often require significant expertise in either education of patients to self-apply the sensors or hooking them up in the sleep center. Although HSAT studies are not as complex as those of PSG, they do require experienced personnel to avoid a high percentage of technically inadequate studies. Golpe et al. (45) found much higher rates of failed studies when the patients set up HSAT in the home (33%) versus having HSAT devices applied at the sleep center (7%). If the HSAT study is negative and the patient is sleepy, most patients will need a PSG. If the HSAT is positive, many patients will need a PSG CPAP titration, unless an alternate approach is available (APAP titration or APAP treatment). One could argue that a split study might be more cost-effective than diagnosis by HSAT followed by a PSG titration. The relative cost of the two approaches will depend on the number of negative HSAT studies, the number of HSAT studies that need repeating, and the treatment algorithm once a diagnosis of OSA is made. In the private sector, in the United States, auto-titration studies are not reimbursed and durable medical equipment (DME) suppliers receive the same reimbursement for CPAP and APAP devices, even though APAP devices are more expensive. These reimbursement issues limit the use of alternate approaches to CPAP treatment. However, as the cost differential between APAP and CPAP devices has decreased considerably, many DME providers are willing to supply APAP devices if specifically ordered by a physician.

Standards and Indications
Unattended HSAT

Clinical guidelines for portable monitoring (CGPM) were published by the AASM in 2007 on the basis of an evidence review and consensus (8). The guidelines state that HSAT "may" be used as an alternative to PSG for the diagnosis of OSA in patients with a high probability of moderate-to-severe OSA (provided certain conditions are met); in cases where PSG is not possible by virtue of immobility, safety, or critical illness; or to monitor the response to non-CPAP treatment of OSA (including oral appliance, upper airway surgery, and weight loss). The CGPM state that *unattended* HSAT "may" be indicated for the diagnosis of OSA in patients with a high pretest probability of having OSA *IF* guidelines for patient selection and procedures for HSAT performance and interpretation are followed (8) (Tables 44-6 and 44-7).

HSAT is not indicated for screening asymptomatic populations. The CGPM also outlined recommendations concerning technical aspects of HSAT and study interpretation. These guidelines state that at a minimum, airflow, respiratory effort, and oximetry should be recorded (Type 3 not Type 4 studies were recommended). More recently, an AASM task force published current practice guidelines for diagnostic testing for adult OSA (4). The task force recommended that PSG *or home sleep apnea testing* with a technically adequate device be used for the diagnosis of OSA in *uncomplicated adult patients* presenting with signs and symptoms that indicate an increased risk of moderate-to-severe obstructive apnea. The selection of "uncomplicated" patients is described in the following section.

Candidates for HSAT

The CGPM states that a comprehensive sleep evaluation must precede HSAT. Ideally, each patient should be seen by a board-certified/board-eligible sleep physician before sleep testing. If this is not possible, a physician extender may perform an evaluation consisting of questionnaires or an interview. The evaluation should occur before HSAT, but if this is not possible, the clinical evaluation can occur at the time of testing. Characteristics of patients who are not good candidates for HSAT are listed in Table 44-6.

Review of the medical record to exclude patients with comorbidities that may degrade HSAT accuracy is important. In the CGPM, comorbidities excluding patients from HSAT include severe pulmonary disease, neuromuscular disease, or congestive heart failure (CHF). The rationale is that such patients may exhibit hypoventilation without discrete respiratory events, or Cheyne–Stokes breathing. Recent guidelines for diagnostic testing for adult OSA published by a task force of the AASM (4) recommended PSG (rather than HSAT) for the diagnosis of OSA in complicated adult patients with *significant cardiorespiratory disease, potential respiratory muscle weakness due to neuromuscular condition, awake hypoventilation or suspicion of sleep-related hypoventilation, chronic opioid medication use, and a history of stroke or severe insomnia.*

Table 44-6 Indications and Conditions for Use of Unattended Home Sleep Apnea Testing (Type 3)

INDICATIONS:
- Diagnosis of OSA in "uncomplicated" adult patients with increased risk (high probability) of having moderate-to-severe sleep apnea (without comorbidities or other sleep disorders)
- Diagnosis of OSA in patients in whom laboratory PSG is not possible by virtue of immobility, safety, or critical illness
- To document the efficacy of non-PAP treatments for OSA (oral appliances, upper airway surgery, weight loss)

CONDITIONS:
- HSAT must be performed in conjunction with a comprehensive sleep evaluation supervised by a BC/BE sleep physician
- No comorbid medical conditions that may degrade HSAT accuracy
  - Severe pulmonary disease
  - Neuromuscular disease (potential respiratory muscle weakness)
  - Congestive heart failure
  - Chronic opioid medication use
  - Awake or suspected sleep-related hypoventilation (Obesity Hypoventilation Syndrome)
  - History of cerebrovascular accident
  - Severe insomnia
- No clinical suspicion of other sleep disorders
  - Central sleep apnea
  - Narcolepsy
  - Periodic limb movement disorder
  - Parasomnias
  - Circadian rhythm sleep disorders
- Not for screening asymptomatic populations
- Use of an acceptable device. Scoring manual: meets criteria for 95800, 95801, 95806. Clinical guidelines for portable monitoring stated at a minimum airflow, effort, and oximetry. 2017 clinical guidelines: airflow, dual thoracoabdominal respiratory inductance plethysmography, and oximetry

HSAT, home sleep apnea testing; PAP, positive airway pressure; PSG, polysomnography; OSA, obstructive sleep apnea.
Based on Kapur, V. K., Auckley, D. H., Chowdhuri, S., et al. (2017). Clinical practice guideline for diagnostic testing for adult obstructive sleep apnea: An American Academy of Sleep Medicine clinical practice guideline. *Journal of Clinical Sleep Medicine, 13*(3), 479–504; Collop, N. A., Tracy, S. L., Kapur, V., et al. (2011). Obstructive sleep apnea devices for out-of-center (OOC) testing: Technology evaluation. *Journal of Clinical Sleep Medicine, 7*(5), 531–548; Department of Health and Human Services. (2008, March 13). *Decision memo for continuous positive airway pressure (CPAP) therapy for obstructive sleep apnea (OSA)* (CAG#0093R2). Baltimore, MD: Centers for Medicare & Medicaid Services.

One can argue that if HSAT devices use the same sensors used for PSG, then both types of testing should have a similar ability to detect central apnea, Cheyne–Stokes breathing (Fig. 44-2), or hypoventilation (manifested by a low SaO_2 without discrete events). According to the AASM scoring manual (13), a diagnosis of hypoventilation should be based on measurement of arterial PCO_2 or an accurate surrogate. Hence, neither routine PSG nor HSAT can definitively document hypoventilation. Even if HSAT can detect Cheyne–Stokes breathing, central apneas not of the Cheyne–Stokes type, or arterial desaturations without discrete events, patients with these findings would not be good candidates for auto-titration or treatment with an auto-titrating device. These patients would benefit from an attended PSG titration. Patients with a low baseline SaO_2 will often need both supplemental oxygen and CPAP. In these situations, a split sleep study may be more cost-effective than HSAT followed by a PSG titration. Most HSAT devices would miss significant cardiac arrhythmias because typically a heart rate signal is derived from the oximeter rather than ECG. If patients with significant insomnia undergo

HSAT, the MT may tremendously overestimate TST, thus reducing the sensitivity of detecting sleep apnea. HSAT is also not indicated in patients in whom other sleep disorders are present and that would be better evaluated by PSG (coexistent OSA and parasomnias).

Recommended HSAT Methodology

The AASM scoring manual (13) provides recommendations for the sensors and devices to be used in HSAT. The device should be Food and Drug Administration approved and meet criteria for 95800, 95801, or 95806. Devices meeting criteria for 95806 are the most commonly used. Raw tracings must be viewable in detail with the ability to edit events. Airflow recording with both oronasal thermal flow and nasal pressure is ideal, but at least one of these sensor types is recommended. *Recommended* alternatives to these airflow sensors include use of the sum of dual (thoracoabdominal) respiratory inductance plethysmography belts (RIPsum) to estimate tidal volume or the first-time derivative of the sum to estimate flow (RIPflow). Using dual polyvinylidene

Table 44-7 Recommended Methodology for Home Sleep Apnea Test

Equipment (Scoring Manual and Accreditation Standards)

- FDA approved with unique identifier for each unit
- Meets criteria for 9580, 95801, 95806
- Monitor at least three parameters: airflow, effort, and oximetry
  (or, peripheral arterial tonometry, actigraphy, oximetry)
- Ability to record oximetry and a measure of heart rate
- Ability to display raw data for review, manual scoring, or editing of automated scoring
- Ability to calculate an REI on the basis of monitoring time as a surrogate for the AHI determined by PSG
- Airflow—at least one: nasal pressure, oronasal thermal airflow sensor, or alternate sensor (Recommended: RIPflow, RIP-sum; Acceptable: PVDF sum)
- Respiratory effort—Recommended: dual thoraco abdominal RIP belts, Acceptable: single RIP belt, single or dual PVDF belts, single or dual piezoelectric belts, single pneumatic effort belt
- Device must provide an REI that approximates AHI by PSG.

Personnel and Setting

- HSAT should be performed by an AASM-accredited sleep center
  - Standard policies and procedures for HSAT
  - Quality assurance program
  - Interscorer reliability program
- Experienced sleep technician/technologist either places sensors or directly educates the patient on sensor application
- Review of all raw data and interpretation by BC/BE sleep physician

Scoring of Study

- Raw data are scored manually or edited if automated scoring
- Scoring criteria according to AASM scoring manual

Follow-Up

- Sleep MD or referring MD/extenders discuss results with patient and plan treatment
- Sleep center has a method to document adequate follow-up
- If HSAT study is technically inadequate or fails to establish a diagnosis of obstructive sleep apnea in a patient with a high pretest probability, a diagnostic PSG should be performed.

The reader should review current accreditation standards for updates.
AASM, American Academy of Sleep Medicine; AHI, apnea–hypopnea index; FDA, Food and Drug Administration; HSAT, home sleep apnea testing; PSG, polysomnography; PVDF, polyvinylidene fluoride; REI, respiratory event index; RIP, respiratory inductance plethysmography.
Based on AASM accreditation standards, Kapur, V. K., Auckley, D. H., Chowdhuri, S., et al. (2017). Clinical practice guideline for diagnostic testing for adult obstructive sleep apnea: An American Academy of Sleep Medicine clinical practice guideline. *Journal of Clinical Sleep Medicine,* *13*(3), 479–504; Collop, N. A., Tracy, S. L., Kapur, V., et al. (2011). Obstructive sleep apnea devices for out-of-center (OOC) testing: Technology evaluation. *Journal of Clinical Sleep Medicine,* *7*(5), 531–548; Department of Health and Human Services. (2008, March 13). *Decision memo for continuous positive airway pressure (CPAP) therapy for obstructive sleep apnea (OSA)* (CAG#0093R2). Baltimore, MD: Centers for Medicare & Medicaid Services.

fluoride (PVDF) effort belts, a PVDF sum can be determined and this can be used as an *acceptable* alternate sensor for airflow. Dual thoracoabdominal RIP belts are *recommended* to detect respiratory effort, whereas the use of a single RIP belt is acceptable. Single or dual PVDF or piezoelectric belts are *acceptable* as is the use of a single pneumatic belt. If sleep is recorded (on the basis of EEG and EOG) an AHI equal to apneas and hypopneas/TST (hours) is reported. If sleep is not recorded, the REI is reported as the number of apneas and hypopnea per hour of MT. Here, MT is recording time minus time the patient is believed to be awake (diary, actigraphy). The rules for scoring an apnea are the same

as those for PSG. When sleep is recorded, the hypopnea rules for HSAT are the same as those for PSG. When sleep is not recorded (arousals cannot be scored), hypopneas are scored using HSAT when all of the following are present: (a) a drop in the peak signal excursion by greater than or equal to 30% of preevent baseline using a recommended or alternate airflow sensor, (b) the duration of the greater than or equal to 30% drop in signal excursion is greater than or equal to 10 seconds, and (c) there is a greater than or equal to 3% oxygen desaturation from preevent baseline (recommended) or greater than or equal to 4% oxygen desaturation from preevent baseline (acceptable).

3 minutes

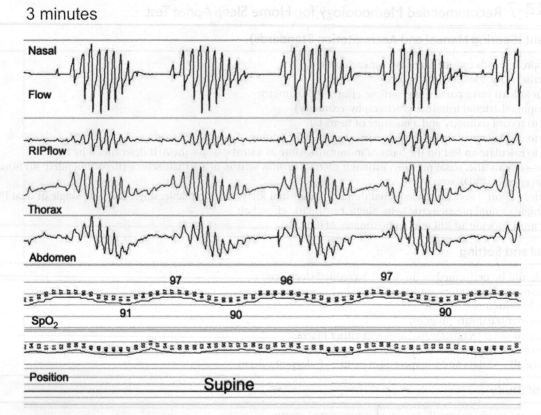

Figure 44-2 A 3-minute tracing from a home sleep apnea testing device that displays RIPflow which is an estimate of airflow (here also measured by nasal pressure after a square root transformation). The thorax and abdomen channels are RIP effort belt signals at those locations. The figure shows an example of Cheyne–Stokes breathing central apnea. RIP, respiratory inductance plethysmography.

The scoring manual also provides guidelines for HSAT devices using PAT. The device must meet the CPT definition of 95800 or 95801. There must be the ability to calculate an REI as a surrogate for an AHI on the basis of PSG.

HSAT should be performed under the auspices of an AASM-accredited sleep center. Adequately trained staff should either place the monitoring equipment on the patient or instruct them on the application of the sensors. This is essential to avoid a high percentage of technically inadequate studies. The raw HSAT tracings must be reviewed and edited for accuracy if an automated scoring system is used. For quality assurance, standard operating procedures for the HSAT process must exist. To verify adequate scoring, interscorer reliability on scoring of HSAT studies should be performed on a routine basis and documented. If the HSAT recording is technically inadequate or if the study results are negative in a patient with a high pretest probability of having OSA, an attended PSG should be performed.

Note that the current practice guidelines for diagnostic testing for adult OSA (4) also defined what the task

force considered a technically adequate HSAT device (a minimum of the following sensors: nasal pressure, chest and abdominal RIP, and oximetry; or PAT with oximetry and actigraphy). The scoring manual recommends dual RIP effort belts, but states that a single belt is acceptable.

In version 2.5 of the AASM scoring manual (Tables 44-8 and 44-9), there are recommended parameters that must be reported and optional parameters that may be monitored at the discretion of the clinician or investigator. Parameters to be reported include the REI based on MT. The REI = (# respiratory events × 60)/MT in minutes. An additional recommended parameter is the oxygen desaturation index (ODI) which is the (# oxygen desaturations ≥3% or ≥4% × 60)/MT in minutes. The definition for ODI should be specified (desaturation defined as a ≥3% or ≥4% drop in the SaO_2). The ODI should use 4% or 3% on the basis of the desaturation used for scoring hypopneas. MT is recording time minus time identified as wake on the basis of diary, actigraphy, or other methods (should be noted in report).

Table 44-8 General Parameters to Be Reported

Type of device	Recommended
Type of airflow sensor(s)	Recommended
Type of respiratory effort sensor(s) (single or dual)	Recommended
Oxygen saturation	Recommended
Heart rate (electrocardiogram or derived from oximeter)	Recommended
Body position	Optional
Sleep/wake or monitoring time (method of determination)	Optional
Snoring (acoustic or piezoelectric sensor or signal derived from nasal pressure sensor)	Optional

Modified with permission from Berry R. B., Albertario C. L., Harding S. M. (2018). *The AASM manual for the scoring of sleep and associated events: Rules, terminology and technical specifications* [Version 2.5]. Darien, IL: American Academy of Sleep Medicine.

Table 44-9 Recording Data to Be Reported

1. Recording start time (h:min)	Recommended
2. Recording end time (h:min)	Recommended
3. Total recording time in min (including wake and artifact)	Recommended
4. Monitoring time (MT) in min (time used to calculate respiratory event index)	Optional
5. Total sleep time (TST) in min (if recorded)	Recommended
6. Heart rate (average, highest, lowest)	Recommended
7. Number of respiratory events	Recommended
7a. Number of apneas	Recommended
7b. Number of hypopneas	Recommended
7c. Number of obstructive, central, and mixed apneas	Optional
8. Respiratory event index (REI) based on MT = (# respiratory events × 60)/MT in min	Recommended
9. Apnea–hypopnea index (AHI) = ([# apneas + # hypopneas] × 60)/TST in min (only if sleep is recorded)	Recommended
10. REI or AHI in the supine and nonsupine positions	Optional
11. Central apnea index = (# central apneas × 60)/MT in min	Optional
12. A measure of oxygen saturation (one of these three parameters)	Recommended
12a. Oxygen desaturation index 3% or 4% = (# oxygen desaturations ≥3% or ≥4% × 60)/MT in min (Specify measure of desaturation 3% or 4%)	
12b. Arterial oxygen saturation, mean value, maximum value, and minimum value	
12c. Arterial oxygen saturation% of time at or below 88% or other thresholds	
13. Occurrence of snoring (if recorded)	Optional

Modified with permission from Berry, R. B., Albertario, C. L., & Harding, S. M. (2018). *The AASM manual for the scoring of sleep and associated events: Rules, terminology and technical specifications* (Version 2.5). Darien, IL: American Academy of Sleep Medicine.

PRACTICAL CONSIDERATIONS FOR HSAT

There are a number of technical and economic factors to be considered in setting up a successful HSAT program. A system that works in one locale may not work in another. A systematic approach is indicated to avoid a high percentage of technically inadequate studies. The choice of the device and method of device application are major considerations. Devices with more sensors provide additional information (and backup sensors) but are more difficult to apply. Before selecting a HSAT device, one must carefully consider the method of device setup that is planned. The HSAT device software should provide the ability to review the raw data in detail. An accurate autoscoring algorithm that minimizes the amount of editing that is required is highly desirable, given the low reimbursement for the technical component of HSAT monitoring. If the software is similar to that used for PSG, this may be an advantage in reducing training costs. The durability of the device and the cost of expendables (nasal cannula, oximeter probes) should be considered. Devices with a rechargeable battery may help reduce costs because devices using batteries typically need new batteries for each patient. The ability of the device to record multiple nights may also be helpful.

HSAT devices can be placed on the patient in the sleep center, or in the home by a technologist. However, the application of the HSAT device by a technologist in a private home is expensive and has safety issues. Therefore, having the patient come to the sleep center is recommended. Alternatively, patients can be trained on the HSAT device and asked to apply the sensors themselves at home. Adequate training is essential and instructional videos or DVDs, along with simple instruction sheets, can be very useful. As noted earlier, one study found over three times the study failure rate when patients applied HSAT sensors at home by themselves (45). One option is to have the patient come to the sleep center for education on device placement and practice sensor application. If patients are unable to successfully attach the sensors or prefer not to do so, they can simply wear the attached HSAT device at home. HSAT devices can be returned by the patient to the sleep center or mailed, if the commuting distance is long. A rapid turnaround time reduces the number of HSAT devices that need to be purchased. If the HSAT device is simple to operate, mailing the device to the patient's home with instructions and having him or her apply it can work in some patient populations. Device loss can be a major expense. Many sleep centers have patients sign a financial responsibility form stating that they will be charged if the device is not returned or is lost.

There are a number of common sensor application problems that need to be addressed. Patients often have difficulty applying some types of oximeter probes as well as chest and abdominal belts. The physician, or sleep center, should be aware of the options before purchasing a device. During a home study, dislodgement of either the nasal cannula or oximeter probe as well as pulling sensor leads out of the HSAT device during movement are typical causes of technically inadequate studies. Patients can be trained to apply tape at strategic points to reduce these events. Many devices have the ability to inform the patient, or technologist, that sensors are working and the device is recording data. For example, some devices use flashing lights or an audible tone to communicate sensor function (or dysfunction). Others provide information in the morning on the adequacy of data collection. This allows the patient to record another night of data before returning the device. It is also useful to have patients complete a brief sleep diary to record their estimate of how long they slept and if the night of sleep was fairly typical. An occasional patient will sleep very poorly with the sensors attached. If minimal sleep is recorded, a false-negative study is likely. Devices that can record more than one night provide another monitoring night opportunity and may also reduce the influence of first-night variability.

TYPES OF HSAT DEVICES

There are numerous devices available for HSAT monitoring (Fig. 44-3). This discussion is intended to cover only a few examples of typical devices. The discussion is not an endorsement of any one device. The recommended and acceptable sensors for HSAT were previously discussed. As noted previously, devices having more sensors provide more information but are more difficult for patients to apply. It is always a trade-off between information and complexity of sensor application. Most HSAT devices monitor airflow using a cannula with monitoring of nasal pressure (with or without a square root transformation). A snore signal is usually derived from nasal pressure, or a separate snore sensor may be used. Some HSAT devices can simultaneously record oral/nasal thermal flow along with nasal pressure. Respiratory effort is typically detected with one or more piezoelectric, PVDF, or RIP bands. Some HSAT devices utilize reusable effort bands, whereas others have the option of disposable band material. Cleaning of devices between patient use is an important consideration, as well as the cost of expendables. Arterial SaO_2 and pulse rate are typically determined by pulse oximetry. A number of oximetry probe options are available, including clip or adhesive wrap probes (either reusable or disposable). The reusable wrap approach is cheaper but more difficult for the patient to apply. Many HSAT devices also have the capability of recording body position and movement (actigraphy). Actigraphy is used by some devices to exclude portions of the tracing from analysis when there is considerable patient movement (assumes the patient is awake).

The Philips Respironics (Murrysville, PA) Alice Night-One and ResMed's ApneaLink™ Plus (San Diego, CA) are examples of relatively simple devices for the patient to attach at home. They use nasal pressure to detect airflow and snoring, a single effort belt, and oximetry (SaO_2 and pulse rate). The Night-One uses a single thoracic respiratory inductance belt that also holds the monitor in place, and the ResMed device uses a pneumatic effort belt. The Night-One also has a body position sensor and can record data via a bluetooth connection from a Philips Respironics PAP device (flow, pressure, leak) instead of nasal pressure.

The Nox-T3 (Nox Medical) is an example of a more complex HSAT device. Nasal pressure is used to detect airflow, and there are dual RIP thoracoabdominal belts. There is a microphone to record snoring, a body position sensor, and actigraphy. The oximetry uses a probe attached to a watch-like oximetry monitor that communicates with the unit recording data by a Bluetooth communication. This avoids the long cable connecting the main monitoring unit to the oximetry probe. Both RIPsum and RIPflow are calculated and provide a backup flow channel (Fig. 44-2) should the nasal pressure signal not be adequate in quality. In the case of mouth breathing, the nasal pressure signal would be flat, but the RIPflow signal would continue to display deflections.

The WatchPAT (Itamar Medical, Caesarea, Israel) is a unique device based on PAT that detects respiratory events by recording changes in sympathetic tone (rather than airflow) (18, 46–52). The device using this technology is worn on the wrist (Fig. 44-4). The WatchPAT device formerly had two probes—a PAT probe and an oximetry probe worn on separate digits. The new unified device uses a single probe to both record oximetry and determine the PAT signal. The PAT signal is a measure of the blood volume in the digit. When sympathetic tone increases, stimulation of alpha receptors causes vasoconstriction of the blood vessels in the digit, which decreases the fingertip volume and the PAT signal. As surges in sympathetic tone follow respiratory event termination, the combination of a decrease in PAT signal, a fall in SpO_2 followed by an increase, and an increase in heart rate allows determination of respiratory events (Fig. 44-5). Nonrespiratory arousals would not reduce the SpO_2. The device results include an estimate of the AHI and RDI (p-AHI, p-RDI) based on estimated TST. One can specify if the AHI is to be based on a greater than or equal to 3% or a greater than or equal to 4% de saturation. An ODI based on the number of greater than or equal to 4% desaturations is also provided. The device has built-in actigraphy and novel algorithms designed for patients with sleep apnea to assist with estimation of sleep (50). Recently, the combination of actigraphy and the PAT signal has been used to determine estimates of wake, light NREM, deep NREM, and REM sleep because the sympathetic tone characteristics of these sleep stages differ (18, 51) (Fig. 44-6). In the study by Hedner and coworkers (18), the agreement with PSG was around 85% for detection of wake versus sleep and 88% for detection of NREM versus REM sleep. However, the kappa values were in the moderate range. An optional combined body position and snore sensor can be placed on the sternum. If the body position sensor is used the device can determine p-AHI values for supine and nonsupine positions. Using motion of the sternal sensor to detect respiratory effort, the WatchPAT can now provide a central AHI and detect Cheyne–Stokes breathing. The PAT devices have been well validated by studies comparing the results with PSG. A meta-analysis showed a high correlation between the PSG AHI and the WatchPAT AHI (52). However, in

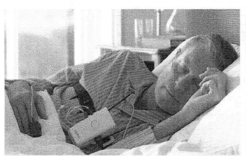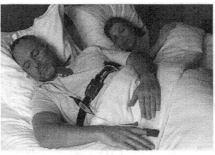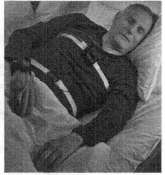

Figure 44-3 Three home sleep apnea testing monitors. In the left panel, an Alice Night-One device (Philips Respironics) is shown. In the center panel, ResMed's ApneaLink™ Plus (ResMed Ltd., San Diego, CA) is shown. Both these devices use nasal cannula to monitor flow and a single effort belt. In the right panel, a Nox-T3 device (Nox Medical, Carefusion) is shown. The device uses chest and abdominal respiratory inductance plethysmography (RIP) belts and derived RIPsum (estimate of tidal volume) and RIPflow (estimate of airflow) tracings that provide additional information to the nasal pressure. An oximeter unit is worn like a watch and communicates with the main recording unit on the chest by bluetooth wireless technology. (Used with permission from Philips Respironics; © ResMed Inc. All rights reserved; Courtesy of Nox Medical. www.noxmedical.com)

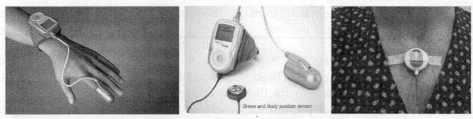

Figure 44-4 The WatchPAT Unified peripheral arterial tonometry monitor. The device is worn on the wrist and has a single probe to record both oximetry and the PAT signal. A combined snore and body position sensor is also available. The sensor is worn below the sternal notch. (Images courtesy of Itamar Medical.)

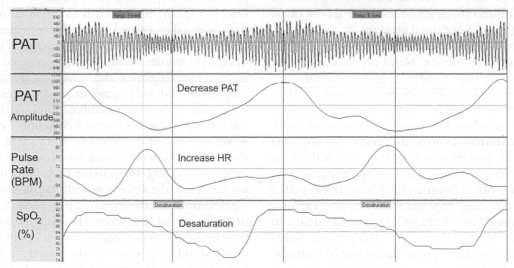

Figure 44-5 An example of respiratory event detection by WatchPAT Unified. A respiratory event is scored when there is a decrease in PAT signal in combination with a fall in the arterial oxygen saturation and an increase in heart rate (HR) (proprietary algorithm). PAT, peripheral arterial tonometry. (Images courtesy of Itamar Medical.)

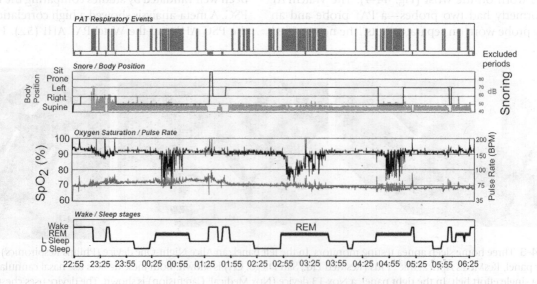

Figure 44-6 An all-night summary of results from a WatchPAT Unified study. A hypnogram (sleep staging) is shown as well as oximetry, PAT events, snoring, and pulse rate. One can see that this patient had rapid eye movement (REM)–associated obstructive sleep apnea. PAT, peripheral arterial tonometry. (Images courtesy of Itamar Medical.)

individual patients, the difference between PSG and WatchPAT AHI values can be over 10 per hour (18). The device is one of the easier to apply. However, the device cannot be used in patients on alpha blockers (Terazosin, etc.). In the past, the device was not recommended for patients in atrial fibrillation, but it can work in these patients unless they have a predominantly paced rhythm. The main downside to using the device is that the PAT probes are relatively expensive. The raw data are available for viewing and editing. However, the algorithm for the identification of respiratory events is proprietary and editing of events, although possible, is problematic. A reviewer can assess the technical adequacy of the recorded data. The WatchPAT device is acceptable to the CMS, and the recent AASM clinical practice guidelines listed devices based on PAT, oximetry, and actigraphy as acceptable (4).

INTEGRATION OF HSAT MONITORING INTO THE OVERALL PATIENT CARE ALGORITHM

Diagnosis of OSA using HSAT is only the first part of the process if the study is positive. It is expected that in populations with a high probability of OSA a high percentage of HSATs will be positive. If PAP is chosen for treatment, there are several alternate pathways to follow. The standard approach would be to perform a PSG PAP titration and subsequent PAP treatment. Patients could also use an AutoPAP device at home (typically for three or more nights) and information obtained could be used to select a pressure for chronic CPAP treatment

(auto-titration) (35–39, 53). A third approach is simply treating the patient with an AutoPAP (auto-adjusting PAP), eliminating the need for titration (40). Issues of cost and reimbursement will vary between settings (VA Health Care System vs. private sector). If a large number of HSAT studies are technically inadequate, or if PSG must be performed because of a high number of negative HSAT studies (to eliminate false negatives), any cost savings from using HSAT will be reduced. On the contrary, there may be less time from suspected diagnosis to treatment using HSAT clinical pathways. If a high percentage of HSAT studies are positive, it is reasonable to question the relative cost–benefit of algorithms using HSAT for diagnosis compared with one using split PSG. An economic analysis by Ayas et al. (54) sought to define the pretest probability of OSA needed for HSAT studies to be cost-effective. The pre-test probability above which portable testing would be less costly than initial diagnostic PSG is 0.47. When an initial split night study was compared to portable testing, the pretest probability above which portable testing was more economically attractive was greater (0.68). Thus, if split studies are used HSAT had an economic advantage only when sleep apnea was very likely.

OVERALL APPROACH TO USING PSG AND HSAT

An overall approach to using a combination of PSG and HSAT is presented in Figure 44-7. A clinical evaluation determines if there is a high probability of

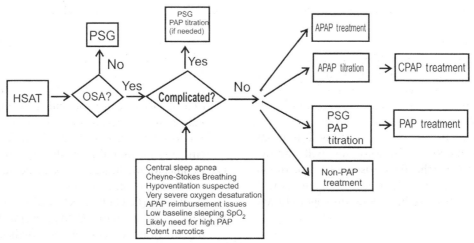

Figure 44-7 A flow diagram showing possible clinical pathways following a home sleep apnea testing study. If the patient has uncomplicated obstructive sleep apnea (OSA), several alternatives are possible, including a polysomnography (PSG) titration and positive airway pressure (PAP) treatment, unattended auto-titration (APAP) followed by continuous PAP treatment based on APAP findings, APAP treatment (auto-adjusting mode), or non-PAP treatments. Patients with central sleep apnea, Cheyne–Stokes breathing, suspected hypoventilation, very severe arterial oxygen desaturation, and a low baseline sleeping SpO_2, those likely to need high pressures (large neck, very high BMI), or patients taking potent narcotics should undergo a PSG PAP titration.

moderate-to-severe OSA, if other sleep disorders for which PSG is indicated are present, and if complicating issues are present that will likely require a PSG titration. Patients with moderate-to-severe CHF (a risk factor for Cheyne–Stokes breathing), those on potent narcotics treatment, hypoventilation, those with severe chronic obstructive pulmonary disease, those with low baseline arterial saturation, or those using supplemental oxygen should undergo a PSG for diagnosis and treatment. If other sleep disorders are suspected in addition to OSA (e.g., a parasomnia), a PSG is the diagnostic test of choice. Although HSAT may be adequate for diagnosis in patients with both obstructive and a significant number of central apneas, most of these patients will need an attended PAP titration. There a split study rather than HSAT is more cost effective. Patients with a high probability of OSA without other complicated factors can undergo HSAT. If OSA is diagnosed, they can have either APAP treatment or APAP titration followed by CPAP treatment. If the HSAT is positive for sleep apnea, but significant amounts of central sleep apnea, Cheyne–Stokes breathing, or severe desaturations are present, a PAP titration with PSG is indicated. Such patients may need supplemental oxygen, bilevel positive airway pressure, or a PAP mode with a backup rate. If the HSAT is negative, a PSG can be performed. The initial clinical evaluation is used to triage patients to HSAT or PSG, and the results of the HSAT study are used to triage the patient to PSG, PSG PAP titration, APAP titration, or APAP treatment.

SUMMARY

Portable sleep monitoring will likely play an increasingly important role in sleep medicine. Like all diagnostic tools, HSAT requires expertise in selecting patients to be studied, proper interpretation of results, and decision making concerning the need for treatment or other diagnostic studies. One can expect technology to improve so that portable monitors are easier to place, less cumbersome, and more reliable. Although some have viewed HSAT as a threat to traditional PSG, HSAT has many limitations. Many patients with OSA and comorbidities will continue to benefit from PSG for the diagnosis and PAP treatment. On the contrary, HSAT may help identify patients with OSA who would otherwise have gone undiagnosed and untreated.

REFERENCES

1. Indications for Polysomnography Task Force ASDA. (1997). Practice parameters for the indications for polysomnography and related procedures. *Sleep, 20,* 406–422.

2. Chesson, A. L., Jr., Ferber, R. A., Fry, J. M., et al. (1997). The indications for polysomnography and related procedures. A standard of practice review. *Sleep, 20,* 423–487.

3. Kushida, C. A., Littner, M. R., Morgenthaler, T., et al. (2005). Practice parameters for the indications for polysomnography and related procedures: An update for 2005. *Sleep, 28,* 499–521.

4. Kapur, V. K., Auckley, D. H., Chowdhuri, S., et al. (2017). Clinical practice guideline for diagnostic testing for adult obstructive sleep apnea: An American Academy of Sleep Medicine clinical practice guideline. *Journal of Clinical Sleep Medicine, 13*(3), 479–504.

5. Littner, M. R. (2005). Portable monitoring in the diagnosis of the obstructive sleep apnea syndrome. *Seminars in Respiratory and Critical Care Medicine, 26,* 56–67.

6. Gay, P. C., & Selecky, P. A. (2010). Are sleep studies appropriately done in the home? *Respiratory Care, 55,* 66–75.

7. American Academy of Sleep Medicine. (2011). *Standards for accreditation of out of center sleep testing (OCST) in adult patients.* Darien, IL: Author.

8. Collop, N. A., Anderson, W. M., Boehlecke, B., et al.; for the Portable Monitoring Task Force of the American Academy of Sleep Medicine. (2007). Clinical guidelines for the use of unattended portable monitors in the diagnosis of obstructive sleep apnea in adult patients. *Journal of Clinical Sleep Medicine, 3*(7), 737–747.

9. Collop, N. A., Tracy, S. L., Kapur, V., et al. (2011). Obstructive sleep apnea devices for out-of-center (OOC) testing: Technology evaluation. *Journal of Clinical Sleep Medicine, 7*(5), 531–548.

10. Department of Health and Human Services. (2008, March 13). *Decision memo for continuous positive airway pressure (CPAP) therapy for obstructive sleep apnea (OSA) (CAG#0093R2).* Baltimore, MD: Centers for Medicare & Medicaid Services.

11. CMS Manual System. (2008, July 3). *Pub 100-03 Medicare national coverage determinations. Transmittal 86.* Baltimore, MD: Centers for Medicare and Medicaid Services. Retrieved March 29, 2018, from https://www.cms.gov/transmittals/downloads/R86NCD.pdf

12. Centers for Medicare and Medicaid Services. (2009, March 3). *Decision memo for sleep testing for obstructive sleep apnea (CAG-00405N).* Baltimore, MD: Author.

13. Berry, R. B., Albertario, C. M., Harding, S. M., et al.; for the American Academy of Sleep Medicine. (2018). *The AASM manual for the scoring of sleep and associated events: Rules, terminology and technical specifications* [Version 2.5]. Darien, IL: American Academy of Sleep Medicine.

14. Flemons, W. W., Douglas, N. J., Kuna, S. T., et al. (2004). Access to diagnosis and treatment of patients with suspected sleep apnea. *American Journal of Respiratory and Critical Care Medicine, 169,* 668–672.

15. Chiao, W., & Durr, M. L. (2017). Trends in sleep studies performed for Medicare beneficiaries. *Laryngoscope, 127,* 2891–2896.

16. Ferber, R., Millman, R., Coppola, M., et al. (1994). Portable recording in the assessment of obstructive sleep apnea. ASDA standards of practice. *Sleep, 17,* 378–392.

17. Flemons, W. W., Littner, M. R., Rowley, J. A., et al. (2003). Home diagnosis of sleep apnea: A systematic review of the literature. An evidence review cosponsored by the American Academy of Sleep Medicine, the American College of Chest Physicians, and the American Thoracic Society. *Chest, 124,* 1543–1579.

18. Hedner, J., White, D. P., Malhotra, A., et al. (2011). Sleep staging based on autonomic signals: A multi-center validation study. *Journal of Clinical Sleep Medicine, 7*(3), 301–306.

19. Quan, S. F., Howard, B. V., Iber, C., et al. (1997). The Sleep Heart Health Study: Design, rationale, and methods. *Sleep, 20,* 1077–1085.

20. Iber, C., Redline, S., Kaplan Gilpin, A. M., et al. (2004). Polysomnography performed in the unattended home versus the attended laboratory setting—Sleep Heart Health Study methodology. *Sleep, 27,* 536–540.

21. Collop, N. A. (2008). Portable monitoring for the diagnosis of obstructive sleep apnea. *Current Opinion in Pulmonary Medicine, 14,* 525–529.

22. Collop, N. A. (2009). Portable monitoring. *Sleep Medicine Clinics, 4,* 435–442.

23. Chediak, A. D. (2008). Why CMS approved home sleep testing for CPAP coverage. *Journal of Clinical Sleep Medicine, 4,* 16–18.

24. Ross, S. D., Sheinhait, I. A., Harrison, K. J., et al. (2000). Systematic review and meta-analysis of the literature regarding the diagnosis of sleep apnea. *Sleep, 23,* 519–532.

25. Dingli, K., Coleman, E. L., Vennelle, M., et al. (2003). Evaluation of a portable device for diagnosing the sleep apnoea/hypopnoea syndrome. *European Respiratory Journal, 21,* 253–259.

26. Calleja, J. M., Esnaola, S., Rubio, R., et al. (2002). Comparison of a cardiorespiratory device versus polysomnography for diagnosis of sleep apnoea. *European Respiratory Journal, 20,* 1505–1510.

27. ATS/ACCP/AASM Portable Monitoring Taskforce Steering Committee. (2004). Executive summary on the systematic review and practice parameters for portable monitoring in the investigation of suspected sleep apnea in adults. *American Journal of Respiratory and Critical Care Medicine, 169,* 1160–1163.

28. Agency for Healthcare Research and Quality. (2004). *Effectiveness of portable monitoring devices for diagnosing obstructive sleep apnea: Update of a systematic review.* Retrieved from https://www.cms.gov/Medicare/Coverage/DeterminationProcess/downloads/id24TA.pdf

29. Agency for Healthcare Research and Quality. (2007). *Technology assessment: Home diagnosis of obstructive sleep apnea-hypopnea syndrome.* Retrieved from https://www.cms.gov/Medicare/Coverage/DeterminationProcess/downloads/id48TA.pdf

30. Agency for Healthcare Research and Quality. (2007). *Obstructive sleep apnea-hypopnea syndrome: Modeling different diagnostic strategies.* Retrieved from http://www.cms.gov/determinationprocess/downloads/id50TA.pdf

31. Standards of Practice Committee ASDA. (1994). Practice parameters for the use of portable recording in the assessment of obstructive sleep apnea. *Sleep, 17,* 372–377.

32. Chesson, A. L., Jr., Berry, R. B., & Pack, A. (2003). Practice parameters for the use of portable monitoring devices in the investigation of suspected obstructive sleep apnea in adults. *Sleep, 26,* 907–913.

33. Whitelaw, W. A., Brant, R. F., & Flemons, W. W. (2005). Clinical usefulness of home oximetry compared with polysomnography for assessment of sleep apnea. *American Journal of Respiratory and Critical Care Medicine, 171,* 188–193.

34. Mulgrew, A. T., Fox, N., Ayas, N. T., et al. (2007). Diagnosis and initial management of obstructive sleep apnea without polysomnography: A randomized validation study. *Ann Intern Med, 146,* 157–166.

35. Berry, R. B., Hill, G., Thompson, L., et al. (2008). Portable monitoring and autotitration versus polysomnography for the diagnosis and treatment of sleep apnea. *Sleep, 31,* 1423–1431.

36. Antic, N. A., Buchan, C., Esterman, A., et al. (2009). A randomized controlled trial of nurse-led care for symptomatic moderate-severe obstructive sleep apnea. *American Journal of Respiratory and Critical Care Medicine, 179,* 501–508.

37. Skomro, R. P., Gjevre, J., Reid, J., et al. (2010). Outcomes of home-based diagnosis and treatment of obstructive sleep apnea. *Chest, 138,* 257–263.

38. Kuna, S. T., Gurubhagavatula, I., Maislin, G., et al. (2011, May 1). Noninferiority of functional outcome in ambulatory management of obstructive sleep apnea. *American Journal of Respiratory and Critical Care Medicine, 183*(9), 1238–1244.

39. Rosen, C. L., Auckley, D., Benca, R., et al. (2012). A multisite randomized trial of portable sleep studies and positive airway pressure autotitration versus laboratory-based polysomnography for the diagnosis and treatment of obstructive sleep apnea: The HomePAP study. *Sleep, 35*(6), 757–767.

40. Berry, R. B., & Sriram, P. (2014). Auto-adjusting positive airway pressure treatment for sleep apnea diagnosed by home sleep testing. *Journal of Clinical Sleep Medicine, 10*(12), 1269–1275.

41. Levendowski, D., Steward, D., Woodson, B. T., et al. (2009). The impact of obstructive sleep apnea variability measured in-lab versus in-home on sample size calculations. *International Archives of Medicine, 2*, 2.

42. Smith, L. A., Chong, D. W., Vennelle, M., et al. (2007). Diagnosis of sleep-disordered breathing in patients with chronic heart failure: Evaluation of a portable limited sleep study system. *Journal of Sleep Research, 16*, 428–435.

43. Flemons, W. W., & Littner, M. R. (2003). Measuring agreement between diagnostic devices. *Chest, 124*, 1535–1542.

44. Santos-Silva, R., Sartori, D. E., Truksinas, V., et al. (2009). Validation of a portable monitoring system for the diagnosis of obstructive sleep apnea syndrome. *Sleep, 32*, 629–636.

45. Golpe, R., Jimenez, A., & Carpizo, R. (2002). Home sleep studies in the assessment of sleep apnea/hypopnea syndrome. *Chest, 122*, 1156–1161.

46. Ayappa, I., Norman, R. G., Seelall, V., et al. (2008). Validation of a self-applied unattended monitor for sleep disordered breathing. *Journal of Clinical Sleep Medicine, 4*, 26–37.

47. Bar, A., Pillar, G., Dvir, I., et al. (2003). Evaluation of a portable device based on peripheral arterial tone for unattended home sleep studies. *Chest, 123*, 695–703.

48. Pillar, G., Bar, A., Betito, M., et al. (2003). An automatic ambulatory device for detection of AASM defined arousals from sleep: The WP100. *Sleep Medicine, 4*, 207–212.

49. Ayas, N. T., Pittman, S., MacDonald, M., et al. (2003). Assessment of a wrist-worn device in the detection of obstructive sleep apnea. *Sleep Medicine, 4*, 435–442.

50. Hedner, J., Pillar, G., Pittman, S. D., et al. (2004). A novel adaptive wrist actigraphy algorithm for sleep-wake assessment in sleep apnea patients. *Sleep, 27*, 1560–1566.

51. Herscovici, S., Pe'er, A., Papyan, S., et al. (2007). Detecting REM sleep from the finger: An automatic REM sleep algorithm based on peripheral arterial tone (PAT) and actigraphy. *Physiological Measurement, 28*, 129–140.

52. Yalamanchali, S., Farajian, V., Hamilton, C., et al. (2013, December). Diagnosis of obstructive sleep apnea by peripheral arterial tonometry: Meta-analysis. *JAMA Otolaryngology—Head and Neck Surgery, 139*(12), 1343–1350.

53. Masa, J. F., Jimenez, A., Duran, J., et al. (2004). Alternative methods of titrating continuous positive airway pressure: A large multicenter study. *American Journal of Respiratory and Critical Care Medicine, 170*, 1218–1224.

54. Ayas, N. T., Fox, J., Epstein, L., et al. (2010). Initial use of portable monitoring versus polysomnography to confirm obstructive sleep apnea in symptomatic patients: An economic decision model. *Sleep Medicine, 11*, 320–324.

chapter 45
Actigraphy

SU JEONG LINSTROM   LISA J. MELTZER

LEARNING OBJECTIVES

On completion of this chapter, the reader should be able to:

1. Appreciate the use, function, and purpose of actigraphy in sleep medicine.
2. Discuss some of actigraphy's strengths and weaknesses, as well as threats to validity.
3. Understand how actigraphy data are applied in a clinical setting.

KEY TERMS

Actigraphy
Accelerometer
Validity

An actigraph is a small device typically worn on the non-dominant wrist. These devices are used to estimate sleep and wake patterns for multiple nights in a wide range of patients. For multiple reasons, the use of actigraphy has become very popular over the past 20 years (1–3). First, actigraphy can collect information for extended periods in the patient's natural environment. Second, actigraphy is relatively noninvasive, most devices being the size of a wristwatch. Third, the cost of performing an actigraphy study is significantly less than that of polysomnography (PSG). Although there are a number of different devices available on the market, the decision about which one to use should be made on the basis of the validity of the device, the cost of the equipment, and the populations to be studied. These issues vary by individual clinicians, researchers, and/or sleep centers; thus, this chapter will not focus on which actigraph to use, but rather provide an overview of actigraphy, when to use actigraphy, how actigraphy works, the validity of actigraphy compared with PSG, and the utility of actigraphy in clinical and research settings.

WHAT IS ACTIGRAPHY?

Most actigraphs are wristwatch-sized devices that use a piezoelectric accelerometer to measure activity levels of the person wearing the device. The use of motion as a measure is common in medical devices. For example, pacemakers have a mechanism that adjusts the rate in response to the patient's activity level, whereas pedometers use motion as a way to monitor the number of steps a person takes. The use of activity monitoring to estimate sleep–wake patterns has been around for many years (4). Early devices were self-contained activity counters with integrated circuits and memory that provided off-line data retrieval (5). Over the years, actigraphs have become more compact and lightweight, with greater memory for data storage and a longer battery life (3). In addition to the newer models of actigraphs being noninvasive and compact, many include a watch capability on the device, so it is also functional to the user. These devices do not interfere with everyday activities, and most brands are also water resistant or even waterproof.

WHEN TO USE ACTIGRAPHY

In 2018, the American Academy of Sleep Medicine (AASM) published updated guidelines for the use of actigraphy in the assessment of sleep and sleep disorders (6), and in 2014, the *International Classification of Sleep Disorders*, 3rd edition provided additional details about the use of actigraphy for the diagnosis and treatment of sleep disorders (7). Specifically, actigraphy should be used (a) for a minimum of 7 days before a multiple sleep latency test to ensure sufficient sleep duration and an appropriate sleep schedule; (b) for a minimum of 7 days with unrestricted sleep opportunity to verify idiopathic hypersomnia (with a 24-hour total sleep time ≥ 660 minutes); (c) to verify insufficient sleep syndrome if there is doubt about the accuracy of a clinical history or sleep diaries; and (d) to demonstrate an irregular circadian rhythm (i.e., delayed sleep–wake phase, advanced sleep–wake phase, and non-24-hour sleep–wake rhythm).

Actigraphy provides many benefits over PSG. During an overnight PSG, patients often have to travel to a center that may be at a distance from their home. In addition, they are sleeping in an unfamiliar setting, removed from the comfort of their own beds, and required to wear numerous sensors that are placed on the head and body. The sensations from the sensors may be overstimulating and difficult to tolerate for some patients (e.g., children with autism spectrum disorders or older adults). Furthermore,

PSG most often records only one night of sleep, which may not be representative of the person's typical sleep because of the "first-night effect," (8). Actigraphy, in contrast, can be worn in the patient's natural home/sleep environment and for an extended period.

However, actigraphy is not a substitute for PSG. PSG uses multiple channels to measure the different physiologic stages of sleep as well as the respiratory state of the patient during the night. These measurements are essential in accurately diagnosing sleep-related breathing disorders, movement-related sleep disorders, and narcolepsy. Actigraphy may be able to measure the disruptions in sleep caused by sleep-related breathing disorders or movement-related sleep disorders; however, it cannot accurately identify the causes of these awakenings. Information from actigraphy can be a useful tool in clinical and research settings, but it should not be used as a simple substitute for PSG.

HOW DOES ACTIGRAPHY WORK?

Activity counts are measured per epoch in actigraphy. Although some devices have a fixed epoch length of 1 minute, other devices allow the user to set the epoch length to 15 seconds, 30 seconds, 1 minute, or 2 minutes. Each device has a different way to digitize the signal. For some devices, the user can choose the data mode; for other devices, the data mode is automatically selected. When the user can select the data mode, there are three choices: time above threshold (TAT), zero crossing mode (ZCM), and proportional integration mode (PIM). TAT measures the amount of time per epoch the activity waveform is above the set threshold; ZCM measures the number of times per epoch the waveform crosses a threshold set close to

zero; PIM, also known as digital integration, measures the area under the curve for each epoch (see reference [3, 5] for more information). Newer devices allow for multiple modes to be used simultaneously. Different studies have provided support for different measurement modes (1). Owing to the variance in results, it is questionable whether there is one best method of measuring the digitalized signal from the actigraphy. Further study should be conducted on a wider range of user populations to see if one mode or a combination of modes yields the most accurate results.

When the actigraphs are returned by the patient, the devices are downloaded to a computer using a device-specific interface. Each brand of actigraph has proprietary software that uses device-specific scoring algorithms (e.g., Sadeh and Cole-Kripke) or wake sensitivity (e.g., medium, high, and low) thresholds to determine whether each epoch should be scored as sleep or wake. The selection of which algorithm to use should be based on the sample being studied (3, 9, 10). Once the data have been scored, the program will generate an actigram (a picture of the patient's sleep during the study; see Figs. 45-1 and 45-2 for examples) as well as summary variables such as total sleep time, actigraphic sleep-onset time, wake after sleep onset, and actigraphic sleep-offset time. Variables such as bedtime, wake time, and sleep-onset latency should be reported only if the patient also keeps a concurrent daily sleep diary (discussed further later) or uses the event marker feature included with some devices. Along these lines, sleep efficiency (SE) should be calculated only if a diary is included (providing bedtime and wake time; SE = minutes of sleep from actigraphic sleep onset to actigraphic sleep offset/minutes from bedtime to wake time × 100).

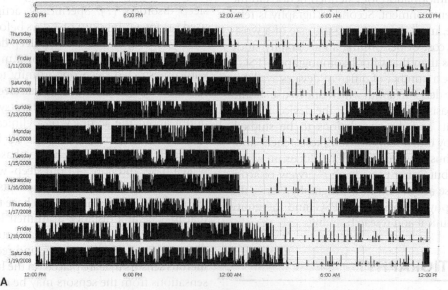

Figure 45-1 A: Actigram of a 17-year-old male who reported excessive daytime sleepiness (EDS). This patient typically fell asleep between 12 and 1 a.m., waking between 6 and 7 a.m., except on weekends, when he would sleep from 3 a.m. until 12 noon.

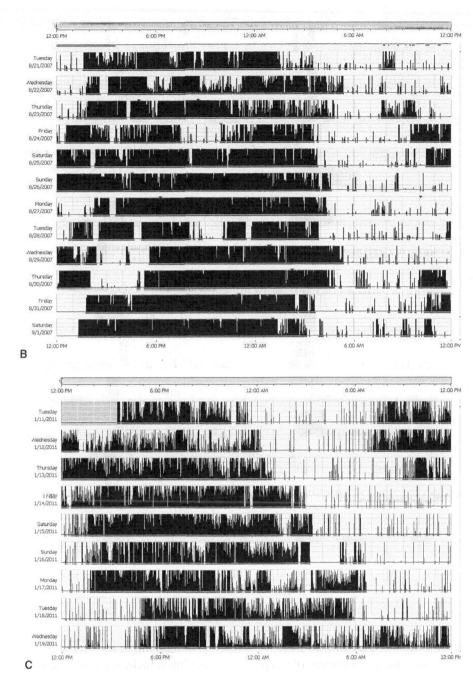

Figure 45-1 (*continued*) **B:** Actigram of a 14-year-old male who reported EDS and the inability to fall asleep before 3 a.m. This patient typically fell asleep around 3 a.m. and woke up around 1 p.m. **C:** Actigram of a 22-year-old female who reported EDS and an irregular sleep pattern. Actigraphy showed a circadian rhythm sleep disorder, free-running type, with her sleep-onset time starting at midnight and then progressively getting later each night over the course of the study.

VALIDITY OF ACTIGRAPHY

Although actigraphy has several benefits over PSG (e.g., relatively low cost, nonintrusive device that can be used for extended periods to estimate sleep–wake patterns), there are several concerns about validity that should be considered. The two primary areas of concern are (1) specificity to detect wake and (2) artifact.

Actigraphy in Comparison with PSG

Several studies have compared the validity of sleep/wake data from actigraphy with a PSG or a videosomnography (2, 10–17). When compared epoch by epoch, the sensitivity, or the ability of actigraphy to detect sleep when PSG scores sleep, is very good (typically >85%). However, the specificity, or the ability of actigraphy to detect wake when PSG scores wake, has been very low

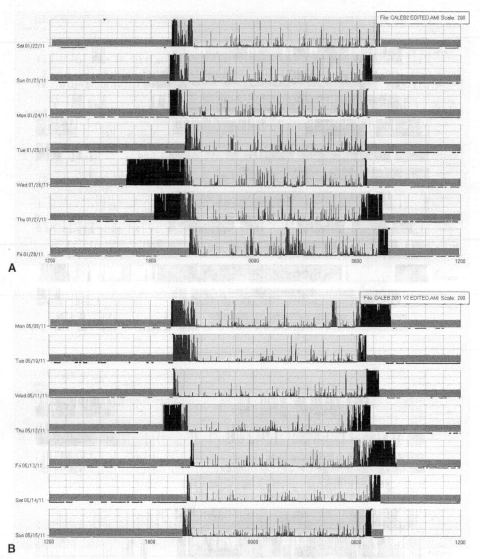

Figure 45-2 A: Actigram of a 7-year-old boy with high levels of activity during sleep. B: Actigram of the same 7-year-old boy following 3 months of iron supplementation showing reduced activity during sleep.

(typically below 70% but reported as low as 24% to 44%). During a PSG, an accurate measurement of sleep and wake can be detected through multiple channels of electroencephalography, whereas wrist actigraphy relies on a single channel of information (movement), which results in this larger margin of error. Most commonly, this error results in an overestimation of total sleep time and an underestimation of wake after sleep onset.

Artifact

Artifact is the other primary threat to validity. Because actigraphy relies on the use of activity to estimate sleep–wake patterns, there are several instances where sleep and wake may be scored inappropriately. For example, actigraphy may identify a person lying in bed watching television as sleeping if there is a low level of activity.

On the other hand, if the user were asleep as a passenger in a moving vehicle, the movement of the car would be detected as sufficient activity to estimate that the person is awake. Environmental causes of awakenings, such as a restless or snoring bed partner, or a pet jumping on the bed, can also alter the results. Finally, atypical days (due to illness, holidays, vacations, etc.) can also result in artifact because the study day would not be representative of that patient's typical sleep–wake patterns.

A daily sleep diary is needed to reduce artifact. Using such a diary (example in Fig. 45-3) allows patients to record times when they removed the device, times with low activity when the person was awake, and times with high activity when the person was asleep. In addition, diaries can include questions about bed partners (or pets) that may have resulted in increased activity during sleep, medications used for sleep, subjective sleep quality, as well as

Fill this form out JUST BEFORE going to bed

Today is _____ Today's Date ____/____/____

What time is it now? _____ a.m./p.m.   Did you go to work/school today? ____ Yes ____ No

Were you sick today? ____ Yes ____ No   If yes, with what? _____

Write times the following occurred (and circle a.m. or p.m.)	START	END
Removed the actigraph	a.m. p.m.	a.m. p.m.
Nap (or accidentally fell asleep)	a.m. p.m.	a.m. p.m.
Very quiet activity (e.g., going to the movies)	a.m. p.m.	a.m. p.m.

Fill this form out FIRST THING in the morning

Today is _____ Today's Date ____/____/____

	Circle a.m. or p.m.
Last night—got into bed at:	a.m. p.m.
Last night—tried to fall asleep at:	a.m. p.m.
Last night it took_____minutes to fall asleep	Min
After falling asleep—woke up____ times during the night (circle one choice)	0 1 2 3 4 5 or more
Woke up this morning at:	a.m. p.m.
Finally got out of the bed this morning at:	a.m. p.m.

Figure 45-3 Example of a daily sleep diary to be used with actigraphy studies.

whether it was a typical day/night of sleep. Daily sleep diaries are also necessary for clinicians or researchers to identify bedtime (time attempted to fall asleep) and wake time (time patient awakened for the day), allowing the calculation of sleep-onset latency. As mentioned, some devices have an event marker feature that allows patients to push a button at bedtime/wake time. However, one study found that 27% of actigraphy data were not valid because of participants' nonadherence to using the event marker (18). A more recent study found strong agreement between actigraphy and diaries for sleep-onset and sleep-offset times, but poor agreement for sleep-onset latency, nocturnal awakenings, and wake after sleep onset (19). A combination of event markers and daily sleep diaries is recommended.

Special Populations

An important consideration for the validity of actigraphy is the population being studied. With the AASM guidelines for the use of actigraphy with special populations (6), studies have examined the validity of actigraphy on different clinical populations, including infants, toddlers, or preschoolers (11, 20, 21); children and adolescents with or without sleep-disordered breathing (9, 10, 13, 20, 21, 22); and older adults (23). Although there have been mixed findings in the literature about the use of actigraphy in patients with insomnia, several papers suggest the benefit of actigraphy in this population (1, 24–26).

Other devices are being developed with applications beyond sleep–wake estimates, including the detection of periodic limb movements (PLMs) in sleep. Studies have found that actigraphic devices specially designed for PLMs were useful in detecting PLMs in adults (16, 17, 27–29). However, traditional actigraphy was shown to be a poor measure of PLMs in children (30). Despite the developments to improve and expand the use of actigraphy in specific populations, further testing is needed to ensure the validity on a wider demographic of users.

Length of Actigraphy Study

The duration of an actigraphy study should be carefully considered. For most people, sleep patterns differ from weekday to weekends; thus, a minimum of 7 to 10 days of actigraphy would be needed to capture these differences. Another consideration is the amount of data lost to artifact. As previously mentioned, some days/nights from an actigraphy study may not be valid if the participant does not wear the device or does not complete the sleep diary, the device has a technical failure, or the night is atypical. One study reported that because of the loss of data from artifact, a minimum of seven nights of data collection is needed to gain information for five nights of sleep (31). The final consideration is billing, with a minimum of three nights required (see next section) in order to bill for an actigraphy study.

CLINICAL APPLICATION

In 2009, actigraphy became a category 1 current procedural terminology code. The description for this service is "testing, recording, analysis, interpretation, and report (minimum of 72 hours to 14 consecutive days of recording requires the patient to wear a home monitor for 24 hours a day for 3 to 14 days)." Although Medicare may provide reimbursement for this service, most other insurances do not, stating that actigraphy is investigational, experimental, or not medically necessary (3).

Despite the lack of insurance coverage, the information about sleep/wake patterns gathered from actigraphy can be an essential tool in clinical settings. As previously stated, wrist actigraphy is minimally invasive and does not interfere with normal routines, and is recommended for use in the diagnosis of different sleep disorders (7). Beyond diagnostic utility, the following provides a description of the most common clinical uses of actigraphy in the sleep center: (1) to identify potential causes of daytime sleepiness (e.g., frequent night wakings and prolonged sleep-onset latency) and (2) to monitor the patient's adherence to treatment recommendations (e.g., maintaining a consistent sleep schedule).

Excessive daytime sleepiness (EDS) is a common complaint in sleep clinics. Once physiologic sleep disorders (e.g., obstructive sleep apnea and PLMs in sleep) are ruled out by a clinical interview or overnight PSG, other potential causes for EDS need to be evaluated, including circadian rhythm sleep disorders, poor sleep hygiene, or insufficient sleep. By monitoring sleep–wake patterns for 1 to 2 weeks, the clinician can examine whether a patient has a consistent sleep schedule and is getting enough sleep. For example, Figure 45-1 includes three actigrams of patients complaining of EDS. Figure 45-1A is a 17-year-old boy who reported EDS but denied symptoms of sleep-disordered breathing or movement during sleep. His actigraphy study revealed that he was obtaining 6 or less hours of sleep on school nights, with significant oversleep on the weekends. This was suggestive of insufficient sleep and poor sleep hygiene rather than an underlying physiologic sleep disorder. Figure 45-1B is a 14-year-old boy reporting EDS and the inability to fall asleep before 3 a.m., regardless of bedtime. His actigraphy study revealed circadian rhythm sleep disorder, delayed sleep-phase type, with a sleep schedule of approximately 3 a.m. to 1 p.m. Figure 45-1C is a 22-year-old female who reported EDS because of an erratic sleep schedule. Her actigraphy study revealed circadian rhythm sleep disorder, free-running type. Actigraphy can also help determine the need for an overnight PSG when sleep center availability is limited or the patient may not tolerate a PSG. For example, as seen in Figure 45-2A, a 7-year-old boy with autism complained of EDS but denied symptoms of sleep-disordered breathing. His mother reported that

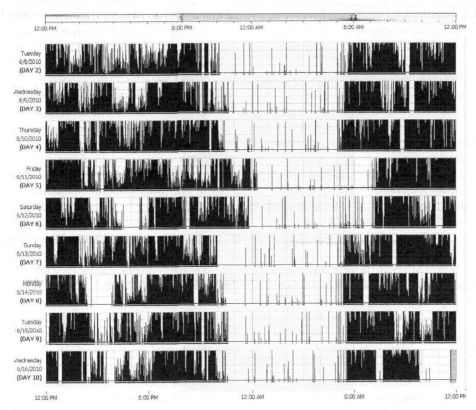

Figure 45-4 Actigram of a 57-year-old female with circadian rhythm sleep disorder, delayed sleep-phase type after chronotherapy treatment. The patient was able to maintain a consistent sleep schedule from 10/11 p.m. to 6/7 a.m.

he was "twitchy" during sleep, but this child would not tolerate a PSG. The high level of activity during sleep resulted in the recommendation for a serum ferritin level to be drawn, which was found to be low (20 ng per mL).

Actigraphy can also help monitor treatments and clinical recommendations. For example, actigraphy can help determine whether a treatment (e.g., iron therapy) is effective. As seen in Figure 45-2B, following 3 months of supplemental iron therapy, along with a clinical report of improvements in daytime functioning, there was a significant reduction in activity during sleep for the same 7-year-old boy with autism. For a patient with circadian rhythm sleep disorder, delayed sleep-phase type, actigraphy can help monitor whether the patient is adherent to adjusting his or her sleep–wake schedule as recommended (e.g., moving schedule forward by 3 hours each day). For example, Figure 45-4 is a 57-year-old female following chronotherapy to regulate her sleep–wake schedule. Her actigraphy study showed a consistent sleep schedule, with a bedtime of 10 p.m. on weekdays and 11 p.m. on weekends, and a wake time of 6 a.m. on weekdays and 7 a.m. on weekends. Figures 45-2B and 45-4 are excellent examples of "normal" actigraphy studies. In addition, if the actigraph has a light sensor, the clinician is able to monitor whether the patient is obtaining a sufficient amount of light in the morning and restricting light late in the day.

CONCLUSION

Actigraphy is a noninvasive way to estimate sleep–wake patterns through the measurement of activity levels. Although actigraphy has been reported as a valid estimate of sleep–wake patterns, additional work is needed to increase the ability of actigraphy to detect wake after sleep onset (3, 9). In a clinical setting, actigraphy can assist with the diagnosis of sleep disorders (7), as well as provide considerable information about potential reasons for daytime sleepiness and whether a patient is adherent to treatment recommendations. Actigraphy is not a substitute for PSG, but when used properly (e.g., with a daily sleep diary and event marker), it is a useful tool for evaluating the sleep–wake patterns of patients.

REFERENCES

1. Sadeh, A. (2011). The role and validity of actigraphy in sleep medicine: An update. *Sleep Medicine Review, 15*(4), 259–267.
2. Meltzer, L. J., Montgomery-Downs, H. E., Insana, S. P., et al. (2012). Use of actigraphy for assessment in pediatric sleep research. *Sleep Medicine Review, 16*, 463–475.

3. Ancoli-Israel, S., Martin, J. L., Blackwell, T., et al. (2015). The SBSM guide to actigraphy monitoring: Clinical and research applications. *Behavioral Sleep Medicine, 13*(Suppl. 1):S4–S38.

4. Tryon, W. W. (1991). *Activity measurement in psychology and medicine*. New York, NY: Plenum.

5. Ancoli-Israel, S. (2005). Actigraphy. In M. H. Kryger, T. Roth, & W. C. Dement (Eds.), *Principles and practice of sleep medicine* (4th ed., pp. 1459–1467). Philadelphia, PA: Elsevier Saunders.

6. Smith, M. T., McCrae, C. S., Cheung, J., et al. (2018). Use of actigraphy for the evaluation of sleep disorders and circadian rhythm sleep-wake disorders: An American academy of sleep medicine clinical practice guideline. *Journal of Clinical Sleep Medicine. 14*(7), 1231–1237. doi: 10.5664/jcsm.7230.

7. American Academy of Sleep Medicine. (2014). *International classification of sleep disorders: Diagnostic and coding manual* (3rd ed.). Westchester, IL: Author.

8. Toussaint, M., Luthringer, R., Schaltenbrand, N., et al. (1995). First-night effect in normal subjects and psychiatric inpatients. *Sleep, 18*(6), 463–469.

9. Meltzer, L. J., Walsh, C. M., Traylor, J., et al. (2012). Direct comparison of two new actigraphs and polysomnography in children and adolescents. *Sleep, 35*(1), 159–166.

10. Quante, M., Kaplan, E. R., Cailler, M., et al. (2018). Actigraphy-based sleep estimation in adolescents and adults: A comparison with polysomnography using two scoring algorithms. *Nature and Science of Sleep, 10*, 13–20.

11. Belanger, M. E., Bernier, A., Paquet, J., et al. (2013). Validating actigraphy as a measure of sleep for preschool children. *Journal of Clinical Sleep Medicine, 9*(7), 701–706.

12. Marino, M., Li, Y., Rueschman, M. N., et al. (2013). Measuring sleep: Accuracy, sensitivity, and specificity of wrist actigraphy compared to polysomnography. *Sleep, 36*(11), 1747–1755.

13. Meltzer, L. J., Wong, P., Biggs, S. N., et al. (2016). Validation of actigraphy in middle childhood. *Sleep, 39*(6), 1219–1224.

14. Benson, K., Friedman, L., Noda, A., et al. (2004). The measurement of sleep by actigraphy: Direct comparison of 2 commercially available actigraphs in a nonclinical population. *Sleep, 27*(5), 986–989.

15. Pollak, C. P., Stokes, P. E., & Wagner, D. R. (1998). Direct comparison of two widely used activity recorders. *Sleep, 21*(2), 207–212.

16. Tonetti, L., Pasquini, F., Fabbri, M., et al. (2008). Comparison of two different actigraphs with polysomnography in healthy young subjects. *Chronobiology International, 25*(1), 145–153.

17. Weiss, A. R., Johnson, N. L., Berger, N. A., et al. (2010). Validity of activity-based devices to estimate sleep. *Journal of Clinical Sleep Medicine, 6*(4), 336–342.

18. Ustinov, Y., & Lichstein, K. L. (2011). Actigraphy reliability. *Sleep, 34*, A330.

19. Thurman, S. M., Wasylyshyn, N., Roy, H., et al. (2018). Individual differences in compliance and agreement for sleep logs and wrist actigraphy: A longitudinal study of naturalistic sleep in healthy adults. *PLoS One, 13*(1), e0191883.

20. Insana, S. P., Gozal, D., & Montgomery-Downs, H. E. (2010). Invalidity of one actigraphy brand for identifying sleep and wake among infants. *Sleep Medicine, 11*(2), 191–196.

21. Sitnick, S. L., Goodlin-Jones, B. L., & Anders, T. F. (2008). The use of actigraphy to study sleep disorders in preschoolers: Some concerns about detection of nighttime awakenings. *Sleep, 31*(3), 395–401.

22. Hyde, M., O'Driscoll, D. M., Binette, S., et al. (2007). Validation of actigraphy for determining sleep and wake in children with sleep disordered breathing. *Journal of Sleep Research, 16*(2), 213–216.

23. Mehra, R., Stone, K. L., Ancoli-Israel, S., et al. (2008). Interpreting wrist actigraphic indices of sleep in epidemiologic studies of the elderly: The Study of Osteoporotic Fractures. *Sleep, 31*(11), 1569–1576.

24. Martin, J. L., & Hakim, A. D. (2011). Wrist actigraphy. *Chest, 139*(6), 1514–1527.

25. Natale, V., Leger, D., Martoni, M., et al. (2014). The role of actigraphy in the assessment of primary insomnia: A retrospective study. *Sleep Medicine, 15*(1), 111–115.

26. Sanchez-Ortuno, M. M., Edinger, J. D., Means, M. K., et al. (2010). Home is where sleep is: An ecological approach to test the validity of actigraphy for the assessment of insomnia. *Journal of Clinical Sleep Medicine, 6*(1), 21–29.

27. Sforza, E., Johannes, M., & Claudio, B. (2005). The PAM-RL ambulatory device for detection of periodic leg movements: A validation study. *Sleep Medicine, 6*(5), 407–413.

28. King, M. A., Jaffre, M. O., Morrish, E., et al. (2005). The validation of a new actigraphy system for the measurement of periodic leg movements in sleep. *Sleep Medicine, 6*(6), 507–513.

29. Kobayashi, M., Namba, K., Ito, E., et al. (2014). The validity of the PAM-RL device for evaluating periodic limb movements in sleep and an investigation on night-to-night variability of periodic limb movements during sleep in patients with restless legs syndrome or periodic limb movement disorder using this system. *Sleep Medicine, 15*(1), 138–143.

30. Montgomery-Downs, H. E., Crabtree, V. M., & Gozal, D. (2005). Actigraphic recordings in quantification of periodic leg movements during sleep in children. *Sleep Medicine, 6*(4), 325–332.

31. Acebo, C., Sadeh, A., Seifer, R., et al. (1999). Estimating sleep patterns with activity monitoring in children and adolescents: How many nights are necessary for reliable measures? *Sleep, 22*(1), 95–103.

chapter 46

Positive Airway Pressure Therapy: Basic Principles

MATTHEW W. ANASTASI

Alveoli
Compliance
Modes

LEARNING OBJECTIVES

On completion of this chapter, the reader should be able to:

1. Describe the anatomy and function of the upper airway.
2. Define the principles of positive airway pressure (PAP) therapy.
3. Explain how PAP therapy restores patency in the upper airway.
4. List the various PAP treatment modalities.

KEY TERMS

Pharynx
Epiglottis
Nasal cavity
Hard palate
Soft palate
Continuous positive airway pressure (CPAP)
Automatic positive airway pressure (APAP)
Automatic bilevel positive airway pressure (ABPAP)
Bilevel positive airway pressure (BPAP)
Adaptive servo-ventilation (ASV)
Volume-assured pressure support (VAPS)
Obstructive sleep apnea (OSA)
Sleep-related breathing disorders (SRBDs)
Sleep-disordered breathing (SDB)
Snoring
Hypopnea
Apnea
Titration
Brainstem
Crescendo–decrescendo breathing
Cheyne–Stokes respiration
Interface
Headgear

OVERVIEW

Positive airway pressure (PAP) therapy is the gold standard and most widely used treatment for obstructive sleep apnea (OSA). PAP therapy is recommended by the American Academy of Sleep Medicine (AASM) in the treatment of moderate-to-severe OSA in adults and as an option for the treatment of mild OSA (1). PAP is a generic term applied to all therapies that use air pressure delivered through the upper airway of patients with sleep-related breathing disorders (SRBDs) with the purpose of creating a "pneumatic splint" to support the anatomic structures of the upper airway by opening and thus allowing an uninterrupted flow of air to the lungs during sleep.

In this chapter, we will establish a framework for how the anatomy of the upper airway contributes to SRBDs and introduce the different types of PAP therapy that have been developed to restore normal breathing. We will also provide an understanding of how these devices interact with the upper airway to produce salutary health benefits on sleep apnea and diseases comorbid with the disorder.

BASIC PRINCIPLES OF PAP THERAPY

The term Apnea is derived from the ancient Greek etymology meaning "absence of breathing," and results in *cessation* of breathing due to closure of the upper airway. Hypopnea, from the Greek for "under breathing", refers to a reduction in breathing due to a narrowing of the upper airway. Both apneas and hypopneas are breathing events that result from obstruction of the airway and can be treated safely using PAP therapy. Snoring is also an obstructive breathing event that can have clinical implications. It is associated with OSA but can occur independently as a result of airway vibrations that typically range from 60 to 80 dB in intensity. As a point of reference, a vacuum cleaner typically emits a decibel level of 70 and a chainsaw, 100. Hearing damage can result from prolonged exposures greater than 80 dB. A grandmother of four in the United Kingdom was recently recorded with a snoring level of 111.6 dB!

Respiratory effort–related arousals (RERAs) are another important clinical manifestation of obstructive sleep-disordered breathing (SDB) that are treated with PAP therapy. These events, like snoring events, don't rise to the level to meet the clinical definition of an apnea or hypopnea, but are characterized by a reduction in airflow that leads to a pattern of arousals from sleep, which mean they are significant for sleep disturbances. Central apneas and central hypopneas are events that can be differentiated from obstructive apneas and obstructive hypopneas in their cause: Central events originate not because of a narrowing or obstruction in the upper airway, but instead result from a neurologic signal from the central nervous system to stop breathing or reduce breathing that can occur in coordination with conditions like heart failure and stroke, and involves an area of the brain called the "brainstem" that triggers breathing. Sleeping at altitude can also cause central events in a breathing pattern called "periodic breathing." The use of opioid-based medications can also trigger central events and a "crescendo–decrescendo" pattern of central events called Cheyne–Stokes respiration.

Although the first modern use of the word "apnea" can be traced to 1719, and the symptoms of the disease first appeared in a fictional description of a Charles Dickens character in the Pickwick Papers in 1836 (2), it was not until 1965 that sleep apnea was first documented in the medical literature and it was another 16 years (1980) until the first noninvasive ventilation device, a positive-pressure breathing circuit connected to the nose using plastic tubing and silicone sealant, was used on a patient by Dr. Colin Sullivan. By the end of the 1980s, continuous positive airway pressure (CPAP) had been developed into a more sophisticated treatment for sleep apnea, and by the 1990s, bilevel positive airway pressure (BPAP) had been in use (3), followed by auto-titrating devices that are continuing to evolve and use more sophisticated treatment algorithms to respond to breath-by-breath changes in patient respiration (Fig. 46-1).

A classification system for sleep apnea is used in the diagnosis and is useful in guiding treatment through the clinical pathway: Mild sleep apnea is defined as the

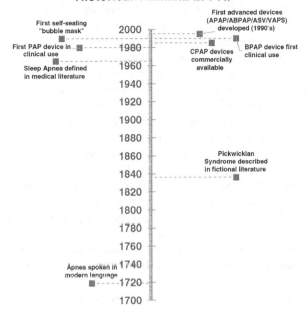

Figure 46-1 Historical timeline of positive airway pressure therapy. ABPAP, automatic bilevel positive airway pressure; APAP, automatic positive airway pressure; ASV, adaptive servo-ventilation; BPAP, bilevel positive airway pressure; CPAP, continuous positive airway pressure; VAPS, volume-assured pressure support.

occurrence of 5 to 14 respiratory events per hour, on average, throughout the sleep period; moderate sleep apnea is defined as 15 to 30 events per hour; severe sleep apnea is defined as greater than 30 events per hour (Fig. 46-2).

It is not unusual for a sleep technologist to observe hundreds of respiratory events during a single night of sleep. Typically, the total number of obstructive and central apneas and hypopneas is combined to yield an apnea–hypopnea "index" (AHI), which is the average number of events per hour during a sleep period based on a polysomnography (PSG) recording. For patients with a high pretest probability of sleep apnea as a result of associated subjective and objective sleep-related symptoms, but who do not reach the clinically defined minimum for diagnosis by AHI, RERAs are often scored and added to the index to yield a respiratory disturbance index (RDI). RDI can be utilized to make a diagnosis of sleep apnea and qualify some patients for related

Mild: ≥ 5 ≤ 15 per hour
Moderate: >15 ≤ 30 per hour
Severe: > 30 episodes per hour

Figure 46-2 Classification system for sleep apnea severity. AHI, apnea–hypopnea index.

follow-up care. For insurance reimbursement purposes, an AHI or RDI greater than or equal to 15 events per hour is required. However, criteria for reimbursement coverage also extend to an AHI or RDI between 5 and 14 events per hour if a patient demonstrates documented objective or subjective sleepiness symptoms or suffers from comorbid conditions such as hypertension, stroke, or heart disease. PAP therapy has been shown to have good clinical outcomes in patients with moderate-to-severe sleep apnea or in patients with mild sleep apnea with associated comorbidities or disorders.

During therapeutic PSG, a sleep technologist fits a mask to the nose and/or mouth of a patient with known sleep apnea and uses it in concert with a medical PAP device that delivers room air at a pressure set by the technologist or determined through an internal device algorithm using the appropriate mode and settings to normalize a patient's breathing. Picture a box with a fan inside: On one end of this box is an opening covered by a filter that draws in room air from the outside. Inside this box is also a chamber filled with heated water through which the air travels before being sent through plastic tubing to a mask interface and ultimately to the lungs where oxygen enters the blood through sacs called "alveoli."

Depending on the physiologic, logistic, and psychological needs of the patient, there are a variety of PAP therapy modes to choose from. Most populations with SRBDs experience a reduced or blocked flow of air because of an obstruction by muscles and tissues of the upper airway behind the mouth and throat. For these patients, a fixed flow of positive air, called CPAP, is typically applied. Alternatively, a PAP device with independently fixed inspiratory and expiratory positive airway pressures (IPAP and EPAP, respectively), known as BPAP, can also be effective. BPAP uses two pressures, and IPAP is applied during inhalation and is higher than the EPAP, which is applied during exhalation. In a version called auto-CPAP or auto bilevel, an internal algorithm within the machine can be used to "auto-titrate" effective pressures.

More advanced titration approaches are needed to treat more complex forms of sleep apnea that involve a reduced airflow as a result of underlying neurologic conditions, lung disease, chronic obstructive pulmonary disease (COPD), or medication effect. Adaptive servo-ventilation (ASV) and volume-assured pressure support (VAPS) are two primary examples. The ASV device algorithm automatically adjusts IPAP, EPAP, and pressure support (PS), which is the difference in pressure between IPAP and EPAP (i.e., IPAP minus EPAP equals PS) settings in response to patient breathing within a set range which is established by a technologist on the basis of a physician's order. The aim of VAPS is to maintain an optimal level of the patient's tidal volume (VT), which is the volume of air displaced through normal inhalation and exhalation. This value is approximately 400 to 500

mL for a normal adult but must be calculated on the basis of the patient's actual height that is used to approximate ideal body weight. The appropriate VAPS setting for VT is equal to 7 mL per kg of ideal body weight. With VAPS, the inspiratory phase switches to exhalation settings only after a preset VT is delivered to the patient (4).

SDB has a significant impact on society. The AASM recently contracted a global research and consulting firm to uncover the economic costs of untreated sleep apnea for payers, employers, and patients (5). Their report estimates that undiagnosed OSA cost the United States approximately $149.6 billion in 2015 alone. Between 2% and 4% of the adult US population is affected by sleep apnea, but of the estimated 22 million with the disorder, 80% are undiagnosed and of those that are diagnosed and treated, compliance on PAP therapy is approximately 50%. This means that less than 10% of those suffering from sleep apnea are being effectively treated! This has significant implications for society because of the known, wide-reaching effects that sleep deprivation, or the lack of quality sleep, has on public health, workplace productivity, and safety. A case can be made that sleep apnea is a hidden health crisis of our time.

ANATOMY AND FUNCTION OF THE UPPER AIRWAY

The upper airway is quite complex (see Fig. 46-3). For the sleep technologist, the most important areas are the nasopharynx, the oropharynx, and the laryngeal pharynx. In terms of preventing snoring, hypopnea, and

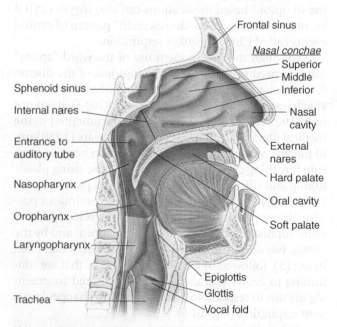

Figure 46-3 Upper respiratory system. (Modified with permission from Moore, K. L., Dalley, A. F., & Agur AMR. (2013). *Clinically oriented anatomy* (7th ed., Figure 7.83). Baltimore, MD: Lippincott Wilkins & Wilkins-Wolters Kluwer.)

OSA, the goal of PAP therapy is to prevent collapse at any point in these three areas of the upper airway.

A useful model of the upper airway is the Starling resistor, invented by Ernest Starling while working on blood vessels in the heart. This model has been applied to analysis of airway collapse in OSA. It represents the complicated upper airway with just three sections—(1) "upstream" or the area of the nose and nasal cavity, (2) the collapsible portions of the upper airway itself, and (3) "downstream" or the trachea and lungs. At its most basic, a formula can be used that allows prediction of airway collapse dependent on the pressure inside the upper airway and the pressure outside of the upper airway. This is the critical closing pressure. The likelihood of reaching this critical pressure and airway collapse is higher when the pressure outside of the upper airway is increased. This occurs when there is submucosal fat or edema present. Collapse is also more likely when the diameter of the airway is reduced, which can also be caused by the accumulation of submucosal fat. Finally, collapse of the upper airway is more likely when flow through the airway is reduced. This can occur upstream when there is nasal congestion or blockage. Reduced flow may also occur downstream when lung function is impaired. When the pressure inside the airway is less than the pressure outside the airway, the critical closing pressure is achieved and the airway collapses.

Unfortunately, the relationship between pressures inside and outside of the upper airway and the effect on airway collapse is not linear. Before closing, the upper airway may oscillate, leading to snoring and flow restriction. The more important nonlinearity is that once the upper airway is closed, increased pressure below the point of closure will not cause the airway to open. This means that once the airway has collapsed, it will stay closed until something in the relationship between pressures is changed. For patients with OSA, this usually means that the airway diameter must be increased, and this occurs when the patient wakes up and muscle tone in the upper airway is increased.

The Starling resistor predicts that several methods will reduce the likelihood of upper airway collapse. One method is to change the anatomy of the upper airway. Surgical options for increasing flow include removal of soft tissue such as tonsils and adenoids that may cause upstream blockage. The diameter of the upper airway may be increased by mandibular advancement, either surgically or with an oral appliance. More recently, methods for increasing muscle tone in the upper airway using surgically implanted stimulators have been shown to be effective in reducing the number of episodes of airway collapse.

The most common method for reducing the likelihood of airway collapse is to increase airway pressure. When the upstream pressure is increased and the external pressure remains the same, the ratio is changed, and

collapse is prevented. PAP therapy provides extra upstream pressure and acts as a pneumatic "splint" to keep the airway open.

Although it is possible to calculate the additional pressure needed to prevent the airway from reaching the critical closing pressure, human airways are not Starling resistors. Pressure requirements change on the basis of elasticity of the upper airway, airway diameter, and flow rate. Tongue position and size are important elements in the equation. These factors change with age, obesity, and tissue swelling. During the night, the pressure requirement may change because of changes in body position. And because pressure is a key part of the discussion and pressure decreases with elevation above sea level, moving from Detroit to Denver will change pressure requirements as well. This makes titration of PAP an important part of the therapeutic process. The airway is complex, but the model of the Starling resistor explains how providing positive pressure at the nose and/or mouth can reduce or eliminate OSA.

MECHANISMS OF PAP THERAPY DELIVERY

Given the complexity of the upper airway, the mechanism by which PAP therapy restores patency is remarkably straightforward. In its simplest form, PAP establishes a positive pressure outside of the airway to the negative pressure inside. This disequilibrium encourages the upper airway (if narrowed or blocked) to expand, thus allowing positive and negative sides to equalize. It's basically a physiologic example of homeostasis, one breath at a time.

PAP therapy introduces positive pressure to the airway by first delivering pressurized air to the nose and/or mouth through what is called an "interface," a mask that covers the nose and/or mouth that is held in place by straps that form the "headgear" (Fig. 46-4). This air is first humidified and typically heated, and the amount of pressure needed to maintain an open airway, measured in centimeters of water (cm H_2O), is established by the technologist (during a manual titration) or machine (using an auto-titrating device) before it is sent to the patient. The measurement cm H_2O refers to the number of centimeters in height that the pressure of the air will push a column of water to, using a detection device called a "manometer." Relatively speaking, each "one" cm H_2O equals much less than "one" atmosphere or pound per square inch (PSI): 1 cm H_2O = 0.0142233 PSI, to be exact! For example, the amount of pressure from a PAP machine at 25 cm H_2O would provide a similar pressure on the lungs during exhalation as standing in the deep end of a pool with the water line up to the chin. If we assume that 25 cm is roughly 10 in or the height above the center of the lungs that air must travel through during exhalation, then 25 cm H_2O is

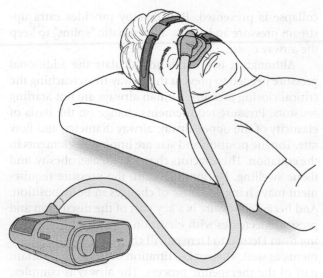

Figure 46-4 Positive airway pressure therapy introduces positive pressure to the airway by first delivering pressurized air to the nose and/or mouth through an *interface*, a mask that covers the nose and/or mouth held in place by straps, referred to as *headgear*. This air is first humidified and typically heated before it is sent to the patient.

comparable to the pressure one must exert to expand the chest against the water in a pool to exhale.

The internal effect of this pressure on the airway follows a similar mechanical progression as illustrated in Figure 46-5. As air enters through the nose, it travels through the nasal cavity and past the structures of the hard palate and soft palate to the areas that are most crowded in the upper airway, such as the epiglottis, and to the trachea, and eventually fills the alveoli of the lungs.

SALUTARY EFFECTS OF PAP THERAPY

The goals of this section are to summarize the negative impact of untreated OSA and describe the beneficial effects of PAP therapy. Achieving the first goal is, as they say in the basketball business, a "slam dunk." In a recent clinical practice guideline (6), the AASM notes the factors that are documented during sleep studies in patients with OSA including fragmented sleep, pressure swings in the thorax, increased sympathetic nervous system activity, and changes in blood gases.

The AASM cites "wide-ranging" consequences of untreated OSA. These include feelings of fatigue and sleepiness during the day, impairment of the ability to stay awake, poor concentration, and diminished quality of life. These "can translate into higher rates of job-related and motor vehicle accidents" (6, p. 480).

Untreated OSA is associated with an increased risk of cardiovascular disease including heart failure, arrhythmias, and stroke. There are also associations with metabolic dysregulation and risk of diabetes. Studies have documented increased health care utilization in patients who have untreated OSA. A limited number of long-term follow-up studies have found increased mortality in patients with OSA who are not treated.

These associations are based on correlation, and as students of statistics frequently hear, correlation does not imply causality. This is an important factor in evaluating the effects of PAP therapy on medical disorders. Patients who choose to use PAP and are adherent to treatment are most likely to adhere to other treatment advice from their physician, such as weight loss, exercise, and avoiding high-cholesterol foods. If these patients have lower

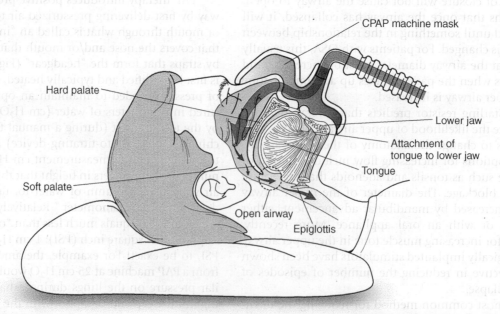

Figure 46-5 Continuous positive airway pressure (CPAP) therapy. Air enters through the nose, travels through the nasal cavity, past the hard palate and soft palate to the areas most crowded in the upper airway, the epiglottis, oropharynx, laryngopharynx, to the trachea, and eventually fills the alveoli of the lungs.

levels of cardiovascular disease, can we say that it is due to the use of PAP therapy and not to the other lifestyle changes that patients have made?

In order to establish a cause and effect relationship and provide strong evidence that untreated OSA causes these consequences, an experiment must be performed. Patients with OSA must be randomly assigned to treatment or no treatment groups. Successful treatment of OSA must result in reduction or elimination of the wide-ranging consequences.

Unfortunately, randomized controlled trials are few and far between. Short-term studies have documented changes in frequency of apnea and blood pressure, but these are not the important consequences that concern patients and physicians. Evidence that PAP therapy reduces cardiovascular events and mortality would be more important, but such studies require long-term follow-up and placing patients in the control, or untreated, group for the duration of the study. In one trial, CPAP provided no benefit for OSA patients in the prevention of cardiovascular events with a mean follow-up of 3.7 years (7). Other trials are ongoing.

In one carefully controlled study (8), a group of patients with central sleep apnea (CSA) who were treated with a form of PAP therapy (ASV) actually had more cardiovascular events than the control group, forcing the investigators to discontinue the study before the intended date.

With regard to sleepiness and quality of life, the results have been more consistent. For example, the "BestAIR" study (9) found that CPAP improved several quality-of-life measures in patients with moderate-to-severe OSA when compared with "sham CPAP."

In an exhaustive review (10), the US Preventive Services Task Force concluded, "There is uncertainty about the accuracy or clinical utility of all potential screening tools. Multiple treatments for OSA reduce AHI, ESS scores, and blood pressure. Trials of CPAP and other treatments have not established whether treatment reduces mortality or improves most other health outcomes, except for modest improvement in sleep-related quality of life" (10, p. 415).

Nevertheless, the position of the AASM has been and continues to be that, "Positive airway pressure (PAP) is the treatment of choice for mild, moderate, and severe OSA and should be offered as an option to all patients" (11, p. 268).

PAP TREATMENT MODALITIES AND SUMMARY

The goals of PAP titration are airway management, breathing stabilization, and patient adherence to therapy. There are many PAP machine settings, generally called "modes," by which PAP therapy can individualize the treatment approach to a patient's breathing abnormality and address each of these treatment goals.

The AASM recommends a starting pressure of 4 cm H_2O to treat sleep apnea with CPAP (12). This starting pressure is then increased in a stepwise procedure in response to a continuation of SDB, until all events and symptoms are abolished. CPAP therapy is typically sufficient to normalize breathing and abolish respiratory events, but there are three main cases when it is advantageous to switch a patient to BPAP after a failed attempt to treat a patient using only CPAP (Fig. 46-6).

After selecting an optimal interface, if a patient is simply not able to tolerate CPAP, especially in cases where exhaling against the pressure is uncomfortable, BPAP mode may be initiated and titrated beginning at 8/4 cm H_2O (IPAP set at 8 cm H_2O; EPAP set at 4 cm H_2O). A second case where a switch to BPAP is recommended occurs when high CPAP is necessary to control events: if higher pressures are not effective in eliminating events, the AASM practice parameters recommend switching to BPAP of 16/8 when a titration reaches 16 cm H_2O. The third scenario for switching to BPAP is in treatment-emergent CSA, which is a phenomenon whereby the CPAP treatment itself is thought to have a causal effect on the transition from obstructive to central apneas or hypopneas. This phenomenon occurs in approximately 10% of sleep apneics treated with CPAP (13).

BPAP is differentiated from CPAP, which provides a constant pressure whether a patient is in the inhalation or exhalation phase of respiration, or airflow. The advantage of BPAP is that it can provide a reduction in pressure, or PS, during exhalation. PS is typically 4 cm H_2O less than IPAP, and at most a 10 cm H_2O difference is recommended between the two pressures for OSA patients, although PS up to 20 cm H_2O is sometimes used for chronic stable hypoventilation patients. PS can address our goals for BPAP therapy by alleviating the pressure that a patient breathes against while keeping inhalation pressure high to address airway obstruction. This makes BPAP a first-line mechanical intervention to address patient compliance. It also allows for improved airway management at high pressures and with treatment-emergent CSA.

BPAP can be set for spontaneous, timed, or spontaneous/timed (ST) modes depending on patient need. In the most common mode, spontaneous, the patient's change from exhalation to inhalation triggers a change in pressure from the device. Less commonly, a timed mode can be set to establish the timing of IPAP/EPAP delivery, which is independent of a patient's own breathing effort. This can lead to patient discomfort. ST mode uses the patient's spontaneous breathing effort to trigger pressure changes but will step in to trigger a breath at a previously set rate if a patient does not self-trigger (14).

CPAP or APAP

Inhalation (breathing in)
CPAP blows constant pressure while you breathe in.

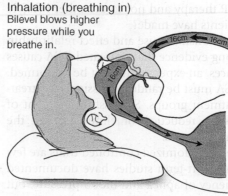

Bilevel PAP (BiPAP)

Inhalation (breathing in)
Bilevel blows higher pressure while you breathe in.

Exhalation (breathing out)
CPAP blows the same pressure while you breathe out.

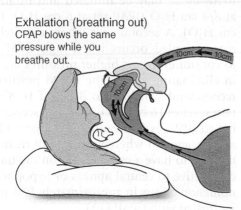

Exhalation (breathing out)
CPAP blows lower pressure while you breathe in, so it's easier to exhale.

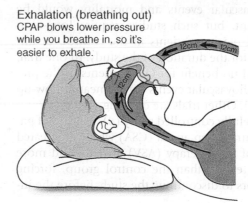

Figure 46-6 Continuous positive airway pressure (CPAP) delivers a continuous prescribed pressure, whereas bilevel positive airway pressure (BPAP) delivers two set of prescribed pressures, one inspiratory positive airway pressure and the other a lower expiratory positive airway pressure. APAP, automatic positive airway pressure.

ST mode is most often used for primary central apnea or central apneas caused by respiratory depression. ST mode may also be used for neuromuscular disease patients, whose respiratory efforts reduce during rapid eye movement (REM) sleep, which may make them unable to trigger inspiration. Timed mode is most often used for patients with severe neuromuscular weakness or spinal cord injury and who are unable to trigger inspiration.

Auto-adjusting CPAP (AutoCPAP) machines measure flow and vibration-based snoring many times per second to tailor treatment pressure to the changing needs of a patient during a therapeutic PSG or home PAP trial. AutoCPAP can be used to determine the optimal fixed treatment pressure for a patient. Typically, AutoCPAP is set to a range of pressures and the machine titrates between these pressures depending on the level of pressure needed at various points throughout the night. This pressure range is usually informed by the results of a previous PAP titration. The advantages of AutoCPAP include the ability to adjust to sleep apnea severity that is greater during Stage R sleep or in certain positions, typically supine. In patients with REM-related or positional

events, higher levels of pressure are needed, and a patient can more comfortably use PAP at a lower effective pressure at other times.

AutoBPAP adds an adjusting PS feature between the IPAP and EPAP settings, which can also be set to a maximum range (usually 10 cm H_2O). With AutoBPAP, an internal algorithm calculates the PS needed in addition to IPAP and EPAP levels (15).

Because higher PAP and high PS can induce treatment-emergent CSA, periodic breathing, and Cheyne–Stokes respiration, devices have been developed to try to even out breathing over several breaths. ASV is an example of this type of device (16). ASV uses an algorithm that senses the patient's breathing patterns and provides subtle changes in pressure to restore normal breathing. The hope is that by stabilizing breathing, the periodic breathing pattern will subside.

VAPS machines adjust PS in order to maintain a target average ventilation. This mode of PAP is often helpful for patients with respiratory insufficiency caused by neuromuscular and restrictive conditions in which respiratory effort varies during sleep or who need PAP during the day. It may also be useful in COPD patients with risk of hypoventilation and for obesity hypoventilation patients who may need compensation on the basis of positional and sleep stage changes.

The upper airway is a critical space in the management of effective breathing and important for the healthy function of an individual. Although the identification of conditions that affect proper breathing is relatively recent in the field of medicine, a variety of effective treatment options are available that can be used in the approach to treatment in an effort to provide precision therapy for OSA.

REFERENCES

1. Epstein, L. J., Kristo, D., Strollo, P. J., et al. (2009). Clinical guideline for the evaluation, management and long-term care of obstructive sleep apnea in adults. *Journal of Clinical Sleep Medicine, 5*(3), 263–276.

2. Dickens, C. (1836). *The posthumous papers of the Pickwick Club*. London: Chapman and Hall. Published in serial form.

3. Sanders, M. H, & Kern, N. (1990). Obstructive sleep apnea treated by independently adjusted inspiratory and expiratory positive airway pressures via nasal mask. *Chest, 98*(2), 317–324.

4. Amato, M. B., Barbas, C. S., Bonassa, J., et al. (1992). Volume-assured pressure support ventilation. *Chest, 102*(4), 1225–1234.

5. Watson, N. F. (2016). Health care savings: the economic value of diagnostic and therapeutic care for obstructive sleep apnea. *Journal of Clinical Sleep Medicine, 12*(8), 1075–1077.

6. Kapur, V. K., Auckley, D. H., Chowdhuri, S., et al. (2017). Clinical practice guideline for diagnostic testing for adult obstructive sleep apnea: An American Academy of Sleep Medicine clinical practice guideline. *Journal of Clinical Sleep Medicine, 13*(3), 479–504.

7. McEvoy, R. D., Antic, N. A., Heeley, E., et al. (2016). CPAP for prevention of cardiovascular events in obstructive sleep apnea. *New England Journal of Medicine, 375*(10), 919–931.

8. Cowie, M. R., Woehrle, H., Wegscheider, K., et al. (2015). Adaptive servo-ventilation for central sleep apnea in systolic heart failure. *New England Journal of Medicine, 373*(12), 1095–1105.

9. Zhao, Y. Y., Wang, R., Gleason, K. J., et al. (2017). Effect of continuous positive airway pressure treatment on health-related quality of life and sleepiness in high cardiovascular risk individuals with sleep apnea: Best Apnea Interventions for Research (BestAIR) trial. *Sleep, 40*(4). doi:10.1093/sleep/zsx040

10. Jonas, D. E., Amick, H. R., Feltner, C., et al. (2017, January). *Screening for obstructive sleep apnea in adults: An evidence review for the U.S. Preventive Services Task Force* (Report No. 14-05216-EF-1) [Internet]. Rockville, MD: Agency for Healthcare Research and Quality (US).

11. Epstein, L. J., Kristo, D., Strollo, P. J., et al. (2009). Clinical guideline for the evaluation, management and long-term care of obstructive sleep apnea in adults. *Journal of Clinical Sleep Medicine, 5*(3), 263–276.

12. Positive Airway Pressure Titration Task Force of the American Academy of Sleep Medicine. (2008). Clinical guidelines for the manual titration of positive airway pressure in patients with obstructive sleep apnea. *Journal of Clinical Sleep Medicine, 4*(2), 157–171.

13. Edwards, B. A., Malhotra, A., & Sands, S. A. (2013). Adapting our approach to treatment-emergent central sleep apnea. *Sleep, 36*(8), 1121–1122.

14. Johnson, K. G., & Johnson, D. C. (2015). Treatment of sleep-disordered breathing with positive airway pressure devices: Technology update. *Medical Devices (Auckl), 8*, 425–437.

15. Berry, R. B., Parish, J. M., & Hartse, K. M. The use of auto-titrating continuous positive airway pressure for treatment of adult obstructive sleep apnea. 2002. In: Database of Abstracts of Reviews of Effects (DARE): Quality-Assessed Reviews [Internet]. York, UK: Centre for Reviews and Dissemination (UK).

16. Donovan, L. M., Boeder, S., Malhotra, A., et al. (2015). New developments in the use of positive airway pressure for obstructive sleep apnea. *Journal of Thoracic Disease, 7*(8), 1323–1342.

chapter 47
Personalizing the Selection of Interfaces

CHERYL THOMAS-YVANAUSKAS

LEARNING OBJECTIVES

On completion of this chapter, the reader should be able to:

1. Recognize the different types of interfaces available.
2. Select the proper interface option to optimize comfort and appropriate fit to enhance patient adherence.
3. Describe the usual obstacles to effective positive airway pressure (PAP) therapy.
4. Describe PAP desensitization and the role of the technologist in optimizing patient outcomes in PAP therapy.

KEY TERMS

Acclimation
Adherence
Desensitization

The clinical guidelines of the American Academy of Sleep Medicine (AASM) indicate that all potential positive airway pressure (PAP) titration candidates (including those candidates before a diagnostic study where the clinical suspicion of obstructive sleep apnea [OSA] is high and a split-night study is a possibility) should receive adequate PAP education, hands-on demonstration, careful mask fitting, and acclimatization before titration (1).

Studies have shown that educational, supportive, and behavioral interventions have shown positive effects on patient adherence (2).

INTERFACE FITTING

It is best to introduce a patient to PAP therapy before the titration night in the sleep center. An education session should include a discussion of the rationale for the use of PAP therapy, side effects, mask fitting, and a hands-on demonstration with acclimatization; this is of particular importance for pediatric patients. Acclimating a patient to PAP therapy with positive feedback, patience, understanding, and empathy will help maximize future outcomes.

A well-fitting comfortable interface is critical for patient adherence. A patient who is uncomfortable with a mask for any reason will not use it regularly. For this reason, it is important that patients be included in the selection of their PAP interface. Among the considerations in selecting an appropriate interface are nasal patency, nasal or facial abnormalities, facial hair, whether the patient wears dentures or is missing teeth, full or shallow cheeks, hand–eye coordination, finger strength, impaired vision, manual dexterity and cognitive abilities, or a history of claustrophobia. There are several varieties of mask styles and sizes from which patients may choose. No single mask is ideal for all patients. The patient may select one type of mask at the beginning of the study that seems to fit comfortably and then during the study awaken and request a different mask. It is important to let patients know that there are alternatives if they have any issues during the study.

BREATHING DURING WAKEFULNESS AND SLEEP

Humans are obligate nose breathers during wakefulness and mainly during sleep independent of sleep stage or position. However, many patients with sleep apnea will state that they are "mouth breathers" during sleep. Mouth breathing during sleep typically occurs when the airway collapses. This is caused by an increase in negative intrathoracic pressure, creating thoracic traction (also known as "thoracic tug") that pulls the jawbone down, leading to mouth opening and an increased breathing effort. For this reason, a nasal mask should be the first mask of choice. A nasal mask is effective at decreasing mouth openings and prevents overuse of oronasal masks, increasing patient adherence (3).

TYPES OF PAP INTERFACES

There are several types of PAP interfaces, including nasal masks, nasal pillow, nasal cushion, oronasal (full-face) masks, oral masks, and total face masks.

When selecting the proper interface, there are several factors to consider: mask size and weight, strap types, the patient's ability to move, and his or her preferred sleep position.

Nasal masks cover only the nose while resting on the upper lip, sides of the nose, and the nasal bridge.

Nasal pillows rest on the inside rim of the nostril. They are light and require minimal headgear. They are appropriate for patients who experience claustrophobia with a nasal mask and may work well for a patient with facial hair that prevents an adequate seal with other types of masks. However, the patient must be able to tolerate the inserts resting in the nostrils.

Nasal cushion masks have minimal contact under the nose cushions that prevent discomfort from or irritation in the nostril or on the bridge of the nose. With any type of nasal interface, there is a chance of air leaking from the patient's mouth. A second option is a nasal mask with a chinstrap. A chinstrap is an elastic fabric band that applies upward pressure on the jaw to keep the mouth closed. These straps often connect to the nasal mask head straps.

Oronasal masks (full face) cover the nose and the mouth while resting on the chin, sides of the nose, and mouth and bridge of the nose. This interface is heavier than nasal masks or pillows but may be required in patients without a patent nasal airway.

Oral masks fit in the mouth between the lips and the teeth. They have a tongue stabilizer, which holds the tongue forward to prevent airway obstruction. Oral masks are not often used in the sleep center. Limitations with this interface include upper airway dryness, rainout associated with heated humidification, and air leakage from the nose.

Total face masks cover the entire face. It is an alternative for patients unable to obtain a good seal with other masks. It is preferably indicated for patients with facial deformities and those suffering from skin breakdown around the facial area.

Also available are combination devices that include an oral appliance and PAP interface (3).

Most manufacturers provide a size guide for sleep centers to use to obtain an accurate mask fit. Using the guide provides a good starting point for finding the right mask for the patient. However, faces and noses are all different, and sometimes it is necessary to try more than one size or type of mask to get an optimal fit. Also, mask sizes differ between manufacturers; a medium-wide mask from one manufacturer may be quite different than a medium-wide mask from another.

ORONASAL (FULL-FACE) MASK VERSUS NASAL MASKS AND UPPER AIRWAY OBSTRUCTION

Upper airway resistance and the likelihood of developing OSA is higher when breathing through the mouth than when breathing through the nose. The oronasal (full-face) mask applies positive pressure equally to the nasopharyngeal and oropharyngeal compartments, thus eliminating the pressure gradient that allows the soft palate and tongue to relax and cause an obstruction. Higher PAPs are required, and leaks are significantly higher in patients wearing oronasal (full-face) mask than nasal mask interfaces. Additionally, oronasal (full-face) masks reflect a lower PAP adherence rate. Sleep efficiency, slow-wave sleep, and rapid eye movement sleep are greater during titration with a nasal mask. Patients wearing the nasal pillows mask and those wearing the nasal masks have both reported improved Epworth Sleepiness Scale score and quality of life. The nasal mask and the nasal pillows are equally as effective when treating patients with OSA requiring high pressures (3). Oronasal masks are associated with higher PAPs, higher residual apnea–hypopnea index (AHI), and poorer adherence than nasal masks. Therefore, patients using oronasal (full-face) masks should be closely monitored. Nasal interfaces should *always* be the first choice. There is evidence that the prolonged use of nasal PAP reduces mouth opening and oral breathing. Therefore, even patients with OSA who claim to be mouth breathers could be initiated with nasal masks. Another clinical implication is that sleep studies for PAP titration must be performed with the same type of mask that the patient will use at home. It is highly suggested that nasal masks or nasal pillows be used instead of oronasal (full-face) masks in OSA patients unless there is a clear indication otherwise (4, 5).

CHINSTRAP AND PAP ADHERENCE

Delivery of PAP requires an adequate seal that prevents leakage. Unintentional air leak in the system results in the development of an open circuit that may reduce the pressure of air delivered to the site of obstruction, with associated recurrence of respiratory events. Air can leak from around a mask that does not fit properly. Leaks can also be caused by mouth opening. A chinstrap may be useful in reducing leak during PAP treatment by supporting the mandible. A study performed at an AASM-accredited Veterans Administration Medical Center sleep center found that chinstrap users had significantly greater PAP adherence, longer nightly duration of PAP usage, lower residual AHI, and lower leak than chinstrap nonusers, at the first follow-up visit (6). An alternate mask for these patients is an oronasal (full-face) mask. Some patients may prefer this kind of mask even without air leakage issues. However, because the full-face mask comes into contact with more of the facial area, it can be difficult to maintain a seal, leading to increased leakage, especially as the pressure is increased. A full-face mask should not be offered as a first choice if the patient has a patent nasal airway.

It is impossible to tell if a mask fits properly when it is not pressurized. Therefore, after ensuring proper measurement, mask selection, and patient comfort, it is critical to initiate a low PAP during the mask-fitting process. Most PAP machines provide a measure of air leakage. A small amount of leakage is expected, and the value varies by manufacturer. Large leaks can cause irritation of the skin or eyes and prevent delivery of an adequate therapeutic pressure. Leaks can often be remedied by reseating the mask on the face and with minor adjustments of the head strap.

The mask should fit snug and the straps firm but not tight. Masks fitted too tightly can cause excessive air leaks, pressure sores, and discomfort. Tight straps may produce abrasions and, in some patients, cause headache, neck pain, and pressure points in the upper gums and teeth. The well-fitted mask should be loose enough to be pulled away from the face about one-half inch and reseated. If a mask has an acceptable leak level only when the straps are tight, then it may not be an appropriate-sized mask for the patient. When you and the patient are convinced that the mask is comfortable, and the leak level is acceptable, the titration can begin (7).

PAP DESENSITIZATION

Following a successful PAP titration, there may be patients who have difficulty adjusting to therapy (8). Common complaints may be the interface or therapeutic pressure. Patients should return to the sleep center for reevaluation. A skilled, knowledgeable, and patient technologist should be able to solicit constructive feedback from the patient to better facilitate a successful treatment plan.

DESENSITIZATION TECHNIQUES

1. Evaluate and measure the patient's face and head carefully and select an appropriate interface and headgear.
2. Allow the patient to handle the mask himself or herself, holding it to the patient's face to assess fit and comfort before connecting the mask to the hose or PAP instrument.
3. Connect the hose to the mask and PAP instrument and allow the patient to hold the mask to the face, gradually introducing pressure at 4 cm H_2O. It is important to allow the patient to have control of the mask.
4. When the patient is comfortable holding the mask as described and breathing with PAP at a low pressure, turn the pressure off and fit the mask and headgear. Show the patient how to disconnect the

hose from the mask and have him or her recline in a recliner or lie supine on a bed.
5. Reinitiate pressure at 4 cm H_2O using heated humidity while the patient is lying down. Offer encouragement, such as "It looks like you are breathing comfortably at this pressure" or "You are doing fine; remember that this is going to help your breathing while you sleep."
6. If the patient is having any difficulty at this low pressure, refrain from increasing the pressure. In some cases, distraction techniques such as watching TV or reading may help the patient tolerate the procedure.
7. If the patient is tolerating the low pressure well, inform him or her that you will gradually increase the pressure. Remind the patient that he or she can disconnect the hose if the pressure becomes intolerable. This allows the patient to remain in control of the process.
8. Verify there are no interface leaks or other issues before beginning to increase PAP.
9. Increase pressure gradually in 1-cm increments in a ramping fashion, carefully monitoring patient reaction and tolerance. In general, pressure should be increased to about 8 cm H_2O during the desensitization process.
10. Check for leaks and adjust interface fit, if necessary, and change interface styles as needed. Utilize a chinstrap or oronasal (full-face) mask if mouth breathing is occurring.
11. If the patient has difficulty tolerating higher pressures, particularly exhaling against the pressure, try using pressure relief or bilevel PAP.
12. Remember to continue to reassure the patient and reinforce his or her success, for example, "You are doing well, keep it up." It is vital to make this a positive experience for the patient.
13. When the patient is able to tolerate 8 cm H_2O for approximately 15 minutes, the desensitization is considered successful. If desensitization is successful, the patient should be able to tolerate a PAP titration study.
14. At the conclusion of the desensitization, ask the patient to summarize his or her experience. Document your assessment as well as the patient's responses.
15. If the patient has difficulty with the mask/interface or does not tolerate the desensitization procedure in the sleep clinic or sleep center, consider sending the patient home with the PAP equipment to continue the process at home for a period of 1 to 2 weeks. Give the patient specific written instructions for the process to follow at home. Some patients become more tolerant of the mask in their own home or surroundings. This can be accomplished

by instructing the patient to wear the mask in the evening while watching TV until he or she can tolerate it for at least 30 minutes. Once the mask is tolerated, desensitization in the sleep clinic or sleep center can be attempted again.

16. If the patient tolerated the mask but had difficulty with the pressure, consider sending him or her home with a PAP device set to approximately 8 cm H_2O and a 30-minute ramp time. Instruct the patient on how to reset the ramp to lower the pressure at any time and encourage him or her to practice outside of the sleep period, perhaps while reclining and watching TV in the evening, until he or she is able to tolerate the pressure at 8 cm H_2O. Once this is accomplished, the patient can be scheduled for a PAP titration study (8).

The desensitization process may be challenging yet very rewarding for the technologist. Through continued support and encouragement, most patients are able to tolerate and benefit from PAP therapy. Desensitization techniques, interface options, pressure relief technology, and humidification along with support, empathy, and understanding from the technologist will have a considerable effect on successful patient outcomes.

TIPS TO HELP YOUR PATIENT ADJUST TO COMMON PAP PROBLEMS

1. **Difficulty wearing a PAP interface**
   Have the patient wear the mask for short periods during the day when watching TV, reading a book, or surfing the Internet. When the patient is comfortable with the mask, have him or her wear the mask and hose with the device turned on during the day while he or she is awake. Once the patient is comfortable with how the mask feels on the face, ask the patient to start wearing the PAP mask every time he or she sleeps, whether it is at night or during a nap (9).

2. **Uncomfortable interface**
   Refit the patient with a different interface, paying attention to the size and style of the mask to ensure a proper fit.

3. **Intolerance of air pressure**
   The inability to tolerate the air pressure may be alleviated by using the ramping feature on the PAP machine. This feature allows therapy to begin with low air pressure, which is then followed by an automatic, gradual increase that eventually sets itself to the prescribed pressure. If this feature does not help, bilevel PAP may be a treatment of choice.

4. **Dry or stuffy nose**
   Check for proper mask fit and for mask leaks. A mask leak can dry out the nose. Check to make sure the patient is using the heated humidifier and it is functioning properly.
   Additionally, the use of a nasal saline spray at bedtime may help prevent nasal passages.

5. **Mask leak, skin irritation, or pressure sores**
   A leaky or an ill-fitting mask may be irritating to the patient's skin, causing pressure sores or directing air into the eyes, triggering dryness or tearing. You may need to refit the patient with a different size or style of mask, particularly if his or her weight has changed significantly. Changing to a different interface style, such as a nasal pillow mask, may be helpful.

6. **Difficulty falling asleep**
   Assure the patient that this is not uncommon, but also confirm whether the patient is practicing good sleep hygiene and using the ramp feature on the PAP device.

7. **Dry mouth**
   Air leaks and oral breathing may dry the mouth of a patient wearing nasal PAP. The use of a chinstrap may alleviate this problem by helping keep the patient's mouth closed.

8. **Unintentional removal of PAP during the night**
   It is not uncommon for a patient to unintentionally remove the PAP interface during sleep. This may be a result of nasal congestion. On such occasions, confirming a good mask fit and adding a heated humidity may help. A chinstrap may also help keep the mask on the patient's face. If this removal is a consistent problem, have the patient set an alarm for a few hours after bedtime to check whether the device is still on. The patient can then progressively set the alarm for later in the night as the device is tolerated longer.

9. **Bothersome noise**
   The newest generation of PAP devices is virtually silent. However, if the patient finds the device disturbing, confirm whether the device's air filters are clean and unblocked. If they are, have the PAP supplier check the device to ensure it is working properly. If it is and if the noise is still bothersome, earplugs can be helpful or a fan or "white noise" machine can disguise the noise of the PAP machine.

CONCLUSION

Biomedical engineers have been working to optimize the PAP interface to enhance comfort and adherence. Various masks are available that use different anchor points on the face and different strategies to hold the mask in place. Innovative methods allowing patients to sleep on their stomachs while using PAP have been developed. Hose holders, special pillows, and pressure relief devices have been developed to assist patients achieve their goals.

The PAP acclimation and choice of interface are integral facilitators of the continued health and well-being of our patients and should therefore be afforded the time and consideration needed to promote successful outcomes.

REFERENCES

1. Kushida, C. A., Chediak, A. C., Berry, R. B., et al. (2008). Clinical guidelines for the manual titration of positive airway pressure in patients with obstructive sleep apnea. *Journal of Clinical Sleep Medicine, 4*(1), 160.

2. Wozniak, D. R., Lasserson, T. J., & Smith, I. (2014). Educational, supportive and behavioural interventions to improve usage of continuous positive airway pressure machines in adults with obstructive sleep apnoea. *Cochrane Database of Systematic Reviews*, (1), CD007736.

3. BaHammam, A. S., Singh, T., George, S., et al. (2017). Choosing the right interface for positive airway pressure therapy in patients with obstructive sleep apnea. *Sleep Breath, 21*(3), 569–575.

4. Budhiraja, R., & Bakker, J. P. (2016). CPAP use: Unmasking the truth about interface. *Journal of Clinical Sleep Medicine, 12*(9), 1209–1210.

5. Andrade, R. G. S., Viana, F. M., Nascimento, J. A., et al. (2018). Nasal vs oro-nasal CPAP for OSA treatment: A meta-analysis. *Chest, 153*(3), 665–674.

6. Knowles, S. R., O'Brien, D. T., Zhang, S., et al. (2014). Effect of addition of chin strap on PAP compliance, nightly duration of use, and other factors. *Journal of Clinical Sleep Medicine, 10*(4), 377–383.

7. Rowland, S., Aiyappan, V., Hennessy, C., et al. (2018). Comparing the efficacy, mask leak, patient adherence, and patient preference of three different CPAP interfaces to treat moderate-severe obstructive sleep apnea. *Journal of Clinical Sleep Medicine, 14*(1), 101–108.

8. American Association of Sleep Technologists. (2012). *Positive airway pressure acclimation and desensitization.* Retrieved from https://www.aastweb.org/hubfs/Technical%20Guidelines/Updated%206.14.2017/PAPacclimation.pdf

9. Brooks, R. (2015). *Top 10 most common CPAP mask problems and discomfort (& how to solve them).* American Association of Sleep Technologists. Retrieved from https://www.aastweb.org/blog/top-10-ways-to-solve-common-cpap-problems-and-discomfort

chapter 48

Titration of Continuous Positive Airway Pressure and Bilevel Positive Airway Pressure

CHERYL THOMAS-YVANAUSKAS   HARRY WHITMORE   RICHARD S. ROSENBERG

LEARNING OBJECTIVES

On completion of this chapter, the reader should be able to:

1. Apply positive airway pressure devices when appropriate to adult and pediatric patients.
2. Optimize pressure settings to eliminate respiratory events and improve sleep pattern.
3. Troubleshoot patient complaints that might interfere with tolerance of treatment.

KEY TERMS

Positive airway pressure (PAP)
Titration
Obstructive sleep apnea
Treatment-emergent central sleep apnea
RERA (respiratory effort–related arousal)
Split-night

No procedure is more challenging for the sleep technologist than positive airway pressure (PAP) titration. Although challenging, PAP titration is also the most potentially rewarding procedure that the technologist will perform in the sleep center. An adequate PAP titration can dramatically improve the health and quality of life for the patient. The technologist must use social skills to prepare the patient for titration and reduce his or her fears. The technologist interacts with the patient to ensure that a proper mask is chosen and is appropriately fit for comfort. Once the titration begins, the technologist must recognize sleep stages, arousals, and sleep-related breathing events "on the fly" to determine

when to increase the pressure to normalize respiration. As changes to the pressure level are made, the technologist must evaluate patient response. All of this must occur within the patient's sleep period, which may be shortened by patient anxiety, resulting in prolonged sleep-onset latency or awakenings.

Most sleep centers have a "split-night" protocol in which the first half of the night is used to make or confirm a diagnosis of obstructive sleep apnea (OSA), and the second half of the night is available for PAP titration. This requires the sleep technologist to closely monitor the patient's sleep and respiratory patterns as well as body position and accomplish the goals of PAP titration in a limited time. Split-night studies are not recommended for pediatric patients less than 12 years of age.

The American Academy of Sleep Medicine (AASM) has provided guidelines for the titration process (1). These guidelines were developed through literature review and consensus. One important conclusion of this review was that appropriate pressure cannot be determined using mathematical models that use height, weight, neck size, airway size, or other measures. The only approved way to determine the pressure needed to normalize breathing is to monitor respiration during a titration study. The primary goal of PAP titration is to eliminate obstructive respiratory events including apneas, hypopneas, respiratory effort–related arousals (RERAs), and snoring. A secondary goal of PAP titration is to improve the patient's sleep architecture. There is a window of acceptable pressures for most patients, rather than one absolutely correct pressure. Pressure that is too low will not treat the patient's respiratory events, and pressure that is too high may cause arousals and central respiratory events. These challenges require the sleep technologist to find an optimal pressure level that normalizes breathing without disrupting sleep.

From the moment the patient enters the sleep center, the technologist begins building a rapport with the patient to ensure a positive experience during PAP titration. A positive initial experience with PAP therapy has been shown to predict future adherence to the treatment (2). Even the best treatment is useless if the patient doesn't use it. The initial impression of the patient to PAP therapy is an essential factor in treatment adherence. The technologist should work to find the best PAP platform for each patient (within the bounds of the sleep center's policies and procedures) and the most comfortable mask and headgear, and if necessary provide heated humidification. Ideally, the titration study provides all the information needed to guide the physician in prescribing the most appropriate treatment for each patient.

Regular meetings between the technologist, the interpreting physician, and the sleep center team provide an opportunity to discuss cases and challenges in determining when to perform a split-night study and address issues that do occur during PAP titrations. The decision to perform a split-night procedure is usually outlined in the sleep center policy manual.

To determine a final pressure for the patient, detailed technologist notes are of utmost importance during PAP titration studies. The technologist is expected to explain why PAP was started, which is typically based on an estimate of the patient's apnea–hypopnea index (AHI). The technologist should always document changes in PAP and the reasons that changes were made. In addition, it is sometimes helpful to note why changes were not made. The technologist may be giving the patient a few minutes to adjust to a change in pressure or waiting to see if sleep-onset central apneas will resolve. A brief note will let the interpreting physician know that the technologist is aware of all aspects of the situations that occur during the titration study and provide insight into the decisions that were made.

PREPARING THE PATIENT FOR PAP TITRATION

Let's take a look at a split-night study scenario. Put yourself in the patient's shoes (or slippers) for a moment. It is 1 a.m. and you have been sleeping soundly in the sleep center. The lights go on suddenly and Bob, the sleep technologist, is at the bedside. He mumbles something about starting treatment. You have no idea what he means. He looks at your face, says "Medium Wide," and begins rummaging in a closet. He pulls out a plastic bag with a contraption inside, connects it to a vacuum cleaner hose, connects the hose to a machine on the bedside table, and tells you to sit up. Looming over you, he presses a plastic mask onto your nose and starts wrapping straps around your head. Can you expect a successful titration? I think not.

Most patients undergoing full-night titrations will have reviewed their diagnostic study with the sleep physician and had a discussion about PAP therapy. Receiving

a diagnosis of OSA can cause anxiety, and patients may not remember what they were told in the office. There should be a copy of the diagnostic report in the patient's chart, which the technologist can review with the patient and answer questions the patient might have. The discussion should include an explanation of why PAP is important, device options, and a review of the masks that are available in your sleep center.

When a split-night study has been ordered, the technologist should review the patient's chart thoroughly before their hookup. The AASM recommends that all potential PAP titration candidates receive adequate PAP education, hands-on demonstration, careful mask fitting, and acclimation before titration (1). Surprises may be OK for birthday parties, but they should be avoided whenever possible in the sleep center. The technologist should inform the patient that if the protocol for a split-night study is met, the technologist will come in during the night to initiate PAP.

ANTICIPATING PATIENT CONCERNS

It is best to introduce a patient to PAP therapy before the night of titration in the sleep center. An education session should include a discussion of the rationale for the use of PAP therapy, side effects, mask fitting, and a hands-on demonstration with acclimatization; this is of particular importance for pediatric patients. However, because of time and reimbursement issues, this is not always possible. The technologist may be providing the first introduction the patient has about the PAP device; if this is the case, the technologist should be as complete as possible and allow plenty of time for questions. It may not be clear what a patient is feeling, and for the titration to be successful, you must maintain a positive, "can do" attitude. Explain that the device uses room air and contains a fan that speeds up to produce increased air pressure when the airway is obstructed. Let the patient know that you will be controlling the pressure from another room. Describe the mask options that are available. Reassure the patient that the mask is clean or new and that procedures are in place to reduce infection. One approach to patient education is:

- If possible, allow the patient to watch a video that follows a patient through diagnosis and treatment.
- Show the patient the equipment and describe how it works.
- Let the patient handle the equipment and the mask. Have the patient hold the PAP mask in place (at the lowest pressure of 4 cm H_2O) without strapping the mask on. Allow the patient to practice breathing through the mask until he or she feels comfortable (a minimum of 2 to 3 minutes). Next, have the patient try PAP with the straps holding

the mask in place. Demonstrate how to release the headgear in the event the patient panics and needs to remove the mask quickly. Allow the patient to remove the mask.

- Explain that he or she will be exhaling against the PAP. Explain that a nasal mask works best with the mouth closed, and that when the patient opens his or her mouth, the air will rush out, making it difficult to talk. Slowly raise the pressure to between 8 and 10 cm H_2O in order to demonstrate a higher level of pressure to the patient.

The most common question encountered before PAP titration is "How will I sleep with that on my face?" Telling the patient "almost everyone sleeps" is often not enough. It is more helpful to address the patient's concerns directly. Ask if the patient is concerned about the mask, the pressure, or the newness of the situation. Patients often ask about going to the bathroom during the night, waking with the mask off, feelings of suffocation, and noise. Some technologists provide answers to these questions even before they are asked. It is also helpful to explain that you will be adjusting the pressure throughout the night with the goal of eliminating the patient's respiratory events. Explain that upon awakening the pressure may feel different from when they fell asleep. Similarly, it is important to be open about the fact that the patient may still have breathing problems during the titration night, as the technologist needs to see respiratory events before increasing PAP. Reviewing this information with the patient before lights out can be beneficial and reduce the patient's apprehension. It is not uncommon for patients to have difficulty falling asleep with PAP in place for the first time.

If it is clear that a patient is tense or anxious, it may be necessary to let the patient take a break from PAP for a brief time and sit up for a while, instead of having him or her continue to try to sleep. By having the patient sit quietly, he or she is likely to calm down and relax, thus increasing the chance that the patient will be able to continue with the PAP titration and be able to sleep. While the patient is sitting up, the technologist can work with the patient to practice using PAP again. The technologist should reduce the pressure before reapplying the mask.

For patients who awaken during the night and have difficulty tolerating PAP while awake, reduce the PAP until the patient returns to sleep. Most PAP devices that the patient will have at home will have a ramp feature to allow him or her to lower the pressure and return to sleep after awakening during the night. Once the patient is asleep, gradually increase to the pressure titrated before the awakening and continue the titration.

With experience, technologists develop techniques and skills to respond to patient concerns and reassure patients in order to get an optimal titration.

Adjustment of PAP

During a full-night titration, adjustment of pressure begins at lights out. For split-night titrations, the sleep center policy and procedures manual should define the criteria that must be met before beginning titration. The AASM practice parameters (3, 4) recommend titration guidelines, but do not set a standard for when to begin the titration portion of a split-night study. The basic recommendation is that PAP titration should be started if an AHI higher than 40 is documented during 2 hours of a diagnostic study. Titration may be considered for an AHI between 20 and 40 on the basis of the clinical judgment of the ordering physician. Because this is a recommendation and not a standard, some centers use different thresholds for initiation of a split-night titration. Some sleep centers set thresholds for the AHI that will cover PAP device reimbursement by Medicare. At the time of this writing, the Medicare requirement is an AHI of 15 or an AHI of 5 or more with associated clinical symptoms such as high blood pressure and daytime sleepiness. Sleep centers should have a policy that delineates the cutoff time for starting a split-night titration. In AASM-accredited centers, the medical director is required to provide clear and detailed instructions for all procedures, including PAP titration, in a Policy and Procedures manual.

Recognizing Inadequate Titration

The core concept of PAP titration is simple: increase the pressure until the goals of titration are met (Fig. 48-1). The primary goal of PAP titration is the elimination of obstructive respiratory events, including apneas, hypopneas, RERAs, and snoring. A secondary goal of PAP titration is to improve the patient's sleep architecture.

Inadequate pressure is defined by the AASM guidelines (1) as two or more obstructive apneas, three or more hypopneas, five or more RERAs, or 3 or more minutes of loud snoring in adults. Scoring of these respiratory events during titration is somewhat different than

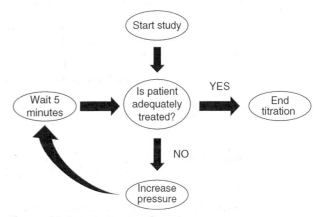

Figure 48-1 Basic titration flow chart.

during the diagnostic portion of the study because the oronasal thermal sensor and the nasal pressure transducer are typically replaced by a flow measure output from the PAP machine. Scoring of both apneas and hypopneas is therefore based on the PAP device flow signal. According to the AASM scoring manual (5), score a respiratory event as an apnea when there is a drop in the peak signal excursion by 90% or more of the preevent baseline and the duration of the *90% or more drop in flow* signal is 10 seconds or more. Two rules for scoring of hypopnea are provided:

Rule 1A Score a respiratory event as a hypopnea when there is a drop in the peak signal excursion by ≥ 30% of the pre-event baseline, the duration of the ≥ 30% drop in flow signal is ≥ 10 seconds, there is a ≥ 3% oxygen desaturation from pre-event baseline or the event is associated with an arousal.

Rule 1B Score a respiratory event as a hypopnea when there is a drop in the peak signal excursion by ≥ 30% of the pre-event baseline, the duration of the ≥ 30% drop in flow signal is ≥ 10 seconds and there is a ≥ 4% oxygen desaturation from pre-event baseline.

When scoring a hypopnea, either rule 1A or 1B should be specified in the PSG report.

Score the hypopnea as obstructive if there is snoring, an increased inspiratory flattening of the PAP device flow signal compared to baseline or there is an associated thoracoabdominal paradox that occurs during the event but not during the pre-event. Score the hypopnea as central if there is no snoring, no increased inspiratory flattening of the PAP device flow signal and no associated thoracoabdominal paradox that occurs during the event but not during the pre-event. (5)

The PAP device flow signal will show flattening of the waveform if there is flow restriction, much like the nasal pressure transducer output. If there is a 10-second or more period of signal flattening or an increasing respiratory effort leading to an arousal from sleep, a RERA can be scored. Increasing effort measured by respiratory inductance plethysmography may also be used to score RERAs. Indicators of inadequate titration are shown in Figure 48-2, which demonstrates a flattened flow signal, even without an arousal, and Figure 48-3, which demonstrates a RERA on the basis of the PAP flow channel. Snoring may be difficult to evaluate with a microphone during titration because the PAP device produces noise, which may mask the snoring. A well-placed sensor on the neck that measures vibration is very helpful

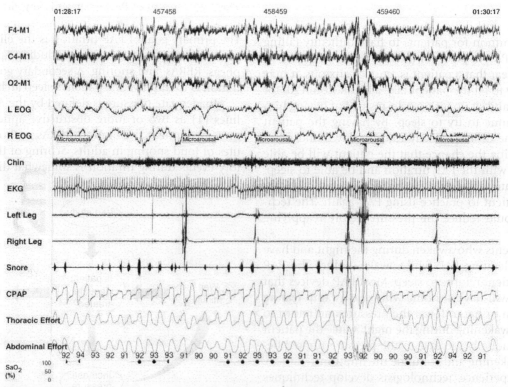

Figure 48-2 A sample of a 2-minute epoch of inadequate titration. CPAP, continuous positive airway pressure; EKG, electrocardiogram; EOG, electrooculography.

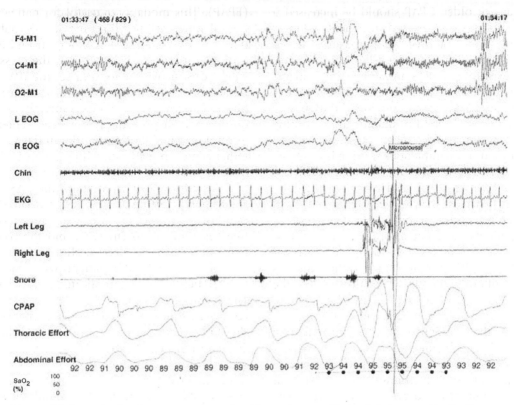

Figure 48-3 A sample of a 30-second epoch with respiratory effort–related arousal indicating inadequate titration. CPAP, continuous positive airway pressure; EKG, electrocardiogram; EOG, electrooculography.

for proper titration. At times, a "sawtooth" pattern in the PAP flow signal provides an indication of snoring.

The AASM guidelines (1) also outline criteria for an optimal, good, adequate, and unacceptable PAP titration. The overall goal of PAP is to control the patient's obstructive respiratory events while maintaining SpO$_2$ above 90%, with acceptable leak parameters at the selected pressure. In an *optimal* PAP titration, the selected pressure keeps the Respiratory Disturbance Index (RDI) below 5 for at least 15 minutes while the patient is supine and in stage R sleep without spontaneous arousals or awakenings. In a *good* PAP titration, the selected pressure keeps the RDI below 10, or reduced by 50% if the baseline RDI was below 15, while the patient is supine and in stage R sleep without spontaneous arousals or awakenings. In an *adequate* PAP titration, the RDI may be above 10 but is reduced by 75% from the baseline study. A PAP titration is also considered *adequate* if it meets the criteria for *optimal* or *good* without evaluation of rapid eye movement (REM) sleep in the supine position. An *unacceptable* PAP titration is one that does not meet any of the above-mentioned criteria (1).

Increasing Pressure

The AASM guidelines recommend 4 cm H$_2$O as the starting pressure for continuous PAP (CPAP) (1). This is a very low pressure that is usually ineffective in treating apnea but allows the patient to fall asleep comfortably. The recommended maximum CPAP is 20 cm H$_2$O for adults and children who are 12 years or older. The maximum recommended CPAP for children under 12 years is 15 cm H$_2$O.

The guidelines recommend increasing pressure in response to inadequate titration in at least 1 cm H$_2$O increments. Larger increases are appropriate during retitration of patients who have previously been determined to have high-pressure requirements, or if there are other reasons to suspect high pressure will be needed. The guidelines recommend waiting a minimum of 5 minutes between changes in PAP, allowing time to confirm that the pressure is inadequate on the basis of the criteria indicated earlier. It is best to increase the pressure during inspiration, because the patient is less likely to notice the change. At times, a change in pressure may cause an arousal or change in sleep stage. Allowing a few minutes for the patient to settle down also provides a better assessment of the patient's response to the increased pressure.

For pediatric patients, CPAP should be increased by at least 1 cm H$_2$O with an interval of no less than 5 minutes. CPAP should be increased if at least one obstructive apnea is observed in patients younger than 12 years or if at least two obstructive apneas are observed in patients

12 years of age or older. CPAP should be increased if at least one hypopnea is observed in patients younger than 12 years or if at least three hypopneas are observed in patients 12 years of age or older. CPAP should be increased if at least three RERAs are observed in patients younger than 12 years or if at least five RERAs are observed in patients 12 years of age or older. CPAP may be increased if 1 minute of loud or unambiguous snoring is observed in patients younger than 12 years or at least 3 minutes of loud or unambiguous snoring is observed in patients 12 years of age or older. Reduction of airway resistance has been demonstrated by increasing PAP; however, do not increase the pressure higher than 5 cm H_2O over what is required to control obstructive events.

Ideally, patients should be recorded in supine REM sleep for at least 15 minutes at the designated optimal pressure during the PAP titration study. If the patient is in REM sleep but not in the supine position while at the designated optimal pressure, the patient may be awakened and instructed to lie in the supine position.

Note that the titration process is circular (see Fig. 48-1). After increasing the pressure, assess the patient to see if the pressure is still inadequate. If the pressure is still inadequate, increase the pressure by at least 1 cm H_2O, wait for 5 minutes, and reassess the patient. The 5-minute rule is a minimum. If the patient has evidence of inadequate titration in the first 2 minutes, wait for at least 5 minutes before making another increase. If the patient does not have evidence of inadequate titration, just wait. The patient may have three RERAs in the first 5 minutes and not have the other two RERAs for 30 minutes. The patient would then meet criteria for inadequate titration at the 30-minute mark, and the pressure should be increased at that point. Remember to document all changes in PAP and the reason for the change on the recording.

The AASM guidelines also recommend exploration of higher pressure levels. In patients who no longer have apneas, hypopneas, RERAs, and snoring, an additional increase in pressure may provide benefits including resolution of flow limitation (as evidenced by elimination of flow signal flattening) and improved sleep continuity. The guidelines recommend increasing pressure by 2 and no more than 5 cm H_2O over the pressure needed for resolution of respiratory events and snoring (1) in the exploratory phase of PAP titration. Part of this exploration should occur during stage R sleep with the patient supine. In most patients, this is the condition during which OSA is at its worst and pressure requirements are greatest. In order to test patients during REM in a supine position, it may be necessary to enter the patient's room and ask that he or she tries sleeping on his or her back.

Switching to Bilevel PAP

Bilevel PAP (BPAP) provides PAP at one level during inspiration (IPAP) and at a lower level during expiration (EPAP). This modality is useful for patients who cannot tolerate CPAP or who complain of trouble exhaling during CPAP therapy (3). To change from CPAP to BPAP during a titration, set the EPAP at the pressure that resolved obstructive events, and set the IPAP 4 cm H_2O higher. BPAP equipment is more expensive than CPAP but may improve compliance, especially in patients requiring a high pressure. Some sleep centers limit the technologist to CPAP during the initial titration study. Other centers provide guidelines for switching to BPAP in their policy and procedures manual.

To perform a BPAP titration, the AASM guidelines recommend starting at an IPAP of 8 cm H_2O and an EPAP of 4 cm H_2O (1). The maximum recommended BPAP is IPAP of 30 cm H_2O, and the recommended maximum difference between IPAP and EPAP is 10 cm H_2O. Increasing BPAP in patients with inadequate titration is slightly more complicated than CPAP titration. The recommendation is that IPAP and EPAP should be increased in response to apneas, whereas only IPAP should be increased in response to hypopneas, RERAs, and snoring (1). As with CPAP, increases of at least 1 cm H_2O with an interval of at least 5 minutes are recommended.

For pediatric patients, BPAP should be increased by at least 1 cm H_2O with an interval of no less than 5 minutes. BPAP should be increased if at least one obstructive apnea is observed in patients younger than 12 years or if at least two obstructive apneas are observed in patients 12 years of age or older. BPAP should be increased if at least one hypopnea is observed in patients younger than 12 years or if at least three hypopneas are observed in patients 12 years of age or older. BPAP should be increased if at least three RERAs are observed in patients younger than 12 years or if at least five RERAs are observed in patients 12 years of age or older. BPAP may be increased if 1 minute of loud or unambiguous snoring is observed in patients younger than 12 years or at least 3 minutes of loud or unambiguous snoring is observed in patients 12 years of age or older. Reduction of airway resistance has been demonstrated by increasing BPAP; however, do not increase the pressure higher than 5 cm H_2O over what is required to control obstructive events.

As is the case with CPAP titrations, during BPAP titrations, patients should be recorded in supine REM sleep for at least 15 minutes at the designated optimal pressure during the BPAP titration study. If the patient is in REM sleep but not in the supine position while at the designated optimal pressure, the patient may be awakened and instructed to lie in the supine position.

As an example, BPAP titration may proceed as follows: the patient begins the night at IPAP 8 cm H_2O and EPAP 4 cm H_2O. Within the first 30 minutes, two obstructive apneas are seen. The technologist raises the pressure to IPAP 9 and EPAP 5 and waits 5 minutes. During the next 5 minutes, two more obstructive apneas are recorded. The pressure is increased to IPAP 10 and EPAP 6. Additional apneas are observed and the pressure is increased to IPAP 11 and EPAP 7. At this point, apneas resolve, but three hypopneas occur in the next 20 minutes. In response to the hypopneas, only the IPAP should be increased. IPAP should be increased to 12 and EPAP remains at 7. Over the next 20 minutes, three more hypopneas are seen. Pressure is increased to IPAP 13 and EPAP remains at 7. At this pressure, hypopneas resolve, but moderate snoring persists. After 3 minutes of continuous loud snoring, the IPAP is once again increased to 14 and EPAP remains at 7. At this pressure, the snoring resolves, and the patient sleeps soundly for the remainder of the night. For home use, BPAP is recommended at IPAP 14 and EPAP 7 for this patient.

Decreasing Pressure

Increasing pressure until the breathing becomes normal is one way to determine the appropriate pressure for a patient. Patients will have a "therapeutic window" of effective PAP. If the pressure is too low, the respiratory events will continue. If the pressure is too high, the patient may develop frequent arousals and/or treatment-emergent central sleep apneas (6).

The determination of the therapeutic window of PAP for a given patient may require a slightly different method than the one outlined earlier. The "staircase method" made famous by the psychophysicist Georg von Békésy, also referred to as an "up-down-up titration," involves starting the pressure low and increasing until it is clearly too high, then reducing the pressure until it is too low. The final step is to once again increase the pressure until it is too high. This process provides a more precise definition of the therapeutic window for each patient. Unfortunately, it takes more time than the standard methods and may not be possible to accomplish during a split-night study.

Indicators that PAP is too high include frequent arousals and the appearance of treatment-emergent central sleep apnea (Figs. 48-4 and 48-5). The most certain indicator of excessive pressure is the patient waking up, complaining that the pressure is too high. When indicators of excessive pressure are seen, the pressure should be reduced in 1 cm H_2O increments until the indicators disappear. A larger decrease in pressure may be necessary when the patient is awake and complaining. In this case, the pressure should be decreased to a level that feels comfortable to the patient. After decreasing the pressure, it is critically important to monitor the patient to be sure that the new pressure setting is adequate, particularly as the patient falls back to sleep. In a few patients, the pressure that adequately treats the OSA may be too high for patient comfort. In other words, the therapeutic window may be very narrow or may not even exist. In these cases, several trials of waiting for the

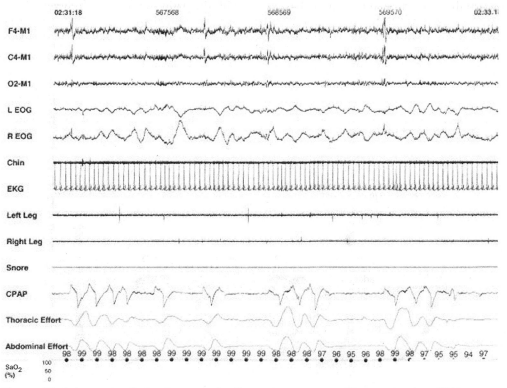

Figure 48-4 A sample of a 2-minute epoch of central apneas caused by overtitration. CPAP, continuous positive airway pressure; EKG, electrocardiogram; EOG, electrooculography.

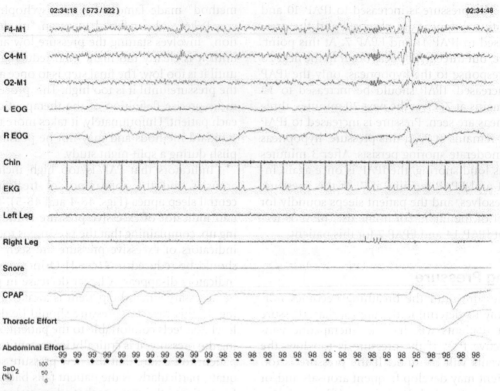

Figure 48-5 Sample 30-second epoch showing central apnea due to overtitration. CPAP, continuous positive airway pressure; EKG, electrocardiogram; EOG, electrooculography.

patient to enter consolidated sleep using a low pressure and then gradually increasing the pressure until it is adequate provides the maximum information for the interpreting physician. Careful technologist documentation is an essential part of this process. These patients will usually tolerate PAP at home using a machine with a "ramp" feature that they can activate as needed. The ramp feature reduces the pressure and then gradually increases it over a preset time, allowing the patient to adjust over time to the higher pressure necessary to control his or her sleep-disordered breathing.

A flowchart that indicates appropriate increases and decreases in pressure, as well as a check for stage R sleep with the patient supine, is shown in Figure 48-6.

Down titrating during a BPAP titration typically involves a 1 cm H_2O decrease in both the IPAP and EPAP at the same time. In cases where an increase in IPAP only in response to hypopnea, RERA, or snoring, seems to lead directly to arousals, a decrease in IPAP alone may be considered. An attempt to monitor the patient in stage R sleep while supine is important during a BPAP titration as well. Figure 48-7 provides a sample flowchart for performing a BPAP titration.

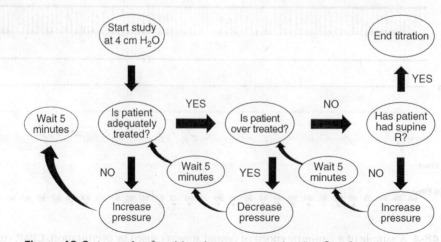

Figure 48-6 A sample of positive airway pressure titration flowchart.

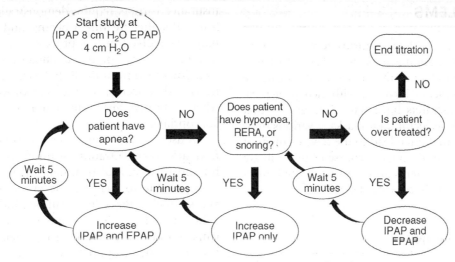

Figure 48-7 Sample bilevel positive airway pressure titration flowchart. EPAP, expiratory positive airway pressure; IPAP, inspiratory positive airway pressure; RERA, respiratory effort–related arousal.

Supplemental Oxygen

Supplemental oxygen should be added to the PAP titration in accordance with physician instructions and the Policy and Procedure manual for the center. For many centers, this occurs if the patient is awake, in the supine position, and the SpO_2 is less than 88%. During the titration, in the absence of obstructive respiratory events, oxygen may be added when the SpO_2 is less than 88% for more than 5 minutes. In both situations, oxygen should be initiated at 1 L per minute and titrated upward to achieve a SpO_2 range of 88% to 94%. O_2 should be increased by 1 L per minute with at least a 15-minute time interval. The minimum starting O_2 rate should be 1 L per minute for both pediatric and adult patients (1).

ALTERNATIVE PAP PLATFORMS

Advances in technology have led to the development of several new PAP devices. Most of these build on the BPAP platform and provide changes in applied pressure that result from measured changes in flow. BPAP decreases applied pressure when patient expiration is detected. Flex-PAP or pressure relief provides a brief decrease in pressure when expiration is detected and, in some patients, may feel more comfortable than CPAP. Auto-titrating positive airway pressure (APAP) therapy devices detect periods of apnea and hypopnea and increase pressure for a time in response.

APAP has been approved for several uses by the AASM:

1. In some centers, APAP is used to titrate pressure during an attended sleep study, with a final fixed CPAP determined for home use.

2. APAP can be used as a treatment device by patients requiring changes in pressure as determined by the device.
3. APAP may be used by the patient at home and a fixed pressure determined on the basis of the information stored in the device. It is recommended that patients using APAP be evaluated on a regular basis to ensure that the treatment is adequate (7).

APAP devices have not been tested and therefore should not be used in OSA patients with significant comorbidities such as chronic obstructive pulmonary disease, in patients with central sleep apnea, or in patients who do not snore. There are several devices that provide auto-titration, and the parameters that can be changed vary from device to device. If APAP devices are used, centers are required to include auto-titration protocols as part of their Policy and Procedures manual.

Adaptive servo-ventilation (ASV) monitors breathing on a breath-by-breath basis and continuously modifies pressure in response to changes. The advantage of ASV over other PAP platforms is that it can respond to hypoventilation (decreased airflow without apnea). There are some data that suggest that ASV may be useful in patients with central apnea or Cheyne–Stokes breathing pattern because it may counteract the waxing and waning of airflow. Most sleep specialists recommend a trial of standard CPAP before switching to ASV and close monitoring of patients once they are on treatment (7).

Troubleshooting

Studies have shown that APAP results in final pressure settings that are not statistically different from attended titrations (6). However, an experienced technologist can have an important impact on treatment by resolving mask and tolerance problems during the night of PAP titration.

MASK PROBLEMS

The most common problem requiring technologist intervention during titration is mask leak. Each mask will have an *acceptable leak* value that arises mainly from the CO_2 port of the mask and increases with increasing pressure. Most manufacturers have published guides that identify acceptable leaks for their masks at various pressures. Two factors that often lead to the development of unacceptable leakages during the course of titration are movement-related problems and pressure-related problems. For further details, see Chapter 47.

HUMIDIFICATION

During normal breathing, room air is warmed, moistened, and cleaned in the nose before it is inhaled into the lungs. PAP devices push air quickly through the nose and sinuses, which can prevent the usual warming, moistening, and cleaning. This often results in a sensation of cold and dryness in the throat for patients using PAP, which is especially problematic in areas where the air is already cold and dry. Saliva production is decreased during sleep and heated humidification is particularly necessary when using a full-face mask. It is important to have adequate humidification to reduce patient arousals and complaints caused by a dry mouth. A heated humidification unit, which is available as an add-on to PAP devices, is typically a "pass over" device in which the air going to the patient passes over a pool of warmed water. The temperature of the water must be regulated to avoid excessive warming and humidification, which causes water to pool in the tubing that connects the machine to the PAP interface.

After the heated humidification process occurs at the PAP device, the air must travel 6 to 8 ft (1.8 to 2.4 m) through a plastic tube before it reaches the mask. If tubing is exposed to room air, it will cool during its journey. Cooling can be reduced by directing the tubing under the bedcovers or by wrapping the tubing in a sheath. Tubing sheaths come in various materials and colors and may provide some benefit for patients. In addition, some manufacturers have developed heated tubing, which has served to improve adherence in some patients.

FOLLOW-UP

Technologists should be involved in the sleep center's efforts to improve PAP adherence. Studies have shown that early intervention may be the most effective method for improving adherence to therapy. Some insurance carriers require demonstration of adherence 3 months after treatment begins, and the technologist may be involved in this process as well. Key elements of follow-up include documentation of usage (usually by a download from the PAP device), response to questions and concerns, replacement of masks and tubing when indicated, and a discussion of alternatives when appropriate.

A useful quality improvement exercise is to provide feedback to the titration technologist on the successful and unsuccessful treatment of patients. Over time, it is possible to evaluate the effectiveness of policies and strategies. Procedures can be modified to improve adherence—keep doing what works and stop doing what doesn't work. Working together, the sleep center team can provide optimal treatment for patients. Proper titration, appropriate equipment adjustments, and timely follow-up are key elements of the evaluation and treatment of patients with OSA.

REFERENCES

1. Kushida, C. A., Chediak, A., Berry, R. B., et al. (2008). Clinical guidelines for the manual titration of positive airway pressure in patients with obstructive sleep apnea. *Journal of Clinical Sleep Medicine, 4*(2), 157–171.
2. Budhiraja, R., Parthasarathy, S., Drake, C. L., et al. (2007). Early CPAP use identifies subsequent adherence to CPAP therapy. *Sleep, 30*(3), 320–324.
3. Epstein, L. J., Kristo, D., Strollo, P. J., Jr., et al. (2009). Clinical guideline for the evaluation, management and long-term care of obstructive sleep apnea in adults. *Journal of Clinical Sleep Medicine, 5*(3), 263–276.
4. Kushida, C. A., Littner, M. R., Morgenthaler, T., et al. (2005). Practice parameters for the indications for polysomnography and related procedures: An update for 2005. *Sleep, 28*(4), 499–521.
5. Berry, R. B., Albertario, C. L., Harding, S. M., et al. (2018). *The AASM manual for the scoring of sleep and associated events: Rules, terminology and technical specifications.* Version 2.5. Darien, IL: American Academy of Sleep Medicine.
6. American Academy of Sleep Medicine. (2014). *International classification of sleep disorders* (3rd ed.). Darien, IL: Author.
7. Morgenthaler, T. I., Aurora, R. N., Brown, T., et al. (2008). Practice parameters for the use of autotitrating continuous positive airway pressure devices for titrating pressures and treating adult patients with obstructive sleep apnea syndrome: An update for 2007. *Sleep, 31*(1), 141–147.

chapter 49

Advanced Positive Airway Pressure Therapies for Sleep-Disordered Breathing

ZACK FREEMAN   SAAD S. AHMAD

LEARNING OBJECTIVES

On completion of this chapter, the reader should be able to:

1. Understand the fundamentals of advanced positive airway pressure devices used in the sleep center setting: adaptive servo-ventilation, spontaneous timed, and volume-assured pressure support.
2. Recognize the indications and limitations of these therapy modes.
3. Understand the operation and algorithm for the titration of both ResMed and Philips Respironics model devices.

KEY TERMS

Central sleep apnea syndrome (CSAS)
Congestive heart failure (CHF)
Sleep-related hypoventilation disorder
Adaptive servo-ventilation (ASV)
Variable-assured pressure support (VAPS)
Spontaneous timed (ST)
Spontaneous breathing
Minute ventilation (MV)
Alveolar ventilation (Va)

INDICATIONS FOR ADVANCED POSITIVE AIRWAY PRESSURE THERAPY MODES

Positive airway pressure (PAP) technology has advanced drastically since continuous positive airway pressure (CPAP) was first offered as a treatment for sleep-disordered breathing (SDB) in 1983 (1, 2). One of the many reasons for these advancements is the increase in the understanding of SDB. Conditions that were once frustrating and baffling to both sleep technologists and physicians are now treatable by specific PAP therapy

modes utilizing advancements in technology and algorithms (2). This chapter focuses on advanced PAP therapy modes applicable to a typical sleep disorders center: adaptive servo-ventilation (ASV), volume-assured pressure support (VAPS), and spontaneous timed (ST). This chapter will cover the indications for their use and the specific devices used in the sleep disorders center at the time of this writing. The two manufacturers of these advanced PAP devices, ResMed and Philips Respironics, each offer training and documentation with every major release in technology; however, the mode types and principles of their instructions have been consistent since their development. The technologist must have a clear understanding of each modality and their indications to properly perform testing using these therapies.

ASV for Central Sleep Apnea Syndrome

ASV is a PAP therapy mode specifically intended for central sleep apnea syndrome (CSAS) (3). The *International Classification of Sleep Disorders (ICSD) 3* identifies eight different forms of central sleep apnea (CSA): Central Sleep Apnea with Cheyne–Stokes Breathing, Central Apnea Due to Medical Disorder without Cheyne–Stokes Breathing, Central Sleep Apnea Due to High-Altitude Periodic Breathing, Central Sleep Apnea Due to Medication or Substance, Primary Central Sleep Apnea, Primary Sleep Apnea of Infancy, Primary Sleep Apnea of Prematurity, and Treatment-Emergent Central Sleep Apnea (4). CSAS is described thoroughly in Chapter 13. ASV was first introduced by ResMed and was first validated as a treatment for CSAS with Cheyne–Stokes breathing in 2001 (5). Philips Respironics soon produced their own version (2, 6). By 2012, ASV was an American Academy of Sleep Medicine (AASM)-recommended treatment option (7). Before the availability of ASV, treatment of CSAS was especially difficult. CPAP, bilevel positive airway pressure (BPAP), BPAP ST, and oxygen therapy were long-standing treatment options for CSAS with varying levels of success (2, 8). The primary function of ASV is to respond to irregular ventilation caused by CSA to maintain proper respiration. ASV is indicated only for CSA (2, 3, 5–7).

VAPS for Hypoventilation Syndromes

VAPS is a type of PAP therapy that is applicable to patients diagnosed with hypoventilation disorders (9, 10). Sleep-related hypoventilation disorders include Obesity Hypoventilation Syndrome, Congenital Alveolar Hypoventilation Syndrome, Late-Onset Central Hypoventilation with Hypothalamic Dysfunction, Idiopathic Central Alveolar Hypoventilation, Sleep-Related Hypoventilation Due to a medication or Substance, and Sleep-Related Hypoventilation Due to a Medical Disorder (4). Therefore, indication for VAPS in the sleep center setting may include patients with diagnosed chronic hypoventilation syndromes such as neuromuscular/restrictive disorders, chronic obstructive pulmonary disorder, or obesity hypoventilation. There is a full explanation of obesity hypoventilation syndromes in Chapter 14. Although there are many similar terms and setting descriptions between ASV and VAPS, the two modalities are not interchangeable (10, 11). VAPS uses variable pressure support to achieve a target tidal volume (Vt), in contrast to ASV that performs a quick constant breath-by-breath response and does not augment the patient's Vt consistently (10, 11). VAPS is an AASM-recommended option for chronic hypoventilation patients receiving PAP therapy adjustment in the sleep center (12).

BPAP ST Mode for Hypoventilation Syndromes

BPAP ST mode refers to a BPAP with an added backup inspiratory rate. Like VAPS, it is indicated for SDB in patients with chronic alveolar hypoventilation syndrome (13, 14). The ST mode can be applied to standard BPAP or VAPS modes, and AASM guidelines recommend its use in patients with alveolar hypoventilation syndromes with central hypoventilation, with a significant number of central apneas or an inappropriately low respiratory rate (RR), and who unreliably trigger inspiration PAP (IPAP)/expiration PAP (EPAP) cycles because of muscle weakness (15). It is also enabled in ASV mode and assists the ASV algorithm with resolving central apnea (3). Regular BPAP in ST mode is not indicated for the treatment of CSAS; however, there is a history of the mode being used for that purpose and it is listed within AASM guidelines as an optional treatment modality when ASV, CPAP, and oxygen therapies are exhausted (15).

FUNDAMENTALS OF THERAPEUTIC MODES

Adaptive Servo-Ventilation

In contrast to standard BPAP that provides static IPAP and EPAP, ASV delivers variable inspiratory pressure support to maintain respiration (3). Although auto CPAP and auto BPAP have varying pressure outputs, those modes increase or decrease on the basis of the detection of upper airway obstruction. ASV uses an algorithm to detect unstable ventilation and compensate with a variable pressure support. Pressure support is the amount of inspiratory pressure above the exhalation pressure. For example, consider a standard BPAP set to IPAP 10/EPAP 6, that is, the expiratory pressure is 6 cm, and the inspiratory pressure is 10 cm. Therefore, the pressure support (Ps) is 4 cm (EPAP 6 cm + 4 cm Ps = 10 cm IPAP). This term is sometimes interchangeable with delta (Δ) pressure, or delta P (ΔP).

Both the Philips Respironics version of ASV, called BiPAP autoSV Advanced, and the ResMed version, VPAP Adapt SV Advanced, follow the same general principle explained in the preceding paragraph, but have different proprietary algorithms.

The BiPAP autoSV monitors the inspiratory peak flow rate (IPFR) of the patient on a breath-by-breath basis. IPFR is the highest amount of liters per minute (L/min) inhaled during a respiratory cycle. Every 4 minutes of monitoring, the device calculates an average peak flow for the patient. This is regarded as a moving 4-minute window, because the most current data continuously override previous data. Once this average peak flow is calculated, the device delivers pressure support to compensate for breathing that falls short of the average peak flow on a per-breath basis. By default, the devices provide an ST backup rate that synchronizes with the patient's spontaneous breathing; however, the setting can be overridden and set to a specific rate. Because a patient's SDB often includes an obstructive component even when predominantly central in nature, the ASV models must also be able to compensate for obstruction. The EPAP can be set to a static setting or an auto setting, in which the EPAP uses Philips Respironics–patented auto PAP algorithm to increase and decrease pressure according to the detection of upper airway obstruction (16).

The ResMed VPAP Adapt SV Advanced algorithm differs in that rather than focusing on peak flow rate, its algorithm focuses on minute ventilation (MV). MV is the total amount of air that moves in and out of the ventilation system, and it is calculated by multiplying the RR by Vt. The device monitors MV on a breath-by-breath basis and uses a moving 3-minute window of monitoring to calculate target MV. The device then delivers pressure support to compensate for breathing that falls short of the target MV. VPAP Adapt SV Advanced incorporates an ST backup rate somewhat differently than its Philips Respironics counterpart. The backup rate is set to a minimum 15 breaths per minute (BPM) and is not adjustable by the clinician. The rate may occur during the first 3 minutes of therapy. The EPAP can be set to a static setting or an auto setting, in which the EPAP uses ResMed-patented auto PAP algorithm to increase and decrease pressure according to the detection of upper airway obstruction (17).

Volume-Assured Pressure Support

Like ASV, VAPS delivers variable inspiratory pressure support to maintain respiration. However, the algorithms and intended purposes are much different. VAPS uses its algorithm to detect insufficient volume or ventilation and compensate with a variable pressure support. Key to the ability of VAPS to adequately perform its function is the input of applicable patient parameters by the technologist performing the titration, so that the algorithm of the device can properly calculate the target volume or ventilation (11, 18). Because the respiratory needs of a patient with hypoventilation can vary through the night, this type of PAP is often helpful for these patients because it is able to constantly adapt throughout the night. These needs can vary significantly according to body position, sleep stage, or sleep versus wake for patients required to use PAP during the day because of the severity of disease (2).

The two versions of VAPS devices available to the sleep center are the ResMed intelligent volume-assured pressure support (iVAPS) mode and the Philips Respironics average volume assured pressure support (AVAPS). ResMed iVAPS utilizes an algorithm on the basis of a target alveolar volume set by the clinician (2). Alveolar volume is inspired air that reaches the alveoli. The volume of inspired air that does not reach the alveoli is referred to as "dead space ventilation." The dead space gas in the conducting airways (the nose, mouth, pharynx, larynx, and lower airways down to, but not including, the respiratory bronchioles) is referred to as "anatomic dead space." The iVAPS algorithm calculates alveolar ventilation by measuring the volume of each breath and subtracting an approximated value of anatomic dead space. From this, a continuous estimate of alveolar ventilation is calculated, and pressure support is then appropriately applied to achieve this target. With Philips Respironics AVAPS, the algorithm depends on a set target Vt (2). Vt is the volume of air that normally moves into and out of the lungs in one quiet breath. The set Vt can be input by the clinician according to ordering provider suggestion, patient comfort, or ideal body weight. Both devices may incorporate ideal body weight into their settings and calculations. The device manufacturer recommends that ideal body weight in kilograms be multiplied by 6 mL per kg (ResMed) or 8 mL per kg (Philips Respironics) to find a target Vt setting (2).

ST Mode

ST mode is a combination of spontaneous mode and timed mode. Spontaneous mode is the term commonly referred to as BPAP. The term "spontaneous" refers to the fact that the patient's own natural breathing triggers the change from EPAP to IPAP. Timed mode refers to a set rate in BPM that triggers the change from EPAP to IPAP. Timed mode would be applicable to patients completely unable to initiate a breath without the assistance of the device. ST then is a combination of the two methods: the patient's natural breathing triggers the change from EPAP to IPAP, unless the patient's natural breathing rate falls below a rate set by the clinician. The rate set during ST mode is referred to as a backup rate, because the timed function is essentially a backup used when the patient's natural breathing falls below a certain rate (19).

CONTRADICTIONS, LIMITATIONS, AND ALTERNATIVES

CSAS has several pathologies, including heart failure. Heart failure is characterized by the heart's inability to pump an adequate supply of blood to the body. Congestive heart failure (CHF) refers to the stage in which fluid builds up around the heart and causes it to pump inefficiently. Severity of CHF is commonly determined by left ventricular ejection fraction (LVEF). LVEF is the percentage of blood that is pumped out of a filled left ventricle with each heart beat. In 2015, a clinical trial called the *Treatment of Predominant Central Sleep Apnoea by Adaptive Servo Ventilation in Patients with Heart Failure (SERVE-HF)* tested the hypothesis that ASV would reduce incidences of heart failure such as all-cause mortality, life-saving cardiovascular interventions, or unplanned hospitalizations for worsening heart failure. The trial was, however, cut short after a discovery that ASV treatment caused a 34% increase in cardiovascular mortality in heart failure patients with a reduced ejection fraction. These findings resulted in ResMed, who had funded the trial, issuing a Field Safety Notice that same year stating that ASV therapy is contraindicated in patients with CHF with an LVEF equal to or less than 45%. Two possible explanations were suggested by the study. One is a theory that has been previously suggested, that CSA may be a compensatory mechanism for patients with heart failure. Another is that PAP can impair cardiac function in certain heart failure patients (20).

This new information led to an update of AASM CSAS treatment guidelines in 2016 regarding the implementation of ASV for patients with heart failure. The updated guidelines state that ASV for the treatment of CSAS related to CHF *should not be used in adults with an ejection fraction equal to or less than 45%*, and *can be used for the treatment of CSAS related to CHF in adults with an ejection fraction over 45%*. ASV is still recommended for CSAS not related to heart failure (Fig. 49-1) (15).

In the sleep lab setting, it is, of course, ideal that a comprehensive policy and procedure manual and

ASV is an appropriate modality for patients with moderate to severe predominantly central sleep apnea who *do not have heart failure*. The following are steps to assess patients for ASV therapy:

- Verify the patient is not at risk for heart failure (HF).
  - Does the patient have signs or symptoms of heart failure?
  - Is there a history of cardiovascular disease?
  - Does the patient take medications used to treat heart failure?
- Consider an echocardiogram to determine left ventricular ejection fraction (LVEF) if there is any suspicion of heart failure.

ASV can also be used appropriately *in some patients with possible or definite heart failure with a documented LVEF of > 45%*. Cardiology assessment is essential including an echocardiogram to assess LVEF.

ASV is **not** appropriate for use in patients with heart failure with a documented left ventricular ejection fraction (LVEF) of ≤ 45%. Cardiology assessment is essential including an echocardiogram to document the LVEF.

Figure 49-1 Assessment of patients with moderate to severe predominant central sleep apnea for consideration for ASV therapy.

thorough patient history exist, leaving the technologist with a clear course of action for patients with CSAS. ResMed's sleep lab titration guide contains a flowchart that may be useful to the technologist lacking a clear direction (13).

Guidelines for the treatment of CSAS related to heart failure indicate ASV for patients failing an initial trial of CPAP and BPAP ST as an optional treatment if there is no response to adequate trials of CPAP, ASV, and oxygen therapies. Oxygen therapy is an indicated treatment for CSAS related to CHF. Of note, these guidelines explain that in studies testing the effectiveness of CPAP and BPAP in CSAS, BPAP ST has been used more frequently; however, data that support BPAP ST being more than just an optional treatment (or not) are limited (15).

Treatment of CHF, including pharmaceutical treatment, is recommended for CSAS related to heart failure in any case. AASM guidelines state that acetazolamide and theophylline, if accompanied by close clinical follow-up and after optimization of standard medical therapy, are options for the treatment of CSAS related to CHF if PAP therapy is not tolerated (15).

VAPS is not recommended for patients with CSAS. Treatment of CSAS requires a variable, breath-by-breath response, so that respiration stabilizes quickly. Breath-by-breath response prevents overshooting or undershooting; VAPS does not have this quick variable response to changes in respiration. It is designed to adjust and maintain a constant Vt with each breath over time (11).

ASV is not recommended to address chronic hypoventilation or for patients with neuromuscular disease having sleep-related hypoventilation. ASV's frequent variable adaptation to respiration is not designed for hypoventilation and could potentially worsen the occurrence as the night progresses (11).

CONCLUSION

The advancement of PAP technology, as well as clinical research and understanding of sleep-related breathing disorders over the past decade, has been vast. This allows sleep clinicians to treat patients and improve quality of life in ways not possible in the past. As technology continues to advance, manufacturers of the said technology strive to provide training for sleep medicine professionals to keep them up to date in advancements. It is the responsibility of the sleep technologist to ensure that they have a sound understanding of the fundamentals of these technologies. Thorough knowledge of key respiratory principles and terminology and the PAP settings that affect these is required. The greater the understanding, the more prepared the technologist will be to provide exceptional patient care.

REFERENCES

1. Sullivan, C. E., Issa, F. G., Berthon-Jones, M., et al. (1981). Reversal of obstructive sleep apnoea by continuous positive airway pressure applied through the nares. *Lancet, 1*(8225), 862–865.
2. Johnson, K. G., & Johnson, D. C. (2015). Treatment of sleep-disordered breathing with positive airway pressure devices: Technology update. *Medical Devices (Auckl), 8*, 425.
3. Javaheri, S., Brown, L. K., & Randerath, W. J. (2014). Positive airway pressure therapy with adaptive servoventilation: Part 1: Operational algorithms. *Chest, 146*(2), 514–523.
4. American Academy of Sleep Medicine. (2014). *International classification of sleep disorders—Third edition (ICSD-3)*. Darien, IL: Author.

5. Teschler, H., Döhring, J., Wang, Y. M., et al. (2001). Adaptive pressure support servo-ventilation: A novel treatment for Cheyne-Stokes respiration in heart failure. *American Journal of Respiratory and Critical Care Medicine, 164*(4), 614–619.

6. Allam, J. S., Olson, E. J., Gay, P. C., et al. (2007). Efficacy of adaptive servoventilation in treatment of complex and central sleep apnea syndromes. *Chest, 132*(6), 1839–1846.

7. Aurora, R. N., Chowdhuri, S., Ramar, K., et al. (2012). The treatment of central sleep apnea syndromes in adults: Practice parameters with an evidence-based literature review and meta-analyses. *Sleep, 35*(1), 17–40.

8. Verbraecken, J. (2013). Complex sleep apnoea syndrome. *Breathe, 9*(5), 372–380.

9. Oscroft, N. S., & Smith, I. E. (2010). A bench test to confirm the core features of volume-assured non-invasive ventilation. *Respirology, 15*(2), 361–364.

10. Selim, B. J., Wolfe, L., Coleman, J. M., et al. (2018). Initiation of noninvasive ventilation for sleep related hypoventilation disorders: Advanced modes and devices. *Chest, 153*(1), 251–265.

11. Philips Respironics. (2018). *Using advanced techniques to maximize PAP therapy: Clinical applications.* Retrieved from http://incenter.medical.philips.com/doclib/enc/9792335/bipapautosvadvanced_protocol.pdf%3ffunc%3ddoc.fetch%26nodeid%3d9792335. Accessed June 17, 2018.

12. Berry, R. B., Chediak, A., Brown, L. K., et al.; NPPV Titration Task Force of the American Academy of Sleep Medicine. (2010). Best clinical practices for the sleep center adjustment of noninvasive positive pressure ventilation (NPPV) in stable chronic alveolar hypoventilation syndromes. *Journal of Clinical Sleep Medicine, 6*(5), 491.

13. Philips Respironics. (2018). *Titration protocol reference guide.* Accessed June 17, 2018.

14. Aurora, R. N., Bista, S. R., Casey, K. R., et al. (2016). Updated adaptive servo-ventilation recommendations for the 2012 AASM guideline: "The treatment of central sleep apnea syndromes in adults: Practice parameters with an evidence-based literature review and meta-analyses". *Journal of Clinical Sleep Medicine, 12*(5), 757.

15. ResMed. (2017). *Sleep lab titration guide.* Retrieved from https://www.resmed.com/us/dam/documents/products/titration/s9-vpap-tx/user-guide/1013904_Sleep_Lab_Titration_Guide_amer_eng.pdf. Accessed June 17, 2018.

16. Philips Respironics. (2018). *Advanced algorithms—Clinical applications.* Accessed June 17, 2018.

17. Thomson, R., Richards G. N., & Woehrle, H. (2012). *Pacewave therapy: An overview of minute ventilation targeted adaptive servo-ventilation (MV ASV).* San Diego, CA: ResMed Science Center.

18. ResMed. (2013). *S9 VPAP^TM ST-A with iVAPS.* San Diego, CA: ResMed. Retrieved from https://www.resmed.com/us/en/consumer/products/devices/s9-vpap-st-a-with-ivaps.html. Accessed June 17, 2018.

19. Ayvazian, L. F. (Ed.). (1988). *Cardiopulmonary anatomy & physiology: Essentials for respiratory care.*

20. Cowie, M. R., Woehrle, H., Wegscheider, K., et al. (2015). Adaptive servo-ventilation for central sleep apnea in systolic heart failure. *New England Journal of Medicine, 373*(12), 1095–1105. Retrieved from https://www.resmed.com/us/en/serve-hf.html

chapter 50

Noninvasive Ventilation in Patients with Respiratory or Neuromuscular Disease

JOHN SEYMOUR

LEARNING OBJECTIVES

On completion of this chapter, the reader should be able to:

1. List the two main types of lung disease and how they impact breathing.
2. Describe the purpose of noninvasive ventilation (NIV) and how it works.
3. Discuss the goals for delivering NIV to a patient with a respiratory or neuromuscular disease.
4. Define modes, settings, and other terms used to implement NIV.
5. Describe the relationship between carbon dioxide levels and ventilation.
6. Discuss the relationship of tidal volume and respiratory rate to alveolar ventilation.
7. Discuss new technologies that can be utilized to track therapy and automatically adjust settings to maintain a desired level of ventilation.

KEY TERMS

Noninvasive ventilation (NIV)
Obstructive sleep apnea (OSA)
Restrictive thoracic disorder
Amyotrophic lateral sclerosis (ALS)
Muscular dystrophy (MD)
Obesity hypoventilation syndrome (OHS)
Chronic obstructive pulmonary disease (COPD)
Continuous positive airway pressure (CPAP)
Inspiration
Expiration
Respiratory rate
Tidal volume
Dead space
Minute ventilation
Alveolar minute ventilation
Hyperventilation
Hypoventilation
Hypocapnia
Hypercapnia

Sleep technologists will see a wide range of patients coming into the sleep laboratory for diagnosis and treatment. These patients will range in complexity from simple obstructive sleep apnea (OSA) patients to complex patients exhibiting periodic breathing. Somewhere in between these extremes of the sleep-disordered breathing spectrum will be those patients with some form of underlying lung disease. Some of these patients will also have the complication of upper airway obstruction.

Respiratory therapists often categorize lung disease into two main types of disease processes. These are restrictive and obstructive disorders. Recognizing the differences in these disease processes will aid the sleep technologist in understanding how noninvasive ventilation (NIV) is used to improve the quality of sleep and life for patients with these diseases.

RESTRICTIVE THORACIC DISORDERS

The term "restrictive thoracic disorder" is used instead of restrictive lung disease because most of the diseases in this category are not really disorders of the lung. These disorders normally involve some problem with the thorax or chest. These patients may have relatively normal healthy lungs but still have a problem breathing. These disorders are characterized by processes that limit the patient's ability to take a normal-sized breath, something that "restricts" the ability to inspire fully. A few of the more common types of restrictive disorders are discussed in the following paragraphs.

Amyotrophic lateral sclerosis (ALS), also known as Lou Gehrig disease, is an example of a restrictive disorder. This disease is characterized by a gradual destruction of motor neurons in the brain and spinal cord. As these motor neurons are gradually destroyed, the patient loses the ability to move voluntarily, speak, swallow, and breathe. Because this is a progressive disease, it is also an excellent example illustrating the need for monitoring therapy after initiation and then adjusting therapy as needed. These patients will get worse after they are seen in the sleep laboratory and their therapy may need to be adjusted to manage their weakening condition.

Muscular dystrophy is the name for a group of genetically inherited muscle diseases that are characterized by a loss of muscle protein. This loss of muscle protein weakens the muscle to the extent that it can no longer do its assigned task. This is also a progressive disorder like ALS and may lead to inability to perform activities of daily living and could ultimately lead to breathing difficulty as the muscles of breathing become affected.

Obesity hypoventilation syndrome (OHS) is another type of disorder that exhibits restrictive characteristics. Patients with this disorder are obese and exhibit daytime alveolar hypoventilation. These patients do not have chronic obstructive pulmonary disease (COPD) as a cause of their alveolar hypoventilation. Consequences of this daytime alveolar hypoventilation include hypercapnia and hypoxemia. The mechanisms causing the hypoventilation are complex and involve reduced chest wall compliance, impaired respiratory drive, and severe OSA. Treatment of the OSA component with continuous positive airway pressure (CPAP) is beneficial to these patients, but if they continue to have persistent hypercapnia and oxygen desaturation, then bilevel therapy or NIV may have to be utilized (1).

All of these patients with restrictive lung disease have the potential to have difficulty maintaining a normal level of ventilation while they are awake. These patients lose voluntary control of ventilation when sleeping and their breathing can become compromised to the point where serious health consequences can occur.

OBSTRUCTIVE LUNG DISEASE

Unlike most of the restrictive thoracic disorders, obstructive lung disease does involve destructive changes to the lung tissue itself. Obstructive lung disease is more commonly known as COPD. COPD is not the only type of obstructive lung disease, but it is the most common one. COPD typically results from cigarette smoking or in some cases industrial exposure to dust or fumes. Asthma is also a type of obstructive lung disease.

Like OSA, there is an obstruction or airflow limitation occurring in these patients, but COPD is very different from OSA. It differs from OSA in two primary ways. The airflow limitation occurs during the expiratory phase of breathing instead of the inspiratory phase as is the case with OSA. The other way by which COPD differs from OSA is that the obstruction to flow occurs in the distal airways and alveoli of the lung instead of the upper airway. COPD is not diagnosed during a sleep study. It is diagnosed with a pulmonary function test called "spirometry."

These patients have trouble exhaling the air out of their lungs. In extreme cases, this will cause the patient to inhale before all the air in the previous breath is exhaled. This causes the patient to gradually hyperinflate his or her lungs over time. Eventually, the patient can get to the point where he or she can no longer inhale properly because there is no more room for air in the lungs.

The patient with COPD and OSA is referred to as an "overlap patient" and like the OHS patient will usually benefit from a resolution of OSA symptoms, but may still experience persistent hypercapnia and oxygen desaturations that may need to be treated using bilevel ventilation or NIV. The patient with COPD in need of NIV presents unique challenges to the sleep technologist. Although these patients need additional alveolar ventilation, the sleep technologist needs to be aware that these patients may present with significant airflow limitation, not on inspiration, but on expiration. It is not simply a matter of turning up the respiratory rate or increasing the amount of pressure delivered in order to increase alveolar ventilation. Although it is always important to deliver the properly sized breath to a patient, in COPD patients with hyperinflated lungs, it is just as important to allow the breath to be exhaled.

NONINVASIVE VENTILATION

NIV has been used successfully for decades in acute care environments to assist patients to avoid intubation in cases of acute respiratory failure. The evidence for using NIV for the successful treatment of chronic respiratory failure caused by neuromuscular disease in home care environments is also well documented. The use of NIV to treat chronic respiratory failure due to COPD has been the focus of several recent studies. The practice of placing these COPD patients on minimal levels of NIV is changing. The focus of recent studies into the use of NIV with COPD patients has been on the use of higher pressures, or high-intensity NIV, in order to increase ventilation to the point where carbon dioxide (CO_2) reductions in blood gasses are produced (2).

One of the main differences in the use of NIV in the acute care environment and for chronic care at home is the different quality of monitoring and intervention by trained health care professionals. This makes the initial setup and effective titration of NIV in the sleep laboratory all the more critical to the successful treatment of the patient with chronic respiratory failure in the home environment. The patient who has an OSA component in addition to chronic respiratory failure has two strikes against him or her when he or she sleeps. Although eliminating the upper airway component is always helpful, these patients will often require the assistance of NIV to mitigate the impact of their chronic respiratory condition on their sleep, health, and quality of life.

GOALS OF NIV TREATMENT

The goal of NIV is to reduce the work of breathing and to normalize or improve the patient's blood gasses. It does not matter if the patient has a restrictive or obstructive disorder; the goal is the same. There are some subtle differences in how NIV is applied for these disorders, but the goal remains the same. Complete normalization of blood gasses is not always attained, but reducing the work of breathing is essential and if not attained it is less likely that the patient will be compliant with the therapy. The consequences of a lack of compliance with NIV therapy can be worse than CPAP noncompliance. If the patients don't use the therapy, there is no benefit.

Anyone who routinely initiates and titrates NIV on patients should experience it for themselves, at least briefly, so they can better relate to what patients feel like. NIV uses pressure support to provide ventilation. Properly adjusted pressure support therapy should follow the patient's breathing pattern and provide assistance with inspiration and allow for comfortable exhalation. Most patients should be able to control both their respiratory rate and tidal volume if the therapy is titrated properly. Easing the work of breathing for someone is one of the most rewarding things a clinician can do.

BASICS OF NORMAL VENTILATION

The basics of normal ventilation should be reviewed before delving into the details of treatment methods. Knowing what is normal ventilation is important before attempting to bring the patient back toward normal ventilation. Some of the terms the clinician should be familiar with include the following: inspiration, expiration, respiratory rate, tidal volume, dead space, minute ventilation, and alveolar minute ventilation.

INSPIRATION

In normal healthy people, *inspiration* is achieved when the diaphragm contracts. This causes the diaphragm to flatten out and drop down in the chest cavity. The result is that the amount of space or available volume in the chest cavity increases. This increase in space causes the pressure in the chest to decrease. If the upper airway is not obstructed, then air will move from outside the chest to fill the lungs. The diaphragm is the primary muscle involved in breathing, but the diaphragm can be supplemented by the use of accessory muscles in the chest to help elevate the rib cage upward and outward to further increase the dimensions of the chest cavity, thus creating more negative pressure to draw more air into the lungs.

EXPIRATION

Expiration is normally passive, with the elastic nature of the diaphragm and lungs providing the recoil to push air out of the lungs. Like inspiration, expiration can also be supplemented by the use of accessory muscles if necessary to facilitate expiration. This is most commonly seen in obstructive lung disease where the distal airways collapse and trap air in the lungs. Patients with obstructive lung disease have to work to inhale and to exhale. They have to actively *push* air out of their lungs in addition to the normal work of breathing to inhale. These patients expend a great deal of energy on just breathing.

RESPIRATORY RATE

The number of times a person breathes each minute is his or her *respiratory rate*. Respiratory rate can vary from person to person, according to their metabolic needs at the time. Normal respiratory rates are about 10 to 12 breaths per minute.

TIDAL VOLUME

The amount of air that is drawn into the lungs on any single breath is called *tidal volume*. The size of the tidal volume can vary greatly from person to person on the basis of his or her size and metabolic activity. Normal tidal volumes are in the range of 6 to 8 mL per kg of body weight. Higher tidal volumes delivered by NIV may be uncomfortable, whereas lower tidal volumes are not efficient for achieving alveolar ventilation.

DEAD SPACE

A portion of each inhaled tidal volume does not participate in gas exchange. This portion of the breath is called *dead space*. There are two types of dead space. Every person has a certain amount of anatomic dead space. This space comprises the larger airways in the lungs and portions of the upper airway. On inspiration, this dead space is the last portion of air from outside of the body that can't reach the gas exchange areas. On expiration, the anatomic dead space is flushed out and filled with air leaving the alveoli. This air has a high CO_2 content and is then pulled back into the alveoli on the next inspiration. The average person has about 150 mL of anatomic dead space (2). Of course, larger people will have larger amount of dead space volumes and smaller people will have smaller dead space volumes.

The other type of dead space is known as "physiologic dead space." This is air that is inhaled and *does* reach the areas where gas exchange is supposed to occur, but for some reason does not fully participate in gas exchange. Proper respiration relies on ventilation matching up with good blood flow to the lungs. Mismatches of ventilation to perfusion can lead to increased amounts of dead space. Physiologic dead space is more of an issue in obstructive lung disorders than it is with restrictive lung disorders. Physiologic dead space is difficult to calculate and in any event it is not always necessary to know what the volume of physiologic dead space is in order to provide adequate therapy.

MINUTE VENTILATION

A person's average tidal volume multiplied by his or her respiratory rate determines his or her *minute ventilation*. Another way to describe minute ventilation is that it is all the air the patient moves in and out of his or her body in a minute.

ALVEOLAR VENTILATION/ALVEOLAR MINUTE VENTILATION

Alveolar ventilation is the effective ventilation. Once dead space is known, then alveolar ventilation is the next calculation that can be made. Alveolar ventilation is calculated simply by taking the tidal volume of the patient and subtracting the dead space from it. This is the alveolar tidal volume. Multiply the alveolar tidal volume by the respiratory rate to determine the alveolar minute ventilation.

RELATIONSHIP OF TIDAL VOLUME TO ALVEOLAR MINUTE VENTILATION

The average amount of anatomic dead space and its relationship to alveolar minute ventilation becomes important when considering assisting a person's breathing with mechanical ventilation. There are numerous ways to get to an adequate level of alveolar ventilation. Start with delivery of an adequate tidal volume that is comfortable to the patient and then assure that this tidal volume is provided at the correct frequency. That frequency or breath rate should be sufficient to provide the minimum alveolar minute ventilation for that patient. See Figures 50-1 and 50-2 for an illustration of the importance of tidal volume and the impact to alveolar ventilation.

These changes to tidal volume and rate have not changed minute ventilation, but in reality, the alveolar ventilation has been reduced by 10% and a rise in CO_2

$$450 \text{ mL} \times 10 \text{ bpm} = 4.5 \text{ L/min}$$

$$\frac{-150 \text{ mL dead space}}{300 \text{ mL} \times 10} = 3.0 \text{ L/min alveolar ventilation}$$

Figure 50-1 The example assumes that the patient weighs 70 kg. A tidal volume of 450 mL would be equal to 6.4 mL per kg of body weight, which is in the normal range for tidal volumes (6 to 8 mL per kg). Delivery of 450 mL would yield a minute ventilation of 4.5 L per minute, but if the anatomic dead space is considered, the effective tidal volume is only 300 mL per breath. The display on the device might indicate a minute ventilation of 4.5 L per minute, but the effective level of ventilation is actually less because of the impact of anatomic dead space.

$$375 \text{ mL} \times 12 \text{ bpm} = 4.5 \text{ L/min}$$

$$\frac{-150 \text{ mL dead space}}{225 \text{ mL} \times 12} = 2.7 \text{ L/min alveolar ventilation}$$

Figure 50-2 If the same 70 kg patient is ventilated with a smaller tidal volume, the impact to alveolar ventilation should be considered. Decreasing the delivered tidal volume to 375 mL and increasing the respiratory rate to 12 breaths per minute may still display a minute ventilation of 4.5 L per minute, but alveolar ventilation has actually decreased.

levels may occur as a result. It can get pretty confusing thinking in terms of alveolar ventilation, dead space, tidal volume, and minute ventilation. The simplest way to approach ventilation is to get the supported breath volume needed correct. Know the patient's weight and use the guideline of 6 to 8 mL per kg as a starting point for determining tidal volume. The tidal volume calculation is based on body size and there is no need to add any extra volume to account for anatomic dead space (see Table 50-1). Tidal volumes larger than 8 mL per kg should be avoided unless ordered by a physician. Larger tidal volumes may produce effective increases in alveolar ventilation and reductions in CO_2, but they do create a risk of discomfort and noncompliance with therapy (3).

CARBON DIOXIDE AND VENTILATION

The common thread between all types of lung disease is that these patients tend to have some degree of hypoventilation. Hypoventilation occurs when a patient either breathes too shallowly or too slowly to remove the CO_2 that he or she is producing. The end result is that CO_2 levels build up in their bodies, producing something called "hypercapnia," or elevated CO_2 levels.

Table 50-1 Conversion Table for Tidal Volume (Vt)

Height (m)	Calculated Ideal Weight (if BMI = 23) (kg)	Target Vt (mL) if 8 mL/kg	Target Vt (mL) if 10 mL/kg
1.50	52.0	410	520
1.55	55.0	440	550
1.60	59.0	470	590
1.65	62.5	500	620
1.70	66.5	530	660
1.75	70.5	560	700
1.80	74.5	600	740
1.85	78.5	630	780
1.90	83.0	660	830

Calculated with an ideal body mass index of 23 kg per m² (BMI = weight/height²).
Guidelines/values developed for use with Philips Respironics products only. Variations may occur with other manufacturers' products. Please consult specific manufacturers' guidelines for specific product information and operational guidelines.

Why is CO_2 so important? Think of CO_2 as the cellular metabolic by-product of life. All of our cells are busy all the time metabolizing or "burning" sugars to produce energy. One of the waste products of this process is CO_2. It is released from the cells into the bloodstream and is carried to the lungs where the lungs try to vent this CO_2 into the air that enters and leaves the lungs. Thinking of this CO_2 as "smoke" from the burning sugar will help in understanding why it is important for it to be removed from the body. When CO_2-rich blood reaches the lungs, it is passively transported from the lungs to the air sacs or alveoli. The lungs then need to exchange this CO_2-laden air with fresh air from outside the body in order to get rid of the CO_2. At a higher rate of ventilation, the CO_2 levels in the blood usually are lower. Conversely, if the amount of air being moved through the lungs is reduced, then the CO_2 level in the blood usually increases. Another way of stating this is that CO_2 levels in the blood are *inversely* proportional to ventilation. This is one of the most important concepts for fully understanding ventilation.

The normal range for CO_2 is between 35 and 45 mm Hg. Simply put, if the patient's measured CO_2 is above the normal range, then he or she is not getting enough alveolar ventilation or is hypoventilating (see Fig. 50-3). If the measured CO_2 is below the normal range, then the patient is getting too much alveolar ventilation or he or she is hyperventilating. Hyperventilation is unusual to see during sleep, except during periods of periodic breathing such as with Cheyne–Stokes respirations. Most of the time hypoventilation/hypercapnia will present clinically.

This brings the discussion full circle back to tidal volumes and the impact they have on alveolar ventilation and CO_2 levels. In critical care, it is common to have CO_2 levels readily available to the clinician with the use of arterial blood gas (ABG) analysis. Respiratory therapists rely heavily on CO_2 measurements to titrate and adjust ventilation. The clinician in the sleep laboratory seldom has access to ABG data. Special lab equipment and qualified clinicians are required to obtain the sample and perform ABG analysis. ABG blood draws are also very painful and would have a negative impact on sleep.

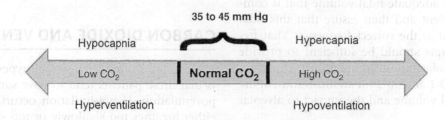

Figure 50-3 *Hypo*ventilation (low ventilation) is associated with *hyper*capnia (high CO_2), and *hyper*ventilation (high ventilation) is associated with *hypo*capnia (low CO_2).

Capnography, or end-tidal CO_2 readings, can be used to estimate what the CO_2 levels are in the blood, but they are never the same as ABG data. The accuracy of end-tidal CO_2 readings obtained during NIV is also impacted by the leak that is a normal component of NIV. Most NIV devices use a leak circuit, just like CPAP, instead of a closed circuit. Capnography may be useful to track how end-tidal CO_2 readings are trending, but clinicians should always be cautious when using capnography as a guide for titration during NIV.

Transcutaneous CO_2 readings are not impacted by the use of NIV and may be a more reliable measure of what the true CO_2 level is in the blood. It can be useful as a trending tool to see if CO_2 levels are decreasing as increases in ventilation are made during a NIV titration.

NONINVASIVE VENTILATION

NIV is the practice of delivering ventilatory assistance without the use of an endotracheal or tracheostomy tube. It is most often delivered via a nasal or full-face mask, but can also be delivered via a mouthpiece in some situations.

NIV or noninvasive positive pressure ventilation can lead to some confusion with terminology. This is compounded by the distinction that insurance providers make between the NIV devices that have the capability to provide a backup rate and those that do not. Discussions about NIV and NIV devices in this chapter will refer to those devices with the ability to deliver a backup breath in the absence of patient effort.

Most NIV devices are not intended to be used as life support devices. The patients who use them should be able to safely discontinue therapy with the device for short periods of time without harm. Some life support devices have NIV modes, but the use of an NIV device in those modes does not make the mode a life support mode.

Most NIV ventilators are designed to be used by adult patient populations and will have age and/or weight restrictions in their intended use statements. Pediatric patients will frequently be placed on life support ventilators that are approved for pediatric patients in NIV modes in order to avoid any use contrary to the intended use statement.

PRESSURE VENTILATION VERSUS VOLUME VENTILATION

There are two common types of ventilation in use today: volume ventilation and pressure ventilation. Volume ventilation delivers a specific tidal volume with each breath. Although the volume is consistent for each breath delivered, the pressure generated in the patient's lungs can and often will change with each breath. This consistent tidal volume allows clinicians using volume ventilation to control the level of ventilation easily using the tidal volume and rate. The use of volume ventilation can sometimes generate high pressures in the lungs that can cause damage in the form of barotrauma.

Pressure ventilation delivers specified pressures during the breathing phase, one pressure for inspiration and one pressure for expiration. These are the inspiratory positive airway pressure (IPAP) and the expiratory positive airway pressure (EPAP) settings. The difference between the EPAP and IPAP settings is the amount of pressure support delivered. Figure 50-4 provides an example of

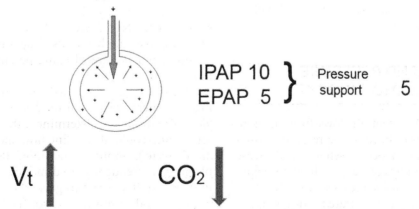

Figure 50-4 With settings of an inspiratory positive airway pressure (IPAP) of 10 cm H_2O and an expiratory positive airway pressure (EPAP) of 5 cm H_2O, the result is a pressure support of 5 cm H_2O.

pressure support of 5 cm H_2O. Pressure ventilation is like a mirror image of sorts to volume ventilation. Pressure ventilation delivers a precise pressure during each inspiration, but the volume delivered by that pressure breath can and often will vary from breath to breath. This possibility of inconsistent tidal volume with pressure ventilation is both good and bad, depending on the situation.

PRESSURE SUPPORT VENTILATION: THE GOOD AND THE BAD

One of the best reasons to use pressure support ventilation is that it is a very comfortable way to support the patient's effort. Because the device is targeting a pressure, it allows the patient to inspire a larger breath if he or she desires. If the patient wants to take a smaller breath, he or she is able to reject the breath when using pressure ventilation. Once the pressure reaches the selected pressure level, the breath is terminated and the patient can exhale. These aspects of pressure ventilation give the patient a great deal of control over how much ventilation he or she receives, making it more comfortable for him or her.

The bad aspect of using pressure ventilation is once again a mirror image of the good aspect. NIV using pressure ventilation does not assure a minimal level of ventilation. Patients change over time. Some get better, but most tend to get worse. Patients with neuromuscular disease will almost certainly get worse. Pressure settings that generate tidal volumes of 500 mL in January may generate only 400 mL in July. Therapy will need to be monitored and adjusted because even though the settings on the device do not change, the resulting ventilation can change on the basis of changes occurring in the patient. Never forget that the patient is a big variable that a clinician has little to no control over. NIV devices are almost exclusively pressure ventilators, but many also are capable of "targeting" a tidal volume or alveolar ventilation with their pressure. This "targeting" will be discussed in more detail later.

HOW DOES NIV AND PRESSURE SUPPORT VENTILATION WORK?

The foundation of NIV is that air flows from areas of higher pressure to areas of lower pressure. As discussed earlier, normal ventilation occurs when we decrease the pressure in our chest by contracting the diaphragm, causing air to flow from outside the chest into the lungs. With NIV, we don't reduce the pressure in the chest, but rather increase the pressure at the opening of the airway in order to affect ventilation. We do this with a flow generator in the NIV device. NIV devices generate a pressure

differential between inspiratory and expiratory phases of the breath. This pressure differential is commonly referred to as "the level of pressure support" or simply as "pressure support." The goal of pressure support is to increase the tidal volume above what one would normally inspire on one's own without assistance. The level of pressure support is controlled by the level of IPAP and EPAP. Some advanced NIV devices allow for setting a pressure support instead of individually setting the EPAP and IPAP.

A pressure support of 5 cm H_2O should generate a larger tidal volume than an unsupported breath, which, in turn, should generate more alveolar ventilation, resulting in lower CO_2 levels. If this level of pressure support does not generate enough of an increase in tidal volume or a decrease in CO_2 (remember that ventilation and CO_2 are *inversely* related), then the IPAP can be increased to increase the pressure support and tidal volume. Increases in pressure support may not always result in increases of tidal volume and ventilation. Remember, the patient is on the other end of the NIV device, and if he or she is uncomfortable with the pressure being supplied, then he or she may resist the ventilation and the end result could be decreased ventilation.

If upper airway obstruction is still present with EPAP of 5, EPAP can be increased as needed, but IPAP will have to be increased the same amount to maintain the same level of pressure support. The level of pressure support is what drives ventilation, and EPAP is used for airway control. These two concepts are the most important ones to understand in order to apply NIV successfully.

NIV TERMINOLOGY

A review of common NIV terminology is warranted before a discussion of therapy concerns about specific patient types. Some of the terms to be familiar with include the following:

(Note to the reader: There are no nomenclature standards for NIV devices. The terms discussed in the following paragraphs are used by a majority of manufacturers, but beware of some potential differences in terms.)

Mode can be described as a timing pattern for breaths. There are several modes available on NIV devices. The mode can determine if there is a backup rate setting and could also define how spontaneous breaths are delivered. Spontaneous timed (S/T) mode is one of the most frequently used modes. Once S/T mode is understood, it is easier to grasp the details of spontaneous (S) mode, pressure control (PC) mode, and timed (T) mode. Most manufacturers provide these modes, but they may use different terminology. Figure 50-5 identifies the various settings in the NIV device.

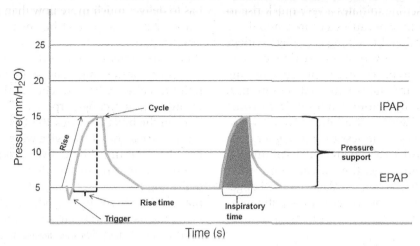

Figure 50-5 The various settings on the noninvasive ventilation device. EPAP, expiratory positive airway pressure; IPAP, inspiratory positive airway pressure.

Bilevel therapy is another way to describe pressure support therapy. This is the application of two different pressure levels during the breath cycle. Ideally, if the pressures are applied at the proper times, they will follow the patient's own breathing pattern and increase pressure to increase the size of the inhaled breath and then decrease to allow for exhalation while maintaining a patent upper airway. Pressures are measured in cm H_2O unless indicated otherwise. Many devices are sold internationally and therefore may support the ability to change pressure settings to hectopascals (hPa).

EPAP is the pressure level set for the expiratory phase of the breath. It is lower than the inspiratory pressure to allow the inhaled breath to be easily exhaled. This pressure is typically titrated to maintain an open upper airway at the transition point between end exhalation and beginning of inspiration. EPAP can also be increased to improve oxygenation in some cases.

IPAP is the higher of the two pressure settings and is used to support the inspiratory phase of the breath. Increasing only IPAP will also increase pressure support at the same time. Doing so will normally increase the tidal volume of the breath. At some point, increasing the IPAP or pressure support may not yield higher tidal volumes because of discomfort or asynchrony.

Pressure support is what drives ventilation in NIV. Pressure support may not be a setting on the device, so it is important to know that it is the difference between the IPAP and EPAP settings. Increase the IPAP if an increase in pressure support is needed. Increases in EPAP will necessitate an increase in IPAP if the pressure support is to be maintained. Increasing the level of pressure support will usually increase the tidal volume for each breath, which, in turn, increases the level of ventilation that normally reduces the CO_2 level in the blood.

Trigger is the transition point between the expiratory phase of the breath and the inspiratory phase. It is the beginning of the breath. During NIV, the patient is at the EPAP during exhalation and the device is waiting for a "trigger" to tell it to transition to IPAP. Devices with trigger settings may refer to them as a "sensitivity setting." When triggering occurs, the device targets the higher pressure level (IPAP) and increases flow to do this. This provides the additional flow necessary for the patient's tidal volume. Almost all of the devices on the market use some type of flow trigger. During use, the device is continually monitoring flow and will determine if the patient is trying to inspire, which will then initiate a transition to IPAP. Flow triggering on NIV devices normally uses settings from 1 L per minute to as high as 9 L per minute. A trigger setting of 1 L per minute means that if the device detects an increase of 1 L per minute of flow over what it is delivering, it will initiate the transition to the inspiratory phase. Low trigger settings, like 1 L per minute, are the most sensitive and may need to be used in pediatric patients or possibly adult patients with neuromuscular disease in order to detect faint inspiratory efforts. In patients with normal inspiratory capability, a setting of 1 L per minute may be too sensitive and may induce false or premature triggering. This will, of course, induce asynchrony and should be avoided. On the other end of the spectrum, a less sensitive trigger setting, like 9 L per minute, may be too difficult for the patient to trigger. Missed trigger events can also induce asynchrony between the patient and the device. Triggering needs to be adjusted to meet each individual patient's needs.

Rise time is the amount of time the device takes to transition from EPAP to IPAP. After the breath is triggered, the pressure starts to rise from EPAP to IPAP. Some devices have time settings for rise time, whereas other devices just use a setting that is correlated to a specific time. In either case, the setting determines how fast the device transitions from low to high pressure.

A short time or low setting initiates a very quick rise to pressure and a longer time produces a more gradual rise to pressure. Manipulating this setting can affect patient comfort with the therapy. A very short rise time can create a very ballistic feel to the change in pressure and the patient may not be comfortable with that sensation. A longer rise time may feel more comfortable to some patients, but longer rise times can affect overall ventilation. Longer rise times mean less time at higher pressures. This could translate to smaller tidal volumes. It may be more important to get the patient comfortable on the therapy than to maximize tidal volume. Longer rise times could be uncomfortable for some patients as well. They may feel a need for a faster breath and prefer shorter rise times.

Rise times are not normally prescribed by physicians. Clinicians should try to determine a comfortable rise time setting for the patient that can be relayed to the home care team. Rise time settings typically range from 0.1 to 0.9 seconds. As an example, think of settings of EPAP 5 and IPAP 15. When inspiration is triggered, the pressure will increase from 5 to 15 cm H_2O. If the rise time is set to 0.1 seconds, the pressure will rise from 5 to 15 in 0.1 seconds. Changes to the rise time will affect how the breath delivery feels to the patient and may also impact the amount of ventilation achieved by the breath (see Fig. 50-6).

Cycling is the opposite of triggering. The device transitions from IPAP back to EPAP at the cycle point. Knowing when to terminate the inspiratory phase of the breath is as important as knowing when to initiate the breath. Reaching the cycle point or "cycling" is done using flow-based algorithms just like triggering does. Cycling settings are percentages. The percentage refers to the peak flow of the current breath. When the patient inspires, the device is targeting a higher pressure by generating more flow. When the patient inhales, the device

has to deliver much more flow than it does during exhalation. When the patient begins to end the breath, the flow needed to deliver the higher IPAP starts to decrease. When the patient starts to decrease his or her inspiratory effort, or the lungs have started to fill, the peak flow point has already been reached and the device will have recorded it for cycling purposes. For example, if the peak flow on the breath reaches 100 L per minute and cycling is set to 40%, then the device will provide flow to maintain the IPAP until the delivered flow reaches 40 L per minute. At that point, the device will "cycle" and stop delivering the IPAP and start delivering a lower flow to maintain the EPAP. If the device does not properly detect when the patient wants to exhale, it will not cycle at the right time. If it cycles too soon, the breath will be too small and the patient may become short of breath and may need to breathe faster. If the device cycles too late, the patient will be trying to exhale against the higher pressure and this will cause asynchrony issues as well. NIV devices have limits on how long the device will stay in IPAP. This limit is usually 50% of the cycle time, so even if the device misses the patient's request to cycle the breath, it will not stay in IPAP excessively long.

Triggering and cycling are extremely important, and device manufacturers spend a lot of time and effort working on algorithms to make sure the devices they make do these things properly. Proper triggering and cycling are key to patient synchrony. Synchrony is essential to patient comfort and adherence to therapy. If the patient attempts to inspire and the device doesn't detect the effort, known as a "missed trigger," it will not provide the extra flow needed for a comfortable inspiration. Determining the right settings for triggering and cycling requires some skill and experience. Some devices offer automated algorithms that do this for the clinician. Is something like this better than manually titrating a trigger and cycle setting? That probably largely depends on the skill level of the clinician. Flow triggering and cycling settings (see Table 50-2) offer the possibility of customization to the patient needs, but they can also be set incorrectly and lead to asynchrony issues for the patient.

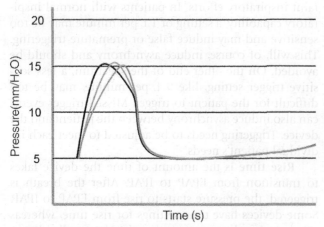

Figure 50-6 The impact of changing rise time on the pressure–time curve. The black line shows a fast rise time of 0.1 seconds. The gray (light) line shows a rise time of 0.2 seconds and the gray (dark) line is a rise time of 0.3 seconds.

Table 50-2	Breath Rates and Corresponding Cycle Times
Breath Rate	**Cycle Time (s)**
8	7.5
10	6
12	5
15	4
20	3

BREATH TYPES: PRESSURE SUPPORT VERSUS PRESSURE CONTROL

One of the subtle things to know about NIV delivery is that there are two different types of breath that can be supplied by NIV devices. There are important differences between a PC breath and a pressure support breath, and these differences can become critical when choosing a mode of ventilation for some patients.

The discussion of the different modes of therapy builds on how these two different breath types are used. Pressure support breaths are the most common type of breath delivered during NIV. A pressure-supported breath is a completely spontaneous breath. The downward spike on the pressure channel may not always be seen because the device may be using flow triggering, and the response time of devices in use today is too fast for a drop in pressure to occur. The length of the breath is essentially determined by the patient, with some limits imposed by the cycling algorithm of the device. This type of breath offers a great deal of flexibility for the patient. The patient is able to initiate the breath and also able to terminate it. The device will essentially monitor the inhaled flow and look for indications whether the patient is trying to cycle or terminate the inspiration. This allows the patient to control the length of the breath and the amount of air he or she inspires, making this a very comfortable breath for the patient. This type of breath may not be best for all patients, however. Patients with a neuromuscular disease may not be able to sustain

an inspiratory effort long enough to attain an adequate tidal volume. In this case, the patient may benefit more from receiving PC breaths. Figure 50-7 demonstrates these various breaths.

Pressure-controlled or timed breaths use device-controlled pressures, just like a pressure support, but the device also controls the amount of time that the inspiratory pressure is delivered. Controlling the amount of time the pressure is delivered requires the use of another control parameter called Inspiratory time (I time). This setting determines the amount of time that the device will remain in the inspiratory phase of the breath. Once the breath is initiated, the device will transition from the lower pressure (EPAP) to the higher pressure (IPAP) and stay at the higher pressure for the set I time. PC breaths are also usually delivered by a timed trigger instead of a patient trigger, so PC breaths are found in modes of therapy that employ a backup rate. These are the breaths that are delivered when the patient's own breathing rate falls below the backup rate that is set on the device.

CYCLE TIME AND RESPIRATORY RATE

One additional concept needs to be addressed before therapy modes are introduced. This is the concept of cycle time. Depending on the mode selected, there are certain control parameters that will need to be set. EPAP, IPAP, and rise time are pretty straightforward. Even respiratory rate and I time appear to be pretty straightforward, but

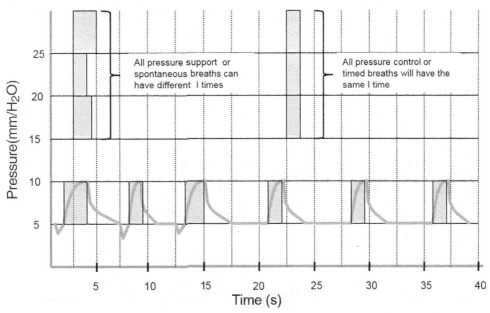

Figure 50-7 The difference between pressure support or spontaneous breaths and pressure control or timed breaths. The first three breaths are pressure support breaths. The breath was initiated by the patient and the device supports that breath with the pressure support set by the clinician. Note the trigger event as the downward spike in pressure just before the pressure rises. The trigger event is shown to highlight the fact that the breath is a spontaneously triggered pressure support breath. Pressure control breaths, shown as the last three breaths, are also sometimes called "timed breaths." I time, Inspiratory time.

there are some subtle concepts that need to be understood. One of the subtleties is cycle time.

When using a mode of therapy with a backup rate feature, an I time and respiratory rate have to be set. When setting a respiratory rate, a cycle time is automatically being set in the background. Calculate the cycle time by dividing 60 seconds by the respiratory rate. Cycle time is the amount of time devoted to a full inspiratory and expiratory phase of the breath. In modes that support a backup rate function, the cycle time is the maximum amount of time allowed between breaths. See Table 50-3 for an inspiratory time conversion table.

S/T mode allows the patient to start a spontaneous breath before the end of the cycle time, but if they fail to do so, a timed breath will be delivered (see Fig. 50-8). Another way of thinking about cycle time is that it is a timer that is counting down. If the patient does not trigger a breath spontaneously before the timer reaches zero, then the device will deliver a timed breath. The timer then restarts with each breath, either timed or spontaneous.

The respiratory rate selected multiplied by the average tidal volume will determine the minimum minute ventilation. It should be understood that the set rate is a minimum rate. Almost all modes of therapy allow for additional breaths if the patient triggers or "asks" for a breath by starting a spontaneous breath. This is why setting an appropriate trigger is important. Most of the time, the respiratory rate is set as a safety net backup to the patient's own rate. The patient should be able to trigger and essentially set his or her own pace for breathing. Higher respiratory rates may be difficult for the patient to be comfortable with, because the rate setting is a minimum and breaths will be delivered when the cycle

Table 50-3	Conversion Table for Inspiratory Time (I Time)		
Set Backup Breath Rate (bpm)	I/E 1/3, Ti/Ttot 25% (s)	I/E 1/2, Ti/Ttot 33% (s)	I/E 1/1, Ti/Ttot 50% (s)
10	1.5	2.0	3.0
11	1.4	1.8	2.7
12	1.3	1.7	2.5
13	1.2	1.5	2.3
14	1.1	1.4	2.1
15	1.0	1.3	2.0
16	0.9	1.3	1.8
17	0.9	1.2	1.7
18	0.8	1.1	1.6
19	0.8	1.1	1.5
20	0.8	1.0	1.5
21	0.7	1.0	1.4
22	0.7	0.9	1.3
23	0.7	0.9	1.3
24	0.6	0.8	1.2
25	0.6	0.8	1.2

Set the I time in seconds: Ti (seconds) = 60/respiratory rate × %Ti.
I/E, inspiratory/expiratory; Ti/Ttot, inspiratory time to total cycle time.

Guidelines/values developed for use with Philips Respironics products only. Variations may occur with other manufacturers' products. Please consult specific manufacturers' guidelines for specific product information and operational guidelines.

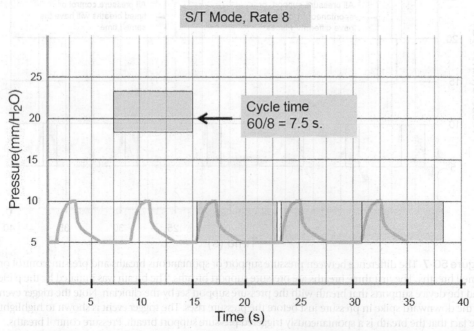

Figure 50-8 A respiratory rate setting of 8 breaths per minute in spontaneous/timed mode shows a cycle time of 7.5 seconds. The gray-shaded area depicts the cycle time of 7.5 seconds.

time expires. If the patient's own respiratory rate is adequate for his or her needs, then the backup respiratory rate is usually set just below the patient's own rate. High backup rates can be a source of asynchrony. The patient can always trigger and get additional breaths, but he or she will not be able to get less breaths than the set backup rate.

SETTING INSPIRATORY TIME

Setting the respiratory rate automatically sets the cycle time. The inspiratory time now needs to be set. With a respiratory rate of 12 breaths per minute, the cycle time is 5 seconds. This means that the breath has to be delivered and exhaled within 5 seconds because the device will deliver the next breath 5 seconds after the last trigger. A normal breathing pattern uses 25% to 33% of the cycle time to inspire the breath. That leaves 67% to 75% of the cycle time for expiration.

I time is only a factor for timed or PC breaths. It has no bearing on spontaneous breaths. The setting for I time has a big impact on tidal volumes if the patient receives a high percentage of pressure-controlled breaths. Many devices that provide NIV will limit the amount of inspiratory time to 50% of the cycle time or less. This is a safeguard to ensure that the patient has sufficient time to exhale the breath before the next one is given. Normal respiratory rates are usually in the low-to-mid-teens, or 10 to 15 breaths per minute. Determine the cycle time and set the I time in the range of 25% to 33% of that cycle time. Patients with COPD have longer expiratory times because of obstruction in the distal airways. These patients may benefit from shorter I times in order to devote a larger portion of the cycle time for exhalation.

Another way to set I time is to review the patient's spontaneous breaths with good tidal volumes. Remember that spontaneous breaths do not use the set I time. The patient may inspire as long or short as he or she needs. See how long the patient inspires with spontaneous breaths (Fig. 50-9). If the spontaneous breath volumes are good, then the I time can be set similar to the patient's own spontaneous I times.

The tidal volumes should be reviewed during spontaneous breaths and, if they are acceptable, then the inspiratory time setting could be lowered to match the spontaneous breathing (see Fig. 50-9). The adjustment in this case would be very minor, and if the longer I time setting is not uncomfortable to the patient, it does not always need to be changed. If the situation was reversed and the set I time was shorter than the spontaneous I times, then the adjustment to match spontaneous I times should always be done.

BUILDING THE BREATH

Knowing how all the settings in NIV come together allows for tailoring those settings to meet the goals of reducing the work of breathing and helping normalize blood gasses. It allows the clinician to build the breath to meet the patient's needs. See Table 50-4 for setting guidelines.

NIV is a series of supported breaths given to the patient. Start by getting the breath adjusted to the patient's needs and then decide how frequently to repeat it. NIV uses pressure support (IPAP–EPAP) applied over time (I time) to generate flow to the patient. This flow is the tidal volume. The applied pressure support is the most important control parameter because many of the delivered breaths will be spontaneous and the patient will have complete control over the I time. When I time must be set, refer to the patient's spontaneous breath I times or keep the I time in the range of 25% to 33% of the cycle time.

The flow channel on a polysomnogram shows flow over time and that is more representative of tidal volume than a pressure–time graph. If the device in use reports tidal volumes, that may be used as well. In most

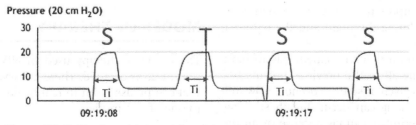

Figure 50-9 The first, third, and fourth breaths are spontaneous (S) breaths, whereas the second is a timed (T) breath. The T breath does not have a downward deflection on the pressure graph, denoting a trigger. The three S breaths stay in the inspiratory phase for a similar length of time. The patient has control over the I time for these S breaths, which appears to be shorter than the I time for the T breath. This may indicate that the I time setting is too long.

Table 50-4 Guidelines for Ventilation Settings

Initial settings	• IPAP = 8–10 cm H_2O • EPAP = 4 cm H_2O • RR = 10–12 bpm
IPAP	Increase IPAP if the patient wants more air, targeting patient tidal volume at 8 mL/kg of ideal weight
EPAP	• Without obstructive sleep apnea (OSA) 4–5 cm H_2O • With OSA: intrinsic PEEP to remove obstructive apnea events • With intrinsic PEP (stable chronic COPD): 5–6 cm H_2O
BPM	Set to 2–3 bpm under the patient's spontaneous frequency
Rise time	• Obstructive patients prefer short rise time: from 1 to 4 (100–400 ms) • Restrictive patients prefer long rise time: from 3 to 6 (300–600 ms)
Ti	• Obstructive patients: set Ti between 25% and 33% • Restrictive patients: set Ti between 33% and 50% • (Refer to table to set I time)

AVAPS Only		
	OHS	**COPD**	**Other Restrictive Diseases (NMD, etc.)**
Vt target	8–10 mL/kg of ideal body weight (refer to table for target tidal volume)		
IPAP window (IPAP min and IPAP max)	Allow a wide range of pressure variation to ensure the right pressure at the right time. IPAP min = EPAP IPAP max = 25–30 cm H_2O	Allow a more restrictive pressure window to combine comfort and efficacy. IPAP min = comfortable IPAP IPAP max = IPAP min + 5 cm H_2O	Allow a more restrictive pressure window to combine comfort and safety. IPAP min = efficient IPAP IPAP max = IPAP min + 5 cm H_2O
AVAPS rate	AVAPS rate setting depends on patient needs and clinical condition: • 0.5 to 3 cm H_2O/min so target tidal volume is reached smoothly • 3 to 5 cm H_2O/min so target tidal volume is reached more rapidly		

Check patient arterial blood gasses ($PaCO_2$ and PaO_2) and oxygen saturation (SpO_2).

Important: Guidelines are intended to serve only as a reference. They shall be used only in conjunction with the instructions and/or protocol set forth by the physician and institution in which the assist device is being used. The guidelines are not intended to supersede established medical protocols.

AVAPS, average volume–assured pressure support; BPM, breaths per minute; COPD, chronic obstructive pulmonary disease; EPAP, expiratory positive airway pressure; IPAP, inspiratory positive airway pressure; NMD, neuromuscular disease; OHS, obesity hypoventilation syndrome; OSAS, obstructive sleep apnea syndrome; RR, respiratory rate.

*Guidelines/values developed for use with Philips Respironics products only. Variations may occur with other manufacturers' products. Please consult specific manufacturers' guidelines for specific product information and operational guidelines.

cases, the majority of breaths will be spontaneous, so the only parameter that matters is the amount of pressure support applied (see Fig. 50-10). This doesn't mean that the I time is not important, because the patient may need timed breaths during the night and the correct I time will matter then.

Always keep in mind that the patient has to have enough time to exhale all of the previous breaths before another breath is given. If settings do not allow full expiration, breath stacking can occur. Breath stacking causes gradually hyperinflated lungs because of an inability to completely exhale breaths. If this occurs, then the ventilation has to be decreased by reducing pressure, reducing I time, or decreasing the rate. Reducing pressure will reduce the inhaled volume. Reducing I time

and respiratory rate will allow more time to exhale before the next breath.

MODES OF THERAPY

The mode of therapy used in NIV is usually the first point that is decided. There are several different modes that can be used, but in reality, the choice comes down to one of two modes.

S Mode

S mode is the simplest of the available modes because it has fewer settings. The only breath that is allowed is one

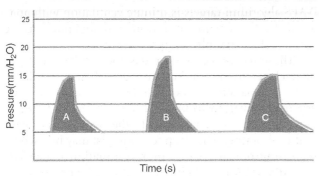

Figure 50-10 The shaded area under the curves represents the pressure support applied over time to the patient airway. This pressure/time representation is a way to demonstrate how to make changes to the settings. In breath A, the tidal volume was insufficient to meet patient needs. An increase in pressure support is shown in breath B. This increase in pressure should create additional flow during the I time and increase the delivered tidal volume. The other choice, shown in breath C, is to increase the I time. This too may increase the tidal volume by applying the pressure for a longer period of time.

that is triggered by the patient. The only parameters that the clinician can adjust are EPAP, IPAP, and rise time. S mode does not support a backup rate feature, so if the patient stops breathing for any reason, the device will not be able to deliver a timed breath. For this reason, it should not be used on patients who cannot or will not trigger a breath on their own consistently.

S/T Mode

S/T mode is the most frequently used mode. This mode of therapy supports a backup rate feature and can deliver all spontaneous, all timed, or a mixture of both spontaneous and timed breaths depending on the rate selected and the spontaneous rate of the patient. If the patient does not trigger breaths on his or her own, the device will deliver timed breaths at the exact rate set on the device. If the patient triggers breaths faster than the set rate on the device, he or she will receive all spontaneous breaths. The patient can also receive a mixture of spontaneous breaths and timed breaths.

The device in S/T mode will use the cycle time window derived from the set respiratory rate to determine which type of breath to deliver. For example, with a rate of 12 breaths per minute, the cycle time is 5 seconds. The device will monitor the patient for 5 seconds after the last breath. If the patient triggers a breath before 5 seconds has elapsed, he or she will get a spontaneous breath. The device will then reset the cycle time window and start the 5-second timer again. If there is no patient trigger after 5 seconds, a timed breath will be given. Remember, these two breaths are

different in that the timed breath has a duration based on the I time setting, and the spontaneous breath is terminated by the patient ending the breath. The rate setting in S/T mode assures that the patient will receive at least that number of breaths, but what type of breath occurs depends on the number of breaths triggered by the patient.

T Mode

T mode is very seldom used. This mode looks just like S/T mode in the settings except that there are no triggering and cycling settings. T mode delivers all timed breaths. Patient triggering and cycling are not allowed. If the rate is set to 12 breaths per minute, then the patient will get a breath from the device every 5 seconds. This mode is seldom if ever used.

PC Mode

The final mode is called PC mode. The settings of this mode are the same as those of S/T, but all the breaths, even spontaneously triggered ones, are delivered for the specified I time. When using this mode, it is critical to get the I time set properly because all breaths delivered will use that I time. This mode is used on patients who are able to trigger breaths, but for some reason are unable to sustain the breath long enough to get an adequate tidal volume. A patient with a neuromuscular disease might be one such person. If the patient triggers a breath but isn't strong enough to sustain the breath, the device may cycle the breath sooner than is acceptable. Not an error of the device, but rather a reflection of the patient's weakened state. For example, assume that a neuromuscular disease patient is being titrated to get to a desired tidal volume in S/T mode. The patient is breathing faster than the set rate on the device, so he or she is getting all spontaneous breaths. If the patient is too weak to sustain an inspiratory effort, the device could terminate breaths too early. If the clinician does not note that the breaths are very short in duration, he or she may be tempted to increase pressures in order to gain more ventilation. In this case, the patient may be better served by changing the mode to PC mode and setting an I time longer than what the patient is achieving during his or her own spontaneous breaths. This could have the result of longer breaths at lower pressures at slower rates that have adequate tidal volumes.

ADVANCED THERAPIES

Unfortunately, even the best titration is just a snapshot in time. There are just too many variables involved that can affect the desired therapy. Medication changes, alcohol use, and weight changes can impact the effectiveness of any titration. Patients with progressive diseases will almost certainly have changes that affect their therapy. At a minimum, NIV patients should have their therapy monitored and appropriate changes made as needed. Most devices in use today provide for monitoring therapy via proprietary software provided by the manufacturer.

Medical device manufacturers have also developed automated technologies that allow the clinician to set a volume target for the device and allow it to operate within pressure boundaries in order to continually titrate therapy so as to maintain the desired level of ventilation. These technologies allow the clinician to set a target for ventilation and the device will continually monitor the delivered therapy and adjust the delivered pressure support in order to stay at or above that level of ventilation.

Average volume–assured pressure support (AVAPS) technology provides settings similar to those of the S/T mode, but instead of a single IPAP setting, there is a minimum IPAP and a maximum IPAP setting. There is also a target tidal volume setting. AVAPS will operate in all the modes outlined earlier: S, S/T, T, and PC. AVAPS will monitor delivered tidal volumes and will raise IPAP if the tidal volume is below the target and decrease IPAP if the tidal volume is above the target. AVAPS keeps a running average of tidal volumes and makes small changes to IPAP in order to avoid arousing the patient with large pressure changes. This mode of therapy essentially continues the titration all the time while the patient is using the device. The IPAP is always at least the IPAP minimum and never more than the IPAP max. Care should be taken to set these pressures to assure a minimum level of pressure support at all times. The IPAP max is then set to limit the maximum pressure the patient will receive, but still high enough to allow the device to achieve the desired tidal volume.

AVAPS with auto EPAP (AVAPS AE) is another mode of therapy that will also titrate EPAP in order to keep the upper airway patent and automatically adjust pressure support on the basis of the tidal volume target. This mode of therapy has settings for minimum and maximum levels of pressure support instead of IPAP. AVAPS AE also has minimum and maximum EPAP settings. This mode of therapy can compensate for changes in the upper airway in addition to changes in the level of ventilation.

Intelligent Volume Assured Pressure Support (iVAPS) technology targets a set alveolar minute ventilation. The device will monitor delivered alveolar minute ventilation and compare it with the target alveolar minute ventilation. iVAPS adjusts pressure support and respiratory rate in order to maintain target alveolar minute ventilation. The alveolar minute ventilation that the

iVAPS algorithm targets is minute ventilation with anatomic dead space subtracted from it. It does not account for any additional physiologic dead space.

These technologies were designed to keep the patient closer to his or her intended therapy while at home. The patient still needs to be monitored and therapy may still need to be adjusted. These technologies may present some challenges to the sleep technologist in the laboratory. The sleep technologist may be used to increasing pressure when more ventilation is needed. If AVAPS or iVAPS is being used, it may be necessary to wait and let the algorithm do the work. Changes may need to be made if pressures are consistently being delivered at either the maximum or minimum pressure settings. If delivered pressures are rising to the maximum setting, it may be necessary to increase the setting in order to allow the algorithm to reach the volume target. If delivered pressures have dropped to the minimum setting, it may mean that the minimum is set too high and the patient could be exposed to unnecessary pressures.

CURRENT TRENDS TREATING COPD

Patients with COPD have historically been "rescued" from ventilatory failure in the intensive care unit by the use of NIV. These patients are then returned to the community, sometimes on NIV and sometimes not, only to return again and again to the hospital in respiratory failure.

Why does NIV work so well in an acute situation and then seem to fail when used chronically in a home care situation? Some physicians feel that one of the reasons is that the NIV is not targeting a high enough reduction in CO_2.

High-intensity noninvasive positive pressure ventilation (HI-NPPV) has recently been utilized in patients with chronic hypercapnic COPD. This form of treatment uses NIV to maximize pressure support and respiratory rate to the highest level that the patient will tolerate. The goal is to gain the greatest reduction in CO_2 levels via ABG analysis. IPAP levels of 30 cm H_2O are common and respiratory rates approaching 20 breaths per minute are as well. The device is essentially taking over for the patient and doing most or all of the work of breathing while the patient is on the device.

This form of NIV has shown good results in CO_2 reduction and improvements in quality-of-life measures. These patients are usually titrated in a hospital or clinic setting in order to ensure that they are comfortable with the therapy and that CO_2 reductions are being achieved. These are not routine NIV titrations. Specific physician directions should be followed when attempting HI-NPPV (4, 5).

SUMMARY

Neuromuscular disease and COPD are two of the most common disorders that are treated with NIV. Each of these disorders can present with or without coincident upper airway obstruction. Although these two disorders are very different in many ways, the goals of NIV therapy are very much the same. The primary goals are to reduce the work of breathing and to normalize blood gasses.

Synchrony is another goal to add to these primary goals. Synchrony occurs when the patient is comfortable and accepting of the therapy that has been applied. Asynchrony is, of course, the opposite of synchrony. Asynchronous events happen all the time during NIV therapy. The job of the clinician setting up and titrating NIV is to minimize the number of these asynchronous events. These events include missed triggers, late triggers, missed cycles, early triggers, and late cycling. Asynchrony can occur because of incorrect I time settings and respiratory rates. Too slow or too fast rise times can also lead to asynchrony events. Too much or too little pressure support can cause asynchrony. If the breath is built properly and delivered with the proper timing, asynchronous events should be minimized.

To provide successful NIV therapy, break it down to the fundamentals. The EPAP is used to control the upper airway and keep it patent. It is the foundation for building a breath that is going to reduce the work of breathing for the patient. Pressure support is used to augment the patient's tidal volume to increase overall ventilation. CO_2 levels can be used as guidance to assure the proper amount of ventilation. ABG measurements of the CO_2 level are the gold standard. Transcutaneous CO_2 monitoring is useful as well. Capnography or end-tidal CO_2 measurements should be used cautiously with NIV. If CO_2 measurements are not available, or even if they are, ventilation can be improved by building a breath for the patient on the basis of the size of the patient. Use 6 to 8 mL per kg of body weight as a guide for the tidal volume and titrate the pressure support to get there. HI-NPPV for COPD patients will override the standard 6 to 8 mL per kg guidance. Follow specific physician instructions if asked to deliver HI-NPPV.

Make sure that the triggering and cycling criteria are set appropriately. Most devices have automated algorithms that perform this function well. Some patients may need manually set flow triggering and cycling. Use caution because these criteria can also be set incorrectly,

making it difficult for the patient to synchronize with the device.

Set the I time to provide a 1:2 to 1:3 inspiratory to expiratory ratio for the cycle time. As the backup rate is increased, the I time usually needs to be decreased in order to maintain the ratio. Remember that the air that goes into the lungs has to be fully exhaled before the next breath is given, or else breath stacking and asynchrony may result.

Respiratory rate is normally set just below the patient's own spontaneous rate. There are exceptions of course. COPD patients on HI-NPPV will probably need higher rates to further reduce CO_2. Weaker neuromuscular patients may have trouble triggering spontaneously and need higher rates in order to maintain their current level of ventilation.

A patient tolerating NIV with adequate tidal volumes is a great start for NIV therapy. Some patients may need more aggressive forms of NIV therapy, but these patients may need frequent follow-up and adjustments and only then will they get to the desired level of ventilation.

REFERENCES

1. Piper, A., & Grunstein, R. (2011). Obesity hypoventilation syndrome, mechanisms and management. *American Journal of Respiratory and Critical Care Management*, *183*(3), 292–298.

2. Pruitt, W. C. (2016). Ventilation and oxygenation. In D. R. Hess, N. R. MacIntyre, W. F. Galvin, et al. (Eds.), *Respiratory care principles and practices* (3rd ed.). Burlington, MA: Jones and Bartlett Learning.

3. Gay, P. C. (2009). Complications of noninvasive ventilation in acute care. *Respiratory Care, 54*(2), 246–258.

4. Struik, F. M., Lacasse, Y., Goldstein, R., et al. (2013). Nocturnal non-invasive positive pressure ventilation for stable chronic obstructive pulmonary disease. *Cochrane Database of Systematic Reviews*, 6. doi:10.1002/14651858.CD002878.pub2

5. Weir, M., Marchetti, N., Czysz, A., et al. (2015). High intensity non-invasive positive pressure ventilation for stable hypercapnic chronic obstructive pulmonary disease patients. *Chronic Obstructive Pulmonary Diseases, 2*(4), 313–320. doi:10.15326/jco pdf.2.4.2015.0145

chapter 51

Oxygen Administration in the Sleep Center

THOMAS RUSSELL

LEARNING OBJECTIVES

On completion of this chapter, the reader should be able to:

1. List the various storage methods for oxygen.
2. Regulate and control the flow of oxygen.
3. Choose an appropriate oxygen administration device.
4. Describe the limitations and inaccuracies of oxygen delivery.
5. List variables affecting oxygen therapy with continuous positive airway pressure/bilevel positive airway pressure.
6. Recognize the potential for creating increased nasal resistance.

KEY TERMS

Hypoxia
Hypoxemia
FiO_2
lpm
psi
Delivered FiO_2
Actual FiO_2
Entrainment
SpO_2%

Ambient or atmospheric air comprises nearly 21% oxygen gas. Oxygen is tasteless, colorless, odorless, and transparent. By itself, oxygen is not flammable but vigorously accelerates combustion. Oxygen is an elemental gas required for life. Various respiratory and/or cardiac problems require augmentation of ambient oxygen concentrations.

This chapter discusses the techniques and concerns of oxygen therapy, specifically, how supplemental oxygen is delivered in the sleep center environment. Common delivery devices and their inherent limitations are discussed.

Effective oxygen administration demands a technologist familiar with the physiology of respiration, ventilation, and gas exchange. Oxygen is considered a drug and therefore administered in accordance with institution policy and procedure. Typically, oxygen therapy is prescribed by a physician and administered by appropriately credentialed personnel. The reader is encouraged to review his or her particular workplace procedures, pertinent policies, and licensure.

Oxygen is one of the most commonly used drugs in hospitals. Interestingly, given the incidence and severity of hypoxemia encountered in the sleep center, the use of oxygen is relatively uncommon. Because hypoxemia occurring during sleep is most often caused by transient upper airway obstruction and/or hypoventilation, treatment is directed toward maintaining upper airway patency using continuous positive airway pressure (CPAP) and/or augmenting ventilation using bilevel positive airway pressure (BPAP). Supplemental oxygen is usually not required and is rarely considered a "stand-alone" therapy (1).

OXYGEN STORAGE AND DISTRIBUTION

The use of medical grade oxygen requires a method of storage and means of delivery. Oxygen is commercially packaged as a compressed gas or in its liquid form. Alternatively, oxygen can be separated and concentrated from room air using an "oxygen concentrator."

Manufactured oxygen is most often void of any humidity and is termed *anhydrous*, meaning without water. The gas is completely dry, which can irritate the upper airway mucous membranes. This is more of an issue with higher oxygen flows not often encountered in the sleep center.

Compressed Oxygen Gas

Medical gas cylinders (tanks) have been in use since 1888. Several medical/anesthetic gases, including pure (99%) oxygen, are packaged in cylinders, which are manufactured of seamless, high-quality, finely tempered steel. For safety, cylinders are color coded. Oxygen tanks are colored white (or green). White is the international color code for oxygen. Despite color coding, the contents of a cylinder should be verified by its tag/label. If there is no tag, *do not use the cylinder*.

Numerous federal and industrial regulatory bodies govern cylinder manufacturing specifications, labeling, transportation, storage, and handling of medical gases.

Oxygen cylinders are available in different sizes that contain various amounts of gas. Cylinder size is designated by single letters. For example, popular oxygen tanks are termed H (large) size and E (small) size. E-sized tanks are usually used for patient transport or in emergencies. H-sized tanks measure over 4½ ft (1.37 m) tall and are used more for stationary/long-term (bedside) applications. Oxygen cylinders are an expensive and bulky form of packaging for a relatively inexpensive substance.

Cylinders contain much more gas than their unpressurized internal volume. By pressurizing the gas into cylinders, H and E cylinders when full contain 244 ft^3 (74.4 m^3) and 22 ft^3 (6.7 m^3) of oxygen, respectively. The reader is reminded that 1 ft^3 (0.30 m^3) equates to 28.3 L. Regardless of the size of the oxygen cylinder, it is filled to a tremendous pressure (2,200 psi). As a comparison, most automobile tires contain less than 50 psi.

A means of controlling the release of oxygen from the cylinder is necessary to permit safe and adjustable delivery to the patient. Typically, this includes three components:

- Cylinder valve
- Pressure-reducing valve
- Flowmeter

In most applications, the pressure-reducing valve and flowmeter are combined into a single assembly called a *regulator*.

Cylinder Valve

Cylinders come with an onboard needle valve, which allows the tank to be opened and closed but does not allow pressure reduction or flow measurement. This valve opens when turned counterclockwise and closes when turned clockwise, much like household water taps. The outlet of the cylinder valve is safety indexed for each type of gas; only a specific oxygen regulator will attach to an oxygen cylinder's valve. H cylinders use a threaded outlet to which a regulator is attached using a hex nut. E cylinders utilize a flat surface that receives a nipple from the oxygen regulator. This special type of regulator is not threaded but is pressed into position using a yoke-styled connection. Remember, only oxygen regulators will fit oxygen tanks. Generally, an appropriate hand tool (wrench) is required to connect and disconnect regulators from the cylinder valve. A special wrench is required to operate E cylinder valves.

Pressure-Reducing Valve

The cylinder valve is only a gross controller of flow, basically on or off. A pressure-reducing valve is used to reduce the extreme pressure within the cylinder to a working pressure, usually 50 psi. Fifty psi is still dangerously high for direct patient use but is a traditional

working pressure for most ancillary oxygen therapy equipment (flowmeters, ventilators, nebulizers, etc.).

There are differing types of pressure regulators (preset, adjustable, and multistage), and most incorporate a round (Bourdon) gauge that measures the gas pressure within the tank. A full tank registers 2,200 psi but gradually drops as the cylinder empties. The registered pressure is accurate only when the cylinder valve is open.

It is possible to calculate how long the contents of an oxygen cylinder will last using a simple formula with the specific conversion factor (CF) for each cylinder size. The CF for E- and H-sized tanks is 0.28 and 3.14 L per psi, respectively.

$$\text{Duration of flow (minutes)} = \frac{\text{Cylinder pressure} \times \text{CF}}{\text{Oxygen flow (lpm)}}$$

Flowmeter

Flowmeters control and indicate the flow rate of oxygen. Given a fixed working pressure of 50 psi, the outlet flow increases in proportion to the opening of a needle valve control. The most common flowmeter uses a Thorpe tube. A small indicator (often a black ball) floats on the flow of gas as it passes through the tapered Thorpe tube. The tube is graduated in increments of liters per minute (lpm). The greater the flow, the higher the float rises within the tube.

Flowmeters are specific to a particular gas. It is wise to ensure oxygen flowmeters are used to measure oxygen flow. Pediatric oxygen flowmeters are available for finer control of gas flow. These flowmeters display flow in increments of 0.5 or even 0.25 lpm. The flow rate is read with the flowmeter in an upright position with the graduation that bisects the ball float indicating the liter flow.

Flowmeters can be used to turn off gas flow; however, if the cylinder is not being used for a prolonged time, it should be turned off using the cylinder valve and the flowmeter left open.

Having two controls (cylinder valve and flowmeter) can cause confusion. For example, the regulator may register near full pressure but then quickly drops to zero when the flowmeter is turned on. This occurs when the regulator is pressurized yet the cylinder valve is turned off. The pressure drops quickly as the relatively small volume of oxygen contained within the regulator bleeds down. This happens when the flowmeter is turned off before the cylinder valve is turned off. For this reason, it is important to watch the flowmeter for a few moments after the flow of oxygen begins to ensure that cylinder pressure is maintained.

Liquid Oxygen

Oxygen can be stored as a liquid. This requires very low temperatures ($-183°$ C) maintained within a thermos-like cryogenic vessel. These systems operate under a pressure of approximately 20 psi. As pressure is reduced, the liquid oxygen is converted into a gas. It is not possible to estimate the contents of a vessel containing liquid oxygen, because the vapor pressure remains constant until the tank is empty. This is analogous to estimating the amount of propane within a tank used with a domestic barbeque. The quantity of liquid gas contained within the vessel is measured in terms of weight, rather than pressure. The storage advantage is obvious when considering that a single cubic foot of *liquid oxygen* is equivalent to about 860 ft^3 (262.1 m^3) of *oxygen gas*. Liquid oxygen vessels can be transfilled, that is, one liquid system can be used to fill another. Patients requiring long-term oxygen treatment often use smaller, portable liquid oxygen vessels. Patients may arrive at the sleep center with portable liquid oxygen systems. Although the patient can easily be switched to the sleep center's oxygen source, the technologist should be aware that the liquid oxygen will slowly vaporize and the vessel will empty even while not being used. This is similar to having a thermos of hot coffee that will slowly cool despite never being opened, the difference being that as liquid oxygen warms, it vaporizes to gas and escapes from the storage vessel.

Liquid oxygen is more expensive than compressed oxygen, and its primary advantage is storage. Most hospitals and other high-volume users store oxygen on-site in its liquid form.

Oxygen Concentrators

These self-contained, somewhat portable devices use electricity to power a compressor and filtration system. Filtering of room air through a molecular sieve bed or permeable plastic membrane produces concentrated oxygen. Oxygen concentrators are not capable of delivering high flows or high concentrations of oxygen and are therefore not suited to emergency situations.

Modern oxygen concentrators are convenient, quiet, and safe and provide a reliable source of relatively inexpensive low-flow oxygen. Because of these benefits, concentrators are a good oxygen source for sleep centers located outside of hospitals. The reader is encouraged to become familiar with their respective oxygen concentrator in terms of flow rate capability and oxygen concentration specifications. Oxygen concentration should be checked as a part of the laboratory equipment quality assurance process.

OXYGEN DELIVERY IN THE SLEEP CENTER

Precautions

Pure oxygen itself presents potential *physical* dangers. First, oxygen cylinders contain very high pressures. It must be ensured that tanks are secured from falling or tipping to avoid tank or regulator breakage. Oxygen cylinders must be stored away from heat sources. Liquid oxygen is of extremely low temperature, and the vaporizing liquid can cause low-temperature burns to the skin. Oxygen itself is not explosive but vigorously supports combustion. Oxygen and materials that are flammable make for a very dangerous mix. For example, collodion, which is both volatile and flammable, should not be used in the vicinity of oxygen.

Oxygen also poses *physiologic* consequences. Prolonged high alveolar oxygen levels (>60%) are associated with the production of free radicals and lung damage (oxygen toxicity). Alveolar oxygen concentrations of more than 80% (with special circumstances) can be associated with regional microlung collapse (absorption atelectasis).

Hypoxic Drive

The predominate stimulus to breathe is carbon dioxide level. There is also a secondary drive to breathe motivated by hypoxemia, and it is termed "hypoxic drive," which is a normal mechanism and can be accentuated at high altitude.

Some chronic lung diseases cause chronic elevation of PaCO$_2$ (hypercarbia). Chronic hypercarbia, it is argued, causes normal sensitivity to carbon dioxide to become blunted, and hypoxia becomes a predominant stimulus to breathe. These patients are said to be dependent on their hypoxic drive; their drive to breathe is diminished when oxygen is administered, and they may become hypopneic or apneic.

Although patients with chronic carbon dioxide retention are predisposed to being more reliant on their hypoxic drive, the dependence is inconsistent. Patients should be closely monitored, and the technologist should be mindful of potential ventilatory drive changes.

Hypoxic drive is a term that is overused, poorly understood, and often misdiagnosed. Hypoxic drive is certainly not a valid argument for withholding oxygen administration when treating hypoxemia.

Aims and Rationale of Intervention

The objective of treatment is to use the least amount of oxygen to bring about the desired therapeutic effect, which is often defined as a predetermined level of oxygen saturation. Various devices are available to deliver oxygen to patients, each with inherent limitations. Choosing the optimum delivery method is dependent on therapeutic goals, clinical status, and delivery device limitations.

It is advisable to establish both criteria and method for oxygen usage *before* performing polysomnography. Such guidelines are set by the physician and are usually based on patient clinical circumstance. The sleeping patient is particularly challenging, because changes in blood oxygen saturation are normal (during rapid eye movement), often transient, and perhaps expected with patients with preexisting respiratory pathology (2). Setting limits of desaturation during polysomnography is a medical determination and must be clear to the technologist.

Patients with sleep-disordered breathing (SDB) who require oxygen therapy when awake will often require oxygen when sleeping despite optimal maintenance of airway patency. In these instances, oxygen may be a useful adjunct to CPAP/BPAP treatment (3).

Procedures describing "how" to add oxygen to CPAP/BPAP treatment should be set forth *in advance of testing*. For example, "when supplemental oxygen is required, the oxygen flow will be added as close as possible to the CPAP interface" or "oxygen requirements will be assessed 10 minutes after each 1 (one) lpm increment change."

In the sleep center, oxygen is most commonly administered in terms of flow rate measured in lpm. The flow of oxygen is controlled at the source, which is commonly located at the head of the bed or within the sleep room. Unfortunately, this requires the technologist to enter the patient's room to make oxygen flow adjustments. Ideally, the oxygen source and flowmeter would be located outside the sleep room, and the oxygen tubing would run to the patient. This can make for long runs of tubing, which should be avoided. It is best to administer oxygen in the sleep center exactly as it is provided at home.

Oxygen can also be delivered in terms of concentration. Concentration is expressed as a percentage, such as 40% oxygen, or a fraction of inspired oxygen, termed FiO_2. For example, FiO_2 of 0.4 means 40% of the inspired air is oxygen (note that FiO_2 has no units of measure).

Both delivery device and liter flow determine FiO_2. In the sleep center, it is rare for the physician to request a specific FiO_2 or liter flow. Oxygen therapy is often ordered in advance by the physician without mention of actual dosage, but based on therapeutic results. For example, "administer oxygen as required to maintain SpO_2% >92%."

OXYGEN DELIVERY DEVICES

Oxygen delivery devices fall into two general categories: *high flow* and *low flow*.

High flow: These systems *theoretically* provide gas flows of specific oxygen concentrations at flow rates greater than the patient's inspiratory flow rate. These systems are touted to provide mid- to high *delivered* FiO_2. However, *in practice*, the patient's inspiratory flow exceeds the delivered flow, and *actual* FiO_2 diminishes proportionally as the patient draws in room air (4).

These devices often require humidification and a full-face mask. For the most part, high-flow systems are impractical for long-term home use and are not often encountered in the sleep center.

Low flow: These systems deliver a specific, relatively low flow of 100% oxygen at less than the patient's inspiratory flow rate. During inspiration, the patient draws in room air mixing with the oxygen, which results in variable inspired oxygen concentrations (5). Actual FiO_2 depends on the amount of room air the patient draws in making up the breath. Mouth breathing and high inspiratory flows result in greater dilution (lower FiO_2).

Other long-term, low-flow oxygen devices include transtracheal oxygen catheters (6) as well as cannulae variants incorporating reservoirs and demand flow capabilities (7). These devices have been developed with the goal of conserving oxygen. Oxygen flow during inspiration is inhaled and therefore useful, but the oxygen flow is essentially wasted during exhalation. Considerable waste occurs because the typical patient exhales three to five times longer than he or she inhales. A number of oxygen conserving devices are available that can be used with patients receiving long-term oxygen treatment. In short, these devices have been shown to deliver similar oxygen concentrations as nasal cannulae but using less oxygen.

Low-flow devices may require supplemental humidity because the oxygen supply is anhydrous; however, typically, humidity is not required with low flows (<4 lpm). When higher flow rates are required, common humidifiers used are bubble or jet type. These types of humidifiers are very inefficient and their value dubious at best. For this reason, simple oxygen delivery devices such as a nasal cannula are not used when higher flow rates of oxygen are necessary to support blood oxygen levels.

Nasal Cannula

The nasal cannula is the most commonly used oxygen delivery device (Fig. 51-1). The nasal cannula is relatively comfortable and often tolerated better than a mask (8, 9). Nasal cannulae are inexpensive and easily positioned with each prong of the cannula within the entrance of each nostril. A small tube runs over each ear, coming together

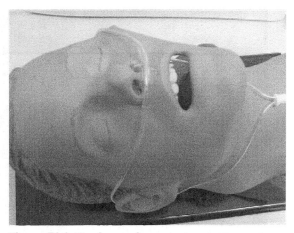

Figure 51-1 Nasal cannula.

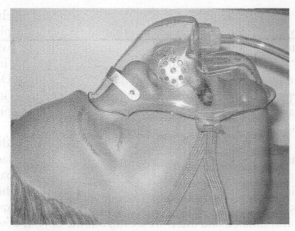

Figure 51-2 Simple oxygen mask.

below the chin, and running to the oxygen source. Most problems are caused by kinked tubing, disconnection, or poor positioning within the nares.

The nasal cannula can provide 24% to 40% oxygen (depending on patient inspiratory flow rate) with oxygen flow rates up to 6 lpm. As a guideline, oxygen flow rates with infants should be limited to a maximum of 2 lpm. Oxygen flows to adults of 4 lpm or less do not require supplemental humidification (10).

Simple Oxygen Mask

The simple oxygen mask is both inexpensive and easily applied (Fig. 51-2). The mask is less well tolerated than the nasal cannula because it is more obtrusive, covering both nose and mouth. Oxygen flows should be greater than 5 lpm to prevent rebreathing. Maximum 12 lpm oxygen flows can be used and bubble-type humidifiers are often used. FiO_2 is variable but thought to be approximately 0.3 to 0.6. Simple oxygen masks are usually used for short-term applications and emergencies requiring higher oxygen concentrations.

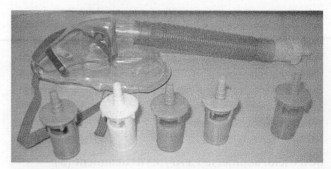

Figure 51-3 Venturi masks (air-entrainment masks).

Venturi Masks (Air-Entrainment Masks)

This mask system incorporates larger mask ports (Fig. 51-3). Assorted jet nozzle attachments are used to deliver specific FiO_2 levels. The nozzles are usually color coded and labeled with their specific oxygen flow requirement and resultant FiO_2. As the oxygen passes through the nozzle, it also pulls in room air. The FiO_2 is dependent on the flow of gas (nozzle size) and the size of the nozzle entrainment port. This approach to delivering oxygen is useful for transportation of patients and in situations where precise FiO_2 levels of less than 0.35 are desired. Limitations include lack of humidity, relatively high expense, and inaccuracies should the jet nozzle entrainment ports become occluded or covered, for example, with bedsheets.

Miscellaneous Oxygen Masks

Other modified simple oxygen masks incorporate reservoirs and/or one-way valves to control the amount of rebreathing and thereby increase FiO_2 (Fig. 51-4). These devices can be dangerous if not properly applied or monitored. It would be most unusual to encounter such devices in the sleep center, and garnering informed assistance before using these devices is recommended.

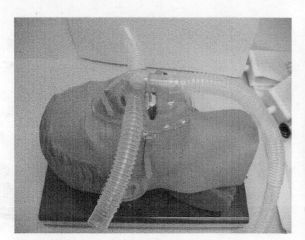
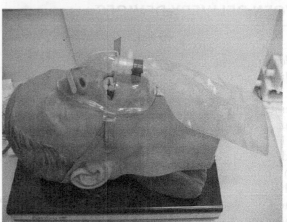

Figure 51-4 Other oxygen masks.

OXYGEN DELIVERY DEVICES AND POLYSOMNOGRAPHY

When patients arrive at the sleep center receiving supplemental oxygen, an effort should be made to maintain the type and style of device, as well as the set flow rate of oxygen. Often, one of the purposes of the polysomnogram is to evaluate nocturnal oxygen requirements. This can pose a problem, as positioning monitoring sensors and tubes or delivering CPAP requires unfettered access to the patient's face, nose, and mouth.

Oxygen is usually administered in the sleep center using a nasal cannula. During diagnostic polysomnography, airflow can be monitored using capnography, a thermocouple or thermistor, or a nasal pressure transducer (11). All these monitoring techniques require the positioning of a probe or cannula into/near the patient's nostrils. Adding an additional cannula for oxygen administration raises various concerns.

Spontaneously Breathing Patients

Many technologists will simply place the oxygen cannula *in addition to* the flow-sensing device. This practice is ill-advised (especially with pediatric patients) for two reasons:

- The added oxygen flow may interfere with airflow-monitoring techniques and result in a dampened airflow signal. The flow-sensing device signal is dampened by the added oxygen flow, artificially changing the actual temperature, pressure, and composition of the patient's breath and breathing.
- Instrumentation occupying the nostrils can significantly increase nasal resistance (12). Given the relatively small cross-sectional area and large variants of patient nare(s), both the size (lumen) and the number of cannulae placed within the nostrils should be minimized. The relationship between increased nasal resistance and SDB has been recently and extensively reviewed (13).

To avoid these shortcomings, bifurcated (dual tube) cannulae allowing individual access to each nostril are commercially available. Because pressure (or end-tidal CO_2) is sampled from only one naris, and oxygen delivered to the other, equally patent nostrils are ideal but rarely encountered. Other cannulae designs provide bifurcated access to each nostril, allowing bilateral oxygen delivery and pressure (or end-tidal CO_2) monitoring. Although this approach minimizes the occupying space of the cannulae, the proximity of the oxygen flow to nasal pressure/gas sampling can result in dampened flow signals.

Patient Using CPAP/BPAP

Flow-monitoring paraphernalia near or within the patient's nose interferes with the placement of CPAP interfaces. Usually, flow-sensing and oxygen delivery devices are removed when instituting CPAP. Flow and pressure signals can be derived from the sleep center CPAP machine remote control DC outputs or from an added inline flow transducer.

Oxygen is usually added directly into the CPAP circuitry and measured in terms of liter flow. However, the *actual* oxygen concentration is determined by several factors: not only the flow rate of oxygen but at which end of the CPAP hose the oxygen is added (near the machine or near the mask), mask leakage, the position of the exhalation port, the type of exhalation port, and the CPAP, inspiratory PAP, and expiratory PAP settings (14, 15).

Some CPAP masks have provisions for adding oxygen, allowing for delivery downstream from the exhalation port. Other masks do not have oxygen inlets, and the oxygen flow must be connected into the CPAP circuit upstream from the exhalation port. Although this has yet to be well studied, it is reasonable to assume there would be an effect on FiO_2. Again, the mask system and approach for plumbing the oxygen flow should be consistent between what is used in the sleep center and that in the patient's home.

One safety-related consideration is keeping the added oxygen flow as distal to the machine as possible. It is generally advisable to keep gases that support or accelerate combustion away from electrical equipment. The only downside is the requirement of having another tube running to the patient.

OXYGEN DELIVERY DEVICES AND INTEGRATION WITH THE POLYSOMNOGRAPH

The author is unaware of any oxygen flow–regulating device capable of producing an electronic output signal allowing integration with a polysomnographic system. For this reason, the technologist almost always annotates the administration of oxygen. The information presented and referenced in the previous section clarifies the need for documenting more than only the liter flow of oxygen. Other factors include the following:

- Oxygen administration device
- Style of oxygen cannulae used
- Other instrumentation occupying the nostrils
- Site of oxygen entry into the CPAP/BPAP circuit
- Type and position of exhalation ports
- Type of CPAP interface (nasal or full-face mask)
- Measures of interface or oral air leak
- CPAP or BPAP settings

This all seems rather laborious, although necessary, because all these factors determine the actual concentration of oxygen delivered to the patient. The underlying objective of this documentation is to achieve accurate duplication in the home environment after the patient leaves the sleep center. It is simple to state CPAP/BPAP and oxygen liter flow rates were required during the sleep study to maintain a certain SpO_2%. However, it is an assumption to extrapolate the sleep center observation to the home without consideration or knowledge of the many determinants of *actual* FiO_2.

The author's suggestion to minimize the documentation is to establish a sleep center protocol so that supplemental oxygen is provided consistently using the same tubing, cannulae, ports, site of interface, and so on. This would require documentation only for deviations from procedure. Ideally, the sleep center standard should be communicated to hospital respiratory therapy services and community durable medical equipment providers.

TROUBLESHOOTING AND REPORTING OUTCOMES

The end point of monitoring oxygen administration is usually the resultant change in blood oxygen levels. Blood oxygen levels are related to FiO_2—not lpm of oxygen. Although there is a relationship between the two, as previously discussed, there are many determinants of actual FiO_2.

Several methods of monitoring and measuring blood oxygen exist; however, detailed review of these techniques is beyond the scope of this chapter. The most common monitoring tool is the arterial oxygen saturation monitor (oximeter), which expresses blood oxygen levels in terms of SpO_2%.

In the sleep center, the pulse oximeter is the device most commonly used for monitoring blood oxygen levels. Most pulse oximeters interface nicely with polysomnographic systems, allowing arterial oxygen saturation to be continually displayed and recorded. As stated earlier, the technologist must manually document (annotate) the specific level of oxygen administration throughout the study.

Another common monitoring technique (arterial blood gases) requires an arterial blood sample to measure the partial pressure of oxygen dissolved within the plasma expressed in units of mm Hg (torr). The blood sample cannot be procured while the patient sleeps. Indwelling arterial lines are uncommon in the sleep lab. Obtaining blood gases when the patient is awake may have some value in patients without SDB (16).

Measuring *transcutaneous* pO_2 is another monitoring method. This approach is noninvasive, and the output is usually used as a trending tool. These monitors also easily interface with the polysomnograph.

Each oxygen measurement/monitoring technique has advantages and inherent limitations. The technologist should become intimately acquainted with the equipment he or she uses.

Although oxygen administration is commonly monitored by SpO_2%, there are numerous caveats. A patient can be hypoxic despite "normal" SpO_2% values. The technologist is urged to explore terms such as oxygen extraction, oxygen delivery, oxygen-carrying capacity, and regional perfusion; see Suggested Readings.

TROUBLESHOOTING OF OXYGEN DELIVERY DEVICES

Should oxygen administration fail to increase oxygen saturation, the first thing to check is the patient. In addition, a check of the monitoring device is prudent; it is important to ensure proper sensor placement and function. The possibility of erroneous or artifactual monitoring cannot be ignored.

Once the patient's oxygen level has been deemed accurate, the next thing to check is your plumbing. Simple checks for flowmeter function, tubing disconnection, cannula misplacement, and kinked tubing should be performed.

Other considerations include mouth breathing or nasal obstruction. If the patient is unable to inhale the oxygen from the delivery device, there may be little or no benefit. Similarly unappreciated, ongoing upper airway obstruction or hypoventilation may confound successful administration of oxygen.

If the patient's oxygen level cannot be maintained when asleep, the technologist may consider waking the patient for assessment. How these decisions are made and when testing ought to be interrupted should be determined in advance. However, a patient not responding to increased FiO_2 may be presenting with a profound physiologic problem that needs immediate attention.

WHEN TO GET HELP!

The sleep technologist should not hesitate to summon help. The ways and means of accessing assistance are varied, depending on the resources available to your sleep center. Once again, the reader is encouraged to explore his or her resources *before* the need becomes a crisis.

Assuming there are no technical problems, the sleep technologist would be generally advised to call for help in the following circumstances:

- The patient's oxygen saturation level cannot be maintained despite reaching the flow limits of the delivery system or the physician's order/guideline.

- The patient is awake and hypoxic, experiencing respiratory distress and/or cardiac instability.
- The patient is hypoxic and unresponsive despite attempts to awaken.

FINAL CONSIDERATIONS

At first glance, a general review of oxygen delivery devices seems rather mundane. Special considerations encountered within the sleep center present complex challenges. There are few studies examining oxygen delivery device function in the sleep center. Most studies have been done in postoperative recovery rooms, in intensive care units, or in ambulatory patients with chronic lung disease. Nonetheless, one cannot ignore the wealth of information available, because many of the principles and relationships apply to the sleep center.

Similarly, documented concerns related to oxygen delivery and delivery devices may also cause problems in the sleep center. For instance, given oxygen is usually provided at low-flow rates through relatively large-bore intranasal cannulae, one must ask how this resistive load affects the *sleeping* patient (17). It is reasonable to assume there is a point where the sum of the cross-sectional area of cannula and sensors will impose an increased nasal resistance. The potential for iatrogenic nasal resistance and resultant upper airway obstruction has yet to be studied.

Inhalation of anhydrous gas flow can be irritating to the nose and may lead to increased nasal resistance. There may be a hypothetical requirement to humidify oxygen at night, in consideration of the natural inclination for increased nasal resistance when supine (18).

As always, when introducing gas flow or catheters into the nasal passage, it is necessary to recognize the link between nasal afferent stimulation and breathing pattern (19).

Newer CPAP modalities and other adjunct therapies pose other questions. It is reasonable to expect FiO_2 fluctuation depending on the amount and extent of interaction during "auto" or "smart" PAP treatment. The introduction of gas flows to systems equipped with adjuncts such as C-Flex is unknown. Similarly, the impact on I → E and E → I phase triggering with bilevel machines is unknown.

REFERENCES

1. Becker, H. F., & Piper, A. J. (1999). Breathing during sleep in patient with nocturnal desaturation. *American Journal of Respiratory and Critical Care Medicine, 159*, 112–118.
2. Plywaczewski, R., Sliwinski, P., Nowinski, A., et al. (2000). Incidence of nocturnal desaturation while breathing oxygen in COPD patients undergoing long-term oxygen therapy. *Chest, 117*(3), 679–683.
3. Kryger, M., Roth, T., & Dement, W. C. (1994). *Principles and practice of sleep medicine* (2nd ed., p. 687). Philadelphia, PA: W.B. Saunders Company.
4. Goldstein, R., Young, J., & Rebuck, A. S. (1982). Effect of breathing pattern on oxygen concentration received from standard face mask. *Lancet, 2*(8309), 1188–1190.
5. Bazuaye, E. A., Stone, T. N., Corris, P. A., et al. (1992). Variability of inspired oxygen concentration with nasal cannulas. *Thorax, 47*(8), 609–611.
6. Christopher, K. L. (2003). Transtracheal oxygen catheters. *Clinics of Chest Medicine, 24*(3), 489–510.
7. Domingo, C., Roig, J., Coll, R., et al. (1996). Evaluation of the use of three different devices for nocturnal oxygen therapy in COPD. *Respiration, 63*, 230–235.
8. Nolan, K. M., Winyard, J. A., & Goldhill, D. R. (1993). Comparison of nasal cannulae with face mask for oxygen administration to postoperative patients. *British Journal of Anaesthiology, 70*(4), 440–442.
9. Costello, R. W., Liston, R., & McNicholas, W. T. (1995). Compliance at night with low flow oxygen therapy: A comparison of nasal cannulae and Venturi face masks. *Thorax, 50*(4), 405–406.
10. AARC Clinical Practice Guidelines. (1992). Oxygen therapy in the home or extended care facility. *Respiratory Care, 37*, 918–922.
11. Hernandez, L., Ballester, E., Farré, R., et al. (2001). Performance of nasal prongs in sleep studies: Spectrum of flow-related events. *Chest, 119*(2), 442–450.
12. Lorino, A. M., Lorino, H., Dahan, E., et al. (2000). Effects of nasal prongs on nasal airflow resistance. *Chest, 118*, 366–371.
13. Rappai, M., Collop, N., Kemp, S., et al. (2003). The nose and sleep disordered breathing: What we know and what we do not know. *Chest, 124*, 2309–2323.
14. Schwartz, A. R., Kacmarek, R. M., & Hess, D. R. (2004). Factors affecting oxygen delivery with bi-level positive airway pressure. *Respiratory Care, 49*(3), 270–275.
15. Yoder, E. A., Klann, K., & Strohl, K. P. (2004). Inspired oxygen concentrations during positive pressure therapy. *Sleep and Breathing, 8*(1), 1–5.
16. Tarrega, J., Guell, R., Antón, A., et al. (2002). Are daytime arterial blood gases a good reflection of nighttime gas exchange in patients on long-term oxygen therapy? *Respiratory Care, 47*(8), 882–886.
17. Weigand, L., Zwilling, C. W., & White, D. P. (1989). Collapsibility of the human upper airway during normal sleep. *Journal of Applied Physiology, 66*, 1800–1808.
18. Desfonds, P., Planes, C., Fuhrman, C., et al. (1998). Nasal resistance in snorers with or without sleep apnea: Effect of posture and nasal ventilation with continuous positive airway pressure. *Sleep, 21*(6), 625–632.

19. Burgess, K. R., & Whitelaw, W. A. (1988). Effects of nasal cold receptors on pattern of breathing. *Journal of Applied Physiology, 64*(1), 371–376.

SUGGESTED READINGS

Branson, R. D., Hess, R. H., & Chatburn, R. L. (1995). *Respiratory care equipment*. Philadelphia, PA: J.B. Lippincott Company.

Hedley-Whyte, J., Burgess, G. E., III, Feeley, T. W., et al. (1976). *Applied physiology of respiratory care*. Boston, MA: Little-Brown.

McPherson, S. P., & Spearman, C. B. (1985). *Respiratory therapy equipment* (3rd ed.). St. Louis, MO: C.V. Mosby Company.

Spearman, C. B., Sheldon, R. L., & Egan, D. F. (1982). *Egan's fundamentals of respiratory therapy* (4th ed.). St. Louis, MO: C.V. Mosby Company.

chapter 52
Dental Sleep Medicine: Oral Appliance Therapy and Titration Management

SHAWN KIMBRO

LEARNING OBJECTIVES

On completion of this chapter, the reader should be able to:

1. Describe the role of the dentist in a comprehensive sleep disorders treatment plan.
2. Describe oral appliance therapy.
3. Identify different types of oral devices and their advantages and drawbacks.
4. Describe the role of the sleep technologist in oral appliance titration and therapy.

KEY TERMS

American Academy of Dental Sleep Medicine
Dental device
Maxillomandibular advancement
Obstructive sleep apnea
Oral appliance therapy
Oral surgery
Sleep-disordered breathing

Management of sleep disorders requires a multidisciplinary approach and diverse perspectives. The role of the dentist has emerged as a key aspect in the care of patients with sleep-disordered breathing (SDB). The recognition and treatment of sleep apnea may be more successful, both in efficacy and in compliance, if dentists and sleep specialists collaborate closely. This includes active participation by sleep technologists who are well-versed in aspects of SDB treatments and management. As practitioners in the health care field, dentists assist patients who are identified with SDB by making recommendations and referrals and by participating in treatment and overall management of the disease. This may include the use of oral appliance therapy (OAT), head and neck surgery, or upper airway surgery.

ORAL APPLIANCE THERAPY

As research into effective therapy options for treating SDB increases, there is growing interest in OAT. Oral appliances, sometimes called "dental devices," are a simple and cost-effective method of treating snoring and mild-to-moderate obstructive sleep apnea (OSA). Snoring is a symptom of OSA and an indication of increased upper airway resistance. The pharyngeal portion of the upper airway, from the soft palate to the base of the tongue, is where snoring and OSA typically occur. During sleep, activity in the upper airway dilator muscles decreases, causing the pharyngeal airway to shrink and sometimes close. Treatments for snoring or OSA aim to maintain upper airway patency during sleep.

The gold standard for treating SDB is continuous positive airway pressure (CPAP). Many patients, however, are unable or unwilling to tolerate CPAP, so other options become necessary. Because oral appliances are portable and cost-effective, they are generally well accepted by patients either as an alternative to CPAP or as a first-line therapy. The appliances are worn in the mouth, similar to orthodontic devices or sports mouth protectors, during sleep to help stabilize the upper airway and promote improved breathing. An oral appliance helps maintain an open and unobstructed airway during sleep by protruding and stabilizing the tongue and mandible.

History

Oral appliances were considered for the treatment of upper airway obstruction as early as 1903 (1). In 1934, Pierre Robin described a functional appliance to move the mandible forward and alleviate tongue obstruction. By the early 1980s, research into SDB found that the vast majority of SDB cases are related to obstruction in the airway. Treatments introduced during this time included the surgical treatment uvulopalatopharyngoplasty (2) and nasal CPAP (3). Some early types of oral appliances were introduced, but they did not come into general use until the 1980s.

In the 1990s, research continued to show the efficacy of OAT in the treatment of SDB. As comparative data became available, physicians became more acceptive of oral devices. In 1991, a group of dentists who were interested in promoting the use of oral appliances as a part of sleep disorders therapy formed the Sleep Disorders Dental Society (now the American Academy of Dental Sleep Medicine [AADSM]). The AADSM's mission also includes the promotion and coordination of research activities and recommendations for the implementation of OAT (4). In 1995, the American Sleep Disorders Association (now the American Academy of Sleep Medicine [AASM]) published a review indicating that oral devices presented an acceptable alternative to CPAP in the cases of simple snoring or mild-to-moderate OSA (5).

Recognizing the need for increased teamwork between physicians and dentists in order to achieve optimal treatment for patients with OSA, the AASM and the AADSM issued the first official joint clinical practice guidelines for the treatment of patients with OAT in 2015 (6). The guidelines note that although positive airway pressure remains the gold standard for the treatment of OSA, the board-certified sleep medicine physician should take the patient's preference into consideration. The guidelines further state that after a sleep physician prescribes OAT, treatment should be provided by a qualified dentist using a customized, titratable device and that efficacy should be confirmed or denied by follow-up sleep testing.

In order to assist technologists that are increasingly encountering oral appliances in the sleep center, the American Association of Sleep Technologists (AAST) released technical guidelines for oral appliance titration in 2018 (7). The guidelines recognize that the patient should be referred back to the sleep center to assess efficacy and that, during the overnight study, the technologist should work with the patient to titrate the oral appliance with the goal of identifying an optimal therapeutic setting.

Types of Oral Devices

Dentists use OAT for many purposes, but there are three primary types used for the treatment of SDB: tongue-retaining devices (TRDs), nonadjustable mandibular repositioning devices, and titratable mandibular repositioning devices.

Tongue-Retaining Devices

TRDs are placed between the upper and lower teeth and usually employ a suction cup or flange to move the tongue away from the back of the throat (Fig. 52-1). Some of these devices contain a bulb in which the tongue is inserted. The resulting repositioning keeps the airway clear from any obstruction caused by the base of the tongue. TRDs can work for patients with large tongues and for those who have few or no teeth. They are also used for patients who cannot adequately advance their mandible. Some TRDs are custom-fitted to the patient's

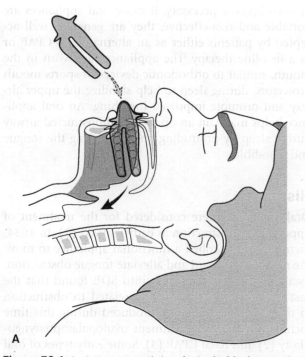
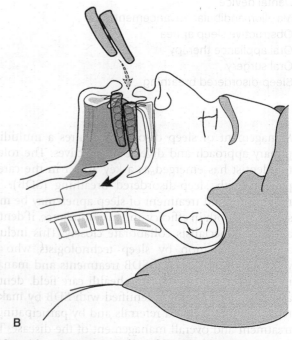

Figure 52-1 **A:** A tongue-retaining device holds the tongue in a forward position, preventing it from falling backward and blocking the airway. **B:** Mandibular repositioning appliances move the mandible and the associated structures, such as the tongue, forward and prevent the tissues from collapsing during sleep.

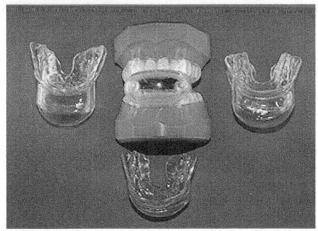

Figure 52-2 Four views of a tongue-retaining device manufactured by Professional Positioners Inc.

Efficacy of Oral Appliances in the Treatment of Obstructive Sleep Apnea

Table 52-1

Treatment Response in 304 Patients	%
RDI <50% of initial RDI	70
RDI <10	51
RDI > initial RDI	13
RDI >20 (patients with initial RDI > 20)	39

RDI = apneas + hypopneas/hour sleep

Adapted from Schmidt-Nowara, W. W., Lowe, A., Wiegand, L., et al. (1995). Oral appliances for the treatment of snoring and obstructive sleep apnea: A review. *Sleep, 18,* 501–510.

teeth by use of dental impressions (Fig. 52-2). TRDs are not used frequently because they can cause an excessive buildup of saliva, difficulty swallowing, irritation of the tongue, and an increased gag reflex.

Mandibular Advancement Devices

Mandibular advancement devices (MADs) are the most commonly used type of oral appliance to treat snoring and OSA. They can be classified into two main categories: nonadjustable (nontitratable) and adjustable (titratable). These devices fit over both the top and bottom teeth and work by repositioning the lower jaw both open and forward (see Fig. 52-1B). MADs are usually more effective in treating OSA than TRDs (8). When the mandible is advanced, the tongue and some soft tissue in the throat move forward to widen the airway space and reduce the likelihood of collapse. Air passes more freely through the airway, reducing snoring and sleep apnea. There are several different kinds of MADs (Fig. 52-3). Most use traditional dental techniques to attach the device to the patient's teeth. Because it is extremely important that the devices fit precisely over the teeth, most MADs require dental impressions and fabrication by a dental laboratory. Because these devices have the potential to cause loss of dental restorations, facial discomfort, and bite changes, participation by a qualified dentist is imperative.

Many patients require significant advancement of the mandible for the MAD to be effective. For these patients, it is beneficial to increase the degree of advancement incrementally by using a titratable device. Gradual advancement over time has been shown to be the most comfortable method of adjustment. One randomized controlled study and another clinical study noted significantly more success after an overnight study that titrated the devices by 17% to 30% (9). Some designs include openings for oral breathing and posterior extensions designed to modify the position of the soft palate or tongue. Side effects include excessive salivation, temporomandibular joint (TMJ) discomfort or pain, discomfort of the teeth or jaw upon awakening, and rare occlusal changes (10).

Efficacy of Oral Devices

OAT is very effective in eliminating snoring and somewhat effective in treating OSA (Table 52-1). A device properly fabricated to the specifications of a dentist who is trained in OAT provides the best likelihood for success. Because oral appliances work best for patients with mild-to-moderate sleep apnea, it is important to evaluate the degree of severity of a patient's condition before the device is installed. If apnea is present to any degree, follow-up polysomnography with the appliance in place is necessary to evaluate efficacy. Research has shown that, despite variations in the design of the oral appliance, clinical results are remarkably consistent (5). Patients with high apnea–hypopnea indices (AHIs) are not good candidates for OAT. Although the use of oral appliances may reduce AHIs in patients with very severe sleep

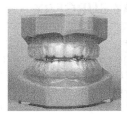 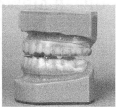 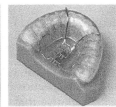 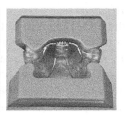

Figure 52-3 Four views of the Klearway appliance for mandibular advancement.

apnea, it is less likely that sleep apnea will be eliminated using only the appliance. Some success in lowering CPAPs to more tolerable levels has been demonstrated by combining an oral appliance with CPAP (11).

Some recent studies have compared OAT with CPAP. These studies show that OAT often, but not always, decreased the AHI, whereas CPAP nearly always resolved SDB entirely. The studies also indicate that patient acceptance of OAT is greater than that of CPAP, resulting in a similar proportion of successfully treated patients. When patients were asked to choose a preferred treatment, the majority chose OAT (12–14).

An important aspect of evaluating the efficacy of any treatment is patient compliance. Studies have demonstrated good long-term compliance with oral appliances (12), from 48% continued usage after 2 years to 86% after 5 years. Proper patient education and instruction is an important aspect of treatment to promote better compliance. The most common reasons for noncompliance include the earlier listed side effects and inadequate treatment outcomes and symptom resolution. Contraindications to oral devices include a diagnosis of central sleep apnea, TMJ disease, or nasal obstruction.

Clinical Protocol for OAT

Indications for OAT include the following:

- Adult patients who request treatment for primary snoring without OSA who do not respond to, or are not appropriate candidates for, treatment with behavioral measures such as weight loss, positional therapy, or alcohol avoidance.
- Adult patients with OSA who are intolerant of CPAP therapy or prefer alternative therapy.

Oral appliances may also be indicated for patients who refuse, or are not candidates for, tonsillectomy and adenoidectomy, craniofacial operations, or tracheostomy (6).

Because upper airway obstruction can lead to serious and life-threatening disease (15), it is crucial to obtain a thorough and accurate diagnosis before implementing any treatment regime. The gold standard for evaluating SDB is attended polysomnography that is interpreted by a board-certified sleep specialist (16). Because CPAP has been found to be superior to oral appliances in reducing the AHI, arousal index, and oxygen desaturation index, it should still be considered the first-line therapy for patients with OSA.

In cases where OAT is chosen, the physician refers the patient to a dentist with advanced training and expertise in the management of oral appliances for SDB. This can be accomplished through a written referral or a prescription and should be accompanied by a diagnostic report of the polysomnogram. It is imperative that there be extensive cooperation between the dentist and the referring physician in both the initiation and the maintenance of OAT.

Factors influencing the type of oral appliance used include a comprehensive dental examination and the dentist's familiarity and comfort level with available devices. When mandibular repositioning devices are used, an initial assessment about the degree of advancement should be made along with a judgment of the final advancement goal. In most cases, a three- to seven-night trial period allows the patient to make a subjective symptom assessment and a preliminary evaluation of tolerance. Final appliance design, fabrication, fitting, and placement then occur, followed by a 1- to 2-month evaluation period. This evaluation period includes adjustments or titration of the appliance, subjective symptom evaluations, and assessment by the dentist of possible dental complications.

In their joint guidelines, the AASM and AADSM recommend that qualified dentists provide oversight of OAT to survey for dental-related side effects or occlusal changes in order to reduce their incidence. Because subjective feedback is inadequate to assess optimal titration of an oral appliance, they also recommend that sleep physicians conduct follow-up sleep testing to improve or confirm treatment efficacy for patients using oral appliances. The follow-up testing should be performed using the standard sensors and data collection parameters recommended by the AASM for polysomnography and may include additional titration of the device. During this titration, a qualified sleep technologist works closely with the patient to adjust the appliance to insure that the airway remains open and reduces the AHI.

A comparison of the risks and benefits of OAT with those of other available treatments suggests that oral devices present a useful alternative to CPAP therapy, especially for patients with simple snoring and patients with OSA who cannot tolerate CPAP therapy (5). A well-made, well-fitted oral appliance will effectively reduce or eliminate snoring and can significantly reduce symptoms of mild-to-moderate OSA. Oral appliances are small, convenient, and easy for most patients to wear. They weigh very little and are easy to travel with. Oral appliances can cost less to the patient than other treatments. Most patients adjust to oral appliances in only a few weeks. Treatment is reversible and noninvasive.

UPPER AIRWAY SURGERY

Upper airway surgery is generally indicated only when other therapies are unsuccessful or intolerable, or for patients with an underlying, specific, surgically correctable abnormality that is causing the OSA (17). Although surgery may be an effective treatment for snoring and OSA, it should be performed only on the appropriate portions of the upper airway. Surgery is site-specific, meaning it requires the identification of specific anatomic areas contributing to airway obstruction. This may vary from patient to patient. A detailed examination of the entire upper airway is necessary before deciding which surgical procedures may be most effective (18). The two most common forms of oral surgery performed by dental professionals for the treatment of SDB are maxillomandibular advancement (MMA) and anterior inferior mandibular osteotomy (AIMO) (19). Other forms of surgery are discussed elsewhere in this text.

Maxillomandibular Advancement

MMA is the most accepted and effective surgical treatment for OSA (20). MMA cuts the bone of the upper and lower jaws, so that soft tissues in the soft palate and tongue are pulled forward. This enlarges and stabilizes the upper airway. The operation is performed under general anesthesia and requires an overnight hospital stay. After the procedure, the patient's jaws are wired shut for several weeks. MMA has a 98% success rate in treating sleep apnea patients for whom this surgery is indicated (21).

Anterior Inferior Mandibular Osteotomy

AIMO involves cutting the chin bone in order to pull forward the tongue and muscles of the hyoid (the U-shaped bone in the anterior neck) to enlarge and stabilize the airway behind the tongue base. Although not as effective as MMA (19), the jaws do not have to be wired shut, and there is no change in bite. AIMO may be performed as an outpatient procedure or in combination with MMA and other procedures.

THE ROLE OF THE TECHNOLOGIST

The sleep technologist must understand the importance of close collaboration between dentists and sleep professionals in treating snoring and OSA. Because technologists may be called upon to assist with referrals and coordinate aspects of a treatment plan, it is important to understand the indications for dental treatment options. As noted earlier, the technologist may be tasked to assist the patient in titrating the oral device during follow-up testing. The technologist also plays an important role in follow-up evaluation and treatment for patients who have undergone oral surgery or other dental interventions.

Remotely controlled mandibular positioners that can be integrated into existing polysomnography systems have entered the market and are used by some sleep centers. These devices allow the technologist to make remote adjustments to mandibular advancement while the polysomnogram is in progress. The technologist should be familiar with the individual types of dental devices used most frequently by the physicians and dentists with whom they work. As research into the growing field of dental sleep medicine continues, the tasks of the technologist will evolve.

SUMMARY

Because there is currently no single universal effective and tolerable treatment for sleep-related breathing disorders, sleep medicine requires physicians and dentists to work closely to manage SDB in patients. In order to facilitate this collaboration, participation by sleep technologists is fundamental. The AADSM[1] is an integral part of the sleep community. The AADSM is the primary organization for the dental profession's involvement in research, assessment, and management of SDB. To insure adherence to practice guidelines and quality standards, the AADSM has an examination and clinical requirements for board certification in Dental Sleep Medicine. Dentists are often at the front line of identifying patients with sleep disorders. As the science of sleep matures, the role of dental sleep medicine is certain to expand.

REFERENCES

1. Robin, P. (1934). Glossoptosis due to atresia and hypertrophy of the mandible. *American Journal of Diseases of Children, 48,* 541–547.
2. Fujita, S. (1987). Pharyngeal surgery for obstructive sleep apnea and snoring. In D. Fairbanks, S. Fujita, T. Ikematsu, et al. (Eds.), *Snoring and obstructive sleep apnea* (pp. 101–128). New York, NY: Raven Press.
3. Sullivan, C. E., Issa, F. G., Berthon-Jones, M., et al. (1981). Reversal of obstructive sleep apnea by continuous positive airway pressure applied through the nares. *Lancet, 1,* 862–865.
4. Lowe, A. A. (1994). Dental appliances for the treatment of snoring and/or obstructive sleep apnea. In M. Kryger, T. Roth, & W. Dement (Eds.), *Principles and practice of sleep medicine* (2nd ed., pp. 722–735). Philadelphia, PA: W.B. Saunders Co.
5. Schmidt-Nowara, W. W., Lowe, A., Wiegand, L., et al. (1995). Oral appliances for the treatment of snoring and obstructive sleep apnea: A review. *Sleep, 18,* 501–510.
6. Ramar, K., Dort, L. C., Katz, S. G., et al. (2015). Clinical practice guideline for the treatment of obstructive

[1]More information about the American Academy of Dental Sleep Medicine can be found on their web site, https://aadsm.org, or by contacting the American Academy of Dental Sleep Medicine, 1101 Warrenville Road, Suite 175, Lisle, IL 60532. Ph: +1 (630) 686 9875; Fax +1 (630) 686 9876.

sleep apnea and snoring with oral appliance therapy: An update for 2015. *Journal of Clinical Sleep Medicine, 11*(7), 773–827.

7. American Association of Sleep Technologists. (2018). *Oral Appliance Titration Technical Guideline.* Retrieved from https://www.aastweb.org/hubfs/OAT%20Technical%20Guideline.pdf

8. Loube, D. I., & Strauss, A. M. (1997). Survey of oral appliance practice among dentists treating obstructive sleep apnea patients. *Chest, 111,* 382–386.

9. Almeida, F. R., Parker, J. A., Hodges, J. S., et al. (2009). Effect of a titration polysomnogram on treatment success with a mandibular repositioning appliance. *Journal of Clinical Sleep Medicine, 5*(3), 198–204.

10. Rose, E. C., Staats, R., Virchow, C., Jr., et al. (2002). Occlusal and skeletal effects of an oral appliance in the treatment of obstructive sleep apnea. *Chest, 122,* 871–877.

11. El-Solh, A. A., Moitheennazima, B., Akinnusi, M. E., et al. (2011). Combined oral appliance and positive airway pressure therapy for obstructive sleep apnea: A pilot study. *Sleep & Breathing, 15*(2), 203–208.

12. Ferguson, K. A., Ono, T., Lowe, A. A., et al. (1996). A randomized crossover study of an oral appliance vs nasal-continuous positive airway pressure in the treatment of mild-moderate obstructive sleep apnea. *Chest, 109*(5), 1269–1275.

13. Ferguson, K. A., Ono, T., Lowe, A. A., et al. (1997). A short-term controlled trial of an adjustable oral appliance for the treatment of mild to moderate obstructive sleep apnoea. *Thorax, 52,* 326–368.

14. Clark, G. T., Blumenfeld, I., Yoffe, N., et al. (1996). A crossover study comparing the efficacy of continuous positive airway pressure with anterior mandibular positioning devices on patients with obstructive sleep apnea. *Chest, 109,* 1477–1483.

15. Guilleminault, C. (1983). Natural history, cardiac impact and long-term follow-up of sleep apnea syndrome. In C. Guilleminault & E. Lugaresi (Eds.), *Sleep-wake disorders: Natural history, epidemiology and long-term evolution* (pp. 107–125). New York, NY: Raven Press.

16. Guilleminault, C., & Mondini, S. (1983). The complexity of obstructive sleep apnea syndrome: Need for multi-diagnostic approaches before considering treatment. *Bulletin of European Physiopathological Respiration, 19,* 595–599.

17. American Sleep Disorders Association. (1996). Practice parameters for the treatment of obstructive sleep apnea in adults: The efficacy of surgical modifications of the upper airway. *Sleep, 19,* 152–155.

18. American Academy of Dental Sleep Medicine (AADSM) Web site. (2018). Scoring of fatigue and sleepiness in patients with obstructive sleep apnea treated with a titratable custom-made mandibular advancement device. Retrieved from https://aadsm.org/award_winning_abstracts_from_a.php

19. Krekmanov, L., Andersson, L., Ringqvist, M., et al. (1998). Anterior-inferior mandibular osteotomy in treatment of obstructive sleep apnea syndrome. *International Journal of Adult Orthodontics and Orthognathic Surgery, 13*(4), 289–298.

20. Hochban, W., Bradendurg, U., & Peter, J. H. (1994). Surgical treatment of obstructive sleep apnea by maxillomandibular advancement. *Sleep, 17,* 624–629.

21. Riley, R. W., Powell, N. B., & Guilleminault, C. (1993). Obstructive sleep apnea syndrome: A review of 306 consecutively treated surgical patients. *Otolaryngology—Head & Neck Surgery, 108,* 117–125.

chapter 53

Technical–Surgical Interventions for Sleep Apnea

EDWIN M. VALLADARES

LEARNING OBJECTIVES

On completion of this chapter, the reader should be able to:

1. Explain technical–surgical therapy for obstructive sleep apnea by way of hypoglossal nerve stimulation.
2. Identify the anatomy of the airway associated with obstructive sleep apnea.
3. Identify upper airway collapse as shown by drug-induced sleep endoscopy.
4. Explain technical–surgical therapy for central sleep apnea by way of phrenic nerve stimulation.
5. Identify the role of the sleep technologist in technical–surgical interventions.

KEY TERMS

Sleep apnea
Obstructive sleep apnea
Central sleep apnea
Hypoglossal nerve stimulation
Phrenic nerve stimulation
Implant
Inspire upper airway stimulation therapy

INTRODUCTION

Continuous positive airway pressure (CPAP) has been the first-line intervention for treating patients with moderate-to-severe sleep apnea since 1981 (1). With approximately 29% to 83% of adult patients unable to meet minimum CPAP therapy adherence criteria (4 hours or more per night for 70% of nights), alternatives to traditional pressure mask–based therapies have long been sought (2–4). As a result, surgical interventions have been developed, but they can't be used without selecting the correct patient for optimal benefit (5). Thus, sleep medicine is moving toward personalized interventions for optimal therapy. Technical–surgical interventions are one such example. I call these therapies technical–surgical interventions because they involve a surgical implantation of a device and technical therapy management.

With the advent of new Food and Drug Administration (FDA)-approved implantable stimulators for treating sleep-disordered breathing in a fraction of non-compliant PAP therapy patients, the landscape of sleep medicine and sleep technology is changing to narrow the gap between compliant and noncompliant patients (6, 7). The Inspire upper airway stimulation (UAS) therapy for treating obstructive sleep apnea (OSA) and the remedē® System for treating central sleep apnea (CSA) are providing new tools for sleep physicians, thus elevating the expertise of sleep technologists and paving the way for personalized medicine.

TECHNICAL–SURGICAL INTERVENTION FOR OSA

In 2014, the FDA approved the Inspire UAS therapy for the treatment of OSA. This therapy provides a feasible option for treating a subset of patients with OSA (7). Although these devices will not be appropriate for all of the PAP-intolerant patients, careful selection criteria make the Inspire UAS therapy a viable option for a small but growing percentage of patients. As of November 2016, Inspire Medical, Inc. had reportedly implanted approximately 1,000 patients (8).

The Inspire UAS therapy is for patients with moderate-to-severe OSA (apnea–hypopnea index [AHI] 15 to 65 per hour) who have not been able to tolerate CPAP therapy and do not have concentric collapse of the upper airway. The Inspire UAS therapy stimulates the hypoglossal nerve during inspiration and moves the tongue base forward to open the upper airway. The UAS therapy stimulates on the basis of signaling from the sensing lead's breathing information. The patient uses an external wireless remote to turn the therapy "on," "off," "pause," and to control stimulation intensity across a limited programmed range (9).

Inspire UAS Therapy: Components, Function, and Indications

The Inspire UAS therapy is composed of a neurostimulator with 1-stimulating lead to provide coordinated tongue protrusion and 1-monitoring sensing lead. The stimulator lead is connected to the hypoglossal nerve (XII), specifically on the medial-XII branch, and the sensing lead is connected to the upper border of the underlying rib in the fourth intercostal region to gate the hypoglossal nerve stimulation to inspiration. The device is accessed through an electronic tablet and interrogation component (see Fig. 53-1) (10). The estimated battery life of the neurostimulator is 10.9 years (11).

The criteria for being implanted are as follows: (1) have tried CPAP and failed, (2) have drug-induced sleep endoscopy (DISE) to rule out concentric collapse at the palate, (3) have an AHI 15 to 65 per hour, and (4) have a body mass index less than 32 kg per m². These criteria narrow the therapy to a subset of noncompliant PAP therapy patients. Contraindications for implanting the Inspire UAS therapy are as follows: central + mixed apneas greater than 25% of total AHI, any anatomic finding that would compromise the performance of the therapy (e.g., concentric collapse), any condition or procedure that has compromised the neurologic control of the upper airway, patients who are unable or do not have the necessary assistance to operate the sleep remote, pregnancy or plan to become pregnant, implantable device that may unintentionally interact with the Inspire system, and patients requiring magnetic resonance imaging (MRI) other than the specified MR conditional labeling (Inspire system implant manual) (11).

Airway evaluation through DISE has become a good predictor of success for UAS therapy (12). DISE is conducted in an operating room where sleep is induced using a sedative, such as Propofol, to mimic airway collapse during sleep and characterize the airway collapse using a fiber-optic laryngoscope. The sedative is used to the lowest dose, which elicits loss of consciousness as measured by loss of response to normal conversational voice stimulation, while monitoring vital signs. Because this is a procedure conducted in an operating room, a team of nurses assists with monitoring the patient's vitals (13). It has been shown that patients with concentric collapse of the palate do not do well with UAS therapy, as opposed to other types of collapse, thereby suggesting that tongue protrusion from UAS is insufficient to overcome airway obstruction in concentric collapse (see Figs. 53-2 and 53-3) (12). Figure 53-3 demonstrates examples of (a) an open airway, (b) lateral wall collapse, and (c) concentric collapse.

Inspire UAS Therapy: Patient Process

A trained otolaryngologist implants the Inspire UAS therapy and is subsequently followed at the sleep clinic by a sleep physician. The patient meets with a trained sleep physician and a trained sleep technologist to activate the device 1 month postimplant. This is the visit when the patient feels the stimulation for the first time

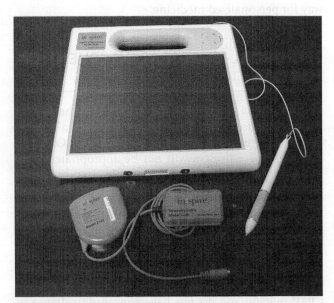

Figure 53-1 Inspire upper airway stimulation therapy components for treatment of obstructive sleep apnea. (Image courtesy of Inspire Medical Systems, Inc. and Edwin M. Valladares, MS, RPSGT, Manager, USC Sleep Disorders Center, Keck Medical Center of USC, University of Southern California.)

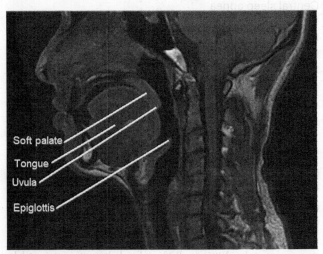

Soft palate
Tongue
Uvula
Epiglottis

Figure 53-2 Anatomy of the upper airway. (Image courtesy of Krishna Nayak, PhD, Professor, Ming Hsieh Department of Electrical Engineering, Viterbi School of Engineering, University of Southern California.)

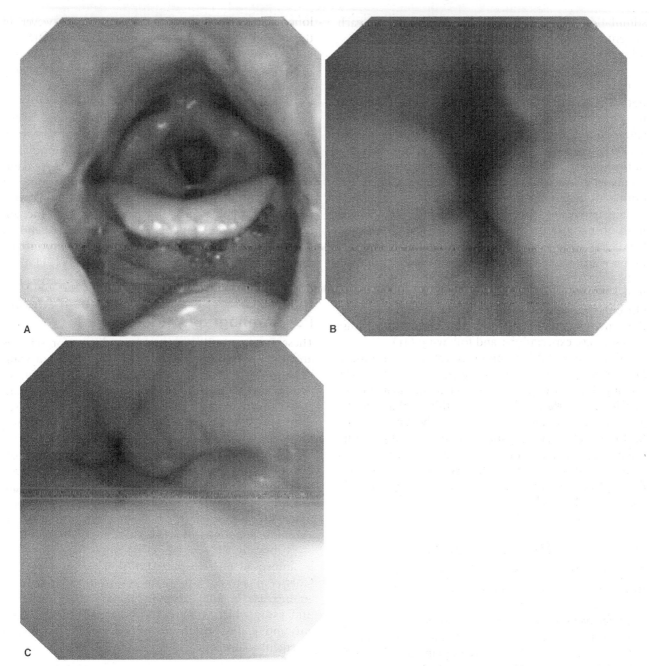

Figure 53-3 Images of the palate during drug-induced sleep endoscopy. **A:** No collapse, **(B)** lateral wall collapse, and **(C)** concentric collapse. (Images courtesy of Eric J. Kezirian, MD, MPH, USC Caruso Department of Otolaryngology—Head & Neck Surgery, Keck School of Medicine of USC; with permission from Valladares, E. M., & Hammond, T. C. (2018). Novel therapies for sleep apnea—The implants have arrived! *The Neurodiagnostic Journal*. Copyright © ASET—The Neurodiagnostic Society, www.aset.org. Reprinted by permission of Taylor & Francis Ltd, http://www.tandfonline.com, on behalf of ASET—The Neurodiagnostic Society.)

and two major parameters are established. The first parameter is the sensing threshold. The sensing threshold is the lowest voltage at which the patient "senses" an impulse from the device. The second parameter is the functional threshold, which is the voltage where the patient's hypoglossal nerve is stimulated enough to protrude the tongue past the lower teeth. The patient is then sent home with a range of "functional threshold + 10 tenths of a voltage" (e.g., 2.1 to 3.0 V). The patient is asked to try to increase the voltage by 0.1 V every three to four nights to become acclimated to the therapy. A month after this activation visit, the patient comes into the sleep lab to be formally titrated by a trained sleep technologist (9, 11). The Inspire UAS therapy has a stimulation range from 0.1 to 5.0 V. Settings for each patient can vary, given differences in upper airway physiology (11, 14).

Inspire UAS therapy titration has an immediate effect on the upper airway when compared with CPAP titration. This immediate effect is due to the change in the physical upper airway evoked by hypoglossal nerve stimulation, as opposed to a more gradual effect from a CPAP setting increase (15). Although supine sleep during a titration is always ideal to eliminate respiratory events as a worst-case scenario, most of the emphasis during an Inspire titration is in identifying the optimal voltage when the patient is sleeping in a comfortable position because the patient has not been able to use CPAP (9). This may result in the patient being sent home with lateral sleep settings. However, stimulation can be raised at a later time once the patient acclimates to the therapy and shows the need for supine titration. Once the patient is sent home with a range of voltages, the patient meets with the sleep physician to further discuss settings, expectations, and follow-up (11).

On June 5, 2017, Inspire Medical, Inc. announced FDA approval for the next generation of Inspire UAS therapy device, the Inspire 3028 neurostimulator (16). The device is 40% smaller and 18% thinner than the original neurostimulator. It has also received conditional MRI labeling, allowing patients to undergo MRI testing safely (16). The patient remote has also been simplified to include features where patients can easily visualize therapy settings, including "on" and "off" buttons via green and white lights.

Inspire UAS Therapy: Clinical Effectiveness and Safety Findings

Inspire Medical, Inc. conducted a multicenter, prospective, single-group cohort design study to evaluate the clinical effectiveness and safety of the Inspire UAS therapy. Their primary measures were the AHI and oxygen desaturation index (ODI). The study implanted 126 participants with a mean age of 54.5 years (83% male). At 12 months, the study showed a 68% decrease in the median AHI, from 29.3 to 9.0 per hour. A similar response was seen in the median ODI with a 70% decrease from 25.4 to 7.4 per hour. Secondary outcomes included the Epworth Sleepiness Scale score (range 0 to 24) to measure subjective sleepiness and the Functional Outcomes of Sleep Questionnaire (FOSQ; range 5.0 to 20.0) to evaluate quality of life and percent of sleep time with oxygen saturation below 90%. Median Epworth decreased from 11 to 6, median FOSQ scores increased from 14.6 to 18.2, and median percent of sleep time with oxygen saturation below 90% decreased from 5.4% to 0.9%. Less than 2% procedure-related serious adverse events were reported (10). Given the relatively recent FDA approval,

long-term studies are yet to be available. However, in the latest 5-year outcomes report published in 2018, patients were reported to have continuous improvement in sleepiness and AHI, with serious adverse events being uncommon (17, 18). Moreover, emerging data continue to show the Inspire UAS therapy's effectiveness (19).

A common question regarding nerve damage caused by neurostimulation is yet to be established. However, decades of information from other neurostimulators (e.g., used in pain management) show that nerve damage is not usually due to long-term stimulation, but the most common issue has to do with lead movement (20). In November 16, 2016, Inspire Medical, Inc. announced that 1,000 patients were implanted (8) and on September 20, 2017, Inspire Medical, Inc. announced a new effort to study 2,500 implanted patients (21).

Inspire UAS Therapy: How Does It Affect Polysomnography Recordings?

These systems, unlike neural stimulators for seizures and depression, do not significantly affect polysomnography (PSG) signals, given their implant location. Artifact can be seen in the submental electromyogram (EMG) more than the electroencephalogram (EEG; see Fig. 53-4). PSG scoring is not significantly hindered and the American Academy of Sleep Medicine (AASM) scoring rules can still be implemented (22). Moreover, scoring of rapid eye movement (REM) sleep is not hindered because EMG artifact is periodic. Other PSG signals are not impacted by these implants; however, it is recommended that piezoelectric belts be used during PSG to eliminate any source of artifact (19, 23).

Clinically, EEG measured sleep has been shown to be improved post–Inspire UAS therapy implant. Hofauer et al. showed a decrease in non-REM 1 sleep and an increase in REM sleep (24). Postmarket trials are under way, which will provide more clarity of functionality and quality. Studies are limited, given that this is an emergent technology.

TECHNICAL–SURGICAL INTERVENTION FOR CSA

The **rem**edē® System is a feasible option for treating a subset of patients with CSA because it received FDA's approval in late 2017 (6). Although not everyone with CSA will require a **rem**edē® System, careful selection criteria can make it a viable and novel alternative, for the most difficult-to-treat patients do not qualify or tolerate PAP therapy.

The **rem**edē® System has become available at a time when the results of the Servo-Ventilation for Central Sleep Apnea in Systolic Heart Failure (SERVE-HF) trial have questioned the role of adaptive servo-ventilation

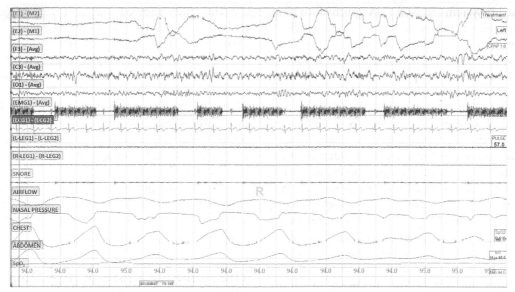

Figure 53-4 Hypoglossal nerve stimulation effect on polysomnography—Epoch (30 seconds) during hypoglossal nerve stimulation acquired using Sandman 10.1 software and Sandman 32+ amplifier. (Image courtesy of Edwin M. Valladares, MS, RPSGT, Manager, USC Sleep Disorders Center, Keck Medical Center of USC, University of Southern California.)

(ASV) in treating patients with CSA and low ejection fraction (25). The **rem**edē® System provides a therapy option for patients who are not able to use ASV. The system utilizes a transvenously placed pacemaker like lead to stimulate the phrenic nerve unilaterally, usually on the left side, to activate breathing on the basis of signaling information from the sensing lead. Stimulation intensity is titrated to a setting where breathing is entrained to a target minute ventilation. The system is minimally invasive and is implanted by specially trained electrophysiologists (EPs). The device is activated at the programmed bedtime when the patient is recumbent and works continuously throughout the entire night without volitional patient effort until the programmed end time or continuous upright posture. Although long-term outcomes for the **rem**edē® System are unknown, its ability to entrain breathing as a nonpressure-based modality makes it an alternative for patients who don't qualify for ASV or are not able to use ASV (26).

The remedē® System: Components, Function, and Indications

The **rem**edē® System is composed of a stimulator called the "implantable pulse generator" (IPG) with 1-stimulating lead and 1-monitoring lead. The stimulating lead is placed transvenously in proximity to the phrenic nerve to allow stimulation through a proprietary algorithm and 1-sensing lead. The stimulator lead is placed in the left pericardiophrenic vein or the right brachiocephalic vein to stimulate the phrenic nerve and produce "diaphragmatic contractions thereby creating negative intrathoracic pressure that mimics normal breathing" (26). The sensing lead is placed in the azygos vein to monitor breathing and to communicate stimulation needs to the system. A preprogrammed computer tablet that is paired with an electronic wand serves as the interface unit, which is used to interrogate and make setting changes to the implanted device (27). All components have specific serial numbers. The IPG has a radiopaque identification marker inside it, allowing for the model number and manufacturing date to be visible through X-ray techniques. The device is accessed through an electronic tablet and interrogation component (see Fig. 53-5) (28). The battery has an estimated life of 41 to 55 months, depending on pulse generation (28).

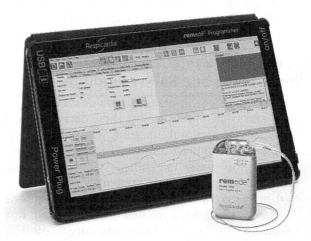

Figure 53-5 Respicardia Inc. **rem**edē® System components for treatment of central sleep apnea. (Image courtesy of Respicardia, Inc.)

The remedē® System received FDA approval to treat adult patients with moderate-to-severe CSA, which is broad and nonspecific to the type of CSA (28). Respicardia, Inc. recommends the use of selection criteria during their pivotal trial. During the pivotal trial, patients were 18 years of age or older, with a PSG test conducted within the last 40 days evidencing an AHI of at least 20 per hour, central apneas being at least 50% or higher of all apneas, 30 or more central apnea events throughout the night, and an obstructive apnea index of 20%. Contraindications for device implantation are active infection and the need for MRI (28). The pivotal study's exclusion criteria also included the following: phrenic nerve palsy, stage D heart failure, cerebrovascular event within the past 12 months, CSA secondary to opioids, and advanced renal disease (26). These criteria make the remedē® System potentially useful in treating patients with heart failure and low ejection fractions, in whom ASV therapy is not recommended (25).

The remedē® System: Patient Process

The remedē® System is implanted by a cardiologist who is an experienced EP in cardiac resynchronization therapy. The system is activated 1 month postimplant to allow time for healing. The device is activated by a trained sleep physician and sleep technologist. In the pivotal study, the device was titrated in the sleep lab 1 month postactivation. A clinical protocol for implantation and activation based on the pivotal trial is currently being finalized.

The system functions independent of the patient's volition. The system is programmed to turn on and off according to the patient's usual sleep schedule. However, for times when the patient goes to bed later or awakens earlier than usual, the IPG does not actively stimulate if the patient is upright, regardless of clock time. The IPG has a programmable setting for pause time that is activated when the patient changes position (27).

The remedē® System: Clinical Effectiveness and Safety Findings

The remedē® System Pivotal Trial evaluated the effectiveness and safety of the therapy. These data were used to apply for FDA approval. The study was a prospective, multicenter, randomized controlled trial, where clinical investigators across the United States and Europe randomized 151 patients to treatment ($n = 73$) or control ($n = 78$) groups. Five participants were excluded from each group, given unrelated deaths ($n = 4$), lost to follow-up ($n = 1$), missed appointments/medical issues ($n = 2$), and patients exiting the study ($n = 3$), with final groups of treatment ($n = 68$) and control ($n = 73$) (26).

The study showed that 35 (51%) of 68 treatment patients achieved a 50% or more reduction in their AHI at the 6-month mark. Moreover, 91% of the 151 patients did not have any serious adverse events at 12 months and 27 of the 73 treatment group patients reported "nonserious therapy-related discomfort." Twenty-six of the 27 patients reporting discomfort had resolution with "simple system reprogramming" (26). At 12 months, patients continue to show sustained efficacy (28). Given recent FDA approval, long-term studies are not yet available.

Like the Inspire UAS therapy, questions regarding nerve damage caused by neurostimulations have not been established. More data are expected to become available as therapy use increases and time passes.

The remedē® System: How Does It Affect PSG Recordings?

Like the Inspire UAS therapy, the remedē® System does not significantly affect PSG signals. Because the remedē® System is implanted closer to the heart when compared with the Inspire UAS therapy, it affects the ECG more than any other signal when stimulation is activated (see Fig. 53-6). As a result, PSG scoring is not hindered and AASM scoring rules can still be implemented, but ECG signals are limited (22). Effects on objective EEG sleep are not available, given this is an emergent technology.

INSURANCE COVERAGE AND COST

Both the Inspire UAS therapy and remedē® System are covered by insurance companies (29, 30). The Current Procedural Terminology (CPT) codes are provided by the respective company to be used when implanting, activating, titrating, and managing the therapy.

The CPT codes for activating and titrating the Inspire UAS therapy in a sleep lab setting are as follows: 95970 for interrogation of the device with no setting changes, 95974 for interrogation for the device with setting changes, and 95810-TC + 95974 for a PSG titration of the Inspire UAS therapy. The CPT codes for activating and titrating the remedē® System in a sleep lab setting are as follows: 0434T for interrogation of the device with no setting changes, 0435T for interrogation of the device with setting changes, and 0436T for PSG and interrogation (CPT code 95810 is not to be used). Because CPT code updates occur from time to time, suitable CPT codes should be periodically verified with the corresponding manufacturer.

A model-based projection for the long-term cost-effectiveness of the UAS has been found to be beneficial when comparing it with nontreatment from a third-party US perspective (31). Inspire Medical has

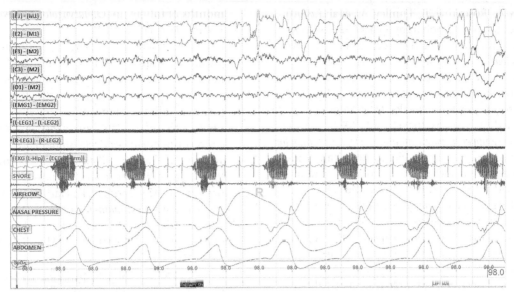

Figure 53-6 Phrenic nerve stimulation effect on polysomnography—Epoch (30 seconds) during phrenic nerve stimulation acquired using Sandman 10.1 software and Sandman 32+ amplifier. (Image courtesy of Edwin M. Valladares, MS, RPSGT, Manager, USC Sleep Disorders Center, Keck Medical Center of USC, University of Southern California.)

reported the approximate cost of its device to be $20,000 plus the cost of surgery (30). A cost-effectiveness analysis for the remedē® System is not available to the knowledge of the authors.

SUMMARY: EFFECT OF TECHNICAL–SURGICAL INTERVENTIONS TO THE FIELD OF SLEEP MEDICINE AND ROLE OF THE SLEEP TECHNOLOGIST

Technical–surgical interventions, such as the Inspire UAS therapy and remedē® System, provide alternative therapies for a subset of OSA and CSA patients who can't benefit from traditional PAP therapies, respectively. These therapies are also expanding the role of the sleep technologist because they are needed to activate, interrogate, and make technical setting changes to these therapies during clinic visits and at night during PSG device titrations. The role of the sleep technologist is evolving as technology intersects with the changing landscape of health care. In an era where less complicated patients are being diagnosed using home sleep apnea testing units, and more complicated patients are being tested in the sleep lab, the role of the sleep technologist is increasingly requiring highly skilled technologists (32). Sleep technologists are required to be ambitious and flexible to learn new facets of our field. Specific training for these devices is provided by the particular device company once a site is identified as having all the required team members (e.g., sleep

physician(s), otolaryngologists for Inspire UAS therapy, and cardiac EP for the remedē® System). These implantable devices also provide sleep physicians more weapons in their arsenal against sleep-disordered breathing, resulting in an even more specialized sleep physician role. Lastly, the increase in available therapies is also paving the way for more personalized sleep medicine care as researchers connect endotypes with specific therapies to maximize efficacy and efficiency for individualized care (14).

REFERENCES

1. Sullivan, C. E., Issa, F. G., Berthon-Jones, M., et al. (1981). Reversal of obstructive sleep apnoea by continuous positive airway pressure applied through the nares. *Lancet, 1*(8225), 862–865.
2. Weaver, T. E., & Grunstein, R. R. (2008). Adherence to continuous positive airway pressure therapy: The challenge to effective treatment. *Proceedings of the American Thoracic Society, 5*(2), 173–178.
3. Wolkove, N., Baltzan, M., Kamel, H., et al. (2008). Long-term compliance with continuous positive airway pressure in patients with obstructive sleep apnea. *Canadian Respiratory Journal, 15*(7), 365–369.
4. Campos-Rodriguez, F., Martinez-Alonso, M., Sanchez-de-la-Torre, M., et al. (2016). Long-term adherence to continuous positive airway pressure therapy in non-sleepy sleep apnea patients. *Sleep Medicine, 17*, 1–6.

5. Senior, B. A., Rosenthal, L., Lumley, A., et al. (2000). Efficacy of uvulopalatopharyngoplasty in unselected patients with mild obstructive sleep apnea. *Otolaryngology—Head and Neck Surgery, 123*(3), 9–82.

6. Respicardia, Inc. (October 10, 2017). *Respicardia's remedē System receives FDA approval.* Press release, CISION PR Newswire. Minnetonka, MN: Author.

7. Inspire Medical Systems, Inc. (May 1, 2014). *FDA approves Inspire upper airway stimulation (UAS) therapy for obstructive sleep apnea.* Press release, American Academy of Sleep Medicine. Minneapolis, MN: Author.

8. Inspire Medical Systems, Inc. (November 16, 2016). *Inspire Medical Systems completes 1,000th implant, names Marilyn Carlson to the Board, and completes series F financing.* Press release. Minneapolis, MN: Author.

9. Coleman, M. (2014). *Inspire upper airway stimulation training for physicians and technologists.* Los Angeles, CA.

10. Strollo, P. J., Soose, R. J., Maurer, J. T., et al. (2014). Upper-airway stimulation for obstructive sleep apnea. *New England Journal of Medicine, 370*(2), 139–149.

11. Inspire Medical Systems, Inc. (2017). *System implant manual* (200-236-101 RevB). Maple Grove, MN: Author.

12. Vanderveken, O. M., Maurer, J. T., Hohenhorst, W., et al. (2013). Evaluation of drug-induced sleep endoscopy as a patient selection tool for implanted upper airway stimulation for obstructive sleep apnea. *Journal of Clinical Sleep Medicine, 9*(5), 433–438.

13. Charakorn, N., & Kezirian, E. J. (2016). Drug-induced sleep endoscopy. *Otolaryngologic Clinics of North America, 49*, 1359–1372.

14. Subramani, Y., Singh, M., Wong, J., et al. (2018). Understanding phenotypes of obstructive sleep apnea: Applications in anesthesia, surgery, and perioperative medicine. *Anesthesia & Analgesia, 124*(1), 179–191.

15. Chen, W., Gillett, E., Khoo, M. C. K., et al. (2017). Real-time multislice MRI during continuous positive airway response to pressure change. *Journal of Magnetic Resonance Imaging, 46*, 1400–1408.

16. Inspire Medical Systems, Inc. (June 5, 2017). *Inspire Medical Systems announces FDA approval of Inspire 3028 neurostimulator for the treatment of obstructive sleep apnea.* Press release. Minneapolis, MN: Author.

17. Woodson, B. T., Soose, R. J., Gillespie, M. B., et al. (2016). Three-year outcomes of cranial nerve stimulation for obstructive sleep apnea: The Star trial. *Otolaryngology—Head and Neck Surgery, 154*(1), 181–188.

18. Woodson, B. T., Strohl, K. P., Soose, R. J., et al. (2018). Upper airway stimulation for obstructive sleep apnea: 5-year outcomes. *Otolaryngology—Head and Neck Surgery, 159*(1), 194–202.

19. Gillespie, M. B., Soose, R. J., Woodson, B. T., et al. (2017). Upper airway stimulation for obstructive sleep apnea: Patient-reported outcomes after 48 months of follow-up. *Otolaryngology—Head and Neck Surgery, 156*(4), 765–771.

20. Eldabe, S., Buchser, E., Duarte, R. V. (2016). Complications of spinal cord stimulation and peripheral nerve stimulation techniques: A review of the literature. *Pain Medicine, 17*(2), 325–336.

21. Inspire Medical Systems, Inc. (September 20, 2017). *Inspire Medical Systems' Inspire therapy for reducing obstructive sleep apnea demonstrates long-term safety and sustained benefit following 5-years of treatment.* Press release. Minneapolis, MN: Author.

22. Berry, R. B., Albertario, C. L., Harding, S. M., et al. (2018). *The AASM manual for the scoring of sleep and associated events: Rules, terminology and technical specifications.* Version 2.5. Darien, IL: American Academy of Sleep Medicine.

23. Inspire Medical Systems, Inc. (2017). *Programmer manual.* (200-081-101 RevD).

24. Hofauer, B., Philip, P., Markus, W., et al. (2017). Effects of upper-airway stimulation on sleep architecture in patients with obstructive sleep apnea. *Sleep Breath, 21*, 901–908.

25. Cowie, M. R., Woehrle, H., Wegscheider, K., et al. (2015). Adaptive servo-ventilation for central sleep apnea in systolic heart failure. *New England Journal of Medicine, 373*(12), 1095–1105.

26. Costanzo, M. R., Ponikowski, P., Javaheri, S., et al. (2016). Transvenous neurostimulation for central sleep apnoea: A randomised controlled trial. *Lancet, 388*, 974–982.

27. Costanzo, M. R., Augostini, R., Goldberg, L. R., et al. (2015). Design of the remedē System pivotal trial: A prospective, randomized study in the use of respiratory rhythm management to treat central sleep apnea. *Journal of Cardiac Failure, 21*, 892–902.

28. Respicardia. *remedē® system implant and clinician use manual.* Issued 2010.

29. Costanzo, M. R., Ponikowski, P., Javaheri, S., et al. (2018). Sustained 12 month benefit of phrenic nerve stimulation for central sleep apnea. *American Journal of Cardiology, 121*(11), 1400–1408.

30. Inspire Medical Systems, Inc. (November 2015). *About obstructive sleep apnea & Inspire upper airway stimulation (UAS) therapy.* Minneapolis, MN: Author.

31. Pietzsch, J. B., Liu, S., Garner, A. M., et al. (2015). Long-term cost-effectiveness of upper airway stimulation for the treatment of obstructive sleep apnea: A model-based projection based on the STAR trial. *Sleep, 38*(5), 735–743.

32. Brooks, R., & Trimble, M. (2014). The future of sleep technology: Report from an American Association of Sleep Technologists summit meeting. *Journal of Clinical Sleep Medicine, 10*(5), 589–593.

chapter 54

Other Therapies for Obstructive Sleep Apnea

ZACK FREEMAN   SAAD S. AHMAD

LEARNING OBJECTIVES

On completion of this chapter, the reader should be able to:

1. Describe the indications for alternative obstructive sleep apnea therapy options.
2. Describe the goals of these alternative therapies.
3. Outline the benefits, challenges, and side effects of alternative therapies.

KEY TERMS

Obstructive sleep apnea (OSA)
Commercial weight loss program
Bariatric surgery
Positional sleep apnea
Positional therapy
American Academy of Sleep Medicine (AASM)
American Society for Metabolic and Bariatric Surgery (ASMBS)
Nasal expiratory positive airway pressure (nEPAP)
Functional residual capacity (FRC)

Positive airway pressure (PAP) is the treatment of choice for obstructive sleep apnea (OSA) regardless of severity (1). However, other therapies are available that may be offered depending on the severity of the OSA, the need for alternative therapy due to intolerance, or the need to provide adjunctive therapy to supplement the primary treatment method. Oral devices and surgical interventions are clinically validated alternative therapies, each detailed in other chapters. This chapter will familiarize the sleep technologist with therapies other than PAP, oral devices, or surgical intervention. Validated treatment options at the time of this writing will be reviewed, as well as popular options that need more research and available options that have been found not to be effective.

WEIGHT LOSS

Obesity affects nearly 38% of adults in the United States (2). Obesity is a significant risk factor for OSA, with prevalence statistically increasing with body mass index. OSA has been shown to exist in approximately 9% of women and 24% of men. Of the morbidly obese, OSA is known to be present in approximately 55% of women and 80% of men. Obesity is known to associate with OSA in a number of ways. Obesity contributes to OSA by altering the upper airway's structure and function. Upper airway collapsibility is increased, as fat deposits narrow the upper airway and abdominal fat masses reduce tracheal tension (3). Obesity also affects the physiologic balances required for normal respiratory function (4). Weight loss is not only a viable option for the treatment of OSA but is also significantly beneficial toward a person's health and quality of life (5–7). Although no specific result can be guaranteed for any patient, decades of accumulated data can lead the practitioner to some perception of possible expected outcomes.

Methods of Weight Loss

There are multiple methods of weight loss, each with different applicable attributes to sleep apnea treatment. When approaching weight loss, the patient must review his or her options and decide which is best for him or her. Health care professionals must be able to assist the patient with information, so that the patient can make the best choices. Weight loss can be achieved by either dietary and lifestyle modification or surgical procedures. As surgery results in a more drastic reduction of weight loss, it accordingly results in a more drastic reduction of apnea–hypopnea index (AHI) (3). When choosing a weight loss program, it is recommended that the patient first consult a health care professional. It may be difficult for health care professionals to assess the patient's interest in engaging with weight loss discussion without the patient expressing interest or asking specific questions; however, it is beneficial for the health care provider to assess the patient's interest and readiness for weight loss (7).

Diet and Lifestyle Changes

Commercial weight loss programs have shown better success with initial weight loss and lower relapse rate than primary care–managed diet or informal diet (8). Many commercial diets come and go, leaving the patient with many to choose from. In 2014, Americans spent approximately $2.5 billion on commercial diet programs (8). A 2015 study published by the U.S. Department of Health and Human Services studied 141 commercial diets and found Weight Watchers and Jenny Craig to give the most evidence for both promising weight loss and long-term outcomes from all the programs (8). It is noted that this study met criteria for recommendations set forth by the U.S. Preventive Services Task Force (USPSTF). The USPSTF is an independent, volunteer panel of national experts in disease prevention and evidence-based medicine that makes recommendations about the effectiveness of specific clinical preventive services for patients without related signs or symptoms. Table 54-1 shows data from this study giving a summary of characteristics and updated costs for commercial programs that had eligible randomized controlled trials available.

Surgical Weight Loss

Bariatric surgery is a term that includes a variety of surgical procedures that reduce the amount of food the stomach can hold and cause malabsorption of nutrients. Bariatric surgery is recognized as one of the most effective treatments for obesity and therefore becomes an effective weight loss method for treating OSA. Bariatric surgeries are shown to be more effective in reducing AHI than intensive lifestyle changes or dieting. The most common bariatric surgery procedures are Roux-en-Y gastric bypass, laparoscopic sleeve gastrectomy, laparoscopic adjustable gastric band (LAGB), and biliopancreatic diversion with duodenal switch (BPD/DS). Each surgery has its own advantages and disadvantages. Table 54-2 is a summary of the advantages and disadvantages according to the American Society for Metabolic and Bariatric Surgery (ASMBS). The ASMBS is the largest medical organization in the world dedicated to obesity-related diseases and conditions and metabolic and bariatric surgery. Studies have shown LAGB and BPD/DS to be the most effective types of bariatric surgery to reduce AHI, with recent evidence showing BPD/DS to be the most effective within these two (9).

Weight Loss Outcomes

Even modest weight loss, described as 10% loss of total body weight, can result in a significant reduction of AHI (5). That is not to say that weight loss is an easy cure for sleep apnea. It has been shown that most patients who undergo bariatric surgeries have significant sleep apnea that requires PAP treatment 1 year after surgery, notably at lower pressures than before the weight loss (6). This information validates the importance of proper evaluation after significant weight loss, as well as the effectiveness of weight loss as an adjunctive treatment.

POSITIONAL THERAPY

Whether a patient with OSA has positional sleep apnea is a significant consideration when reviewing treatment options. Positional sleep apnea is defined as supine AHI two times the nonsupine AHI. Reports on the prevalence of positional sleep apnea vary, but it is estimated that approximately 56% to 75% of patients with OSA exhibit an increase in severity in the supine position (10).

Indications for Positional Therapy

Positional therapy for OSA refers to the implementation of a strategy to keep the patient in a nonsupine position while sleeping. Positional therapy is recommended as a secondary therapy. It is also considered a suitable alternative therapy, but only if the patient has been shown to have positional sleep apnea where the AHI normalizes in a nonsupine sleeping position. The American Academy of Sleep Medicine (AASM) guidelines state that when positional therapy is implemented, a positioning device should be used, an objective positional monitor should be considered, and outcomes should be monitored. Methods to monitor outcomes may be self-reported compliance, objective position monitoring, and symptom resolution (1).

Methods of Positional Therapy

Perhaps the most well-documented method of positional therapy is known as the "tennis ball technique." As the name implies, this method originated from the use of a tennis ball. A tennis ball would be sewn into the front pocket of a t-shirt and then the patient would wear the t-shirt backward to bed. When the patient would attempt to move to the supine position, the discomfort from the tennis ball would prompt the patient to roll off the back. The term has since been associated with any device that includes a mass strapped to the patient's back, causing him or her to not lay supine. Although this method is effective in efficacy, compliance is unsatisfactory. Compliance is estimated to be 40% to 70% in the short term, but as low as 10% in the long term (10).

Newer devices exist with promising results to date, but there are limited data on long-term compliance. These devices strap to a person's chest or neck and give off vibrations or auditory alarms when the patient moves to the supine position (10). When considering a device, one should consider whether it has Food and

Table 54-1   Summary of Commercial Weight-loss Programs

Programs	Intensity[a]	Nutrition	Physical Activity	Behavioral Strategies	Support	Costs	May Meet USPSTF Criteria[b]
Weight Watchers	High	Low-calorie conventional foods, point tracking	Activity tracking	Self-monitoring	Depending on membership level: group sessions, online coaching, online community forum	$19.95–$54.9/mo depending on membership level	Yes
Jenny Craig	High	Low-calorie meal replacements	Encourages increased activity	Goal setting, self-monitoring	One-on-one counseling	$15–$26/d for meals. Membership is $20 for 10 wk, or $359 yearly.	Yes
Nutrisystem	High	Low-calorie meal replacements	Exercise plans	Self-monitoring	Depending on membership level: one-on-one counseling, online community forum	$10.18–$13.93/d depending on membership level	Yes
HMR	High	Very-low-calorie or low-calorie meal replacements	Encourages increased activity	Goal setting	Group sessions, telephone counseling, medically supervised	$301.95/3 wk kit, +groceries needed	Yes
Medifast	High	Very-low-calorie or low-calorie meal replacements	Encourages increased activity	Self-monitoring	One-on-one counseling, online coaching	$443.60–$557.30/mo depending on membership level	Yes
Optifast	High	Very-low-calorie or low-calorie meal replacements	Encourages increased activity	Problem solving	One-on-one counseling, group support, medically supervised	$150/wk	Yes
Atkins	Self-directed	Low-carbohydrate conventional foods or meal replacements	Encourages increased activity	Self-monitoring	Online community forum	Can be free, meal kits and plans up to $200/wk	No
Lose It!	Self-directed	Calorie tracking	Activity tracking	Self-monitoring	Online community forum	$0 to $39.95	No
SlimFast	Self-directed	Low-calorie meal replacements	–	Self-weighting	Online nutrition support, coaching text messages	$75/mo	No

Prices were updated per program web sites in 2018. Two programs were removed as they are no longer available (24–32).
[a]High-intensity programs recommend more than 12 sessions per year; low-intensity programs recommend less than 12 sessions per year or are self-directed.
[b]Assessment of whether the programs may potentially meet U.S. Preventive Service Task Force criteria for intensive behavioral counseling for obesity. HMR, health management resources; USPSTF, United States Preventive Services Task Force.
Information presented in this table was extracted from Gudzune, K. A., Bleich, S. N., & Clark, J. M. (2015). Efficacy of commercial weight-loss programs. *Annals of Internal Medicine, 163*(5), 399.

Table 54-2 Summary of the Advantages and Disadvantages of Various Procedures According to the American Society for Metabolic and Bariatric Surgery (ASMBS)

Procedure	Summary	Advantages	Disadvantages
Roux-en-Y gastric bypass (RYGB)	The two main components to the procedure are (1) a small 30-mL stomach pouch created by dividing the top of the stomach from the rest of the stomach and (2) the first portion of the small intestine is divided with the bottom end of the divided small intestine brought up and connected to the newly created small stomach pouch. The top portion of the divided small intestine is connected to the small intestine further down. This allows the bypassed stomach acids and digestive enzymes from the stomach and the first portion of the small intestine to eventually mix with food. The rerouting of the food stream produces changes in gut hormones that promote satiety.	• Produces significant long-term weight loss (60%–80% excess weight loss) • Restricts the amount of food that can be consumed • May lead to conditions that increase energy expenditure • Produces favorable changes in gut hormones that reduce appetite and enhance satiety • Typical maintenance of >50% excess weight loss	• Is technically a more complex operation than the AGB or LSG and potentially could result in greater complication rates • Can lead to long-term vitamin/mineral deficiencies, particularly deficits in vitamin B_{12}, iron, calcium, and folate • Generally requires a longer hospital stay than the LAGB • Requires adherence to dietary recommendations, lifelong vitamin/mineral supplementation, and follow-up compliance
Laparoscopic sleeve gastrectomy (LSG)	Eighty percent of the stomach is removed. The remaining stomach is a tubular pouch. The new stomach pouch holds a considerably smaller volume than the normal stomach and the surgery has significant effect on gut hormones that impact factors such as hunger, satiety, and blood sugar control.	• Restricts the amount of food the stomach can hold • Induces rapid and significant weight loss that comparative studies find similar to that of the RYGB. Weight loss of >50% for 3 to 5+ y data, and weight loss comparable to that of the bypass with a maintenance of >50% • Requires no foreign objects (AGB), and no bypass or rerouting of the food stream (RYGB) • Involves a relatively short hospital stay of ~2 d • Causes favorable changes in gut hormones that suppress hunger, reduce appetite, and improve satiety	• It is a nonreversible procedure • It has the potential for long-term vitamin deficiencies • Has a higher early complication rate than the LAGB

	Summary of the Advantages and Disadvantages of Various Procedures According to the		
Table 54-2	American Society for Metabolic and Bariatric Surgery (ASMBS) (*continued*)		

Procedure	Summary	Advantages	Disadvantages
Laparoscopic adjustable gastric band (LAGB)	An inflatable band that is placed around the upper portion of the stomach, creating a small stomach pouch above the band, leaving the rest of the stomach below the band. With the smaller stomach pouch, eating just a small amount of food will satisfy hunger. The size of the stomach opening can be adjusted by filling the band with sterile saline, which is injected through a port placed under the skin.	• Reduces the amount of food the stomach can hold • Induces excess weight loss of ~40%–50% • Involves no cutting of the stomach or rerouting of the intestines • Requires a shorter hospital stay, usually <24 h, with some centers discharging the patient the same day as the surgery • Is reversible and adjustable • It has the lowest rate of early postoperative complications and mortality among the approved bariatric procedures • Has the lowest risk of vitamin/mineral deficiencies	• Slower and less early weight loss than other surgical procedures • Greater percentage of patients failing to lose at least 50% of excess body weight compared with the other surgeries commonly performed • Requires a foreign device to remain in the body • Can result in possible band slippage or band erosion into the stomach in a small percentage of patients • Can be mechanical problems with the band, tube, or port in a small percentage of patients • Can result in dilation of the esophagus if the patient overeats • Requires strict adherence to the postoperative diet and to postoperative follow-up visits • Highest rate of reoperation
Biliopancreatic diversion with duodenal switch (BPD/DS)	The first component of the procedure involves a smaller, tubular stomach pouch that is created by removing a portion of the stomach. Next, the duodenum (the first portion of the small intestine) is divided just past the outlet of the stomach. A segment of the distal (the last portion of) small intestine is then brought up and connected to the outlet of the newly created stomach, so that when the patient eats, the food goes through a newly created tubular stomach pouch and empties directly into the last segment of the small intestine. Roughly three-fourths of the small intestine is bypassed by the food stream.	• Results in greater weight loss than RYGB, SG, or LAGB, that is, 60%–70% excess weight loss or greater, at 5-y follow-up • Allows patients to eventually eat near "normal" meals • Reduces the absorption of fat by 70% or more • Causes favorable changes in gut hormones to reduce appetite and improve satiety • Is the most effective against diabetes compared with RYGB, LSG, and AGB	• Has higher complication rates and risk for mortality than LAGB, SG, and RYGB • Requires a longer hospital stay than AGB or LSG • Has a greater potential to cause protein deficiencies and long-term deficiencies in a number of vitamin and minerals, that is, iron, calcium, zinc, fat-soluble vitamins such as vitamin D • Compliance with follow-up visits and care and strict adherence to dietary and vitamin supplementation guidelines are critical to avoiding serious complications from protein and certain vitamin deficiencies

AGB, adjustable gastric band.

Drug Administration (FDA) approval and clinical studies showing effectiveness.

The Zzoma and Night Shift Sleep Positioner are two FDA-approved prescription devices for positional sleep apnea. Zzoma (Fig. 54-1) is a more traditional approach to positional sleep apnea therapy, cleared by the FDA as a treatment option for OSA. The device is worn around the torso placing a large mass on the patient's lower back, preventing the patient from sleeping on the back. The Night Shift Sleep Positioner (Fig. 54-2A, B) is an example of a modern positional therapy device that is cleared by the FDA for the treatment of OSA. This device has many user and practitioner features for objective monitoring and good long-term compliance compared with other methods (11).

The Sleep Position Trainer (SPT) is another modern positional therapy device that is backed by clinical studies that support significant efficacy and adherence. At the time of this writing, the SPT is not available in the United States and is available only in the European Union. SPT is a small, lightweight device that is inserted into a strap worn around the patient's chest. The device creates soft vibrations to prompt the patient to change sleeping positions. It also records compliance and therapy data that can be uploaded to a computer for review by the patient and/or clinician. SPT has been shown to reduce AHI, subjectively improve quality of life, and improve daytime sleepiness by decreasing average supine sleep time. This device has been tested to compare with oral appliance therapy (OAT), which is a validated, widely used alternative treatment option to mild-moderate OSA. OAT has significant adherence rates and reduction in AHI, so it is a significant find that SPT was/is found to match both adherence and effectiveness of OAT in patients with positional sleep apnea (12).

NASAL EXPIRATORY POSITIVE AIRWAY PRESSURE THERAPY

Concept

Provent is the trademarked name for a nasal expiratory positive airway pressure (nEPAP) therapy device to treat OSA. Expiratory positive airway pressure (EPAP) commonly refers to increased expiratory positive pressure delivered via interface from a positive airway device such as continuous airway pressure or bilevel PAP. In this case, however, EPAP refers to increased expiratory PAP delivered by the patient. Provent therapy consists of a single-use valve inserted into each nostril and held

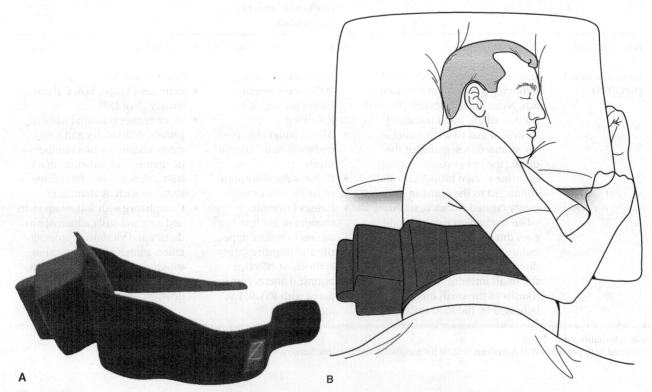

Figure 54-1 A, B: Zzoma Positional Device is a Food and Drug Administration–cleared positional medical device approved for the treatment of sleep apnea. This device uses an advanced version of the "tennis ball technique" to keep the patient from sleeping supine. It is a prescription device and costs $189.95. It is generally an out-of-pocket expense to the patient (11). (View A used with permission from Sleep Specialists LLC, 150 Monument Rd, Suite 207, Bala Cynwyd, PA 19004, http://zzomaosa.com/contacts-us/)

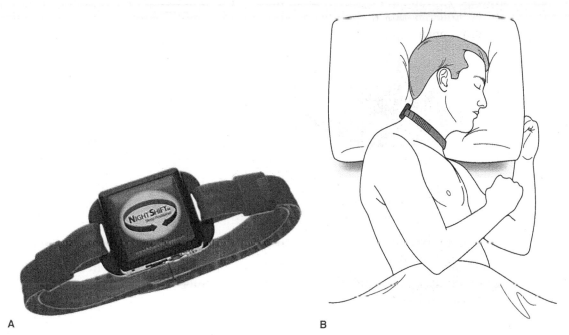

A   B

Figure 54-2 A, B: The Night Shift Sleep Positioner is a Food and Drug Administration–cleared positional medical device approved for the treatment of sleep apnea. This device worn around the neck vibrates when it detects supine sleeping to alert the patient to not sleep supine. This device has a number of features such as interactive adherence and snoring monitoring for the clinician via online portal, and interactive sleep monitoring, snore detection, and behavioral modification for the patient. This is a prescription device and costs $349.00 and is generally an out-of-pocket expense to the patient (33). (View A used with permission from Sleep Specialists LLC, 150 Monument Rd, Suite 207, Bala Cynwyd, PA 19004, http://zzomaosa.com/contacts-us/)

in place by an adhesive similar to that found in adhesive bandages (see Fig. 54-3A). The valve has minimal inspiratory resistance but an increased expiratory resistance. This increased expiratory resistance creates increased end-expiratory pressure that leads to upper airway dilation and increased functional residual capacity (FRC), creating greater lung expansion and volume during exhalation (Fig. 54-3B). FRC is the volume of air present in the bottom of the lungs at the end of expiration. This makes the upper airway more resistant and reduces AHI (13).

Efficacy and Compliance with nEPAP

It is especially important for patients using this therapy to have close clinical follow-up. Provent treatment is shown to have good compliance and has been shown to reduce AHI, reduce snoring and improve subjective daytime sleepiness regardless of OSA severity (13, 14). There are, however, important factors to consider. A significant AHI reduction does not guarantee enough of a reduction to normalize the patient's breathing. This treatment has been shown to effectively treat AHI in approximately 50% of patients (13). It is uncertain why AHI is significantly reduced in some patients but not in others. In addition, there may not be a significant

decrease in oxygen desaturation index, minimum SaO_2 level, or an improvement in sleep architecture in these patients. If OSA leads to adverse consequences because of sleep disruption and intermittent hypoxia, then this treatment would fall short in cases where these factors are not addressed (15). Although no AASM guidelines exist regarding the use of Provent at the time of this writing, there are several publications validating its effectiveness in some patients (13, 14, 16).

MEDICATION THERAPIES

Several pharmacologic agents have been evaluated for the treatment of OSA, and none are shown to be an effective treatment. Selective serotonergic uptake inhibitors, protriptyline, methylxanthine derivatives, and estrogen therapy were studied enough to be named in AASM practice parameters to be not recommended or indicated for OSA treatment (17). Short-acting nasal decongestants are not recommended for the treatment of OSA. Topical nasal corticosteroids, however, may be a useful adjunct to primary therapies for patients with OSA *and* concurrent rhinitis (17).

At the time of this writing, one of the latest proposed medicinal treatments for OSA is medical cannabis, or

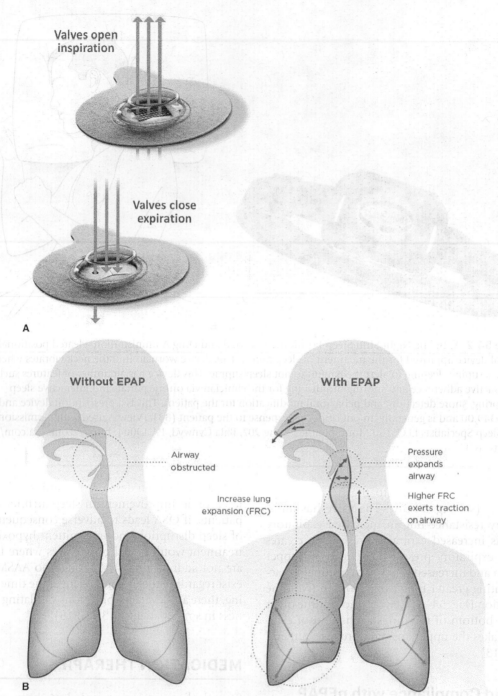

Figure 54-3 A: Provent therapy consists of a single-use valve inserted into each nostril and held in place by an adhesive. The cost is generally $65 to $80 for a 30-day supply. Currently, it is not covered by Medicare or by most private insurances (34). **B:** The Provent one-way resister valves create positive end-expiratory pressure that leads to upper airway dilation with subsequent tracheal traction and increased lung volumes during exhalation, thereby making the upper airway more resistant to inspiration. EPAP, expiratory positive airway pressure; FRC, functional residual capacity. (Images reprinted with permission from Proventtherapy. com, Provent Sleep Therapy, LLC, Manchester, NH.)

more specifically, the synthetic extract dronabinol. Clinical findings indicate a potential for dronabinol to be a treatment option for OSA. Data are limited, and mechanisms of how the chemical may lower the AHI are uncertain. It is hypothesized to be related to increased

vagal afferent activity in the upper airway (18). Dronabinol is not FDA approved for the treatment of OSA. No synthetic extracts from cannabis other than dronabinol have been studied in patients with OSA. At the time of this writing, the AASM position is that medical cannabis should not be used for the treatment of OSA, and further research is needed to better understand the mechanistic actions of medical cannabis and its synthetic extracts, the long-term role of these synthetic extracts on OSA treatment, and the harms and benefits (19).

NONPRESCRIPTION PRODUCTS

There are many nonprescription products that are marketed for the treatment of snoring and OSA. These products may be appealing to patients for many different reasons. They may provide a sense of control, avoid the time and expense associated with consulting a physician or other health care providers, and they may feel they are using a "safe and natural" method. It goes without saying that nonvalidated treatments should not be recommended by health care professionals for several reasons. A substance influences a person's state of health and may be inherently associated with side effects. "Natural" products are not necessarily nontoxic. The preparation of these products lacks, standardization and review, and information detailing the efficacy and safety of these products is not commonly available. The sleep technologist may notice many products marketed to the general product, some more valid than others. Several of these nonprescription products have been evaluated out of concerns for patient safety as well as patient and clinician awareness (20).

External Nasal Dilators

The FDA has approved external nasal dilators (ENDs) for use for temporary relief from transient nasal breathing difficulties. END strips mechanically pull the lateral nasal vestibule walls outward by means of two parallel springs enclosed in an adhesive strip (Fig. 54-4). Studies

show END use appears to be safe and may be useful for mild snoring in some patients. They also show no meaningful improvement in OSA and reveal the potential worsening of OSA severity in some patients. Overall, there is not sufficient evidence to support the use of END for snoring with or without OSA (21).

Internal Nasal Dilators

Internal nasal dilators (IND), like external dilators, are FDA approved for temporary relief from transient nasal breathing difficulties. As the name suggests, these products keep open the lateral nasal vestibule walls from inside the nostrils (Fig. 54-5). Limited studies exist for the effectiveness for sleep-disordered breathing. Indications are that snoring is generally reduced; however, long-term compliance is poor. There is no evidence to support the use of IND in the treatment of OSA (20).

Lubricants

A variety of lubricant sprays or drops for the nose or throat are advertised as a method for the treatment of snoring. The FDA does not approve any of these products to treat or cure any disease. Soft-tissue lubricating agents may have efficacy in reducing snoring, but there are little data regarding their use in OSA patients, and it does not support a clinically significant reduction in AHI. The use of these products should be limited to patients with primary snoring (20).

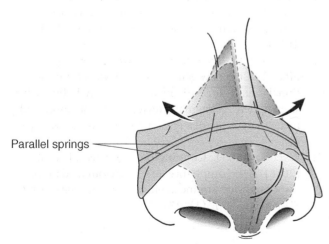

Parallel springs

Figure 54-4 External nasal dilator strips mechanically pull the lateral nasal vestibule walls outward by means of two parallel springs enclosed in an adhesive strip (21).

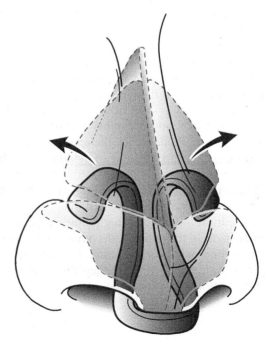

Figure 54-5 Internal nasal dilators that keep open the lateral nasal vestibule walls from inside the nostrils.

Dietary Supplements

Ingredients in oral dietary supplements for snoring reduction include various herbs, enzymes, and melatonin. Being sold as dietary supplements, they are not subject to regulation by the FDA. Extremely limited data suggest a reduction in snoring with oral dietary supplements, and there is no published scientific literature using objective measurements to support the efficacy of dietary supplements for the treatment of snoring or OSA (20).

Chinstraps

Chinstraps have been advertised as treatments for snoring and/or OSA. They are not clinically valid treatment options. An interesting case study was published in 2007 where a patient with severe OSA discontinued CPAP after 1 month, then used only a chinstrap. A repeat study 2 months post-CPAP showed a normal AHI (21). This case study may have been the catalyst for many advertisements advocating this product for snoring and/or OSA. This case study prompted a study published in the *Journal of Clinical Sleep Medicine* that concluded that a chinstrap alone is not an effective treatment for OSA. It does not improve sleep-disordered breathing, even in mild OSA, nor does it improve the AHI in rapid eye movement sleep or supine sleep. It is also ineffective in improving snoring (22).

CONCLUSION

Many of the therapies described in this chapter have the potential to effectively treat OSA or be an effective adjunctive treatment option. It is extremely important that reports from patients about their symptoms be considered with these treatments, and that patients be reevaluated to assess the efficacy of their treatment. No one treatment option is best for all patients. In fact, some treatments available to the patient population are not suited for a single individual or are not effective at all. Despite the constant advancements in PAP technology and adherence methods, other therapies are available and may be well-suited for some individuals. PAP therapy remains the most effective treatment option for OSA. Adherence with PAP therapy is variable but is optimized by a patient-centered approach that includes pretreatment education and ongoing follow-up (23). As a vital participant in the patient's sleep medicine journey, the sleep technologist must be familiar with these other therapies and able to convey some general knowledge of validated treatment options (23).

REFERENCES

1. American Academy of Sleep Medicine. (2009). Clinical guideline for the evaluation, management and long-term care of obstructive sleep apnea in adults. *Journal of Clinical Sleep Medicine, 5*(3), 263.
2. Fryar, C. D., Ogden, C. L., & Carroll, M. D. (2010). Prevalence of overweight, obesity, and extreme obesity among adults: United States, trends 1960–1962 through 2013–2014. *National Center for Health Statistics, 6*(1), 1–6.
3. Fredheim, J. M., Rollheim, J., Sandbu, R., et al. (2013). Obstructive sleep apnea after weight loss: A clinical trial comparing gastric bypass and intensive lifestyle intervention. *Journal of Clinical Sleep Medicine, 9*(5), 427.
4. Strobel, R. J., & Rosen, R. C. (1996). Obesity and weight loss in obstructive sleep apnea: A critical review. *Sleep, 19*(2), 104–115.
5. Peppard, P. E., Young, T., Palta, M., et al. (2000). Longitudinal study of moderate weight change and sleep-disordered breathing. *JAMA, 284*(23), 3015–3021.
6. Lettieri, C. J., Eliasson, A. H., & Greenburg, D. L. (2008). Persistence of obstructive sleep apnea after surgical weight loss. *Journal of Clinical Sleep Medicine, 4*(4), 333.
7. Jensen, M. D., Ryan, D. H., Apovian, C. M., et al. (2014). 2013 AHA/ACC/TOS guideline for the management of overweight and obesity in adults: A report of the American College of Cardiology/American Heart Association Task Force on practice guidelines and the obesity society. *Journal of the American College of Cardiology, 63*(25, Pt. B), 2985–3023.
8. Gudzune, K. A., Bleich, S. N., & Clark, J. M. (2015). Efficacy of commercial weight-loss programs. *Annals of Internal Medicine, 163*(5), 399.
9. Sarkhosh, K., Switzer, N. J., El-Hadi, M., et al. (2013). The impact of bariatric surgery on obstructive sleep apnea: A systematic review. *Obesity Surgery, 23*(3), 414–423.
10. Ravesloot, M. J., White, D., Heinzer, R., et al. (2017). Efficacy of the new generation of devices for positional therapy for patients with positional obstructive sleep apnea: A systematic review of the literature and meta-analysis. *Journal of Clinical Sleep Medicine, 13*(6), 813.
11. Levendowski, D., Cunnington, D., Swieca, J., et al. (2018). User compliance and behavioural adaption associated with supine avoidance therapy. *Behavioral Sleep Medicine, 16*(1), 27–37.

12. Night Shift Sleep Positioner. Retrieved from http://nightshifttherapy.com. Update August 20, 2018.

13. Riaz, M., Certal, V., Nigam, G., et al. (2015). Nasal expiratory positive airway pressure devices (provent) for OSAHS: A systematic review and meta-analysis. *Sleep Disorders, 2015*, 734798.

14. Patel, A. V., Hwang, D., Masdeu, M. J., et al. (2011). Predictors of response to a nasal expiratory resistor device and its potential mechanisms of action for treatment of obstructive sleep apnea. *Journal of Clinical Sleep Medicine, 7*(1), 13.

15. White, D. P. (2009). Auto-PEEP to treat obstructive sleep apnea. *Journal of Clinical Sleep Medicine, 5*(6), 538–539.

16. Kryger, M. H., Berry, R. B., & Massie, C. A. (2011). Long-term use of a nasal expiratory positive airway pressure (EPAP) device as a treatment for obstructive sleep apnea (OSAHS). *Journal of Clinical Sleep Medicine, 7*(5), 449.

17. Morgenthaler, T., Kapen, S., Lee-Chiong, T., et al.; Standards of Practice Committee; American Academy of Sleep Medicine. (2018). Practice parameters for the medical therapy of obstructive sleep apnea. *Sleep, 29*(8), 1031–1035.

18. Carley, D. W., Prasad, B., Reid, K. J., et al. (2017). Pharmacotherapy of apnea by cannabimimetic enhancement, the pace clinical trial: Effects of dronabinol in obstructive sleep apnea. *Sleep, 41*(1). doi:10.1093/sleep/zsx184

19. Ramar, K., Rosen, I. M., Kirsch, D. B., et al. (2018). Medical cannabis and the treatment of obstructive sleep apnea: An American Academy of Sleep Medicine position statement. *Journal of Clinical Sleep Medicine, 14*(4), 679–681.

20. Meoli, A. L., Rosen, C. L., Kristo, D., et al. (2003). Nonprescription treatments of snoring or obstructive sleep apnea: An evaluation of products with limited scientific evidence. *Sleep, 26*(5), 619–624.

21. UCI News. (2016). *UC Irvine Health review finds nasal dilators effective*. Retrieved from https://news.uci.edu/2016/06/30/uc-irvine-health-review-finds-nasal-dilators-effective/

22. Bhat, S., Gushway-Henry, N., Polos, P. G., et al. (2014). The efficacy of a chinstrap in treating sleep disordered breathing and snoring. *Journal of Clinical Sleep Medicine, 10*(8), 887.

23. Wickwire, E. M., Lettieri, C. J., Cairns, A. A., et al. (2013). Maximizing positive airway pressure adherence in adults: A common-sense approach. *Chest, 144*(2), 680–693.

24. WeightWatchers. Retrieved from www.weightwatchers.com

25. Jenny Craig. Retrieved from www.jennycraig.com

26. CBS News. Retrieved from www.cbsnews.com/news/the-best-ways-to-lose-20-pounds/

27. Nutrisystem. Retrieved from www.nutrisystem.com

28. Health Management Resource. Retrieved from www.hmrprogram.com/

29. Medifast. Retrieved from www.medifast1.com

30. Optifast. Retrieved from www.optifast.com

31. Lose It. Retrieved from www.loseit.com

32. SlimFast. Retrieved from www.slimfast.com

33. Zzoma. Retrieved from http://zzomaosa.com/regulatory-compliance/

34. Provent Sleep Apnea Therapy. Retrieved from www.proventtherapy.com

SECTION 7
Patient Management

chapter 55

Sleep Health Educator and Patient Self-Management: The Connection

ROBYN V. WOIDTKE

LEARNING OBJECTIVES

On completion of this chapter, the reader should be able to:

1. Describe the roles and functions of a clinical sleep educator.
2. Describe the importance of patient self-management support in the continuum of care and as it relates to patient adherence.
3. Describe health literacy and how it impacts patient health.

KEY TERMS

Adherence
Self-management
Psychosocial
Shared decision making (SDM)
Care coordination
Health literacy
Behavioral intervention
Cognitive behavioral therapy
Activation
Patient engagement
Motivational enhancement (ME)
Patient outcomes

They may forget your name, but they will never forget how you made them feel.

Maya Angelou

INTRODUCTION

According to Ganguli and Ferris (1), in the United States, health care remains fragmented, poorly communicated, and expensive. This disconnected health care system creates an environment of patients who are unable to self-manage their care. As more health care is shifted to the home and includes not only the patient but the family as well, it is important to develop mechanisms to improve support of self-management programs and patient outcomes for patients with sleep disorders (2).

Sleep health educators can make a meaningful difference in patients and the community. Obstructive sleep apnea (OSA) is a modifiable risk factor for cardiovascular, endocrine, and neurocognitive dysfunction (3). Sleep health educators can improve adherence to treatment and quality of life. In addition to helping sleep disorders patients, the field has a fiduciary duty to promote healthy sleep in the community. Sleep health professionals possess the knowledge to support treatment efforts.

Our counterparts in diabetes and asthma treatment have garnered support of the medical community to provide important self-management support including education, navigation, and care coordination for patients with these conditions. This has not been the case for our profession.[1]

PATIENT EDUCATION

The role of patient education cannot be adequately summarized in a chapter—it is a complex intertwining of characteristics of the patient and clinician, including gender, learning theories, age, and materials as well as the social determinants of health. According to Barnason et al. (4), therapeutic patient education can be defined as "an approach to facilitate patient and family learning about the treatment of disease and the adoption of self-management behaviors and lifestyles to improve physical and psychosocial health outcomes." Sleep health educators can be instrumental in educating sleep disorder patients in order to promote long-term adherence to sleep therapy.

---

[1] https://www.medicare.gov/coverage/diabetes-self-mgmt-training.html

ADHERENCE

Patient adherence to medical recommendations is complex and multifactorial. Simply put, adherence means "sticking to treatment" or following the instructions provided by the medical team. Adherence can be broken down into several components, including the cost of therapy, health literacy, language barriers, difficulty in therapy, age, and access to care (5). Individual predictors of adherence are difficult; thus, tailoring approaches to each person may require a multimodal approach (6, 7) including various teaching techniques, and family and community resources. In 2003, the World Health Organization (WHO) (8) published its report on adherence. In a nutshell, lack of adherence leads to increased health care costs, patient safety issues, and overall poorer quality of life—all of which sleep health professionals should be concerned with.

The WHO (8) states, "Increasing the effectiveness of adherence interventions may have a far greater impact on the health of the population than any improvement in specific medical treatments." And indeed, for patients with OSA, a Cochrane review (9) indicated that there were few clinical advantages to a variety of "comfort"-enhancing features such as humidification and reduction of expiratory pressure. However, another Cochrane review (10) assessed the effectiveness of education and behavioral interventions, and although the data were mixed and the overall quality of the studies assessed was low to moderate, in patients who were naïve about continuous positive airway pressure (CPAP), such interventions resulted in improved usage. Both reviews indicated that more studies were needed to assess these issues.

The literature supports that adherence to sleep apnea therapy is poor, estimated between 23% and 84%, and has not changed much over the past 20 years. However, there are varying definitions for adherence ranging from 4 to 7 hours per night (11, 12). Luga and McGuire (13) conducted a review of the literature regarding medication adherence and health care costs mainly assessing chronic illness such as chronic obstructive pulmonary disease and congestive heart failure. They indicate that medication nonadherence ranges from 25% to 50%, similar to CPAP adherence. Their review concludes that adherence can improve health outcomes and health care cost expenditures. Indeed, a recent article by Truong et al. (14) found that compared with nonadherers, adherence to CPAP was associated with a significantly lower all-cause 30-day hospital readmission rate.

THE ROLE OF THE CLINICAL SLEEP EDUCATOR

The role of the clinical sleep educator within our profession is evolving and there are many designations for individuals who provide these services within a clinic or hospital. Although there may be differing titles, the patient-centered goals are the same: to provide the right care, to the right patient, at the right time (15). In addition, the goal is also to improve adherence to sleep treatment, regardless of the condition, by providing patients with the necessary tools for self-management at home. Although there is no one distinct definition for the role, core competencies exist for the sleep health educator, which include assessing the patient's educational needs and providing education appropriately, the ability to counsel patients with regard to treatment options, providing access to community-based resources, and developing patient education materials (16).

For individuals in this role, it is not only about providing education about a specific topic or condition or training on a device but really truly understanding the patient's preferences, concerns, and limitations. When patients enter the support "wasteland" called home, it is often difficult for them to perform self-management, which is what is expected of them. The sleep health educator can do much to mitigate this issue by providing much-needed support in a variety of ways.

PERSON-CENTERED CARE

Person- or patient-centered care refers to incorporating shared decision making (SDM), care coordination and accessibility, top-down commitment to ensuring alignment with patient-centered goals, family inclusion, consideration of social determinants of health, and information sharing. Almeida et al. (17) in their focus groups found that patients have a variety of factors that influence their response to therapeutic decisions including side effects and impact to bed partners. By providing a more patient-focused approach rather than a one-size-fits-all approach, the patient may be more adherent to therapy. Value in providing patient-centered care has been demonstrated in improved patient satisfaction, clinician satisfaction, financial margins, and enhanced reputation of providers (15). In addition, the Institute of Medicine in their report "Crossing the Quality Chasm" includes person-centered care in their six aims for health care improvement (see Table 55-1) (18). For an excellent overview for sleep apnea patients regarding patient-centered care, see Hilbert and Yaggi (19).

Another consideration for why adoption and adherence to CPAP is low is that patients may be skeptical of their diagnosis. In a recent article by Zarhin (20), it was found that many patients do not believe their diagnosis of OSA because of a lack of daytime symptoms or a lack of trust in the diagnostic procedure. This is an important consideration, which is probably often not thought about.

There are many ways by which the clinical sleep professional can provide support to patients. These

Table 55-1 Six Aims for Health Care Improvement

- Safe: avoiding injuries to patients from the care that is intended to help them
- Effective: providing services on the basis of scientific knowledge to all who could benefit, and refraining from providing services to those not likely to benefit
- Patient-centered: providing care that is respectful of, and responsive to, individual patient preferences, needs, and values, and ensuring that patient values guide all clinical decisions
- Timely: reducing waiting times and sometimes harmful delays for both those who receive and those who give care
- Efficient: avoiding waste, including waste of equipment, supplies, ideas, and energy
- Equitable: providing care that does not vary in quality because of personal characteristics such as gender, ethnicity, geographic location, and socioeconomic status

Reprinted with permission from Institute of Medicine. (2001). *Crossing the quality chasm: A new health system for the 21st century.* Washington, DC: National Academy of Sciences. Courtesy of the National Academies Press.

include such areas as SDM, patient care coordination, alignment of social resources, and care planning for self-management.

SHARED DECISION MAKING

Although SDM is primarily done by physicians, the sleep health professional can provide foundational education to the patient regarding his or her condition and options,

and elicit what is important to him or her. This information gathering and education could be performed in conjunction with or following the physician providing the patient with a diagnosis and treatment options. In 2012, the first three-step model for SDM was proposed (21). In 2017, a revised model was published (see Fig. 55-1). The basic premise remains the same and includes team talk (replaces choice talk), option talk, and finally decision talk. There are competencies that may need to be learned by the sleep health educator regarding the application

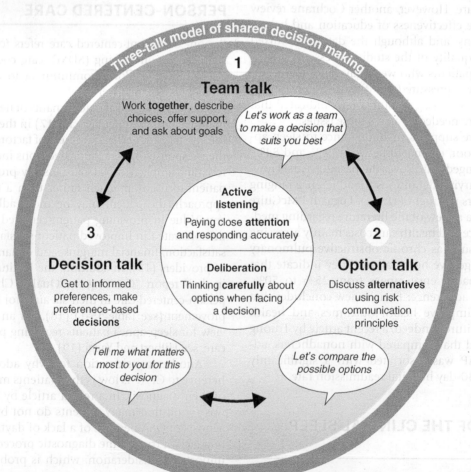

Figure 55-1 A three-talk model for shared decision making. (From Elwyn, G., Durand, M. A., Song, J., et al. (2017). A three-talk model for shared decision making: Multistage consultation process. *British Medical Journal, 359,* j4891. doi:10.1136/bmj.j4891)

of SDM (21–23). The process is fluid and should take the patient from initial preferences to informed preferences. SDM has been demonstrated to improve patient outcomes and satisfaction, although the data are mixed in this regard (24, 25).

PATIENT CARE COORDINATION

Various definitions for care coordination exist. The Agency for Healthcare Quality Research (25) describes care coordination as "the deliberate organization of patient care activities between two or more participants (including the patient) involved in a patient's care to facilitate the appropriate delivery of health care services. Organizing care involves the marshaling of personnel and other resources needed to carry out all required patient care activities and is often managed by the exchange of information among participants responsible for different aspects of care." Figure 55-2 demonstrates some of the dimensions of care coordination. The role of the sleep health educator should be to act as an intermediary as needed.

HEALTH LITERACY

Health literacy is an issue for many patients. According to the Office of Disease Prevention and Health Promotion (26), the definition of health literacy is "the degree to which individuals have the capacity to obtain, process, and understand basic health information and services needed to make appropriate health decisions." Health literacy is dependent on not only the patient's ability to have such capacity but also the communication skills of the clinician, the patient's culture and belief systems, and the demands of the condition and health care system. Health literacy also includes skills such as numeracy. According to Rothman et al., numeracy is "the ability to understand and use numbers in daily life" (27).

The data of the National Center for Education Statistics Health Literacy of America's Adults (28) indicate that only 12% of adults are proficient, and 36% are at basic or below basic health literacy. And further that older individuals as well as those whose English is not the first language pose additional barriers to understanding and hence to the ability to perform self-management in the

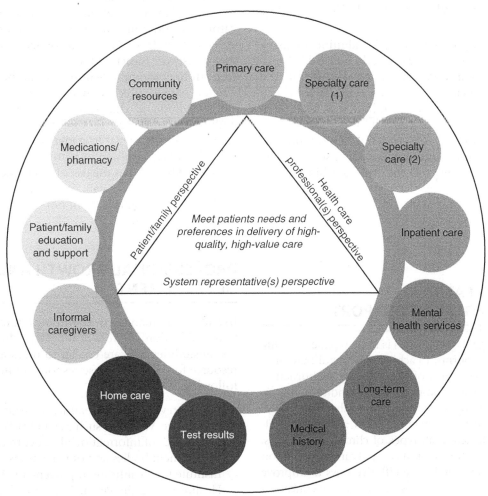

Figure 55-2 Dimensions of care coordination. (Reprinted with permission from Agency for Healthcare Research and Quality. (2014, June). *Care coordination measures Atlas update.* Rockville, MD: Author. Retrieved from http://www.ahrq.gov/professionals/prevention-chronic-care/improve/coordination/atlas2014/index.html)

home environment. The data regarding patients' ability to incorporate numeracy into daily care are similar to those of health literacy, but there are difficulties in determining how best to measure this data (29).

In sleep health care, many numbers are used to communicate with patients, such as the apnea–hypopnea index and percentages of sleep times and stages. Long-term health consequences should be explained to the patient, with particular emphasis on the impact to the individual. Both numbers and health information link back to the patient's health literacy ability. These types of information can be confusing for patients unless explained in a manner that they understand. Thus, part of the role is the ability of the individual to translate these types of data into "plain language." In both written and spoken language, key elements of plain language include (28) the following:

- Organizing information so that the most important behavioral or action points come first;
- Breaking complex information into understandable chunks;
- Using simple language or defining technical terms; and
- Providing ample white space so that pages look easy to read.

In spoken communications, in addition to using such techniques as the "teach-back method," limiting the use of medical jargon can also be helpful. The teach-back method is a health literacy tool that has been found useful to enhance communication. It is a mechanism that allows patients to put into their own words what was told to them. It provides an opportunity for the provider to correct information and ensure that the patient understands what is needed from him or her. The burden is on the clinician to ensure that they have communicated effectively. For more information, see: http://www.ihi.org/resources/Pages/Tools/AlwaysUseTeachBack!.aspx.

PROVIDING PATIENT SELF-MANAGEMENT SUPPORT

Ultimately, the goal of clinicians is to help patients along their therapeutic journey to achieve successful outcomes such as improving quality of life, reducing the burden of illness, and achieving control of their condition. This is typically achieved by way of improved adherence to lifestyle modifications, treatment regimens, and routine follow-up care (6). Across all types of chronic conditions, behavioral intervention, education, and care coordination have been demonstrated to be effective ways to improve long-term adherence to therapy. Alone, patient education has not been shown sufficient to make a difference (6).

Patient engagement and activation in addition to education are relevant to our goals. What is patient engagement and activation? These are actions that individuals must take to obtain the greatest benefit from the health care services available. Activation is a component of engagement and is defined as "understanding one's role in the care process and having the knowledge, skill, and confidence to manage one's health and health care" (6). These concepts are crucial in the patient's ability to perform successful self-management at home. For example, patients diagnosed with OSA are expected to acquire knowledge of their condition, learn how to use and maintain a medical device in the home, and know when to seek help to overcome barriers. They should also understand when therapy is not working and when to contact their provider.

Another approach is to include a bed partner. A recent study found that when education and self-management support includes the bed partner, motivation is enhanced for CPAP use. The bed partner is often forgotten in terms of "needing to know" and also of his or her own sleep disruption, which can have a negative effect on a relationship (30).

One of the tools available for the sleep health educator, with additional training, is the use of motivational enhancement (ME). One does not need an advanced degree to use ME. Structured training, however, is required to learn how to implement it. ME can be defined as "a client-centered, directive method for enhancing intrinsic motivation to change by exploring and resolving ambivalence" (31, 32). This technique has been demonstrated to be beneficial to patients with sleep apnea in several studies, resulting in better long-term adherence (33–35). ME includes the use of open-ended questions, assessment of change talk, and creating discrepancy. Additional information about implementing ME is provided in the appendix.

PROFESSIONAL GROWTH AND DEVELOPMENT

In addition to mandated continuing education to maintain certification, the role of the sleep educator also has responsibilities that are crucial to one's ability to be a resource for patients. These responsibilities include the following:

- Regular review of the literature to ensure up-to-date knowledge. Web sites such as ClinicalTrials.gov can be a wealth of information about current research. Government bodies and organizations such as the Institute for Healthcare Improvement, Agency for Healthcare Quality Research, National Institutes of Health, and the Centers for Disease Control and

Prevention are also excellent sources. MEDLINE contains journal citations and abstracts for biomedical literature from around the world. PubMed provides free access to MEDLINE and links to full text articles when possible (36). Google Scholar is also a good resource. These are only a few of the options available. There are many resources available on patient-centered care; chronic care; and patient education, activation, and engagement. An understanding of these forms of patient care is essential to ensure that the sleep educator develops a well-rounded foundation.

- A thorough understanding of the various therapies used for the treatment of sleep apnea. In addition to positive airway pressure therapy and keeping up to date with innovation around this modality, it is vitally important because new positional aids, surgical approaches, and improvements in oral appliances are constantly being developed. New therapies for insomnia have also come to market, which require new knowledge. The use of online cognitive behavioral therapy programs should also be included in the sleep educator's repertoire. This knowledge should encompass, at a minimum, mechanisms of action, and the limitations and benefits of each type of treatment for a variety of sleep disorders.

- Wearables and consumer apps for tracking sleep are increasing. Thus, an individual in this role should be aware of these technologies and how he or she may both help and hinder a patient's experience. Privacy and data issues are of concern. Understanding the advantages, such as increased patient engagement, and limitations regarding the rigor in which wearables have been developed will be important (37). These fall under a new category of product within the US Food and Drug Administration (FDA)-coined *general wellness products*. This category includes such things as sleep trackers and over-the-counter pulse oximeters. These products do not have to undergo review by the FDA for determination of safety and effectiveness. Many of them are "listed" products, and the FDA retains the right to inspect companies that produce such products (38).

- Measuring treatment-related patient outcomes will become increasingly more important. According to a 2016 article by Abma et al. (39), the best measures are the sleep apnea quality of life index, Maugeri obstructive sleep apnea syndrome questionnaire, Quebec sleep questionnaire, and the OSA patient-oriented severity index. Including these types of measurements during baseline and subsequent follow-up visits provides a wealth of information to assess the utility of the role of the sleep educator. Other measurements such as patient satisfaction, including aspects of communication, caring, and testing, should be collected.

- Finally, research is needed to support the role of the sleep health educator as a necessary component of ongoing coordinated care for sleep patients. Individuals currently engaged in this role are strongly encouraged to disseminate their findings and successes to others in the field.

In summary, there are many theories, tools, and ongoing support mechanisms that are pertinent to the role of the sleep health educator. Only providing "education" about an illness or treatment is not sufficient to aid a patient along his or her therapeutic journey toward self-management. This requires a complex interaction between the practitioner and the patient to ensure similar goals, and a consideration of the patient's preference and values, culture, and social foundations. A broad understanding of the complexities of the role and vigilance in learning and enhancing one's skills and knowledge is critical. This allows the sleep health educator to provide patients with optimal care and follow-up. The role of the sleep health educator is to strive to provide the right care, to the right patient, at the right time and make a positive difference.

REFERENCES

1. Ganguli, I., & Ferris, T. G. (2018). Accountable care at the frontlines of a health system bridging aspiration and reality. *JAMA, 319*(7), 655–656. doi:10.1001/jama.2017.18995

2. Landers, S., Madigan, E., Leff, B., et al. (2018). The future of home health care: A strategic framework for optimizing value. *Home Health Care Management & Practice, 28*(4), 262–278. https://doi.org/10.1177/1084822316666368

3. Lee, W., Nagubadi, S., Kryger, M. H., et al. (2008). Epidemiology of obstructive sleep apnea: A population-based perspective. *Expert Review of Respiratory Medicine, 2*(3), 349–364. doi:10.1586/17476348.2.3.349

4. Barnason, S., White-Williams, C., Rossi, L. P., et al. (2017). Evidence for therapeutic patient education interventions to promote cardiovascular patient self-management: A scientific statement for healthcare professionals from the American Heart Association. *Circulation: Cardiovascular Quality and Outcomes, 10*, e000025. doi:10.1161/HCQ.0000000000000025

5. Brown, M. T., & Bussell, J. K. (2011). Medication adherence: WHO cares? *Mayo Clinic Proceedings, 86*(4), 304–314. doi:10.4065/mcp.2010.0575

6. Grady, P. A., & Gough, L. L. (2014). Self-management: A comprehensive approach to management of chronic conditions. *American Journal of Public Health, 104*(8), e25–e31. doi:10.2105/AJPH.2014.302041

7. Kardas, P., Lewek, P., & Matyjaszczyk, M. (2013). Determinants of patient adherence: A review of systematic reviews. *Frontiers in Pharmacology, 4,* 91. doi:10.3389/fphar.2013.00091

8. Sabaté, E., & World Health Organization. (2003). *Adherence to long-term therapies: Evidence for action.* Geneva, Switzerland: World Health Organization.

9. Smith, I., & Lasserson, T. J. (2009). Pressure modification for improving usage of continuous positive airway pressure machines in adults with obstructive sleep apnoea. *Cochrane Database of Systematic Reviews,* (4), CD003531. doi:10.1002/14651858.CD003531. pub3

10. Wozniak, D. R., Lasserson, T. J., & Smith, I. (2014). Educational, supportive and behavioural interventions to improve usage of continuous positive airway pressure machines in adults with obstructive sleep apnoea. *Cochrane Database of Systematic Reviews,* (1), CD007736. doi:10.1002/14651858.CD007736.pub2

11. Rotenberg, B. W., Murariu, D., & Pang, K. P. (2016). Trends in CPAP adherence over twenty years of data collection: A flattened curve. *Journal of Otolaryngology—Head & Neck Surgery, 45,* 43. doi:10.1186/s40463-016-0156-0

12. Weaver, T. E., & Grunstein, R. R. (2008). Adherence to continuous positive airway pressure therapy: The challenge to effective treatment. *Proceedings of the American Thoracic Society, 5*(2), 173–178. doi:10.1513/pats.200708-119MG

13. Luga, A. O., & McGuire, M. J. (2014). Adherence and health care costs. *Risk Management and Healthcare Policy, 7,* 35–44. doi:10.2147/RMHP.S19801

14. Truong, K. K., De Jardin, R., Massoudi, N., et al. (2018). Nonadherence to CPAP associated with increased 30-day hospital readmissions. *Journal of Clinical Sleep Medicine, 14*(2), 183–189. doi:10.5664/jcsm.6928

15. New England Journal of Medicine Catalyst. *What is patient-centered care?* Retrieved from https://catalyst.nejm.org/what-is-patient-centered-care/. Accessed June 11, 2018.

16. American Association of Sleep Technologists. (2017). *Competencies: Sleep health educator.* https://www.aastweb.org/hubfs/Core%20Competencies/Sleep%20Health%20Educator%20Competencies%20Final%206.13.2017.pdf. Accessed January 11, 2019.

17. Almeida, F. R., Henrich, N., Marra, C., et al. (2013). Patient preferences and experiences of CPAP and oral appliances for the treatment of obstructive sleep apnea: A qualitative analysis. *Sleep Breath, 17,* 659. doi:10.1007/s11325-012-0739-6

18. Institute of Medicine. (2000). *Crossing the quality chasm.* Washington, DC: The National Academy of Sciences.

19. Hilbert, J., & Yaggi, H. K. (2018). Patient-centered care in obstructive sleep apnea: A vision for the future. *Sleep Medicine Reviews, 37,* 138–147.

20. Zarhin, D. (2015). Contesting medicalisation, doubting the diagnosis: Patients' ambivalence towards the diagnosis of obstructive sleep apnoea. *Sociology of Health and Illness, 37,* 715–730. doi:10.1111/1467-9566.12229

21. Elwyn, G., Frosch, D., Thomson, R., et al. (2012). Shared decision making: A model for clinical practice. *Journal of General Internal Medicine, 27*(10), 1361–1367. doi:10.1007/s11606-012-2077-6

22. Elwyn, G., Durand, M. A., Song, J., et al. (2017). A three-talk model for shared decision making: Multistage consultation process. *British Medical Journal, 359,* j4891. doi:10.1136/bmj.j4891

23. Truglio-Londrigan, M., & Slyer, J. T. (2018). Shared decision-making for nursing practice: An integrative review. *The Open Nursing Journal, 12,* 1–14. doi:10.2174/1874434601812010001

24. Lang, E., Bell, N. R., Dickinson, J. A., et al. (2018). Eliciting patient values and preferences to inform shared decision making in preventive screening. *Canadian Family Physician, 64*(1), 28–31.

25. Agency for Healthcare Quality Research. *Chapter 2. What is care coordination?* Rockville, MD: Agency for Healthcare Research and Quality. Retrieved from http://www.ahrq.gov/professionals/prevention-chronic-care/improve/coordination/atlas2014/chapter2.html

26. Office of Disease Prevention and Health Promotion. (2018). *Health Literacy.* Retrieved from https://health.gov/communication/about.asp. Updated November 6, 2018. Accessed June 11, 2018.

27. Rothman, R. L., Montori, V. M., Cherrington, A., et al. (2008). Perspective: The role of numeracy in health care. *Journal of Health Communication, 13*(6), 583–595. doi:10.1080/10810730802281791

28. National Center for Education Statistics. (2018). *Health Literacy of America's Adults.* Retrieved from https://nces.ed.gov/naal/health_results.asp. Accessed June 11, 2018.

29. Office of Disease Prevention and Health Promotion, U.S. Department of Health and Human Services. (2018). *Plain language: A promising strategy for clearly communicating health information and improving health literacy.* Retrieved from https://health.gov/communication/literacy/plainlanguage/IssueBrief.pdf. Accessed June 11, 2018.

30. Luyster, F. S., Dunbar-Jacob, J., Aloia, M. S., et al. (2016). Patient and partner experiences with obstructive sleep apnea and CPAP treatment: A qualitative analysis. *Behavioral Sleep Medicine, 14*(1), 67–84. doi:10.1080/15402002.2014.946597

31. Miller, W. R., & Rose, G. S. (2009). Toward a theory of motivational interviewing. *The American Psychologist*, *64*(6), 527–537. doi:10.1037/a0016830

32. Lussier, M.-T., & Richard, C. (2007). The motivational interview: In practice. *Canadian Family Physician*, *53*(12), 2117–2118.

33. Lai, A. Y. K., Fong, D. Y. T., Lam, J. C. M., et al. (2014). The efficacy of a brief motivational enhancement education program on CPAP adherence in OSA: A randomized controlled trial. *Chest*, *146*(3), 600–610.

34. Olsen, S., Smith, S. S., Oei, T. P. S., et al. (2012). Motivational interviewing (MINT) improves continuous positive airway pressure (CPAP) acceptance and adherence: A randomized controlled trial. *Journal of Consulting and Clinical Psychology*, *80*(1), 151–163.

35. Aloia, M. S., Arnedt, J. T., Strand, M., et al. (2013). Motivational enhancement to improve adherence to positive airway pressure in patients with obstructive sleep apnea: A randomized controlled trial.

Sleep, *36*(11), 1655–1662. https://doi.org/10.5665/sleep.3120

36. United States National Library of Medicine. *MEDLINE⁻/PubMed⁻ resources guide*. Retrieved from https://www.nlm.nih.gov/bsd/pmresources.html

37. Montgomery, K., Chester, J., & Kopp, K. (2018). Health wearables: Ensuring fairness, preventing discrimination, and promoting equity in an emerging internet-of-things environment. *Journal of Information Policy*, *8*, 34–77. doi:10.5325/jinfopoli.8.2018.0034

38. Piwek, L., Ellis, D. A., Andrews, S., et al. (2017). The rise of consumer health wearables: Promises and barriers. *PLOS Medicine*, *13*(2), e1001953. doi:10.1371/journal.pmed.1001953

39. Abma, I. L., van der Wees, P. J., Veer, V., et al. (2016). Measurement properties of patient-reported outcome measures (PROMs) in adults with obstructive sleep apnea (OSA): A systematic review. *Sleep Medicine Reviews*, *28*, 18–31.

chapter 56

Developing and Maintaining Therapeutic Compliance

MELINDA O. TRIMBLE

LEARNING OBJECTIVES

On completion of this chapter, the reader should be able to:

1. Explain the importance of education before and after a sleep study is performed.
2. Identify educational opportunities in patient care.
3. Develop a process for patient education within the sleep center.
4. Identify written materials to reinforce compliance.
5. Identify support mechanisms for questions/concerns about positive airway pressure (PAP).
6. Communicate with the patient's family about the importance of PAP compliance.
7. Explain the techniques to help bed partners adjust to PAP.
8. Reinforce the importance of cleaning procedures.
9. Identify potential problems and setbacks to successful therapy.
10. Describe various techniques to increase compliance.
11. Identify community education resources.
12. Assess patient outcomes.

KEY TERMS

Assessment
Compliance
Education
Intervention
Obstructive sleep apnea (OSA)
Outcomes
Positive airway pressure (PAP)

In an era in which there is increasing knowledge, sophistication, and technologic advances to prevent and/or control many diseases, it is alarming that large numbers of individuals continue to be incapacitated, debilitated by, or succumb to, conditions for which effective treatments or measures of prevention are available (1). Sleep disorders are no exception. Although few would disagree that education is an important component of patient care, the majority of health professionals have received no formal training to prepare them for conducting patient education. Often, it is assumed that anyone with a health care background is qualified to educate a patient.

Sleep health education is an essential component to overall patient care. The provision of education for all sleep disorder patients is critically important. In 2014, the Board of Registered Polysomnographic Technologists created a new certification examination for sleep health professionals as a benchmark to assure that minimum competency levels for patient education are achieved. The Certification in Clinical Sleep Health is offered to health care professionals seeking a nontechnical sleep certification. Certification is not required but is an important component of the evolving field of sleep health.

In the sleep center setting, patient education can be one of the most rewarding and gratifying things a sleep technologist experiences. Unfortunately, this is not true for many sleep technologists. A lack of time to educate patients properly and/or a lack of tools to educate patients can be especially frustrating. In this chapter, we will provide you with tools and methodologies that are useful to teaching regardless of the setting (i.e., hospital, home, or in daily lives).

Establishing a standard of care for positive airway pressure (PAP) therapy and education is essential to enhance therapeutic compliance. Managing sleep apnea patients with consistent, standardized instruction and information about sleep-disordered breathing is an achievable goal. This involves educating patients during the initial contact with a sleep technologist at the time of the sleep study, as well as during subsequent treatment and follow-up.

Patient education is best defined as the process that evolves from an exchange between health professionals and patients. As a sleep technologist, one has many opportunities to provide patient education.

Education may occur on the phone, during a chance encounter, after an office visit, or at the time of a procedure; it may even occur in a more public setting such as a support group or an outreach effort. Although recognizing opportunities for education is important, effective education requires establishing a rapport with the patient and acquiring trust.

Consider the individual who is unable to tolerate daytime sleepiness, who has a nagging worry over near-miss auto accidents, or who is worried about the distress that snoring causes to the family. The patient decides to see a physician and is referred to a sleep center for a consultation with a sleep specialist. The opportunity to build a rapport begins the moment the patient calls to make the appointment. The rapport that is established between the patient and the sleep center staff will establish a foundation of trust and contribute to the successful resolution of the patient's sleep issues. If patients have confidence in the staff and the physician, they are more likely to listen, ask questions, and follow instruction. Likewise, when the patient is referred to the sleep center, that initial contact with the scheduling staff will have an impact on how the patient perceives the entire sleep study process. In addition, if the patient is approached with a genuine concern for his or her well-being, he or she is more likely to become engaged in the efforts to successfully resolve sleep problems.

One of the most common diagnoses established in a sleep center is obstructive sleep apnea (OSA). Although there are no cures for this disorder, there are treatments, and one of the most effective forms of treatment available to date is PAP. There are many reasons why an individual may have trouble acclimating to the PAP device, and understanding the patient's concerns will be key to a successful titration. Consider the pretitration situation where the patient declares, "I will not be able to sleep with that mask on my face or use that machine." The sleep technologist should understand from the patient's perspective the fundamental reason(s) why the patient believes the device would not be tolerated and work to address the issues. As an example, if the patient is claustrophobic, consideration may be given to acclimation sessions. If PAP has been determined to be the primary therapeutic intervention for the patient, all efforts should be exhausted before alternative therapeutic options (if any) are considered. Knowing how well the patient tolerates the device during the titration is imperative, especially if the patient is resistant to using the device at home. Review the titration detail carefully. Look for positive as well as negative responses throughout the titration segment of the polysomnogram. The information gleaned from a titration is critical to establishing the starting point, as well as goals for the patient's adherence to therapy.

PATIENT EVALUATION

Setting Goals

Patient education is an effective approach to improving PAP adherence. The plan for education should include specific goals and outcomes (Fig. 56-1), as these will determine the focus for the patient's adherence. Work with the patient to establish these goals; ensure that they are realistic and appropriate for the patient's unique situation. The sleep technologist's role is to enable the patient to act on his or her own behalf by providing information, assisting with the practical problems of carrying out recommendations, increasing awareness of alternatives, and supporting the patient in the general acceptance and integration of new knowledge (1).

To begin, the sleep professional must get to know the patient. It will be necessary to consider the patient's emotions, his or her personal and professional environments, and beliefs and values. A thorough review of the patient's chart should provide fundamental information about the patient; however, information beyond this

---

Structuring the educational program for the patient

1. How does the patient learn?
2. What is needed for the patient to learn?
3. Are there any priorities to the educational process (i.e., medical urgency)?
4. Include success measurements.

Patient assessment

1. What is the patient's attitude toward learning?
2. What is the patient's ability to learn?
3. What are the patient's priorities?

Putting the plan into action

1. Help the patient put together a plan to meet the goals.
2. Help the patient determine a reasonable time frame to achieve the goals.
3. Allow the patient to have ownership of the process.
4. The patient needs to share the responsibility for his or her success.
5. Use all the patient support resources (e.g., family).
6. Make the plan manageable for the patient according to medical priorities.

Outcome assessment

1. Did the patient reach the set goals?
2. If goals were not reached:
   a. Identify reasons.
   b. Develop appropriate solutions.
   c. Alter plan accordingly to get the patient back on track.

Figure 56-1 Worksheet for setting patient goals.

source will need to be obtained. Talking with the patient will be necessary to identify any concerns the patient has about his or her own health condition as well as determine the value the patient places on personal health. With this basic understanding, the sleep technologist can begin to develop an appropriate patient-centered therapy adherence plan.

An assessment of resources and a determination of professional and personal support available to the patient will be necessary for plan development. Coordination of educational efforts will minimize the risk of redundancy and contradictions and prevent components of the plan from being overlooked. It is necessary to determine who from the sleep center will be involved in the adherence plan and identify specific responsibilities for each person. Every staff member has the opportunity to be involved in the patient's compliance. If not involved directly, the staff member should at least be familiar with the structure of the adherence plan.

Family and friends can influence the success or failure of a patient's medical outcome. As the sleep technologist becomes involved with the patient's therapy, the role of the family becomes increasingly apparent. The sleep technologist will need to understand the family's general lifestyle. A series of questions such as "Who talks to whom?" and "How does the family interact with each other?" will be important to assess the dynamics and the appropriateness of the family's involvement. If there are family or friends available for support and if it is appropriate that they be involved in the patient's therapy, permission to involve them will need to be obtained from the patient. The impact of OSA extends beyond the individual and may have significant effects on the family. As such, the family should be included in the education process whenever possible to ensure the best outcome for the patient.

More than 70 sleep disorders have been classified in the *International Classification of Sleep Disorders*—Third Edition (*ICSD*-3), with varying options for treatment. Whether the therapy is behavioral, psychological, pharmacologic, or surgical, education is a key component to the patient's success for improving the quality of life. For some, it may be a fairly expeditious process with relatively few steps; for others, it will be a lengthy process and the steps will be minute and numerous. Understanding the patient, coordinating resources, and assessing his or her response to the prescribed therapy will be vital to structuring realistic achievable goals toward adherence to therapy.

Learning Needs

No matter how dire the situation, patient compliance is always a choice. It is a very important concept for the sleep technologist to understand the process of patient education, and it is critical to recognize what is necessary

for patients to learn and understand about their sleep disorder and the prescribed therapy to achieve long-term adherence.

Learning begins when the patient starts to ask questions and, conversely, when the patient does not have answers for the questions being asked by the health care professional. Initially, the patient will need to be made aware of the sleep disorder, its prognosis, possible treatment options, and consequences of noncompliance. Also, it will be helpful for the patient to understand who participates in the education plan and the roles and responsibilities of each individual. It should be clearly communicated that the health care professionals involved in this treatment compliance plan work on behalf of the patient and want to establish a partnership to ensure adherence and improve the patient's quality of life.

Participants for such a plan may include, but are not limited to, the

- patient
- durable medical equipment (DME) company staff
- sleep technologist
- clinical sleep specialist
- family
- primary care physician (PCP)
- payer (insurance company)
- sleep disorders center staff
- support group

Establishing a coordinated partnership with the patient is a group effort. Effective communication needs to be developed collectively among the participants as well as individually with the patient. The patient should realize that even with complete adherence there might be circumstances that necessitate assistance or direction. A change in health status, a trip out of the country, or equipment problems will be issues that can be readily addressed by the respective sleep professional(s).

Learning Priorities

With most medical conditions, the prognosis generally dictates the path and the priorities for learning. The spectrum of sleep disorders is extremely broad, and consequences range from the merely troublesome day or two of mild jet lag to the tragic loss of life when someone falls asleep at the wheel of an automobile (2).

Health and safety risks associated with the patient's condition will be a priority in the learning process. For the sleep patient, this may involve the PCP in the assessment of health and the sleep specialist to evaluate the patient's complaints and symptoms. If an individual does not understand or comprehend the significance of the health condition, it will be difficult to convince that individual to proceed with diagnostic testing or to comply with treatment recommendations. Therefore, it is important that the patient understands why a PAP machine has been prescribed and what the therapy will involve.

Sleep professionals need to determine what type of information is appropriate for the patient, as well as what type of changes the patient will need to make in everyday life. The goal of the adherence plan should be to assist the patient in learning the skills and knowledge necessary to develop behaviors that will maximize a positive health outcome.

Learning Assessment

Although an adherence plan involves many sleep professionals, one of the most influential roles is that of the sleep technologist responsible for the PAP titration. The sleep technologist has a very narrow window of opportunity to introduce the patient to PAP, titrate to an optimum therapeutic pressure, and influence the patient's willingness to consider PAP as a treatment option. This time constraint makes the interaction between the sleep technologist and the patient all the more essential to achieving long-term compliance.

Acquiring specific information as part of an assessment will maximize the opportunity for a successful titration and increase the probability of compliance. An appropriate assessment will provide the sleep technologist with insight to the patient's motivation, which is necessary before he or she can effectively communicate with the patient (Table 56-1). There are certain factors that influence a patient's motivation and how the patient responds to sleep testing and treatment; these factors may be classified as individual, social, and environmental.

Individual Factors: Determine the Patient's Learning Potential

Determining the knowledge level of the patient is part of the patient assessment and critical to education and the learning process. Generally, a sleep technologist can identify an individual's level of knowledge through observation and conversation. If the patient's level of knowledge is unknown, it will be difficult for the sleep technologist to know if the patient understands the health condition, has sufficient knowledge to assume responsibility for treatment, or understands the consequences of not following the treatment recommendations. In addition to knowledge, skill level and attitude contribute to an individual's ability to learn. The sleep technologist needs to ascertain whether or not the patient has the appropriate skill level to adhere to the treatment regimen. If not, the sleep technologist may need to adjust or modify the teaching techniques used, so that the patient is able to understand the concepts needed to use the treatment device.

Social and Environmental Factors: Determine if These Factors Facilitate or Hinder Medical Care

Social factors such as family, religious beliefs, cultural values, and employers have the potential of facilitating

Table 56-1 Assessment Questions for PAP as a Therapeutic Intervention: Potentially Helpful Questions When Assessing the Patient with Sleep Apnea

Sample Questions	Helpful Information for Technologist
What can you tell me about your condition?	Helps indicate the patient's basic knowledge and level of understanding about the purpose of the overnight study and the potential treatment of the condition
Do you have help or support at home?	A lack of family support may reduce the patient's ability to achieve his or her goals or his or her potential for PAP adherence
Do you think you can use the PAP device?	Helps assess the patient's knowledge level, attitude, and willingness to improve his or her condition
How did you do with the mask?	Helps identify potential problems with the interface device. It is important to work through these types of problems as early as possible to improve the chances of success
Do you need help choosing a homecare company?	Most patients will not have worked with a homecare company. Helps the patient to understand homecare service process in advance to avoid frustration later
Do you have questions about your treatment plan?	Allows the patient the opportunity to ask questions and gives technologist information about the patient's attitude and comprehension of the information and treatment plan that has been recommended
What are your expectations?	Helps the patient set realistic goals

PAP, positive airway pressure.

or hindering patients from reaching their desired goals. As an example, a patient returned for a follow-up to the sleep center and during the appointment was asked if he had been using his continuous positive airway pressure (CPAP) machine. He stated that he had not and upon further questioning, it was discovered that the reason he was not using it was that the noise bothered his wife. With this knowledge, the sleep technologist can start helping the patient by determining if the noise issue involves the mask or the device and suggest changing to a different mask or moving the device further away from the bed.

It is vital for the sleep technologist to understand the reaction of family members to the patient's condition and treatment. If family members appear hesitant or apprehensive about learning the skills needed to assist with care of the patient at home, then the success of the treatment may be compromised. Some family members may not be responsive or may not wish to take an active role.

Issues such as these can be identified only after the sleep technologist has had the opportunity to observe and communicate with the family. If issues are identified, support and guidance should be provided to assist the family in creating solutions. The sleep technologist must understand the significant impact that social factors (e.g., family) may have on the desired goals and create an educational plan according to the patient's priorities.

The impact of environmental factors such as geographic location, employer and job requirements, work and social schedule, and living arrangements should also be considered. The sleep technologist will need to understand the availability of resources to the patient. Does the patient's work schedule hinder his ability to arrange follow-up appointments? Is transportation available to allow for participation with a support group? Considerations such as these will need to be made because the sleep technologist works with the patient to look at solutions for these issues in order to establish and meet treatment goals.

Understanding the patient's priorities will allow the sleep technologist to determine which factors may facilitate the patient's progress and which factors may hinder it.

EDUCATIONAL OPPORTUNITIES

Education should start at the initial visit. The sleep technologist and the board-certified sleep specialist should codevelop the educational process used within the sleep center. This will ensure a consistent educational process. Patient education should be a multitiered process consisting of pretest, test, posttest, and PAP setup instruction and information.

Pretest

When possible, the patient should have the opportunity to visit the sleep center before the sleep study.

This offers the patient the opportunity to become familiar with the facility and the test process and minimizes any apprehension about sleeping in an unfamiliar environment. Written instructions should be provided before the study to ensure that the patient is appropriately prepared and the information being recorded will be valid. Basic instructions are listed in Table 56-2.

The admission process as well as the testing process should be fully explained to the patient. While the patient is at the sleep center, there is an opportunity for him or her to experience the PAP device. This helps acclimate the patient to the device in case it is necessary to apply PAP during the study. The patient can also be introduced to a PAP interface to assure proper fit before titration, and notes can be made in the patient's chart to notify the night sleep technologist of any potential problems the patient may have acclimating to the device. If problems arise, the sleep technologist should make every effort to work through the issues before the test. Potential issues may include hard-to-fit faces, claustrophobia, nasal obstruction, and edentulous mouths.

This is the patient's opportunity to ask any questions before testing and the sleep technologist's opportunity to address any concerns. The sleep technologist should make the most of this time to ensure that the patient is comfortable with the facility and the procedure.

Test Night

When the patient arrives on the night of the study, the sleep technologist should orient and/or reorient the patient to the facility, the procedure, the hookup, and the PAP titration if applicable. In many instances, the patient will not have had a pretest visit to the sleep center and the sleep technologist will be the sole educator for the patient before testing. The sleep technologist should always ensure that the patient understands the

Table 56-2 **Pretest Instructions**

- Arrival and departure time
- Facility policies regarding guests
- Comfortable and appropriate bed clothing
- Personal toiletry items
- Items to enhance the patient's comfort (e.g., pillow)
- Bring scheduled medications
- List of medications taken in the past week
- Instruct not to nap on the day of the study
- Abstain from caffeine after 12 noon

procedure(s) being performed. The patient should have ample opportunity to ask questions or express concerns. It is particularly important to fit the patient with a mask and acclimate him or her to PAP therapy pretest if there is a possibility for a split-night study.

Posttest

Educating patients after a sleep study can sometimes present a challenge. The patient may become overwhelmed by information about a new diagnosis, treatment options, DME provider selection, insurance questions, and overall lifestyle changes. To alleviate information overload, it is helpful for patients to leave the sleep center with written materials. It is important to recognize and respect a patient's hesitancy toward therapy. The more positive, informative, and helpful the educator is with the instruction, the more receptive the patient will be to accept therapy, initially and in the future. In the event the patient is unable to remain in the sleep center for poststudy education, it is imperative that the sleep technologist contact the patient for follow-up and/or mail educational materials to the patient's home. Patients who do not receive poststudy information are at a disadvantage for achieving success with PAP therapy. The sleep technologist should follow the sleep center's policy on what information is to be provided to the patient following the use of PAP therapy during the sleep study.

DME Setup

The peak of most patients' acceptance and enthusiasm for PAP therapy occurs immediately after a successful titration or physician visit. Capitalizing on this enthusiasm promotes improved adherence to therapy and ongoing success. Patient participation in selecting the DME provider and equipment may enhance adherence through shared ownership of the choices, although in some cases, sleep center protocols, location, and insurance guidelines may dictate the DME selection process. Patients should receive written information with the name of the DME provider and a contact number where they may call for questions, concerns, or delivery schedules. A smooth flow of information among the sleep center, DME provider, and patient will reduce delays in the initiation of therapy.

Acclimating to PAP and the mask interface may be enhanced by desensitization techniques to minimize pressure discomfort, claustrophobia, and aversion to the mask. For these reasons, it is especially important to be understanding and reassuring. If the patient is hastily fitted and as a result gets panicky, he or she may be reluctant to try PAP at a later date. For many patients, there is a negative connotation or stigma of "failing a PAP trial" during a sleep study. This negativity should be countered with positive feedback from the sleep technologist at the time the comments are made. Offer the patient reassurance and praise for PAP attempts and remind him or her that many patients require additional time for adjustment to PAP.

Minimizing discomfort and hastening adaptation to the mask pressure can be approached in various ways. Desensitization or acclimation techniques are beneficial during initial mask fitting before a split-night or titration study (Table 56-3). The goal of these techniques is to reduce the failure of adaptation to PAP.

Table 56-3 Desensitization and Acclimation Strategies

Complaint	Solution
I cannot breathe	Increase the pressure
I cannot exhale	Start with a very low pressure or ramp with the patient in an upright position. Instruct the patient to exhale into the mask as soon as he or she feels the pressure and then slowly inhale through his or her nose.
It is smothering me. . .	Start with a very low pressure or ramp with the patient in an upright position. Instruct the patient to exhale into the mask as soon as he or she feels the pressure and then slowly inhale through his or her nose.
The pressure is too high. . .	Reduce to a lower pressure or ramp
I cannot stand anything against my face. . .	Work with alternate interface styles to obtain a mask that will aid in patient comfort. Do not apply headgear or air pressure until the patient is comfortable. With the patient in an upright position, instruct him or her to hold the mask against the face and practice breathing. While performing this exercise, provide a distraction (e.g., television) to minimize the patient's focus on the mask. Have the patient perform this exercise at home. Schedule additional acclimation sessions as necessary.
The mask is uncomfortable. . .	Verify mask fit. Readjust headgear. Replace mask as necessary.

TREATMENT REGIMEN

It is the sleep technologist's responsibility to advise the patient that a follow-up appointment with the referring physician is necessary to receive study results. The patient should always have the opportunity to review the sleep study with the sleep physician. This may or may not be done in the sleep center setting. If the patient was placed on a PAP device, the physician may also request the patient have a follow-up visit with the sleep technologist at the sleep center to work through any problems the patient may be having with PAP therapy. This is an opportunity for the technologist to review the patient's adherence to therapy and explore any issues the patient may be having with the interface and PAP device. Some sleep centers establish PAP clinics. PAP clinics provide the patient an opportunity to work one-on-one with the sleep technologist to assure adherence, offer the patient an avenue to express concerns, and work through problems with the device. A follow-up visit after the sleep study is extremely beneficial to adherence and patient success with therapy.

Adherence

The most frequently used definition of adequate adherence to therapy (previously designated as compliance) was first proposed in 1993 in one of the earliest studies with objective measurement of CPAP use (3). In this study, the authors defined a minimal use criterion (>4 hours per night) and an optimal use criterion (>7 hours per night) and found that CPAP use met minimal criteria on about 50% of nights and optimal criteria on about 20% of nights. By consensus of the authors, regular users were those who used CPAP at least 4 hours per day on at least 70% of nights; 46% of patients met this criterion. Thus, the most frequently used definition of adherence is use for a minimum of 4 hours per night, 5 to 7 nights per week. This definition has been adopted by the Centers for Medicare and Medicaid Services as the minimum objective adherence/compliance a patient must demonstrate for continued reimbursement for PAP therapy (4).

PAP adherence is a long-term, comprehensive process. It is important for the patient to learn as much as possible about his or her condition to successfully and proactively manage it.

Follow-Up Telephone Calls

Follow-up telephone calls to a patient beginning PAP therapy can enhance adherence. The 24- to 72-hour period after initiation of PAP therapy is the most critical time to be in contact with the patient. Some patients may be tired, frustrated, hesitant, or even angry about their struggles with PAP therapy. Others may feel fully rested

and even be ecstatic about their therapy. In either situation, a follow-up call should be instructional, helpful, and full of encouragement. Follow-up calls should be made at intervals of approximately 1 to 2 days, 1 week, 2 weeks, 6 weeks, 6 months, and yearly. During the call, the patient should be asked about hours of usage, problems with the mask or pressure, equipment cleaning, nasal problems, and any continued presence of snoring or excessive daytime sleepiness. Sometimes, patients are hesitant to discuss certain issues such as bed partner complaints or embarrassment about using the equipment. Expressing empathy, respect, and support builds positive relationships with patients that facilitate education. It is helpful to be understanding, empathetic, and to listen to all the patient's concerns and problems at the beginning of the phone call and then give suggestions and solutions to those problems. Some patients need and want lots of help, whereas others want only the bare necessities. It takes an intuitive listener and educator to be able to fulfill the needs of all types of patients. Ultimately, better patient communication can increase both patient and clinician satisfaction, improve efficiency, enhance adherence to therapy, and improve patient health outcomes.

Personal Empowerment

Quality of life is contingent upon a patient's willingness to take responsibility for positive choices for better health and living. Patients need to believe in their ability to achieve and maintain effective therapy. Goal setting gives patients an incentive to aim for, increasing adherence on a nightly basis and over the long term. Personal empowerment aids in mastering the challenges of PAP therapy acceptance. Turning struggles and conflicts into learning opportunities is a way of providing positive feedback to the patient. It is important to encourage patients to become their own advocates for promoting good health, achieving their goals, and maximizing adherence to therapy.

Technology

Modern technology has provided various tools and options that may enhance adherence and increase breathing comfort for patients on PAP therapy. These may be used as augmentation measures for an adherent patient or to identify and assist a nonadherent patient to become adherent. PAP manufacturers have developed technology that provides relief on exhalation, making PAP therapy more comfortable.

Occasionally, there are patients who cannot tolerate PAP therapy, even when enhanced by this technology. When all avenues with standard PAP therapy have been exhausted, a physician-ordered bilevel positive airway pressure (BPAP) trial could be attempted. Patients who qualify for BPAP treatment are those who are at high surgical risk, have multiple medical problems in addition to sleep apnea, or require unusually high PAP levels to overcome their apnea. Rescue/trial BPAP is a final attempt to achieve successful therapy. The BPAP settings may be determined from the patient's current CPAP or a separate BPAP titration study.

In clinical practice, it is important to measure, assist, track, and enhance adherence. Various manufacturers have created tools that assist patients, sleep technologists, physicians, and home health care providers with feedback or efficacy data to determine effective therapy and to measure outcomes. Compliance meters and data-card tracking devices can be very useful in measuring PAP adherence. Judging one's sleep time is always subjective and generally inaccurate. Patients tend to either underestimate or overestimate the amount of time they spend using PAP therapy. A data tracking system provides accurate information when addressing an adherence issue. When tracking adherence, it is important to first inform patients about the capabilities of the device and then instruct them on how to use it for their situation.

Patients can react negatively to data tracking if they perceive it as negative feedback from the clinician. An example is the patient who feels that he or she is using the PAP device all night, every night. Then, upon reviewing the data download, the usage is recorded as poor. Perhaps the patient is unknowingly removing the PAP mask early in the night while believing it is near morning when this occurs. If adherence feedback is perceived as a reprimand or therapy failure, usage may actually reduce. Consequently, care should be taken not to discourage the patient, but to help solve the problem and offer a solution. In contrast, some patients believe that they have not been using their machine as much as expected, although the data download confirms adequate use. In these cases, the patients can be reassured about their accomplishments and praised for their efforts.

Most PAP machines now have "true" adherence monitors that measure the actual time during which patients are breathing with the device in place. A simple hour meter that records only the running time of the machine is not useful for determining or enhancing adherence. Data storage and retrieval technology is available from several PAP system manufacturers. For example, PAP machine manufacturers have developed technology that tracks usage hours, pressure, mask leak, and apnea–hypopnea index on selected machines. Detailed reports can be generated to share information with the patient's health care team.

Some devices provide the ability for the patient to track usage when the feature is enabled. Information for monitoring adherence is also available through wireless modules used with PAP devices within the home environment. The wireless module transmits therapy data from the device to a centralized server for access by the sleep professional through the Internet and provides the sleep professional with timely, objective data for assessing the patient's adherence to therapy.

Questionnaires

Questionnaires and rating scales can be useful for measuring a patient's transition from diagnosis to treatment and for tracking long-term results. Baseline information should be collected before the initial sleep study. Subsequent questionnaires and rating scales can then be used during follow-up visits to determine how much symptomatic improvement the patient is experiencing.

The Functional Outcomes of Sleep Questionnaire is a clinically validated, self-reporting measurement developed by Terri Weaver designed to assess the improvement of excessive sleepiness on the basis of multiple activities of daily living. This 30-item questionnaire, intended specifically for people with sleep disorders, allows sleep professionals to follow improvements in the patient's quality of life after treatment.

The Epworth Sleepiness Scale (ESS) is a very simple, self-administered questionnaire, used to assess a patient's own perception of sleepiness. The ESS was developed by Murray Johns, MD, from the Epworth Hospital in Melbourne, Australia. This questionnaire helps sleep professionals to recognize and measure excessive daytime sleepiness. Again, it is preferred that the ESS be completed before a sleep study and then repeated at subsequent clinical visits to measure improvement.

Education/Support Meetings

People with sleep disorders often report being labeled as lazy, depressed, or even as hypochondriacs. They are offered little sympathy about their tiredness. Many have been to doctors and complained of being tired "for years" to no avail. Having a diagnosis and a way to treat their disorder can be very empowering for them. Support groups can alleviate the feeling of isolation and provide emotional support and understanding between patients and their families. This also opens the door for discussion and validation of their treatment with bed partners and other family members. Promoting communication and positive support, a sleep technologist can bridge the gap between patients and their families.

Assisting patients to integrate into the network of PAP education and support groups is suggested. Keeping in contact with sleep professionals and networking with other PAP users can help patients maintain their long-term commitment to treatment. One such group is the A.W.A.K.E. (alert, well, and keeping energetic) network developed by Lucy Seger, RPSGT.

PAP Information Line

A dedicated toll-free telephone information line for patients with PAP questions can be a very helpful tool.

First and foremost, the phone line gives patients a lifeline to PAP educators and reassurance that help is available to them with their therapy. Knowing that there are professionals staffing the phone line is therapeutic in itself. Sometimes a patient will have questions; at other times simple reassurance or a pat on the back may be all that is needed. The phone line may also minimize calls to the sleep center, physician's office, and the medical equipment provider.

Messages should be checked frequently and calls returned in a timely manner, because patients who need help will get discouraged after a short period of time and adherence will reduce. Providing a toll-free number gives the traveling patient, or the patient who lives elsewhere during a part of the year, a familiar resource to access.

Behavioral Change and Sleep Hygiene

Behavioral change is an important part of beginning any new therapy. Beginning PAP therapy can force changing a treasured or habitual lifestyle. Patients may perceive this change as an intrusion on bedtime and morning routines. Some of the required changes include washing the mask and humidifier in the morning, filling the humidifier chamber with distilled water, and washing their face before bed to remove makeup and oils from the skin to promote a good mask seal. Patients may also have to adjust to the emotional aspect of using a medical device such as a PAP machine in their home. These changes, although minor, may seem insurmountable to the patients. The patients should be reminded that these additional changes to their daily/nightly routine will help reduce skin irritation and prevent premature breakdown of the mask and equipment.

Patients should also be informed of the risks of using alcohol, tobacco, and sleeping pills before bedtime. These may increase upper airway instability during sleep and should be avoided. Finally, encouraging weight loss is important to promote better health and to possibly reduce the necessary PAP level. In some cases, considerable weight loss may even eliminate the need for PAP therapy. A repeat sleep study should be recommended after considerable weight loss, such as from bariatric surgery. Change is difficult for most people. However, implementing good sleep hygiene techniques along with PAP therapy can improve a patient's and bed partner's sleep. Most compliant patients will agree that the benefits of PAP therapy outweigh its inconveniences.

Techniques for promoting good sleep:

- Maintain a regular sleep schedule.
- Implement a bedtime routine.
- Use your bedroom for sleep and intimacy only.
- Go to bed only when drowsy.
- If you are unable to fall asleep, leave the bedroom and do something quiet in another room.

- Avoid clock watching.
- Perform a repetitious activity or something to distract your mind.
- Avoid caffeine 2 to 4 hours before bedtime.
- Avoid nicotine close to bedtime.
- Avoid alcohol 2 to 4 hours before bedtime.
- Avoid large meals before bedtime.
- Avoid strenuous exercise 4 or more hours before bedtime.
- Limit napping during the day, and do not nap after 3 p.m.
- Minimize light, noise, television, and radio use in the bedroom.

Potential Problems, Setbacks, and Solutions
Initial Mask Fit

The initial mask fit for a patient is one of the most important tasks a technologist will undertake. Remaining cheerful and enthusiastic helps the initial mask fit begin on a positive note. It is imperative that a poor fit not dampen the patient's enthusiasm to using PAP at a later date.

Problem:
The patient's mask does not fit well. It may leak, cause sore spots, or hurt the face.

Solution:
- Adjust mask/interface straps, forehead pads, or nasal cushions.
- Do not overtighten the mask.
- Refit with a different mask or nasal pillow.
- Refit mask to a different size.
- If all else fails, a full-face mask trial may be attempted. Because of safety issues (possible aspiration) and potential leak problems, a full-face mask should be used only as a last resort, with physician approval.

Adapting to Pressure Complaints

Problem:
The patient complains of too much air, too high a pressure, difficulty exhaling, or that the air is coming too fast.

Solution:
- Verify correct PAP setting using a manometer (significant discrepancies may be present among various PAP equipment pressure readouts).
- Instruct the patient to exhale while initially applying mask to face.
- Initiate relaxation skills and desensitization techniques.
- Use ramp or delay features.

- Increase ramp or delay time.
- Add cool or heated humidifier (this requires a written prescription from the patient's physician).
- Use pressure relief technology to enhance patient comfort.
- Consider an ENT (ear, nose, and throat) consultation to check for possible nasal obstruction (this option would be determined by the patient's physician).

Claustrophobia

Problem:
The patient complains of not being able to breathe, not being able to exhale, or having a sense of suffocation.

Solution:
- Ask the patient to hold the mask to face without air pressure while he or she sits on the edge of the bed and provides distractions such as television, music, or conversation.
- Start with a very low pressure or ramp.
- Instruct the patient to exhale into the mask as soon as he or she feels the pressure and then slowly inhale through the nose.
- Try alternate mask styles to aid in patient comfort.
- Apply the headgear once the patient is comfortable.
- Instruct the patient to lie down with the mask on.
- Instruct the patient to gradually increase usage time with each attempt.

Noise Complaints

Problem:
The machine is too loud!

Solution:

- Recommend that the patient and/or bed partner wear earplugs.
- Use a white noise machine (a device that produces continuous background sounds, such as ocean waves).

Air Hunger Complaints

Problem:
The patient states that he or she cannot get enough air or feels as if suffocating.

Solution:
- Check for mask/interface leak.
- If using a ramp feature, increase the starting pressure.

- Mouth opening with PAP while awake does not necessarily indicate a need for a chin strap—this is necessary only when mouth opening occurs during sleep.
- If using an autoPAP machine, increase the starting pressure (this requires verbal or written approval from the patient's physician).
- Consider an ENT consultation for surgical options (as determined by the patient's physician).

Removing PAP Unknowingly during Sleep

Problem:
The patient wakes up to find the mask off and does not remember removing it.

Solution:
- Check the efficacy data (if available) to determine actual PAP usage.
- Review desensitization techniques to make sure the patient is comfortable with wearing the mask.
- Check for proper mask fit (for same reason as above).
- Ask the patient if he or she suffers from nasal congestion. This could be a possible cause for mask removal and should be addressed with the patient's physician.
- Avoid using a chin strap, because using a chin strap is unlikely to prevent the patient from removing the mask.
- Activate the disconnect alarm (if available).
- Encourage the patient to keep trying. Sometimes, the mask is removed inadvertently during deep sleep. As the patient's sleep patterns normalize and the patient becomes accustomed to the treatment, the problem may resolve on its own.
- Avoid using a full-face mask, because using a full-face mask does not preclude the patient from removing it during sleep. Full-face masks are more susceptible to leaks and may pose a potential aspiration hazard.

Mask Leak

Problem:
Air leakage around the mask interface

Solution:
- Make sure the patient is not overtightening the mask.
- Adjust mask/interface straps, forehead pads, or nasal cushions for proper fit.
- Refit to a different mask or nasal pillows.
- Refit mask to a different size.
- Apply mask to the face while air is blowing through the circuit to help seal the mask on contact.

Mouth Breathing

Mouth opening during sleep may cause significant pressure drops, leading to a resumption of obstructive breathing, as well as mouth dryness and discomfort. Instruct the patient to try to keep the mouth closed when applying the PAP mask. If the PAP level is properly set for the patient, in most cases, the mouth will remain closed during sleep. A common cause for mouth breathing may be unresolved nasal congestion or obstruction. Problems with mouth breathing may also be seen in elderly patients, in patients who wear dentures, and in those with a history of stroke. Mouth breathing may also be an indication of inadequate titration, with pressures set either too high or too low.

Strategies to combat mouth breathing during sleep include the following:

- Verifying correct PAP level using a manometer
- Using a heated humidifier (to reduce nasal congestion)
- Increasing the temperature of the humidifier
- Using a chin strap
- Using a pressure relief technology to reduce pressure upon exhalation
- Using a full-face mask (this should be used only as a last resort, with physician approval)
- Addressing any unresolved problems (such as nasal obstruction) with the patient's physician

Eye Discomfort

Problem:
The patient reports that his or her eyes feel dry, air is blowing into the eyes, or the eyes are bloodshot.

Solution:
- Make sure the patient is not overtightening the mask.
- Adjust mask/interface, forehead pads, or nasal cushions.
- Refit to a different mask or nasal pillow.
- Refit mask and change to a different size.
- Advise the patient to consult the physician if the problem remains unresolved.

Skin Irritation

Problem:
The patient develops an unremitting rash, pressure sore, or skin irritation at the mask contact points.

Solution:
- Make sure the patient is not overtightening the mask.
- Check for proper mask fit.

- Refit to a different mask or nasal pillow.
- Review proper mask cleaning techniques with the patient.
- Remind the patient to clean the mask daily.
- Advise the patient to consult the physician about any unresolved skin problems.

Complaints of Feeling Tired/Fatigued

Problem:
The patient reports using the PAP on a regular basis but continues to complain of sleepiness or fatigue.

Solution:
- Reassess the patient's sleep–wake habits to make sure he or she has adequate sleep time.
- Ask if the patient has been snoring on PAP.
- Check for proper mask fit and the condition of the mask to make sure it is not leaking.
- Reassess the patient's sleep hygiene.
- Reassess PAP usage during the entire night.
- Evaluate possible environmental factors such as noise.
- Ask about bed partner or pet disturbances in the bedroom.
- Ask if the patient is taking naps during the day.
- Ask about leg movements or bruxism.
- Inquire if the patient is using alcohol before bed.
- Ask about mouth opening during the night and/or a very dry mouth.
- Advise the patient to consult the physician if the problem is unresolved.

Communication with Family Members

Although PAP therapy mostly affects the patient, it can also have a great impact on other family members. Patients and their families may lack open communication. Having the patient and family members learn together about sleep-disordered breathing and PAP therapy can help bridge that communication gap. If a patient or family member makes negative comments about sleep-disordered breathing or PAP therapy, it is important to acknowledge the comment and then to counter the negativity with a positive aspect that PAP therapy has brought to that patient and family. Bringing the focus back to a positive note should be a recurring theme. Never underestimate the power of encouragement from family members. Remember, often it is a family member or bed partner who encouraged the patient to seek medical attention in the first place. Family and bed partner support after diagnosis is just as important as before diagnosis. Patients with families who are supportive and aware of the benefits of PAP therapy often use their PAP more consistently.

Bed Partners

Adjustment periods are not exclusive to the PAP patient. The patient's entire household will need time to adjust to PAP therapy, bed partners more so than other family members. Bed partners, as well as patients, may feel therapy is an intrusion on a cherished bedtime routine. Also, bed partners may need time to adjust to a medical device in the bedroom. A common complaint from bed partners is noise from the device. This noise is produced either by the blower or by the air exchange through the mask ventilation port. The noise is actually very minimal, but to a sensitive sleeper, or a bed partner who is just returning to the bedroom, it may seem loud. A good solution for noise intrusion is the use of earplugs or using a white noise machine. In other cases, the bed partner may actually complain that the patient is now too quiet without the familiar sound of snoring (although this is unusual, most bed partners welcome the change from loud, obnoxious snoring). Another common complaint is of air blowing toward the bed partner from the exhalation port. Using a blanket or pillow as a barrier between the patient and the bed partner can help deflect the flow of air. Occasionally, there is a complaint that the machine indicator light is too luminous in the bedroom. This light can disturb the patient and the bed partner. On some PAP machines, the light can be turned off; on others, the light remains on for a short time and then turns off automatically. If the light does not turn off automatically, then covering the light with electrical tape will eliminate the brightness. Always caution patients not to cover the entire PAP unit because that would interfere with its function and present a potential hazard.

When patients are better rested and the routine of PAP therapy has been established, sometimes there is a reversal of complaints. Now it is the patient who complains about the bed partner's snoring or movements. The dynamics between a patient and a bed partner can fluctuate throughout this transition period.

Equipment Cleaning

Daily:
- Emphasize daily mask cleaning.
- Caution the patient about the risks of skin irritation or infection due to poor mask fit or from using a dirty mask.
- Clean the mask and tubing as per the manufacturer's directions.
- Clean the mask in the morning with warm, mild soapy water, rinse well, and allow to air-dry.
- Do not use chemicals, soaps with perfume-like smells, or antibacterial soaps that can cause a breakdown of the mask cushions.
- Disinfect the mask and tubing with water and white vinegar mixture as per the manufacturer's directions.

Monthly:
- Clean filters more frequently if soiled or if pets sleep in the bedroom.
- Clean nondisposable filters with warm mild soapy water, rinse well, and allow to air-dry.
- Discard and replace paper filters monthly.

Humidifiers:
- Replace the distilled water daily.
- Clean in the morning with warm, mild, soapy water, rinse well, and allow to air-dry all day.
- Do not use chemicals or soaps with perfume-like smells.
- Clean and disinfect the humidifier with water and white vinegar mixture as per the manufacturer's directions.
- Use only distilled water in the humidifier. (Do not use tap water in the humidifier because it will result in mineral buildup in the water chamber.)

General Considerations
Travel

Travel requires advanced planning and leaving home well rested for the PAP patient. Optimal driving time is during the hours when alertness is at its peak. PAP patients are advised to avoid alcohol and sedating medications while traveling. Driving with a companion can help both the patient and the companion keep each other awake. It is recommended that when patients travel they bring their PAP along with them on their trip. Even after one night without wearing PAP, patients may feel tired and experience a return of symptoms and the risks associated with untreated sleep-disordered breathing. These risks, combined with sleepiness, may make a vacation or business trip unpleasant and potentially hazardous. PAP equipment should be packed in the passenger compartment to minimize temperature extremes. The PAP travel bag should include a heavy-duty extension cord for hard-to-reach outlets and an extra fuse if specific PAP equipment requires it. Voltage converters and wall receptacle adapters are available for traveling internationally. Additionally, an external power source and supplies will need to be packed if traveling where electricity is not available.

A PAP machine is a medical device and usually comes with its own travel or carrying bag. To make sure the PAP equipment does not become lost or damaged, it is recommended to carry it on a plane; never check it as baggage. The limit of one carry-on bag for airline travel does not usually apply to medical supplies or equipment. It is recommended to separately pack the equipment manual and a copy of the prescription and/or letter of medical necessity from the physician. This information will help travelers in the event that the PAP device is lost or broken and will assist them at airport checkpoints and customs.

Because of limited packing space, many patients may not be able to bring a humidifier while traveling. When using a humidifier while traveling, it is important to either carry distilled water to the destination or obtain distilled water upon arrival. A temporary alternative when the humidifier is not available is an over-the-counter normal saline nasal spray or gel. Also, a water-soluble gel to help with nasal dryness can be used; both of these products are available without a prescription.

When patients travel internationally, it is important that they learn about the voltage output and types of wall receptacles used in the countries they plan to visit. Most PAP machines adjust to international voltages, either manually through voltage converters or automatically. It is also important to bring the appropriate wall receptacle adapter(s) in order to be able to plug the unit in.

When traveling and changing altitudes, such as living at sea level and traveling to 5,000 ft (1,524 m), it may be necessary to adjust the PAP levels to adapt the equipment to atmospheric pressure changes. Increasing the pressure setting is required at elevations above 2,500 ft (762 m) to maintain treatment efficacy. If these modifications are not made, the patient may begin to snore and experience partial airway obstruction. Usually, the patient can make these adjustments with simple instructions from the PAP manual. Typically, adjustments for three levels are available. A low-level elevation is considered below 2,500 ft (762 m), a medium level is 2,500 to 5,000 ft (762 to 1,524 m), and a high-level elevation is greater than 5,000 ft (1,524 m) above sea level. Always remember to instruct the patient to reset the altitude when returning from high elevations. Many PAP machines now adjust automatically for altitude changes.

Many patients enjoy camping and boating, but traveling without a power source can be a challenge. Patients should be encouraged to investigate an appropriate alternate source of power for their device. Some patients may also want an alternate source of power in the event of a power outage. A battery backup system with an inverter or a 12-V cigarette lighter adapter can be used with most PAP machines. If using a humidifier, a pure sine wave inverter is recommended. Patients should refer to their manuals for specific instructions. It is important to note that using an unapproved electrical source could void any warranty and possibly damage PAP equipment.

Hospital Admissions and Surgery

If patients using PAP are scheduled to have surgery, they should be instructed to check with the hospital about being able to bring their PAP equipment with them to the hospital. Most medical facilities have a biomedical department that will inspect the PAP equipment

for electrical safety and cleanliness before allowing its use in the hospital. Nearly all PAP machines are double-insulated for electrical safety. Patients should be encouraged to share information about their sleep-disordered breathing and pressure requirements with the attending physician. Using PAP before and after surgery, or during a hospital stay, will ensure continuity of treatment and enhance the recovery process.

Logistical Challenges at Home

The placement of the PAP machine and tubing in a patient's bedroom is different in every home. The machine should be placed on a stable and safe surface, keeping at least 6 ft (1.8 m) away from a heat source, air conditioner, or room humidifier. Some patients place the machine on the bedside table and others place it near the floor. Tubing lengths of 6 to 12 ft (1.8 to 3.7 m) can be used with the circuit to facilitate movement in bed. Tubing lengths greater than 12 ft (3.7 m) are not recommended because of pressure drops within the circuit.

If the machine is near the floor, it is recommended that it be elevated at least 4 to 6 in (10.2 to 15.2 cm). If not, the machine could draw fibers and dust from the carpet and flooring, which could impede the air intake. It is also not recommended to place the PAP machine higher than the patient's head. There is a potential for condensation to accumulate in the tubing and flow back to the patient's face. Also, if the machine is above the patient's head, there is the risk of it falling and striking them. It is important to keep the machine air intake unobstructed and free from blockage that would impair its function. An example of this would be an item of clothing or a towel draped over the device.

Placement of the tubing should enhance the patient's movement in bed. This is a very individual choice. One option is to bring the tubing up between the mattress and the headboard, or up over the headboard, so it is centered behind the patient's head. Usually, two sections of tubing (12 ft [3.7 m]) are required for this placement. There are also a variety of holders and hooks available that support the tubing above the patient, connected to an extension arm that fits between the mattress and the box spring. These alternate placements reduce tension on the tubing and provide greater flexibility for unrestricted movement and body position changes during the night. Patients who try various placements are more likely to arrive at a satisfactory solution for their PAP situation than those who do not experiment.

PAP therapy can bring about unexpected challenges with pets that share a bedroom with the PAP user. Dogs and cats that sleep in the same bed as the PAP user may become mischievous or fearful of their owner because of the apparatus or the sound of the device. The exhalation port is a particularly intriguing or frightening aspect of the machine for some pets. Also, cats and dogs are curious about the equipment when it is not in use. The mask can be especially tempting because it smells like its owner. It is not uncommon to have a dog chew a face mask or a cat to chew through the PAP tubing.

OUTCOME ASSESSMENT

Assessing outcomes for effective patient education and PAP compliance will involve a comparative analysis to previously collected data. The sleep technologist will need to compare, deduce, examine, differentiate, and question all data collected over the course of the patient's care and training. A quality assurance program may be set up to track different aspects of the educational process. The program itself should also be evaluated. The program evaluation should be conducted with an awareness of the program's setting as well as the cost to maintain the program. Persons directly and indirectly related to the program should be reviewed as well. Because a program will need to operate within the department's budget, management will play a big role in the development as well as the operation of the program.

One to 3 Days

Long-term adherence to CPAP therapy can be predicted as early as 3 days after the initiation of CPAP therapy. The pattern of adherence to CPAP at 3 and 7 days strongly predicted longer-term (1 month) adherence. Eighty-four percent of those who used CPAP for more than 4 hours a day at day 3 used CPAP for an average of more than 4 hours a day at day 30 compared with only 26% of those who used CPAP for less than 4 hours a day at day 3 (3).

The most critical time during PAP initiation is the first 1 to 3 days. Patients may be tired, frustrated, hesitant, or even angry about the struggles with PAP therapy. Others may acclimate quickly and be fully rested and even ecstatic about their results. When patients are struggling with their treatment, it is important to be understanding and empathetic and to offer possible solutions for their problems. Remind them that even sleeping a small amount of time on PAP is a step in the right direction. Likewise, when patients are doing well, it is important to congratulate them on their success and encourage continued use of PAP. Remind all patients that they can call for help and reassurance and always reiterate the importance of any available educational opportunities and A.W.A.K.E. meetings.

Four Days to 8 Weeks

This period in PAP therapy is transitional. Patients who were initially successful with wearing PAP may express disappointment that they do not feel the exuberance

that they did in the first few days of therapy. These patients need to be told that this is a normal transition of PAP therapy called "the rebound effect." The rebound effect occurs when a patient who has been sleep-deprived because of sleep-disordered breathing uses PAP and catches up on lost slow-wave and rapid eye movement sleep. This rebound effect may cause the patient to feel much rested during the first 1 to 3 days; they may even feel euphoric. After the first few days, this effect tapers off and the patient returns to a normal sleep architecture.

Patients may also complain about waking up at night during this transition period. They are often not aware of the frequent arousals that occur during untreated sleep-disordered breathing. But after the elimination of the problem, nighttime awakenings may become bothersome. Patients need to be reassured that it is normal to awaken during the night while rolling over, adjusting blankets, or repositioning during the night. If awakenings happen frequently and the patient feels tired, then intervention is needed. If the patient is intolerant of PAP, has been working with the PAP educators, and has exhausted all suggestions, he or she should be instructed to return to the physician to discuss progress and other treatment options. For the patient who has adjusted to PAP therapy, once again, remind him or her that he or she can call for help and reassurance. Also reiterate the importance of any available educational opportunities and A.W.A.K.E. meetings.

Six Months

At 6 months, most PAP patients are quite confident with their therapy. Patients should be reminded that most insurance companies allow for a new mask every 6 months (the mask cushion should be replaced every 3 months; this is generally covered by insurance). Continue to remind the patients that they can call for help and reassurance and always reiterate the importance of any available educational opportunities and A.W.A.K.E. meetings.

One-Year and Long-Term Follow-Up

After 1 year, expect the PAP patient to be very confident with therapy. Many patients become very educated about sleep-disordered breathing and PAP during this time. Increases in available educational materials, Internet access, and the media have helped patients become more knowledgeable and compliant. Patients should be encouraged to continue their pursuit of knowledge about their disorder and remain updated in PAP technology. Again, remind the patient that most insurance companies will cover a new mask. The equipment company holds a long-term prescription for this purpose. Many physicians suggest that their patients schedule a follow-up with their sleep physician or their PCP at 1 to 2 years or as needed. Communications with patients at the 1-year mark offer the opportunity to reiterate support and provide informational resources such as educational opportunities and A.W.A.K.E. meetings.

Success with PAP therapy often requires a team effort from the patient, the physician, and the sleep technologist and/or sleep educator. The sleep professional's role cannot be underestimated in reassuring his or her patients that any effort to lengthen their use of PAP therapy will improve their chances of success. Comprehensive education, patient communication, feedback, application of desensitization strategies, and long-term follow-up will improve outcomes and result in improved quality of life for the sleep-disordered breathing patient.

CONCLUSION

Effective patient education and PAP adherence requires more than giving the patient information and having them recite it back to you. To be effective, patient education must be based on a well-developed educational program that takes into account all of the patient's needs. The educational program must be provided in a manner that facilitates the patient's ability to carry out

recommendations. Remember, communication in patient education is a two-way process. It is essential that the sleep technologist and the patient be able to communicate effectively. The sleep technologist must have the ability to recognize patient cues and respond accurately as well as to provide support and feedback. Such skills promote a sense of trust that helps maintain an open relationship with the patient. This is crucial if the sleep technologist hopes to elicit accurate information from the patient and identify any misconceptions or misunderstanding he or she may have (1).

REFERENCES

1. Falvo, D. R. (1994). *Effective patient education: A guide to increased compliance.* Gaithersburg, MD: Aspen.
2. Chokroverty, S. (1994). *Sleep disorders medicine: Basic science, technical considerations, and clinical aspects.* Stoneham, MA: Butterworth-Heinemann.
3. Kribs, N. B., Pack, A. I., Kline, L. R., et al. (1993). Objective measurement of patterns of nasal CPAP use by patients with obstructive sleep apnea. *American Review of Respiratory Disease, 147,* 887–895.
4. Arfoosh, R., & Rowley, J. A. (2010). Adherence to positive airway pressure therapy. *Sleep Medicine Clinics, 5(3),* 321–334.

chapter 57

At-Home Positive Airway Pressure Follow-Up: Therapy Assessment Tools, Interventions, and Equipment Maintenance

LAURA S. LEHNERT

LEARNING OBJECTIVES

On completion of this chapter, the reader should be able to:

1. Describe mask-fit process for home usage of interface.
2. Recognize side effects of positive airway pressure (PAP) and how to intervene once the patient is on PAP therapy.
3. Perform patient therapy assessment using auto-PAP report tools.
4. Maintain and replace equipment

KEY TERMS

Mask
PAP (positive airway pressure)
HSAT (home sleep apnea test)
Compliance
Acclimation
Wireless
Side effects
Assessment
Equipment
Residual apnea–hypopnea index (AHI)

Today's consumer-driven industry and access to information via the Internet, expectations of personalized and quick service, an increased number of people with health care coverage, efforts to contain health care costs, and demand to improve outcomes are all factors that have impacted the diagnosis, treatment, and management of sleep-disordered breathing. Patient education and mask-fitting evaluation once performed during laboratory polysomnography (PSG) can now be overlooked as home sleep apnea testing (HSAT) and treatment with auto-positive airway pressure (APAP) devices become more prevalent. Furthermore, even a single-night PSG titration may not determine optimal pressure or address long-term PAP compliance (adherence) issues (1). Collaboratively, clinical health care teams are assessing and managing patients remotely to provide education on pre-PAP treatment with post-PAP follow-up.

MASK-FIT PROCESS FOR HOME USE

There are several opportunities for mask education and fit assessment to occur: during a desensitization period before PSG, HSAT, or APAP test setup; during discussions of results of the study before ordering the PAP machine; or during PAP setup and follow-up PAP management encounters. Equipment manufacturers provide mask-fit kits with sizing gauges and, in some cases, multiple-size cushions. This prevents cross-contamination and provides patients the opportunity to size themselves at home. If issues arise, the manufacturers' 30-day mask-fit guarantee facilitates a change to a more suitable style following an assessment.

Mask procurement, however, can happen in various ways. Patients can order through the Internet, or possibly receive one from a friend or family member, or even pick one up at yard sale. The ideal situation is that patients have been assessed by a health care professional and recommended or given an appropriate mask option. When patients have made a decision as to which mask type they want before a clinical fitting or assessment, it is important to listen to reasons why they made the choice and then provide further education. Patients who have been educated on treatment intervention and the disease state have increased adherence than those who did not receive education and support (2).

Whether by phone or in person, review the patient history and determine physical attributes (facial hair, facial features), claustrophobia, airflow limitations (restrictive or obstructive lung disease, hypoventilation, rhinitis, or sinusitis), physical limitations, and mental or emotional issues. Try to observe the physical attributes rather than asking if patients are "mouth-breathers." Try to observe when the patient is unaware and in his or her natural state. Avoid giving the diagnosis. Observe or discuss if mouth breathing is situational or observable. Self-diagnosis by patients or by health professionals can lead to suboptimal mask choice, suboptimal pressures, and increased side effects and abandonment of therapy. Striving to achieve a positive experience within the first week on therapy can affect the patient's perception, side effects, and tolerance. An estimated 50% of patients do not use therapy a year later because of mask discomfort, nasal dryness/irritation, and intolerance of pressure. Predictors of patient adherence include the type of mask used (3–6). Pre- and post-PAP mask education should include a review of mask types and common side effects.

TYPES OF COMMONLY USED MASKS

There are a variety of masks and interfaces available to patients using PAP therapy. Each type of interface has pros and cons, and the interface selection should be personalized on the basis of the patient's individual needs.

1. **Nasal pillows (intranasal)**
   Pros: smallest footprint, offers easy application, addresses claustrophobia, and can be worn with facial hair.
   Cons: can contribute to flow limitations, may not fit well with those with small nostrils, may dislodge, may be worn upside down, may cause soreness in nostrils, may increase sinus issues, and may increase turbulence/leaks at pressures above 12 cm H_2O and difficulty exhaling.
2. **Nasal mask (nose only)**
   Pros: moderate footprint, moderate application, softer flow, ease of exhalation, stable, secure straps, less dryness, closer fit styles can be worn with facial hair, some with no forehead straps help address claustrophobia.
   Cons: some claustrophobia, increased pressure points, sinus issues, application issues, more straps.
3. **Full-face mask (oral–nasal)**
   Pros: occasionally addresses claustrophobia, option for observable mouth-breathers, unresolved mouth leaks, severe physical sinus obstruction.
   Cons: largest footprint, more straps, increase claustrophobia, higher pressure needs, higher leaks, increase oral–nasal dryness, less stable, requires tighter fit, noisy, limits sleeping positions, aerophagia and elevated residual apnea–hypopnea index (AHI), highest rate of abandonment.

SIDE EFFECTS OF MASK USAGE

Common side effects to therapy are pressure sores, aerophagia, dryness, sinusitis and rhinitis, headaches, irritated eyes, ear pain, mouth breathing, and claustrophobia.

The strategy to mitigate these side effects is the alignment of PAP with humidification and a properly fitting mask. Leaks are dependent on mask fit and pressure.

Common Mask Side Effects
Pressure sores
Aerophagia
Dryness
Sinusitis/rhinitis
Headaches
Irritated eyes
Ear pain
Mouth breathing
Claustrophobia

Mask leaking issues should be explored in conjunction with reviewing pressure and humidification. If PAP is suboptimal, it can cause intolerance, mouth venting, destabilize the mask fit, cause leaks, increase dryness, headaches, ear pain, and aerophagia. If humidification is suboptimal, it can lead to headaches, nasal constriction/inflammation leading to a high-pressure response, patients reporting not receiving enough air, and mouth venting (7, 8). If mask fit is suboptimal, it can result in excessive mask leak, eye irritation, erratic machine pressure detection and response, patient discomfort, and increased dryness. This negative feedback loop can lead to artifact and inaccurate results that can cause multiple mask changes, misdiagnosis of complex breathing, suboptimal pressure changes, ongoing side effects, and poor compliance.

Aerophagia can occur because of therapy intolerance whether the patient is getting too much air or feeling as though he or she is struggling to get sufficient air (9). Patients may report complaints of excessive burping, choking, chest pain, stomach pain, and inability to get air in or out, and may exhibit higher leaks. This is associated more often with full-face mask, PAP intolerance, pressures too high or too low, and the acclimation period.

Pressure sores are a result of a poor-fitting mask or overly tightened mask in an attempt to maintain a good seal. Corrected leaks (to satisfy leak data) should not impact patient comfort or tolerance of therapy. Having to wear a mask extremely tight to maintain a seal can result in sores on the neck, head, or face, limitation in sleep positions, and frequent disruption of sleep. An alternate mask should be tried first.

A full-face mask used with a chinstrap to hold down the mask should be avoided. It is best to try to identify the source of the issue. Avoid oversaturating the patient with air. This can result in frequent use of ramping to decrease pressure, increased arousals and awakenings, poor sleep continuity, low PAP usage, and discomfort. The goal is to improve sleep and compliance with a "less is best" approach to mask type for long-term comfort. Nasal mask types should be recommended as first option because full-face masks have the highest negative impact with lowest adherence (10, 11). Mouth breathing can be a result of untreated or undertreated sleep apnea, overtreated sleep apnea, and sinus flow limitations. Given time, mouth venting often will reduce with effective pressure and humidification. Strive for the lowest optimal level of PAP to correct sleep-disordered breathing while improving sleep continuity, reducing sleep disruptions, and mitigating side effects. Nasopharyngeal problems are frequently found in patients with obstructive sleep apnea syndrome before starting treatment, with a tendency to increase with treatment (12). However, with regular PAP use, nasal inflammation and infection can revert (13).

Claustrophobia can be associated with larger mask profiles, full-face masks, headgear, and intolerance to PAP. Complaints may occur with pillow masks or nasal masks that constrict sinus airflow. It is important that time and effort are spent to ensure comfort during the initial phase of treatment and to develop strategies for ongoing success (14). Consider all available avenues of patient support and education: literature, Internet educational tools, video demonstrations, phone and remote support, automated feedback apps, and/or clinic visits.

INTERVENTIONS AND TOOLS TO SUPPORT HOME PAP USE AND FOLLOW-UP

When patients are at home using therapy, they have ability to track their PAP usage either by cloud-based technology or data displayed on their machine. This access allows patients to be engaged in their therapy and monitor progress. Although patients are given user manuals and provided education during PAP setup, frequently they will have questions later about comfort, function, and management.

Many health care teams are providing clinical, phone, and virtual support during follow-up including a discussion of PAP usage information. Current advances in technology allow for PAP data results to be accessed wirelessly and by data card download if needed. This allows the clinician to review the data reports while communicating with the patient and quickly provide feedback, address issues, suggest changes, titrate pressures, and follow-up on improvements. Team-based clinical protocols will allow timely intervention and better patient management when managing high patient volumes.

PAP Reports

PAP reports provide useful tools for patient therapy assessment. The reports are broken into various categories, depending on the manufacturer. Each subset of the report offers benefit to evaluate overall therapy success and these reports should be used in tandem. However, when artifacts (leaks, flow limitations) are introduced, the data may be unreliable because the machine may not accurately determine the event (10). Ninety percent or 95% pressure may not be an accurate representation of patient need at these settings and may lead to overtitration, which can further exacerbate side effects. The sleep team will need to use critical thinking to address these situations within set protocols, which should be periodically reviewed for best strategies to assist patients with adherence to therapy.

Subsets of the PAP report demonstrate that various parameters can provide information regarding the effectiveness of PAP therapy for the patient and point toward issues that may need to be addressed.

Usage and compliance data reports provide a quick graphic view of days and hours of usage. This is useful in identifying gaps, patterns, and fragmentation (see Fig. 57-1).

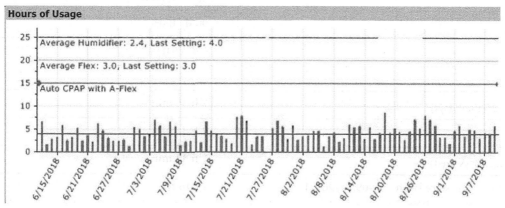

Figure 57-1 Graphs can be used as a quick view of assessment of adherence to therapy. Graph depicts hours of therapy use over a period of 90 days. CPAP, continuous positive airway pressure.

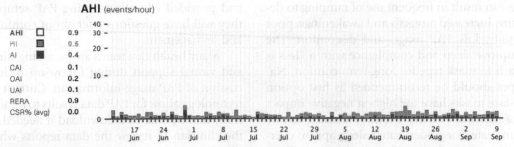

Figure 57-2 Graph depicts apnea–hypopnea index (AHI) on positive airway pressure therapy over a period of 90 days.
AI, apnea index; CAI, central apnea index; CSR, Cheyne Stokes Respiration; HI, hypopnea index; OAI, obstructive apnea index; RERA, respiratory event related arousal; UAI, unclassified apnea index.

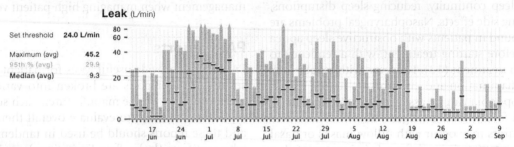

Figure 57-3 Graph depicts leak on positive airway pressure therapy over a period of 90 days and corresponds to the apnea–hypopnea index graph in Figure 57-2.

The trends, patterns of use data therapy report consists of histograms that show multiple parameters such as AHI (see Fig. 57-2), leak (see Fig. 57-3), and pressure (see Fig. 57-4) within the selected time frame. This is useful in tracking patterns of improvement in all measures over time (i.e., tracking leaks and AHI against pressure adjustments, pressure or leaks with mask change).

The detailed report and daily data report shows a single-night timeline of use that is helpful in assessing what precedes sleep disruptions and the frequency of disruptions, ramp use, fragmentation, pressure variations, and leak patterns.

The compliance report and summary data report provides an overall summary of use, leaks, mean or median pressure, 90% or 95% pressure, heat/humidity settings, comfort setting, and compliance criteria (see Figure 57-4).

Compliance or summary reports with a histogram and daily detail reports can also be of great benefit.

Listening to Patient Feedback and Adjusting Treatment Plan

It is important to first listen to patients' feedback and then to hear or identify issues related to data downloads

Usage	06/12/2018–09/09/2018
Usage days	90/90 d (100%)
≥4 h	90 d (100%)
<4 h	0 d (0%)
Usage hours	687 h 21 min
Average usage (total days)	7 h 38 min
Average usage (days used)	7 h 38 min
Median usage (days used)	7 h 33 min
Total used hours (value since last reset—09/09/2018)	1,646 h

Figure 57-4 An example of a 90-day compliance report showing hours of use and average therapy use over the 90-day period.

as they align with their feedback. If the patient is doing well, congratulate and share in the excitement. If they are struggling, then collaborate with the patients and the sleep team to determine the best improvement strategies. Using wireless access to the PAP device, staff will be able to adjust and follow-up quickly as soon as the next day.

TROUBLESHOOTING STRATEGIES

The most common problems and side effects of PAP therapy are related to the interface, to the PAP machine components, or to effects of issues related to these facets of therapy. Patients on PAP therapy often need assistance with equipment as well as education to be successful with therapy. Every visit offers an opportunity to review adherence data and discuss any difficulties the patient may be experiencing. Understanding the download report and utilizing it to assist the patient is essential. Sharing results with the patient and working with him or her to alleviate any issues discovered can make the difference between an adherent patient and a nonadherent patient.

The following are strategies to address common problems or side effects.

Sinus Issues/Dry Mouth

- Adjust humidification by adjusting either temperature or humidity.
- Consider changing mask type or size.
- Recommend heated tubing system, saline irrigation, sinus sprays, tubing covers, use of humidifier preheat function.
- Assess if pressure appears to reach maximum quickly, if so increase ramp time.
- If using nasal pillows, consider a different size or type or switch to a mask interface.
- Review daily detailed reports and trend usage data.

Water in Tubing

- Use a heated tubing system, tube covers.
- Move PAP device away from direct sources of cold air and/or place tubing under covers.
- Keep tubing lower than the bed.
- Adjust tube temperature up or humidity down or use auto-humidification settings.

Tangling in Tubing/Equipment When Turning

- May benefit from head of the bed-mounted tube holders

Skin Irritation or Breakdown

- If the patient is wearing mask too tight, ask the reason for this. May need to adjust pressure and/or perform a mask refit
- To help healing, may need antibiotic or barrier cream, protective pads (gel or cloth), and a new cushion

Not Enough Air

- Check if airflow is impeded in the beginning of or during the night and if it appears to be related to sinus issues, obstructive events, or lung issues.
- Consider ramp or pressure adjustments, check mask type, check for restricted airflow, and use humidifier prewarm feature and humidity adjustments. If adjustments and time do not resolve the issues, the patient may need a mask refitting with continuous positive airway pressure (CPAP)/bilevel positive airway pressure (BiPAP) desensitization.
- Review trend and daily reports.

Too Much Air/Choking Sensation

- Adjust max pressure down, add or adjust ramp, check leaks, if on full-face mask, consider change to a nasal interface. If adjustments and time do not resolve, may need mask fitting with CPAP/BPAP desensitization.
- Review trend and daily reports.

Mouth Breathing

- Review frequency and leak value.
- Check sinus flow limitations, mask type, and pressure. May need acclimation time, increased or decreased pressure, or change in ramp pressure; increase humidification and use prewarm feature.
- If adjustments and time do not resolve, may need mask fitting with CPAP/BPAP desensitization.
- Review trend and daily reports.

Mask Shifting/Leaks

- Check the reason behind the mask not staying in place and where it is leaking.
- Check for proper mask application, tightness of fit, intolerance to PAP, maintenance and replacement needs, and whether the patient is using oxygen in line (attached to mask).

- Recommend different-size cushions or headgear, headgear clips, tube holders, and an oxygen port distal to the mask to prevent drag.
- A mask refit with possible desensitization may be necessary.

Residual AHI Elevated

- Identify the source of issue (acclimation period, periodic breathing, discomfort).
- Check for high-pressure variability, appropriateness of high or low PAP settings, comfort issues, or unstable mask.
- Review comorbid issues, rule out full-face mask effect (elevated residual AHI, leaks, high pressure, dry mouth, fragmented sleep). Adjust and closely follow.
- Refer to all data reports during the assessment. Follow trend data to monitor the results of changes made.
- If central apneas appear, allowing a couple of weeks of therapy and an acclimation period may allow resolution; monitor to determine if trending toward improvement.
- During therapy follow-up, if resolution is not achievable through virtual means, then a mask fitting or desensitization session is recommended. Be sure to have the patients bring their PAP equipment and mask with them for a full assessment of the equipment and an educational support session.

MASK FITTING/DESENSITIZATION

Mask fitting and sometimes desensitization may be necessary for patients who are having difficulty acclimating to PAP therapy. Finding the right PAP interface and using desensitization, a behavioral technique commonly used to treat fear and anxiety, may improve a reluctant patient's ability to adapt to therapy. Desensitization should be performed while the patient is lying quietly in a dimly lighted room and gradually exposed to the PAP interface and PAP. Assuring the patients that they are in control and allowing them to manage the PAP interface during the desensitization process are frequently successful techniques.

During the mask fitting, the sleep technologist should do the following:

- Observe the patient's breathing pattern and natural effort using the nose or mouth.
- Listen for sinus flow and discuss comfort issues.
- Listen to patient complaints and concerns.
- Share download reports and discuss corrective measures to address any issues.

Optimally, desensitization should be accomplished with the patient in a reclining position or lying down. Discuss any anxieties that might prevent certain mask options and provide education on the pros and cons of various interface options. Ask patients if they are open or willing to try an alternate mask and the plan to assist them to succeed with therapy. The following is a step-by-step guideline for the desensitization process:

- First ask the patient to apply his or her mask and observe. Determine if it is incorrectly placed, then test the mask fit with pressure applied.
- Adjust mask fit or consider an alternate mask.
- Do not initiate testing pressure at 90% or 95% especially if switching from a full-face to a nasal mask or in the presence of leaks or pressure intolerance. Pressure needs with nasal mask are often less, and high pressure can cause mouth leaks if pressure is not adjusted down. This can also hinder a mask change and result in a misdiagnosis of mouth breathing.
- If baseline AHI is mild to moderate, consider starting pressure at 4 cm H_2O or to patient comfort.
- If baseline AHI is severe, consider starting pressure at 6 cm H_2O or to patient comfort.
- Assess airflow restrictions exacerbated by physical hindrance from the mask. Check comfort, assess pressure points. If possible, test in multiple laying positions for stability of fit.
- Start pressure low or to comfort with gradual stair stepping of pressure increases until a "breaking" point is reached. If indicated, switch to BPAP and repeat. BPAP also offers comfort-setting adjustments for normal, restrictive, and obstructive lung conditions. Do not start BPAP at the highest ending CPAP level. Mouth breathing can occur if pressure is too low, too high, restrictive, or in an inappropriate modality. This process will provide an estimate of patient tolerance threshold.
- Recommend mask type and pressure adjustments and follow-up with data downloads.
- Encourage the patient to set usage goals and provide conditioning techniques to help him or her acclimate to therapy.

EQUIPMENT MAINTENANCE, CLEANING, AND MANAGEMENT

Patients may be overwhelmed with maintaining and cleaning PAP equipment. It can cause inconvenience or worry and lead to avoidance of use. There are various recommendations provided by manufacturers, durable medical equipment (DME) personnel, clinical teams, and on the Internet. Each patient's circumstance should be taken into consideration as to what procedures will work best for them; if they don't wish to clean equipment on a routine basis, they may have to replace supplies more often to prevent Infections and assure good fit.

Organisms such as fungus, yeast, and mold grow in warm, dark, moist environments, which could potentially cause irritation in the lungs. Although there haven't been scientific reports of direct association with upper respiratory infection or pneumonia, patients should be cautious. To avoid cross-contamination, do not share equipment (15).

Humidification makes PAP therapy far more comfortable, but humidifier chambers can be a source of infection. Good hygiene can reduce the risk of sinus inflammation and infection. The use of distilled water is recommended; however, if using tap or filtered water, look for signs of calcification (chalky white appearance), which can pit the water chamber and trap bacteria. Do not leave water in the humidifier for prolonged periods of time and avoid topping it off. Some current devices will, once the machine is turned off, allow for low amounts of airflow in the system to dry out the tubing. When traveling, or when storing PAP equipment, be sure the water chamber is dry.

Filters have been shown to reduce the spread of bacteria within the device. They protect both the patient and the function of the machine. If the intake is occluded, it can cause increased device noise. Do not let the air inlet become obstructed.

Masks tend to collect mucous and oils and shape may shift, which can contribute to overtightening, skin irritation, or leaks. *Headgear* can become overstretched, disconnect too easily, and become dirty. *Tubing* can become warped and punctured or harbor bacteria. Masks may dislodge if they are overstretched or defective. Wires in a heated tubing system can break, which cause it to register as a standard hose when connected to PAP device.

Supplies for cleaning: Use wipes, dish soap water, vinegar and water, a soft cloth or towel, and a sink or basin. Avoid the use of alcohol, lanolin, or perfumes. Clean the outside of the machine, filters, and the hose, mask, and humidifier chamber. Refer to manufacturer recommendations for cleaning found online or in the equipment manual.

Daily: Wipe or wash the mask cushion to remove oil buildup, which will cause skin irritation. Pour out any remaining water in the humidifier chamber and let it air-dry. Allow tubing to dry out.

Weekly: Unplug the PAP machine from power and wipe the outside of the machine. Disconnect the mask, headgear, tubing, and water chamber. Soak these for 20 to 30 minutes in a basin with warm water and dish soap soak and wash each item. Black foam filters can be washed (do not oversqueeze to dry because this can cause the fibers to compress and obstruct the PAP intake). Some water chambers are dishwasher safe. Allow all parts to dry before reassembly.

Occasionally sanitize: Cleanse the unit with a solution of vinegar and water (vinegar:water ratio of 1:1 to 1:3). Replace or clean equipment more frequently during an infection. *Sanitizing devices* claim to disinfect by using ultraviolet light or activated oxygen. Some hook up directly to the PAP machine but require specific adapters. This is typically an out-of-pocket cost but may be covered by health savings accounts.

RESUPPLY: CENTER FOR MEDICARE AND MEDICAID GUIDELINES

PAP resupply is important. Masks, filters, tubing, and PAP machines wear out and need replacement. The DME supplier and provider should ensure that the patient understands the need for replacement equipment and the approximate resupply schedule. The Centers for Medicare and Medicaid (CMS) provides resupply guidelines in National Coverage Determination (NCD) and Local Coverage Determination (LCD) documents. Insurers also provide guidelines for resupply for their participants.

Note that CMS and most insurers require the supplier to contact the patient before providing replacement PAP supplies, even if they have received a physician order for resupply. Table 57-1 shows a typical resupply schedule for various supplies used for PAP therapy. Table 57-2 provides a sample Medicare coverage resupply schedule with current procedural terminology coding. The technologist must be aware of resupply requirements in order to appropriately care for the patient and assist with PAP adherence issues. It is important to note that the LCD always takes precedence over the NCD guidelines and that each facility or DME supplier must review and follow the guidelines in place for their jurisdiction. Commercial insurers may have specific guidelines that differ from the CMS guidelines; therefore, it is important to review insurer requirements for patients with commercial insurance.

Table 57-1 A Typical Resupply Schedule for PAP Equipment

Quick View Supply Schedule

Monthly	3 mo	6 mo
Cushions	Mask frame	Headgear
Disposable filters	Tubing	Chinstrap
		Nondisposable filter
		Water chamber

Table 57-2 Medicare Coverage Guidelines for Replacement Sleep Supplies (16)

Heated tubing	1/3 mo	A4604
Combo oral/nasal interface	1/3 mo	A7027
Oral cushion for oral/nasal combo	2/1 mo	A7028
Nasal pillow for oral/nasal combo	2/1 mo	A7029
Full-face mask interface	1/3 mo	A7030
Full-face mask cushion	1/1 mo	A7031
Nasal interface (mask or pillow type)	1/3 mo	A7034
Nasal cushion	2/1 mo	A7032
Pillow cushion	2/1 mo	A7033
Headgear	1/6 mo	A7035
Chinstrap	1/6 mo	A7036
Standard heated tubing	1/3 mo	A7037
Filter, disposable	2/1 mo	A7038
Filter, nondisposable	1/6 mo	A7039
Water chamber	1/6 mo	A7046

CMS Local Coverage Determination. *Positive Airway Pressure (PAP) Devices for the Treatment of Obstructive Sleep Apnea (L33718)*. Retrieved from https://www.cms.gov/medicare-coverage-database/details/lcd-details.aspx?LCDId=33718&ContrID=140. Accessed September 9, 2018.

REFERENCES

1. Berry, R. B., Parish, J. M., & Hartse, K. M. (2002). The use of auto-titrating continuous positive airway pressure for treatment of adult obstructive sleep apnea. *Sleep*, 25(2), 148–158.
2. American Association of Sleep Technologists. (2012). Sleep technology: Technical guideline. Positive airway pressure acclimation and desensitization. Retrieved from https://www.aastweb.org/hubfs/Technical%20Guidelines/Updated%206.14.2017/PAPacclimation.pdf
3. Weaver, T., Collop, N., & Finlay, G. (n.d.). Adherence with continuous positive airway pressure (CPAP). *UpToDate*. Retrieved from https://www.uptodate.com/contents/adherence-with-continuous-positive-airway-pressure-cpap. Accessed November 3, 2014.
4. Borel, J. C., Tamisier, R., Dias-Domingos, S., et al. (2013). Type of mask may impact on continuous positive airway pressure adherence in apneic patients. *PLoS One*, 8(5), e64382.
5. BaHammam, A. S., Singh, T., George, S., et al. (2017). Choosing the right interface for positive airway pressure therapy in patient with obstructive sleep apnea. *Sleep Breath*, 21(3), 569–575.
6. Dibra, M. N., Berry, R. B., & Wagner, M. H. (2017). Treatment of obstructive sleep apnea, choosing the best interface. *Sleep Medicine Clinics*, 12(4), 543–549.
7. Tuggey, J. M., Delmastro, M., & Elliott, M. W. (2007). The effect of mouth leak and humidification during nasal non-invasive ventilation. *Respiratory Medicine*, 101(9), 1874–1879.
8. Nillus, G., Domanski, U., Franke, K.-J., et al. (2008). Impact of controlled heated breathing tube humidifier on sleep quality during CPAP therapy in cool sleeping environment. *European Respiratory Journal*, 31(4), 830–836.
9. Kushida, C. A., Chediak, A. C., Berry, R. B., et al. (2008). Clinical guidelines for the manual titration of positive airway pressure in patients with obstructive sleep apnea. *Journal of Clinical Sleep Medicine*, 4, 161.
10. Rigau, J., Montserrat, J. M., Wöhrle, H., et al. (2006). Bench model to simulate upper airway obstruction for analyzing automatic continuous positive airway pressure devices. *Chest*, 130(2), 350–361.
11. Ebben, M. R., Narizhnaya, M., Segal, A. Z., et al. (2014). A randomized controlled trial on the effect of mask choice on residual respiratory events with continuous positive airway pressure treatment. *Sleep Medicine*, 15(6), 619–624.
12. Brander, P. E., Soirinsua, M., & Lohela, P. (1999). Nasopharyngeal symptoms in patient with obstructive sleep apnea syndrome. Effect of nasal CPAP treatment. *Respiration*, 66(2), 128–135.
13. Gelardi, M., Carbonara, G., Maffezzoni, E., et al. (2012). Regular utilization reduces nasal inflammation assessed by nasal cytology in obstructive sleep apnea syndrome. *Sleep Medicine*, 13(7), 859–863.
14. Wolkove, N., Baltzan, M., Kamel, H., et al. (2008). Longer-term compliance with continuous positive airway pressure in patients with obstructive sleep apnea. *Canadian Respiratory Journal*, 15(7), 365–369.
15. Brandon, P. *CPAP cleaning tips: A step by step maintenance guide, keeping CPAP equipment clean ensures optimal function and health*. Retrieved from https://www.verywellhealth.com/how-to-clean-cpap-3015322?_ga=2.205906707.1424601836.1547150439-551719944.1473879967. Accessed February 24, 2018.
16. CMS National Coverage Determination (NCD) for Continuous Positive Airway Pressure (CPAP) Therapy For Obstructive SLEEP APNEA (OSA) (240.4). Retrieved from https://www.cms.gov/medicare-coverage-database/details/ncd-details.aspx?NCDId=226&ncdver=3&CoverageSelection=Both&ArticleType=All&PolicyType=Final&s=All&KeyWord=sleep+apnea&KeyWordLookUp=Title&KeyWordSearchType=And&bc=gAAAACAAAAAA&. Accessed September 9, 2018.

chapter 58
Treatment for Insomnia

ROBERT N. TURNER

LEARNING OBJECTIVES

On completion of this chapter, the reader should be able to:

1. Describe insomnia treatment techniques and interventions.
2. Discuss individual differences in insomnia therapy.
3. List some of the medications used to treat insomnia.

KEY TERMS

Insomnia
Sleep hygiene
Cognitive therapy
Pharmacotherapy
Stimulus control therapy
Sleep restriction therapy
Relaxation therapy
Bright light therapy

Treating insomnia can be challenging.

Some patients presenting to the sleep disorders clinic have had trouble initiating and maintaining sleep for months or years; consequently, poor sleep–wake habits are often firmly established. Many "self-medicate," using alcohol or over-the-counter sleep aids for relief of insomnia. Dependency upon sedative-hypnotics also occurs. Others present with personality styles generally associated with enduring, maladaptive patterns of thinking and relating to others and their world. A multitude of interplaying patient characteristics, social and environmental factors as well as medical conditions can contribute to a persistent sleep–wake disturbance. Thus, it is essential to identify the disorder correctly as an initial step in specifying rational interventions for insomnia.

On a broader, conceptual scale, one may question whether nondrug treatments for insomnia are worthwhile or necessary. Although pharmacotherapy has been the mainstay of treatment for decades, patients accept cognitive-behavioral or other nondrug interventions when adequately prepared. Some patients express fears of "becoming addicted" to sleeping pills and prefer to rely on themselves rather than depend upon a medication to sleep. Furthermore, it has become well known that sedative-hypnotics may not be effective in the long-term treatment of insomnia and, if compounds have a short half life, some can induce "rebound insomnia" when discontinued.

On the contrary, sedatives can be helpful to those with various types of insomnia, and many of these compounds are immediately effective in promoting sleep onset and sleep maintenance. If a patient presents with a disorder of hyperarousal, pharmacotherapy and/or relaxation training may be a rational first-line treatment, providing some quick relief to an overactive sympathetic nervous system (SNS). Both patients and physicians are accustomed to treating insomnia in this manner, although this is not necessarily helpful in the long run or to the patient's best benefit.

Before addressing techniques associated with the treatment for chronic insomnia, some general observations, derived through clinical work with an outpatient population, are worth mentioning. Many of these issues have not been subject to rigorous systemic evaluation and may not be significant in every case. The following is not an all-inclusive list but highlights important concerns and some practical matters:

- The initial diagnostic session generally serves as the foundation for subsequent treatment and may provide some relief to the patient, who has finally initiated steps to manage the problem(s). Building rapport and fostering an alliance with the patient during the first meeting is unquestionably essential.
- Some patients actually gain from their misery and suffering, a psychological process called "secondary gain." These people may receive substantial attention and special consideration from family members because of the misery that insomnia causes.
- Patients present to the sleep disorders clinic with wide-ranging and sometimes unrealistic ideas concerning their care. Some expect immediate relief from their long-standing insomnia and may complain bitterly if treatment does not coincide with their expectations.

- Many will actively participate in their treatment *if they understand* the rationale for interventions. Resistance to therapeutic measures requires exploration with the patient.
- Because people with insomnia also present with personality disorders and various psychiatric conditions, it is advantageous for the clinician to utilize strategies from several psychotherapeutic orientations, such as psychodynamic, family systems, interpersonal, and cognitive-behavioral. This is especially important in the treatment for patients with "comorbid" insomnias (e.g., depression, anxiety) because concurrent treatment for the primary condition along with sleeplessness can provide substantial benefit to the patient. If the clinician neglects to address the comorbid disorder and focuses *entirely* upon the patient's insomnia, another interpersonal (or relational) disappointment will certainly be experienced by some patients.
- It is important to understand the principles of sleep hygiene, stimulus control, sleep restriction, relaxation training, and psychotherapy. With sleep hygiene measures, two or three recommendations per session provide the patient time to accommodate to change. Simply furnishing a set of sleep hygiene instructions and/or stimulus control measures rarely provides much benefit to any patient.
- Among many primary care providers, pharmacotherapy continues to be the mainstay for treating insomnia. Using cognitive-behavioral interventions with medication management has not, as of yet, become a "usual and customary" procedure.
- Nonpharmacologic treatments can benefit people with insomnia associated with medical conditions, especially if combined strategies are implemented (e.g., relaxation training and stimulus control have been helpful to several patients with chronic pain).
- Listening empathetically and responding appropriately to patient concerns requires the clinician to remain authentic throughout the process. Patients recognize insincere responses and may feel irritated (at best) by hasty responses. Responding apathetically, challenging beliefs abruptly, or ignoring individual concerns are detrimental to the treatment process.
- It is best for the treating practitioner to remain available to patients, yet establish and maintain firm psychological boundaries throughout therapy. Otherwise repeated "critical" telephone calls can occur between sessions.

When necessary, referring patients to appropriate specialists is essential. However, presenting this to patients requires careful consideration. Some with insomnia firmly believe that they cannot be helped. This notion needs to be addressed rather than providing reinforcement when presenting the need for referral.

COGNITIVE AND BEHAVIORAL TREATMENTS

Once a detailed evaluation of underlying factors that could be contributing to difficulty initiating and/or maintaining sleep has been completed, a variety of techniques are available that have been shown to offer improvements (1).

The American Academy of Sleep Medicine's (AASM) practice parameters for psychological and behavioral treatment of insomnia recommend its use in patients with chronic insomnia (2).

Sleep restriction therapy is based upon the homeostatic regulation of sleep, facilitating sleep initiation and maintenance through partial sleep deprivation. It is important to note that sleep restriction should not fall below 5 hours per night. Additionally, extreme caution should be used with patients for whom sleepiness presents a risk in their profession (e.g., drivers, heavy equipment operators). Restricting the amount of time spent in bed is based upon findings from baseline sleep diaries. The goal is to achieve 85% sleep efficiency (SE). Sleep diaries are reviewed on a weekly basis and if SE goal is met, time in bed is increased by 20 minutes for a week. If SE goal is not met and SE is less than 80%, time in bed is reduced by 20 minutes. Time in bed is kept stable if SE falls between 80% and 85%. Weekly adjustments in the sleep schedule are made until optimal sleep time is reached (3).

Stimulus control therapy includes several instructions that target sleep-incompatible behaviors. Instructions to patients are as follows: Go to bed only when sleepy; get out of bed when unable to sleep, go to another room and return to bed only when sleep is imminent; stop all nonsleep-promoting activities (i.e., watching TV or problem solving); and get up at a regular time every morning despite any problems with sleep during the previous night.

Relaxation therapies center upon reducing cognitive and/or somatic arousal. Progressive muscle relaxation techniques, diaphragmatic breathing, and biofeedback training have all been used among patients with insomnia. Cognitive interventions such as meditation or imagery may also be employed (4). These procedures may be most beneficial to those who experience excessive muscular tension and/or ruminative thought patterns. Relaxation procedures are often described initially and the patient's chosen and preferred relaxation strategy is encouraged. It is important for these methods to be employed over time (2 to 4 weeks at minimum) and practiced daily.

Cognitive therapy focuses upon changing dysfunctional, arousing thoughts and beliefs regarding sleep and insomnia. Catastrophic thinking is challenged; maladaptive thoughts, which may perpetuate insomnia, are addressed; and faulty, unrealistic beliefs are discussed. Worry and rumination over the loss of sleep, unrealistic thoughts regarding the effects of partial sleep deprivation, and irrational expectations about sleep requirements are all relevant issues requiring careful examination and modification. Common examples of irrational beliefs might include "I cannot sleep at all," as well as "My day will be ruined if I do not sleep for at least 8 hours tonight." Because dysfunctional attitudes and thoughts about sleep can promote arousal, both anticipatory and performance anxiety can also occur, adding to difficulties with sleep onset. Offering suggestions to modify and replace these unrealistic or dysfunctional thoughts with rational ideation should be based upon scientifically proven sleep facts. Cognitive-behavioral therapy has been found to benefit various patients with insomnia (5, 6).

Sleep hygiene education focuses upon practices and patterns that can promote or disrupt sleep. The goal is to optimize sleep–wake patterns and habits. Encouraging patients to adopt a regular time of going to bed (with 1- to 2-hour variations) and, more importantly, instructing the patient to get up at about the same time every day are helpful. Avoiding stimulants such as caffeine or tobacco several hours before bedtime, limiting alcohol near bedtime, exercising regularly, providing a time to wind down at least 1 hour before bedtime, and managing stress are other useful suggestions. Environmental variables, such as noise, light, sleep surface, and ambient temperature, can also be addressed. Specific instructions including moving the bedroom clock out of sight, not exercising too close to bedtime, and stopping intense efforts to try to sleep often result in clinical improvement. The latter remains particularly important because the more one tries to sleep, the more aroused one becomes. It is, therefore, less likely that sleep will ensue easily (7).

Bright light therapy can be useful for those with circadian rhythm sleep disorders, such as delayed sleep phase syndrome or advanced sleep phase syndrome (8). Patients with delayed sleep phase syndrome benefit from bright light therapy in the morning to phase-advance their sleepiness time to an earlier time (e.g., from 3:00 a.m. to 12:00 midnight). Patients with advanced sleep phase syndrome benefit from bright light therapy in the evening (about 6:00 to 8:00 p.m.) to phase-delay their sleep time from the early evening to a more appropriate time (e.g., about 10:00 or 11:00 p.m.). However, the utility of bright light therapy among patients with primary insomnia has not, as of yet, been clearly and firmly established.

Paradoxical intention approaches are recommended only sparingly and probably are best implemented by very well-trained clinicians who *have developed a strong working alliance with the particular patient* (9). In utilizing these approaches, the clinician *prescribes the symptom;* with insomnia patients, this translates to essentially telling the patient to try to sleep poorly and utilizing measures contradictory to treating insomnia. These approaches can be helpful among those who generally function adequately or "need to rebel." Some reasonably mentally healthy patients find these humorous. Others, however, consider these interventions cynical, insincere, and insulting or "just plain crazy." It cannot be overemphasized that the treating clinician needs to be reasonably certain of some positive benefit to the patient when utilizing the *paradoxical intention approaches.*

Biofeedback therapy has also been applied to the treatment for disturbances in initiating and maintaining sleep (10). Years ago, several researchers investigated its utility from varying perspectives. Hauri (11) evaluated frontalis electromyogram, electroencephalogram theta, and sensorimotor rhythm biofeedback in the treatment for insomnia. Overall, patients who were more aroused appeared to benefit more than those who were less aroused.

Other strategies rely upon scores of possible folk remedies or beliefs. Aromatherapy and acupuncture can be included here. These interventions may have little or no empirical support, yet could potentially facilitate treatment for some patients. Additional examples of these varied "treatments" may include listening to soft music, prayer, and meditation. If previously helpful, these are worth exploring and using, along with the more recognized and scientifically validated therapies.

PHARMACOTHERAPY

Sedative-hypnotics have long been used in the treatment for insomnia. Older preparations included the bromides, chloral hydrate, glutethimide, and numerous other compounds. Barbiturates were also used throughout the 1950s. The departure of these agents from clinical use probably evokes little nostalgic remorse because several serious problems occurred with many of them. Among other concerns, gastric disturbances, the development of tolerance to their therapeutic effects, risks of dependence and abuse, lethality in overdose due to a limited therapeutic margin of safety, and the potential for convulsions or seizures upon withdrawal were noteworthy reasons for avoiding some of these older hypnotics. The potential for barbiturate abuse and overdose also became well publicized after the death of Marilyn Monroe. Another compound, thalidomide, was responsible for severe birth defects, such as children born without limbs. The latter disaster apparently stimulated more stringent regulations in drug testing in the United States.

With the advent of sleep laboratory technology and methodology, direct objective evaluation of hypnotics became possible. The earliest studies began in the mid-1960s with Oswald and Priest (12) describing rapid eye movement (REM) sleep rebound and nightmares following drug withdrawal. Kales and associates (13, 14) published important work describing methodology and hypnotic efficacy and later reported on the ineffectiveness of several medications over 2 weeks of use (15, 16). The latter research group has also been credited with describing rebound insomnia (17) following discontinuation of several hypnotics, particularly Dalmane. Through these and numerous other studies, several research designs were developed and used in evaluating dosage, efficacy, tolerance, withdrawal, and potential dependence issues of sleep-promoting medications.

Over 30 years ago, the first benzodiazepine (*chlordiazepoxide*, or Librium) was introduced. Thereafter, several other benzodiazepine compounds were developed and many were subject to systematic sleep laboratory evaluation. The most commonly used agents in this category, as well as nonbenzodiazepine hypnotics, are included in Table 58-1. Generally, the benzodiazepines can facilitate sleep onset and increase sleep duration. However, they vary considerably in dosages and elimination half-lives. Consequently, undesired effects such as daytime sedation, memory impairment, and accidents, as well as potential problems with tolerance, dependence, abuse, and withdrawal, all require consideration before implementation. In addition, these compounds can be effective for a week or two, yet safety beyond six consecutive weeks of use has not consistently been established. Rebound insomnia can occur especially when using agents with short elimination half-lives.

Some adverse effects (including daytime impairment, infections, risks of diseases) or other unfavorable outcomes *may or may not* be published. In addition, labels and package inserts are written by manufacturers. These remain critical issues (18). Although pharmacologic treatment of insomnia is pervasive, AASM clinical practice guidelines provide only a weak recommendation for their use in chronic insomnia (19). This is due to a lack of certainty in the outcomes for all patients. However, the benefit and use of pharmacologic agents is ultimately left to the judgment of the clinician. A number of agents used in treating chronic insomnia did not have enough literature to receive positive or negative recommendations from the AASM. These include

Table 58-1 Food and Drug Administration–Approved Medications for Insomnia

Generic Name	Trade Name	Usual Dosage (mg)	Half-Life (h)
Benzodiazepines			
Flurazepam	Dalmane	15–30	47–100
Quazepam	Doral	7.5–15	2–73
Estazolam	Prosom	1–2	10–24
Temazepam	Restoril	7.5–15	3.5–18.4
Triazolam	Halcion	0.125–0.5	1.5–5.5
Nonbenzodiazepines			
Zolpidem	Ambien	5–10	2.6
Zaleplon	Sonata	10	~1
Eszopiclone	Lunesta	1, 2, 3	6
Melatonin agonists			
Ramelteon	Rozerem	8	1–2.6
Orexin receptor agonists			
Suvorexant	Belsomra	10	10–22
Tricyclic antidepressants			
Doxepin	Silenor	3, 6	15.3
Antihistamines			
Diphenhydramine	Benadryl	25–50	8–17
Doxylamine	Unisom	25–50	10–12

estazolam, flurazepam, oxazepam, quetiapine, gabapentin, and paroxetine (19).

Estazolam has an intermediate half-life and a rapid absorption rate. Promoting sleep onset and maintenance, this compound is often taken approximately 15 to 30 minutes before bedtime. Patients with impaired hepatic or renal function and the elderly may use this drug, yet caution is usually exercised because a reduced capacity to eliminate this compound and an increased sensitivity to the active metabolites always require consideration.

Flurazepam was one of the first benzodiazepines evaluated through sleep research methodologies. This compound has a long half-life (time necessary to clear half of a given agent from blood plasma) and a rapid absorption rate. It can be useful with younger patients, yet caution is warranted with the elderly because the elimination half-life is considerably longer than in younger patients. The half-life of this compound is so long that its sedative-hypnotic effect often extends into the waking hours, thus causing daytime confusion, disorientation, risk of falls, daytime sedation, and numerous other problems. Most of these undesirable side effects are caused by the remaining active metabolites of certain types of benzodiazepines following bedtime administration. In addition, case reports of exacerbation of sleep-disordered breathing following ingestion of some of these benzodiazepine compounds have also appeared.

Quazepam also has a long half-life and a rapid absorption rate. Taken 60 to 90 minutes before bedtime, this compound facilitates both sleep onset and sleep maintenance. Accumulation of metabolites may also pose a risk for elderly or other patients, as well as those with pulmonary diseases. This agent is not recommended for use during pregnancy or while breastfeeding.

Temazepam has a slow absorption rate and an intermediate half-life. Generally taken 30 to 60 minutes before desired sleep onset, peak plasma levels occur between 1 and 3 hours later. Daytime sedation occurs rarely. The gelatinous form of this agent was removed from the market in the United Kingdom because of abuse.

Triazolam has a rapid absorption rate, a short half-life, and generally does not promote daytime sedation following use. This compound is usually taken 15 to 30 minutes before bedtime and typically promotes sleep onset but does not significantly improve sleep maintenance. Daytime sedation typically does not occur, but anxiety and amnesia following use have been reported.

Zolpidem, zaleplon, and *eszopiclone* are nonbenzodiazepines. All of these hypnotics (relatively) selectively target the γ-aminobutyric acid (GABA) receptor sites that are involved with sleep. They leave the other GABA sites that are involved with muscular relaxation or coordination relatively unaffected and do not affect inhibitory sites that reduce seizure activity. They all have short half-lives, promote relatively normal sleep architecture, and do not seem to reduce REM sleep or inhibit slow-wave sleep. They are not often associated with sedation following use, do not usually promote respiratory depression, and all seem to have a low abuse potential. Rebound insomnia would not appear to be a significant issue following discontinuation of use. Presently, these agents are commonly used in the short-term treatment for insomnia.

Ramelteon is a melatonin agonist, which binds to the MT_1 and MT_2 receptors in the suprachiasmatic nucleus of the hypothalamus. No appreciable affinity for the $GABA_A$ receptor sites has been reported. The 8-mg dosage is taken approximately 30 minutes before bedtime and peak plasma concentration reportedly occurs within 30 to 90 minutes. Sleep architecture does not appear to be adversely affected.

Doxepin (3 and 6 mg dosages) is an H_1 receptor antagonist with a half-life of approximately 3.5 hours. It has been approved for the treatment for insomnia and can be helpful for patients with sleep-maintenance difficulties. Higher dosages have been used for the treatment for depression and anxiety.

Suvorexant is a dual orexin receptor antagonist. It blocks both OX1R and OX2R. It promotes sleep through the inhibition of orexin A and B. It has a longer-lasting effect and should be taken only if the patient has at least 7 hours before he or she gets out of bed for the day.

Antidepressants are also very commonly used in the treatment of patients with insomnia and depression, but these agents have not been specifically approved by the Food and Drug Administration (FDA) for the treatment of insomnia. The tricyclics (*amitriptyline, trimipramine,* and *nortriptyline*) reduce sleep latency and improve sleep continuity, yet these agents are associated with various anticholinergic side effects (dry mouth, constipation, urinary hesitancy, dry eyes), as well as hypotension, cardiac rate, and conduction problems, and both confusion and poor memory. In addition, the risk of overdose is substantial with this group of medications. The selective serotonin reuptake inhibitors—paroxetine, fluvoxamine, sertraline, fluoxetine—and other compounds would appear to have largely replaced these agents in clinical usage but do not consistently promote sleep among many patients.

The sedating antidepressants include *trazodone, mirtazapine,* and *nefazodone.* Each of these can facilitate sleep onset and/or sleep continuity, yet none have been subject to careful multicenter evaluations in sleep laboratory settings with large numbers of patients. The antipsychotics (*quetiapine and olanzapine*) can also promote sleep but have not been adequately evaluated through extensive clinical trials with insomnia patients. None of these compounds are presently approved by the FDA for the treatment of insomnia. Studies of these compounds with nonsymptomatic subjects and those with psychophysiologic insomnia may represent an important research opportunity, which could provide practitioners with objective information supporting the use of these agents in the treatment for insomnia.

The popular media have suggested the use of over-the-counter sleep aids such as melatonin, valerian root, chamomile, passionflower, hops, ginseng, lemon balm, kava kava, lavender, St. John's wort, and skullcap, as well as other products for the treatment for insomnia. These compounds are not FDA regulated. Representative objective data detailing therapeutic benefits of these agents have not, as of yet, consistently appeared in the professional literature. Their usefulness, therefore, remains questionable. However, melatonin has been shown to have some slight hypnotic effects, but its main scientifically demonstrated action is that of a phase advancer when taken in the evening several hours before bedtime.

Over-the-counter sleep aids typically contain antihistamines such as diphenhydramine or doxylamine. On occasion, these agents can be helpful for some people but do not seem to be effective when used regularly. Side effects can include daytime drowsiness, blurred vision, forgetfulness, clumsiness, and dry mouth.

TREATMENT DELIVERY

Regardless of the type of insomnia, short-term or chronic, it is recommended that consideration be given to psychological and behavioral interventions as well as any pharmacologic treatment (2). Following completion of the sleep history and other relevant measures to arrive at a correct diagnosis, a realistic therapeutic strategy may be formulated. Even if the patient's insomnia co-occurs with another primary sleep disorder (e.g., sleep apnea, restless legs syndrome, other sleep disorders), behavioral and/or pharmacologic approaches to treatment may be implemented provided that the other condition is treated as well.

In treatment planning and delivery, Spielman's theoretical approach (20) requires consideration. He suggests that the development of insomnia depends upon three factors: predisposing factors that must be present for insomnia to develop in a given patient, precipitating factors that trigger these patients to develop insomnia, and perpetuating factors that maintain the insomnia once it has started. Predisposing, precipitating, and perpetuating issues are germane to adequate therapy. Vulnerability to biologic (circadian, hyperarousal, neurophysiologic) and psychological (worry, apprehension, rumination, dysphoria, others) factors, as well as other underlying patient characteristics, may predispose the

patient to bouts of insomnia. Precipitating factors may include an acute illness, the loss of a loved one, sudden changes of the sleep–wake cycle, mood disturbances (depression, anxiety due to stressors), and numerous other potential activating internal and/or external triggers. Worry, fears, irrational beliefs about sleep, clock watching, irregular sleep–wake schedules, caffeine use, engagement in stimulating activities immediately before bedtime, and other poor sleep hygiene practices may perpetuate the insomnia once it develops.

In general, the initial focus of treatment will depend upon the patient's presentation and an appropriate analysis of these three (predisposing, precipitating, perpetuating) factors. Because hyperarousal may be an underlying and essential predisposing feature, measures to reduce arousal are often important components in the first treatment session. Rather than focusing only on the sleep–wake disturbance, some forms of relaxation therapy (abbreviated progressive muscle relaxation, autogenic training, guided imagery, diaphragmatic breathing, and others) may be an important first step. Adjunctive medication therapy, targeted to decrease SNS activity, may also be necessary. These measures are important for those who are physiologically aroused (high muscle tension) but may not significantly benefit patients who are not experiencing biologic activation. In addition, encouraging patient expressions of concerns regarding arousal are helpful in beginning treatment. Reducing hyperarousal, rather than merely promoting sleep (through behavioral measures or sedation) remains important because increased SNS activation could potentially increase the patient's risk of hypertension, myocardial infarction, or coronary artery disease.

Systemic, consistent algorithms for the cognitive-behavioral treatment for *all* forms of insomnia have not yet been firmly established among the different sleep centers. However, Morin (21) described an approach in treating primary insomnia. Very briefly, the first session would serve to provide education about sleep and to address the treatment program. Sleep restriction and stimulus control procedures would be discussed during the second session, and the third session would focus upon problems encountered with measures described during the second session. Cognitive therapy would be introduced during the following session and continued, along with an evaluation of the patient's compliance with behavioral measures, during the fifth counseling hour. Session six would serve to review compliance and continue with cognitive therapy and sleep education. Sessions seven and eight would focus on reviewing treatment components and addressing measures to avoid the reappearance of insomnia.

Edinger and associates have systematically researched treatment protocols for primary insomnia. One study (22) evaluated a brief, two-session therapy program and found significant treatment effects with primary care patients. Another investigation (23) found a four-session, biweekly cognitive-behavioral treatment program efficacious in the treatment of sleep-maintenance insomnia. A good manual describing therapeutic strategies for the treatment for primary insomnia was also published (24).

For more than 20 years, practitioners and researchers have conducted group treatment for insomnia. Facts about sleep and wakefulness, sleep hygiene and stimulus control measures, relaxation therapy, and at least some elements of cognitive-behavioral therapy for insomnia (CBTi) can be addressed in a suitable group setting. One study (25) found improvements in sleep onset, total sleep time, and SE, a reduction in wake time after sleep onset, and improved sleep quality among selected people with insomnia. A reduction in dysfunctional beliefs and attitudes about sleep and negative daytime symptoms was also reported. CBTi delivered in group settings has been shown to be effective (26). It is of vital importance that the practicing clinician (group leader) keep in mind general principles of group therapy described by Yalom (27) before ambitiously implementing this approach with insomnia patients. Further studies have shown that online and phone treatment with CBTi are also effective (28).

Individualized treatment planning for patients with primary and comorbid insomnia is essential. Standard interventions (stimulus control, relaxation, etc.) do not benefit *all* patients equally. Therefore, flexibility in treatment delivery approaches is important because there are several good ways of treating afflicted patients. What follows is one approach.

Following initial interview and assignment of correct diagnosis, an individualized sleep log is written *with the patient* during the first assessment/treatment visit. This *simple* self-monitoring diary is written on standard paper with sleep-related variables as headers and days of the week along the left margin. Headers include date, bedtime, sleep-onset latency, frequency of awakenings during the night, and arising time. An additional category or two remains open for other variables, such as medication usage, sleepiness in the morning, dog in the bed, or other relevant information. Constructing the sleep log in the patient's presence can serve as an important *engagement* technique and the author has found it to be helpful in building rapport.

At the bottom of the handwritten sleep diary, two or three stimulus control items or other relevant suggestions are provided. Most commonly, patients are instructed to begin utilizing at least 1 hour of wind down time every evening, to go to bed only when sleepy, and get up at the same time daily. Recommendations for patients with affective or anxiety disorders often include increasing pleasurable activities on a daily basis, utilizing

relaxation techniques, and eating regularly. Patients are instructed to complete the diary over the course of 1 or 2 weeks (time between visits often depends upon insurance coverage, patient financial resources, practical patient issues, or scheduling matters).

Some clinicians have understandably questioned why treatment measures are included during the assessment period (i.e., completing the sleep log and using stimulus control or other intervention measures). Although it is clearly understood by most practitioners that the ideal manner to evaluate sleep onset or sleep maintenance insomnia includes first completing the sleep log for a week or two without intervention(s), many patients are very frustrated with perceived or actual sleep difficulties and are unwilling to experience additional nights of misery and insomnia without actively doing something about it.

During the second visit, the patient's sleep diary is reviewed and focus is often placed upon what the patient has accomplished and sustained since the last visit. Troubleshooting begins during this session. Basic information about normal sleep processes is usually provided during this visit. Addressing negative thoughts and feelings about sleep and conversing about not watching the clock, eliminating naps, and reducing caffeine and alcohol intake can occur. Patients are also often introduced to common principles of cognitive therapy (such as activating events and their association with internal beliefs, and resulting consequences [thoughts, feelings, and behaviors]).

Subsequent visits focus upon reducing the tendency to "take problems to bed" or other worries about sleep onset and sleep maintenance. Reducing the pattern of trying to sleep and further addressing negative thoughts and feelings associated with poor sleep are also addressed. Treatment gains and relapse prevention are the final therapeutic steps for treating the patient's insomnia, and we usually begin focusing more attention on other problem areas during forthcoming sessions.

IMPLEMENTATION OF PHARMACOTHERAPY

Brief pharmacotherapy can be useful with many patients, especially those with short-term insomnia. Although sedating antidepressants are widely used, zolpidem, eszopiclone, and zaleplon are also employed (29). As with other medications, the smallest effective dose is usually prescribed initially. The choice of hypnotic and appropriate dosage will depend on several patient factors, such as age, duration of the insomnia, associated medical and/or psychiatric conditions, potential for compliance and appropriate use, and the type of insomnia (i.e., onset or maintenance).

Because many people have become accustomed to using sedative-hypnotics and have developed physical or psychological dependence upon these agents, it is important to assist the patient in medication reduction and eventual cessation. An individualized approach combining a slow taper of the compound along with cognitive-behavioral and other appropriate interventions seems to benefit many. The tapering schedule will vary depending upon the compound. Distress about sleeplessness and daytime consequences occurs frequently, and the treating clinician can expect the patient to express fears or concerns about expected insomnia. Reassurance can be helpful, but active involvement (including taking between-session calls) with patients is often necessary.

Among patients who have not used hypnotics, combining pharmacotherapy and cognitive-behavioral therapy is advantageous because sedating agents can initially promote sleep, while modifying thoughts, feelings, and behaviors in therapy aids in sustaining these changes. Although these ideas are intuitively attractive, there are data that do not clearly support this notion. For instance, Hauri (30) found sleep hygiene and behavioral therapy most helpful when patients did not use hypnotics. Another study (28) among older adults found similar short-term treatment gains with both nonpharmacologic and medication therapies, yet treatment effects were better maintained with cognitive-behavioral therapies over 12 and 24 months. In addition, the authors of the latter paper addressed the notion of initiating drug therapy first and providing behavioral therapy when medications are discontinued.

With secondary insomnia, traditional clinical lore has suggested that insomnia would cease once the primary condition was adequately treated. Although this may be true with some cases, it has not been found to be correct on a consistent basis. As an example, a young patient with major depressive disorder or generalized anxiety disorder can continue to experience significant insomnia even when considerable progress has been made in psychotherapy. Adequately treated patients with chronic pain conditions can also complain of sleeplessness. Thus, treatment for comorbid insomnia represents a significant challenge for practitioners and always requires consideration.

Both patient and clinician factors require consideration in the treatment for any sleep–wake disorder. Patients must possess the internal resources to change (and the capacity to tolerate treatment challenges), be sufficiently motivated to feel better, and possess significant distress about their sleeplessness. These very real issues are extremely important because many people with chronic insomnia feel out of control and are initially unable to modify their thoughts, feelings, and behaviors. Furthermore, patients need to be willing to comply with recommended interventions. And, family members often need to be alerted to potential changes with the patient. The latter is critical in some situations because a growing sense of self-esteem, independence, and self-efficacy can actually produce turmoil within family systems.

Among other characteristics, clinician factors have included empathy, interpersonal warmth, and both understanding and acceptance of the patient. Although these issues would appear to be obvious, the capacity to develop and maintain an effective treatment relationship (even briefly) is not always easy with the wide variety of patients presenting with insomnia. The treating clinician also needs to understand basic cognitive-behavioral principles in sleep medicine and likewise benefits from an adequate understanding of psychodynamic, cognitive, interpersonal, and family-systems models of therapy. Those providing treatments to the wide range of patients with insomnia also need to realize that treatment failures can and do occur, yet have little or nothing to do with therapeutic relevance or quality. The patient's lack of success with interventions often reflects noncompliance, motivational problems, or assorted other factors.

INSOMNIA AND SLEEP APNEA

Patients experiencing insomnia with sleep apnea obviously present with at least two sleep–wake disorders, and both typically require adequate treatment. Cognitive-behavioral treatments can be effective; utilizing wind down time, going to bed only when very sleepy, and putting continuous positive airway pressure (CPAP) on before "nodding off" have been helpful for some. Recommending the patient arise at the same time daily, avoiding naps, and desensitizing with CPAP before starting treatment with CPAP have been useful. These challenging patients can be helped if practitioners allocate sufficient time and energy.

REFERENCES

1. Edinger, J. D., Leggett, M. K., Carney, C. E., et al. (2017). Psychological and behavioral treatments for insomnia II: Implementation and specific populations. In M. Kryger, T. Roth, & W. C. Dement (Eds.), *Principles and practice of sleep medicine* (6th ed.). Philadelphia, PA: Elsevier.
2. Morgenthaler, T., Kramer, M., Alessi, C., et al. (2006). Practice parameters for the psychological and behavioral treatment of insomnia: An update. An American Academy of Sleep Medicine report. *Sleep, 29*(11), 1415–1419.

3. Kyle, S. D., Miller, C. B., Rogers, Z., et al. (2014). Sleep restriction therapy for insomnia is associated with reduced objective total sleep time, increased daytime somnolence, and objectively impaired vigilance: Implications for the clinical management of insomnia disorder. *Sleep, 37*(2), 229–237.

4. Ong, J. C., Manber, R., Segal, Z., et al. (2014). A randomized controlled trial of mindfulness meditation for chronic insomnia. *Sleep, 37*(9), 1553–1563.

5. Morin, C. M., Bastien, C., & Savard, J. (2003). Current status of cognitive-behavior therapy with insomnia: Evidence for treatment effectiveness and feasibility. In M. L. Perlis & K. L. Lichstein (Eds.), *Treating sleep disorders: Principles and practice of behavioral sleep medicine* (pp. 262–285). New York, NY: John Wiley & Sons.

6. Harvey, A. G., Bélanger, L., Talbot, L., et al. (2014). Supplemental material for comparative efficacy of behavior therapy, cognitive therapy, and cognitive behavior therapy for chronic insomnia: A randomized controlled trial. *Journal of Consulting and Clinical Psychology, 82*(4), 670–683.

7. Carney, C., & Manber, R. (2009). *Quiet your mind & get to sleep: Solutions to insomnia for those with depression, anxiety, or chronic pain.* Oakland, CA: New Harbinger.

8. van Maanen, A., Meijer, A. M., van der Heijden, K. B., et al. (2016). The effects of light therapy on sleep problems: A systematic review and meta-analysis. *Sleep Medicine Reviews, 29*, 52–62.

9. Broomfield, N. M., & Espie, C. A. (2003). Initial insomnia and paradoxical intention: an experimental investigation of putative mechanisms using subjective and actigraphic measurement of sleep. *Behavioural and Cognitive Psychotherapy, 31*(3), 313–324.

10. Hauri, P. J. (1997) Insomnia. Can we mix behavioral therapy with hypnotics when treating insomniacs? *Sleep, 20*(12):1111–1118.

11. Hauri, P. (1981). Treating psychophysiological insomnia with biofeedback. *Archives of General Psychiatry, 38*, 752–758.

12. Oswald, I., & Priest, R. G. (1965). Five weeks to escape the sleeping pill habit. *British Medical Journal, 2*, 1093–1095.

13. Kales, A., Scharf, M., Tan, T. L., et al. (1969). Sleep patterns with short term drug use. *Psychophysiology, 6*, 262.

14. Kales, A., Tan, T., Scharf, M., et al. (1969). Effects of long and short-term administration of flurazepam (Dalmane) in subjects with insomnia. *Psychophysiology, 6*, 260.

15. Kales, A., Allen, C., Scharf, M. B., et al. (1969). Hypnotic drugs and their effectiveness. *Archives of General Psychiatry, 23*, 226–232.

16. Kales, A., Kales, J. D., Bixler, E. O., et al. (1975). Effectiveness of hypnotic drugs with prolonged use: Flurazepam and pento-barbital. *Clinical Pharmacology and Therapeutics, 18*, 356–363.

17. Kales, A., Scharf, M. B., & Kales, J. D. (1978). Rebound insomnia: A new clinical syndrome. *Science, 201*, 1039–1041.

18. Schwartz, L. M., & Woloshin, S. (2009). Lost in translation-FDA drug information that never reaches clinicians. *New England Journal of Medicine, 361*, 1717–1720.

19. Sateia, M. J., Buysse, D. J., Krystal, A. D., et al. (2017). Clinical practice guideline for the pharmacologic treatment of chronic insomnia in adults: An American Academy of Sleep Medicine clinical practice guideline. *Journal of Clinical Sleep Medicine, 13*(2), 307–349.

20. Spielman, A. J., Nunes, J., & Glovinsky, P. B. (1996). Insomnia. *Neurologic Clinics, 14*, 513–544.

21. Morin, C. (1993). *Insomnia: Psychological assessment and management.* New York, NY: Guilford Press.

22. Edinger, J. D., & Sampson, W. S. (2003). A primary care "friendly" cognitive behavior insomnia therapy. *Sleep, 26*, 177–182.

23. Edinger, J. D., Wohlgemuth, W. K., Radtke, R. A., et al. (2004). Dose response effects of behavioral insomnia therapy: Final report. *Sleep, 27*, A265.

24. Perlis, M. L., Jungquist, C., Smith, M. T., et al. (2005). *Cognitive behavioral treatment of insomnia: A session-by-session guide.* New York, NY: Springer.

25. Jansson, M., & Linton, S. J. (2005). Cognitive behavioral group therapy as an early intervention for insomnia: A randomized control trial. *Journal of Occupational Rehabilitation, 15*(2), 177–190.

26. Davidson, J. R., Dawson, S., & Krsmanovic, A. (2017). Effectiveness of group cognitive behavioral therapy for insomnia (CBT-I) in a primary care setting. *Behavioral Sleep Medicine*, 1–13. doi:10.1080/15402002.2017.1318753

27. Yalom, I. D. (1995). *The theory and practice of group psychotherapy* (4th ed.). New York, NY: Basic Books.

28. Ulmer, C. S., Bosworth, H. B., Voils, C. I., et al. (2018). 0403 Tele-self CBTI: Provider supported self-management cognitive behavioral therapy for insomnia. *Sleep, 41*(Suppl 1), A153.

29. Mccall, C., & Mccall, W. V. (2012). What is the role of sedating antidepressants, antipsychotics, and anticonvulsants in the management of insomnia? *Current Psychiatry Reports, 14*(5), 494–502.

30. Hauri, P. J. (1997). Can we mix behavioral therapy with hypnotics when treating insomniacs? *Sleep, 20*(12), 1111–1118.

chapter 59

Telemedicine in Sleep Medicine

FAYÇAL ABDENBI

LEARNING OBJECTIVES

On completion of this chapter, the reader should be able to:

1. Provide an overview of telemedicine applications in sleep medicine and the technologist's role.
2. Describe how to use telemedicine to manage patients on positive airway pressure and other therapies.
3. Identify the major opportunities for and challenges to telemedicine implementation.
4. Describe the factors that make a program successful and less successful.
5. Design a viable model for telemedicine implementation where you work.

KEY TERMS

Telemedicine
Telecommunication
Telemonitoring
Information technology (IT) infrastructure

Sleep disorders, in general, and sleep-disordered breathing (SDB), more particularly, affect a substantial number of subjects and may be increasing in prevalence (1, 2), with a potentially serious health impact (3). Several studies have shown that daytime sleepiness is a risk factor for motor vehicle accidents (4) and may have significant socioprofessional consequences (5). The Sleep Heart Health Study has shown that in patients with excessive daytime sleepiness or difficulty initiating or maintaining sleep, health-related quality of life is impacted (6).

Although physicians understand the importance of sleep and its impact on a patient's health, many sleep disorders remain unrecognized and untreated in clinical practice (7). Improving awareness of various types of sleep disorders and their impact on patients and public health can lead to a higher demand not only for documentation but also for diagnosis, treatment, and follow-up.

Many sleep disorders, particularly sleep apnea, are chronic conditions and require continuous treatment and monitoring of therapy success. However, barriers such as long distances between these services and the patients' home or long waiting lists can prevent sufferers from getting quick or easy access to those medical services. In such cases, telemedicine and remote patient–physician interaction could be useful to establish diagnostic and therapeutic strategies and improve access to medical services.

Telemedicine is a bidirectional interaction between patients and health care providers (8), which consists of delivering remote health care services by using telecommunications technologies. In such a system, health care professionals can diagnose (telediagnostics), treat (teletherapy), and monitor (telemonitoring) the patients from a distance without the need of their physical presence, while the patients' data are transmitted from one site to another via Internet or smartphones. We will review some of the applications of telemedicine in sleep medicine and the technologist's role in it.

USE OF TELEMEDICINE FOR SLEEP DIAGNOSTICS

In the context of a highly prevalent disease such as SDB (2) having a significant impact on health, sleep laboratories are facing an increased demand for sleep testing with scarcity of sleep specialists. Such factors can keep the sleep laboratories busy and overloaded with a prolonged waiting list of patients requiring a screening and diagnosis. This has triggered more usage of portable equipment for home sleep apnea testing (HSAT), which is becoming more accurate, more sensitive, and more specific in detecting respiratory events.

With a HSAT setup, the patient will perform the sleep recording at home by applying the sensors to himself or herself at bedtime following the sleep technologist's instructions, which are usually provided at the time of the consultation. When the patient returns the equipment to the sleep center, the sleep technologist will perform a data download from the device and score the study. The right therapeutic decision will then highly rely on the accuracy of the sleep technologist's scoring.

Using telemedicine techniques could help extend diagnostic services to wide sectors of the population (9). Coma-del-Corral et al. (10) have examined the technical feasibility of performing respiratory polysomnography (PSG) along with real-time transmission of sleep sounds and images of the patients to their sleep unit (80 km distance) in a group of 40 subjects with a clinical suspicion of obstructive sleep apnea (OSA) syndrome. At the sleep unit, the technologists were continuously monitoring in real time the recording and the patient images transmitted. They have observed good agreement between the data transmitted in real time and that stored in the polygraph. This virtual sleep unit extends the possibilities of providing specialized health care to a geographically distant population and can lead to reducing the patient's travel time and expense as well as optimizing the sleep center's resources.

In a prospective study, Borsini et al. (11) have explored the feasibility of establishing a network of satellite units for the diagnosis of sleep disorders connected to a reference Central Sleep Unit using respiratory PSG with remote data transmission. Of 499 studies, only 20 recordings (4%) were invalid because of cannula or oximeter disconnection. The study concluded that remote diagnosis strategy using portable respiratory PSG was useful in diagnosing OSA patients with a low probability of missing data and with safe transmission from remote centers to the Central Sleep Unit.

The role of the sleep technologists in such models is crucial because they are needed to perform regular monitoring of the remote sleep study and to check the quality of the signals. In case of bad signal quality, the technologist may call the patient to reposition a sensor correctly. However, the current practice of telemedicine in sleep medicine seems to be primarily for monitoring compliance to continuous positive airway pressure (CPAP) therapy rather than for diagnostic procedures (12). The main reason could be that telemonitoring with HSAT systems is not as needed as with PSG. Thus, the sleep medicine field seems somehow to have limited application for telemedicine technologies (13) and is only benefiting from a small part of it.

USING TELEMEDICINE TO MANAGE POSITIVE AIRWAY PRESSURE THERAPY

CPAP is the most effective treatment for OSA, and its related outcomes can only be achieved if the patient is adherent. Without optimal CPAP use, the patients may fail to achieve the full cardiovascular and symptomatic benefits of therapy. However, a key obstacle for sleep specialists is how to optimize their patients' adherence

to therapy. Many studies have reported that a main predictive factor for long-term CPAP compliance is patient adherence in the first weeks of treatment. Kribbs et al. have reported that only half of OSA patients remain compliant with CPAP by 3 months after therapy initiation (14).

The use of telemedicine also seems to have an impact by optimizing the time of early interventions. In a recent study, telemedicine has shown similar side effects and satisfaction rates when compared with standard care and can lead to lower total costs because of savings on travel (15).

In a study by Fox et al. (16), two OSA patient groups were randomized to either telemedicine or standard care. CPAP data were monitored daily and patients were contacted when there was suboptimal usage or other issues. Despite the compliance level, which was not very high in both groups, the telemedicine intervention led to significantly increased CPAP usage at 3 months by nearly 90 minutes per night compared with the standard care.

Hwang et al. conducted a randomized trial (17) where moderate-to-severe OSA patients were prospectively included and randomized to receive standard care or telemedicine. In both arms, an educational session was planned after CPAP initiation, and medical visits were planned. Delay to the first intervention was significantly shorter in the telemedicine group (29 ± 25 vs. 47 ± 30 days, $p = 0.02$). These first interventions were triggered by the detection of problems by the telemedicine system in nearly 40% of patients. This early detection and troubleshooting was associated with a significantly improved compliance at 3 months in the telemedicine group (5.7 ± 1.6 vs. 4.2 ± 1.9 h/night). Such results suggest that early intervention with telemedicine can be an important tool for the improvement of long-term CPAP acceptance.

The current technology enables the health care provider to monitor relevant data such as CPAP, leakage, apnea–hypopnea index, and adherence to therapy as well as raw data (flow and pressure curves). These data along with personal usage information are shared with the health care provider by means of a modem (using either GSM or WiFi technology). According to each country's regulation, there are differences in the way a health care provider can get access to these data and use them. In some countries (e.g., France), the usage data are regularly sent to the home care provider (HCP) who receives payment from the national health insurance system as long as the patient is using his or her device and is compliant. The data are also shared with the physician who can discuss potential problems with the patient at an early stage. Thus, appropriate cases can be followed in the sleep unit with specialized technical support, whereas less complex cases can be titrated or followed using home-based settings.

Telemedicine can be useful in improving patient adherence if linked to adequate patient education about the disease and support of therapy usage primarily during the early phases of therapy.

OPPORTUNITIES FOR AND CHALLENGES TO TELEMEDICINE IMPLEMENTATION

The high demand for diagnosis and treatment of SDB is generating more pressure on sleep laboratories and prolonging the waiting list. Hospitals and clinics can leverage telemedicine capabilities to better absorb and manage high patient flow, whereas insurance bodies look at options to reduce patient follow-up costs.

Telemedicine can be an opportunity to improve clinical outcomes and the patient's overall experience. Physicians can prescribe therapy and the HCP will have access to the prescription using the same web platform. Patients' therapy data can be monitored via remote access to check their therapy adherence, and if needed, the health care provider can remotely adjust the device settings according to the physician's recommendations.

Telemedicine can potentially help reduce health care costs by facilitating clinician identification of the patients who need special attention and further face-to-face visits and interacting with those who are responding well to the therapy at home. Thus, travel time for the patient can be reduced and the time spent by the health care professional can be significantly shortened (18).

Implementing telemedicine will require very detailed investigations to understand the regulations in the selected geographical area. Indeed, telemedicine practice is controlled by strict rules and policies related to data protection and privacy, and its implementation has some technical considerations. For instance, encrypted communication and storage systems are required to comply with privacy regulations and ensure patient confidentiality. Such investigations can take quite a significant time and effort because there are several parties involved and many procedures to consider before establishing the appropriate contracts with each party. New regulations, if not existing, should be prepared and created to allow adoption of telemedicine services.

The resistance that some health care professionals and some patients have to telemedicine as an alternative to in-office care can limit its expansion for the management of sleep apnea patients. The perception and acceptance of telemedicine will differ on the basis of local context. Patients can perceive telemedicine as an intrusion in their life because they are monitored, and

their usage data are collected and transmitted every day. The implementation of such a new model needs to be explained well to the patients and their family in order to eliminate any concerns.

Some reluctant clinicians might see this as an additional challenge that adds a burden to their clinical routine. Indeed, this means implementing new ways of working, learning how to navigate with new web interfaces protected by passwords, and managing patients requiring immediate or specific attention.

FACTORS THAT CAN MAKE A PROGRAM SUCCESSFUL

The health field involves a number of different groups and stakeholders: patients, doctors, hospital administrations, HCPs, health authorities and insurance companies, medical device companies, and others. All these groups are not necessarily looking at telemedicine from the same angle and may have different interests. Given the diversity of health care systems and differences in reimbursement models, implementing a telemedicine program requires a methodological approach to ensure success and performance. Successful adoption of a telemedicine program will require a number of changes in terms of policies and regulations and a significant investment of time and money. Implementation will also affect the routine practice of the medical staff. Thus, it is better to identify the right model to optimize your investment and increase the overall satisfaction with this experience.

Here are a few questions to have in mind before implementing a telemedicine program:

1. What is not working with my current model?
2. How would a telemedicine program help me and my team perform better? Is it the right strategy for my team and me?
3. Is it for all my patients?
4. Am I comfortable with the technology?
5. Am I ready to adopt new skill sets related to such technologies?
6. What investments are required? Do I need a new information technology (IT) infrastructure (software and hardware)?
7. Can my current facility or space fit for a telemedicine program (size, design layout, etc.)?
8. Who will be leading this program?
9. What contracts do I need?
10. Do I have the right partners to help me understand the regulations in terms of data transfer, data storage, data privacy, and data security?
11. Will there be any impact on my team organization and setup?

12. What equipment does the patient need at home?
13. How is my hotline organized?
14. What can I do in case of connectivity or IT issues? Do I have a backup plan?

Once you have reached a clear understanding of your model, you can identify facilities with a similar setup, visit them, and spend time understanding their experience. You can learn from your peers what did work and what did not and leverage this information to fine-tune your model.

Taking the time to run a trial period under real-life conditions and including all stakeholders is key to the success of the program. This will allow experience with the new model and give you and your team time to adopt it and become familiar with all related aspects. Special attention should be paid to the technical aspects of the model.

As part of a patient–provider relationship, your patients should have the choice between virtual visits and traveling to your site for an in-person visit. Nevertheless, the patient should be informed about the equivalence of both methods.

CONCLUSION

Sleep apnea is underdiagnosed, and only a fraction of sufferers have received diagnosis and treatment. Among barriers to diagnosis are access to care, awareness and knowledge about sleep disorders, and their treatment and related costs. In sleep medicine, telemedicine is applicable at each stage of patient management, from diagnosis to the monitoring of treatment. There are benefits to patients, physicians, and the health care system as a whole to embrace telemedicine in order to remove these barriers and improve health care access. Adoption of telemedicine for sleep medicine can work for the following:

- Patient–physician consultation in case of suspected sleep disorders
- Remote diagnostic testing
- Remote CPAP adherence monitoring
- Remote coaching to assist patients with adjusting CPAP device features and for troubleshooting common issues such as mask fit

Currently, the use of telemedicine in sleep medicine seems to be widely applied to the last two areas. In regions where distance between the patients and the sleep laboratories is a barrier, bidirectional communication is a useful feature, where telemedicine can be helpful in managing patient therapy by changing the applied CPAP remotely to adapt to the patient's status (weight change, switching from one type of mask to another, etc.). With imagination, many additional uses can be found for telemedicine in sleep medicine.

REFERENCES

1. Young, T., Peppard, P. E., & Gottlieb, D. J. (2002). Epidemiology of obstructive sleep apnea. *American Journal of Respiratory and Critical Care Medicine, 165,* 1217–1239.
2. Peppard, P. E., Young, T., Barnet, J. H., et al. (2013). Increased prevalence of sleep-disordered breathing in adults. *American Journal of Epidemiology, 177*(9), 1006–1014.
3. Gottlieb, D. J., Yenokyan, G., Newman, A. B., et al. (2010). Prospective study of obstructive sleep apnea and incident coronary heart disease and heart failure: The Sleep Heart Health Study. *Circulation, 122,* 352–360.
4. Gander, P. H., Marshall, N. S., Harris, R. B., et al. (2005). Sleep, sleepiness and motor vehicle accidents: A national survey. *Australian and New Zealand Journal of Public Health, 29,* 16–21.
5. Léger, D., Guilleminault, C., Bader, G., et al. (2002). Medical and socioprofessional impact of insomnia. *Sleep, 25,* 625–629.
6. Baldwin, C. M., Griffith, K. A., Nieto, F. J., et al. (2001). The association of sleep-disordered breathing and sleep symptoms with quality of life in the Sleep Heart Health Study. *Sleep, 24,* 96–105
7. Jaiswal, S. J., Owens, R. L., & Malhotra, A. (2017). Raising awareness about sleep disorders. *Lung India, 34*(3), 262–268.
8. Flodgren, G., Rachas, A., Farmer, A. J., et al. (2015). Interactive telemedicine: Effects on professional practice and health care outcomes. *The Cochrane Database of Systematic Reviews,* (9). doi:10.1002/14651858. CD002098.pub2
9. Cooper, C. B. (2009). Respiratory applications of telemedicine. *Thorax, 64,* 189–191.
10. Coma-del-Corral, M. J., Alonso-Álvarez, M. L., Allende, M., et al. (2013). Reliability of telemedicine in the diagnosis and treatment of sleep apnea syndrome. *Telemed Journal and E-Health, 19*(1), 7–12.
11. Borsini, E., Blanco, M., Bosio, M., et al. (2016). "Diagnosis of sleep apnea in network" respiratory polygraphy as a decentralization strategy. *Sleep Science, 9*(3), 244–248.
12. Singh, J., Badr, M. S., Diebert, W., et al. (2015). American Academy of Sleep Medicine (AASM) position paper for the use of telemedicine for the diagnosis and treatment of sleep disorders. *Journal of Clinical Sleep Medicine, 11*(10), 1187–1198.

13. Randerath, W., Bögel, M., Franke, C., et al. (2017). Position paper on telemonitoring in sleep-related breathing disorders [in German]. *Pneumologie, 71*(2), 81–85.

14. Kribbs, N. B., Pack, A. I., Kline, L. R., et al. (1993). Objective measurement of patterns of nasal CPAP use by patients with obstructive sleep apnea. *The American Review of Respiratory Disease, 147*(4), 887–895.

15. Isetta, V., Negrín, M. A., Monasterio, C., et al. (2015). A Bayesian cost-effectiveness analysis of a telemedicine-based strategy for the management of sleep apnoea: A multicentre randomised controlled trial. *Thorax, 70*(11), 1054–1061.

16. Fox, N., Hirsch-Allen, A. J., Goodfellow, E., et al. (2012). The impact of a telemedicine monitoring system on positive airway pressure adherence in patients with obstructive sleep apnea: A randomized controlled trial. *Sleep, 35*(4), 477–481.

17. Hwang, D., Chang, J. W., Benjafield, A. V., et al. (2018). Effect of telemedicine education and telemonitoring on continuous positive airway pressure adherence. The tele-OSA randomized trial. *American Journal of Respiratory and Critical Care Medicine, 197*(1), 117–126.

18. Munafo, D., Henver, W., Crocker, M., et al. (2016). A telehealth program for CPAP adherence reduces labor and yields similar adherence and efficacy when compared to standard of care. *Sleep Breath, 20*(2), 777–785.

SECTION 8
Pediatrics

chapter 60
Pediatric Polysomnography

JULIE DEWITTE · EMMANUEL (JOEL) PORQUEZ

LEARNING OBJECTIVES

On completion of this chapter, the reader should be able to:

1. Determine the special needs of the pediatric patient in performing sleep studies.
2. Identify the recommended hours of sleep in children and its importance for sleep stage development.
3. Implement age-appropriate techniques when applying electrodes to ensure a quality recording.
4. Understand the need for flexibility when performing pediatric sleep studies and the use of extra equipment, particularly CO_2 monitoring.

KEY TERMS

Polysomnography
Adenotonsillectomy
Capnography
End-tidal CO_2
Transcutaneous CO_2

HISTORY OF PEDIATRIC MEDICINE AND SLEEP DISORDERS

Consider that at the beginning of the 20th century children's health care was basically nonexistent. The physicians used the adult criteria for children, and at the turn of the 20th century, no more than 50 pediatric providers existed in the United States. Of these 50 providers, less than 12 limited their practice to be exclusive with children. The second half of the 20th century saw changes in priorities for pediatric disorders with the development of multi- and interdisciplinary approaches to diagnosing and treating children.

In 1953, eye movements in infant sleep were documented, and in 1958, rapid eye movement (REM) sleep and nonrapid eye movement sleep cycles were noted to occur throughout the sleep period. In 1972, Dr. Guilleminault managed uncontrolled hypertension in a 10-year-old boy by tracheostomy. This was the first identification of successful treatment of a comorbidity of obstructive sleep apnea in a human, and most remarkably, it occurred in a pediatric patient, not in an adult patient.

In 1971, *A Manual for Standardized Techniques and Criteria for Scoring of States of Sleep and Wakefulness in Newborn Infants* was published and it took another 42 years to develop criteria for all pediatric ages. Today there are criteria for infants older than 2 months till the attainment of puberty and updated criteria for infants younger than 2 months in the American Academy of Sleep Medicine's (AASM) *Manual for the Scoring of Sleep and Associated Events*.

Since the 2002 inception of sleep medicine as an independent specialty, the growth and awareness of sleep disorders has evolved; however, pediatric sleep disorders have not been a primary focus. Pediatric sleep medicine is an evolving field that requires further development and awareness (1).

THE PEDIATRIC PATIENT AND POLYSOMNOGRAPHY

Although originally developed for adults, polysomnography (PSG) was later adapted for the pediatric age group. Until recently, pediatric PSG has not been well standardized in obtaining sleep data, scoring, or interpretation. This changed in 2007 with the publication of the AASM scoring manual describing pediatric scoring criteria and the physiologic parameters typically measured.

PSG is considered the gold standard for testing children with suspected sleep-disordered breathing, which includes central and obstructive sleep apnea or hypoxemia. There are many nonrespiratory indications for pediatric PSG, including nocturnal seizures versus parasomnia, narcolepsy, and periodic limb movement disorder (2).

The criteria for acquiring data and pediatric scoring are quite different for infants younger than 2 months as well as for children and adolescents younger than 18 years. The pediatric sleep specialist may opt to use adult criteria for scoring respiratory events in children 13 years of age or older (3).

PSG is important in detecting and determining the severity of obstructive sleep apnea. Adenotonsillectomy may lead to significant improvement in sleep-disordered breathing in most pediatric patients; however, residual disease is present in a large proportion of children after surgery, particularly among older (>7 years) or obese children (4).

The acquisition process for pediatric PSG requires specially trained sleep technologists and extra equipment to obtain sleep data. Staffing ratios may be modified to meet the special needs of the pediatric population and may require one-to-one care, especially with infants, toddlers, and challenging patients.

Unlike adult studies, pediatric polysomnograms may require a lengthier setup time and a family-centered approach to meet the needs of the parent and child as well as modifications to standard sleep center policies and procedures. The goal is to obtain a quality study for physician interpretation with as little discomfort to the child as possible. Consideration must be given to the family bedtime routine, special needs, and possible stress levels of all involved. Simulating the child's home sleep environment may be helpful in facilitating sleep in an unfamiliar place. For instance, if the child typically cosleeps with the parent, it may be beneficial to allow this for children who are 12 months and older. Cosleeping ordinarily should not be permitted in the sleep center for infants less than 12 months of age, unless allowed to facilitate sleep onset, because of increased risk of sudden unexpected infant death to which sudden infant death syndrome (SIDS) is a subcategory. When appropriate, health care providers should be encouraged to discuss unsafe sleeping practices with the parents (recommended and nonrecommended sleeping positions, loose or soft bedding around the infant, etc.). Thoroughly document any unsafe sleeping practices identified during the sleep study (5).

Car seats should not be allowed in the sleep center as a sleeping device for infants. There is a high risk of death associated with infants sleeping in car seats because of asphyxiation. Infants are at risk for sliding down in the car seat and becoming entangled in the safety straps. Another potential risk is positional asphyxia (6). Sleep center personnel should teach parents about unsafe sleep practices and modifiable risk factors for the prevention of SIDS as outlined in the sleep center policy manual.

Infants and children generally have earlier bedtimes than teenagers and should sleep longer than adults. In 2016, the AASM published a consensus paper in the *Journal of Clinical Sleep Medicine* with sleep recommendations on the basis of evaluation of scientific evidence (Table 60-1) (7).

During the sleep study, it is best to coordinate "lights off" as close to the child's normal bedtime as possible to optimize data collection. Therefore, the setup process of placing electrodes should start earlier. Most sleep centers serving the pediatric age group schedule a technologist for a 12-hour shift, usually from 7 p.m. to 7 a.m. A technologist working earlier in the day can assist with setting up younger patients and infants who have an earlier bedtime or assist with those patients who might require extra assistance. Infants younger than 2 months typically have sleep-onset REM sleep, so it is important to get them to bed by their usual bedtime in order to capture all REM periods during the acquisition.

Technologists performing pediatric PSG should have experience in caring for pediatric patients of all ages. It is especially helpful for the technologist to have basic knowledge of common pediatric disorders such as Down syndrome, autism, and seizure disorders, as well as pulmonary diseases such as asthma and chronic lung disease. Sleep technologists who are experienced with pediatrics have learned various techniques that accommodate not only the age of the child but also their cognitive level. For instance, a child with Down syndrome may not tolerate anything placed on their face; however, if the child is given a small hand mirror so that they can see their reflection, applying electrodes becomes much easier because the child gets distracted. Another technique that may be useful is to allow the child to be involved with placing electrodes. Allowing the child to touch and feel the electrodes and even hand them to you may be beneficial because children like to help out with certain tasks. You can ask them which color of wire they want to put on first or if they want a sticker put on their stuffed animal or on the parent. It is generally a good idea to avoid asking "yes" or "no" questions because the child will probably say "no" to everything. Continued emphasis that they will not be hurt often puts the child at ease.

Table 60-1	Recommended Sleep Duration in the Pediatric Population

Age	Recommended Amount of Sleep in 24 Hours (Naps Included) (h)
0–3 mo	Not enough scientific evidence for consensus
4–12 mo	12–16
1–2 y	11–14
3–5 y	10–13
6–12 y	9–12
Teenagers, 13–18 y	8–10

From Paruthi, S., Brooks, L. J., D'Ambrosio, C., et al. (2016). Recommended amount of sleep for pediatric populations: A consensus statement of the American Academy of Sleep Medicine. *Journal of Clinical Sleep Medicine*, 12(6), 785–786.

There are various disorders seen only in pediatric sleep centers, which can add extra challenges to obtaining a high-quality acquisition. Technologists must have a great deal of patience and incorporate a family-centered approach to care in all situations. Age-specific care is highly important for the technologist to understand when caring for pediatric patients because there are different levels of age-specific care (e.g., neonate/infant, toddler/preschool, and adolescent). The sleep technologist must fully understand these different levels to appropriately interact with the patient (8). The family should also be involved in all aspects of the PSG process.

SLEEP CENTER ENVIRONMENT

There is no escaping the fact that a night in the sleep center will be different from a normal night's sleep at home. It is important for the technologist to understand that the relationship with the child and the family begins when they enter the sleep center. A distraught, unhappy child may be a challenge to all involved. Favorite items brought from home, such as a blanket, bedtime book, or stuffed animal, may provide relief during the process. Toddlers, on the contrary, may fare better if their focus is directed to other activities during the setup: watching an appropriate video, coloring, or reading a book with the parent. Practice age-specific care at all times. Nighttime awakenings, diaper changes, or feeding require parental attention, and sleep center staff should assist with navigation of the sensor wires during these times (9).

Children of different ages have different fears and concerns. Normal childhood anxieties include fear of strangers, separation anxiety, and fears not based in reality, such as monsters and ghosts. Given the normal childhood anxieties of being separated from their caregiver and fear of strangers, a young child would be terrified of waking up in an unfamiliar environment without the immediate reassurance of a parent. Although a child may developmentally progress past these age-appropriate fears, there can be a regression in stressful situations. In patients with complex medical histories who have frequent hospital encounters, this effect can be compounding. Younger children should be reassured that they will not be separated from their caregiver and that nothing will hurt them. Children seek safety, comfort, and protection from their caregiver. Older children, particularly adolescents, need to be assured of privacy and may not want the parent sleeping in the same room. However, a caregiver is required to stay in the sleep center with the patient for the duration of the study if they are under the age of 18. The caregiver is typically provided a recliner or bed to sleep on and discouraged from cosleeping.

DESENSITIZATION

For children with particular disabilities or behavioral issues, a desensitization appointment before the PSG may be beneficial to the success of the study. Desensitization for these patients is especially important before a continuous positive airway pressure (CPAP) titration. The desensitization assessment process will assist the technologist performing the study to be prepared in advance with helpful techniques.

A simple prestudy tour of the sleep center is helpful for all pediatric patients. The family should be given information explaining the PSG procedure, preparation for the study, and follow-up information. The prestudy tour will help reduce anxiety (for both the child and the parent) and assist the parent in bringing the proper necessities on the night of the study (bedclothes, DVD of favorite movie, etc.).

The desensitization process provides a brief practice session with some sensations the child would be exposed to during the study. A more extensive desensitization session might be needed especially if the child is in the sleep center for a positive airway pressure (PAP) titration. The process might be performed at a date before the scheduled sleep study or on the day of the study. This hopefully will ensure that the child will tolerate the study and maximize outcomes. Conducting the desensitization session in one of the rooms used for sleep studies will also help the child become more comfortable with the surroundings and the procedure. During the setup, allowing the child to apply sensors to the parent or to the doll may diminish apprehension or fascination with the unusual objects being presented.

Begin desensitization starting with the child's feet and working up to the head because most children seem to have the hardest time with head/face sensations. Let them feel the sensation of having an electrode site prepped and how it feels to have the electrode taped to their skin. Let the child feel and hold the nasal cannula before placing it by their nose. When fitting the CPAP mask, let the child hold and touch the mask so they know it will not harm them. Guide the patient's hand, while holding the mask, up over their nose and involve the parent by having them assist with this process. Allow the child to become comfortable with the mask before turning on the air pressure. Try to apply the headstraps as the last step so the child has some sense of control while adapting to the air pressure. The family can assist in the desensitization process by practicing at home, particularly with the nasal cannula and CPAP mask, which seem to be the most difficult items for children to tolerate. The desensitization process must remain flexible depending on the child's progress.

A Child-Friendly Environment

A child-friendly sleep center is important to the success of your pediatric program. A comforting environment for both the parent and the child is essential. Colorful wallpaper borders with a pediatric theme, rocking chairs, and toys are helpful. The rooms should be private with enough space to allow one parent to stay in the room with the child. Ensuring that the room is soundproof will eliminate noise from outside of the room (e.g., other patients crying), which can affect the sleep environment and quality of the acquisition. The parent should have a separate bed within the room, which could be a recliner chair or foldaway bed. Having snacks, diapers, and pediatric gowns available is helpful to parents who may have forgotten to bring these items with them to the sleep center. The appropriate bed size or crib should be available, keeping in mind the necessity of side rails for toddlers and children with special needs. Patients with physical disabilities may need a lift to assist with transfers from the wheelchair to the bed and should have easy access to a wheelchair-accessible restroom. Some patients may require equipment for nocturnal gastrostomy feedings. Caregivers should be informed in advance to bring any formula or medications to the sleep center that the patient normally takes at home. Inform the caregiver that they will also need to administer any medications, because this is not within the scope of practice of sleep technologists. If the patient is asthmatic and requires a nebulizer treatment, the parent will need to bring the equipment.

Staff members working in a pediatric sleep center must always be aware of environmental safety hazards, which include sharp objects and hazardous chemicals. All electrical outlets should have safety cover plugs. Equipment used during the acquisition process such as pulse oximeters, capnographs, and noninvasive ventilation units should all be kept out of the patient's reach and secured so that the child cannot pull it off of the shelf and injure themselves. Many items used during the sleep study can be a choking hazard, so a child should not be left unattended during the setup process. Toddlers could put items in their mouth because of their natural

curiosity and desire to explore their new environment. Beds and cribs must have side rails to avoid falls. Remember to look at the environment from a child's eyes and observe what could fall, be pulled down, or chewed. Even the fun stickers that are handed out as a reward to the child can be a choking hazard. A crash cart that is equipped for infants and pediatric patients should be available along with properly sized pediatric resuscitation equipment (10).

Nap Studies

Infants younger than 3 months have a cyclic sleeping pattern of 3 to 4 hours asleep with wakefulness for 1 to 2 hours. As the infant matures, the sleep cycles lengthen, with less sleep occurring during the daytime, usually around 6 months of age (11).

For evaluation of infants, a daytime nap study is appropriate to evaluate breathing and oxygen saturation as long as they sleep sufficiently. An adequate nap study will typically include about 4 hours of sleep with consolidated sleep and observation of REM sleep.

ESSENTIAL RECORDING ELEMENTS

Pediatric Considerations

As previously discussed, the sleep center environment, parents, and children should be prepared appropriately to obtain a successful pediatric PSG. Efforts should be made to meet the needs of the parents and child. Anticipating the child's needs can reduce stress and anxiety for everyone involved.

Before the patient's arrival, prepare the room and determine the type of bed the patient needs, either a crib for infants and toddlers or a bed with side rails for young children or those with special needs. It is important to have a parent bed or recliner in the same room throughout the study. A rocking chair is also useful for parents of infants and toddlers who may need to be held during the hookup, comforted, or fed during the night.

Capnography

In 2007, the *AASM Manual for the Scoring of Sleep and Associated Events* first clearly described the technical requirements for pediatric PSG. For patients younger than 13 years, carbon dioxide (CO_2) monitoring, either transcutaneous or end-tidal, is recommended by the AASM. Capnography is a noninvasive way to measure the adequacy of ventilation during sleep. Both methods are acceptable noninvasive methods for assessing alveolar hypoventilation. Measuring CO_2 is a useful assessment tool in children with chronic lung disease, those on ventilatory support, or when initiating supplemental oxygen during a PSG. Some patients may be dependent on their hypoxic respiratory drive, and the initiation of oxygen without monitoring CO_2 may lead to worsening hypoventilation. Sleep is normally associated with an increased transcutaneous CO_2 (tcCO_2) level of approximately 4 to 6 mm Hg (12).

End-Tidal CO_2

End-tidal CO_2 (EtCO_2) can be measured using a sidestream nasal cannula or directly from a tracheostomy or an endotracheal tube. EtCO_2 measurements are subject to breath-to-breath fluctuations and may be affected by varying respiratory patterns such as tachypnea, sighs, or mouth breathing. Measurement of end-tidal fluctuations can also be used as an "alternative" channel for scoring respiratory events according to the AASM scoring manual. For mouth-breathers, signals may be obtained by placing the sampling cannula over the patient's mouth. Vigilance by the technologist is necessary to keep the sampling lines open because these lines may become occluded on account of humidity and patient secretions, which may affect accuracy.

Because of breath-to-breath variability, EtCO_2 values should be assessed as a percentage of total sleep time with hypercapnia rather than isolated peak values during the night. The values obtained using EtCO_2 monitoring must be evaluated very carefully and require a good signal plateau to be accurate. A poor-quality signal plateau will show a lower than actual CO_2 reading, which may occur in patients with nasal obstruction, mouth breathing, nasal cannula delivery of supplemental oxygen, technical issues with placement of EtCO_2 cannula, and severe chronic obstructive lung disease (13).

Transcutaneous CO_2

Monitoring of tcCO_2 is accomplished using a CO_2 measurement obtained through the skin, and it closely mimics arterial CO_2. The transcutaneous electrode warms the skin surface, increasing local capillary perfusion, and measures the CO_2 as it diffuses from the dermis across a gas-permeable membrane. Where end-tidal monitoring has breath-to-breath variability, transcutaneous measurements tend to respond more slowly (2 minutes or more) and demonstrate a trending pattern. tcCO_2 monitoring is valuable in patients who have interstitial lung disease (a group of rare lung diseases) where EtCO_2 is not accurate (14). tcCO_2 monitoring is also beneficial during PAP titration. With children using CPAP, the use of tcCO_2 monitoring is preferred because

the end-tidal sampling cannula is typically removed during a PAP titration.

Care must be taken to prevent possible skin burns caused by the heat emitted by the electrode. Most tcCO_2 monitors allow for variable temperature settings, which impacts the duration that the sensor can be safely left on one skin site and making it less likely to cause harm. It is essential to follow the manufacturer's safety recommendations regarding temperature settings, particularly when testing young children. Adherence to the manufacturer's instructions for proper calibration and electrode maintenance will maximize optimal electrode performance, accuracy, and safety.

Audio and Video Recordings

The ability to record high-quality audio and video recordings during an acquisition is essential for observation of sleep behaviors and to accurately evaluate the child's activity. An infrared light source is essential when viewing and recording the patient inside a dark room. There are several behavioral parameters that can be monitored via video during a PSG that include body position, respiratory patterns, breathing sounds (e.g., snoring, stridor, catathrenia), possible seizure activity, bruxism, and other parasomnias. The technologist must remain attentive and ready to adjust the camera as needed to capture the patient's behavior. The technologist must also document their observations to further assist the physician in making a diagnosis. Videotaping unusual parental interactions may also present opportunities for education, particularly in relation to inappropriate practices (e.g., placing the infant in a prone position and bottle propping).

Video data must be synchronized with the PSG data. With today's technology, the majority of acquisition systems have the ability to record the video digitally. Cameras with pan–tilt–zoom capability (as opposed to a single, fixed focal point) enable the technologist to frame the patient for a better recording image and follow active sleepers as they move in the bed or crib. Zooming in can be useful for highlighting the respiratory patterns and observing nasal flaring, retractions, mouth breathing, or paradoxical respiratory effort. High-resolution video should be used to record the child's behavior, keeping in mind that high-resolution recording will result in larger electronic file size and increase data storage requirements.

Electrode and Sensor Placement Adjustments

As infants vary in shapes and sizes, these little patients require slight adjustments when placing specific electrodes. Placement adjustments must be properly documented. Smaller head size often requires slight modifications when placing electrodes on the scalp and face. The distance between the chin electromyogram (EMG) leads in small children should be reduced from 2 to 1 cm. Electrooculographic (EOG) leads may need to be placed 0.5 cm from the outer canthus instead of 1 cm as recommended in adults (3, p. 33).

Standard 10-mm electroencephalogram (EEG) electrodes may also be too large for neonates; therefore, using 6-mm electrodes is recommended. A poorly positioned effort belt may lead to positional artifact because of slippage or may miss paradoxical breathing if the belts are too loose or too tight.

Electrode and Sensor Placement

Using an age-appropriate child-friendly approach may help in overcoming some of the challenges of placing electrodes and sensors. Because the child is a minor (<18 years of age), it should not be separated from its caregiver. Electrodes and sensors should be applied in a position that is comfortable for the child and technologist. Usually, the ideal position for an older pediatric patient is sitting up. Sitting allows the child to maintain a sense of control and security, whereas laying a child down creates a sense of vulnerability. It is imperative that the setup position is ergonomically comfortable for the technologist and may require raising the bed or having a taller chair available for the child and/or caregiver to sit on. Sensor application for an infant is normally performed with the infant lying down in a crib or being held by the parent or guardian.

The order in which electrodes are placed may also lower the child's anxiety and improve the level of cooperation by earning the patient's trust. Start with the least threatening sensors like leg leads and respiratory effort belts. This allows the child to see and touch the equipment and can satisfy its curiosity. Some children realize that nothing will hurt them after touching or holding the electrodes. Sensors that are poorly tolerated, like the EEG, EMG, EOG leads, nasal pressure/EtCO$_2$ cannula, and thermistor, should be placed at the end of the setup process, saved to the very last, or placed when the child falls asleep.

Electrodes well-placed with optimal contact to the skin are essential for obtaining artifact-free signals. Proper electrode placement also minimizes the need for adjusting filters unnecessarily or rereferencing channels. Skin oils, as well as dead or dry skin cells, can act as barriers to electrical conduction. If the infant has cradle cap, lotion, or possibly baby oil on their skin, it may interfere with electrical conduction and electrode adherence. Electrode sites are prepped using a fine-particle mild abrasive skin preparation product. Gentle scrubbing in one direction will avoid possible irritation of the skin. After prepping, skin should be wiped with a gauze pad before placing the electrode. Extra care should be taken in handling infants and while placing electrodes on the head because the anterior fontanelles on top of the head are often soft. When prepping the scalp, the technologist must remember not to press too hard and to prep and attach electrodes as gently as possible. The anterior fontanelle is often small by 6 months of age and usually closes between 10 and 20 months (15).

The International 10–20 system for electrode placement is the same in children as it is for adults. A nontoxic water-soluble color marker is typically used for marking the scalp when measuring the head. Allowing the child to participate by choosing a color will engage the child and create a sense of control, keeping the process fun.

EEG electrodes should be applied to the scalp using a conduction paste, which has both adhesive and conductive qualities. The conduction paste should be hypoallergenic and water soluble. To secure the electrode to the scalp, a small square of gauze with a dab of conduction paste can be used to cover and adhere the electrode to the patient's scalp. The use of collodion is usually not advised for the pediatric population. Collodion has a strong odor, is highly flammable, and must be used in a well-ventilated room. Because children often move a lot, there is a risk of accidents and spills. Collodion should especially be avoided in children diagnosed with respiratory illnesses like asthma.

Once the technologist has completed the setup, securing the electrode wires will reduce the possibility of leads being removed throughout the night. Infants and toddlers can be active sleepers, so proactively securing electrodes and sensors anticipating possible movements, such as rolling or standing in a crib, is time well spent. Parents handling their child during diaper changes, bottle feeding, and burping can also affect electrode placement and increase the likelihood of electrodes coming off. Electrode wires should be gathered together in ponytail fashion at the base of the neck and bundled with tape, Posey straps, or wire covers. Socks can be used to cover the hands of infants, allowing them to move freely and not grab the electrode wires. Wrapping the child's head with gauze is another way to secure the EEG electrodes, which makes the wires less accessible to curious fingers. Wrapping of the head should not be excessive, because undesirable effects such as sweat artifact and electrode popping may result. Excessive wrapping of the head may also make it difficult to reach the scalp. Alternatively, a piece of tubular stretch mesh stockinette can be placed over the scalp area of the child's head. The mesh material permits better air circulation, keeps the head cooler, and allows easier access to the electrodes.

Pediatric Recording Parameters

The physiologic parameters measured during a pediatric PSG are similar to those of adult studies with a few exceptions. The elements of a pediatric montage are

Table 60-2 Suggested Polysomnography Montage

Signal	Measured Parameters
EEG derivations	F4-M1, F3-M2
	C4-M1, C3-M2
	O2-M1, O1-M2
EOG derivations	E1-M2
	E2-M2
ECG	Lead II
Chin EMG	Mentalis and submentalis muscles
Leg EMG	Anterior tibialis muscle
Nasal pressure	Nasal air pressure transducer
Oronasal airflow	Oronasal thermal sensor
Respiratory effort: chest and abdominal wall motion	Dual thoracoabdominal RIP belts or esophageal manometry
Capnography	End-tidal and/or transcutaneous
Snore	Snore sensor
Oxygen saturation	SpO2
Body position	Body position sensor
Audio and video recordings	Time synchronized with polysomnography data

ECG, electrocardiogram; EEG, electroencephalogram; EMG, electromyogram; EOG, electrooculography; RIP, respiratory inductance plethysmography.

outlined in Table 60-2. In addition to the *recommended* EEG derivations F4-M1, C4-M1, and O2-M1, the contralateral electrodes, F3, C3, and O1, are referenced to M2 and added as backup sites in the event a *recommended* electrode becomes dislodged during the study. The extra electrodes provide the technologist with the flexibility to rereference electrodes and often prevents having to enter the child's room unnecessarily. Similarly, there is redundancy seen when measuring airflow. Airflow sensors include nasal pressure transducer, oronasal thermal airflow, RIPsum and RIPflow, and EtCO2. The technologist may not need to immediately replace a sensor that comes off when utilizing alternative respiratory sensors.

Equipment Adjustments Based on the Age of Child

Sleep centers performing pediatric sleep studies must have various types and sizes of equipment readily available. Sensors should be specifically designed for pediatric patients rather than modified adult sensors. Ill-fitting sensors may be poorly tolerated and produce a lesser-quality signal. Adult cannulas for measuring nasal pressure or EtCO2 monitoring may have prongs that are too long and wide to accurately sample lower pressure or CO2 fluctuations sometimes seen in pediatric patients. Adult respiratory effort belts are usually wider than pediatric belts and may yield dampened signals. Pediatric oximeter sensors are designed specifically for a child's small finger or toe to provide a "snug" fit. Proper use and fit of pediatric oximetry sensors will reduce motion artifact and the chance of the sensor falling off.

Similar to adult PSG, having a well-thought-out plan with deliberate application of electrodes ensures a high-quality acquisition. Making recording parameter changes to clean up recording artifacts is not recommended. For example, increasing the low-frequency filter to 1 Hz will reduce slow-wave artifact and respiratory sway artifact that degrades slow-wave EEG signals, but this is not recommended. Excellent electrode and sensor application is the best approach. The PSG system should have the ability to adjust sensitivity/gain settings to accommodate the high-amplitude EEG signals characteristic of pediatric waveforms. This is an acceptable, often necessary, setting change to record a readable EEG in infants and young children.

The AASM recommends a minimum sampling rate of 200 Hz and ideally 500 Hz (see Table 60-3) for EEG. For more detailed EEG analysis, higher sampling rates and high-frequency filter (HFF) settings are desirable. For accurate EEG representation, the sampling rate should be at least three times the frequency of the fastest signal to be recorded. For recording seizure activity, higher sampling rates of 500 to 1,000 Hz are recommended in conjunction with HFF settings of 70 to 75 Hz.

The frequency of waveforms often increases as the child grows and develops. From infancy to childhood, EEG patterns will vary at different growth phases. Differentiating age-related morphology makes scoring pediatric sleep more challenging. Primarily, the background rhythms in pediatric EEGs are of higher amplitude than those seen in adults and are prone to waveform blocking and signal channel overlap. Reducing sensitivity settings may be necessary to preserve waveform reconstruction.

Expanded Montage

A sleep EEG montage corresponds to the underlying area of the cerebral cortex specific to sleep stage activity. Although it is common to capture seizure activity during a PSG, the modified EEG montage used in a PSG is often missing channels helpful in differentiating seizures versus nonepileptic events (16). The addition of temporal leads T3 and T4 improves the accuracy of detecting temporal lobe seizure, and using 7 and 18 channels of

Table 60-3 AASM-Recommended Technical Specifications (3)

| Type | Sampling Rates | | Low-Frequency Filter (Hz) | High-Frequency Filter (Hz) |
	Desirable (Hz)	Minimal (Hz)		
EEG	500	200	0.3	35
EOG	500	200	0.3	35
EMG	500	200	10	100
ECG	500	200	0.3	70
Snore	500	200	10	100
Nasal pressure	100	25	0.1	15
Airflow	100	25	0.1	15
Thoracoabdominal movements	100	25	0.1	15
EMG	200	500	10	100
Oximetry	25	10	N/A	N/A
Body position	1	1	N/A	N/A
Esophageal pressure	100	25	N/A	N/A
Capnography[a]	100	25	N/A	N/A

[a]Not specified by the AASM.
AASM, American Academy of Sleep Medicine; ECG, electrocardiogram; EEG, electroencephalogram; EMG, electromyogram; EOG, electrooculography.

EEG has the best sensitivity for seizure detection. However, frontal lobe seizure detection is not affected by the number of channels used (17).

As a minimal testing requirement, the American Clinical Neurophysiology Society guidelines require all 21 electrodes of the International 10–20 system and standard adult montages be used (18, 19). PSG equipment should be able to record the expanded EEG montage as well as standard channels for the detection of sleep apnea, periodic limb movements, and parasomnias. A qualified neurologist should determine the appropriate seizure montage to be used and ideally interpret the EEG.

With patience, perseverance, and perhaps the help of a caregiver or additional technologist, sensors and electrodes can be successfully applied to almost all patients. However, for some patients, it may be neither possible nor realistic to apply or maintain all the electrodes and sensors needed for a standard PSG. Cerebral palsy patients, for example, may have spastic motor activity, sustained muscle contractions, and uncontrolled head movements that prohibit complete sensor application. Children with autism, Down syndrome, and Asperger syndrome often have sensory integration dysfunction. They can be hypersensitive to sensory stimulation, particularly tactile, touch involved with head measurements, pressure of scalp scrubbing, the wetness of the prep product. To reduce trauma to the patient, caregiver, and technologist, an alternate montage may yield limited but useful data. Patients with mental retardation may have associated circadian desynchrony because of the inability to process normal zeitgebers. For these patients, EEG data have limited utility; therefore, a respiratory-oriented montage may yield more relevant data. The sleep center should have policies and procedures regarding the use of alternate montages, indications, physician orders, and the minimum channels required to record data.

Biocalibrations

Before lights out, biocalibrations should be performed to confirm accurate sensor responsiveness. Table 60-4 shows the recommended biocalibration commands and corresponding sensors.

Cooperation will vary greatly depending on the child's level of comprehension, temperament, and mental and physical development. Some children may not be able to complete all or any of the biocalibrations. Creativity and use of age-appropriate terminology may be needed to elicit the desired biocalibration response.

Table 60-4 Biocalibration Commands and Affected Sensors

Command	Sensor
Eyes open, eyes closed	O1 and O2
Eyes up, eyes down	REOG and LEOG
Eyes left, eyes right	REOG and LEOG
Jaw clench or smile	Chin EMG
Count aloud or snore	Snore microphone
Nose breathe, mouth breathe	Thermistor and nasal pressure
Big breath and hold	Respiratory effort belts Thermistor and nasal pressure
Move left foot, move right foot	Left and right leg EMG

EMG, electromyogram; LEOG, left electrooculography; REOG, right electrooculography.

For example, a few rounds of "peek-a-boo" can produce open and closed eyes. Moving a penlight or flashlight beam on the ceiling or a toy in the child's vision field can help track their eyes in the desired direction. Biting down like your chewing gum may simulate jaw-clenching. With pediatric patients, the usual adult biocalibrations are used; however, infants require a thorough documentation of observations because they are incapable of following biocalibration instructions.

Recording Duration

As mentioned earlier, within the pediatric age group, recommended sleep duration ranges from 12 to 16 hours per day for infants, 10 to 12 hours for children, and 8 to 10 hours for teenagers. "Lights out" for a pediatric polysomnogram should start at or near the child's normal bedtime as much as possible. Because the pediatric patient goes to bed earlier and sometimes sleeps later, it is common for the PSG to last more than 7 hours, and the child's last REM cycle should be captured before ending the study.

Behavior Observations and Documentation

As with all other aspects of pediatric PSG, sleep behaviors may vary as the child grows and develops. Behavioral observations are an important aspect of the PSG and provide additional information about the child's sleep quality and respiratory patterns. Observations and time of occurrence should be documented by the technologist and captured on video. Observations commonly include respiratory changes (paradoxical breathing, mouth breathing, snoring, wheezing, gasping), positional changes, and parasomnias. Behavioral characteristics are used in determining infant wake and sleep cycles because their brain waves are not fully developed. For example, wakefulness is identified when the eyes are open or there is obvious crying; scanning eye movements and brief eye closure may occur with crying. Sleep is identified when the eyes are closed, fewer body movements are occurring, and possibly sucking or snoring sounds are present. It is important to be vigilant with infant observations and thoroughly document all behaviors such as grimacing, hiccups, and startle jerk.

SUMMARY

Pediatric overnight PSG is a common procedure and remains the gold standard for identifying sleep-disordered breathing in children. Although challenges often occur with either the patient or the caregiver, the pediatric PSG can be successfully performed with minimal stress when the technologist is properly prepared for the unexpected. Keys to success are (1) anticipation and advance preparation for the child and caregiver's basic needs based on the child's age, development, and any special needs; (2) a family-centered approach: engaging the child and caregiver in the process, including prestudy education, a sleep center tour, the hookup process, and using age-appropriate distractors; (3) extra attention to securing sensors; and (4) a high level of vigilance and responsiveness to recognize and replace sensors when appropriate and accurately documenting behavioral observations.

REFERENCES

1. Kryger, M. H. (2014). Differential diagnosis of pediatric sleep disorders. In S. H. Sheldon, R. Ferber, M. H. Kryger, et al. (Eds.), *Principles and practice of pediatric sleep medicine* (2nd ed., pp. 13–16, chap. 2). Philadelphia, PA: Elsevier Saunders.
2. DelRosso, L. M. (2017). Case 4: Overview of pediatric polysomnography: A newborn infant with snoring and witnessed apnea (Section 2). In L. M. DelRosso, R. B. Berry, S. E. Beck, et al. (Eds.), *Pediatric sleep pearls* (pp. 10–11). Philadelphia, PA: Elsevier.
3. Berry, R. B., Albertario, C. L., Harding, S. M., et al.; for the American Academy of Sleep Medicine. (2018). *The AASM manual for the scoring of sleep and associated events: Rules, terminology and technical specifications* (Version 2.5). Darien, IL: American Academy of Sleep Medicine.

4. Bhattacharjee, R., Kheirandish-Gozal, L., Spruyt, K., et al. (2010). Adenotonsillectomy outcomes in treatment of obstructive sleep apnea in children: A multicenter retrospective study. *American Journal of Respiratory and Critical Care Medicine, 182*(5), 676–683.

5. Moon, R. Y.; Task Force on Sudden Infant Death Syndrome. (2016). SIDS and other sleep-related infant deaths 2016 updated recommendations for a safe infant sleeping environment. *Pediatrics, 138*(5). doi:10.1542/peds.2016-2940

6. Batra, E. K., Midgett, J. D., & Moon, R. Y. (2015). Hazards associated with sitting and carrying devices for children two years and younger. *Journal of Pediatrics, 167*(1), 183–187.

7. Paruthi, S., Brooks, L. J., D'Ambrosio, C., et al. (2016). Recommended amount of sleep for pediatric populations: A consensus statement of the American Academy of Sleep Medicine. *Journal of Clinical Sleep Medicine, 12*(6), 785–786.

8. American Association of Sleep Technologists. (2017, June). *Sleep technology: Core competency.* Chicago, IL: Author.

9. Beck, S. E., & Marcus, C. M. (2009). Pediatric polysomnography. *Clinical Sleep Medicine, 4*(3), 393–406.

10. Zaremba, E. K., Barkey, M. E., Mesa, C., et al. (2005). Making polysomnography more "child friendly:" A family-centered care approach. *Clinical Sleep Medicine, 1*(2), 189–198.

11. Wagner, M. H. (2017). Case 10: A 2-month-old infant with sleep-onset REM period on polysomnography (Section 3). In L. M. DelRosso, R. B. Berry, S. E. Beck, et al. (Eds.), *Pediatric sleep pearls* (pp. 27–28). Philadelphia, PA: Elsevier.

12. Kacmarek, R. M., Stoller, J. K., & Heuer, A. J. (2013). Analysis and monitoring of gas exchange. In *Egan's fundamentals of respiratory care* (10th ed.). St. Louis, MO: Elsevier.

13. DelRosso, L. M. (2017). Case 6: A 14-year-old with an abnormal end-trial CO_2 waveform during polysomnography (Section 2). In L. M. DelRosso, R. B. Berry, S. E. Beck, et al. (Eds.), *Pediatric sleep pearls* (pp. 16–19). Philadelphia, PA: Elsevier.

14. Katz, E. S., & Marcus, C. L. (2014). Diagnosis of obstructive sleep apnea. In S. H. Sheldon, R. Ferber, M. H. Kryger, et al. (Eds.), *Principles and practice of pediatric sleep medicine* (2nd ed., p. 225). Philadelphia, PA: Elsevier Saunders.

15. Larsen, P. D., & Stensaas, S. S. (n.d.). *Pediatric neurologic exam—6 months.* Retrieved from http://library.med.utah.edu/pedineurologicexam/html/06month.html. Updated August 2016. Accessed November 22, 2018.

16. Foldvary-Schaefer, N., De Ocampo, J., Mascha, E., et al. (2006). Accuracy of seizure detection using abbreviated EEG during polysomnography. *Journal of Clinical Neurophysiology, 23*(1), 68–71.

17. Foldvary, N., Caruso, A. C., Mascha, E., et al. (2000). Identifying montages that best detect electrographic seizure activity during polysomnography. *Sleep, 23*(2), 221–229.

18. Jasper, H. H. (1958). The Ten-Twenty Electrode System of the International Federation. *Electroencephalography and Clinical Neurophysiology, 10*, 371–375.

19. Kuratani, J., Pearl, P. L., Sullivan, L., et al. (2016), American Clinical Neurophysiology Society guideline 5: Minimum technical standards for pediatric electroencephalography. *Journal of Clinical Neurophysiology, 33*, 320–323.

chapter 61

Pediatric Scoring

TIM A. STATZA

LEARNING OBJECTIVES

On completion of this chapter, the reader should be able to:

1. Describe the stages of sleep in infants and children.
2. Recognize the differing characteristics in polysomnogram tracings between an infant, a child, and an adult study.
3. State the age criteria for infant and pediatric scoring rules.
4. Explain the importance of technologist notes during pediatric studies.
5. Recognize respiratory events in the pediatric patient.
6. Know what to look for in pediatric patients when marking arousals.
7. Identify cardiac dysrhythmias common to the pediatric patient.
8. Describe common artifacts in pediatric sleep studies.
9. Explain the limitations of limited channel sleep studies in children.
10. List the elements of the summary report in pediatric polysomnograms.
11. Describe common challenges in scoring pediatric studies.

KEY TERMS

Hypnagogic hypersynchrony
Dominant posterior rhythm (DPR)
Tracé alternant
Tracé discontinue
Stage W (Wakefulness)
Stage R (REM)
Stage N (NREM)
Stage T (Transitional)
Dysrhythmias
Supraventricular tachycardia

Sleep disorders are extremely common during childhood. Unfortunately, even with the prevalence of sleep problems and despite being either preventable or treatable, childhood sleep disorders often go underrecognized and undiagnosed. There are many reasons for this, but the fact remains that children are not receiving the attention they need when it comes to sleeping. Proper restorative sleep for children is critical for their development, and quality sleep for a child is just as important, if not more so, than it is for adults. Even though sleep disorders are prevalent in children, the majority of the literature regarding sleep testing primarily covers adult disorders. Despite the massive amount of research on pediatric sleep disorders, which grows by the day, the pediatric content in most sleep medicine textbooks receives very limited coverage. Published in 1968, *A Manual of Standardized Terminology, Techniques, and Scoring System for Sleep Stages of Human Subjects* standardized sleep stage scoring in adults; pediatrics was not addressed in the manual. In 1971, a committee cochaired by Drs. Anders, Emde, and Parmelee authored *A Manual for Standardized Techniques and Criteria for Scoring of States of Sleep and Wakefulness in Newborn Infants*. Not addressed in that publication were standards for evaluating sleep in older infants, toddlers, children, and preadolescents.

In the last few decades, standards for pediatric sleep testing have received increased attention. In 2007, the American Academy of Sleep Medicine (AASM) published *The AASM Manual for the Scoring of Sleep and Associated Events: Rules, Terminology, and Technical Specifications*. This manual includes sections on sleep staging and respiratory rules for pediatric patients. In 2011, the AASM published *Respiratory Indications for Polysomnography in Children: An Evidence-Based Review* to help sleep specialists determine the appropriateness of ordering a sleep study in children. Standards for staging and scoring pediatric studies have evolved since 2007. With several revisions in the last few years and updated regularly, the *AASM Scoring Manual* is frequently redefining and issuing improved rules for pediatrics.

Sleep architecture changes significantly over the first two decades of life. Sleep patterns and sleep behaviors evolve and are modified by both "intrinsic" (e.g., normal development) and "extrinsic" (e.g., environment and parenting practices) processes as we progress from infancy to childhood and through adolescence. This chapter will discuss the developmental issues inherent when performing pediatric sleep studies as related to both sleep staging and respiratory event scoring. It will review the current scoring rules implemented by the AASM and how to apply these rules for pediatric patients. This chapter will focus on differences between adults and children as they apply to performing and scoring pediatric polysomnography. Techniques used to identify staging and events specific to children will be included. The goal is to provide an overall enhanced appreciation regarding the complexities involved with pediatric sleep scoring.

THE PEDIATRIC DIFFERENCE

Even though most of what is written about sleep medicine concerns adults and their disorders, children experience the same broad range of sleep disorders encountered in adults, including sleep apnea, insomnia, parasomnias, delayed sleep–wake phase disorder, narcolepsy, and restless legs syndrome. In fact, a pediatric sleep center will encounter a diverse population of disorders on a more regular basis than the typical breathing and arrhythmia disorders seen in an adult sleep center. Sometimes labeled the same in adults and children, the clinical presentation, evaluation, and management of some disorders may differ significantly. For example, an adult with obstructive sleep apnea (OSA) may present with excessive sleepiness and lethargy, whereas a child with OSA could present with hyperactivity and restlessness, sometimes labeled incorrectly as attention-deficit hyperactivity disorder. Although snoring and sleep apnea are common indications for referral to a sleep specialist, many children also have a behavioral or nonrespiratory sleep disorder either as another comorbid diagnosis or as a primary sleep disorder. In addition and similar to adults, children are increasingly prescribed medications that affect their sleep, making treatment more complicated (1).

Scoring pediatric sleep studies is a challenging experience, but so can be performing sleep studies on pediatric patients. Most adult sleep centers are not properly suited to treating young children. A pediatric sleep center needs an atmosphere designed with the child in mind. There should be child-pleasing surroundings and decorations that help soothe and distract. Well-trained sleep center staff are necessary to care for the pediatric population. To be prepared, staff must be well informed regarding the variances in development not only physically, but also mentally with the age and medical condition of each patient. Competent pediatric sleep technologists understand proper distraction techniques, and they are provided the tools needed to perform this function well for each patient. It is also helpful to have the parent or caregiver involved to make the testing go smoothly. There should be accommodations for the parent or caregiver to stay in the room with the child. Furthermore, consider the testing equipment. It is best if the monitoring equipment is contained outside the bedroom or in a cabinet hidden from view, as it can seem intimidating to a child. As much as possible, keep equipment and supplies away from the reach of the curious child.

The physical and anatomic differences between younger children and older adults are obvious, but also consider mental development before performing a sleep study. It is best practice to have the child seen by a pediatric sleep specialist who can review the history and symptoms in a clinical setting. The sleep specialist has the opportunity to assess for and prioritize the various sleep concerns before ordering appropriate testing. Pediatric sleep studies can be "customized" on the basis of the child's symptoms. An enuresis alarm, esophageal pressure monitoring, pH recording, and seizure montage are some of the additional monitoring tools often added for pediatric testing. At this time, it may be determined that a sleep diary or actigraphy monitoring is essential to collect additional information on sleep behavior. Some children and their families find it helpful to visit the sleep center before the actual study. This is often possible during the clinic visit and should be encouraged. Making the surroundings friendly and familiar to the child increases compliance during the night of the study.

It is best practice to have a prescreening tool in place to assess the child's needs and developmental level. Information gathered at the clinic visit and during the scheduling portion is helpful in predicting what to expect on the night of the study. By the day of the study, staff should be aware of the patient's needs for testing and preparation in staffing adjusted so it is appropriate for difficult or medically complex children. On the night of the study, schedule the family to arrive at the sleep center early enough so that the study begins as close as possible to the child's normal bedtime. Children are encouraged to bring any favorite toys, pillows, and even videos that will make their stay in the sleep center more comfortable. To help children and parents feel more comfortable, show them the area where the parent or caregiver is to stay overnight. During the stay, involving the parent or caregiver as much as possible will enhance the experience of the child and create a more peaceful experience.

Many adult sleep centers have a protocol of performing a split-night test, in which the first part of the night is diagnostic to determine if the patient has sleep-disordered breathing or other events affecting sleep. If the study uncovers events that warrant positive airway pressure (PAP) treatment, then a titration study is performed the second part of the night. In pediatrics, there is a concern that a shortened study may underestimate the degree of sleep-disordered breathing in children. Most often, respiratory events increase in frequency or become more severe as the night progresses and the child spends more time in rapid eye movement (REM) sleep. It is highly recommended to perform a baseline study for an entire night to get a full appreciation of the child's sleep-disordered breathing. In addition, from a practical standpoint, many children with OSA do not require PAP treatment. Instead, children with sleep apnea typically receive referrals to an otolaryngologist for consideration of an adenotonsillectomy. If it is decided that a titration study is needed, it will be performed on another night, preferably after the child has undergone a desensitization period with the PAP mask. Then when the child returns for his or her PAP study, it will allow the technologist a full night to properly titrate the patient and find the correct pressure.

Proper application of the electroencephalogram (EEG) electrodes and other monitoring leads is critical to acquiring a quality sleep study in children, and it lays the foundation for quality scoring. There are many techniques available to help the child feel comfortable and be cooperative while applying electrodes. In spite of this if the child adamantly refuses to allow the sensors to be applied, the technologist may, depending on the type of study to be performed, allow the child to first fall asleep without applying the full montage. At times, adding the additional electrodes and sensors after the child has entered deep delta sleep results in better impedances, improving the quality of the study collected for scoring.

Performing patient calibrations is another important step in performing quality sleep studies and aids the technologist in proper scoring. Because of their lack of a clear alpha pattern, it is especially important to obtain a lengthy sample baseline of wake EEG in children. This recording portion is helpful during staging of the study as a reference to aid in determining wake versus sleep. Calibrations can be difficult, if not impossible, in the noncompliant or very young child. There are a variety of methods that can be used depending on the situation. One technique to obtain calibrations in this population is with the assistance of another technologist or parent. For instance, to check electrooculogram (EOG) waveforms, the assistant or parent can move an object back and forth for the child to track with the eyes, and leg movement calibrations can be done with the assistant flexing the child's foot when instructed.

One important respiratory measurement collected routinely in pediatric studies and typically not recorded in adult studies is carbon dioxide (CO_2) monitoring obtained through either end-tidal CO_2 nasal cannula or placement of a transcutaneous CO_2 monitor. Because of airflow concerns, using transcutaneous CO_2 monitoring at times may be more beneficial, especially with infants or children on positive pressure ventilation. In addition to providing another assessment of air exchange, end-tidal CO_2 measurements allow for the detection and quantification of hypoventilation, often more commonly seen in children than in adults.

IDENTIFYING SLEEP STAGES IN INFANTS AND CHILDREN

Newborn infants or neonates do not have the fully developed sleep stages as those seen in adults. Infants have a *dominant posterior rhythm* (DPR) EEG pattern slower than that seen with adults who have an 8- to 13-Hz alpha rhythm (Fig. 61-1). The DPR in most normal children develops as they grow, changing from a 3.5- to 4.5-Hz

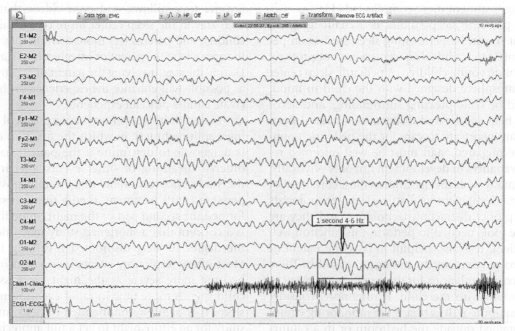

Figure 61-1 Dominant posterior rhythm in a 3-month-old.

rhythmic activity at 3 to 4 months postterm to a 5- to 6-Hz activity by 6 months of age. EEG activity is generally 7 Hz by 1 year of age. Vertex sharp waves develop at 2 months and are more noticeable in children after the age of 3. Sleep spindles can be seen by 2 months postterm. K-complexes seen as early as 3 months are usually present by 6 months of age, as is slow-wave activity. At 2 years of age, both sleep spindles and K-complexes appear similar to those seen in adults. Infants 2 months or older postterm typically can be staged using W, N1, N2, N3, and R stages (Table 61-1) (2, 3).

There is a period when some infants will not have developed all the well-defined characteristics of nonrapid eye movement (NREM) sleep stages as seen in N1, N2, and N3. Sleep spindles, K-complexes, or slow-wave sleep may not be easily recognizable in the EEG waveform for these infants. During this time, the epochs that do not meet the criteria for stages W, N1, N2, or N3 are scored as stage N (NREM). The rules state that if all the epochs of NREM sleep in an infant study show no sign of sleep spindles, K-complexes, or high-amplitude slow-wave sleep, then score all these epochs as stage N. If there are any epochs that have sleep spindles and K-complexes, score these epochs as stage N2. If some epochs contain more than 20% slow-wave activity, score these as stage N3, and otherwise score the NREM sleep as stage N (4).

Scoring Sleep Stages

Although EEG characteristics will be different because of the age of the patient, sleep staging in pediatrics follows the adult rules for stages N2, N3, and R. One difference in children will be the greater amount of high-amplitude slow-wave sleep, especially in younger children. Slow-wave sleep decreases as we age. Compared with the preteen child, there will be a noticeable reduction in slow-wave activity as the child ages into his or her late teenage years and beyond. Younger children entering sleep will show a slowing of their DPR and will often have *hypnagogic hypersynchrony* or theta activity. Unless there are events causing disturbances either from the patient or externally,

children do not stay in stage N1 for long periods. Within minutes, they progress into deeper stages of sleep. The younger the child, the sooner this tends to happen.

Sleep staging in children is similar to that of adults, except that the younger child will have a slower DPR or baseline pattern. The DPR indicates wakefulness and it varies from child to child because of the wide range of maturity levels seen in a pediatric sleep center. Again for this reason, patient calibrations used as a reference can be extremely helpful in determining what pattern of EEG is predominant in the wakeful child (Table 61-2).

Once you are comfortable with recognizing the DPR wakefulness EEG pattern in your patient, look for a slowing and attenuation or lowering of amplitude in the EEG waveform to detect sleep onset. If you see this change in waveform pattern for more than 50% of the epoch, then score that epoch as stage N1. To further help recognize the beginning of stage N1 or sleep onset, watch closely for the EEG waveform to become clearer and sharper as artifact is decreased or drops out as the child relaxes upon entering sleep. This is seen more noticeably in infant polysomnography and, along with other signs, can indicate relaxation into sleep (see Fig. 61-2 that determines sleep and sleep hypnagogic hypersynchrony).

SLEEP IN INFANTS UNDER 2 MONTHS POSTTERM

Pediatric sleep staging rules can be applied to infants 2 months postterm or older. For infants less than 2 months postterm who have not yet developed recognizable sleep spindles, there is another set of sleep staging criteria created by Anders et al. and detailed in

Table 61-1 Pediatric Sleep Stages

Stage W (Wakefulness)
Stage N1 (NREM1)
Stage N2 (NREM2)
Stage N3 (NREM3)
Stage N (NREM)
Stage R (REM)

NREM, nonrapid eye movement; REM, rapid eye movement.

Table 61-2 Sleep Staging Rules

1. Score stage W when alpha or DPR occupies >50% of the occipital channel or when eye blinks or reading eye movements are present.
2. Score stage N (NREM) when there are no identifiable sleep spindles, K-complexes, or high-amplitude slow-wave activity.
3. Score stage N2 when sleep spindles or K-complexes are present.
4. Score stage N3 when >20% slow-wave activity is present.
5. Score REM when electroencephalogram activity shows low-voltage mixed frequency or a DPR, low-chin electromyogram activity, and rapid eye movements.

DPR, dominant posterior rhythm; NREM, nonrapid eye movement. Reprinted with permission from Berry, R. B., Albertario, C. L., & Harding, S. M. (2018). *The AASM manual for the scoring of sleep and associated events: Rules, terminology and technical specifications* (Version 2.5). Darien, IL: American Academy of Sleep Medicine.

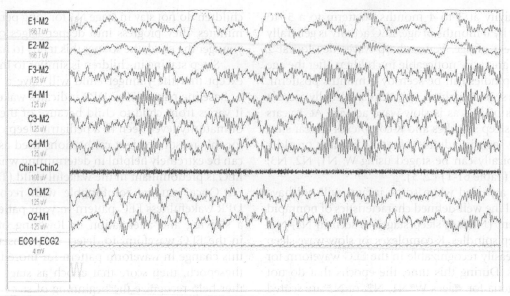

Figure 61-2 Hypnagogic hypersynchrony occurs normally in infants and children. It consists of paroxysmal bursts of theta waves often seen during drowsiness and sleep onset.

their publication from 1971, *A Manual of Standardized Terminology, Techniques and Criteria for Scoring of States of Sleep and Wakefulness in Newborn Infants.* This guide was developed over 40 years ago and until recently was still acceptable to use in practice for scoring infants. It described sleep staging in infants using the terminology *quiet, active,* and *indeterminate* sleep. Today these terms are replaced with stage *N (NREM), stage R (REM)*, and *stage T (Transitional)*, and rules for infants are now covered in the *AASM Scoring Manual.*

Infant Patterns of EEG

Sleep staging is based on five criteria: eye movements, EEG, body movements, submental electromyogram (EMG), and cardiorespiratory pattern (Table 61-3).

Table **61-3** Infant Sleep Scoring

	Stage R (REM) Sleep	Stage N (NREM) Sleep
Behavior	Movements, smiles, grimaces	Movements rare
Respirations	Irregular	Regular
Eye movements	Present	Absent
Electroencephalogram	Low voltage, mixed frequency	High-voltage slow or TA
Electromyogram	Suppressed	High

NREM, nonrapid eye movement; REM, rapid eye movement; TA, tracé alternant.

Newborn infants manifest four general EEG patterns. These include *low-voltage irregular* (LVI), *tracé alternant* (TA), *high-voltage slow waves* (HVS), and *mixed* (M). LVI is mostly theta activity (5 to 8 Hz) and slow activity (1 to 5 Hz) and can range between 14 and 35 μV in amplitude. TA is 3 to 8 seconds of high-voltage (0.5 to 3 Hz) slow waves separated by 4 to 8 seconds of lower-voltage mixed-frequency waves (see Fig. 61-3 for an example of stage N with a TA EEG). HVS is continuous rhythmic 50 to 150 μV waves at a frequency of 0.5 to 4 Hz. M contains both HVS and LVI waves (5). Infants born prematurely often have a pattern of EEG called *tracé discontinue.* This waveform is similar to TA; however, it shows longer periods of very low-amplitude activity in between HVS (see Fig. 61-4 for an example of *tracé discontinue*).

Wakefulness

Body movements, crying, or quiet awake when the infant is inactive and the eyes are open and alert can distinguish wakefulness in the newborn infant. Body movements, vocalizations, and facial or limb twitches can also occur during sleep, so it is important to know if the eyes are closed and for how long. Infants will not close their eyes and remain awake. Synchronized digital video is helpful in determining whether the infant is awake or asleep, although video recording is not the only method of documenting patient activity. Technologist notations regarding patient activity, along with documentation of any other issues, are important for accurate scoring.

Upon review of the completed study, there may be problems with the video or sound not discovered or corrected during the actual recording, such as a broken

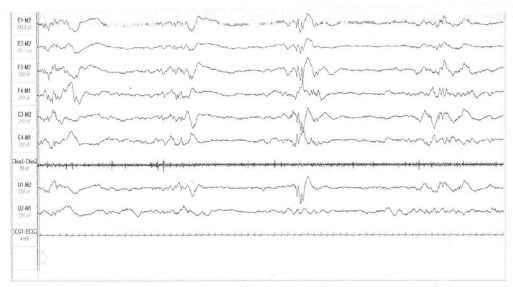

Figure 61-3 Electroencephalogram waveform showing immaturity and tracé discontinue pattern in a 7-week premature infant. This tracing shows short bursts of high-amplitude waves separated by long periods of very low-amplitude activity.

microphone, reduced lighting, poor camera angle, or something obstructing the camera view. It is imperative that the technologist monitoring the study frequently observe and note whether the infant's eyes are open or closed; the level of any snoring, vocalizations, and body movements; along with any other details specific to the study, such as whether the infant is receiving oxygen or settings of a ventilation device. Because it may be impossible to distinguish sleep from quiet wakefulness, without the technologist's documentation, determining sleep is often difficult (Fig. 61-5). The EEG pattern of the infant in quiet wakefulness will not show the alpha rhythm seen in older children and adults. Instead it will be a low-amplitude, mixed-frequency waveform with no delta waves. The voltage is usually less than 75 μV. The chin EMG is usually high, and the EOG will show eye movements. When more than 50% of the epoch displays this nonsleep state, it is scored as *wake* (6).

Infant Stage R (REM)

Sleep onset is often very difficult to establish because of the variable DPR among newborns (see Fig. 61-6). When infants become drowsy, they become inactive and the eyes become unfocused, blinking and closing for

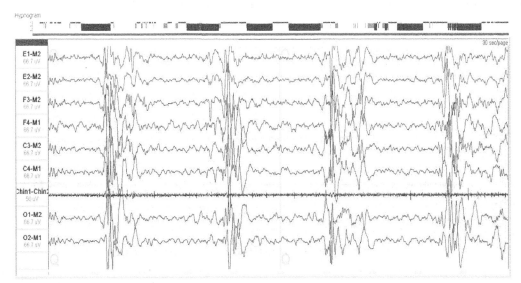

Figure 61-4 Maturation of the electroencephalogram waveform showing development of tracé alternant pattern in a 4-week-old postterm infant. This tracing shows short bursts of high-amplitude delta waves interrupted by periods of low-amplitude mixed-frequency activity.

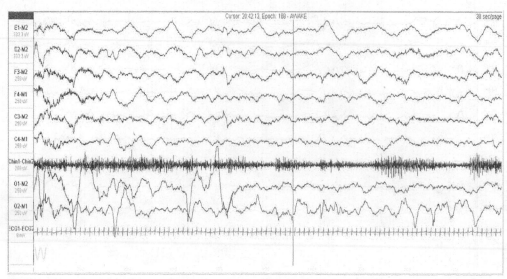

Figure 61-5 Awake movement and increased electrical activity seen in electroencephalogram. Awake waveforms are darker and thicker than seen in a sleep state. Utilize video to determine quiescence.

longer periods until they fall asleep. Most infants will enter sleep in *stage R (REM)* characterized by eye movements, along with other facial movements in the way of smiles, frowns, and sucking. The EEG channels show theta waves of low voltage in an irregular mixed pattern. The eyes are closed, although sometimes not completely, and the EOG channels will show out-of-phase movement similar to the REM period seen in an adult study. The chin EMG is usually reduced, but can be variable. Respirations will become irregular, and short central pauses are common with short, rapid breathing at other times. Body movement is present at times throughout this stage. When an epoch displays these characteristics in the EEG, EOG, EMG, and respiratory channels for more than 50% of the epoch, it is scored

as *stage R* sleep (see Fig. 61-7 that demonstrates the eye movements, low-voltage mixed-frequency EEG, and reduced EMG tone seen in stage R). This stage will make up approximately 50% of a newborn's sleep time. After about 3 months of age, an infant begins to enter into sleep in an NREM state, the same as is seen in older children and adults (4).

Infant Stage N (NREM)

An EEG pattern with HVS, TA, or M waveforms categorizes *stage N (NREM)*, with one of these patterns primarily present depending on the maturity of the newborn. The EOG will show no REMs. The chin EMG is higher in tone than during *stage R* sleep. The breathing pattern is regular and cyclical, much like the breathing pattern

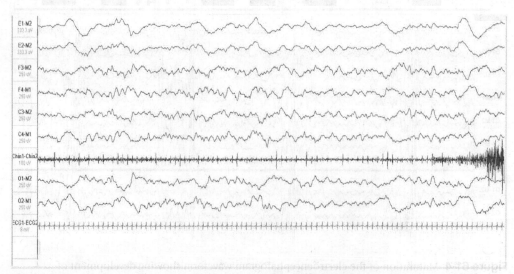

Figure 61-6 Sleep-onset electroencephalogram electrical activity quiets down and waveform clears, becoming thinner and less dark. Waveform frequency slows. Infant has eyes closed.

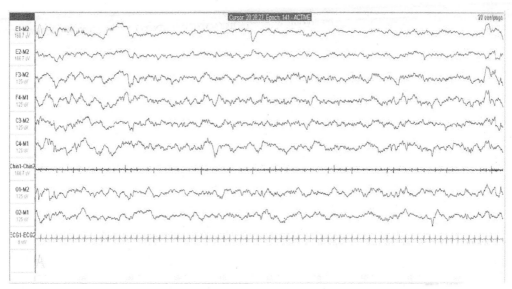

Figure 61 7 This polysomnographic tracing of stage R sleep in a 5-week postterm infant shows electroencephalogram—low-voltage mixed-frequency waves, electrooculogram—rapid eye movements, and electromyogram—(chin) low muscle tone.

seen in deep sleep in an adult study. There are no body movements, outside of respiration, except for phasic activity such as startles or sucking (6). When an epoch displays these characteristics in the EEG, EOG, EMG, and respiratory channels for more than 50% of the epoch, it is scored as stage N (NREM) (see Fig. 61-8) (4). Notice that during this time there is a lack of eye movement and slower higher-voltage EEG.

Infant Stage T (Transitional)

Epochs that do not meet the criteria for one of the two sleep states, R or N sleep, are scored as *stage T (transitional sleep)*. This is a transitional sleep state more likely to be seen when the infant is alternating between stages R and N sleep, at sleep onset, or during arousals. Stage T can also be scored when a combination of different sleep states is seen in one epoch, with none being the

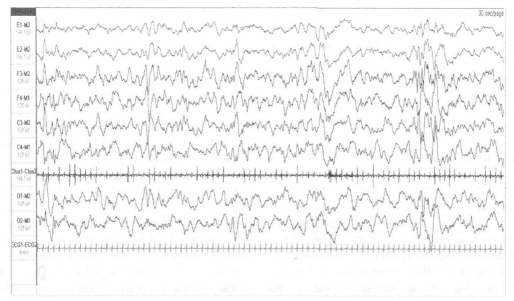

Figure 61-8 Stage N sleep in a 5-week postterm infant, which includes absence of eye movements, sustained muscle tone, and regular breathing and heart rate patterns. Few body movements are noted in this state. The electroencephalogram pattern evolves from tracé discontinue to tracé alternant and then into mature nonrapid eye movement sleep by age 6 months postterm.

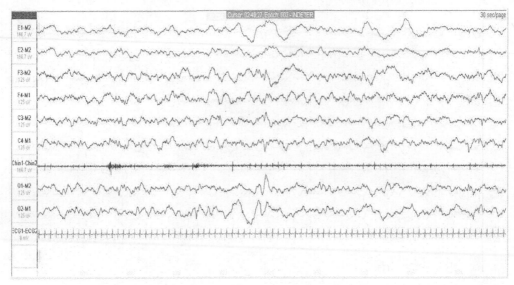

Figure 61-9 Example of transitional sleep. Electroencephalogram is disorganized, and the epoch cannot be classified as stage R or stage N sleep. Commonly seen in a transition period, such as from stage N to stage R sleep.

dominant state (see Fig. 61-9 for an example of transitional sleep) (4).

For a technologist inexperienced with scoring infant studies, it is best to start with determining sleep and wake activity, staging as much sleep time as possible. Next try to recognize stage R versus stage N activity. It is normal to sometimes not realize what stage R or REM looks like for that particular patient until the later part of the study. As with any study, if this happens, go back to the beginning to look for any possible missed REM periods. Once comfortable with finding wake, stage N, and stage R, then look to mark *stage T* during the epochs just before each stage change. When staging infant sleep, it is important to determine wake and sleep states, while keeping in mind that the infant most likely is having the study performed to check for a breathing disorder. Therefore, respiratory events are extremely important, and proper staging is needed to recognize and score events correctly.

SCORING PEDIATRIC RESPIRATORY EVENTS

When scoring respiratory events in children, it is necessary to know the developmental level of the child and apply the appropriate rules for pediatrics. The AASM defines an abnormal respiratory event in the adult patient as one lasting greater than 10 seconds. In that period, the adult may miss two or three respiratory cycles, whereas young children have a higher respiratory rate and can easily have missed four to six or more breaths in the same 10-second period. This is one reason why respiratory events in children, and especially in infants, have different standards. Because young infants have

a more compliant chest wall than do older children or adults, paradoxic movements of the chest wall and abdomen may be normal. Therefore, constantly maintaining good airflow signals is important during the study.

Respiratory event scoring rules from *The AASM Manual for the Scoring of Sleep and Associated Events* have been established for infants and children under 18 years. However, at the discretion of the sleep specialist, children 13 years and older can be scored using the established adult standards.

Apnea

Many pediatric laboratories enhance their ability to detect deficits of airflow and respiration by applying several different sensors, including thermistors, nasal pressure transducers, capnography, and esophageal pressure monometers, and use the sum channel of respiratory inductance plethysmography. Oronasal thermal sensors are recommended for use in detecting and classifying apneas, and a nasal pressure signal is used if the thermal sensor is unreliable. In pediatrics, if airflow is absent for the duration of two baseline breaths or more while respiratory efforts continue, then the event is considered to be an *obstructive apnea* (Table 61-4). If there is no airflow for two breaths or more with an associated arousal, an awakening, or a greater than or equal to 3% desaturation, and if respiratory efforts are absent, then the event is considered to be a *central apnea*. If the patient is under 1 year of age, also score a central apnea if the event lasts for at least two missed breaths and is accompanied by a drop in heart rate to under 50 for at least 5 seconds or under 60 for 15 or more seconds. Central apneas greater than 20 seconds

Table 61-4 Apnea Rules

Score an obstructive apnea when

(1)	The event lasts for the duration of two missed breaths
(2)	There is a >90% fall in the signal amplitude
(3)	There is continued or increased inspiratory effort throughout the event

Score a mixed apnea when

(1)	The event lasts for the duration of two missed breaths
(2)	There is a >90% fall in the signal amplitude
(3)	There is no respiratory effort during one portion of the event and presence of inspiratory effort in another portion, regardless of which portion comes first

Score a central apnea when

(1)	Inspiratory effort is absent
(2)	The event lasts 20 s or longer
(3)	The event lasts for the duration of two missed breaths and is associated with an arousal, an awakening, or a >3% desaturation

Reprinted with permission from Berry, R. B., Albertario, C. L., & Harding, S. M. (2018). *The AASM manual for the scoring of sleep and associated events: Rules, terminology and technical specifications* (Version 2.5). Darien, IL: American Academy of Sleep Medicine.

Table 61-5 Hypopnea Rules

Score a hypopnea when

(1)	There is a ≥30% decrease in the nasal pressure or other airflow signal
(2)	The event duration is at least two missed breaths
(3)	The decreased signal amplitude lasts at least the minimum duration of the event
(4)	The event is associated with an arousal, an awakening, or a ≥3% desaturation

Reprinted with permission from Berry, R. B., Albertario, C. L., & Harding, S. M. (2018). *The AASM manual for the scoring of sleep and associated events: Rules, terminology and technical specifications* (Version 2.5). Darien, IL: American Academy of Sleep Medicine.

centers distinguish between obstructive and central hypopneas. Generally, if the respiratory efforts remain in phase (assuming good belt position), and there is no snoring or flattening of the pressure transducer airflow signal, score the event as a *central hypopnea*. If the respiratory efforts are out of phase, or if snoring or pressure transducer flattening is present, score the event as an *obstructive hypopnea*.

In contrast to adults, children may sleep through respiratory events and therefore may not have an arousal associated with a respiratory event (7). Children tend to have a higher threshold for arousal. Another important difference is that children have a more compliant respiratory system, allowing them to maintain their oxyhemoglobin status without the oxygen desaturations or arousals seen more prominently with adults.

Respiratory Effort–Related Arousal

Perhaps because their need for sleep is greater than their need to wake up to breathe, younger children do not arouse from sleep as easily from respiratory events. Unlike with adults, respiratory effort–related arousal (RERA) events in childhood are less common. For the child to have a scorable arousal from sleep, the respiratory event is usually significant enough to meet the criteria for either apnea or hypopnea. The AASM scoring rules for a RERA include the requirement of a respiratory sequence that does not meet the scoring rules for apnea or hypopnea. In pediatrics, scoring RERAs differs from that for adults in duration requirement. In children, events are a sequence of greater than or equal to two breaths, instead of 10 seconds for adults (4). The important aspect in scoring a RERA is that the event, although not an apnea or hypopnea, still involves an associated arousal (Table 61-6). In children younger than teenage, RERA events are less likely.

should be scored even if there are no desaturations, as long as the apnea is not associated with movement or a sigh. Central apneas less than 20 seconds are considered normal in children and are *not* scored unless they cause an associated arousal, an awakening, or a greater than or equal to 3% desaturation. *Mixed apnea* is scored if the event meets apnea criteria and contains a portion with no respiratory effort and a portion with respiratory effort, regardless of which occurs first.

Hypopneas

Ideally, the waveform from a nasal air pressure transducer signals the detection of hypopneas; however, the waveform from an oronasal thermal sensor is used if the nasal pressure signal is unreliable. A respiratory event where there is a reduction in the waveform of greater than or equal to 30% for a period of two baseline breaths or more accompanied by an arousal, an awakening, or a desaturation of more than 3% should be scored as a hypopnea (Table 61-5). The decrease in nasal pressure during the event should last for greater than or equal to 90% of the complete respiratory event when compared with the waveform amplitude before the event. Some

Table 61-6 Respiratory Effort–Related Arousal Rules

Score RERA using a nasal pressure sensor when

(1) The event does not meet criteria for an apnea or hypopnea and leads to an arousal

(2) The event duration is at least two missed breaths

(3) The nasal pressure waveform demonstrates flattening, or effort channels show increasing respiratory effort

(4) Snoring, noisy breathing, increased end-tidal or transcutaneous PCO_2, or visual evidence of increased work of breathing is present

Score RERA using an esophageal pressure sensor when

(1) Inspiratory effort progressively increases during the event

(2) The event duration is at least two missed breaths

(3) Snoring, noisy breathing, increased end-tidal or transcutaneous PCO_2, or visual evidence of increased work of breathing is present

RERA, respiratory effort–related arousal.
Reprinted with permission from Berry, R. B., Albertario, C. L., & Harding, S. M. (2018). *The AASM manual for the scoring of sleep and associated events: Rules, terminology and technical specifications* (Version 2.5). Darien, IL: American Academy of Sleep Medicine.

Younger children more frequently have periods of nonarousal respiratory episodes that do not meet the criteria to be scored as a RERA, apnea, or hypopnea (see Fig. 61-10 for an example of a nonarousal respiratory episode). Often seen in pediatric patients are periods of increased work of breathing with substernal retractions, snoring, an increase in end-tidal CO_2, and a flattening in the nasal pressure waveform for a period of at least two breaths. There is no scorable cortical arousal seen in the EEG waveform, and desaturations are less than 3%. By AASM rules, these episodes do not meet the criteria for an apnea, hypopnea, or RERA and cannot be scored as a respiratory event. During these episodes, careful review using the data from sensors such as pulse oximeter, nasal pressure transducer, esophageal monometer, and respiratory inductance plethysmography can identify subtle events that could possibly be scored as hypopneas in these periods.

Partial airway obstruction, characterized by an increasing respiratory effort similar to obstructive events, but without a significant drop in oxygen saturation or a 30% drop in airflow, may signify upper airway resistance. Even without a desaturation, these occurrences may be fragmenting the patient's sleep, resulting in hypersomnolence, difficulty attending school, or other daytime sequelae. These episodes, although not scorable as a RERA, may be contributing to the child's symptoms, and therefore the epochs should be noted and brought to the attention of the sleep specialist for careful analysis.

Sleep-Related Hypoventilation

Distinct extended periods of sleep where CO_2 level is increased and/or respiratory effort is lower in amplitude than resting wakefulness baseline can indicate sleep-related hypoventilation in pediatric studies (Table 61-7). Neuromuscular weakness and other congenital disorders such as chronic lung disease can contribute to

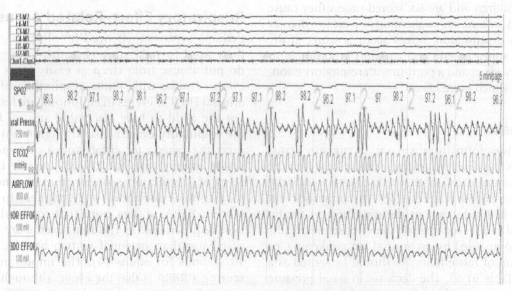

Figure 61-10 Nonarousal-related episode. Periods of reduction in nasal pressure waveform. Patient has increased work of breathing with snoring, and desaturations of only 1% to 2% with no scorable electroencephalogram arousal.

Table 61-7 Hypoventilation Rule

Score hypoventilation when

End-tidal or transcutaneous PCO_2 indicates a CO_2 level of >50 mm Hg for >25% of the total sleep time

Reprinted with permission from Berry, R. B., Albertario, C. L., & Harding, S. M. (2018). *The AASM manual for the scoring of sleep and associated events: Rules, terminology and technical specifications* (Version 2.5). Darien, IL: American Academy of Sleep Medicine.

hypoventilation. This is one of the reasons pediatric studies utilize end-tidal CO_2 monitoring (see Fig. 61-11 for an example of hypoventilation). When the PCO_2 is greater than 50 mm Hg for more than 25% of the total sleep time, it is considered hypoventilation. Mark epochs from start of these periods to end and submit for further evaluation from the interpreting physician.

APNEA OF PREMATURITY, APNEA OF INFANCY, AND PERIODIC BREATHING

Short central apneas are common in children of all ages during REM sleep, during transitions between sleep stages, or following an arousal. Children can have central apneas after a sigh or movement that lasts more than 10 seconds without a related oxygen desaturation.

Distinguished by central apneas lasting 20 seconds or longer, shorter central apneas associated with bradycardia, significant oxygen desaturation, and/or neurologic sequelae, *apnea of prematurity*, as its name suggests, occurs in premature infants and is quite common. These respiratory events usually resolve when the infant reaches full-term gestational age. If the infant is not premature, the condition is then called *apnea of infancy*. These events can be very frightening to parents and can be very serious when associated with frequent bradycardia or oxygen desaturations.

Another breathing disorder commonly seen in newborns is *periodic breathing*. Characterized by three or more central respiratory pauses of 3 seconds or more each and with less than 20 seconds of regular respiration between each apnea, periodic breathing can occur in normal newborns, particularly during active sleep (Table 61-8). It is more likely in premature infants and usually decreases as the infant's respiratory control system matures. Depending on the age and development of the infant, periodic breathing episodes during sleep are considered normal if they occur only for a small percentage of the total sleep time. Higher percentages of periodic breathing during sleep time or those causing desaturations and/or arousals may require treatment. Begin scoring periodic breathing events starting from the beginning of the first apneic event and continuing until the end of the last event that meets the criteria (Fig. 61-12 shows an episode of periodic breathing).

Arousals

Subcortical arousals may occur more often than we capture with EEG electrodes attached on the scalp, yet arousals are extremely important in discovering the cause of poor-quality sleep. In pediatrics, there is no rule difference in scoring arousals; therefore, score them following the same directions as for adults (Table 61-9). The rules state that the duration of the EEG waveform shift must be at a minimum of 3 seconds. The variation observed in children having arousals is that they will often have subtle events with periods of EEG shifts less

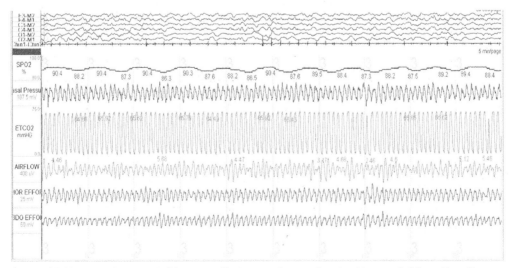

Figure 61-11 Central congenital hypoventilation syndrome showing increased CO_2 and cyclic desaturations.

Table 61-8 Periodic Breathing Rule

Score periodic breathing when

Three or more episodes of central apneas lasting >3 s are separated by ≤20 s of normal breathing

Reprinted with permission from Berry, R. B., Albertario, C. L., & Harding, S. M. (2018). *The AASM manual for the scoring of sleep and associated events: Rules, terminology and technical specifications* (Version 2.5). Darien, IL: American Academy of Sleep Medicine.

than 3 seconds in length. By AASM rules, these do not count to be scored as an arousal.

From the patient, an arousal can be caused by a respiratory or movement disorder. Careful examination utilizing all EEG channels is best to score arousals in pediatric patients. Respiratory events, leg movements, video, and additional channels are important indicators of the presence of an arousal. If you suspect arousal events, use the video and waveforms to identify what is occurring. Then look closely at the EEG waveform for the earliest increase in artifact or an increased frequency within alpha range of 8 to 13 Hz in the EEG waveform. In an infant, darkening or thickening of the waveform can indicate arousal from sleep. Mark the event from the point of the EEG change and until the end when the EEG waveform returns to its previous sleep pattern. If this period in the waveform meets the criteria, then score it as an arousal.

Cardiac Dysrhythmias in Children

Cardiac dysrhythmias are uncommon in children, but as in adults, the technologist monitoring the sleep study

should be familiar with the different types and their electrocardiogram (ECG) characteristics. The technologist must be able to recognize life-threatening conditions and must feel comfortable with responding appropriately according to his or her specific sleep center protocols.

Dysrhythmias are conditions where the heart rhythm is irregular, too fast (tachycardia), or too slow (bradycardia). A heart rate less than 80 bpm for the first month of life, less than 70 bpm in an infant 1 to 2 months of age, or less than 60 bpm for an older infant is considered bradycardia. A brief period of sinus bradycardia is common following a respiratory event. Tachycardia is defined as a heart rate of more than 190 bpm for a newborn or more than 160 bpm for an infant. Both of these conditions occur commonly for brief periods during phasic REM sleep, when the heart rate increases and then decreases before recovering to normal baseline (8). They can also occur during apnea episodes or arousals, as the heart slows down and then works harder to recover. Cardiac decelerations can also occur, defined as a drop in heart rate from baseline where the rate does not achieve the minimum level necessary to be considered bradycardia. These are usually of sinus origin seen in association with a respiratory event.

Other dysrhythmias in children are similar but less common than those witnessed in adults. Children can have premature ventricular contractions (PVCs) occurring during the night. PVCs, where the heart produces an extra ectopic beat that originates in the ventricles rather than the sinus node, are common in normal children and adults. However, PVCs that occur in series or appear to have more than one focus (different appearances to the waveform) should be brought to the attention of the physician.

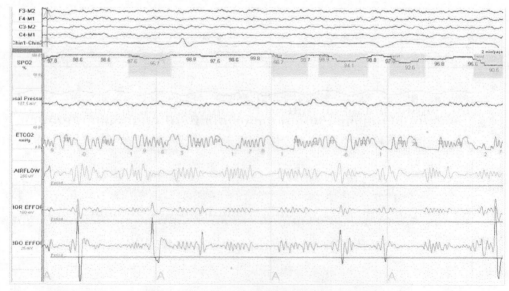

Figure 61-12 Periodic breathing in a full-term infant at 4 weeks of age.

One dysrhythmia that occurs more commonly in children is supraventricular tachycardia. It produces a heart rate greater than 220 bpm and can produce increased respiratory rate, anxiety, fussiness in the infant, or discomfort. Most episodes last only a few seconds and should be noted by the technologist. Prolonged or frequent episodes indicate the need for intervention, and the technologist should treat this condition as indicated in his or her protocols.

MOVEMENT, ARTIFACT RECOGNITION, AND BEHAVIORAL NOTATION

Bruxism, rhythmic movement disorder, myoclonus, and other movement disorders are all seen in pediatric sleep studies. Movement disorders are not specific to pediatric polysomnography and are scored using the same rules as in adult studies. These are mentioned here because the main difference is that in children there is the potential for seeing more of them. These events can and will occur anytime during studies performed in a pediatric sleep center. Expect to see them and know how to differentiate between a movement disorder and other causes of artifact. For specifics on the variety of disorders, their characteristics, and scoring of these events, turn to the chapters on movement disorders and adult scoring. Also, refer to the *AASM Scoring Manual* for rules on how to mark each event accordingly.

As displayed in the sleep study waveforms, artifacts seen in the pediatric study are similar to those associated with adults. Sweat, movement, muscle contraction, and 50/60-Hz artifacts are as common in pediatric sleep studies as they are in adult studies. Along with these artifact types, children generate artifacts from crying, rocking, sucking, and feeding that will appear at different times throughout the study. Although it is often helpful during a study to have a parent stay in the room with the child, the parent can cause artifact by touching or rubbing the child to provide comfort. Sometimes, the snoring of a parent can be mistaken as coming from the child. Artifact from laptop computers and cell phones, and noise from TVs used by the parents can also interfere with the recording. Not only can the noise and light cause problems, but the devices can cause artifact. Some parents arrive at the sleep center expecting to talk on their phone during the night or wanting to use their laptop. It is important to address this before the night of the study and while scheduling, so that the parent or guardian is aware of the sleep center policy.

Children find it very difficult to get back to sleep, and correcting artifacts during the recording usually means disrupting their sleep and potentially awakening them. Some artifacts do not need immediate attention and can wait until the child is in deep sleep to avoid waking the child. It takes an experienced, knowledgeable technologist who has reviewed the child's history and symptoms to determine when to correct the artifact. For instance, a leg lead that has fallen off a sleeping patient with suspected narcolepsy does not require replacement immediately if it has fallen off just after lights out. In that case, it is best to wait and capture sleep and REM latencies. The redundancy built into the studies with several EEG channels collecting brain waves and a thermistor, capnography, and nasal pressure, all assessing the presence of airflow, allows the technologist to use his or her best discretion on when it is appropriate to disturb the patient in order to correct artifact. It is essential that the technologist document patient movements and parental actions that may indicate the source of the artifact. Children are often restless during a sleep study, making application of the electrodes challenging. If the electrodes are not attached properly, it will lead to a long night of adjusting or reattaching to try to correct the artifacts that occur when the child moves, pulls, or touches the electrodes. Properly applying electrodes and achieving low impedances from the start is the best way to reduce artifacts throughout the study.

Table 61-9 Arousal Rule

Score an arousal when

(1)	There is an abrupt shift in electroencephalogram frequency lasting at least 3 s that is preceded by at least 10 s of stable sleep
(2)	During REM, the shift in electroencephalogram frequency is accompanied by an increase in submental electromyogram lasting at least 1 s

Reprinted with permission from Berry, R. B., Albertario, C. L., & Harding, S. M. (2018). *The AASM manual for the scoring of sleep and associated events: Rules, terminology and technical specifications* (Version 2.5). Darien, IL: American Academy of Sleep Medicine.

LIMITED CHANNEL STUDIES

Although there are some pediatric patients who could benefit from home sleep apnea testing or pneumograms, these limited channel studies are not as useful in the pediatric population as they are with adults. Generally, these devices measure airflow by thermistor, chest wall movement by impedance, ECG, heart rate, and oximetry, with additional channels sometimes added such as snore, EMG, or EEG. Without a technologist present to correct artifacts and document activities such as feeding, movement, or breath sounds, quality can be variable in children. Video, sound, extended EEG, EMG, or

EOG are often not collected, making it difficult to assess arousals and sleep.

Studies such as pneumograms are portable and brought to the patient's bedside in the hospital setting. There are fewer sensors compared with an in-laboratory sleep study, so setup time is considerably less. As with home sleep apnea tests, these studies usually measure airflow, respiratory effort, ECG, heart rate, and oxygen saturation. Less technologist time is required to perform these studies because they are usually not directly monitored. They also take less time to process because of the limited number of channels recorded. However, the data obtained from these studies are quite limited (9). Utilizing only effort sensors and a single airflow sensor in infants' obstructive events often cannot be identified with certainty, although central apneas and periodic breathing are often seen in this patient population. Actual staging of sleep is not performed, so wakefulness, stage R, and stage N are inferred by observing cardiorespiratory stability. In infants, sleep is inferred by looking at the time spent absent of artifact and where the respiration is even and rhythmic. If the breathing is more irregular or respiratory events such as apneas with desaturations are more severe, one could conclude this is REM sleep, but it could also be wake activity in an infant in respiratory distress.

Sleep latency is approximated, and an activity log documented by a parent may be helpful in some cases; however, the limited number of channels does not offer a comprehensive view of sleep cycles or assessment of sleep stages, and REM latency cannot be determined with any certainty. These studies are helpful in discovering some types of respiratory events but are not useful in diagnosing narcolepsy or parasomnias such as night terrors. The benefit of this type of testing is that it is portable and can screen a patient, such as a newborn who is having desaturation events, by being set up quickly at the bedside in the event a bed in the sleep center is not available or on a night when the sleep center is unstaffed.

PREPARING THE SUMMARY REPORT

Report Values

The content of any sleep study report can change from center to center. It is up to each center to decide what criteria are useful and how it wants to display data in its reports. The report generated for the interpreting physician should include any specific equipment used and variables collected during the study. It should state and define the center's criteria for scoring events. Documentation should include detailed technologist notes explaining procedures during the testing along with all interventions made during the study such as adding or adjusting oxygen, initiation or adjustment of PAP, ventilator adjustments, or any other changes made, along with an explanation for the change. For the duration of his or her stay in the sleep center, patient behaviors such as crying, screaming, talking, feeding, parent comforting, intensity of any snoring, and any other interventions before, during, and after the study should be included in the technologist documentation along with the report for interpretation. Any comment the technologist makes regarding breathing effort, respiratory rate, or heart rate, along with deviations from their norm, should include the time of occurrence and epoch numbers.

Final reports for infant studies will include some of the same data parameters as older child and adult reports. Apnea and hypopnea indexes, along with low, average, and high heart rates and oxygen saturations, as well as the patient's body position status during the study, are incorporated. Include total recording time, together with a breakdown of total and percentage of stage R, N, and T sleep times (10). In the report of an infant study, the total number of periodic breathing episodes, percentage, and index are calculated. The number and duration of bradycardia and desaturation events should be reported. Baseline, low, average, high, and the amount of time spent in certain heart rate and oxygen level ranges are also important. As with adult studies, report events by position and in what state of sleep they occurred.

A carefully performed, documented, scored, and interpreted study can provide invaluable data for diagnosing and treating sleep disorders in infants and children. Review the parameters to be reported for polysomnography contained in the AASM manual to decide what other information to include in a computer-generated report. Given that there are a great deal of data to present, it may be a good idea to have several varied report templates customized for different types of studies. In this way, the report is concentrated on the data collected for that type of patient, and useful for diagnoses, leaving unnecessary information out of the report.

REFERENCES

1. Wise, M. S., Nichols, C. D., Grigg-Damberger, M. M., et al. (2011). Executive summary of respiratory indications for polysomnography in children: An evidence based review. *Sleep, 34*(3), 389–398.
2. Sheldon, S., Riter, S., & Detrojan, M. (1999). *Atlas of sleep medicine in infants and children* (pp. 99–135). New York, NY: Futura Publishing.
3. Grigg-Damberger, M. M., Gozal, D., Marcus, C. L., et al. (2007). The visual scoring of sleep and arousal in infants and children. *Journal of Clinical Sleep Medicine, 3*(2), 201–240.
4. Berry, R. B., Albertario, C. L., Harding, S. M., et al.; for the American Academy of Sleep Medicine. (2018). *The*

AASM manual for the scoring of sleep and associated events: Rules, terminology and technical specifications [Version 2.5]. Darien, IL: American Academy of Sleep Medicine.

5. Anders, T., Emde, R., & Parmelee, A. (Eds.). (1971). *A manual of standardized terminology, techniques and criteria for scoring of states of sleep and wakefulness in newborn infants.* Los Angeles, CA: Brain Information Service/Brain Research Institute.

6. Crowell, D. H.; the CHIME Study Group. (2003). *An atlas of infant polysomnography* (pp. 63–77). New York, NY: Parthenon Publishing.

7. Marcus, C. L. (2001). Sleep-disordered breathing in children. *American Journal of Respiratory and Critical Care Medicine, 164,* 16–30.

8. American Thoracic Society. (1996). Standards and indications for cardiopulmonary sleep studies in children. *American Journal of Respiratory and Critical Care Medicine, 153,* 866–878.

9. Ramanathan, R., Corwin, M. J., Hunt, C. E., et al. (2001). Cardiorespiratory events recorded on home monitors: Comparison of healthy infants with those at increased risk for SIDS. The CHIME Study Group. *Journal of American Medical Association, 285,* 2199–2207.

10. Iber, C., Ancoli-Israel, S., Chesson, A., et al. (2007). *The AASM manual for the scoring of sleep and associated events: Rules, terminology and technical specifications.* Westchester, IL: American Academy of Sleep Medicine.

chapter 62

Sleep-Related Breathing Disorders in Children

BRIAN J. SCHULTZ   LEE J. BROOKS

LEARNING OBJECTIVES

On completion of this chapter, the reader should be able to:

1. Describe sleep-related breathing disorders in children.
2. Review currently available treatment options.
3. Discuss the relationship between sleep-related breathing disorders and comorbidities.
4. Discuss the effects of sleep-related breathing disorders on quality of life.

KEY TERMS

Apnea of prematurity (AOP)
Brief resolved unexplained event (BRUE)
Obstructive sleep apnea syndrome (OSAS)
Sudden infant death syndrome (SIDS)
Apparent life-threatening event (ALTE)
Adenotonsillectomy
Congenital central hypoventilation syndrome (CCHS)

Respiratory problems, most notably apnea, are the most common reason for a child to be referred to a sleep center. The presentation, consequences, and treatment of sleep-disordered breathing (SDB) in children are different from those in adults. Premature infants are at risk for central apneas, whereas obstructive events are more common in children and adolescents. Children with neurologic, neuromuscular, craniofacial, and genetic disorders are at particular risk for respiratory compromise and may need ventilatory assistance in the form of continuous positive airway pressure (CPAP) or bilevel positive airway pressure (BPAP). Children with SDB may have neurocognitive, neurobehavioral, cardiovascular, growth, metabolic, and quality of life (QOL) consequences. Many of these sequelae can be alleviated with appropriate clinical management.

APNEA OF PREMATURITY

The respiratory control systems of the newborn may be immature, resulting in instability of ventilation and pauses in respiration. Hypoxia and hypercarbia, impaired ventilatory response, and inhibitory reflexes are exaggerated. Even normal term newborns may exhibit occasional respiratory pauses of 30 seconds or more (1, 2). Premature infants may be even more unstable, with more frequent and longer respiratory pauses (2) often associated with bradycardia, hypoxemia, and/or hypercarbia. These are accentuated by the newborns' rapid respiratory rate and smaller oxygen capacities.

Apnea of prematurity (AOP) is often seen in infants less than 33 weeks' gestation. These events may be noted in the preterm nursery. AOP is usually central in nature, although obstructive and mixed events can also occur. By the time premature babies have reached term, the prevalence and severity of events is similar to that of healthy term babies (2), although very premature babies (24 to 28 weeks' gestation) may have persisting apnea beyond full term (3).

If the events are clearly documented in the neonatal intensive care unit, treatment is often initiated without a sleep study. Full polysomnography (PSG) is needed if obstructive events are being considered, but a pneumogram measuring chest wall movement by impedance, airflow by thermistor, heart rate, oximetry, and perhaps esophageal pH may be requested to document central apneas and establish their relationship, if any, to gastroesophageal reflux (GER).

AOP is usually treated with methylxanthine therapy (caffeine or theophylline). Caffeine can significantly reduce apneas within the first week of treatment (4). Theophylline significantly improves periodic breathing and central apneas in premature infants in both active (rapid eye movement [REM]) and quiet (non-REM) sleep but does not affect bradycardia or obstructive events (5). If the patient continues to have significant obstructive events, positive airway pressure, either CPAP or BPAP, can be used. CPAP can reduce obstructive events and the severity of apnea-related desaturations (6). Caffeine in combination with CPAP therapy may reduce

732

the number of days for which respiratory support is required. The combination of these treatments may also have neurodevelopmental benefits (7). Long-term effects of caffeine use in newborns have not been shown to increase obstructive sleep apnea (OSA) but may increase periodic limb movements in sleep (8).

Sleeping position may affect the frequency and severity of cardiorespiratory events. Healthy preterm infants sleeping supine have a higher respiratory rate, lower oxyhemoglobin saturation, and reduced ventilatory response to hypercapnia compared with those in the prone position (9). Although the total number of events remained low, infants sleeping supine had nearly twice the number of obstructive events than the ones sleeping prone (10).

However, infants sleeping prone have deeper, quiet sleep and fewer arousals with increased central apnea (10, 11). The risk of sudden infant death syndrome (SIDS) is increased in the prone position. Therefore, it is recommended that healthy term newborns sleep in the supine position (12).

BRIEF RESOLVED UNEXPLAINED EVENT

Brief resolved unexplained event (BRUE) is "an event occurring in an infant younger than 1 year when the observer reports a sudden, brief, and now resolved episode of one or more of the following: (1) cyanosis or pallor; (2) absent, decreased, or irregular breathing; (3) marked change in tone (hyper- or hypotonia); and (4) altered level of responsiveness" (13). Patients are classified on the basis of history and physical examination. Suggested care of low-risk patients may include a 12-lead electrocardiogram, pulse oximetry monitoring, child abuse evaluation, and pertussis testing. The family should receive education about BRUEs and where cardiopulmonary resuscitation training is offered. There are no specific treatment recommendations for high-risk BRUEs.

Some of these events have been classified as an apparent life-threatening event (ALTE). ALTE is defined as "An episode that is frightening to the observer and is characterized by some combination of apnea (central or occasionally obstructive), color change (usually cyanotic or pallid but occasionally erythematous or plethoric), marked change in muscle tone (usually marked limpness), choking, or gagging" (12). The cause of an ALTE is identified in only about half of the patients. Possible diagnoses include seizures, cardiac arrhythmias, laryngomalacia, tracheomalacia, and child abuse. A patient presenting with an ALTE is usually hospitalized to ascertain a cause for the event. Laboratory tests may include a blood count, metabolic panel, chest roentgenogram, electrocardiogram, and physiologic monitoring during sleep.

An overnight PSG is needed if obstructive events are suspected. A pneumogram, measuring chest wall movement by impedance, airflow by thermistor, heart rate, oximetry, and perhaps esophageal pH, may be requested to document central apneas and establish their relationship, if any, to GER. Visual cues such as work of breathing, positioning, and type of bedding are important and should be documented during an infant's overnight study. Episodes of cyanosis or pallor should be documented and warrant a call to the physician covering the lab. If esophageal pH or impedance monitoring is performed, the technologist should document feeding times, volume, and type. Apple juice feedings are preferred because milk may act as a buffer, limiting the ability of the pH probe to detect reflux. If a cause of the event is found, it should be treated, but in many cases no cause is found (14, 15). When no specific cause of the event is found in an infant greater than 37 weeks' gestational age, the patient is considered to have "apnea of infancy." These patients are often sent home on cardiorespiratory monitors (16).

A relationship between ALTE and SIDS has not been proven. SIDS is defined as "The sudden death of any infant under 1 year of age, which remains unexplained after a thorough case investigation, including performance of a complete autopsy, examination of the death scene, and review of the clinical history" (17). The prevalence of SIDS in the United States is about 0.6 per 1,000 infants, with a peak incidence at about 2 months of age (18).

Several studies have noted an increased risk of SIDS in patients sleeping in the prone position, leading to international public health campaigns encouraging families to put their infants to sleep in the supine position (19). Since the 1992 "Back to Sleep" (20) campaign in the United States, the prevalence of supine sleeping has increased, and the incidence of SIDS has decreased dramatically (21). The number of ALTE cases has increased during this time, however, with an increased prevalence of GER, possibly because more babies are sleeping in the supine position (22, 23).

CHILDHOOD OSA

The majority of children studied in a sleep center will have been referred for suspected obstructive SDB, which in children can range from primary snoring to OSA. Nearly 12% of children snore "on most nights," with obstructive sleep apnea syndrome (OSAS) occurring in 1% to 4% of school-age children (24). OSAS in children is characterized by prolonged partial upper airway obstruction (obstructive hypopnea) and/or intermittent complete obstruction (obstructive apnea) that disrupts normal ventilation and sleep patterns (25). Risk factors for snoring and OSAS include anything that affects the size or compliance of the pharynx, such as adenotonsillar hypertrophy, obesity, disorders affecting tone, and craniofacial and neuromuscular disorders (25, 26). Parents usually report nighttime snoring, snorting, gasping, nighttime awakenings, enuresis, diaphoresis, and/or apnea. Reported daytime symptoms such as irritability, hyperactivity, poor school performance, mouth breathing, headaches, and sleepiness are common. Even primary snoring, in the face of a normal polysomnogram, has been associated with neurocognitive impairments, resulting in poor school performance for math, science, and spelling (27). Newborn infants may initially present with what seems to be severe apnea on a PSG. This may, in part, be due to their higher respiratory rate, resulting in more events being scored. However, their breathing typically improves as they grow older (28).

Clinical Evaluation

The clinician should have a high index of suspicion for OSA in any child with risk factors including obesity, enuresis, or difficulty paying attention in school. The family should be queried about snoring and restless or nonrestorative sleep. Tonsil size should be noted. However, only about half of children with a suggestive history and physical examination have OSA confirmed when assessed objectively in the sleep center (28–30).

Polysomnography

Overnight PSG is the "gold standard" for confirming the diagnosis of OSA in children. An overnight PSG is also necessary to evaluate the severity of OSAS because this will affect treatment. The PSG should take place over a full night because nap studies have been shown to underestimate the severity of the disorder, perhaps because insufficient REM sleep is achieved (31). Alternative monitoring such as at-home or abbreviated sleep studies are not recommended for children because they have not proven to accurately predict the severity of the disorder.

Children are more difficult to study because of noncooperation and increased movement during sleep, which may result in poor signal quality. An overnight PSG in children requires a staff who is comfortable dealing with children and their families. In addition to the standard adult PSG montage, end-tidal carbon dioxide ($ETCO_2$) or transcutaneous carbon dioxide is monitored to quantitate hypoventilation. A higher level of staffing, often one-to-one for children who are medically or developmentally complex, may be required.

Sequelae of OSAS

Sequelae of OSAS in children can be categorized as cardiovascular, metabolism/growth, and learning/behavior. Cardiovascular sequelae of OSAS in children are similar to those of adults. Children are at risk for hypertension, cor pulmonale, and reduced ventricular

function (32–34). Obesity is a confounding variable, contributing to both OSA and decreased cardiovascular function. OSA is a clear risk factor for hypertension even after obesity is accounted for (35). Cardiac function improves after treatment of the OSA (36).

Children with OSA may be obese and may also present with failure to thrive, which improves after adenotonsillectomy (36). This is reflected in a reduction in the work of breathing (37), or improvements in growth hormone (GH), which is secreted during slow-wave sleep. Following adenotonsillectomy, children with OSAS experience a resurgence of GH and an increase in body mass index, body fat mass, and fat-free mass (38). OSA may increase the child's risk of diabetes and the metabolic syndrome, independent of obesity, most likely acting through the hormone adiponectin (39).

Children with OSA may exhibit hyperactivity, aggressiveness, emotional problems, and improper behaviors (40). Sometimes, these behaviors may be misdiagnosed as attention-deficit hyperactivity disorder (41). These behaviors usually improve after treatment (42–44). Children with OSA and even primary snoring may have reduced verbal and performance IQ as well as reduced sustained and selective memory IQ scores (45). It is unclear whether these neurocognitive scores improve after adenotonsillectomy (46–48).

SDB has been shown to adversely affect QOL measures in children, including daytime sleepiness, daytime function, and reduced alertness. QOL significantly improves after adenotonsillectomy (48, 49), even if their sleep has not fully normalized (50).

Nocturnal enuresis can be associated with OSAS in children (51, 52). Enuresis is a common problem, seen in over 15% of school-aged children (53), and may occur in the sleep center. If enuresis occurs during the PSG, the technologist should make a note of it. Adenotonsillectomy often provides substantial improvement of bed-wetting (54).

TREATMENT

Surgery

In contrast to adults, for whom positive airway pressure (PAP) is the first-line treatment, children usually respond well to adenotonsillectomy. The apnea–hypopnea index (AHI) almost always improves after adenotonsillectomy, although it may not completely normalize, particularly in the face of severe disease or obesity (28, 49, 55). Adenotonsillectomy usually results in improvement in the consequences of OSAS, including cardiovascular function (36) and behavior (42).

Maxillomandibular advancement surgery should be considered for those children with craniofacial defects, including midfacial or mandibular hypoplasia and for some with severe OSAS (56–58).

Oral Appliance Therapy

Dental devices that reposition the jaw and/or tongue may be useful in children with mild OSA. These should be initiated and followed by a dentist/orthodontist with training and experience using these devices in children. Follow-up is especially important in view of the growing teeth and jaw. Rapid maxillary expansion has also been successfully used in select groups of children (59), including newborns with micrognathia (28).

PAP Therapy

If adenotonsillectomy is not effective, if there are contraindications to surgery or simply for patient preference, CPAP is a reasonable alternative (60, 61). Obesity, craniofacial anomalies, recurrent idiopathic OSAS post adenotonsillectomy, Down syndrome, and Prader–Willi syndrome are common indications for CPAP therapy. CPAP adherence is a factor in treating adults and children. Teaching the parent and child how the CPAP system works and fitting an appropriate mask are crucial in the steps to successful adherence to therapy. Behavioral techniques can increase the likelihood of CPAP adherence (62). There are a growing number of small PAP masks more suitable for children.

BPAP provides a lower pressure on expiration than inspiration. It was designed with the hope that a lower pressure on expiration would enhance patient adherence but has not proven to be the case in adults (63) or children (64). BPAP may be used to deliver noninvasive ventilation to children who need it, including patients with neuromuscular weakness or neurologic disease.

Weight Loss

Weight loss should be encouraged in all obese patients, but can be difficult to achieve. School-aged children with obesity and OSA are more likely to eat fast food, consume fewer fruits and vegetables, and be less active in organized sports compared with healthy children (65).

Medications

Adenotonsillectomy is the treatment of choice for OSAS in children, but alternative choices to treat residual or mild apnea have shown some promise. Nasal corticosteroids and/or oral anti-inflammatory medications such as montelukast (66-68) have been shown to reduce AHI and improve sleep in several studies, indicating a possible nonsurgical therapy for patients with mild OSA (69, 70). Long-term studies have not been done.

Oxygen

Oxygen may be useful in children with chronic lung disease but should be used with caution in children with OSA, where it may simply mask hypopneic events (71). Supplemental oxygen will increase the nadir and baseline saturation levels of patients with OSAS but does not reduce the number or duration of obstructive or central apneas. It may be suitable for temporary relief of OSA symptoms (72), but the possibility of reducing respiratory drive must be considered and ETCO$_2$ should be carefully monitored.

Congenital Central Hypoventilation Syndrome

Congenital central hypoventilation syndrome (CCHS), originally termed Ondine's curse, is a rare disease that usually presents in newborns but occasionally in adults. Patients suffering from CCHS will hypoventilate when asleep but may breathe normally during wakefulness. They have a reduced ventilatory response to hypercarbia and hypoxia and may not perceive dyspnea (73). The disease is genetic, often with a polyalanine expansion of the PHOX2B gene that controls autonomic function. However, 10% of cases are due to nonpolyalanine repeat expansion mutation.

Some patients may do well with noninvasive ventilation, for example, BPAP during sleep, with supplemental oxygen or even room air during wakefulness. More severe patients will need ventilator assistance around the clock, often requiring mechanical ventilation through a tracheostomy. Diaphragm pacing may also be used (75).

Rapid-Onset Obesity with Hypothalamic Dysfunction, Hypoventilation, and Autonomic Dysregulation

CCHS patients often require yearly polysomnograms to assess oxygenation and ventilation during sleep and adjustment of ventilator settings. Pulse oximetry and PCO$_2$ monitoring (end-tidal or transcutaneous) are necessary elements of PSG in these patients.

Some children appear healthy and normal at birth and then rapidly gain weight and progress into the various stages and sequelae of rapid-onset obesity with hypothalamic dysfunction, hypoventilation, and autonomic dysregulation (ROHHAD) over the next several years. Weight gain of 20 to 30 lb over a period of less than a year is one of the first indications of this rare disorder. Snoring and OSA may follow, warranting a PSG. All children will need ventilation at night because of hypoventilation and lack of respiratory control. Similar to CCHS patients, more severe cases will require around-the-clock ventilation. CCHS and ROHHAD are associated syndromes in that both have autonomic dysfunction. Unlike CCHS, children with ROHHAD are missing the *PHOX2B* gene defect.

SUMMARY

Breathing disorders are the most common reason for a child to be referred to a sleep center. OSA is the most prevalent disorder, which, if left untreated, can result in serious cognitive, neurologic, and metabolic sequelae. AOP is seen in many preterm infants; however, methylxanthine therapy can be used to treat the central apnea until they reach term and breathing normalizes. Infants may present with a BRUE, yet a cause may not be found. The relationship between ALTE and SIDS is unknown. CCHS and ROHHAD are rare but serious disorders that usually require respiratory support that may be initiated and followed in the sleep center. Caring for children in the sleep center requires a friendly environment and good rapport between the sleep technologist, the child, and the family.

REFERENCES

1. Marcus, C. L. (2001). Sleep-disordered breathing in children. *American Journal of Respiratory and Critical Care Medicine, 164,* 16–30.
2. Ramanathan, R., Corwin, M. J., Hunt, C. E., et al.; Collaborative Home Infant Monitoring Evaluation (CHIME) Study Group. (2001, May 2). Cardiorespiratory events recorded on home monitors comparison of health infants with those at increased risk for SIDS. *JAMA, 285*(17), 2199–2207.
3. Eichenwald, E. C., Aina, A., & Stark, A. R. (1997). Apnea frequently persists beyond term gestation in infants delivered at 24 to 28 weeks. *Pediatrics, 100*(3, Pt. 1), 354–359.
4. Skouroliakou, M., Bacopoulou, F., & Markantonis, S. L. (2009). Caffeine versus theophylline for apnea of prematurity: A randomized controlled trial. *Journal of Pediatrics and Child Health, 45*(10), 587–592.
5. Finer, N. N., Peters, K. L., Duffley, L. M., et al. (1984). An evaluation of theophylline for idiopathic apnea of infancy. *Developmental Pharmacology and Therapeutics, 7*(2), 73–81.
6. Kurz, H. (1999). Influence of nasopharyngeal CPAP on breathing pattern and incidence of apnoeas in preterm infants. *Biology of the Neonate, 76*(3), 129–133.
7. Davis, P. G., Schmidt, B., Roberts, R. S., et al. (2010). Caffeine for apnea of prematurity trial: Benefits may vary in subgroups. *Journal of Pediatrics, 156*(3), 382–387.
8. Marcus, C. L., Meltzer, L. J., Roberts, R. S., et al. (2014). Long-term effects of caffeine therapy for apnea of prematurity on sleep at school age. *American Journal of Respiratory and Critical Care Medicine, 190*(7), 791–799.
9. Martin, R. J., DiFiore, J. M., Korenke, C. B., et al. (1995). Vulnerability of respiratory control in healthy preterm infants placed supine. *Journal of Pediatrics, 127*(4), 609–614.
10. Bhat, R. Y., Hannam, S., Pressler, R., et al. (2006). Effect of prone and supine position on sleep, apneas, and arousal in preterm infants. *Pediatrics, 118*(1), 101–107.
11. Kahn, A., Groswasser, J., Sottiaux, M., et al. (1993). Prone or supine body position and sleep characteristics in infants. *Pediatrics, 91*(6), 1112–1115.
12. American Academy of Pediatrics, Task Force on Infant Sleep Position and Sudden Infant Death Syndrome. (2000). Changing concepts of sudden infant death syndrome: Implications for infant sleeping environment and sleep position. *Pediatrics, 105,* 650–656.
13. Tieder, J. S., Bonkowsky, J. L., Etzel, R. A., et al.; Subcommittee on Apparent Life Threatening Events. (2016). Brief resolved unexplained events (formerly apparent life-threatening events) and evaluation of lower-risk infants. *Pediatrics, 137*(5). doi:10.1542/peds.2016-0590
14. American Academy of Pediatrics. (2003). Apnea, sudden infant death syndrome, and home monitoring. *Pediatrics, 111*(4, Pt. 1), 914–917.
15. Kahn, A., Rebuffat, E., Franco, P., et al. (1991). Apparent life-threatening events and apnea of infancy. In C. E. Hunt & R. T. Brouillette (Eds.), *Respiratory control disorders* (pp. 178–189). Baltimore, MD: Baltimore Press.
16. Davies, F., & Gupta, R. (2002). Apparent life threatening events in infants presenting to an emergency department. *Emergency Medical Journal, 19,* 11–16.
17. Beck, S. E., & Brooks, L. J. (2011). Home apnea monitoring. In M. J. Light, D. N. Homnick, M. S. Schechter, et al. (Eds.), *Pediatric pulmonology.* Elk Grove Village, IL: American Academy of Pediatrics.
18. Willinger, M., James, L. S., & Catz, C. (1991). Defining the sudden infant death syndrome (SIDS): Deliberations of an expert panel convened by the National Institute of Child Health and Human Development. *Pediatric Pathology, 11*(5), 677–684.
19. McNamara, F., & Sullivan, C. E. (2000). Obstructive sleep apnea in infants: Relation to family history of sudden infant death syndrome, apparent life-threatening events, and obstructive sleep apnea. *Journal of Pediatrics, 136*(3), 318–323.
20. Esani, N., Hodgman, J. E., Ehsani, N., et al. (2008). Apparent life-threatening events and sudden infant death syndrome: Comparison of risk factors. *Journal of Pediatrics, 152*(3), 365–370.

21. Farrell, P. A., Weiner, G. A., & Lemons, J. A. (2002). SIDS, ALTE, apnea, and the use of home monitors. *Pediatrics in Review, 23*, 3–9.

22. Fleming, P. J., Gilbert, R., Azaz, Y., et al. (1990). Interaction between bedding and sleeping position in the sudden infant death syndrome: A population based case-control study. *British Medical Journal, 301*(6743), 85–89.

23. AAP Task Force on Infant Positioning and SIDS. (1992). *Pediatrics, 89*(6), 1120–1126.

24. Positioning and sudden infant death syndrome (SIDS): Update. American Academy of Pediatrics Task Force on Infant Positioning and SIDS. (1996). *Pediatrics, 98*(6, Pt. 1), 1216–1218.

25. Lumeng, J. C., & Chervin, R. D. (2008). Epidemiology of pediatric obstructive sleep apnea. *Proceedings of the American Thoracic Society, 5*(2), 242–252.

26. American Thoracic Society (1996). Standards and Indications for Cardiopulmonary Sleep Studies in Children. *American Journal of Respiratory and Critical Care Medicine, 153*, 866–878.

27. Dyken, M. E., Lin-Dyken, D. C., Poulton, S., et al. (2003). Prospective polysomnographic analysis of obstructive sleep apnea in Down syndrome. *Archives of Pediatrics and Adolescent Medicine, 157*, 655–660.

28. Cielo, C. M., Taylor, J. A., Vossough, A., et al. (2016). Evolution of obstructive sleep apnea in infants with cleft palate and micrognathia. *Journal of Clinical Sleep Medicine, 12*(7), 979–987. doi:10.5664/jcsm.5930

29. Brockmann, P. E., Urschitz, M. S., Schlaud, M., et al. (2012). Primary snoring in school children: Prevalence and neurocognitive impairments. *Sleep and Breathing, 16*(1), 23–29.

30. Suen, J. S., Arnold, J. E., & Brooks, L. J. (1995). Adenotonsillectomy for the treatment of obstructive sleep apnea in children. *Otolaryngology—Head and Neck Surgery, 21*(5), 525–530.

31. Masters, I. B., Harvey, J. M., Whales, P. D., et al. (1999). Clinical versus polysomnographic profiles in children with obstructive sleep apnoea. *Journal of Pediatrics and Child Health, 35*(1), 49–54.

32. Carroll, J. L., McColley, S. A., Marcus, C. L., et al. (1995). Inability of clinical history to distinguish primary snoring from obstructive sleep apnea syndrome in children. *Chest, 108*, 610–618.

33. Marcus, C. L., Keens, T. G., & Ward, S. L. (1992). Comparison of nap and overnight polysomnography in children. *Pediatric Pulmonology, 13*(1), 16–21.

34. Amin, R. S., Kimball, T. R., Bean, J. A., et al. (2002). Left ventricular hypertrophy and abnormal ventricular geometry in children and adolescents with obstructive sleep apnea. *American Journal of Respiratory and Critical Care Medicine, 165*(10), 1395–1399.

35. Marcus, C. L., Greene, M. G., & Carroll, J. L. (1998). Blood pressure in children with obstructive sleep apnea. *American Journal of Respiratory and Critical Care Medicine, 157*, 1098–1103.

36. Brown, O. E., Manning, S. C., & Ridenour, B. (1988). Cor pulmonale secondary to tonsillar and adenoidal hypertrophy: Management considerations. *International Journal of Pediatric Otorhinolaryngology, 16*, 131–139.

37. Leung, L. C., Ng, D. K., Lau, M. W., et al. (2006). Twenty-four-hour ambulatory BP in snoring children with obstructive sleep apnea syndrome. *Chest, 130*(4), 1009–1017.

38. Ugur, M. B., Dogan, S. M., Sogut, A., et al. (2008). Effect of adenoidectomy and/or tonsillectomy on cardiac functions in children with obstructive sleep apnea. *ORL: Journal for Oto-Rhino-Laryngology and Its Related Specialties, 70*(3), 202–208.

39. Marcus, C. L., Carroll, J. L., Koerner, C. B., et al. (1994). Determinants of growth in children with the obstructive sleep apnea syndrome. *Journal of Pediatrics, 125*(4), 556–562.

40. Nieminen, P., Löppönen, T., Tolonen, U., et al. (2002). Growth and biochemical markers of growth in children with snoring and obstructive sleep apnea. *Pediatrics, 109*(4), e55.

41. Kelly, A., Dougherty, S., Cucchiara, A., et al. (2010). Catecholamines, adiponectin, and insulin resistance as measured by HOMA in children with obstructive sleep apnea. *Sleep, 33*(9), 1185–1191.

42. Gottlieb, D. J., Vezina, R. M., Chase, C., et al. (2003). Symptoms of sleep-disordered breathing in 5-year-old children are associated with sleepiness and problem behaviors. *Pediatrics, 112*(4), 870–877.

43. Crabtree, V. M., Ivanenko, A., & Gozal, D. (2003). Clinical and parental assessment of sleep in children with attention-deficit/hyperactivity disorder referred to a pediatric sleep medicine center. *Clinical Pediatrics (Phila), 42*(9), 807–813.

44. Ali, N. J., Pitson, D., & Stradling, J. R. (1996). Sleep disordered breathing: Effects of adenotonsillectomy on behavior and psychological functioning. *European Journal of Pediatrics, 155*(1), 56–62.

45. Chervin, R. D., Archbold, K. H., Dillon, J. E., et al. (2002). Inattention, hyperactivity, and symptoms of sleep-disordered breathing. *Pediatrics, 109*(3), 449–456.

46. Avior, G., Fishman, G., Leor, A., et al. (2004). The effect of tonsillectomy and adenoidectomy on inattention and impulsivity as measured by the Test of Variables of Attention (TOVA) in children with obstructive sleep apnea syndrome. *Otolaryngology—Head and Neck Surgery, 131*(4), 367–371.

47. Kennedy, J. D., Blunden, S., Hirte, C., et al. (2004). Reduced neurocognition in children who snore. *Pediatric Pulmonology, 37*(4), 330–337.

48. Kohler, M. J., Lushington, K., van den Heuvel, C. J., et al. (2009). Adenotonsillectomy and neurocognitive deficits in children with sleep disordered breathing. *PLoS One, 4*(10), e7343.

49. Marcus, C. L., Moore, R. H., Rosen, C. L., et al. (2013). A randomized trial of adenotonsillectomy for childhood sleep apnea. *The New England Journal of Medicine, 368*(25), 2366–2376.

50. Friedman, B. C., Hendeles-Amitai, A., Kozminsky, E., et al. (2003). Adenotonsillectomy improves neurocognitive function in children with obstructive sleep apnea syndrome. *Sleep, 26*(8), 999–1005.

51. Blunden, S., Lushington, K., Kennedy, D., et al. (2000). Behavior and neurocognitive performance in children aged 5–10 years who snore compared to controls. *Journal of Clinical and Experimental Neuropsychology, 22*, 554–568.

52. Constantin, E., Kermack, A., Nixon, G. M., et al. (2007). Adenotonsillectomy improves sleep, breathing, and quality of life but not behavior. *Journal of Pediatrics, 150*(5), 540–546.

53. Mitchell, R. B., & Kelly, J. (2005). Quality of life after adenotonsillectomy for SDB in children. *Otolaryngology—Head and Neck Surgery, 133*(4), 569–572.

54. von Gontard, A., Heron, J., & Joinson, C. (2011). Family history of nocturnal enuresis and urinary incontinence: Results from a large epidemiological study. *Journal of Urology, 185*(6), 2303–2307.

55. Su, M. S., Li, A. M., So, H. K., et al. (2011). Nocturnal enuresis in children: Prevalence, correlates, and relationship with obstructive sleep apnea. *Pediatrics, 159*, 238–242.

56. Brooks, L. J., & Topol, H. I. (2003). Enuresis in children with sleep apnea. *Journal of Pediatrics, 142*(5), 515–518.

57. Weissbach, A., Leiberman, A., Tarasiuk, A., et al. (2006). Adenotonsillectomy improves enuresis in children with obstructive sleep apnea syndrome. *International Journal of Pediatric Otorhinolaryngology, 70*(8), 1351–1356.

58. Bhattacharjee, R., Kheirandish-Gozal, L., Spruyt, K., et al. (2010). Adenotonsillectomy outcomes in treatment of obstructive sleep apnea in children: A multicenter retrospective study. *American Journal of Respiratory and Critical Care Medicine, 182*(5), 676–683.

59. Smatt, Y., & Ferri, J. (2005). Retrospective study of 18 patients treated by maxillomandibular advancement with adjunctive procedures for obstructive sleep apnea syndrome. *Journal of Craniofacial Surgery, 16*(5), 770–777.

60. Prinsell, J. R. (1999). Maxillomandibular advancement surgery in a site-specific treatment approach for obstructive sleep apnea in 50 consecutive patients. *Chest, 116*, 1519–1529.

61. Won, C. H., Li, K. K., & Guilleminault, C. (2008). Surgical treatment of obstructive sleep apnea: Upper airway and maxillomandibular surgery. *Proceedings of the American Thoracic Society, 5*(2), 193–199.

62. Pirelli, P., Saponara, M., & Guilleminault, C. (2004). Rapid maxillary expansion in children with obstructive sleep apnea syndrome. *Sleep, 24*, 761–766.

63. Downey, R., III, Perkin, R. M., & MacQuarrie, J. (2000). Nasal continuous positive airway pressure use in children with obstructive sleep apnea younger than 2 years of age. *Chest, 117*(6), 1608–1612.

64. Marcus, C. L., Ward, S. L., Mallory, G. B., et al. (1995). Use of nasal continuous positive airway pressure as treatment of childhood obstructive sleep apnea. *Journal of Pediatrics, 127*(1), 88–94.

65. Rains, J. C. (1995). Treatment of obstructive sleep apnea in pediatric patients. Behavioral intervention for compliance with nasal continuous positive airway pressure. *Clinical Pediatrics, 34*(10), 535–541.

66. Marcus, C. L., Rosen, G., Ward, S. L., et al. (2006). Adherence to and effectiveness of positive airway pressure therapy in children with obstructive sleep apnea. *Pediatrics, 117*(3), e442–e451.

67. Spruyt, K., Sans Capdevila, O., Serpero, L. D., et al. (2010). Dietary and physical activity patterns in children with obstructive sleep apnea. *Journal of Pediatrics, 156*(5), 724–730.

68. Brooks, L. J. (1993). Treatment of otherwise normal children with obstructive sleep apnea. *Ear, Nose and Throat Journal, 72*(1), 77–79.

69. Brouillette, R. T., Manoukian, J. J., Ducharme, F. M., et al. (2001). Efficacy of fluticasone nasal spray for pediatric obstructive sleep apnea. *Journal of Pediatrics, 138*(6), 838–844.

70. Kheirandish-Gozal, L., Bhattacharjee, R., Bandla, H. P., et al. (2014). Antiinflammatory therapy outcomes for mild OSA in children. *Chest, 146*(1), 88–95.

71. Kheirandish-Gozal, L., & Gozal, D. (2008). Intranasal budesonide treatment for children with mild obstructive sleep apnea syndrome. *Pediatrics, 122*(1), e149–e155.

72. Goldbart, A. D., Goldman, J. L., Veiling, M. C., et al. (2005). Leukotriene modifier for mild sleep-disordered breathing in children. *American Journal of Respiratory and Critical Care Medicine, 172*(3), 364–370.

73. Kheirandish, L., Goldbart, A. D., & Gozal, D. (2006). Intranasal steroids and oral leukotriene modifier therapy in residual sleep-disordered breathing after tonsillectomy and adenoidectomy in children. *Pediatrics, 117*(1), e61–e66.

74. Aljadeff, G., Gozal, D., Bailey-Wahl, S. L., et al. (1996). Effects of overnight supplemental oxygen in obstructive sleep apnea in children. *American Journal of Respiratory and Critical Care Medicine, 153*(1), 51–55.

chapter 63

Nonrespiratory Pediatric Sleep Disorders

KRISTINE BRESNEHAN SERVIDIO

LEARNING OBJECTIVES

On completion of this chapter, the reader should be able to:

1. Describe the essential features of nonrespiratory sleep disorders in children.
2. Give examples of how nonrespiratory sleep disorders manifest differently in children at various age ranges.
3. Explain the uses and limits of polysomnography in the evaluation of pediatric sleep disorders other than sleep apnea.
4. Describe the role that clinical observations have in the diagnosis of nonrespiratory sleep disorders in children.

KEY TERMS

Sleep
Insomnia
Narcolepsy
Enuresis

Approximately 25% of all children experience some type of sleep problem during childhood (1). Although some pediatric sleep disorders are treatable, many become chronic if left untreated (1). Chronic insufficient sleep is increasing because of competing priorities such as homework, television, social activities, and poor sleep hygiene (1). Sleep disorders are preventable through education regarding normal sleep behavior, routines, self-soothing techniques, and sleep hygiene. Sleep problems in children have a direct effect on parents' sleep, stress levels, and family interactions. Most importantly, sleep is necessary for children to function optimally (1).

Although insufficient quantity and quality of sleep in children usually result in excessive daytime sleepiness, children may not exhibit the same symptoms as adults. Sleepiness in children often manifests as mood disturbances, hyperactivity, poor impulse control, and neurocognitive dysfunction. Mood disturbances such as irritability, temper tantrums, and poor emotional

regulation are some of the many signs of insufficient sleep. Cognitive dysfunction may appear as inattention, poor concentration, decreased reaction time, impaired vigilance, poor decision making and problem solving, learning problems, and poor academic performance. Behaviorally, the child may be overactive, noncompliant, have poor impulse control, and demonstrate oppositional behavior and increased risk taking (2).

Sleep disturbances in children are most often reported by the parents or caregivers because of the negative impact that they have on the family. It makes sense that pediatricians are often the first to hear a complaint regarding pediatric sleep disorder. Pediatricians, in collaboration with the Sleep Disorders Center, should take an aggressive role in the early detection and treatment of sleep disorders.

AGE-RELATED FEATURES OF NONRESPIRATORY PEDIATRIC SLEEP DISORDERS

Depending on the child's age and maturity, nonrespiratory sleep disorders can manifest themselves in different ways. Some sleep disorders are more frequent at certain ages, and it is helpful to the sleep technologist to be aware of the signs and symptoms of common nonrespiratory sleep disorders seen in each age range. The technologist must also have an understanding of normal sleep patterns for each of the age groups to understand the impact that a sleep disorder can have on the individual's sleep requirements.

Normal Sleep Patterns for Newborns and Infants

Newborns (0 to 2 Months)

Hours of sleep: 16 to 20 hours per 24 hours. No nocturnal/diurnal pattern in the first few weeks; sleep is distributed throughout the day and night (1).

Infants (2 to 12 Months)

Hours of sleep: nighttime 9 to 12 hours and daytime naps 2 to 4.5 hours. Regular rhythm of periods of sleepiness and alertness will emerge by 2 to 4 months.

Common sleep disorders in this age group include the following:

Colic

Body rocking and headbanging

Sleep-onset association disorder

Colic is one of the most common causes of sleep disturbance in the 3- to 6-month-old infant. Colic appears to be related to digestion and is an often misunderstood condition. The most common form of colic is circadian in nature and begins at approximately 2 to 3 months, resolving spontaneously at approximately 5 to 6 months.

The pediatrician must differentiate colic from milk intolerance or gastroesophageal reflux disease. An important feature of the differential diagnosis is that in colic, the crying has a clear circadian rhythm. The baby does not cry after daytime feedings, but becomes irritable in the evening and fusses inconsolably until around the same time in the late evening or night (2). Parents will often misperceive the "vomiting" that occurs as a result of swallowing air while crying, to be a symptom of a stomach upset. Infants with central or obstructive sleep apnea syndrome may also have frequent arousals with crying, but this occurs during all sleep periods, day or night (1).

CASE EXAMPLE **Severe Colic in a 4-Month-Old Infant**

A 4-month-old baby girl is accompanied by her parents to the sleep center. The baby appears content, but the parents complain of fatigue and lack of sleep. They report that at approximately 9 p.m. every evening their usually good-natured baby becomes a different child. She begins fussing, squirming, and drawing her legs up in pain. The parents have tried medication for possible reflux, medication for allergies, changing the formula from milk to soy, all to no avail. They take turns walking and patting her, which often leads to more crying and screaming. The only thing that seems to calm her is a drive around the neighborhood with her in the car seat. She falls asleep at about midnight and is fine for the rest of the night. The next morning, she is back to her usual happy self. The sleep physician ordered a polysomnogram to rule out apnea and reflux.

Normal Sleep Patterns for Toddlers and Preschool Children
Toddlers (12 Months to 3 Years)

Hours of sleep: 12 to 13 hours per 24 hours. Daytime naps: from two to one nap by age 18 months lasting 30 minutes to 2 hours.

Preschool-Age Children (3 to 5 Years)

Hours of sleep: 11 to 12 hours per 24 hours. Daytime naps: from 1 to none.

Sleep problems occur in 25% to 30% of children in the preschool-age group. This is a time when many developmental changes occur. Naps decrease from two to one by 3 years of age and then to none by age 5. Timing and duration of naps can affect nighttime sleep. The child gives up the bottle and moves to a big bed. At around 3 years, the child develops imagination and fantasy, which can lead to increased night fears. Bedtime routines need to be consistent with a progression toward relaxation. Transitional objects such as blankets, dolls, and stuffed animals help the child learn to self-soothe for sleep onset and after arousals. Parental reassurance that the child is safe is more effective than actions, which reinforce the idea that a "monster" exists (1).

Common sleep disorders in the preschool-age group include the following:

Sleep-onset association disorder/nighttime waking

Limit-setting sleep disorder/bedtime resistance

Rhythmic movement disorders like headbanging, body rocking, and body rolling

Nighttime fears and nightmares

Normal Sleep Pattern for School-Aged Children (5 to 11 Years)

Hours of sleep: 10 to 11 hours per 24 hours.

School-age children may not obtain sufficient sleep, which can lead to behavioral and learning problems. The child may be misdiagnosed with attention-deficit disorder or learning disabilities, particularly in classroom subjects that require complex problem solving or sustained attention (2).

Some of the more common nonrespiratory sleep disorders in the school-age child are as follows:

Sleepwalking and sleep terrors

Bruxism

Insufficient sleep

Inadequate sleep hygiene

Periodic limb movement disorder (PLMD)

Disorders of arousal parasomnias are more frequent in childhood than in adolescence. Estimates of sleep terrors range from 1% to 6%, sleepwalking up to 17% with a peak at 8 to 12 years, and confusional arousals up to 17.3% (1). School-age children with chronic sleep deprivation rarely articulate the need to nap or rest because they don't know what it feels to be adequately rested.

Bruxism is a movement-type sleep disorder characterized by repetitive grinding or clenching of the teeth during sleep. It is accompanied by scraping and clicking sounds. Bruxism has two distinct patterns, diurnal and nocturnal. Although bruxism is closely related to stress, the two etiologies appear to be different (1). Allergies, cerebral palsy, intellectual disability, alcohol, stimulant medications, and seizure can contribute to bruxism. Adult-type bruxism usually begins in childhood or adolescence; however, most cases of bruxism are self-limiting and may even disappear with the eruption of secondary teeth. Diagnosis rarely involves a sleep study. Bruxism can lead to excessive wear of the teeth, periodontal tissue damage, jaw pain, and headache. Dental appliances, sleeping position, pharmacotherapy, or psychological treatment may be used to alleviate the symptoms (2).

Inadequate sleep hygiene is caused by activities that increase arousal, like caffeinated soda, stimulating television, and play. Napping during the day, nighttime awakenings from periodic limb movements (PLMs), loud noises, and bright lights lead to disorganized and often insufficient sleep for the youngster.

Normal Sleep Pattern for Adolescents (Ages 12 to 18)

Hours of sleep: 9 to 9.5 hours needed but 7 to 7.25 hours obtained.

Sleep disorders seen in this age group include the following:

Insufficient sleep

Inadequate sleep

Insomnia

Delayed sleep phase syndrome

Restless legs syndrome (RLS)/PLMD

Narcolepsy

Kleine–Levin syndrome

Around puberty, hormonal changes cause a daily delay in melatonin secretion. This delay results in a delayed sleep onset of approximately 2 hours. Despite the circadian rhythm delay, the adolescent still needs 9 to 9.25 hours of sleep. With early school start times, extracurricular activities, more independence, part-time jobs, and increasing socialization, adolescents manage an average of 7 to 7.5 hours of sleep, causing them to be chronically sleep deprived. Insomnia may be caused by new social pressures, academic pressures, increased responsibilities, or a bedtime too early for the adolescent's circadian rhythm (3). Parents and adolescents may attribute the symptoms of RLS or PLMD to growing pains or sports injuries. A polysomnogram is useful in identifying the movements and the extent of related arousals.

Chronic sleep restriction can cause mood disturbances, depression, poor academic performance, attention or memory deficits, risk-taking behavior, and increased involvement in traffic accidents (3). All the previously listed sleep disorders lead to excessive day time sleepiness. However, narcolepsy has more complex symptomatology.

Narcolepsy is caused by impaired sleep–wake regulation of the central nervous system (CNS). The patient complains of excessive daytime sleepiness, cataplexy (the abrupt loss of muscle tone provoked by strong emotion), hypnagogic hallucinations (vivid auditory or visual "dreams" often frightening), and sleep paralysis (inability to move or speak for a few seconds at sleep onset or offset). Although narcolepsy is reported for all age groups, it is most often reported by teenagers and young adults (4).

Kleine–Levin syndrome (5), or recurrent hypersomnia, is characterized by acute episodes of excessive sleepiness, hyperphagia, and hypersexuality lasting up to several weeks at a time. Kleine–Levin syndrome usually occurs during adolescence and is more common in males. Sleep and behavior are normal between episodes (5).

TECHNICAL CONSIDERATIONS

Technical considerations related to polysomnographic (PSG) testing in the child begin with a consideration of the environment in the sleep center. The sleeping environment should provide separate beds for parent, baby, child, or adolescent. Keep in mind that the parent is usually suffering from sleep deprivation as a result of the child's problem.

1. A foldaway bed, not a recliner, must be provided to ensure that the parent is rested well enough to take the child home after the polysomnogram.
2. Room temperature should be comfortable for an average adult.
3. The crib slats should be no greater than $2^{3}/_{8}$ in (6.03 cm) apart.
4. The crib mattress should be firm, tight fitting in the crib, and no comforters or pillows should be used.

5. The American Academy of Pediatrics recommends that the baby be placed on the back, during sleep, to reduce the risk of sudden infant death syndrome (4).

6. Infants can be swaddled or wear mittens, during setup, to prevent them from inadvertently pulling off leads.

7. Place belts under pajama top, bring wires and leads to the side of the infant, and bind them together. Point head leads toward the top of the head and bind together. This placement will allow the infant or child to sleep supine or on one side without lying on wires.

8. Toddlers and children enjoy participating in the setup with the support of a parent. Props, such as flashlights, music, dolls, and stickers, can be used to make the "sleepover event" into a game. Have the toddler sit on the parent(s) lap during setup to help reduce anxiety.

9. Adolescents need to feel informed regarding the purpose of each lead.

10. The pediatric sleep technologist should observe parent–child interactions and document them in the log. An audiovisual recording should be made during setup, polysomnogram recording, and takedown to document all interactions for the sleep specialist.

CLINICAL OBSERVATIONS

The clinical observations made by the technologist during the PSG recording are extremely valuable in the diagnosis of pediatric sleep disorders. The technologist serves as the eyes and ears of the sleep physician and therefore thorough documentation is essential.

The initial assessment of a pediatric sleep disturbance will include the following:

Detailed sleep history from the parents, a home video, if possible, and a sleep diary

Medical history, with a developmental assessment of school functioning

Family history, a psychosocial history, and a behavioral assessment

Physical examination

This information will direct the sleep technologist to focus on the observations most valuable to the sleep physician. The use of video recordings during PSG is important in documenting both parent and child behavior. However, the sleep technologist's written observations can provide the sleep physician with information regarding how the child feels, what he or she believes is happening, what he or she needs, and whether the family can support his or her needs.

The technologist should document anything out of the ordinary such as the following:

Unusual behavior of the child

Headbanging or rocking

Sleepwalking

Prolonged crying

Hypersomnolence

Hypersexuality

Hallucinations

Sleep paralysis or cataplexy

Unusual behavior of a family member (swearing, yelling, and rough handling)

Unusual eating habits (eating during sleep time and overeating)

Unusual sleeping positions (arched back and sitting up)

Unusual verbalization (screaming, prolonged crying, and words inappropriate for age)

Signs of abuse; bruises (black eyes)

Bed-wetting (sleep stage and parents' and child's reactions)

Numerous visits to the bathroom or resistance to bedtime

Clinical Observations in the Infant to Preschool Population (Ages 0 to 5)

Bedtime in the sleep center should be identical to the bedtime in the child's home, and the nighttime routine should approximate the routine at home as closely as possible. Obviously, the environment is different, but the parent should nevertheless be encouraged to attempt to simulate the environment and bedtime routine. Have the child bring his or her favorite blanket, pillow, pajamas, bedtime snack, and snuggle toy. Document the bedtime routine, use of a night light, bedtime stalling, and the interaction between the parent(s) and the child at or around sleep onset. Some of the most common sleep disorders in this age group are sleep-onset association disorders in which the child's innate self-quieting skills are replaced by a need for the physical presence of the parent and/or some parental bedtime behavior in order to initiate sleep. The best course in documentation is to describe an observed activity quoting the dialogue between parent and child. The technologist should not write an opinion or make any judgment regarding the activity or event.

Clinical Observations in the School-Age Child

While scheduling the sleep study, the technologist should identify and document any special needs the child may have during the test. On the basis of the child's normal bedtime, plan the setup to allow for as representative a night's sleep as possible. The child should be offered a tour of the lab and given an overview of the procedure. The technologist should involve the parent or caregiver in the study setup and explain the procedure. The child's nightly routine should be followed as closely as the situation will allow, and the technologist should take careful and elaborate notes. The parent or caregiver must spend the night in the lab, either in a separate bed or in another bedroom.

Following the onset of sleep, it is important for the technologist to be especially vigilant at the beginning of the night when slow-wave sleep ensues. Many of the disorders seen during this stage of development occur in stage N3 sleep. Any awakening from slow-wave sleep should be carefully observed and thoroughly described. The primary disorders that may occur at this age during deep sleep include confusional arousals, sleepwalking, and sleep terrors. As is the case with any partial arousal disorder, it is the responsibility of the technologist to provide for the safety of the child. Review the electroencephalogram (EEG) before the episode and after the episode for epileptiform and/or postictal activity and document the activity on the study log (5).

It is important to remember that the technologist's responsibility to observe the patient continues after the polysomnogram is completed. The behaviors observed following lights on might be a crucial component in the evaluation of the patient. Before lights on, determine roughly the amount of sleep the child actually obtained during the night and compare this with the normative value for the child's age. The technologist should observe and record at lights on to document paralysis, automatic behaviors, confusion, or amnesia. This documentation should include the reaction of the child and any behaviors that might be seen up to the time when the child actually leaves the facility.

Clinical Observations in the Adolescent

When scheduling the sleep study, the teen should be asked if he or she has any special needs or prefers a technologist of the same sex. The teen should be offered a tour of the lab and given an overview of the procedure. Privacy is very important to the adolescent patient, and this need must be respected. The patient may also have concerns and misperceptions about the polysomnogram procedure, but may not always express these concerns directly. The technologist should explain the purpose of each measurement device during the setup. The technologist can ask if the adolescent has any questions and answer them with patience. The principles of behavioral observations in adolescents are similar to those in other children as well as adults (3).

SLEEP DISORDERS

The *International Classification of Sleep Disorders*, third edition divides sleep disorders into seven categories as follows (6):

1. Insomnia
2. Sleep-related breathing disorders
3. Central disorders of hypersomnolence
4. Circadian rhythm sleep–wake disorders
5. Parasomnias
6. Sleep-related movement disorders
7. Narcolepsy

Although the neurobiology of sleep is a constant, psychosocial and cultural practices, such as cosleeping, can change the natural sleep behavior of a developing brain. Other variables, like the child's temperament and medical problems, can affect his or her response to zeitgebers (i.e., environmental cues) for signaling circadian rhythms. For example, the easygoing child may bend to varying bedtimes, whereas the more anxious child may need a consistent bedtime to foster a more predictable and secure environment. A blind child will never respond to the light versus dark zeitgeber. Parenting styles, education levels, mental health issues, family stress, and lifestyle also have an effect on both the real and the perceived pediatric sleep pattern. Sleep habits are influenced by normal developmental changes. For example, toddlers experience separation anxiety, which may lead to bedtime resistance. The pediatric sleep technologist observes the family dynamics and behaviors for the sleep physician and, therefore, must be knowledgeable in all the disorders listed earlier (7).

Sleep-related breathing disorders and parasomnias are discussed in other chapters in this textbook. Nonrespiratory sleep problems most frequently studied by the pediatric sleep technologist are hypersomnia, circadian rhythm disorders, and epilepsy. Insomnia, per se, is relatively rare in the pediatric population (8).

INSOMNIA

Insomnia is defined as a persistent difficulty with sleep initiation, duration, consolidation, or quality that occurs despite adequate opportunity to sleep and results in some form of daytime impairment (1). Because the child cannot articulate the sleep complaint, the pediatrician often makes a referral to a sleep specialist when the parent or caregiver voices concern over the child's sleeplessness (1). A polysomnogram may be ordered to evaluate the duration of sleep and the underlying causes for the sleep complaint. Some of the most frequently encountered causes of sleep-onset insomnia and prolonged nocturnal awakenings in children are as follows:

1. Sleep-onset association disorder
2. Circadian rhythm disorders
3. Inadequate sleep hygiene
4. PLMS and RLS
5. Limit-setting behaviors
6. Obstructive sleep apnea syndrome

Sleep-Onset Association Disorder

Approximately 25% to 50% of 6- to 12-month-olds and 30% of 1-year-olds experience sleep-onset association disorder. The child cannot fall asleep without a habituated set of conditions that require parental intervention to initiate sleep. Parental interventions include the following: being held, rocked, breastfed; watching television; or listening to music. When the condition is present, sleep onset is normal. When the association is absent, sleep latency is increased at sleep onset and after nocturnal arousals. The child has no underlying medical or mental disorder, and the symptoms do not meet the criteria for any other sleep disorder. Transitional objects such as a pacifier, special blanket, or stuffed animal allow the child to self-soothe and fall asleep without parental response (1).

CASE EXAMPLE **Feeding as a Sleep-Onset Association in an Infant**

A 9-month-old breastfed baby boy is referred to the sleep center for numerous arousals and excessive crying at night. His mother nurses him until he falls asleep. She puts him in the crib, next to her bed, and goes to sleep. The baby's father sleeps in another room to obtain adequate sleep. The baby boy wakes up every 2 to 3 hours and cries until his mother gets up and nurses him back to sleep.

CASE EXAMPLE **Use of the DVD Player as a Sleep Aid in a Pre-school Child**

A 4-year-old boy is being evaluated in the sleep center for daytime sleepiness. He has a regular bedtime and rise time of 9 p.m. to 6 a.m. He states that he cannot fall asleep without the movie, *Toy Story*, playing on his bedroom

television. If he wakes up during the night, his mother starts the movie again, and he returns to sleep, after watching for 20 to 30 minutes. This pattern may repeat itself several times during the night. The patient went to his grandmother's house for the summer. But the grandmother did not have the movie. The 4-year-old hardly slept for the first week, but during the second week, he slept very well and felt great during the day. When he returned home, he resumed his Toy Story movie habit and his daytime sleepiness returned. The sleep physician ordered a sleep diary and behavioral therapy.

CASE EXAMPLE **Pet Dog Presence with Physical Contact as a Sleep Aid for an Adolescent**

A 14-year-old boy insists on having his pet collie sleep in his bed every night. He tosses and turns until the dog is lying firmly against his side. If the dog gets out of bed to drink or go outside, the boy wakes up. He cannot return to sleep until the dog comes back and gets into her usual place, beside the boy. When the collie was hospitalized, the boy was unable to fall asleep until past 3 a.m. and was late for school. This pattern continued until the adolescent's dog was returned home.

Inadequate Sleep Hygiene

Inadequate sleep hygiene, which frequently results in insufficient sleep, can be divided into two sleep-related behaviors.

1. Practices that increase arousal
2. Practices that reduce sleep organization

Practices that increase arousal before bedtime are stimulating TV or movies, games, team sports, and excessive caffeine intake. Practices that reduce sleep organization are afternoon napping, inconsistent sleep schedule, light, noise, bed type, cosleeping, and use of the bedroom for activities other than sleep.

Inadequate sleep hygiene is the most common cause for difficulty initiating and maintaining sleep (6). The patient has a complaint of excessive sleepiness, delayed sleep onset, and nighttime awakenings for at least 3 months. The patient's usual sleep episode is shorter than expected for his or her age. A therapeutic trial of a longer sleep episode eliminates the symptoms (9).

The sleep physician will request that the parent complete a sleep diary, which can identify the above-mentioned behaviors. Generally, a polysomnogram is not ordered. Behavioral therapy is the typical treatment.

CASE EXAMPLE Irregular Sleep Schedule with No Bedtime Routine in a Toddler

A 2-year-old boy and his parents are in the sleep clinic for evaluation of problem behaviors occurring both day and night. The child falls asleep in his car seat. When his mother wakes him to go into the grocery store, he has temper tantrums in the store. He often falls down screaming and kicking when his mother refuses him a treat. He kicks strangers in the legs when they approach him. His height, weight, and head circumference are, respectively, in the 60%, 50%, and 50%, for his age. The parents state that he eats well but is a very restless sleeper. He often gets out of the family bed and plays for hours until a parent takes him back to bed. The child falls asleep when he is sleepy and is placed in the family bed when the parents go to bed. He has never had a regular bedtime because the father works rotating shifts. The parents estimate that he sleeps 6 to 7 hours each day. After a complete physical workup, the sleep physician ordered a sleep diary and PSG to rule out other causes for his sleep problems, such as sleep apnea, seizure, and restless legs. When the PSG revealed no pathology, family behavioral therapy was suggested.

CASE EXAMPLE Insomnia Caused by Inadequate Sleep Hygiene

A 17-year-old obese female is referred to the sleep center for difficulty initiating and maintaining sleep. She complains that it often takes her 30 to 45 minutes to fall asleep and she awakens frequently. She is an A-B student, active in drama, math club, and band. She gets up at 6 a.m. to attend band practice at 7 a.m. She drinks a caffeinated power drink as she leaves home. School starts at 8 a.m. So she has another caffeinated soft drink and some breakfast bars at school. From 4 to 6 p.m., she has drama and math club. The family has dinner, with iced tea, at 7 p.m. The 17-year-old makes phone calls until 9 p.m., then has a caffeinated power drink, and does homework until 11 p.m. She showers and does her hair before going to bed at midnight. She rarely sleeps in on the weekends because she is participating in one or more of her extracurricular activities. She feels tired in the morning, but the power drinks perk her up. Lately she has been falling asleep at lunch break. The sleep physician ordered a sleep diary and a PSG to rule out sleep apnea and seizures. The PSG revealed a prolonged sleep onset, but no pathology. The study was allowed to continue past her normal wake-up time and she slept until 9:00 a.m. Sleep hygiene training was recommended for the family.

Limit-Setting Type

Limit-setting sleep disorder is characterized by difficulty initiating sleep. The child stalls or refuses to go to sleep at the set bedtime. After lights out, the child will get up for a drink, another kiss, or to ask "one last question." Once the child is asleep, sleep quality and duration are normal.

When limits are not set or enforced consistently, the child's sleep is delayed and the sleep period may be insufficient for his or her needs. Bedtime resistance occurs in 10% to 30% of toddlers and preschoolers and 15% of 4- to 10-year-old children (1). Permissive or conflicting parenting styles, environment (such as cosleeping with parents or grandparents), and circadian cycles can contribute to limit-setting sleep disorder.

CASE EXAMPLE Insomnia Caused by Limit-Setting Sleep Disorder

A 2-year-old girl is brought to the clinic for what the parents describe as refusing to go to bed on time. Her mother says she began fighting sleep when they got her a "big girl bed." She has a nap around 1 to 2 p.m., dinner around 5 p.m. She then has her bath and bedtime stories until around 8 p.m., which is lights out time. She climbs out of bed several times for the next 2 hours asking for a drink, another hug, or an "important question." She had surgery for a hernia at the age of 6 months and her mother has a fear of upsetting the child. Limit-setting therapy was recommended.

HYPERSOMNIA

Insufficient sleep quantity

Fragmentation or poor sleep quality

Inappropriate timing of the sleep period

Narcolepsy and idiopathic hypersomnia

Insufficient Sleep

Insufficient sleep quantity may be the result of difficulty in initiating sleep, prolonged periods of wake time during the night, or the need to terminate the sleep period early. Ultimately, the child obtains less sleep than needed and experiences excessive daytime sleepiness (3).

Sleep Fragmentation

Sleep fragmentation is usually the result of repetitive brief arousals. Practices such as caffeine use before bedtime, and bright light, and loud noises in the bedroom frequently lead to arousal during sleep. Sleep fragmentation can also be caused by disorders of arousal such as sleepwalking, confusional arousals, and sleep terrors. These arousals occur most often during slow-wave (N3) sleep, which is most prominent in the first third of the night. The child's transition from N3 to a lighter stage appears to be incomplete and phenomena such as automatic behavior, altered perception of the environment, and amnesia regarding the event result in disturbed sleep (5).

Delayed Sleep–Wake Phase Disorder

Inappropriate timing of the sleep period is often the result of delayed sleep–wake phase disorder (DSWPD). The adolescent or child has a persistent shift in the sleep–wake schedule, which conflicts with school, or lifestyle. Sleep onset may be delayed, causing the adolescent to complain of insomnia. This delay is seen in combination with difficulty waking in the morning to participate in the daily routine. Typically, DSWPD begins during adolescence when the "night owl" preference becomes exaggerated by social, academic, or work demands. It affects about 5% to 10% of adolescents (1). The sleep physician will request a sleep diary, and actigraphy may be utilized to confirm a phase delay. A polysomnogram may be appropriate in some patients to rule out other pathology. Behavior modification may be used to move bedtime forward until a more desirable circadian rhythm can be established.

CASE EXAMPLE   Insomnia Caused by DSWPD

A 15-year-old male came to the sleep clinic accompanied by his father. The patient says that he avoids all caffeine, does not nap in the day, and still cannot fall asleep at night. Bedtime is 10 p.m. every night. He waits for his parents to go to bed at 11 p.m., then gets up and plays on the computer for a couple of hours. He tries to go back to bed but cannot sleep, so he gets up again. He has been prescribed various different sedative–hypnotic medications. He was also prescribed medication to improve his daytime alertness, but developed headaches, so this was discontinued. He feels that the sedating medications do not help him fall asleep and that he has even more difficulty getting out of bed in the morning when he takes his medications. He likes school but is in constant trouble for falling asleep in class, losing his temper when the kids tease him for being sleepy or sneaking into the library for a nap. He frequently misses morning classes and has missed so many classes that he will have to repeat the ninth grade. During summer break, the adolescent is allowed to stay up until he feels sleepy. He generally falls asleep around 3 a.m. and gets up at 11 a.m., feeling refreshed, and has no need for naps.

Narcolepsy

Primary disorders of excessive daytime sleepiness involve more complex pathophysiology, which presents as excessive daytime sleepiness. A salient feature of narcolepsy is hypersomnia (4). Type I narcolepsy is primarily characterized by excessive daytime sleepiness and cataplexy, and is associated with a deficiency in hypothalamic hypocretin (orexin) signaling (7). Type II narcolepsy is characterized by excessive daytime sleepiness and abnormal manifestations of rapid eye movement (REM) sleep without cataplexy (6).

The four hallmark clinical features of narcolepsy (also called the "narcoleptic tetrad") are as follows:

1. Excessive daytime sleepiness
2. Cataplexy
3. Sleep paralysis
4. Hypnagogic hallucinations

Excessive daytime sleepiness is the irresistible urge to fall asleep when environmental stimulus is relatively reduced. Children may appear inattentive, lazy, sleepy, or hyperactive. Narcolepsy–cataplexy is most commonly caused by a loss of hypocretin (Hert-1)-producing cells in the hypothalamus. Low cerebral spinal fluid Hert-1 levels can be used to diagnose the condition. Whether narcolepsy is an autoimmune disorder is still unclear, but the evidence of autoimmune destruction of Hert-1-producing cell is documented (7). Children of narcoleptics have a 40 times greater risk for developing narcolepsy than the general population. Narcolepsy is also associated with head trauma, brain tumors, and demyelinating disease. Narcolepsy onset is most common in the second decade of life, and incidence of onset falls with each subsequent decade (5).

Nighttime symptoms of narcolepsy may include sleep disruption, sleep paralysis, and hallucinations. Daytime symptoms may include falling asleep at school, inattentiveness, poor concentration, distractibility, academic problems, and automatic behavior. Children may report that daytime naps help in maintaining alertness. Narcolepsy symptoms in children are frequently misdiagnosed as psychiatric or behavioral disorders, including attention-deficit hyperactivity disorder (ADHD), depression, conversion reaction, and psychosis.

Other symptoms of narcolepsy include *hypnagogic/ hypnopompic hallucinations*, which are often described as "dreams," but are actually vivid auditory or visual hallucinations. They occur during transitions from wakefulness to sleep (hypnagogic) and from sleep to wakefulness (hypnopompic). It is reported that 50% to 70% of narcoleptics experience these hallucinations during both day and nighttime sleep periods.

Sleep-onset REM is defined as stage R occurring within the first 15 minutes of sleep. However, neonates enter sleep through stage R about 50% of the time. Sleep-onset REM periods can occur in children who are sleep deprived or who have sleep apnea; therefore, the interpretation of sleep-onset REM periods during the multiple sleep latency test (MSLT) in the pediatric population can be deceiving. Because of this phenomenon, it is particularly important to assess sleep patterns and perform a polysomnogram the night before performing an MSLT in children (2).

Cataplexy is defined as the loss of muscle tone provoked by strong emotion such as laughter, surprise, anger, or sadness. During cataplexy, the individual is conscious and remembers the event. Loss of muscle tone can be localized to the face, eyes, and jaw or can cause complete body collapse. Cataplexy usually develops within a year of the excessive daytime sleepiness symptom. In children with narcolepsy, cataplexy is uncommon.

After a thorough medical history and tests to rule out underlying medical conditions, alcohol, and drug use, the sleep physician will order an overnight sleep study followed by the MSLT to evaluate symptoms of narcolepsy. In children with narcolepsy, the polysomnogram should indicate a sleep latency of less than 10 minutes and a sleep efficiency of greater than 90%. The MSLT begins 1½ to 2 hours after awakening. The test consists of five 20-minute nap opportunities spaced at 2-hour intervals during the day. An MSLT with a mean sleep latency for all naps of less than 8 minutes, and with at least two sleep-onset R periods, is consistent with narcolepsy (5).

CASE EXAMPLE **Narcolepsy in an Adolescent**

A 16-year-old male was seen in the clinic for what his parents reported as severe sleepiness to the point of falling down. They reported that the "young man falls asleep any time he is not eating or walking around." At first, the parents thought the adolescent wasn't sleeping well because of a history of bad dreams. They monitored his nighttime routine and found that he was consistently falling asleep by about 10 p.m. and waking up at 7 a.m., with the alarm clock. He would stare at the ceiling for a few minutes and then get out of bed. Nevertheless, he falls asleep doing homework, watching television, and texting his friends. When his friends tease him about his clumsiness, he does not laugh. He closes his eyes and makes a face. After a physical workup, the sleep physician ordered a polysomnogram followed by an MSLT.

Idiopathic Hypersomnia

Idiopathic hypersomnia can be differentiated from narcolepsy by the lack of refreshment from napping, the absence of cataplexy, sleep paralysis, hypnagogic hallucinations, and sleep-onset REM periods. After a rigorous evaluation to rule out organic causes, encephalopathy or a CNS space-occupying lesion, substance abuse, and psychiatric conditions, a polysomnogram is generally ordered to rule out apnea, PLMD, seizure activity, or a phase delay syndrome. An MSLT is necessary to rule out narcolepsy. The underlying cause of idiopathic hypersomnia is unknown (1).

PARASOMNIAS

Parasomnias are generally classified as follows:

1. Disorders of arousal from non-REM sleep
2. Parasomnias usually associated with REM (R) sleep
3. Other parasomnias

Common characteristics of these disorders include an incomplete transition from stage N3 to a lighter stage of sleep, automatic behavior, altered perception of the environment, and amnesia for the event. Disorders of arousal tend to occur in the first third of the night when stage N3 is most prominent. Essentially, parasomnias occur in the transition between stage N3 and stage R sleep and wakefulness. The EEG presents a mixture of theta, delta, and alpha frequencies. Additional information on the parasomnias can be found in other chapters in this textbook.

Sleep Enuresis (Bed-Wetting)

Enuresis is the involuntary voiding of urine during sleep that occurs at least twice a month in a child age 5 or older. If the child has never been dry for a period of 1 year, the condition is called "primary enuresis." Primary enuresis constitutes 80% of all bed wetters. Secondary enuresis is the recurrence of bed-wetting after at least a year of being dry. The child wets during the first third of the night, which coincides with the longest period of stage N3 sleep. The child has no recollection of the event. Enuresis is slightly more common in boys than in girls (2).

A number of factors may contribute to enuresis:

A family history of enuresis

Delayed maturation

A stressful life event such as divorce or the birth of a sibling

Delayed arousal from sleep

Small functional bladder capacity

Some organic causes for enuresis are as follows:

Chronic constipation, which can irritate the bladder

Sleep apnea

Urinary tract infection

Diabetes causing excess urine production

Seizure causing loss of bladder control

After the pediatrician has ruled out the organic causes for bed-wetting, a polysomnogram may be useful to determine the phase of sleep during which the enuresis occurs and whether it is related to sleep apnea or nocturnal seizures. Every year, about 15% of bed wetters become dry without treatment. The pediatrician can treat persistent enuresis using both medication and behavioral therapy (1).

Sleep-Related Seizure Disorders

PSG performed with an expanded EEG montage is very useful in the evaluation of nocturnal seizures. Sleep deprivation, illness, fever, irregular sleep schedules, obstructive sleep apnea, and medications used for the treatment of behavioral or psychiatric problems can exacerbate seizures. A nocturnal seizure can occur at any time during a polysomnogram, but seizures are more commonly seen at the beginning or end of slow-wave sleep and just after awakening in the morning (10).

Acute or chronic sleep deprivation increases the probability of a seizure in susceptible individuals. The most frequently seen EEG abnormality, in children with seizure disorders, is isolated spikes prominent in the temporal and central EEG placements and 3-Hz spike-wave discharges. Sleep-related seizure disorder is part of the differential diagnosis for primary enuresis and non-REM parasomnias (2). Seizures can be isolated to either sleep or waking. However, seizures can occur in both states (10).

CASE EXAMPLE **Status Epilepticus of Sleep in an Adolescent with a History of Frequent Generalized Tonic–Clonic Seizures after Awakening for School in the Mornings**

A 15-year-old male with a long history of generalized tonic–clonic seizures is referred to the sleep center by his neurologist for evaluation of nonrestorative sleep. He has approximately one generalized tonic–clonic seizure per month, always in the morning within the first few minutes after his dad awakens him for school. These seizures do not seem to be related to the adolescent's sleep schedule, which is highly regular. He goes to bed at 9:30 p.m. and is awakened for school at 7 a.m. He never resists going to bed. He admits to feeling sleepy in class almost every day, but had always thought this was due to his anticonvulsant medications. The polysomnogram revealed electrical status epilepticus throughout 90% of non-REM sleep, but the patient's EEG was essentially normal during REM sleep.

SLEEP-RELATED MOVEMENT DISORDERS

Restless Legs Syndrome

RLS is diagnosed on the basis of the clinical history of the child. The child may describe the symptoms as creepy/crawly, itchy bones, spiders in my legs, or growing pains. The symptoms are usually worse in the evening or during the night and can be relieved by movement or rubbing the legs. Primary RLS is idiopathic in nature. Secondary RLS can be related to a number of factors such as iron deficiency anemia, neurologic disorders, medical disorders (uremia, diabetes, cancer, etc.) drugs, or chemicals. RLS is usually worse in the evening and during the night, which may lead to difficulty falling asleep and maintaining sleep. All these symptoms can reduce sleep time and be associated with mood, behavioral, and academic problems. RLS is found in 5% to 15% of the general adult population, and first-degree relatives are six to seven times more likely to have early-onset RLS. Leg movements are usually not reported before sleep onset or during wake time; however, the technologist should make note of them in the sleep study log.

The essential diagnostic features of RLS in pediatric patients include additional criteria over and above the criteria used to diagnose adults. In adults or children older than 12 years, specific criteria are used to diagnose RLS. They include a reported urge to move the legs accompanied by an uncomfortable or unpleasant sensation in the legs, worsening of the urge to move or unpleasant sensations during periods of inactivity, the urge to move or unpleasant sensation is relieved by movement, and symptoms are worse or occur only in the evening or at night (1).

In pediatric patients under age 13 years, the child must meet all the essential criteria and relate a description that is consistent with leg discomfort. If the child is unable to relate a description that is consistent with leg discomfort, he or she must meet all the essential criteria and meet two of three additional criteria. The additional criteria include a sleep disturbance for age, a biologic parent or sibling with definite RLS, or PSG-documented PLMS (Periodic Limb Movements in Sleep) index of 5 or more per hour of sleep.

Periodic Limb Movement Disorder

PLMD should be diagnosed by a polysomnogram identifying five or more PLMS per hour of sleep. A PLM is defined as lasting 0.5 to 5 seconds, separated by 4- to 90-second intervals. PLMS often do not disturb sleep; however, limb movements that occur within 3 seconds of an arousal or an awakening are associated with a sleep disturbance. Because about 80% of RLS patients also have PLMD, these findings support the diagnosis of RLS. It is believed that central dopamine may be involved in the pathophysiology of primary PLMD. Secondary PLMD can be the result of the same factors that cause secondary RLS (7).

Headbanging and Body Rocking

Studies indicate that approximately two-thirds of 9-month-old infants use body rocking to self-soothe at sleep onset and after nighttime arousals. Half of all babies continue this rhythmic behavior to 18 months (1). Headbanging usually begins at around 9 months of age (2). The child may be lying prone and lifting the head and banging it down on the bed, on hands and knees rocking and banging the head against the crib, or sitting upright and banging the head against the crib. Other rhythmic movements include head rolling and body rolling side to side. PSG findings indicate that these movements can occur in all stages of sleep or in wakefulness. There is no seizure activity involved. In the absence of underlying medical problems, this behavior is normal, common, and is outgrown by 2 or 3 years of age (7).

SUMMARY

Performing a polysomnogram on a pediatric patient is a team process. It begins with the sleep specialist identifying issues, building trust with the parents, and communicating carefully. Acquiring an adequate study necessitates the involvement and support of both child and caregiver. The technologist should involve the parents in all aspects of the sleep study to maintain their trust and cooperation. The technologist should exercise patience and tact when performing the setup and answer questions from both parents and child. An understanding of the signs, symptoms, and characteristic clinical presentation of children with sleep disorders helps the technologist to be alert for specific behaviors that should be documented.

REFERENCES

1. Mindell, J., & Owens, J. (2015). Sleep in infancy, childhood and adolescence. In *A clinical guide to pediatric sleep* (3rd ed.). Philadelphia, PA: Wolters Kluwer.
2. Sheldon, S., Ferber, R., Kryger, M., et al. (Eds.). (2014). *Principles and practice of pediatric sleep medicine* (Chapter 6: Sleep during adolescence, Chapter 10: Sleep and colic, Chapter 13: Sleep related enuresis, Chapter 14: Bedtime problems and night wakings, Chapter 15: Attention deficit hyperactivity, and sleep disorders, Chapter 18: Narcolepsy). Philadelphia, PA: Elsevier Saunders.
3. Carskadon, M. (Ed.). (2002). *Adolescent sleep patterns: Biological, social, and psychological influences*. Cambridge, MA: Cambridge University Press.
4. Kryger, M., Roth, T., & Dement, W. (Eds.). (2017). *Principles and practice of sleep medicine* (Chapter 90: Narcolepsy: Genetics, immunology, and pathophysiology, Chapter 100: Klein Levin syndrome) (6th ed.). Philadelphia, PA: Elsevier, Saunders.
5. Kryger, M., Avidan, A., & Berry, R. (2014). *Atlas of clinical sleep medicine* (2nd ed.). Philadelphia, PA: Lippincott, Williams & Wilkins.
6. American Academy of Sleep Medicine. (2014). *International classification of sleep disorders: Diagnostic and coding manual* (3rd ed.). Darien, IL: Author.
7. Chokroverty, S. (2008). *100 questions and answers about sleep and sleep disorders* (2nd ed.). Sudbury, MA: Jones and Bartlett.
8. Loughlin, G., Carroll, J., & Marcus, C. (Eds.). (2000). *Sleep and breathing in children* (pp. 347–362). New York, NY: Marcel Dekker.
9. Jenni, O., & Bourgeois, M. (2005). Understanding sleep-wake behaviour and sleep disorders in children: The value of a model. *Current Opinion in Psychiatry, 19*, 282–287.
10. Eisermann, M., Kaminska, A., & Moutard, M. (2013). Normal EEG in childhood from neonates to adolescents. *Neurophysiologie Clinique, 43*, 35–36.

chapter 64
Parasomnias in Children

MATTHEW J. BALOG   STEPHEN H. SHELDON   DARIUS LOGHMANEE

LEARNING OBJECTIVES

On completion of this chapter, the reader should be able to:

1. Describe the evaluation of children with suspected parasomnias.
2. Explain the differences between sleep–wake transition disorders, parasomnias associated with nonrapid eye movement (NREM) sleep, and parasomnias associated with REM sleep.

KEY TERMS

Sleep
Children
Parasomnias

Parasomnias are dysfunctions associated with transitions into sleep, partial arousals during sleep, or following arousals from sleep (1, 2). Exclusive to sleep and wake-to-sleep transitions, these phenomena include arousals with abnormal motor, behavioral, autonomic, or sensory symptoms. Parasomnias can be noticeably dissimilar in clinical manifestations, but most share biologic characteristics. Symptoms typically begin early in childhood, gradually transform, and resolve themselves, which suggest a maturation etiology. Although often benign, these sleep disorders can be disruptive and even dangerous to the patient (3). In some cases, psychopathology plays a crucial role in sleep disorders; however, in other cases, recurrent parasomnia episodes induce psychopathology (4). Few pathologic abnormalities or objective diagnostic criteria can be identified, despite the presence of intense and often striking symptoms. Although symptoms are significant, spontaneous remission is typical.

Transitional parasomnias, partial arousals during sleep, or undesirable events or experiences following arousals from sleep may gradually appear or have a sudden and unexpected onset. Frequency can vary from a single isolated episode to multinightly events and persist for a protracted period (5). Patients appear medically

and developmentally normal, with no obvious clinical abnormalities present during wakefulness, although unusual motor activity, behavior, or undesirable events or experiences occur during or immediately surrounding the sleep period. In general, sleep disorders in children and adolescents is a topic that is, and remains, neglected in public health and professional education and training. Despite the growing knowledge that has been accumulated in recent years, it has been poorly distributed, therefore, relatively little has been put into practice (6).

ETIOLOGY

The etiology of arousal disorders, partial arousal disorders, and transitional parasomnias is unknown. Because of the natural history and progression of symptoms, a maturation etiology is theorized. Any hypothetical basis of the cause for these phenomena, however, must focus on common features. Classification of these disorders in the child and adolescent separates them into several broad categories (Table 64-1): (1) sleep–wake transition disorders, (2) somniloquy, (3) parasomnias associated with nonrapid eye movement (NREM) sleep, (4) parasomnias associated with REM sleep, (5) sleep-related enuresis (SRE), and (6) sleep-related bruxism. Classification is based on observable behaviors (1).

EVALUATION

Evaluation begins with a comprehensive medical history and physical examination. These are essential and usually result in an accurate diagnosis without elaborate testing. Attention should be placed on a detailed description of the abnormal sleep behaviors. A comprehensive history should include, but not be limited to, the following:

- Time of occurrence
- Symptoms manifested
- Discussion of results of caretaker's intervention
  - Do symptoms quickly improve with intervention?
  - Do symptoms worsen with intervention?
- Length of spell
- Intensity of autonomic nervous system discharge

Table 64-1 Comparison of Parasomnias

Parasomnia	Characteristics	Sleep Period	Polysomnography
Somniloquy	• Not associated with any patho-logic states • May be related to other parasomnias	Any sleep stage	• Increased activity in the snore mic and chin EMG • Artifact in the EEG may be present
Confusional arousals	• Partial awakenings from SWS • Confusion and disorientation are prominent	Usually seen in the first half of the sleep period, but may occur at any time during the night	• EEG shift from N3 sleep to wake rhythm • Vocalization postarousal may occur
Somnambulism	• Abrupt arousal from SWS, which can produce sitting up in bed to a full ambulatory session	• First third to first half of the sleep period	• EEG shift from N3 • Significant body movement • Muscle artifact in EEG
Isolated sleep paralysis	• Inability to move skeletal mus-cles, but the patient is fully awake	• Beginning of a sleep period, or upon awakening	• Reduction in general EMG activity with wake EEG rhythm • EOG movements may be present
REM sleep without atonia	• Considerable motor activity • Elaborate, purposeful move-ments, which may be accom-panied by vocalizations	• REM sleep	• Increased muscle tone and movements while exhibiting REM sleep in other aspects (EEG, EOG)
Sleep-related enuresis	• Involuntary and repeated void-ing of urine	• Any sleep stage, but usually in the first few hours of sleep	• Arousals may be more preva-lent before the voiding event
Bruxism	• Forceful clenching or grinding of teeth, which produces an un-mistakable sound • EEG arousals may or may not be present	• Generally N1 and N2 sleep	• Increased activity in chin or masseter EMG • Muscle artifact in EEG, typ-ically in the temporal region, but may be found in other channels

EEG, electroencephalogram; EMG, electromyogram; EOG, electrooculogram; REM, rapid eye movement; SWS, slow-wave sleep.

• Presence or absence of agitation during the spell
• Symptoms following waking
• Presence or absence of stereotypic activity

It is important to begin by assessing neurodevelopmental landmarks. The presence of daytime waking behavioral or developmental abnormalities may suggest other underlying disorders. Sleep–wake schedules, habits, and the typical pattern of the appearance of these sleep behaviors require delineation. Morning wake time, evening bedtime, and nap time rituals require description. Sleep logs or sleep diaries are frequently helpful. Video recordings of the episodes often reveal identifiable characteristics and can be very helpful in understanding the nature of the episodes. Evaluating for the presence of excessive daytime sleepiness, unintentional sleep episodes/sleep attacks, restless sleep, limb

movements during sleep, and/or snoring may assist in determining precipitating factors (2). A careful evaluation of family history is also quite important as many parasomnias demonstrate a familiar pattern.

Comprehensive physical examination with emphasis placed on neurologic function and developmental assessment is required. Developmental delays, chronic medical or surgical history, or symptoms suggestive of neurologic disorders might indicate an organic cause for symptoms. Comorbid states are often present. Primary sleep disorders such as obstructive sleep apnea (OSA) or periodic limb movement disorder (PLMD) must be first addressed, and treatment may often result in resolution of the symptoms. In some instances, a urine drug screen might be helpful if there is concern that symptoms may be a side effect of or adverse reaction to medication.

Home video recording of the spells may provide important diagnostic information. Under certain circumstances, video polysomnography (PSG) is indicated (7, 8). Using an expanded electroencephalogram (EEG) electrode array during PSG provides additional information and increases sensitivity for identifying neurologic pathology. Concurrent video recording of the patient during PSG may demonstrate symptoms and document movements (9).

If PSG is conducted, it is often helpful to have the patient drink fluids and avoid urination before lights out as bladder distension may precipitate some partial arousals from sleep (10). Analysis of the PSG should place special emphasis on identification of primary sleep-related pathology that may be a factor in the precipitation of spells or fragmentation of sleep (e.g., OSA, PLMD). Increased amplitude of slow waves, synchronization of slow-wave activity (Fig. 64-1) occurring sporadically or just before a spell, as well as arousal rhythms occurring during slow-wave sleep (SWS), and intrusion of 4 to 7 Hz EEG activity may be noted in older patients (2).

Other common PSG findings include movement arousals without state change, frequent arousal rhythms on EEG without state change (Fig. 64-2), and theta–delta sleep pattern (hypersynchronous theta activity intruding into SWS at an age where this hypersynchrony should not still be present; Fig. 64-3). These findings are associated with, but not diagnostic of, disorders of arousal from NREM sleep (2).

Sleep–Wake Transition Disorders

Most commonly noted at the beginning of the major nocturnal sleep period, sleep–wake transition disorders may also occur following arousals, awakenings, or during naps. They may involve stereotypic movements, including but not limited to hypnic jerks, or "sleep starts," body rocking, head rolling, or head banging. Movements may persist into NREM sleep and may occur following arousals or during waking from sleep. The etiology of these movements is unknown.

Rhythmic movements surrounding sleep are very common and have been reported in about two-thirds of normal children (11). Predominantly seen in infants and young children, rhythmic movements generally have a frequency of 0.5 to 2 seconds lasting less than 15 minutes. Prevalence is especially high in infants with a 59% incidence rate, which drops to 5% by 5 years of age (12). A strong correlation between rhythmic movement disorders and attention-deficit/hyperactivity disorder has been noticed (12). Institutionalized children, as well as children with neurologic sequelae from brain injury, show an affinity for rhythmic movements. Rhythmic movements typically resolve spontaneously by 4 years of age; however, sleep-disordered breathing (SDB) may act as a trigger for the reemergence of these episodes in adults who experienced rhythmic movements as children (13, 14). If, however, a patient's head banging continues for a prolonged period, steps should be taken to protect the child from causing any injury to himself or herself. At the same time, efforts should be made to help the child fall asleep without relying on rhythmic movements to calm down. PSG is generally not indicated, because diagnosis can be made by history and physical examination alone; however, when associated with other symptoms that might suggest a primary sleep disorder, a polysomnogram may reveal typical rhythmic movements.

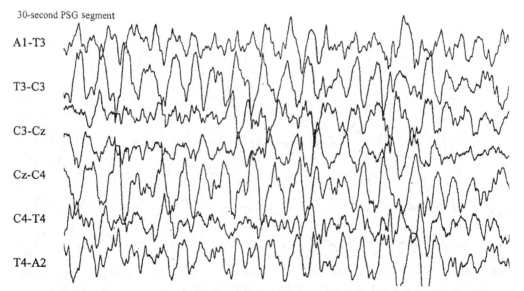

Figure 64-1 Hypersynchronous delta activity. This segment demonstrates an episode of hypersynchronous delta activity during slow-wave sleep. This delta hypersynchrony occurred immediately before a partial arousal with agitation and confusion. PSG, polysomnography.

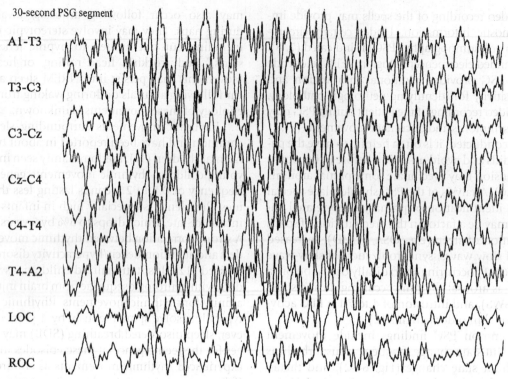

Figure 64-2 Arousal rhythm in slow-wave sleep (SWS). This segment is from the same patient as depicted in Figure 64-1. There is an arousal rhythm lasting about 10 seconds, occurring without state change during SWS. PSG, polysomnography.

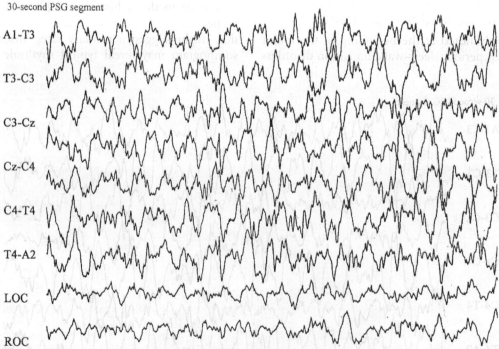

Figure 64-3 Theta–delta sleep. This segment of a 30-second polysomnography (PSG) epoch was recorded from an 8-year-old child with a history of agitated sleepwalking. There is considerable 4 to 7 Hz activity superimposed upon 0.5 to 1 Hz activity.

Rhythmic movements may be seen in NREM sleep but are rare in REM sleep (15). Focal, paroxysmal, or epileptiform activity is notably absent. Rarely, prolonged EEG recording may be required to rule out a seizure disorder. Sleep architecture, progression of states, and state percentages as proportions of the total sleep time are normal for age.

SOMNILOQUY

Somniloquy, typified by talking during sleep, is almost universal, with some studies suggesting a prevalence of 84.4% during childhood (16). Somniloquy is most frequently of little concern to parents or health care practitioners, but rare episodes of vocal outbursts, loud talking, or unintelligible speech may occasionally be significant enough to disturb the sleep of other family members (17). Somniloquy is not associated with pathology but can occur during sleep terrors, confusional arousals, or sleepwalking.

Diagnosis is based on typical manifestations of either apparent coherent speech or incoherent mumbling during sleep. The child is typically amnestic for the event, and somniloquy is most often self-limited. PSG is rarely indicated unless other clinical manifestations are present. When noted outside of the context of a primary sleep disorder, treatment is unnecessary.

PARASOMNIAS ASSOCIATED WITH NREM SLEEP

Parasomnias during NREM sleep (typically, SWS) are considered to be part of a continuum of undesirable manifestations of arousal or partial arousal that occur during sleep. Symptoms typically begin in childhood and resolve spontaneously. Rarely do they persist into adolescence or adulthood. Manifestations can be alarming and, in certain circumstances, injury might occur. Spontaneous resolution and benignity of most signs and symptoms suggest a maturational etiology. Stereotypic movements characteristic of some parasomnias most likely arise from a disinhibition of subcortical central pattern generators. Genetic predisposition, an inherent instability of NREM sleep, and underlying sleep disturbances such as OSA may predispose to the activation of confusional arousals, sleepwalking, or sleep terrors. Inherited anatomic risk factors, present at birth, and even subtle SDB can lead to sleep disruption, instability of NREM sleep, and an increase in the number of parasomnia activities (18). Many of these parasomnias can be recognized by history alone, but some require nocturnal PSG to guide further evaluation and treatment (19).

Arousal and partial arousal disorders can cause simple symptoms, such as briefly sitting up in bed with rapid return to sleep or bizarre, dramatic symptoms. Nonetheless, these phenomena share several common features, which seem to occur during or following abrupt arousals from SWS. Confusion, disorientation, and amnesia for the event are common.

Arousal disorders occur more frequently during periods of anxiety or stress, with bladder distension, following periods of sleep deprivation, in the context of fever, or with hypersomnolence due to sleep deprivation or prolonged sleep fragmentation. Stress can increase the number and frequency of brief partial arousals in normal children. SWS rebound (increased time spent in SWS following sleep deprivation) can exacerbate partial arousals. These events may also be precipitated by external environmental stimuli. Computer-assisted identification of nonvisible arousals, cyclic alternating patterns, or respiratory cycle–related EEG changes may complement what can be accomplished by human scorers. Addition of autonomic arousal measures, such as heart rate variability, pulse transit time, and peripheral arterial tonometry, into standard reports may help discover more subtle sleep fragmentation (20).

CONFUSIONAL AROUSALS

Confusional arousals consist of partial awakenings from SWS usually occurring in the first half of the sleep period, but may happen at any time during the night (2, 21, 22). Episodes are sudden and startling, and may be precipitated by environmentally induced awakenings. Children may appear fully awake during the spell, but may not respond appropriately to commands or may resist being consoled. Confusion and disorientation are prominent. Attempts to abort the spell may make the symptoms more severe. These differ from agitated sleepwalking in that the patient is more aware of the environment, and the EEG may abruptly progress from SWS to wake following a very brief period of partial arousal.

Factors that increase SWS, such as rebound from sleep deprivation, or those that impair arousal may result in confusional arousals. Hypersomnia secondary to narcolepsy, OSA, PLMD, or idiopathic hypersomnia may exacerbate symptoms. Confusional arousals are often seen in patients with narcolepsy syndrome following prolonged daytime naps with resultant sleep inertia. As with other parasomnias, stress, anxiety, and fever may precipitate attacks. Organic pathology is rarely present. Injuries during confusional arousals may occur if the youngster leaves the bed or if dangerous objects are left within reach.

The prevalence of confusional arousals has been noted to be as high as 39.8% for children between 2.5 and 6 years of age, with the yearly incidence decreasing as the child ages (2). There appears to be an equal distribution between males and females. Although clear genetic mechanisms for transmission are unknown, a strong familial pattern has been noted.

Symptom onset is usually before 5 years of age. Patients may thrash about or fall from the bed. Combativeness may occur, and attempts at consolation may result in the worsening of symptoms. Episodes are usually brief, lasting for only a few minutes; however, on rare occasions, they may be prolonged and last for several hours (23). As with other NREM parasomnias, patients are amnestic for the spell.

Diagnosis is based on the identification of classical symptoms of confusion, disorientation, agitation, and/or combativeness upon arousal, typically occurring during the first third to first half of the sleep period. Comorbid medical or psychiatric disorders are typically absent. Occasionally, the description of a confusional arousal may require differentiation from partial complex seizures with automatisms.

PSG, although rarely indicated, might reveal sudden arousal from SWS, brief episodes of hypersynchronous delta activity, theta–delta sleep, recurrent microsleep episodes, or poorly reactive alpha activity. Focal, paroxysmal, or epileptiform activity is absent in the EEG.

The presence of obstructive SDB or periodic limb movements might precipitate a spell. Symptoms are most frequent during middle childhood and then undergo spontaneous remission. Clinical course is usually benign. Physical injury might occur and the child must be protected from trauma during the episode.

SOMNAMBULISM

Somnambulism, or sleepwalking, may vary in presentation from simple sitting up in bed to agitated running during sleep (2, 24–27). A complex series of automatic behaviors are present and may seem purposeful. As with other NREM parasomnias, sleepwalking episodes occur following an abrupt arousal from SWS during the first third to first half of the sleep period. When accompanied by agitation, spells may be quite alarming and injuries may occur. Because of the possibility of injury, agitated sleepwalking should be addressed quickly to protect the child from harm.

Somnambulism has been reported to occur in up to 15% of the population; however, a recent meta-analysis of 51 studies with a total sample size of 100,490 revealed an overall prevalence of 6.9% (28, 29). Symptoms are most common during childhood and reduce significantly during adolescence. Episodes can vary broadly in frequency, intensity, and length. Parental reports may be quite inaccurate, and the true incidence is unknown. There appears to be an equal sex distribution, as well as a significant familial pattern. The genetic locus for sleepwalking is identified at chromosome 20q12-q12.12 in a multiplex family (30). There is a 60% incidence when both parents were affected as children, 45% when one parent was affected, and 22% when there was no family history of sleepwalking (28).

Sleepwalking typically has its onset between 4 and 8 years of age, although onset may occur at any time after the child develops the ability to walk. Symptoms range from quietly walking around the home to extremely agitated, semipurposeful automatisms and frantic running. Performance of complex tasks, such as unlocking doors, taking food from the refrigerator, and eating, is common. Children have been noted to leave the house and wander the neighborhood. Despite the apparent purposeful movement, these behaviors are often meaningless and unusual. Vocalizations may occur. Eyes are typically open, and the youngster may appear awake. Choreiform movements (repetitive and rapid, jerky, involuntary movements that appear well coordinated) may occur during spells. Enuretic episodes may occur and the child may urinate (or attempt to urinate) at unusual places around the house. During a somnambulistic episode, the child is extremely difficult to wake, although complete arousal is possible. If awakened, confusion and disorientation are often present.

Motor activity can quickly cease and the child may lay down on the floor or return to sleep at unusual places around the home. On the contrary, the child may return to bed without ever becoming alert.

Many factors similar to those previously mentioned may expedite sleepwalking spells. Fever, sleep deprivation, and sudden changes in environment are notable for increasing the frequency of spells. Any disorder that can produce significant disruption of SWS may precipitate events. In addition, sleepwalking can often be precipitated by urinary bladder distension in the susceptible patient. Environmental noise may also trigger an event. Several medications can exacerbate the disorder, including thioridazine, fluphenazine, perphenazine, desipramine, and chloral hydrate.

PSG typically reveals an arousal from stage N3 sleep, most commonly seen during the first half of the sleep period. Most of the background EEG activity is obscured by muscle artifact; however, seizure activity is notably absent.

Clinically, somnambulism can be differentiated from other disorders of arousal, such as confusional arousals and night terrors. Leaving the bed and calm nocturnal wanderings are less common with confusional arousals. Sleep terrors are more typically associated with the appearance of intense fear and panic and are less likely to be associated with the child leaving the bed. Intense autonomic discharges and an initial scream herald a sleep terror and are usually not present in sleepwalking. Nocturnal seizure disorders typically reveal epileptiform discharges during spells; however, the interictal EEG may be normal. REM sleep behavior disorder (RBD) has been rarely described in children, but characteristically occurs during REM sleep in adults and is associated with clear verbalizations, more purposeful movements, and dream reenactment.

SLEEP TERRORS

The term *sleep terror* is preferred to night terror to clearly differentiate this disorder from nightmares (10, 31, 32). Nightmares are considered "anxiety dreams" and are clinically quite different from sleep terrors in etiology and presentation. The onset of a sleep terror is sudden, abrupt, striking, and frightening. These arousals are associated with profound autonomic discharges and behavioral manifestations of intense fear.

Similar to other NREM parasomnias, prevalence of sleep terrors is unknown. They may occur in up to 3% of prepubertal children. Males are typically affected more frequently than females, and there appears to be a clear familial pattern. Onset of symptoms is usually between 2 and 4 years of age. Precipitating factors are similar to other NREM parasomnias and include fever, bladder distension, sleep deprivation, and central nervous system (CNS) depressant medication. Symptoms tend to reduce during puberty and rarely persist into adolescence. Psychopathology can be associated with sleep terrors in adolescents and adults, but is unusual in children.

Sleep terror episodes usually begin suddenly as the child sits upright in bed and emits a powerful, piercing scream. Severe autonomic discharge occurs, manifest as eyes opening widely and pupils dilating, tachycardia, tachypnea, diaphoresis, and increased muscle tone. During the sleep terror, the child is unresponsive, and efforts to restrain the child or console the youngster might exacerbate autonomic and motor activity. If awakened, the child is confused and disoriented, and there is amnesia for the event. In contrast to confusional arousals, episodes of sleep terrors are usually brief, lasting only a few minutes, and subside spontaneously.

Diagnosis is based on identification of the above-mentioned symptoms and exclusion of organic pathology. PSG is rarely indicated; however, if conducted, it may reveal sudden arousal from SWS during the first third to first half of the major nocturnal sleep period. Sleep terrors, however, can occur at any time during the night. Partial arousals without motor manifestation occur more frequently in children with sleep terrors compared with normal children. Autonomic discharge, in the form of tachycardia, can be seen during these partial arousals without full-blown symptoms.

Sleep terrors are clinically differentiated from partial complex seizures by their characteristic history and clinical course. Epileptic events may also be distinguished from disorders of partial arousal by the presence of a combination of clinical features and stereotypic behaviors and the fact that they may occur during wakefulness. Identification of epileptiform activity, however, does not completely rule out the presence of a partial arousal, because they may occur concomitantly in the same patient. Patients should also be evaluated for causes of sleep fragmentation such as SDB or PLMD as the arousals associated with these disorders can trigger episodes.

THERAPEUTIC CONSIDERATIONS

There is no clear consensus regarding when NREM sleep parasomnia requires treatment. Symptoms are most often mild, occur less than once per month, and result in injury to neither the child nor the parents. In these *mild* cases, reassurance may be all that is necessary. A comprehensive explanation of the nature of these parasomnias and reassurance that the child is normal mentally and developmentally should be provided. Parents should be encouraged to let the event run its course and to intervene minimally. Interventions should be focused on preventing injury and guiding the child back to bed. Vigorous intervention may prolong and exacerbate the episode.

Parents can be warned of a sleepwalking spell by a simple alarm system, such as fixing a bell to a door. Sleep deprivation should be avoided, and regular sleep–wake schedules should be maintained. Brief daytime naps might be attempted, and a period of quiet activity or relaxation techniques should be instituted before bedtime. Fluids after the evening meal should be limited, and the child should be encouraged to void before bedtime. If episodes of sleepwalking occur at the same time every night, waking the child 20 to 30 minutes before the regular time of occurrence can often prevent sleepwalking episodes from occurring. Fevers, if present, should be appropriately treated; the cause of the fever should be identified and appropriately handled.

Severity of partial arousals is considered *moderate* when symptoms occur more than once a month, but less that once per week, and do not result in harm to the patient or to others. In these cases, reassurance and a behavioral approach (including behavior training, sleep hygiene, psychotherapy, and/or hypnosis) have been successful (2).

In *severe* cases, when episodes occur almost nightly or are associated with injury, nondrug approaches are considered first. Drug treatment, when used, should be prescribed for a short period and should be used in conjunction with a behavioral approach. Medications should be discontinued when behavior therapy begins to take effect.

When necessary, a benzodiazepine might be considered; however, prolonged use of medications increases the potential for side effects and complications as well as chronic disruption of sleep architecture. Melatonin has shown to be useful in significantly improving parasomnia activity as well as seizure activity in children with intractable epilepsy and controlled seizures (33). The young child generally responds well to both behavioral and medicinal approaches. The adolescent and adult patient with partial arousal disorders typically respond poorly to any form or combination of therapy.

PARASOMNIAS ASSOCIATED WITH REM SLEEP

Manifestations of REM sleep parasomnias are quite dissimilar to those occurring during NREM sleep. Most of these disorders can be differentiated by clinical evaluation alone. Frequency of REM sleep parasomnias varies considerably in children from those that are common (nightmares) to those that are rare (RBD).

NIGHTMARES

A nightmare occurs during REM sleep and is manifested by a frightening dream followed by a prolonged period of wake (10, 21, 34, 35). Clear recall of the dream with varying degrees of anxiety may be present. Nightmares are characterized by a sudden arousal from REM sleep to a fully awake state. The youngster is fully oriented to the environment and sensorium is clear. Mild autonomic nervous system discharges may occur.

Nightmares most commonly occur during the last half to last third of the sleep period, although they may occur at any time during the night. A vivid story is often present, there is often complex mentation, and recall is appropriate for the child's developmental level. Nightmares are primarily associated with an emotional response rather than the intense autonomic activity exhibited with sleep terrors. Children are usually easily comforted following a nightmare, but return to sleep is delayed. Nearly all youngsters experience a nightmare at one time or another. Some studies show approximately 75% of children as having experienced at least one nightmare (23). Prevalence data are not clear, but some studies have shown the peak prevalence for the

occurrence of nightmares to be between 6 and 10 years of age (23). Age of onset appears to parallel the development of dream expression.

Movements, other than phasic twitches and/or other phasic activity, are rare. Arousal from sleep with vivid dream recall is typical. Clinical symptoms are generally mild. Diagnosis is based on identification of the milder characteristics, such as time of occurrence, vivid story line, and prolonged return to sleep. Laboratory investigations are rarely necessary because nightmares and sleep terrors can usually be differentiated on clinical grounds alone.

PSG findings associated with nightmares typically depict an abrupt waking from REM sleep, followed by a somewhat prolonged period of wake after sleep onset. Mild tachycardia may be present, associated with a degree of anxiety. Increased eye movement density and increased phasic muscle twitches may be present during REM sleep, but are not diagnostic. Focal, paroxysmal, and epileptiform activity are notably absent.

Occasional nightmares during childhood are common; however, if they are frequent, persist for prolonged periods, or are associated with daytime behavioral problems, underlying medical or psychologic causes should be sought.

Treatment is based on reassurance and identification of stressors. Maintenance of appropriate sleep hygiene is important. Relaxation before bedtime and identification and elimination of stressors are very helpful. Occasionally, further psychologic and/or psychiatric evaluations are needed if symptoms are frequent, severe, or associated with other clinical manifestations.

ISOLATED SLEEP PARALYSIS

Isolated sleep paralysis is characterized by a period of inability to voluntarily move skeletal muscles at the beginning of a sleep period (hypnagogic) or immediately after awakening (hypnopompic) (36, 37). Consciousness is maintained, but the youngster feels paralyzed and is unable to open the eyes or speak. This phenomenon is typically due to persistent active inhibition of alpha motor neurons that persist after cortical waking. A sensation of difficulty breathing may occur, and episodes are typically frightening. Episodes of sleep paralysis may be prolonged or brief and subside spontaneously. Isolated infrequent episodes of sleep paralysis can occur in normal individuals. Frequent events are present in patients with narcolepsy and in familial sleep paralysis.

Onset of isolated sleep paralysis typically occurs during adolescence, but symptoms may begin before the onset of puberty. Children have difficulty describing the event. They may appear asleep during the spell and are often anxious or frightened upon waking. Complaints may center on difficulty waking. Parents may be unaware of their occurrence, and symptoms can be mistaken for resistance to waking. Typically, children who resist waking arouse cranky and may pull away from the parent trying to wake them; conversely, during a spell of sleep paralysis, children appear "floppy" and cannot resist parental interventions.

The clinical course varies. Most episodes are isolated and are provoked by sleep deprivation, excessive sleepiness, stress, irregular sleep–wake schedules, or acute changes in sleep phase. Sleep paralysis might run a more chronic course in patients with narcolepsy syndrome or in the familial form of the disorder. Sleep deprivation is a common trigger of isolated sleep paralysis in otherwise healthy teenagers (38).

Diagnosis is based on the identification of presenting symptoms; however, symptoms may not be clear. Approximately 20% of young adults with anxiety disorder may manifest isolated sleep paralysis (39). Sleep paralysis associated with narcolepsy can be differentiated from the isolated form by the absence of chronic excessive daytime sleepiness, sleep attacks, cataplexy precipitated by emotions, and hypnagogic hallucinations. Atonic generalized seizures or "drop attacks" occur during wakefulness and may or may not be associated with changes in levels of consciousness. Syncope occurs during wakefulness as well and is commonly associated with altered levels of consciousness.

PSG is typically not indicated, but if a spell occurs in the laboratory, it might reveal decreased skeletal muscle tone in the presence of a normal waking EEG pattern and conjugate eye movements.

REM SLEEP WITHOUT ATONIA

REM sleep without atonia, described in adults as RBD, has also been described in childhood (40–43). REM sleep without atonia differs from sleep terrors and NREM parasomnias by considerable motor activity and state dissociation during REM sleep. REM sleep without atonia may be characterized by elaborate, purposeful movements accompanied by vocalizations. There is a paradoxical increase in muscle tone and frequent limb movements during REM sleep, which has been considered state dissociation. Occasionally, violent behaviors occur, with patients punching, kicking, and/or leaping out of bed. This motor activity is associated with dream recall as patients seem to be acting out their dreams (44). An injury to the patient or bed partner is common in adults with RBD.

RBD usually begins during late adulthood and progresses over a variable period. Children may also be affected, but little is known of its prevalence, frequency, or natural history. Further understanding of this disorder

may reveal the incidence and prevalence to be higher than currently suggested. Many cases are idiopathic in nature. RBD, although rare in the pediatric population, can be seen in children who carry the diagnosis of narcolepsy with cataplexy (45). Neurologic disorders, such as Parkinson disease, have been reported in approximately 40% of affected adults (10). Signs and symptoms have also been reported in posttraumatic stress disorder.

PSG reveals increased muscle tone and frequent limb movements that persist throughout sleep, especially in REM sleep. There is increased phasic muscle activity and excessive limb movements. No epileptiform activity is noted on the EEG. Interestingly, symptoms of RBD in both children and adults respond rapidly to benzodiazepines.

OTHER PARASOMNIAS

Sleep-Related Enuresis

SRE, or bed-wetting, is characterized by recurrent and involuntary voiding of urine that occurs during sleep (46–48). Bed-wetting is fairly common during childhood, which affects 5 to 7 million children in the United States alone (46). These episodes can occur during any stage of sleep, but usually during the first few hours when the bladder is filled to maximum daytime capacity (46). As children age, the incidence of bed-wetting diminishes. The underlying cause may be related to delayed maturation of bladder mechanisms, a hindrance in the development of portions of the CNS required for maintenance of continence (47, 48). The age range for an abnormal SRE episode is the source of some debate. The generally accepted lower limit where concern and possibly intervention should occur is 5 years (48).

SRE can be separated into primary and secondary enuresis. Primary enuresis can further be separated into primary nonmonosymptomatic and primary monosymptomatic enuresis. Primary nonmonosymptomatic enuresis is characterized by nighttime enuresis with daytime micturition problems, whereas primary monosymptomatic enuresis is defined as nighttime enuresis without daytime micturition problems (47). In each of the primary enuresis types, the child generally does not have many consecutive nights without a bed-wetting incident, whereas in secondary enuresis, the child has been dry for a period of 6 months before wetting the bed at least twice a week for a period of at least 3 months (49). Secondary SRE, as well as daytime wetting, is more commonly linked with organic or psychologic issues than is primary SRE (50).

Primary sleep enuresis is seen in greater proportions of boys than girls among all age groups, with a ratio of 3:1 (49). There is evidence that suggests a genetic predisposition to enuresis. Studies show that regions linked to chromosomes 22q, 13q, and 12q across different families may be responsible for issues of enuresis. Current prevalence is 77% in children with two enuretic parents and 44% when only one parent has a history of childhood bed-wetting (46, 48). Enuresis may be associated with small bladder size, increased bladder contractibility, decreased antidiuretic hormone secretion, and OSA, as well as other sleep-fragmenting disorders (10, 23, 48–51).

OSA should especially be considered if the child is overweight and does not respond well to standard enuresis treatment programs (52). Organic factors such as urinary tract infections, sickle cell anemia, sickle cell trait, spinal cord lesions, and tumors, as well as seizure disorders may result in enuresis in the child (53).

PSG is not indicated in diagnosing nocturnal enuresis as patient history and physical examination are all that is needed, but a sleep study may be helpful in ruling out contributory primary sleep disorders (53).

Treatment options start with the diagnosis and management of any organic or pathologic condition. Treatment of SDB and sleep fragmentation often alleviates the enuretic episodes (50). Other options vary but include alarms, medication, fluid restriction, psychotherapy, hypnosis, biofeedback, retention control exercises, or a combination of therapies (53). Because the spontaneous cure rate for children aged 5 to 16 is roughly 15% per year, treatment options are often not suggested. If treatment is utilized, patience and vigilance are required, as initial changes in the model of bed-wetting generally begin after 3 to 6 weeks of treatment (50). Parents should be understanding and avoid showing disappointment or disciplining the child for any relapse as some bed-wetting will happen throughout the course of treatment.

Sleep Bruxism

Sleep bruxism can be characterized by rhythmic jaw movements, which produce grinding or clenching of teeth during sleep and which may or may not cause arousals (11). These movements are caused by involuntary contractions of the masseter, temporalis, and pterygoid muscles. Recent thinking has suggested that bruxism is regulated centrally by several neurotransmitters (54). When grinding occurs, there is an unmistakable noise produced. This noise is a reliable means of making a diagnosis.

Predisposing factors have been reported to include minor abnormalities of the teeth, malocclusion, stress, and anxiety. Some evidence shows that the protrusion of the jaw in conjunction with the rhythmic movements of teeth grinding also occurs during arousals associated with occlusive SDB.

Although the exact prevalence is unclear, bruxism is a fairly common occurrence during childhood, with studies reporting that 14% to 20% of children experience some teeth grinding (11). The average age of onset is 10.5 years. The condition, most prevalent in children and young adults, seems to have an equal sex distribution as well as a familial pattern without clear genetic transmission (10).

Episodes of rhythmic jaw movements occur either periodically or paroxysmally in bursts, which vary in duration, but are most commonly 5 to 15 seconds. These movements are generally repeated throughout the night. Daytime symptoms are common and include jaw pain, craniofacial pain, painful teeth, morning headaches, chronic wear to the crowns of the teeth, periodontal tissue damage, and bleeding from the gums. Resorption of the alveolar bone, hypertrophy of the masseter and temporalis muscles, and dysfunction of the temporomandibular joint can occur. Evidence suggests that sleep bruxism generally occurs in sleep stages N1 and N2 (55).

The diagnosis of bruxism is made by the identification of the loud, unmistakable sound of teeth grinding in the absence of other medical or psychiatric disorders that may produce abnormal movements during sleep. Obstructive SDB should also be assessed especially in the presence of morning headaches, frequent nocturnal awakenings, snoring, restless sleep, daytime sleepiness, hyperactivity, attention span problems, and performance difficulties.

PSG shows paroxysmal, rhythmic muscle activity manifested by about 1 Hz muscle artifact over the temporalis muscle. This rhythmic activity may also be seen in the chin muscle electromyogram or masseter muscle groups. If it is associated with occlusive SDB, the muscle activity occurs during the arousal immediately after the obstructive respiratory event.

Because therapeutic interventions have not been overwhelmingly successful in preventing bruxism long term, the most important therapeutic measure is appropriate dental management to minimize damage to teeth, especially in young adults (10, 54). A mouth guard may be worn at night, which will not alleviate the symptoms, but is more of a preventative dental intervention. If stress, anxiety, or other pressures are prominent, efforts should be taken to alleviate or minimize the causes of these troubles as this may prove helpful. Treatment of dental and/or other anatomic abnormalities through surgical intervention may not alter the bruxing behavior. Of course, if bruxism is associated with SDB of any kind, this should be managed first and foremost.

SUMMARY

Despite the broad spectrum of clinical manifestations of pediatric parasomnias, most of these occurrences share some biologic and etiologic characteristics. Children experiencing these disorders will tend to show no obvious clinical or developmental abnormalities when awake despite having disrupted sleep patterns. Parental accounts of the child's sleeping habits may or may not be accurate or helpful in some instances, yet PSG is not always the best clinical course in making a diagnosis. As such, parasomnias may not be consistently noted in the sleep laboratory. As is the case for most pediatric sleep disorders, children with parasomnias require a thorough history and a physical examination by a health practitioner with experience in sleep disorders so that the most appropriate plan for evaluation and treatment could be determined.

REFERENCES

1. American Academy of Sleep Medicine. (2014). *International classification of sleep disorders* (3rd ed., pp. 225–227). Darien, IL: Author.

2. Rosen, G. M. (2014). Disorders of arousal. In S. H. Sheldon, R. Ferber, & M. H. Kryger (Eds.), *Principles and practice of pediatric sleep medicine* (2nd ed., pp. 313–320). Philadelphia, PA: Elsevier/Saunders.

3. Avidan, A. Y., & Kaplish, N. (2010). The parasomnias: Epidemiology, clinical features, and diagnostic approach. *Clinics in Chest Medicine, 31*(2), 353–370.

4. Bloomfield, E. R., & Shatkin, J. P. (2009). Parasomnias and movement disorders in children and adolescents. *Child and Adolescent Psychiatry Clinics of North America, 18*(4), 947–965.

5. Golbin, A. Z. (1979). *Pathological sleep in children.* Leningrad, Russia: Medicine.

6. Stores, G. (2009). Aspects of sleep disorders in children and adolescents. *Dialogues in Clinical Neuroscience, 11*(1), 81–90.

7. de Lissovoy, V. (1961). Head banging in early childhood: A study of incidence. *Journal of Pediatrics, 58*, 803.

8. Golbin, A. Z. (1976). Movements as an active factor in organization of sleep. *Human Physiology (USSR), 3*, 354.

9. Kravitz, H., Rosenthal, V., Teplitz, Z., et al. (1960). A study of head-banging in infants and children. *Diseases of the Nervous System, 21*, 203.

10. Sheldon, S. H. (2005). The parasomnias. In S. H. Sheldon, R. Ferber, & M. H. Kryger (Eds.), *Principles and practice of pediatric sleep medicine* (pp. 305–315). Philadelphia, PA: Elsevier/Saunders.

11. Cogen, J. D., & Loghmanee, D. A. (2014). Sleep-related movement disorders. In S. H. Sheldon, R. Ferber, & M. H. Kryger, *Principles and practice of pediatric sleep medicine* (2nd ed., pp. 333–336). Philadelphia, PA: Elsevier/Saunders.

12. Attarian, H., Ward, N., & Schuman, C. (2009). A multigenerational family with persistent sleep related rhythmic movement disorder (RMD) and insomnia. *Journal of Clinical Sleep Medicine, 5*(6), 571–572.

13. Parkes, J. D. (1983). *Sleep and its disorders* (p. 195). London, UK: W.B. Saunders.

14. Chiaro, G., Maestri, M., Riccardi, S., et al. (2017). Sleep-related rhythmic movement disorder and obstructive sleep apnea in five adult patients. *Journal of Clinical Sleep Medicine, 13*(10), 1213–1217. doi:10.5664/jcsm.6778

15. Rechtschaffen, A., Goodenough, D., & Shapiro, A. (1962). Patterns of sleep talking. *Archives of General Psychiatry, 7*, 418.

16. Petit, D., Touchette, E., Tremblay, R. E., et al. (2007). Dyssomnias and parasomnias in early childhood. *Pediatrics, 119*(5), 1016–1025. doi:10.1542/peds.2006-2132

17. Saskin, P., Whelton, C., Moldofsky, H., et al. (1988). Sleep and nocturnal leg cramps. *Sleep, 11*, 307.

18. Cao, M., & Guilleminault, C. (2010). Families with sleepwalking. *Sleep Medicine, 11*(7), 726–731.

19. Kotagal, S. (2009). Parasomnias in childhood. *Sleep Medicine Review, 13*(2), 157–168.

20. Paruthi, S., & Chervin, R. D. (2010). Approaches to the assessment of arousals and sleep disturbances in children. *Sleep Medicine, 11*(7), 622–627.

21. Guilleminault, C. (1987). Narcolepsy and its differential diagnosis. In C. Guilleminault (Ed.), *Sleep and its disorders in children* (p. 182). New York, NY: Raven Press.

22. Ferber, R. (1989). Sleepwalking, confusional arousals, and sleep terrors in the child. In M. H. Kryger, T. Roth, & W. C. Dement (Eds.), *Principles and practice of sleep medicine* (p. 641). Philadelphia, PA: W.B. Saunders.

23. Mindel, J. A., & Owens, J. A. (2015). *A clinical guide to pediatric sleep: Diagnosis and management of sleep problems* (3rd ed.). Philadelphia, PA: Wolters Kluwer.

24. Broughton, R. (1968). Sleep disorders: Disorders of arousal? *Science, 159*, 1070.

25. Kales, A., Jacobson, A., Paulson, M. J., et al. (1966). Somnambulism: Psychophysiological correlates. I. All-night EEG studies. *Archives of General Psychiatry, 14*, 586.

26. Bawkin, H. (1970). Sleep-walking in twins. *Lancet, 2*, 446.

27. Kales, J. D., Kales, A., Soldatos, C. R., et al. (1979). Sleep walking and night terrors related to febrile illness. *American Journal of Psychiatry, 136*, 1214.

28. Sheldon, S. H., & Glaze, D. G. (2005). Sleep in neurologic disorders. In S. H. Sheldon, R. Ferber, & M. H. Kryger (Eds.), *Principles and practice of pediatric sleep medicine* (pp. 269–292). Philadelphia, PA: Elsevier/Saunders.

29. Stallman, H. M., & Kohler, M. (2016). Prevalence of sleepwalking: A systematic review and meta-analysis. *PLoS One, 11*(11), e0164769. doi:10.1371/journal.pone.0164769

30. Licis, A., Desruisseau, D., Yamada, K., et al. (2011). Novel genetic findings in an extended family pedigree with sleepwalking. *Neurology, 76*, 49–52.

31. Broughton, R. (1978). Childhood sleep walking, sleep terrors and enuresis nocturna: Their pathophysiology and differentiation from nocturnal epileptic seizures. In L. Popoviciu, B. Asgian, & G. Badiu (Eds.), *Sleep* (pp. 103–111). Basel, Switzerland: S. Karger.

32. Kales, A., Soldatos, C. R., Bixler, E. O., et al. (1980). Hereditary factors in sleepwalking and night terrors. *British Journal of Psychiatry, 137,* 111.

33. Elkhayat, H. A., Hassanein, S. M., Tomoum, H. Y., et al. (2010). Melatonin and sleep related problems in children with intractable epilepsy. *Pediatric Neurology, 42*(4), 249–254.

34. Mack, J. E. (1970). *Nightmares and the human conflict.* Boston, MA: Little, Brown.

35. Foulkes, D. (1982). *Children's dreams: Longitudinal studies.* New York, NY: Wiley.

36. Hishikawa, Y. (1979). Sleep paralysis. In C. Guilleminault, W. C. Dement, & P. Passouant (Eds.), *Narcolepsy* (pp. 97–124). New York, NY: Spectrum.

37. Penn, N. E., Kripke, D. F., & Scharff, J. (1981). Sleep paralysis among medical students. *Journal of Psychology, 107,* 247.

38. Otto, M., Simon, N. M., Powers, M., et al. (2006). Rates of isolated sleep paralysis in outpatients with anxiety disorders. *Journal of Anxiety Disorders, 20,* 687–693.

39. Kotagal, S. (2008). Parasomnias of childhood. *Current Opinion in Pediatrics, 20*(6), 659–665.

40. Sheldon, S. H., & Jacobsen, J. (1998). REM-sleep motor disorder in children. *Journal of Child Neurology, 13,* 257–260.

41. Schenck, C., Bundlie, S. R., Ettinger, M. G., et al. (1986). Chronic behavioral disorders of human REM sleep: A new category of parasomnia. *Sleep, 9,* 293.

42. Schenck, C. H., Hurwitz, T. D., & Mahowald, M. W. (1988). REM sleep behavior disorder. *American Journal of Psychiatry, 145,* 652.

43. Schenck, C. H., Bundlie, S. R., Smith, S. A., et al. (1986). REM behavior disorder in a 10-year-old girl and aperiodic REM and NREM sleep movements in an 8-year-old brother. *Sleep Research, 15,* 162.

44. Sheldon, S. H., & Loghmanee, D. A. (2014). REM behavior disorder. In S. H. Sheldon, R. Ferber, & M. H. Kryger (Eds.), *Principles and practice of pediatric sleep medicine* (2nd ed., pp. 321–323). Philadelphia, PA: Elsevier/Saunders.

45. Cipolli, C., Franceschini, C., Mattarozzi, K., et al. (2011). Overnight distribution and motor characteristics of REM sleep behavior disorder episodes in patients with narcolepsy-cataplexy. *Sleep Medicine, 12,* 635–640.

46. Butler, R. J. (1998). Annotation: Night wetting in children: Psychological aspects. *Journal of Child Psychology and Psychiatry, 39,* 453–463.

47. Gontard, A. (1998). Annotation: Day and night wetting in children—A paediatric and child psychiatric perspective. *Journal of Child Psychology and Psychiatry, 39,* 439–451.

48. Kumar, H., & Vardhan, S. (2014). Other parasomnias. In S. H. Sheldon, R. Ferber, & M. H. Kryger (Eds.), *Principles and practice of pediatric sleep medicine* (2nd ed., pp. 325–329). Philadelphia, PA: Elsevier/Saunders.

49. American Academy of Sleep Medicine. (2014). *International classification of sleep disorders* (3rd ed., pp. 270–276). Darien, IL: Author.

50. Sheldon, S. H. (2005). Sleep-related enuresis. In S. H. Sheldon, R. Ferber, & M. H. Kryger (Eds.), *Principles and practice of pediatric sleep medicine* (pp. 317–325). Philadelphia, PA: Elsevier/Saunders.

51. Brooks, L. J. (2005). Enuresis in children with sleep apnea. In S. H. Sheldon, R. Ferber, & M. H. Kryger (Eds.), *Principles and practice of pediatric sleep medicine* (pp. 231–233). Philadelphia, PA: Elsevier/Saunders.

52. Barone, J. G., Hanson, C., DaJusta, D. G., et al. (2009). Nocturnal enuresis and overweight are associated with obstructive sleep apnea. *Pediatrics, 124*(1), e53–e59.

53. Capdevila, O. S. (2014). Sleep related enuresis. In S. H. Sheldon, R. Ferber, & M. H. Kryger (Eds.), *Principles and practice of pediatric sleep medicine* (2nd ed., pp. 99–103). Philadelphia, PA: Elsevier/Saunders.

54. Lobbezoo, F., Van Der Zaag, J., Van Selms, M. K. A., et al. (2008). Review article: Principles for the management of bruxism. *Journal of Oral Rehabilitation, 35,* 509–523.

55. Lavigne, G. J., Khoury, S., Abe, S., et al. (2008). Review article: Bruxism physiology and pathology: An overview for clinicians. *Journal of Oral Rehabilitation, 35,* 476–494.

chapter 65

Interventions in the Pediatric Sleep Laboratory

CARLA A. EVANS   CAROL WOOD   CARLA UY   KAREN WATERS

LEARNING OBJECTIVES

On completion of this chapter, the reader should be able to:

1. Discuss the nuances of continuous positive airway pressure titration in children.
2. Explain the importance of monitoring carbon dioxide when titrating oxygen in children.
3. Describe when and how to initiate noninvasive ventilation in children.

KEY TERMS

Sleep apnea
Hypoventilation
Continuous positive airway pressure
Oxygen
High-flow oxygen therapy
Noninvasive ventilation
Invasive ventilation

This chapter reviews interventions relevant to sleep-disordered breathing (SDB) in children. All these disorders can be diagnosed in the sleep laboratory and can be simply grouped as disorders of

1. upper airway obstruction (i.e., obstructive sleep apnea [OSA]),
2. restrictive lung function and/or poor muscle tone (i.e., hypoventilation), and
3. impaired respiratory drive (i.e., central sleep apnea [CSA], or hypoventilation).

Interventions that will be discussed include continuous positive airway pressure (CPAP), supplemental oxygen, and noninvasive and invasive ventilation. All forms of respiratory support therapy need to be adjusted to suit the patient requirements, and regular reviews and titrations are to be performed in the sleep laboratory to accommodate for growth and monitoring of disease progression.

DETERMINING WHICH RESPIRATORY SUPPORT TREATMENT TO USE

Optimal gas exchange is dependent upon three variables: (1) brain and central nervous system (CNS) function, (2) the structural design of the airways, and (3) muscle tone. If there is a fault with any one of these variables, then a child is at risk for developing SDB. On the basis of the child's clinical history and physical examination, one can hypothesize the nature of the SDB the child will develop. Diagnostic polysomnography and blood gas testing allow clinicians to diagnose the problem and to determine the treatment to be initiated. Treatment recommendations may include CPAP, oxygen therapy, and/or ventilation (Fig. 65-1).

Central Respiratory Control

A number of conditions interfere with normal regulation of breathing by the brain and the CNS. Respiration is initiated in the pre-Bötzinger complex in the pons and medulla oblongata in the brainstem and further regulated by the carotid and aortic bodies. These areas submit electrical pulses to the diaphragm through the phrenic and thoracic nerves in the spinal column. Conditions associated with the spinal column or head, such as trauma, tumors, or malformations (e.g., an Arnold–Chiari malformation), can interfere with respiratory drive, respiratory rhythm, or respiratory regulation. The hypoxic response is primarily driven by the carotid bodies, whereas the response to carbon dioxide (CO_2) is primarily driven by brainstem structures. These combined abnormalities result in susceptibility to CSA and/or hypoventilation and a need for the child to be treated with positive pressure or volume ventilation in order

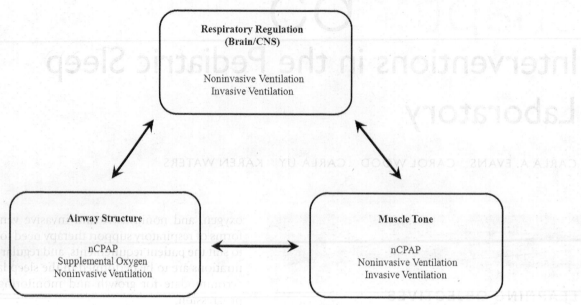

Figure 65-1 The pathophysiology of sleep-disordered breathing. On the basis of the origin of the sleep-disordered breathing, the appropriate respiratory therapy can be determined. CNS, central nervous system; nCPAP, nasal continuous positive airway pressure.

to regulate the respiratory rate and/or tidal volume. If a child requires only nocturnal support, then noninvasive ventilation (NIV) is the optimal treatment. On the basis of modern technology, NIV is predominately positive pressure ventilation. If the individual requires assistance during wake and sleep and has a chronic condition, then invasive ventilation should be considered. Depending on the severity of the lack of respiratory drive, invasive ventilation can be pressure or volume ventilation.

Structural Compromise of the Airway

Structural abnormalities in the airway can interfere with optimal gas exchange by predisposing to narrowing or collapse of the airway. Obstruction to airflow can occur at any point along the airway from the nares to the alveoli. Examples of the physical obstruction in the upper airway include adenoid and/or tonsil hypertrophy, choanal atresia/stenosis, a cleft palate, or an enlarged tongue (macroglossia). These may be identified on physical examination or through more invasive testing procedures including nasendoscopy. Children at risk for upper airway obstruction may also be assessed using the Mallampati classification (1). Other causes of structural narrowing include micrognathia, a congenitally narrow airway, or childhood obesity whereby increased adipose tissue surrounds the muscular soft tissue of the upper airway. The primary example of a congenital floppy airway is laryngomalacia in infants, usually presenting soon after birth.

Surgical interventions can often alleviate these problems, but CPAP may be required for stabilization or long-term therapy when surgery is either contraindicated or not curative. The most easily corrected cause of obstruction is adenotonsillar enlargement, but other commonly performed surgical procedures include mandibular distraction and supraglottoplasty.

Gas exchange abnormalities can also be caused by structural abnormalities in the lower airway such as restrictive lung disease and/or chest wall abnormalities (i.e., kyphoscoliosis, cystic fibrosis, and bronchiectasis). It is important to note that morbidly obese children (particularly adolescents) may be at an increased risk of nocturnal hypoventilation because of the excessive adipose tissue deposited on the truck and abdomen restricting pulmonary function. If hypoventilation is present, treatment with NIV (with or without oxygen therapy) should be considered. It is common for children with lung disease (i.e., neonatal lung disease and cystic fibrosis) to be treated with supplemental oxygen, but in some cases, CPAP or NIV is also required because of associated conditions such as OSA or airway malacia.

Poor Muscle Tone

Gas exchange is also influenced by the effectiveness of respiratory muscle function. Many congenital myopathies are associated with progressive muscle weakness; the classic example is Duchenne muscular dystrophy. Mild loss of muscle tone can also affect the upper airway and predispose to upper airway obstruction, and treatment with CPAP therapy may be sufficient in these cases.

More severe loss of muscle power, such as in spinal muscular atrophy or at the later stages of Duchenne muscular dystrophy, requires ventilation because of loss of diaphragmatic and/or intercostal muscles, with additional compromise in sleep due to loss of respiratory accessory muscle activity.

Congenital Heart Disease

The use of CPAP or NIV for patients with congenital heart disease (CHD) is often for the management of respiratory issues occurring secondary to the underlying cardiac condition. CHD can affect the respiratory system by causing obstructive and/or diffusion defects.

Direct anatomic compression of the airway can occur in association with cardiac abnormalities, secondary to the enlargement of cardiac structures or abnormal vascular structures (such as vascular rings). As an example, tetralogy of Fallot is associated with the narrowing of the pulmonary artery as well as ventricular septal defect, and leads to the deviation of the aorta to the right and thickening of the right ventricle. This in turn can lead to pulmonary artery dilation, bronchial or tracheal compression, and atelectasis, resulting in respiratory distress (2).

In terms of diffusion defects, ventricular or atrial septal defects can result in increased pulmonary blood flow because of left to right shunts (3). The increase in pulmonary blood flow can result in loss of elasticity in pulmonary vessels and increase the resistance in the pulmonary bed (4), thus impacting on gas exchange.

The use of CPAP or NIV should be aimed at relieving airway compression, increasing lung volume, equalizing transalveolar pressures (in addition to cardiac medications), and expanding surface area available for gas exchange to occur in the pulmonary bed (5).

CPAP THERAPY FOR CHILDREN

The most common reason for initiating CPAP in a child is to treat upper airway obstruction, predominantly OSA. But under what circumstances and how severe does the upper airway obstruction have to be before CPAP is warranted? There is no consensus on this matter, but from clinical experience, a number of factors can be evaluated to help with this decision. From diagnostic polysomnography, the main variables used include the following:

1. The obstructive apnea–hypopnea index (AHI)
2. Oxygen desaturation index and oxygen saturation nadir (SpO_2)
3. Evidence of CO_2 retention
4. Increased arousal frequency and fragmentation of sleep architecture
5. Increased work of breathing

OSA in children is diagnosed as an AHI greater than or equal to one event per hour (6, 7); however, CPAP is generally commenced only on children who have at least a moderate OSA or have a mild OSA with comorbidity(ies). A symptomatic child with mild OSA may be recommended CPAP if he or she has poor sleep quality, that is, an inability to fall asleep due to the obstruction, an elevated arousal index (>10 events per hour), and/or poor sleep architecture. Clinically, if the child has a high work of breathing, failure to thrive (8), poor development (9, 10), poor daytime performance and/or behavior, and/or respiratory distress, then CPAP may also be considered. Using CPAP alleviates the high work of breathing, thus conserving calorie consumption and allowing weight gain (11), and improves sleep quality and thus daytime function and behavior (12). Nasal steroids, body positioning, and surgical intervention (i.e., adenotonsillectomy) may be used without CPAP for milder cases of OSA, or used in conjunction with CPAP to help alleviate OSA in more severe cases (13, 14).

The most common correctable pathologies underlying OSA in children are adenoid and/or tonsil hypertrophy and obesity. The most common age for presentation with adenoid and tonsil hypertrophy as the cause of OSA is 2 to 5 years, and this subsequently declines with age. Conversely, the risk of OSA associated with obesity increases with age (15). Although most children with mild-to-moderate OSA respond to adenotonsillectomy (16), a proportion of children fail to respond to this surgery. Persistence of disease in a number of these children is reflected by the fact that a history of past adenotonsillectomy increases the risk of current OSA more than 2-fold, whether or not there is an underlying abnormality such as myelomeningocele (17, 18). Clinical practice has demonstrated that treatment with CPAP is a viable option for the majority of children who fail surgery. Treatment with CPAP is also increasingly recognized as effective for the management of perioperative airway obstruction (19–22). Criteria for such intervention are becoming clearer as the predictors for perioperative problems are clarified (23, 24).

A number of common syndromes and conditions increase the risk and severity of OSA, and therefore increase the likelihood of requiring CPAP. These include Trisomy 21, achondroplasia, Pierre Robin sequence, Prader–Willi syndrome, cerebral palsy, and obesity. In these instances, although surgical intervention remains appropriate, it is likely to alleviate but not "cure" the OSA, and CPAP treatment may still be required for effective long-term management of the upper airway obstruction. Nonetheless, it is important to note that a proportion of children who present with OSA, particularly those presenting during infancy, show improvement as they get older (10). Our experience suggests that if we can provide respiratory support during early development, many of these children are able to cease treatment. The caveat in this circumstance is that the presence of disease during childhood may be an indicator of small central and upper airways that will persist throughout life and into adulthood (25, 26). At the more severe end of the spectrum or where the diagnosis of upper airway obstruction is made in later childhood, the prognosis for cure appears to be poor.

Commencing CPAP Therapy

The data presented here regarding the commencement of CPAP in children are derived largely from clinical practice and experience. An intervention that can be specific for children includes behavioral strategies to assist with compliance. If hospital or home nursing resources are available, another strategy can be CPAP acclimatization in the presence of medical and nursing care. This provides family support, aids with adherence, and optimizes CPAP pressure. Otherwise, many of the other steps for commencing CPAP therapy follow adult practice (27). A few published studies address the issues surrounding CPAP initiation and adherence for children, and there has been limited formal evaluation of the acceptance by pediatric patients of different devices (28). However, what is known is that with proper training good adherence can be achieved in children (29, 30) and that it can be maintained with careful follow-up.

The strategies to commencing CPAP vary according to the age and development of the child. For infants (less than ~6 months old), the therapy can generally begin immediately, with no need for prior behavioral programs. Instead, intervention strategies and education should be primarily geared toward the parents/primary caregiver because of their primary role in achieving adherence with therapy. The adaptation process for CPAP is approximately 3 to 7 days; however, in some cases, infants take to the therapy almost immediately.

For older children, success in implementing CPAP therapy is improved if it is commenced in a graduated manner. To maximize adherence, the children must first become adapted to the nasal mask. This takes approximately a week and is done in the home environment. Role-playing with the child (e.g., acting as an elephant, "Buzz Lightyear," or an astronaut) assists with this. Allowing the child to wear the mask for 10 to 15 minutes when awake minimizes the "scare factor." Once the mask is accepted, the child is admitted to hospital and a CPAP pressure is introduced. Others report successful introduction of CPAP in an immediate manner, with or without the addition of behavioral intervention programs (31).

In adolescents, in general the process is the same as for adult patients. Reports now suggest that adults utilizing CPAP also benefit from access to a multidisciplinary approach to aid adherence with therapy (32). Practice guidelines derived from evidence in the literature suggest that once a diagnostic study has demonstrated the presence of OSA, the patient is fitted with the mask interface, and the process is explained to the patient. A trial of CPAP can be undertaken with the patient awake and participating. An overnight sleep study for pressure titration can be undertaken almost immediately. Pressures are adjusted during the study and the patient is discharged the next day on the pressure setting deemed optimal on the basis of a single night of determination. Although this may be appropriate for the older adolescent, a hospital admission to commence therapy may still be appropriate for younger or developmentally delayed teenagers.

In all age categories, CPAP therapy is commenced on a low pressure (e.g., 5 cm H_2O) to allow the child to get used to the sensation of the therapy and therefore maximize the likelihood of adherence. The first stage is to achieve overnight adherence with low-pressure therapy. A clinical review permits appropriate pressure changes to follow, for example, in the presence of ongoing snoring, pressures need to be increased. It is also important to note, depending on the age and complexity of a child's condition, that commencing CPAP at home with the assistance of a community nurse may also help the child and parents adjust to using CPAP as part of their bedtime routine.

PRINCIPLES OF TITRATION

For disorders with upper airway obstruction, the goal of pressure support is to splint the airway open in order to relieve the obstruction and achieve normal ventilation. When performing polysomnography for CPAP pressure determination, the channels that should be closely monitored in order to achieve an optimum CPAP pressure are nasal airflow, respiratory effort, oxygenation (SpO_2), and CO_2 (33). Monitoring of CO_2 during titration studies requires the use of transcutaneous ($TcCO_2$) rather than end-tidal measurements ($EtCO_2$). With the exception of children with lung or cardiac disease, the aim of a CPAP pressure determination study is to achieve a normal oxygen saturation (i.e., $SpO_2 \geq 95\%$) and CO_2 concentration (i.e., $35 \leq TcCO_2 \leq 45$ mm Hg). The pulmonologist and/or cardiologist should set discretionary guidelines for children with underlying/associated lung and/or cardiac disease.

Titrating CPAP during Polysomnography

Once the patient has adapted to the use of the pressure support, a full CPAP titration polysomnogram is undertaken in the sleep center. It is recommended that titration studies follow the American Academy of Sleep Medicine (AASM) guidelines (34). In general, pressure titration studies commence with minimal positive pressure (e.g., 4 cm H_2O) and do not exceed 15 cm H_2O for children less than 12 years old. The priorities for pressure adjustment are to eliminate discrete obstructive respiratory events, eliminate signs of increased work of breathing, and eliminate signs of airflow limitation.

Discrete obstructive events and labored breathing on the polysomnogram are seen as a loss of nasal airflow and increased respiratory effort with, or without, oxygen desaturations and/or arousals. The general practice is to increase the CPAP in 1 cm H_2O increments if at least one obstructive apnea or two hypopneas are seen in children aged 12 or less or at least two apneas or three hypopneas are present in children greater than age 12. Each pressure change should be separated by at least 5 minutes of recording.

Once discrete obstructive events are eliminated, the next step is to put an end to nasal airflow limitation, residual snoring, and respiratory effort–related arousals (RERAs). The CPAP for children aged less than 12 years is to be increased if there are at least three RERAs or 1 minute of loud or unambiguous snoring. The CPAP is to be titrated higher for children 12 years or older who experience at least five RERAs or 3 minutes of loud or unambiguous snoring. CPAP is increased in approximately 1 cm H_2O increments until this is achieved.

Once optimal pressure is achieved, there should be no snoring or stridor, and there should be normal nasal airflow and respiratory effort, stable oxygenation without intermittent desaturations, and normal CO_2. Allowing 30 to 60 minutes before additional incremental increases in CPAP will provide sufficient time for the patient to blow off any excess CO_2 and allow adequate sleep for analysis by the assessing physician. To allow the sleep physician to assess and confirm the optimal pressure, an ideal study includes pressure adjustments to a level slightly above the optimal CPAP. Acute signs that the CPAP has been increased too high include increased frequency of arousals, recurrence of the use of accessory muscles, fall in baseline oxygenation and CO_2 retention, and the occurrence of central (rather than obstructive) respiratory events (9). AASM standards indicate that an optimal CPAP is achieved when the respiratory disturbance index (RDI) is less than five events per hour for at least 15 minutes, SpO_2 is above 90%, and a rapid eye movement (REM) period in the supine position is recorded (34). The titration is considered good when the RDI remains greater than 10 events per hour and SpO_2 is above 90%. The titration may be adequate if the RDI has been reduced by 75% from diagnosis or titration was not assessed during supine REM sleep. AASM standards indicate that a titration

is unacceptable when any of the above-mentioned criteria remain unmet.

For long-term users of CPAP, the prescribed pressure requires regular review to ensure that ongoing optimal therapy is maintained (35). This is particularly true in children where growth increases the likelihood of change in airway structure, muscle tone, and tidal volume. Infancy, in particular, is a period of rapid growth, and therefore may require more frequent review, for example, repeating a sleep study at the age of 3 months, 6 months, and 1 year. As children become older, these can be spaced further apart, until annual reviews are undertaken. However, in other practices, retitrations are undertaken only as clinically indicated, by growth, weight changes, or changes in nocturnal or diurnal symptoms.

Advancements in CPAP technology continue to refine how pressure is delivered. CPAP devices come with expiratory pressure relief options or can be set to automatically adjust pressure to optimize airflow. Care must be taken in the selection of devices used in young or small children to ensure that tidal volume and flow rates generated are detected by the device. Some model devices are generally produced with adult specifications and children may not trigger them, so care is required to ensure that their specifications and functions will translate to pediatric patients.

Common Problems and Solutions Experienced with Children on CPAP

The most common problems experienced are pressure sores generated by the CPAP mask, air leak, and drying of the nasopharynx. The range of pediatric masks is increasing, but one of the most common difficulties in children is finding an appropriately sized nasal mask. Caregivers, including technologists and parents, must be vigilant to assure there is no facial skin breakdown. Careful observation of the face when the mask is removed every day is essential, just as with mask care for NIV. Rotating among two or more commercially available mask types can help minimize the risk of pressure sore. It is helpful to allow the child to choose his or her own mask from a suitable group. This implied consent gives the patient some control over his or her own care and improves cooperation.

Pressure sores generated from masks are a common problem in pediatrics, whether for long periods of acute treatment or for regular nocturnal support. They occur more often because of either the straps being adjusted too tightly onto the face and/or an ill-fitting mask. Acute and chronic pressure effects are increasingly recognized in children, including the potential for mid-face hypoplasia (36, 37). Suggestions to alleviate pressure sores include adding padding and/or applying a dressing to the affected area at night. Massaging the facial areas improves circulation when the mask is removed every morning.

A poorly fitting mask can also be associated with a mask leak. It is important to correct any leaks during the pressure titration polysomnogram as these lead to loss of pressure and, in turn, affect the optimum pressure settings. No air should escape around the perimeter of the mask. Mask leaks can also cause eye irritation and reduced user adherence.

Pressure loss can be generated by a mouth leak. Nasal masks are often the primary mask type used in pediatrics, and full-face masks are used only after careful evaluation by the sleep team. Pediatric sleep physicians can be hesitant to use full-face masks in young, developmentally delayed, or physically impaired children because of the risk of vomiting into the mask as well as the inability of the child to remove the mask himself or herself. Alternate solutions to alleviating mouth leaks in children include using a pacifier, wedging a rolled washcloth between the chin and the chest, and/or adding humidification.

The delivery of dry and/or cold air can precipitate or exacerbate nasal mucosal swelling and/or inflammation. Humidification is useful as it keeps the nasopharynx warm and humidified, preventing drying of the nasal passages. Maintaining humidification of the nasal passages minimizes the likelihood the user will open his or her mouth on inspiration. Humidification also minimizes inflammation of the nasal epithelium and consequent nose bleeds. For young children, the impact of CPAP without humidification can be significant in fluid balance and for this reason we never use CPAP without humidification in children aged less than 24 months.

Other problems that may be associated with CPAP are gastrointestinal wind and excessive salivation. Children, particularly infants, often swallow air when CPAP is commenced, perhaps exacerbated by sucking on a pacifier, poor tone in the lower esophageal sphincter, or if the pressure is set too high. Infants can develop abdominal distension, but this is usually a temporary problem that settles over the first 7 to 10 days of CPAP use. Children may also experience increased drooling, and occasionally this becomes excessive. Finally, removal of the mask during sleep times is a common problem that may be helped by adding mittens to the hands or using infant sleeping bags, making it difficult for the infant to grasp at the mask or head strap.

Equipment for infants should be soft with minimum capacity for causing pressure sores. In infants, it is especially important to ensure that the fit of the mask and head strap does not lead to air leak into the eyes. Infants should always be placed supine or in a lateral position to permit direct visualization and to ensure that the nostrils do not become occluded by the mask. It is also important that the tubing does not pull the mask up or off the face; in infants, the weight of the tubing can displace small masks and head straps upward; one way to alleviate this problem is to slacken the weight of the tubing by anchoring it to the side of the crib.

Another possible consequence to the use of CPAP or NIV long term is structural changes to the face. Young children who use a noninvasive device long term are at risk for developing mid face hypoplasia (36). Although evidence for this remains elusive, the concern is that during body development the nasal mask can push on the mid face, altering the growth patterns to affect the shape of the face. It is, therefore, important to monitor the development of the face for long-term users of CPAP or NIV and consider alternating between different masks, so that points of maximum pressure vary.

If leaks or other problems associated with CPAP are evident during the polysomnogram, it is important for the sleep technologist to document and report this to the physician, so appropriate steps can be made to alleviate the problem(s) and maximize user adherence.

NASAL INSUFFLATION

Klein et al (1986) suggested the use of insufflation (passage of warm humidified air through a thin nasopharyngeal tube at 2 to 10 L per minute; mean 3.5 L per minute) to treat upper airway obstruction in children. They pointed out that airway obstruction in children commonly presents with prolonged periods of partial upper airway obstruction, rather than the longer discrete obstructive events seen in adults, and demonstrated a marked reduction in the work of breathing in children treated with this modality (38). One significant benefit of transnasal insufflation is that it is better tolerated than CPAP, with 23.5% to 63.2% reductions in the AHIs in studies of adults (39). The flow rates used in studies of adults and children were 15 to 20 L per minute (40). At these flow rates, the insufflation increases nasal pressure by approximately 2 cm H_2O and inspiratory airflow by approximately 100 mL per second. Airway obstruction may not be completely eliminated with this technique, but it is particularly useful for patients who have trouble tolerating CPAP and may be more effective in treating children because it is most effective for those with partial obstruction or hypopneas rather than discrete apneic events (41). We have found the use of insufflation useful with flow rates of 7 to 10 L per minute in infants and children where CPAP is not tolerated and/or where upper airway obstruction is moderate, rather than severe.

NIV FOR CHILDREN

Noninvasive therapy is recommended for children with nocturnal hypoventilation or CSA. Unlike children with

OSA, surgical procedures are rarely an option for treatment of hypoventilation or CSA. A range of disorders can underlie hypoventilation and vary from congenital disorders affecting the CNS control of breathing to progressive or acquired disorders affecting the heart, lungs, and/or respiratory musculature. Children may suffer from severe restrictive lung disease, chest wall deformities, myopathies, and congenital or acquired abnormalities of the CNS. An increasing number of children are also being commenced on NIV because of the long-term adverse effects of chemotherapy on the lungs for treatment of oncologic diseases, and as a support mechanism for children waiting for lung transplantation. Whether the condition affects tidal volume, respiratory rate, and/or gas exchange in the lower airway, if the end result is inadequate minute ventilation, then NIV may assist lung inflation and/or produce an artificial breath rate to normalize gas exchange.

Sleep-associated changes in respiratory control and respiratory dynamics mean that hypoventilation will usually manifest first during sleep and only later progress to include daytime respiratory compromise. Broadly speaking, NIV is commenced when respiratory failure is demonstrated during sleep. A number of factors determine the time to commence NIV. Children with CSA will start on NIV if the polysomnography shows the following:

1. Bradypnea sufficient to compromise ventilation
2. Pathologic or extreme central apneic events
3. Evidence of respiratory failure—usually nocturnal

The changes occurring in blood gases are usually progressive, rather than being related to frank respiratory events. The common definition of acute respiratory failure is a CO_2 greater than 50 mm Hg and PaO_2 lesser than 50 mm Hg, thus acknowledging that hypoxia and hypercapnia occur simultaneously in disorders that compromise ventilation.

NIV can be started in the intensive care unit if children are acutely unwell but can also be commenced in a ward environment following a planned admission. It is recognized that children presenting with recurrent respiratory failure, or respiratory failure in the presence of an underlying (especially progressive) disorder, have frequently experienced acute or chronic respiratory failure (42, 43). That is, they regularly experience respiratory deterioration during sleep times, but acute respiratory failure can develop rapidly during a superimposed respiratory infection or with acute deterioration in their underlying condition. Recognition of the risk of sleep-associated respiratory deterioration has led to more proactive screening and identification of the disorder before these florid deteriorations occur. Children who are recommended NIV following polysomnography generally require NIV long term. Polysomnography can also be undertaken to screen children before surgery for scoliosis and, if required, NIV commenced to maximize their lung health before the scheduled surgery. Children who commence NIV in an acute setting may have a newly identified disorder and require only short-term therapy, or may need to continue on to long-term therapy after review in the period of recovery.

Hypoventilation of central origin leads to maximum blood gas abnormalities during slow-wave sleep when ventilation is almost exclusively under automatic control (no cortical influences). Congenital central hypoventilation syndrome (CCHS) may be attributable to a Phox2B mutation or to other CNS disorders that affect ventilatory control, such as a hypoxic insult or a brainstem pathology including the Arnold–Chiari malformation with or without syringomyelia, hypoxic insults, spinal cord trauma, or tumors. At best, the absence of CO_2 sensitivity results in a dependence on hypoxic ventilatory drive.

Peripheral hypoventilation describes failure of the respiratory pump to allow adequate gas exchange (i.e., chest wall and/or respiratory musculature movement). Conditions that pose a risk of peripheral hypoventilation are often linked with restrictive lung disease and include kyphoscoliosis, cystic fibrosis, bronchiectasis, myopathies, and morbid obesity. Peripheral hypoventilation results in both hypoxia and hypercapnia that are most apparent during REM sleep when there is skeletal muscle atonia, particularly affecting activity of the respiratory accessory muscles. Such loss of accessory muscle activity can shift marginal respiratory function to respiratory failure in children who can otherwise maintain adequate respiratory function while awake or in slow-wave sleep by recruiting respiratory accessory muscles.

One major advantage of NIV is fewer and shorter hospital admissions and maintenance of a better quality of life in children with neuromuscular disorders (43, 44). Follow-up of a group of patients, the majority of whom had neuromuscular disease, suggested that the commencement of NIV for nocturnal hypoventilation arrests deterioration rather than improving the underlying disease processes, with gains attributable to reversal of respiratory failure and improvement in sleep (45).

Commencing NIV Therapy

Although it is clear that NIV can reverse alveolar hypoventilation, the criteria for establishing ventilation are not universal. It is generally agreed that NIV should commence in the presence of daytime hypercapnia or during an acute or chronic exacerbation. Nocturnal hypoventilation likely heralds imminent daytime hypoventilation, but there is no current consensus about when to start screening children with progressive disorders. Further studies will need to determine what level of nocturnal dysfunction will be associated with improvement if nocturnal ventilation is established.

Our processes for commencing NIV therapy in children follow the same strategies as for CPAP outlined earlier. Although NIV may be commenced in the intensive care unit, elective treatment can also start in a general medical ward with overnight monitoring of SpO_2 and CO_2. Unlike CPAP, there are multiple settings (i.e., inspiratory positive airway pressure [IPAP], expiratory positive airway pressure [EPAP], and backup rate) that may require adjusting and fine-tuning when a child is commenced on NIV. Therefore, it would not be practical to commence NIV within the home setting. In the hospital setting, adjustments to ventilation can take place in a closely supervised environment with titration sleep studies performed only after the child has adapted to the therapy and shows stability of blood gases. Noninvasive therapy requires more frequent adjustments during periods of growth, especially puberty, and our policy has been to undertake studies at more frequent intervals during this time.

Principles of Titration

The primary principle for titrating NIV is to achieve normal gas exchange, indicated by normal oxygenation, CO_2, pH, and bicarbonate measures on blood gases. There are a number of primary settings utilized in NIV in order to achieve normal gas exchange and user comfort (Fig. 65-2). The first setting to be considered is the "mode"; this dictates how the respiratory rate is regulated. The "mode" determines if the respiratory rate is regulated solely by the user, the device, or a combination of both. The "spontaneous" mode allows the user to have a spontaneous respiratory rate 100% of the time. "Timed" mode allows the NIV device to regulate the respiratory rate at all times and overrides the user's spontaneous respiratory rate. Because of user discomfort and asynchrony between the user and the device, in our

clinic, this setting is rarely used. The final, but the most commonly used mode is "spontaneous/timed," which allows the user to breathe spontaneously but delivers breaths to meet a fixed, minimum rate if the patient does not trigger the machine within a prescribed time period.

EPAP is a positive airway pressure delivered on expiration. It can act as CPAP, providing an air splint to prevent collapse of upper and/or lower airways. EPAP is also termed "positive-end expiratory pressure" or PEEP. IPAP is the positive inspiratory pressure being delivered. To deliver ventilation, not CPAP, the IPAP should be at least 4 cm H_2O higher than the EPAP. This pressure difference between IPAP and EPAP is termed "the delta (Δ) swing" or "pressure support." The larger the delta swing, the greater the lung expansion and collapse. Increased pressure support increases pulmonary expansion and can increase CO_2 clearance.

The "backup respiratory rate" setting is activated only on "spontaneous/timed" and "timed" modes to control the minimum respiratory breath allowed by the user. The "inspiratory time" (alternatively known as "IPAP max") is a setting that works in parallel with the backup respiratory rate. This determines the maximum inspiratory time and the maximum duration of IPAP delivery before the pressures return to EPAP. The "rise time" setting is used for comfort and is the time taken to increase the pressure from EPAP to IPAP. Our clinical experience suggests that small infants and patients with stiff lungs tolerate a shorter rise time, whereas children with muscle weakness prefer a longer rise time.

AVAPS (Average Volume–Assured Pressure Support, also known as iVAPS) is another form of NIV but delivers a set tidal volume rather than fixed pressures. It helps patients maintain a fixed tidal volume by controlling the pressure support. In AVAPS, a minimum and maximum IPAP are set and the device fluctuates within this range

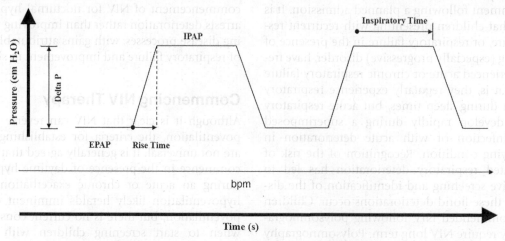

Figure 65-2 Fundamental settings of noninvasive ventilation. bpm, beats per minute; EPAP, expiratory positive airway pressure; IPAP, inspiratory positive airway pressure.

to deliver a set tidal volume. EPAP is a set pressure. This mode allows for improvement in synchrony between the patient and the device. As the patient's effort reduces (usually at night), the device will deliver higher pressure to ensure that the prescribed volume is delivered. AVAPS is becoming increasingly used in children (46).

In order to correctly commence NIV, one must first identify the cause of the hypoventilation/CSA. If the pathophysiology is caused by impaired brain/CNS function, whereby the CNS fails to regulate respiratory rate and blood gases, then a backup rate is mandatory to ensure that the patient breathes at the minimum prescribed rate. Backup respiratory rates are also required for patients with hypoventilation caused by myopathies and/or kyphoscoliosis, where the patient may not be able to generate sufficient negative pressure to trigger the device.

If hypoventilation and poor gas exchange are related to restrictive lung disease, then NIV titration focuses on correct titration of the IPAP and EPAP settings. In the majority of cases, a backup respiratory rate is also used to help regulate CO_2. Earlier generations of devices were designed for adults who weighed at least 25 kg, and if a child cannot trigger the device, then a mandatory respiratory rate may need to be used to deliver adequate support. Obese adolescents diagnosed with nocturnal hypoventilation and patients with cystic fibrosis tend to be the only instances in pediatric practice where a backup respiratory rate is not routinely required.

Titrating NIV Pressures during Polysomnography

In the context of our protocols, which aim to optimize ventilation before the pressure determination sleep study, monitoring in the sleep center generally results in only small additional changes. This minimizes the number of changes required in the course of a single study while still aiming to achieve the following: (1) SpO_2 greater than or equal to 95% and (2) $TcCO_2$ between 35 and 45 mm Hg and maximize synchrony between the user and the device (Fig. 65-3). Titrating NIV pressures should be in keeping with the AASM guidelines (34).

Ideally, the recording should include a period of quiet wakefulness off NIV to document the respiratory rate, SpO_2, and $TcCO_2$ during wakefulness. Once this is achieved and the patient has fallen asleep, the first step is to normalize oxygen saturation, which is usually achievable by adjusting EPAP. Changes in oxygenation can be seen almost immediately. If upper airway obstruction is seen, the EPAP is adjusted to overcome this, in the same manner as for CPAP.

Once the desired oxygen saturation is achieved, the next step is to eliminate CO_2 retention. This can be achieved by two methods: (1) increase IPAP to increase the delta swing and/or (2) increase the respiratory rate. After each adjustment to improve CO_2 clearance, approximately 30 minutes should be allowed for the changes to have an effect before the next pressure change or adjustment in respiratory rate.

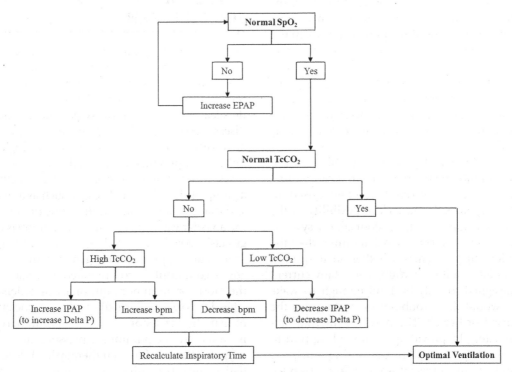

Figure 65-3 Titrating noninvasive ventilation settings to optimize blood gases. bpm, beats per minute; EPAP, expiratory positive airway pressure; IPAP, inspiratory positive airway pressure; SpO_2, oxygen saturation; $TcCO_2$, transcutaneous CO_2.

As a rule, setting the backup respiratory rate 1 to 2 bpm slower than the child's spontaneous respiratory rate during sleep regulates CO_2 while maximizing synchrony. As children grow, their spontaneous respiratory rate decreases with age, and backup respiratory rates need to be reviewed. Any alterations to respiratory rates should be accompanied by adjustment of the "inspiratory time" setting. The "inspiratory time" setting can be calculated using the following steps:

α (seconds) = 60 seconds/backup respiratory rate

β (seconds) = $\alpha \times 1/3$

Inspiratory time (seconds) = β + 0.2 seconds

The rationale for this formula is based on (1) the number of breaths per minute (i.e., 60 seconds), (2) the inspiratory to expiratory ratio (I:E ratio) of 1:2; thus, for every respiratory cycle, one-third of that time is spent on inspiration, and (3) to assist with comfort and compliance 0.2 seconds is added to allow extra time for the patient to breathe spontaneously before the machine initiates premature expiration.

The primary cause(s) of asynchrony during the polysomnogram are an incorrect backup respiratory rate and/or incorrect inspiratory time (usually too long). Asynchrony can also occur if the child fails to trigger either inspiration or expiration.

Common Problems and Solutions Experienced with Children on NIV Therapy

Children on NIV therapy can experience the same or additional problems as those on CPAP. Other than the common problems with mask interfaces seen in children on CPAP therapy as outlined previously, the major issues we confront are due to limitations of the technology relative to the requirements of children. In particular, these include sensitivities that are not appropriate for the smaller-sized patients, lack of alarms for caregivers, and limited portability of the devices; young children are frequently required to sleep in transit or away from the family home.

The limited number of products suitable for children that are currently being manufactured can require compromise in the mode of ventilation being used, or desired respiratory rates due to lack of flexibility in the technology, rather than the child. Poor alarm systems may limit the ability of caregivers to determine when the child is experiencing problems—whether on account of his or her limited mobility or young age. Many current alarms are designed to only be loud enough to wake the user who would then troubleshoot and correct the problem himself or herself. The need for internal batteries ensures safety, by providing continued support in the event of an AC power failure and during transport. Travel demands occur in several ways. Infants sleep for long periods and family demands may limit the ability of parents to stay home whenever the child sleeps.

With increasing numbers of children being supported with NIV in the community, we regularly see these children present with respiratory failure during acute illnesses. During these acute exacerbations, many children can be managed with a short-term increase in either pressure settings or the duration of their NIV (in each 24-hour period) and therefore avoid admission to the intensive care unit and intubation (47). In general, once a child commences therapy with nocturnal ventilation, his or her need is ongoing, although some disorders improve over time. Adults who commence nocturnal ventilation have reduced annual mortality, but equivalent information is not available for children.

The domains in which we are required to support the delivery of NIV therapy continue to expand. During acute illnesses, patients who live long distances from hospitals may be faced with the need to provide support while seeking medical assistance and ambulance transport. Traditionally, our medical transportation services intubate children in order to secure their airway for transport, but there are increasing demands to provide NIV during transport. Finally, as quality of life improves and these children actively participate in a broad range of family activities, we have increasingly frequent requests for NIV therapy during travel for leisure. One exciting development has been the need to oversee the transition of children who receive respiratory care, including ventilatory support, into adult services.

SUPPLEMENTAL OXYGEN THERAPY FOR CHILDREN

Disorders affecting lung diffusion include abnormalities of the small airway structure or function, and abnormalities of the alveolar wall or its components. In children, this includes various disorders, but the most common disorders leading to a need for oxygen include neonatal lung disease, cystic fibrosis, and chronic lung disease associated with aspiration secondary to neurologic conditions. Other examples include a selection of "orphan" lung diseases, which individually are rare, but together comprise a group of chronic lung diseases, such as abnormalities of surfactant proteins, and infiltrations or abnormalities of the alveolar wall, such as interstitial fibrosis or lymphangiectasis. For these disorders, where children are unable to maintain appropriate oxygen saturations, oxygen therapy is commonly recommended. Cardiac problems are the most common nonpulmonary disorders that lead to a need for oxygen, particularly those associated with pulmonary hypertension, where the pulmonary vasculature is (and therefore pulmonary pressures are) responsive to oxygen. The use of oxygen therapy in children under palliative care is becoming more common to alleviate symptoms toward the end of life (48). Occasionally, children with OSA who do not tolerate CPAP are recommended oxygen to alleviate the oxygen desaturations associated with the respiratory events.

High-Flow Oxygen Use in Children

Traditionally, oxygen therapy is delivered only at low flows less than 2 L per minute via nasal prongs or 4 L per minute via Hudson mask. The drying effect of the higher flows of the oxygen can irritate the nasal mucosa and cause distress and discomfort to the children as well as effecting secretion clearance and mucociliary functions. Recent technical advancements have led to the development of devices that deliver high-flow oxygen/air mix (47, 49). Adding heated humidification to the circuits allows for enhanced patient comfort and this is used in a variety of settings, including palliative care and periods of acute respiratory distress.

The underlying diagnosis is the major determinant of whether the disorder is progressive or will improve with growth and development. For example, during infancy, chronic neonatal lung disease requiring oxygen supplementation tends to improve with age. In contrast, adolescents requiring oxygen because of a progressive lung disorder, such as cystic fibrosis, will inevitably deteriorate over time. Ideally, oxygen therapy should be utilized only to maintain oxygen saturation (as clinically appropriate). In all cases where oxygen therapy is being provided, care should be taken to ensure that CO_2 retention is not precipitated in patients who are reliant on their hypoxic drive to maintain their ventilation (50). If this cannot be achieved, then NIV may be required, whether oxygen is required in addition or not.

Commencing Oxygen Therapy

The goal of oxygen therapy is to maintain adequate oxygenation and to do so without precipitating hypoventilation by removing hypoxic ventilatory drive. A diagnostic study (e.g., oximetry, $TcCO_2$ monitoring, or polysomnography) should be undertaken to evaluate the degree of hypoxia that is anticipated and to confirm a need for oxygen supplementation. The most common indicators of a need for oxygen supplementation are low baseline oxygen saturation levels. Other indicators may include tachypnea, deterioration in oxygen saturation levels during REM sleep, or the absence of REM sleep.

For infants who were transferred out of an intensive care unit, it is often helpful to "recommence" treatment by undertaking a diagnostic study and reviewing their absolute need for oxygen supplementation, as well as ensure that there is no accompanying evidence of CO_2 retention indicating hypoventilation. Passive hypercapnia is used in some of these infants on the basis that they will drive their CO_2 down as their lung function improves. The purpose of the review is to ensure that the hypercapnia is not unstable and to ensure that there is no additional CO_2 retention during REM sleep.

The signals in the sleep study, which provide most information, are sleep stages (proportion and progression), airflow, respiratory rate, respiratory effort, oxygenation (SpO_2), and CO_2 ($EtCO_2$ or $TcCO_2$ monitoring). It is important to monitor these children with full polysomnography as hypoxia is often accompanied by fragmented sleep with arousals, and adequate oxygenation may lead to an increase in REM sleep.

Principles of Titration

Oxygen therapy is a very common therapy in hospital environments, so detailed titration of oxygen requirements is necessary only in situations where oxygen use is expected to continue in the home environment. The supplemental oxygen concentration should be titrated with simultaneous oximetry and CO_2 monitoring to document when specified oxygen saturation is achieved and to determine if there is any CO_2 retention. Hypoventilation resulting from the removal of the hypoxic drive is relatively common in infancy and childhood. This makes it imperative for CO_2 monitoring when supplemental oxygen therapy is commenced, especially in children with chronic conditions. Children with potentially progressive disorders require regular review to ensure that hypoventilation is detected and treated should their disease progress.

Children requiring less than 2 L per minute supplemental oxygen can use a nasal cannula. Higher oxygen concentrations require the use of a face mask, although as mentioned earlier, there is increasing use of high-flow mixtures of air and oxygen up to 60 L per minute delivered via nasal cannulae (48). An oxygen concentrator is often used to deliver oxygen therapy for patients who require up to 5 L per minute in the home. Children who require very small flow rates (<0.5 L per minute) can use oxygen cylinders. Children with daytime oxygen requirements are also provided oxygen cylinders to permit mobility. It is helpful to use the appropriate mechanism during the sleep study (i.e., wall oxygen or a concentrator, with a low-flow regulator if required), so that monitoring is undertaken at an equivalent flow as achieved in the home environment.

Titrating Oxygen during Polysomnography

Our protocols for monitoring during an overnight sleep study begin with the infant/child breathing room air to record baseline ventilation. Oxygen flow rates are then increased at timed intervals (usually 2-hour increments), although ideally each period of monitoring should include both nonrapid eye movement (NREM) and REM sleep. Depending on the age of the child and any observations of prior oxygen requirements, titration can follow low-flow or high-flow regimes: (1) for infants, increments of 0.25, 0.5, 0.75, and 1.0 L per minute or (2) for older children 0.5, 1.0, and 2.0 L per minute. However, a physician may also specify certain flow rates on the basis of individual patient needs. Ideally,

2 hours of recording should be achieved at each flow rate in order to capture a full sleep cycle and the presence of CO_2 retention, changes in oxygenation saturation between NREM and REM sleep, and/or ongoing sleep fragmentation. Where there is any question about hypoventilation, it is extremely helpful to have a period of monitoring with saturation in the high 90% range to allow exclusion of hypoventilation secondary to loss of a hypoxic ventilatory drive.

Common Problems and Solutions Experienced with Children on Oxygen Therapy

In children, the most common problems associated with oxygen therapy are noncompliance with the nasal cannula, skin breakdown associated with the use of adhesive tape, and/or drying of the nasal passages and mouth. For skin problems, we apply a "second skin" type of adhesive tape to the cheeks to minimize direct contact with the adhesive tape. With an oxygen flow rate greater than 4 L per minute, patients can experience symptoms of a dry mouth and nasal airways, and to alleviate these symptoms, the oxygen can be delivered through a heated humidification device.

TRACHEOSTOMY AND INVASIVE VENTILATION

When to Consider Tracheostomy

Making a decision to proceed to tracheostomy is difficult and usually requires several medical teams. This should include the practicalities of other therapies, including whether alternative surgery can help avoid this outcome (51). Initial clinical responses to mask treatments are very favorable, but treatment failures do occur and tracheostomy remains an important clinical treatment option. Episodes of life-threatening obstruction can mean that despite the recognized morbidity and mortality related to the procedure, tracheostomy is required for safe management of the airway. Children who require greater than 16 hours respiratory support per day on a long-term basis should be considered for insertion of tracheostomy to facilitate safer delivery of the pressure and reduce the impact (pressure area skin breakdown) of wearing a nasal/face mask for that period of time, as well as permitting normal developmental activities such as eating.

When to Consider Invasive Ventilation

Our usual first line of treatment is nocturnal pressure support ventilation through a mask interface. In disorders where respiratory failure is secondary to a lung (rather than systemic) disorder, nocturnal ventilation is regularly used as a bridge to lung transplantation. Once full-time ventilation is required, then a tracheostomy is often required for the ventilatory interface. This may be from the outset, for example, traumatic quadriplegia or CCHS with full-time ventilation requirements, or may evolve over time in a child with progressive lung disease. Commencing full-time ventilation through a tracheostomy inevitably requires the involvement of a multidisciplinary team. Discharging children on full-time ventilation requires recruitment and training of overnight caregivers, modifications to the home environment, and the ongoing maintenance of equipment and supplies of consumables. The availability of such resources can vary among states and countries, and establishing the capability and proficiency in coordinating such care has proven to be the ambit of centers of expertise, where experienced staff can support and train the families and their caregivers in a way that will prepare and support the children as they are discharged into the community.

Children on ventilation are reviewed, at a minimum, annually, with more frequent review during times of rapid growth, the first year of life and puberty when scoliosis and restrictive lung disease may show rapid progress. The main goal is to ensure that the treatment is matching their requirements as they change with growth and development. Changes to ventilation often comprise only a minor part of comprehensive medical care. We monitor with blood gases as well as overnight sleep studies, again taking the approach that any adjustments made in the sleep center are for fine-tuning.

For children with progressive underlying disorders, the transition from nocturnal to full-time ventilation may need to be accompanied by evaluation for lung transplant. Although the initial progression may only be during acute lower respiratory tract infections, frank discussions regarding long-term prognoses often need to be held repeatedly. Eventually, a decision may need to be made about the introduction of tracheostomy. In some cases, prospective medical management requires that the devices be utilized in the palliative care setting (52) and our preference for palliative care is to use noninvasive respiratory support through a nasal interface (53). The benefits are that ventilatory support can permit ongoing care in the home, providing parents with a means to intervene and reduce respiratory distress as needed.

SUMMARY

The overarching goal of these therapies is to maximize children's participation in the community despite their underlying respiratory problems. Concrete outcomes include reduced hospital admissions, improved quality of life, and the encouragement of social and emotional development. Continuing advances in the technology available to assist these children has enabled us to steadily improve our capacity to achieve these goals.

REFERENCES

1. Hiremath, A. S., Hillman, D. R., James, A. L., et al. (1998). Relationship between difficult tracheal intubation and obstructive sleep apnoea. *British Journal of Anaesthesia, 80*(5), 606–611.

2. Apostolopoulou, S. C. (2017). The respiratory system in pediatric chronic heart disease. *Pediatric Pulmonology, 52*(12), 1628–1635.

3. Schidlow, D. N., Freud, L., Friedman, K., et al. (2017). Fetal interventions for structural heart disease. *Echocardiography, 34*(12), 1834–1841.

4. Schroeder, M. L., Delaney, A., & Baker, A. (2015). The child with cardiovascular dysfunction. In M. Hockenberry & D. Wilson (Eds.), *Wong's nursing care of infants and children* (pp. 1251–1321). St Louis, MO: Mosby Elsevier.

5. Healy, F., Hanna, B. D., & Zinman, R. (2012). Pulmonary complications of congenital heart disease. *Paediatric Respiratory Reviews, 13*(1), 10–15.

6. Redline, S., Tishler, P. V., Schluchter, M., et al. (1999). Risk factors for sleep-disordered breathing in children. *American Journal of Respiratory and Critical Care Medicine, 159*(5), 1527–1532.

7. Goodwin, J. L., Kaemingk, K. L., Fregosi, R. F., et al. (2003). Clinical outcomes associated with sleep-disordered breathing in Caucasian and Hispanic children—The Tucson Children's Assessment of Sleep Apnea study (TuCASA). *Sleep, 26*(5), 587–591.

8. Witmans, M., & Young, R. (2011). Update on pediatric sleep-disordered breathing. *Pediatric Clinics of North America, 58*(3), 571–589.

9. Amin, R. S., Kimball, T. R., Bean, J. A., et al. (2002). Left ventricular hypertrophy and abnormal ventricular geometry in children and adolescents with obstructive sleep apnea. *American Journal of Respiratory and Critical Care Medicine, 165*(10), 1395–1399.

10. Arens, R., & Marcus, C. L. (2004). Pathophysiology of upper airway obstruction: A developmental perspective. *Sleep, 27*(5), 997–1019.

11. Marcus, C. L., Carroll, J. L., Koerner, C. B., et al. (1994). Determinants of growth in children with the obstructive sleep apnea syndrome. *The Journal of Pediatrics, 125*(4), 556–562.

12. Blunden, S. L., & Beebe, D. W. (2006). The contribution of intermittent hypoxia, sleep debt and sleep disruption to daytime performance deficits in children: Consideration of respiratory and non-respiratory sleep disorders. *Sleep Medicine Reviews, 10*(2), 109–118.

13. Brouillette, R. T., Manoukian, J. J., Ducharme, F. M., et al. (2001). Efficacy of fluticasone nasal spray for pediatric obstructive sleep apnea. *The Journal of Pediatrics, 138*(6), 838–844.

14. Georgalas, C., Thomas, K., Owens, C., et al. (2005). Medical treatment for rhinosinusitis associated with adenoidal hypertrophy in children: An evaluation of clinical response and changes on magnetic resonance imaging. *Annals of Otology, Rhinology and Laryngology, 114*(8), 638–644.

15. Kohler, M. J., Thormaehlen, S., Kennedy, J. D., et al. (2009). Differences in the association between obesity and obstructive sleep apnea among children and adolescents. *Journal of Clinical Sleep Medicine, 5*(6), 506–511.

16. Brietzke, S. E., & Gallagher, D. (2006). The effectiveness of tonsillectomy and adenoidectomy in the treatment of pediatric obstructive sleep apnea/hypopnea syndrome: A meta-analysis. *Otolaryngology—Head and Neck Surgery, 134*(6), 979–984.

17. Morton, S., Rosen, C., Larkin, E., et al. (2001). Predictors of sleep-disordered breathing in children with a history of tonsillectomy and/or adenoidectomy. *Sleep, 24*(7), 823–829.

18. Waters, K. A., Forbes, P., Morielli, A., et al. (1998). Sleep-disordered breathing in children with myelomeningocele. *The Journal of Pediatrics, 132*(4), 672–681.

19. Carroll, J. L. (2003). Obstructive sleep-disordered breathing in children: New controversies, new directions. *Clinics in Chest Medicine, 24*(2), 261–282.

20. Rosen, G. M., Muckle, R. P., Goding, G. S., et al. (1994). Postoperative respiratory compromise in children with obstructive sleep apnea syndrome: Can it be anticipated? *Pediatrics, 93*(5), 784–788.

21. Waters, K. A., Everett, F. M., Bruderer, J. W., et al. (1995). Obstructive sleep apnea: The use of nasal CPAP in 80 children. *American Journal of Respiratory and Critical Care Medicine, 152*(2), 780–785.

22. Witt, P. D., Marsh, J. L., Muntz, H. R., et al. (1996). Acute obstructive sleep apnea as a complication of sphincter pharyngoplasty. *The Cleft Palate-Craniofacial Journal, 33*(3), 183–189.

23. Jaryszak, E. M., Shah, R. K., Vanison, C. C., et al. (2011). Polysomnographic variables predictive of adverse respiratory events after pediatric adenotonsillectomy. *Archives of Otolaryngology—Head and Neck Surgery, 137*(1), 15–18.

24. Wilson, K., Lakheeram, I., Morielli, A., et al. (2002). Can assessment for obstructive sleep apnea help predict postadenotonsillectomy respiratory complications? *Anesthesiology, 96*(2), 313–322.

25. McNamara, F., Harris, M. A., & Sullivan, C. E. (1995). Effects of nasal continuous positive airway pressure

on apnoea index and sleep in infants. *Journal of Paediatrics and Child Health, 31*(2), 88–94.

26. Tasker, C., Crosby, J. H., & Stradling, J. R. (2002). Evidence for persistence of upper airway narrowing during sleep, 12 years after adenotonsillectomy. *Archives of Disease in Childhood, 86*(1), 34–37.

27. O'donnell, A. R., Bjornson, C. L., Bohn, S. G., et al. (2006). Compliance rates in children using noninvasive continuous positive airway pressure. *Sleep, 29*(5), 651–658.

28. Marcus, C. L., Rosen, G., Ward, S. L. D., et al. (2006). Adherence to and effectiveness of positive airway pressure therapy in children with obstructive sleep apnea. *Pediatrics, 117*(3), e442–e451.

29. Rains, J. C. (1995). Treatment of obstructive sleep apnea in pediatric patients. *Clinical Pediatrics, 34*(10), 535–541.

30. Koontz, K. L., Slifer, K. J., Cataldo, M. D., et al. (2003). Improving pediatric compliance with positive airway pressure therapy: The impact of behavioral intervention. *Sleep, 26*(8), 1010–1015.

31. Järund, M., Dellborg, C., Carlson, J., et al. (1999). Treatment of sleep apnoea with continuous positive airway pressure in children with craniofacial malformations. *Scandinavian Journal of Plastic and Reconstructive Surgery and Hand Surgery, 33*(1), 67–71.

32. Engleman, H. M., & Wild, M. R. (2003). Improving CPAP use by patients with the sleep apnoea/hypopnoea syndrome (SAHS). *Sleep Medicine Reviews, 7*(1), 81–99.

33. Fauroux, B., Lavis, J.-F., Nicot, F., et al. (2005). Facial side effects during noninvasive positive pressure ventilation in children. *Intensive Care Medicine, 31*(7), 965–969.

34. Kushida, C. A., Chediak, A., Berry, R. B., et al. (2008). Clinical guidelines for the manual titration of positive airway pressure in patients with obstructive sleep apnea. *Journal of Clinical Sleep Medicine, 4*(2), 157–171.

35. Tan, E., Nixon, G. M., & Edwards, E. A. (2007). Sleep studies frequently lead to changes in respiratory support in children. *Journal of Paediatrics and Child Health, 43*(7/8), 560–563.

36. Li, K. K., Riley, R. W., & Guilleminault, C. (2000). An unreported risk in the use of home nasal continuous positive airway pressure and home nasal ventilation in children. *Chest, 117*(3), 916–918.

37. Villa, M. P., Pagani, J., Ambrosio, R., et al. (2002). Mid-face hypoplasia after long-term nasal ventilation. *American Journal of Respiratory and Critical Care Medicine, 166*(8), 1142–1143.

38. Klein, M., & Reynolds, L. (1986). Relief of sleep-related oropharyngeal airway obstruction by continuous insufflation of the pharynx. *The Lancet, 327*(8487), 935–939.

39. Haba-Rubio, J., Andries, D., Rey, V., et al. (2011). Effect of transnasal insufflation on sleep disordered breathing in acute stroke: A preliminary study. *Sleep and Breathing, 16*(3), 759–764

40. McGinley, B., Halbower, A., Schwartz, A. R., et al. (2009). Effect of a high-flow open nasal cannula system on obstructive sleep apnea in children. *Pediatrics, 124*(1), 179–188.

41. Nilius, G., Wessendorf, T., Maurer, J., et al. (2010). Predictors for treating obstructive sleep apnea with an open nasal cannula system (transnasal insufflation). *Chest, 137*(3), 521–528.

42. Ward, S., Chatwin, M., Heather, S., et al. (2005). Randomised controlled trial of non-invasive ventilation (NIV) for nocturnal hypoventilation in neuromuscular and chest wall disease patients with daytime normocapnia. *Thorax, 60*(12), 1019–1024.

43. Yates, K., Festa, M., Gillis, J., et al. (2004). Outcome of children with neuromuscular disease admitted to paediatric intensive care. *Archives of Disease in Childhood, 89*(2), 170–175.

44. Fauroux, B., & Lofaso, F. (2005). Non-invasive mechanical ventilation: When to start for what benefit? *Thorax, 60*(12), 979–980.

45. Katz, S., Selvadurai, H., Keilty, K., et al. (2004). Outcome of non-invasive positive pressure ventilation in paediatric neuromuscular disease. *Archives of Disease in Childhood, 89*(2), 121–124.

46. Johnson, K. G., & Johnson, D. C. (2015). Treatment of sleep-disordered breathing with positive airway pressure devices: Technology update. *Medical Devices (Auckland, NZ), 8*, 425–437.

47. Ramnarayan, P., Lister, P., Dominguez, T., et al. (2017). FIRST-line support for Assistance in Breathing in Children (FIRST-ABC): Protocol for a multicentre randomised feasibility trial of non-invasive respiratory support in critically ill children. *BMJ Open, 7*(6), e016181.

48. Chiang, J., & Amin, R. (2017). Respiratory care considerations for children with medical complexity. *Children, 4*(5), 41.

49. Hernández, G., Roca, O., & Colinas, L. (2017). High-flow nasal cannula support therapy: New insights and improving performance. *Critical Care, 21*(1), 62.

50. Brouillette, R. T., Jacob, S. V., Waters, K. A., et al. (1996). Cardiorespiratory sleep studies for children can often be performed in the home. *Sleep, 19*(Suppl. 10), S278–S280.

51. Cohen, S. R., Simms, C., Burstein, F. D., et al. (1999). Alternatives to tracheostomy in infants and children with obstructive sleep apnea. *Journal of Pediatric Surgery, 34*(1), 182–186; discussion 187.

52. Waters, K., Everett, F., Harris, M. A., et al. (1994). Use of nasal mask CPAP instead of tracheostomy for palliative care in two children. *Journal of Paediatrics and Child Health, 30*(2), 179–181.

53. Collins, J. J., & Fitzgerald, D. A. (2006). Palliative care and paediatric respiratory medicine. *Paediatric Respiratory Reviews, 7*(4), 281–287.

chapter 66
Infant Polysomnography

PATRICK SORENSON

LEARNING OBJECTIVES

On completion of this chapter, the reader should be able to:

1. Describe the indications for infant polysomnography (PSG).
2. Describe the electrode and sensor application techniques to achieve an optimal PSG in the infant patient population.
3. Describe the disorders found in medically complex infant patients.
4. Describe the essential documentation during a polysomnogram.
5. Describe how to assess for central apnea and periodic breathing.
6. Define the methods for working with a caregiver.
7. Discuss the performing studies in the neonatal intensive care unit.

KEY TERMS

Apnea
Treatment
Serotonin
Gestational age (GA)—age since end of last menstrual cycle
Chronologic age (CA)—age since birth
Corrected age—GA + CA
Home cardiorespiratory monitors
Central nervous system (CNS)

INTRODUCTION

The polysomnographic (PSG) technologist performing studies on an infant population in no small measure provides this service not only with prior extensive experience in the field of PSG, in general, but also with expertise specifically in pediatric PSG with a knowledge base of the factors that can positively and negatively affect the scoring and interpretation of a polysomnogram on an infant. The consequences of both positive and negative production aspects can be significant in the diagnosis of the infant. This chapter seeks to provide the biologic, environmental, interpersonal, and technical underpinnings necessary to provide the technologist performing PSG on an infant population with the information necessary to achieve and maintain a positive and rewarding experience not only for the technologist themselves but as a critical member of a team of infant specialists providing other medical providers and caregivers accurate and helpful information most expeditiously.

Chapter 60 (Pediatric Polysomnography) also addresses aspects of infant PSG such as age classifications that can determine how and when an infant's PSG can and should be done and interpreted, as well as general PSG knowledge. These areas are addressed only tangentially within this chapter, and the reader is encouraged to seek additional information to gain a comprehensive understanding of infant PSG. It is further recommended for a new technologist to seek a mentoring relationship with a provider who is well versed in infant PSG. Although studying the sleep of infants can be more challenging than studies of an adult, working with infants can be a highly rewarding aspect of one's career.

INDICATIONS FOR INFANT PSG

An understanding of why most infants undergo PSG testing is critical to the technologist's approach to the study. Infants being tested fall into the following two main categories:

1. To assess for sleep-related breathing problems because of concerns following observations by caregivers, referred to as symptoms, or medically documented evidence causing concerns for the infant's medical providers, referred to as signs. There may also be signs that central nervous system (CNS) abnormalities or immaturity may play a part in the signs and symptoms of concern. Symptoms are often confirmed by signs before the physician orders the PSG.
2. To confirm signs and/or symptoms of improvement or worsening or to assess changes, if any, following

treatment referred to as efficacy of treatment. PSG evaluation to assess improvement may also simply include maturation of the infant, and worsening may include a progression of a disease process or syndrome that may or may not yet be confirmed by genetic or other types of testing.

STAFFING AND SPECIAL CONCERNS FOR INFANT PSG

Technologists working with the infant population should *want* to work with this population. Many PSG technologists enjoy working with this population and seek out these younger patients. However, technologists who, for whatever reason, clearly do not desire to work with this population should not be forced to. The results of an infant sleep study are directly dependent on the role and effort invested by the technologist. The technologist should be thoroughly dedicated to working with this potentially challenging population, maintain the knowledge necessary to produce an optimal PSG on an infant, and possess the desire and ability to work diligently to produce an artifact-free recording. Just imagine trying to accurately evaluate a PSG on an infant with artifactual oxyhemoglobin saturation data and/or no airflow signal. Without the technologist's full dedication to ensuring the integrity of each channel, the recording will be suboptimal and the scoring and interpretation will not be accurate.

Infants are not a population where guesswork should be employed. For an accurate diagnosis, only a PSG technologist invested in the study can consistently perform at this level of expertise. PSG technologists working with this age group must be certified in infant and pediatric cardiopulmonary resuscitation (CPR). This kind of work is not for all PSG technologists and that aspect should be recognized by management—even as early as the hiring process.

TECHNOLOGISTS' ROLE—WORKING OPTIMALLY WITH CAREGIVERS

Producing PSGs on the infant population certainly has its own challenges, and working with the infant's parent or parents can, at times, be challenging. Caregivers often bring a level of stress to the situation, and this stress can manifest itself in difficult interactions with the technologist. However, with a few simple strategies, these stressors can be minimized or eliminated. Most, if not all, of these difficult interactions are because of occurrences that have little or nothing to do with the technologist but are related to other aspects of care of their infant. Emotions can be heightened for many reasons; some of these include complications during the birth, fear and alarm following the witnessing of an apparent life-threatening event (ALTE) or a brief resolved unexplained event (BRUE) that may or may not have the required contacting emergency medical professionals, the loss of some control over the care of their newborn by medical staff, and birth order of the infant where the first-born infant can elicit additional anxiety. The PSG may be seen as a stressful medical procedure caused by unfamiliarity with the process and the perceived or real consequences of a positive study.

Although there can be many more reasons for heightened anxiety of the caregiver, the PSG technologist can work to reduce these anxieties by clearly understanding the patient's history and what is to be ruled out with a sleep study and exhibiting sensitivity for the caregiver's state of mind. To address the caregiver's anxiety, it is important to thoroughly review with the caregivers the exact procedures that will occur during the study and the technologist's role. Explaining the procedures and function before touching the infant and checking the caregivers' complete understanding is essential. Keep the initial explanation on a basic level unless the caregivers ask for a more in-depth explanation, which the technologist can provide if requested. Remember that results are not available until the study is completely scored and evaluated by the medical staff and that the technologist cannot make any statements about whether the findings are abnormal or normal. Remind caregivers that your primary purpose is to obtain an optimal study according to the protocols set forth by the medical director of the sleep center.

Technologists should be knowledgeable regarding the clinic's policies and procedures so that they can be cited quickly and with authority. For example, if your laboratory has a cosleeping policy for infants, the policy should be stated to the caregivers during the initial instructions and not at the time of lights out. Another example is a policy about when and how to feed the infant during the study. In this regard, the technologist should retain sensitivity to the mother and infant while still being able to describe the clinical picture for the clinicians and scoring personnel.

Technologists' Role—Assuring Accurate Documentation

Staging an infant's sleep may be difficult, particularly during the infants' transitions to-and-from sleep, which often includes entering the sleep state in rapid eye movement (REM). This may appear as wakefulness due to respiratory rate and eye movements. The technologist must provide a clear description of what is happening with the infant and, particularly, to include comments of whether the eyes are open or closed because an infant usually cannot maintain wakefulness with eyes closed; even brief eye closure indicates drowsiness.

Additional comments on the recording should indicate the technologist's clinical impressions using comments such as "looks awake," "looks asleep," "feeding," "burping infant," "bouncing infant," and *anything else* that can help determine the sleep state more clearly.

HELPFUL TIPS

During video recording of an infant, focus the video camera on the closed eyelids to show eye movements under the closed or partial eyelids during REM sleep. This helps confirm that the infant is in REM. Be sure to zoom out and readjust the view to include the infant's entire body and head after the close-up of the head.

Try to make the caregivers a part of the study by questioning them regarding the infant's history and their approach to initiating sleep in the home for their infant. An infant-specific pre- and postsleep questionnaire can yield a great deal of information. The presleep questionnaire should address information such as sleep habits, medications, exposure to nicotine in utero or postnatally in the home, and the infant's age. A postsleep questionnaire assesses the typicality of the infant's sleep and breathing in the laboratory when compared to the home if the infant is old enough to have established and recognizable patterns. The infant's respiratory pattern, both awake and asleep, may be the sole reason the sleep study was ordered. At times, color changes during feeding may also be the reason for the referral, and close observation during both sleep and wakefulness is important in this population. Medical personnel caring for the infant on an inpatient unit is an excellent additional source for this information because parental caregivers may not be present during an inpatient study or they might not have noticed something the medical staff observed.

NORMAL SLEEP DEVELOPMENT

An infant is defined as a child from birth to 2 years of age. Age difference from birth to 2 years, although comparatively short over the life span, shows many differences even within a matter of a few months or even weeks or days. Therefore, it is important for the technologist to report the gestational age (GA) along with chronologic age (CA) to derive the infant's corrected age. The infant's GA is the age of the child at birth expressed in weeks from the first day of the mother's last normal menstrual period to the day of birth. The CA is the amount of time since the birth. From the GA and CA, the corrected age is derived. Obtaining the corrected age of the infant assists the clinician in determining the maturity of the CNS, and this maturity is linked to the electroencephalogram (EEG) waveforms obtained during the polysomnogram.

Since EEG features, both normal and abnormal, are closely linked to the corrected age of the infant, reporting the corrected age will affect the production and interpretation of the infant polysomnogram. The age of the infant can influence many facets of the study. An infant born at less than 36 weeks GA is considered preterm, an infant born between 36 and 40 weeks CA is considered term, and an infant born at 40 weeks is considered full-term. Since infants at less than 4 months corrected age sleep (<53 weeks corrected age) demonstrate an ultradian rhythm (repeated cycles across a 24-hour period) rather than a circadian rhythm (cycles driven by environmental cues), a sleep study on an infant can be performed at any time day or night. After 4 months corrected age, the infant begins to have more consolidated night sleep with a series of naps, and environmental cues begin to have an effect.

Neonates cycle through REM and non-REM (NREM) sleep differently than an older child or adult [1]. In the first few months of life, they have not yet become fully entrained on a day–night cycle, and more of the control of sleep is internal. Full-term infants can spend as much as 50% of their total sleep time in REM sleep. At this age, this is often referred to as "active sleep" [1]. The infant often enters the sleep cycle in REM. By about 4 months of age, as the infant approaches the adult mode of sleep-state cyclicity, sleep-state progression matures and NREM sleep typically precedes REM sleep. Breathing abnormalities, including obstructive sleep apnea syndrome (OSAS), may be exacerbated or only seen in REM sleep. For this reason, sleep staging is an important aspect of infant PSG evaluation to assess the sleep-state dependence of breathing abnormalities and to ensure that all stages have been documented during the study [2].

Normally, brief arousals occur as the sleeper transitions between each stage of sleep, usually without a return to full wakefulness [1]. These endogenous transitional arousals are common as sleep begins to differentiate in the REM and NREM progression of the infant both quantitatively and qualitatively as the infant matures. As an individual transitions to REM through the lighter phases of NREM sleep during the night, a continuum of behaviors, including stretching, brief vocalizing, crying, or changing of position, are common. Cortical arousals during infant PSG are scored because these may also be the consequences of abnormal breathing events during sleep, but the significance of cortical arousals in infants remains uncertain because there is the suggestion that apnea in children may not always be terminated with frank cortical arousal [2].

PSG PARAMETERS

The data used for the staging of infant sleep include the combined measurement of the EEG to record brain activity, the electrooculogram (EOG) to record bilateral eye movements, and the electromyogram (EMG) to record facial and intercostal muscle tone. The placement of the EEG leads should always be on the basis of the International "10–20" system of electrode placement so that the clinician can determine the maturity of the CNS as well as the exact location of any abnormalities. EEG placement for scoring sleep in infants is similar to that used in an adult population. For a sleep study, electrodes are placed at M1, M2, F3, F4, C3, C4, O1, and O2 for ease of sleep staging due to the increased amplitude obtained in referential lead derivations. The exploratory leads are referenced to the opposite mastoid. The central leads show activity at the vertex such as vertex sharp waves and sleep spindles, which develop by about 2 to 3 months postterm and K-complexes that do not start to develop until about 5 to 6 months postterm and are usually not fully formed until around 2 years of age. In infants, sleep spindles migrate to the vertex where they generally start more anteriorly and are often asymmetric until they are seen consistently centrally and become symmetric to both hemispheres. Activity in both hemispheres changes rapidly in the first months of life until around 4.5 to 6 months when the infant approaches the adult pattern of sleep-state cyclicity.

Even infants have a posterior dominant rhythm (PDR) seen mainly in the occipital channels, which in younger children starts at about 4 Hz and gradually increases as the child ages. The PDR in infants typically contains intermixed slower EEG activity (3). This frequency provides information to the clinician to help determine wakefulness versus sleep. Children with developmental delays may retain a slower PDR longer than typically developing children. Because of the special criteria used to define sleep states in infants younger than 6 months and the unique EEG features for this population, an extended EEG montage, or PSG channel derivation, is preferred. This extended montage should include bilateral EEG electrodes, utilizing the addition of bipolar channels to more accurately evaluate the EEG of the two hemispheres of the brain. EEG features specific to infants, such as tracé alternant and "delta brushes," as well as certain epileptiform activity can provide useful information regarding the maturity of the brain and alert clinicians to potential problems in brain activity.

Certain normal features of the infant EEG, such as rudimentary sleep spindles, are better seen using an extended EEG montage that includes some derivation referencing frontal to central to parietal to occipital leads in a bipolar array. The addition of T3–T5 and T4–T6 can provide more complete information regarding the

maturity and function of the temporal lobes. This is referred to as a bilateral parasagittal montage with the addition of the temporal leads bilaterally and should be considered the minimum number of EEG leads. Other options would include a transverse EEG montage or the more inclusive "double banana" used more often during formal EEG evaluation. Because developing sleep spindles may not be symmetric and begin to develop more anteriorly migrating to the vertex as the infant matures, the bilateral parasagittal with midtemporal leads derivation provides a more comprehensive monitoring of both hemispheres of the brain. Two more aspects in monitoring the EEG of infants are that the lead placement should be precise and the head accurately measured, and EEG lead placement should not be "estimated" or "eyeballed." In an infant, imprecise placements can and often do yield erroneous information. Additionally, no matter how young and fragile the infant appears, gentle prep of each site, using a mild abrasive, and avoiding the more abrasive preps that are commercially available, the technologist can and should obtain balanced impedances of less than 5 kΩ (3). To expect an accurate representation of the infant's EEG, without performing these two critical functions, is tantamount to doing a disservice to the patient.

The accurate scoring of sleep stages also requires the proper application of EOG sensors bilaterally to monitor REMs that normally occur during the phasic portion of REM sleep, as well as the slow eye movements that occur with the onset of sleep seen even at younger ages. The REMs of an infant appear more pronounced than those of older children or adults, and the placement of both leads at the outer canthi bilaterally rather than offsetting them is left up to the discretion of the technologist. The placement of eye leads should be as close to the sclera as possible, as long as the tape used does not encroach on the sclera or the lashes of the eye. The EOG leads are referenced to the same mastoid to more easily discern true eye movements from the higher voltages produced by the CNS and picked up in the EOG leads and the mastoid, a site felt to be electrically neutral but known to produce signal voltages sufficient to have an effect on the recording channel once amplified. The impedances for these leads should be at or below 5 kΩ, and the more abrasive skin prep should certainly be avoided around this sensitive area (3).

An EMG recording of facial muscle tone assists the clinician in more accurately determining the presence of REM sleep when skeletal muscle tone, particularly the muscles of the face, is normally inhibited. For infants, chin EMG leads should be placed adjacently and close together on the anterior aspect of each cleft of the chin following sufficient prep. In this manner, the channel will accurately represent the atonia of REM sleep in this population. Since oral and nasal secretions are common in this age group, covering the chin EMG leads with a moisture resistant tape will usually assure the integrity of the channel and is removed easily following the study.

To comprehensively assess the adequacy of respirations and ventilation and identify and differentiate between central and obstructive apnea and its severity, the recording should also include effort movements of the chest wall and abdomen with ideally a summation channel output, airflow at the nose and mouth, transcutaneous oxygen saturation data with a validating plethysmograph waveform from the monitor (also known as a "pleth wave" or pulse wave), and end-tidal carbon dioxide ($EtCO_2$) measures (3).

A summation channel is simply an output representing the combination of the chest and abdominal effort channels and acts as a fourth airflow signal should airflow or $EtCO_2$ sensors become dislodged during the study. A pulse waveform assists to assess the reliability of oxygenation data because oxygen saturation monitors can yield artifactual data at times usually when the infant is feeding or moving. It may be difficult to attach an oxyhemoglobin probe to infant digits, and this recording can be difficult to obtain. On small infants, the oxyhemoglobin probe may be placed on the side of the foot. If the technologist notices a poor output from the oxyhemoglobin sensor, a second probe may be added allowing the technologist to choose the signal that is most optimal without waking the infant. Capnography, a graphic representation of $EtCO_2$, is recommended for infant PSG because it can assess airflow and ventilation simultaneously. It detects the retention of CO_2 associated with sleep-related breathing abnormalities in this population (3). Calibrated $EtCO_2$ measurements can effectively detect CO_2 retention associated with apnea or prolonged hypoventilation.

Standard PSG also includes additional parameters that can provide important information relevant to the patient's electrophysiologic status. An electrocardiogram (ECG) monitors cardiac rate and rhythm and is useful in evaluating the consequences of breathing disorders on the heart. An EMG recording of the intercostal muscles detects expansion of the chest wall to assess for the presence of respiratory effort to help differentiate between central versus obstructive apnea. An infant PSG could include EMG of the anterior tibialis muscles to identify periodic limb movement disorders, although these disorders are rare in infants and leg EMG channels are not routinely monitored in children younger than about 2 years unless specified by the medical director or ordering physician. Limb movements in infants are generally a startle response to exogenous stimuli or endogenous stimuli and unrelated to low ferritin levels or known nervous conditions. Further, treatment modalities used for these disorders in the adult populations would be inappropriate for infants.

To assess for the presence of gastroesophageal reflux, and its potential cardiorespiratory consequences, continuous esophageal pH measurement can be performed in conjunction with PSG to assess the temporal relationship, if any, to reflux and apneic events. A pH probe is placed either just above the gastroesophageal junction or, using the newer pH probes that detect acidity in both the liquid and aerosol states, placed anywhere in the aerodigestive tract (from the esophagus to the nasopharynx) by the clinician and is normally less invasive.

Video recording with highly sensitive sound assessment is essential because it provides invaluable information on sleep behavior, snoring, respiratory effort, and sleep positions associated with a particular respiratory pattern. PSG on infants must be attended by a trained technologist who ensures the integrity of the recording, provides descriptions regarding unusual events or behaviors, and makes notations on the recording regarding physiologic changes such as snoring and color changes such as cyanosis, pallor, and erythema.

ASSOCIATED CONDITIONS FOR PSG IN INFANT POPULATIONS

Sudden Infant Death Syndrome

Sudden infant death syndrome (SIDS), previously referred to as "crib death," is a major disorder associated with sleep during the first year of life. It is the leading cause of death in infants between 1 week and 1 year of age. In the United States, mortality rates have steadily declined from more than 5,000 infant deaths per year in the early 1990s to just over 2,500 deaths per year by 1999. This decline is largely attributed to avoidance of placing infants prone or on their sides to sleep. By the year 2000, the incidence of SIDS around the world varied from about 0.1 to 1 case per 1,000 live births (4). According to the Centers for Disease Control and Prevention, the incidence of SIDS (see Fig. 66-1) in the United States as of 2016 was 38.0 deaths per 100,000 live births, which is greatly reduced from a rate of 130.3 per 100,000 live births in 1990. SIDS is best defined as the sudden and unexpected death of an infant for which sufficient cause cannot be found by a death scene investigation, review of the history, and a postmortem examination. As this definition implies, it is a diagnosis of exclusion; there are no findings on autopsy that are entirely specific for SIDS. Because of the breadth of the definition and the lack of specific postmortem lesions, it is probable that SIDS has multiple causes (4).

Closely linked to any discussion of SIDS is that of ALTEs. An ALTE is defined by the American Thoracic Society (ATS) as "an episode of apnea, color change (pallor, cyanosis or erythema), and hypotonia that the

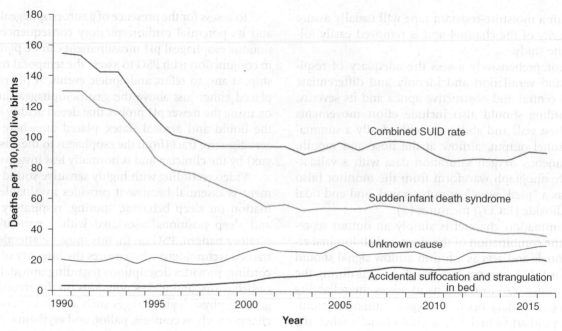

Figure 66-1 This graph shows the trends in sudden unexpected infant death (SUID) rates in the United States from 1990 through 2016. Sudden infant death syndrome rates declined considerably from 130.3 deaths per 100,000 live births in 1990 to 38.0 deaths per 100,000 live births in 2016. (Source: Centers for Disease Control and Prevention, US Department of Health and Human Services, National Vital Statistics System, Compressed Mortality File. Retrieved from https://www.cdc.gov/sids/data.htm)

observer believes to be life-threatening to the infant and for which some intervention (stimulation, shaking, and/or cardiorespiratory resuscitation) is felt to be required" (5). Recently, the American Academy of Pediatrics recommended the replacement of the term ALTE with BRUE. Although the relationship between ALTE and SIDS is poorly understood, many believe that ALTE may indicate a risk for cardiorespiratory instability, which could lead to death.

SIDS almost always takes place when the infant is presumed to have been asleep, either during the day or night. However, more than 70% of its victims are found in the early morning hours after nighttime sleep (4). SIDS is widely considered to have a developmental component because infants in the first month of life are generally spared. The incidence then peaks in infants from 2 to 4 months of life, which coincides with significant changes known to occur in sleep organization and in the modulation of brainstem centers involved in respiratory and arousal state control by the forebrain (6). Crib death is uncommon after infants are 6 months old, with 90% of SIDS victims affected in the first 6 months of life. It is rare after the first birthday. This particular pattern of incidence is unique to SIDS.

There are many risk factors for SIDS, most of which cannot be easily eliminated. However, there are several risk factors that lend themselves to intervention. They are (1) prone positioning, (2) maternal smoking, and (3) bottle-feeding (see Box 66-1).

Historically, numerous international epidemiologic studies pointed to an increased risk of SIDS when infants are put to sleep in the prone position (7–9).

A U.S. study confirmed this relationship, although the relative risk of prone versus supine posture in this study was lower than it had been in the foreign studies. Many mechanisms have been proposed to explain the relationship to sleep position, but most have not been tested or have not withstood critical examination. One hypothesis is that a subgroup of prone-positioned infants actually "burrow" their faces into their bedding rather than keep their heads turned to one side. These infants are theorized to die because of suffocation or rebreathing of CO_2 (10). An analysis of one supine-sleeping campaign in Norway published in 1998 showed that the SIDS rate dropped from 3.5 deaths per 1,000 live births to 0.3 deaths per 1,000 live births 4

BOX 66-1: Risk Factors for Sudden Infant Death Syndrome

Male sex
African-American race
Teenaged mother
Exposure to opioids and cocaine in utero
Anemia during pregnancy
Late or no prenatal care
Bottle-feeding
Prematurity
Low birth weight
Prone position
Winter season

years after an intervention program designed to avoid prone sleeping (7). Similar public education campaigns to inform parents about the risk factors associated with SIDS in the United States have yielded a clear decline in the incidence of SIDS. Other risk factors besides prone and side infant sleeping positions include exposure of infants to cigarette smoke (11), potentially hazardous crib-related sleeping environments, infant feeding, and perhaps the absence of a pacifier (9).

Maternal cigarette smoking during pregnancy is associated with increased risk in a dose-dependent manner: the more cigarettes smoked, the greater the risk (11). This dose dependency suggests a relationship between a factor that may be causing SIDS and prenatal maternal cigarette smoking. In addition, there is evidence that postnatal exposure to cigarette smoke (passive smoking) further increases the risk. Some studies have found breastfeeding to be partly protective against SIDS, but other studies have found no effect. Any beneficial effect may be related to the fact that breastfed babies have fewer infections than do bottle-fed babies because infections may increase the risk of SIDS.

Normal Control of Breathing and Heart Rate

Much of the control of breathing resides in the most primitive part of the brain, the brainstem. It is there that the central rhythm generator (CRG) is postulated to exist, and information flows from the peripheral chemoreceptors and the mechanoreceptors to the brainstem, modulating the output from the CRG. The presence of an "off switch" mechanism is also postulated because phrenic nerve output to the diaphragm is absent during expiration. The off switch terminates inspiration by inhibition of the CRG. Input from higher centers of the brain, such as the cortex, is also integrated within the brainstem. Hence, the ability to voluntarily control breathing also exists.

Control of the heart rate occurs primarily through the autonomic nervous system, which is divided into sympathetic and parasympathetic branches. Sympathetic stimulation of the heart increases the heart rate, whereas parasympathetic stimulation acts to decrease the heart rate. The vagus nerve is the parasympathetic conduit from nuclei (ambiguous nuclei and tractus solitarius) in the brainstem to the heart. "Vagal" stimuli, such as coughing, choking, or expiring against a closed glottis (the Valsalva maneuver), can induce bradycardia. The bradycardia that follows obstructive apnea may also be vagally mediated.

SIDS and Control of Breathing

The importance of the brainstem in the control of breathing and, possibly, SIDS is further supported by the fact that apnea in premature infants is associated with immaturity of the brainstem. Premature infants with apnea have prolonged brainstem conduction times for auditory-evoked responses compared with premature infants without apnea. Also, some SIDS victims have gliosis (representing scarring) of cellular bodies in the medulla oblongata, specifically in the area of the arcuate nucleus that controls respiratory and cardiac function (11, 12). Finally, newer research on the etiology of SIDS indicates that the syndrome likely comprises heterogeneous disorders that lead to death that is not explained following a thorough postmortem investigation and review of the child's history. It has been reported by Kinney et al. (12) that approximately 40% of SIDS deaths were associated with serotonergic abnormalities in brainstem regions with homeostatic regulation where there were elevated serotonin (5-hydroxytryptamine) levels. This finding suggests that SIDS may be associated with peripheral abnormalities in the pathway for transportation of serotonin. Serotonin is one of the most important neurotransmitters in the regulation of the sleep–wake cycle, and its expression is related to the maintenance of wakefulness. The deficit in serotonin suggests that abnormalities in this pathway prevent the sleeper from awakening under certain conditions and is a compelling explanation for the infant's inability to arouse from sleep despite conditions such as elevated CO_2 levels requiring the infant to arouse to resolve the adverse condition (12).

Although the specific neuronal dysfunction that leads to both central apnea and periodic breathing has yet to be determined, it appears as though factors in the maturation of central chemoreceptors and mechanoreceptors play a pivotal role in the alterations of respiratory drive in preterm infants. Some preterm infants exhibit an unexpected and paradoxical decrease in ventilatory response to increases in CO_2 values. Also, preterm infants often respond to a fall in inspired oxygen concentrations with a transient increase in ventilation followed by a return to baseline or even a depression of ventilation. The diminution of respiratory drive during hypercarbia and the biphasic response to hypoxia can potentially predispose a vulnerable child to apnea and its sequelae (13).

As intriguing as these hypotheses may be, the precise cause of SIDS is still not known. SIDS may have several causes, but all are likely to be related to a developmental immaturity or malfunction of the brain, leading to either cardiac or respiratory death.

There is no test that accurately predicts the risk of SIDS, perhaps because it has multiple causes and because most tests are performed weeks or months before death, during a period of life in which the infant is undergoing rapid change. Some laboratories may assess an infant with a pneumocardiogram consisting of a two- to four-channel recording usually consisting of transthoracic impedance (chest movements) and heart rate, as well as oxygen saturation data and an airflow channel in the more sophisticated models. The pneumocardiogram is usually performed overnight in a controlled, but unattended setting. Its value is markedly diminished because it provides limited ability to differentiate between central and obstructive apnea and does not provide thorough information regarding the severity and physiologic consequences of the breathing disturbance. It is widely accepted that the pneumocardiogram is not effective at screening for the risk of SIDS (14). In this regard, home sleep apnea testing (HSAT) fares no better, despite the addition of effort and electrocardiograph channels.

PSG performed according to the standards accepted by the ATS (5) and the AASM (3) provides the clinician with a more thorough evaluation of pediatric sleep and breathing disorders than a pneumocardiogram or HSAT. PSG for cardiopulmonary indications includes simultaneous recording of physiologic variables, including sleep state, respiration, cardiac rhythm, muscle activity, gas exchange, and snoring data. The technologist, in attendance during PSG, is trained to evaluate and document behavioral and physiologic changes as well as quality of sleep. Thus, a more accurate diagnosis of obstructive sleep apnea (OSA) is possible with PSG, in contrast to the lack of this capability in the limited-channel sleep apnea studies.

Although PSG is not always indicated after an uncomplicated ALTE or BRUE, it may be helpful to define the frequency of the type of apnea and the extent of cardiac, blood gas, and sleep alterations in certain infants with apnea or an ALTE. PSG is especially useful for the detection of occult hypoxemia. Test results may also suggest the further direction of the workup; for example, if abnormal amounts of obstructive apnea are noted, consultation with an otolaryngologist may be indicated. In addition, data acquired from these studies are often helpful in the later interpretation of waveforms from home monitors. However, the major concern after an ALTE episode is the related risk of recurrent events or death.

THE PEDIATRIC SLEEP FACILITY

Laboratory Supervision

A pediatrician with training and experience in pediatric respiratory disorders and/or sleep medicine should be responsible for supervision of a sleep laboratory whose primary activity is performing PSG in infants and children with cardiorespiratory disorders. If this is not possible, because of limited PSG resources, it is recommended that a pediatrician with expertise in pediatric pulmonology, neonatology, neurology, or pediatric sleep medicine oversee laboratory operations in

studying children in sleep centers. A pediatric specialist can ensure that the PSG is performed, scored, and interpreted appropriately for the age and condition of the child.

Setting

Infants should be studied in a dedicated pediatric facility with a laboratory decor that is both age-appropriate and nonthreatening. If a separate pediatric laboratory is not available, an area of the laboratory should be dedicated for infants. Accommodations for a parent to sleep near the infant are recommended because immediate parental access to the infant is often necessary to reduce fear and anxiety and provide ordinary childcare while the study is in progress. Safe and comfortable bedding is necessary when performing PSG on infants and children, and the technologist should be aware that they may be modeling appropriate or inappropriate sleeping practices. Mattresses should be made of material that is easy to clean and disinfect if soiled.

Personnel

A pediatric sleep laboratory should be staffed with personnel trained to deal with infants and their caregivers. Because PSG evaluation can be seen as stressful, particularly in this age group, laboratory personnel should have knowledge of infant behavior and developmental stages to effectively deal with children and provide medical information in a nonthreatening manner. Because of the differences in the sleep characteristics of children when compared with adolescents and adults, only qualified individuals who know the unique characteristics of sleep breathing in children of different ages should evaluate the PSG (3).

INFANT BREATHING DISORDERS

Apnea

Apnea is best defined as the absence of airflow at the nostrils and mouth. The three main categories of apnea are central, obstructive, and mixed. Central apnea occurs when respiratory effort ceases; there is no chest movement and hence no airflow. Diagnosis of central apnea must take into account a multitude of factors. It is ordinarily significant when it exceeds 20 seconds in duration. Because infants normally have a more rapid baseline respiratory rate and a reduced respiratory reserve, and, therefore, less protection from hypoxia, shorter central events can be more clinically significant in this age group. Central apnea can yield significant physiologic compromise such as bradycardia or color change associated with declining oxyhemoglobin levels.

For infants, central sleep apnea must be distinguished from other causes of respiratory pauses, including the more common periodic breathing pattern and the obligatory respiratory pauses that often follow a deep yawn or sigh. Although a rare cause of central apnea, seizures will also change the respiratory pattern seen on a recording. In the more severe cases, central apneas can be treated with medication. The presence of frequent central sleep apnea is a usual cause for respiratory monitoring during sleep. Premature infants are at increased risk for central apneas. Central apnea accounts for 10% to 25% of all apneas in premature infants (15).

Obstructive Sleep Apnea Syndrome

In children, OSAS is a disorder of breathing during sleep that is characterized by prolonged partial upper airway obstruction (hypopnea) and/or intermittent complete obstruction (apnea) that disrupts normal ventilation during sleep and normal sleep patterns. Clinically, obstructive apnea is the lack or diminution of airflow, despite the continuation of respiratory efforts. The obstruction can be functional or anatomic. When obstruction is present, respiratory efforts continue, and tugging or retraction of the skin can be seen. OSAS accounts for only 10% to 20% of all apneas in preterm infants (2). It has been estimated that 7% to 9% of children snore regularly, with an estimated prevalence of OSAS of 0.7% in 4- to 5-year-old children. Most affected children breathe normally while awake. However, a minority with marked upper airway obstruction also have noisy, mildly labored breathing while awake.

Obstruction lasting the length of two missed breaths or longer is regarded as significant in infants. In some infants with clinically significant OSAS, little or no snoring may be heard by the caregiver, unlike the clinical manifestations of OSAS in older children and adults (3). To accurately diagnose OSAS in an infant, clinical descriptions of the infant's noises by the technologist doing the study are critical because of the consistent presence of paradoxical breathing in the infant related to the way the infant breathes. Infant breathing is primarily costal in nature and the chest wall at this age is pliable, yielding paradoxical efforts seen mainly in REM sleep. The clinician needs to rely on the airflow channels, the intercostal EMG channels, and the technologist's descriptions to accurately classify sleep-related breathing abnormalities as obstructive.

Obstructions can be caused by the presence of an anatomic abnormality, neurologic condition, or medical condition. Reduction of the airway size leads to increased respiratory effort, which can create negative airway pressure and, paradoxically, worsen the obstruction. The most common anatomic factors leading to OSAS include large tonsils or adenoids, obesity, micrognathia (small jaw), or other anatomic anomalies. Muscular hypotonia is one of the most common neurologic factors contributing to OSAS in infancy. Normal muscle tone inhibition during REM sleep can change respiratory patterns, with more breath-to-breath variability increasing the risk of full or partial airway obstruction. Hypotonia can be commonly seen in Down syndrome, muscular dystrophy, and other genetic disorders. Allergies or even mild upper respiratory tract infections can serve to swell mucous membranes and thereby contribute to obstruction. Some of the less common risk factors include laryngomalacia, pharyngeal flap surgery, sickle cell disease, structural malformations of the brainstem, and certain metabolic and genetic disorders.

Apneas and hypopneas lead to a drop in oxygen saturations and an increase in blood CO_2 and often will cause a full or partial arousal pattern in sleep EEG recordings. When these events occur multiple times at night, there are several anticipated effects. The presence of frequent arousals leads to fragmented and inefficient sleep as yet not clearly defined for infants. This can lead to increased daytime sleepiness.

Adenoid and tonsillar removal is contraindicated for most cases of infant OSA. Other ways to relieve the obstructed breathing could include a tongue-lip adhesion, continuous positive airway pressure using a large cannula that does not create a seal but stimulates breathing, or perhaps tracheostomy may be necessary.

Mixed sleep apnea is the combination of central and obstructive apnea, with the central component usually followed by obstruction. Because of this, therapies that are effective for central apnea are also effective in treating mixed apnea. For example, during infancy, medications can be used to treat both forms of apnea.

Periodic Breathing

In the normal neonate, particularly the premature infant, breathing can be irregular. Periodic breathing is defined as episodic pauses in respiratory movements, each lasting 4 to 10 seconds alternating with several appropriate breaths. Periodic breathing is most easily seen by reviewing the breathing pattern in compressed view. Figure 66-2A-E provides examples of periodic breathing at increasingly compressed views. Apnea is considered a more serious condition because the respiratory pause is long-lasting and is frequently associated with more significant decreases in heart rate below 80 bpm and declining oxyhemoglobin values. Although periodic breathing is usually considered benign, for very small infants, even short apneic pauses can cause significant bradycardia and oxygen desaturations.

Periodic breathing can occur during wakefulness, active sleep (REM), and quiet sleep (NREM), but its prevalence is increased in active sleep. In quiet sleep, periodic

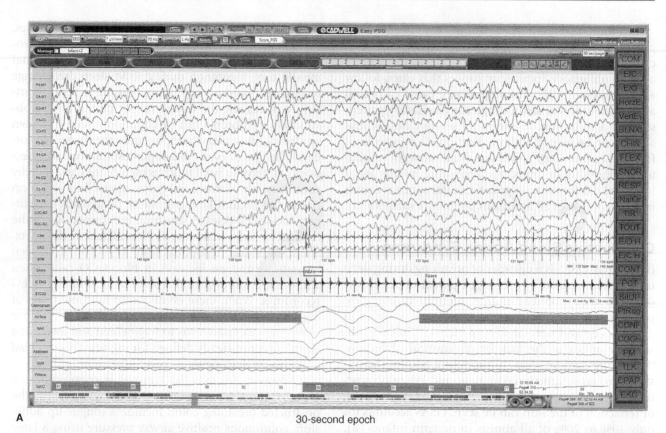

A   30-second epoch

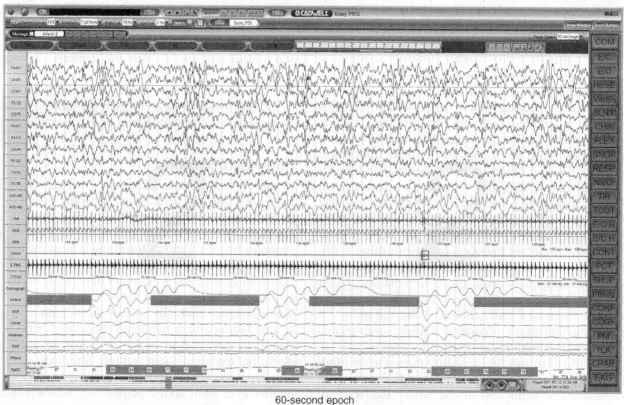

B   60-second epoch

Figure 66-2 The following are examples of periodic breathing in an infant at increasing epoch time spans. Note the difficulty in making this determination using a shorter window. **A:** 30-second epoch. **B:** 60-second epoch.

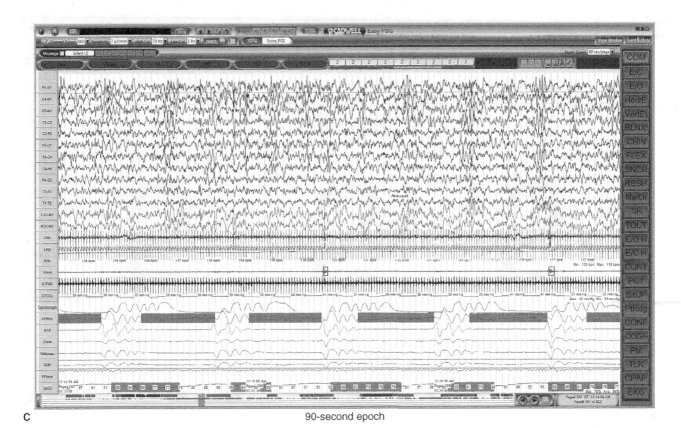

C
90-second epoch

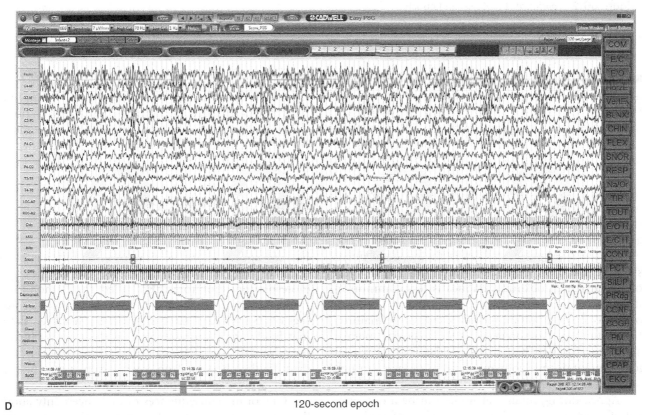

D
120-second epoch

Figure 66-2 (*continued*) C: 90-second epoch. D: 120-second epoch.

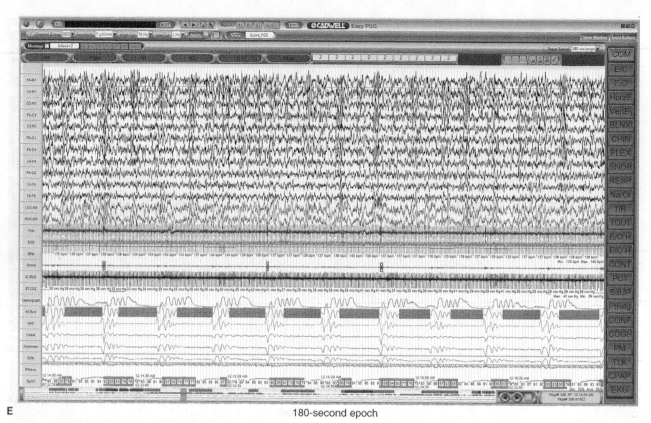

180-second epoch

Figure 66-2 (*continued*) **E:** 180-second epoch.

breathing becomes regular, that is, breathing and apneic intervals are of similar duration. In active sleep, the frequency of respirations and, subsequently, periodic breathing becomes irregular. The most well-defined periodic breathing observable in small infants is in quiet sleep during the EEG pattern known as tracé alternant, commonly seen in infants younger than 44 weeks' conceptional age (16). Tracé alternant is an episodic EEG pattern in which complex bursts of moderate- to high-amplitude slow waves are superimposed on a continuous background of polymorphic theta and faster rhythms (16).

All types of apneas are seen in the neonatal intensive care unit (NICU) and at home during the first year of life, although obstructive apnea is less common in infants. The causes of apnea in the NICU are numerous. The most important include apnea of prematurity (idiopathic), gastroesophageal reflux, hypoxia, anemia, and intraventricular hemorrhage. Sedative drugs passed to the infant during labor and delivery, or later through breast milk, can also lead to apnea.

Apnea during infancy at home can be a component of an ALTE. These episodes were often referred to as "near miss" SIDS in the past. Those that require vigorous stimulation or CPR are severe ALTEs and demand special attention because there is an increased risk of subsequent death. Episodes that occur while the infant is awake are more likely to be associated with gastroesophageal reflux, seizures, incoordination of swallowing and breathing during feedings, and crying with breath holding (17). In contrast to the neonate in the NICU and the infant at home, the older child is predominately affected by OSAS.

HOME CARDIORESPIRATORY MONITORS

Because apnea and/or respiratory instability has been the most prominent hypothesis for several decades, cardiorespiratory monitors (also called apnea monitors) are frequently prescribed for high-risk infants. Recordings of a small number of SIDS deaths, however, show that bradycardia is present for several minutes before the advent of central apnea (18). The cause of this bradycardia then becomes the crucial issue. It may be secondary to hypoxemia after apnea.

One of the consequences of our uncertainty about the cause or causes of SIDS is that a rational approach to prevention is difficult. Cardiorespiratory monitors theoretically should be useful in prevention of either cardiac or respiratory death, but the efficacy of these devices has not been scientifically proved or disproved, and monitored infants have died despite quick parental response to the alarm (14). Conversely, there are hundreds of anecdotal reports that infants have been saved after a caregiver is alerted by a monitor alarm.

Cardiorespiratory monitors for use at home provide two immediate purposes: (1) to alert the caregiver to a cardiorespiratory abnormality and (2) to serve as diagnostic devices (19). Ultimately, they are intended to prevent death. The standard monitor in the United States is an impedance-type monitor that detects chest movements and ECG tracings through electrodes placed on the chest. The monitors contain alarms for conditions such as apnea, tachypnea, bradycardia, tachycardia, and, sometimes, oxygen desaturation. The settings at which each alarm may ring are typically adjustable. Because the monitors detect chest wall movement, they are not much sensitive for obstructive apneas, since chest wall movements may continue through the apnea (20).

Many monitors can record data in memory for later downloading and analysis. In this manner, the conditions leading up to an alarm can be evaluated for clinical significance and "false alarms" eliminated. Often, alarms will be programmed to save data recorded just before, during, and after an alarm. However, the alarm memory will also indicate the total recording time, which is a useful gauge of parental compliance with monitoring. Ensuring compliance may be important because some studies suggest that the majority of infant deaths with prescribed monitors occur during periods of noncompliance or inappropriate use (21, 22). Hence, encouraging parents to use the monitor is vital.

False alarms are often apnea alarms for which the monitor fails to detect the breathing movements that are actually present. Inspection of the recorded waveforms may show a complete lack of breathing movements, but without any associated change in the heart rate or oxygen saturation. The presence of the ECG allows confirmation of bradycardia and recognition of some arrhythmias. This is how the monitor functions as a diagnostic device.

Several studies have shown that false apnea alarms and loose lead alarms can be frequent and can substantially outnumber true alarms (20, 21). False alarms can be reduced by attention to electrode placement so that the electrodes "see" maximal chest or abdominal wall movements. This often means that parents must be properly trained in lead placement. However, there will always be some false alarms. Appropriate attention to the monitor settings can help eliminate false alarms set off by patient crying or movement.

Discharge and Parents' and Caregivers' Training

It is essential that parents and other caretakers be fully trained in how to respond to an alarm. This includes being able to distinguish a false alarm from a true event

and to be prepared to administer CPR if necessary. CPR is a complex skill that we expect parents to be able to perform effectively at a time when they are worried or panicked. In fact, there is evidence that parents forget CPR training within a matter of weeks (23). Affording the parents the opportunity to have repeated CPR training sessions may be lifesaving because many repeat ALTEs occur within weeks after discharge from the hospital on a home monitor.

Monitors are traditionally intended only for infants in various high-risk groups, which include those with severe ALTEs and preterm infants who continue to have apneas and bradycardias as discharge from the NICU approaches. As monitoring is begun, it is often helpful to have clear clinical criteria for the discontinuation of monitoring at a later date. Monitoring is often perceived by families as an important safety net, and it can often be difficult to stop monitoring even when the clinical indications for monitoring are no longer present. Because parents are understandably often incorrect in their assessment of alarms, it follows that discontinuation is much easier and surer when the infant is on a memory-equipped monitor.

The time of hospital discharge is an emotionally taxing time for parents. The anxiety produced by having a child on a monitor at home is magnified by the likelihood that parents' sleep will be more disrupted to attend to false alarms during the night. A support system comprising personnel from the monitor supply company and medical professionals responsible for the infant's care can lessen this burden (21). The most important criterion for the discontinuation of a home apnea monitor is the absence of any significant events for 2 consecutive months. A significant real event is a real alarm for which the infant, in the judgment of the clinician, required stimulation.

REFERENCES

1. Anders, T., & Keener, M. (1985). Developmental course of nighttime sleep-wake patterns in full-term and premature infants during the first year of life. *Sleep, 8,* 173–192.
2. Kelmanson, I. A. (2006). *Sleep and breathing in infants and young children* (chaps. XIV–XVII). New York: Nova Biomedical Books.
3. Berry, R. B., Albertario, C. L., Harding, S. M., et al.; for the American Academy of Sleep Medicine. (2018). *The AASM manual for the scoring of sleep and associated events: Rules, terminology and technical specifications* (Version 2.5). Darien, IL: American Academy of Sleep Medicine.
4. Glotzbach, S., Ariagno, R., & Harper, R. (1995). Sleep and the sudden infant death syndrome. In R. Ferber & M. Kryger (Eds.), *Principles and practice of sleep medicine in the child* (p. 231). Philadelphia, PA: W. B. Saunders.

5. American Thoracic Society. (1996). Standards and indications for cardiopulmonary sleep studies in children. *American Journal of Respiratory and Critical Care Medicine, 153*, 866–878.

6. Tildon, J. T., Meny, R. G., & O'Brien, J. (1991). Sudden infant death syndrome. In R. Dulbecco (Ed.), *Encyclopedia of human biology* (pp. 315–322). San Diego, CA: Academic Press.

7. Skadberg, B. T., Morild, I., & Markstad, T. (1998). Abandoning prone sleeping: Effect on the risk of sudden infant death syndrome. *Journal of Pediatrics, 132*(2), 340–343.

8. Mitchell, E. A., Thach, B. T., Thompson, J. M. D., et al.; for the New Zealand Cot Death Study. (1999). Changing infant's sleep position increases risk of sudden infant death syndrome. *Archives of Pediatrics & Adolescent Medicine, 153*, 1136–1141.

9. Oyen, N., Markestad, T., Skaerven, R., et al. (1997). Combined effects of sleeping position and prenatal risk factors in sudden infant death syndrome: The Nordic epidemiological SIDS study. *Pediatrics, 100*, 613–621.

10. Kemp, J. S., Kowalski, R. M., Graham, M. A., et al. (1992). Positional ventilatory impairment in a serial study of 23 SIDS cases. *Pediatric Research, 31*, 360A.

11. Haglund, B., & Cnattingius, S. (1990). Cigarette smoking as a risk factor for sudden infant death syndrome: A population-based study. *American Journal of Public Health, 80*, 29–32

12. Kinney, H. C., Burger, P. C., Harrell, F. E., Jr., et al. (1983). Reactive gliosis in the medulla oblongata of victims of the sudden infant death syndrome. *Pediatrics, 72*, 181–187.

13. Rigatto, H. (1995). Control of breathing during sleep in the fetus and neonate. In R. Ferber & M. Kryger (Eds.), *Principles and practice of sleep medicine in the child* (p. 35). Philadelphia, PA: W. B. Saunders.

14. Meny, R. G., Blackmon, L., Fleischmann, D., et al. (1988). Sudden infant death and home monitors. *American Journal of Diseases of Children, 142*, 1037–1040.

15. Miller, M. J., & Martin, R. J. (1998). Pathophysiology of apnea of prematurity. In R. A. Polin & W. W. Fox (Eds.), *Fetal and neonatal physiology* (pp. 1129–1143). Philadelphia, PA: W.B. Saunders.

16. Pedley, T. A., Lombroso, C., & Hanley, R. (1981). Introduction to neonatal electroencephalography: Interpretation. *American Journal of EEG Technology, 21*, 15–29.

17. Spitzer, A. R., Boyle, J. T., Tuchman, D. N., et al. (1984). Awake apnea associated with gastroesophageal reflux: A specific clinical syndrome. *Journal of Pediatrics, 104*, 200–205.

18. Kelly, D. H., Pathak, A., & Meny, R. (1991). Sudden severe bradycardia in infancy. *Pediatric Pulmonology, 10*, 199–204.

19. Weese-Mayer, D. E., Brouillette, R. T., Morrow, A. S., et al. (1989). Assessing validity of infant monitor alarms with event recording. *Journal of Pediatrics, 115*, 701–708.

20. Nathanson, I., O'Donnell, J., & Commins, M. F. (1989). Cardiorespiratory patterns during alarms in infants using apnea/bradycardia monitors. *American Journal of Diseases of Children, 143*, 476–480.

21. Ahmann, E., Wulff, L., & Meny, R. G. (1992). Home apnea monitoring and disruptions in family life: A multidimensional controlled study. *American Journal of Public Health, 82*, 719–722.

22. Carroll, J. L., & Siska, E. S. (1998). SIDS: Counseling parents to reduce the risk. *American Family Physician, 57*, 1566–1572.

23. Dracup, K., Doering, L. V., Moser, D. K., Evangelista, L. (1998). Retention and use of cardiopulmonary resuscitation skills in parents of infants at risk for cardiopulmonary arrest. *Pediatric Nursing, 24*(3), 219–225.

SECTION 9
Sleep Center Management

chapter 67
Sleep Center Facilities and Equipment

TODD EIKEN

LEARNING OBJECTIVES

On completion of this chapter, the reader should be able to:

1. Describe the key components of a conventional sleep center facility.
2. Outline the advantages and disadvantages of converting traditional hospital rooms to patient rooms for sleep testing as against facility renovation.
3. Explain the importance of ensuring patient privacy and confidentiality through facility design.
4. Describe the general applications of video/audio recording in the sleep center.
5. Outline the available options for camera, lighting, microphone, and sound processing equipment.
6. Describe the data archiving options available for polysomnographic (PSG) data files.
7. List the general categories of instrumentation in the sleep lab.
8. Explain the primary options and variables associated with PSG acquisition systems.
9. Describe the sensor options available for each common PSG physiologic parameter.

KEY TERMS

Ancillary equipment
Data acquisition
Data analysis
Data archive
LAN
Control room
Analog
Digital
Ethernet
Screen resolution
USB
Image resolution
PSG time synch
Omnidirectional
Unidirectional

THE SLEEP CENTER PHYSICAL PLANT

The primary components of a sleep center facility consist of designated areas intended to separate patients from each other, separate patients from employee areas, and allow for designated activities to take place, such as patient setup, equipment cleaning and storage, continuous positive airway pressure (CPAP) patient education and data download, and polysomnographic (PSG) data acquisition, analysis, and review (Fig. 67-1).

Current Trends in Sleep Center Construction

As awareness of sleep disorders, obstructive sleep apnea in particular, continues to grow within the medical community, an increasing number of sleep centers are being established. This great demand for testing has resulted in sleep centers being established outside of the conventional hospital setting. Facilities such as professional/medical office buildings, bed and breakfast inns, hotels, and even condominiums have been converted for use as sleep disorder testing facilities. This departure from the conventional hospital setting does not always allow the inclusion of all the previously described primary components of a conventional full-service sleep disorders facility.

The use of computer networking within sleep testing facilities allows increased efficiency for analysis and interpretation tasks utilizing remote connectivity. PSG data files can be moved between computers, and scoring as well as interpretation tasks can be performed outside of the sleep center. Network cabling must be installed within the facilities between patient rooms and control rooms, and servers must be stored and powered. Wireless network communications can considerably reduce the network cabling requirements within a sleep center facility, but attention must be given to data encryption and security.

As the number of sleep testing beds increases within a particular community, competition among facilities can often become an ongoing operational factor. Facility design considerations, particularly features intended to increase patient comfort, can become a pivotal marketing point within advertising strategies and can

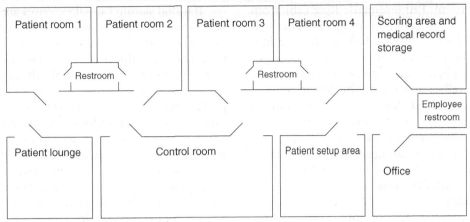

Figure 67-1 Efficient, cost-effective layout for a first-stage sleep center facility. Two of these four rooms could be eliminated from the design, thereby reducing costs even further.

significantly impact a center's testing volumes, as well as the facility's reputation within the local community.

General Location Considerations

The first step in converting existing space into a functional sleep center is to determine the benefits of using existing space as against renovating the space. Within a hospital setting, the most common "first-stage" design for a sleep testing area involves three adjacent standard hospital rooms. The two outside rooms are furnished with a variety of home furnishings intended to reduce the sterile hospital environment, such as a TV, bedside stand, and perhaps a recliner and wall art. The room in the middle of the two outside patient rooms serves as the control area. This area houses the diagnostic equipment for the two beds, and provides storage for supplies, a desk for the technologists, filing cabinets, and chart storage. This scenario is a very efficient and quick way to establish a sleep testing program with very little, if any, facility renovation. However, only two patients can be monitored per night, and the many other primary components described, which could enhance patient satisfaction and testing quality, cannot be utilized in this scenario because of space limitations.

Environmental noise is a very important factor to consider when choosing an area to establish a sleep center facility. Noise can play a major role in prolonging sleep latency and disrupting the patient's sleep during a PSG. When identifying a space within the community for a freestanding facility, one should consider the proximity of the facility to highways and freeways, which produce significant noise. Proximity to an airport should also be considered. When identifying space within an existing facility such as a hospital, environmental noise should also be considered. Common sources of undesirable noise within a hospital facility include the following:

- Emergency room areas
- Helicopter landing areas
- Psychiatric ward
- Heating and cooling room
- Outside trash dumpsters

Occasionally, during a sleep study, oxygen may need to be administered to the patient. Within a hospital setting, oxygen, as well as room air and suction, is typically supplied to each patient room throughout the facility through a complex system of piped medical gases. If a center is to be established within an existing hospital facility, it is likely that existing medical gases can be delivered to patient rooms within a sleep center and accessed through wall-mounted regulators. However, in a non-hospital facility, consideration should be given to the method of providing supplemental oxygen to patients. If renovating the facility for piped gases is determined to be cost prohibitive, oxygen can be delivered to most patients through the use of an oxygen concentrator. When an oxygen concentrator is utilized, backup oxygen tanks should be available in the sleep center in case of a power failure. It is important to be aware that the maximum liter flow of an oxygen concentrator is typically lower than that available from a piped gas flow regulator system. In addition, portable suction devices may be used outside of a conventional hospital setting.

The issue of cabling is certainly a very important consideration when designing a sleep center space. Cabling is required to transfer the physiologic PSG signals from the patient room to the control room. Some sleep testing–related hardware items have maximum cable length specifications that need to be considered. Clinical CPAP systems that incorporate a flow generator unit in the patient room and a remote pressure control in the control room will require cabling between the two locations. Intercom systems and closed circuit video/audio systems may also require cabling between the patient and the control room. Extraordinarily long cables can occasionally result in a reduction of signal strength, as well as the introduction of electrical interference into the signal. Common sources of electrical interference include fluorescent light fixtures and elevator areas. The type of cable, as well as maximum cable length requirements for the mentioned devices, may differ among manufacturers. Advances in technology allow many computer-based monitoring instruments in a sleep center facility to communicate using a wireless networking method, thereby eliminating the need for physical cabling. This may be advantageous and cost-effective for some facility designs.

When evaluating existing space for a sleep center, future expansion potential should be considered as well. In light of the prevalence of sleep disorders, sleep apnea in particular, once a sleep center has been established and is operational, the number of patients referred for testing will usually increase to the point of a scheduling backlog. In established sleep center facilities, expansion of the number of testing beds will be the only option to reduce the scheduling backlog. Therefore, the presence of nearby space that could be renovated in the future for patient room expansion will definitely be advantageous. Also, additional space within the control room to house additional diagnostic equipment should be considered.

Consideration for handicapped and disabled patients should be made when identifying areas within a sleep center facility that will be used by patients. This includes reasonable accommodations for wheelchair access within the patient rooms, hallways, and doorways, support bars within restroom and shower facilities, and patient beds equipped for raising and lowering the head and foot sections.

Many cities and towns require facilities to be built in a manner that allows for fast evacuation of people in case of fire and incorporates specific building materials that are either fire retardant or capable of slowing the spread of fire, such as a door. When establishing a sleep center within an existing space, local fire codes should be reviewed to ensure that the space meets the specific code requirements, such as location of fire sprinklers. Building codes will specify the requirements for lighted exit signs and backup lighting necessary in case of a power failure or an emergency.

As a sleep center is typically open for operations 24 hours a day, security for patients as well as the staff is important, especially in freestanding facilities. Security personnel employed within a hospital facility will usually address these issues for hospital-based sleep centers. In the case of freestanding facilities, issues including door locks, security systems, intercoms, and a communication protocol with law enforcement must be considered.

If initial startup capital expenses are of concern, utilizing existing space within a facility is certainly the least expensive route. However, if absolutely no facility renovation can be performed, many of the described primary components of a conventional full-service sleep center will, in most cases, need to be sacrificed. This may impact a program's ability to meet the standards defined by various sleep center certification or accreditation entities. Some programs that exist today choose to "specialize" in diagnosing and treating only a portion of the many sleep disorders that have been identified to date, such as sleep apnea and periodic movements of sleep. This scenario not only may reduce costs as well as reliance on some of the primary sleep center facility components but may also reduce the number of patients a sleep center can accept for testing. Utilizing existing space and performing a moderate amount of facility renovation to meet instrumentation and environmental requirements and to allow for the inclusion of primary sleep center facility components will result in the most cost-efficient startup scenario, and will allow the program to meet all of the patient's diagnostic and treatment needs. Building an entirely new facility is, of course, the most expensive scenario but allows the facility to be built in a manner that meets all possible facility and patient population needs and considerations, as well as allowing for the incorporation of unique facility features that can be marketed to the community.

Functional Considerations and Descriptions of Sleep Center Facility Components

Patient Room

The patient room is one of the most important components of the sleep center. Its design and construction can affect not only the quality of data acquired during a PSG procedure but also the facility's reputation within a community. Design considerations should be made to facilitate not only the night testing procedures but daytime testing procedures as well. In addition, patients will most likely occupy the room for periods of time when no testing is being performed, and ensuring patient satisfaction within a room during this time is just as important as during testing periods. Facility design should include analysis of the type of patients evaluated at the sleep center.

As a general rule, there is no minimum size requirement for a patient room, although 140 ft^2 is often recommended. The preeminent issues relating to room size include the ability of a medical emergency team to have easy access to the patient from either side of the bed and the ability of the patient to move safely in the space available. The American Academy of Sleep Medicine

(AASM) accreditation standards require that the room be of sufficient size to accommodate emergency personnel access with a minimum of 24 in (60.96 cm) of available clear space on three sides of the bed (1). Consider the need for a code cart, often referred to as a "crash cart," that is readily accessible to health care workers and strategically placed in a hospital sleep center.

An important goal in designing a patient room is to eliminate a sterile, hospital-based atmosphere and have the room look and feel like either a hotel or a home bedroom. One of the most effective ways to accomplish this is through the selection of bedroom furnishings. A patient room should include a bed, preferably a full-size bed that has an adjustable head and foot section (Fig. 67-2A). A headboard and footboard made of finished wood is also effective in providing a home-like feel. In addition, in the interest of minimizing patient injury, the bed should have side rails that can be used for patient safety during testing conducted for parasomnia disorders or abnormal behaviors during sleep.

Bedside stands are an important furniture component of the patient room. Aside from selecting a more home-style designed stand, the stands should have enough room to store any diagnostic or treatment devices required during testing such as a CPAP flow generator. Some bedside stands incorporate a small drawer that can be very useful for storing commonly used disposable supplies in the room for easy access by the technologist during the night. Other common items placed on a bedside table include a telephone, reading lamp, and tissues. If space permits, it can be useful to incorporate a bedside stand on each side of the bed to accommodate all of the possible items commonly placed on a bedside stand (Fig. 67-2B).

Seating for the patient and guests should be available in each patient room. Some obese patients and visitors may be hesitant to sit on a chair that they perceive may collapse beneath them. Furniture may need to be able to withstand weight of 500 lb (227.27 kg) to 800 lb (363.64 kg). Because the patient will be seated in the chair during hookup, the design of the chair should allow the technologist ease in applying the sensors and electrodes. When selecting patient seating, consider the patient's comfort and dignity.

It is certainly desirable to have windows in a patient room. If a patient is undergoing a multiple sleep latency test (MSLT) during the day, it is often useful to allow daylight into the room between nap trials to aid the patient in staying awake. However, windows can be a problem during daytime testing, because it can be difficult to totally eliminate the daylight from the room during MSLT nap trials. A type of blind often referred to as a blackout blind should be considered for better control of daylight within the patient room. This blind incorporates tracks on the bottom and sides of the window, thereby blocking out all light coming in through the window. It can be useful during the night as well, because it will block moonlight or street lights in the same manner.

It will be important for the patient to have a closet or armoire available in the room to store and hang daytime clothing. In addition, this space can be used to store extra blankets or pillows that the patient may request during an all-night test.

Other optional furnishings to consider that add to the home-style setting include wall art, waste receptacles, and remote-controlled televisions. If you choose to allow patients to watch television, pay special attention to designing the sleep center patient room with acoustic/sound attenuation in mind. One of the easiest things that can be done in this regard is to construct each wall of a patient room to extend up to, and connect with, the ceiling. This method greatly reduces the amount of noise that can travel above typical hanging or suspended ceiling tiles. Placing insulation in the ceiling can provide some noise reduction. Some of the

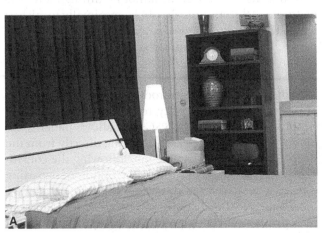

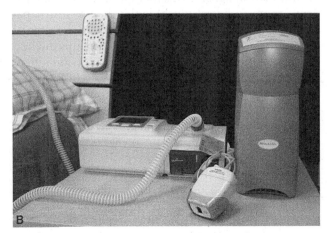

Figure 67-2 **A:** Patient bedroom. **B:** Two bedside stands provide room for the positive airway pressure device and acquisition system amplifier and also a lamp.

more expensive commercially available ceiling tiles have sound attenuation ratings. Disregarding this construction consideration can lead to noise from one patient room disturbing another patient, or even control room noise traveling to patient rooms. Floor carpeting is certainly advantageous in reducing environmental noise, as is the use of inner wall insulation. A thick fire door for the patient room entrance can also reduce noise.

A number of electrical lighting options should be considered for the patient room. Certainly, a general ceiling-mounted light, which illuminates the entire room, should be in place and controlled at the room entrance. A reading lamp located on a bedside stand can also be used. However, many existing sleep centers shy away from allowing patients the opportunity to control any aspect of the environment such as light, as they may inadvertently disrupt testing procedures by turning the lights on and off during the test. Some patients are not able to tolerate total darkness. In such cases, a small night-light plugged into a wall receptacle can be useful. Also, connecting the general ceiling-mounted light to a dimmer control will allow a very small amount of light to illuminate the room for certain patient needs. Incandescent black light illumination is an additional lighting option that can significantly enhance coexisting infrared illumination for video recording. A light fixture with a blacklight bulb, installed somewhere near the patient and connected to a dimmer control, will work quite well to accomplish this method of increasing video display quality.

One of the most important facility considerations related to a patient room is temperature control. A patient's comfort relative to room temperature can, in many cases, make or break the ability to perform a quality sleep study. In order to most effectively control this aspect of the testing environment, individual thermostat controls assigned to each patient room are the most advantageous. This method will allow one patient's room to be set much cooler than a nearby patient's room, thereby allowing both patients a degree of comfort to facilitate a quality test. However, this method can be rather expensive. In cases where individual temperature controls are not an option, every effort should be made to assign the fewest patient rooms to each thermostat control. More than three patient rooms assigned to one temperature control will most certainly result in conflicting patient temperature preferences from time to time, resulting in one or more patients experiencing disrupted, poor-quality sleep during the test. Consideration should also be given to the placement of the thermostat control. If possible, mounting a control outside of a patient room is most desirable. Otherwise, a technologist may be required to enter the room of one patient to adjust the temperature of a different patient's room, potentially disrupting the sleep of both patients. Making sure that any ceiling or wall-mounted vent used for heating or cooling is not near, or directed specifically toward, the patient can minimize the impact of room temperature on the patients.

Alternatively, placement of fans in the patient rooms allows a degree of flexibility in cooling the room when individual controls are not an option. Many patients sleep at home with a fan, and one should be available on request.

The technologist should also be cognizant of technical considerations for the integrity of the PSG such as sweat artifact caused by overly warm room temperatures and carefully monitor the room temperature. In addition, thought should be given to maintaining an adequate supply of blankets to accommodate the needs of individual patients when individual thermostat controls are not available.

Restrooms

Restrooms for patients and staff are an obvious necessity in a sleep center facility. The most desirable and comfortable design for patients and staff allows for multiple restrooms designated for both patients and staff. This design eliminates the potential scenario of a patient interrupting a PSG procedure to use the restroom, but not being able to do so because the restroom is being occupied by a staff member, thereby increasing the duration of the test interruption. The AASM accreditation standards require that the sleep facility has clean bathrooms with a minimum ratio of one bathroom for every three testing rooms; these bathrooms must each contain a toilet and a sink. Toilet fixtures can be floor mounted or wall mounted. A floor-mounted toilet can support up to 800 lb (363.64 kg) and toilet-to-floor supports can be added as required. Patients often lean on a sink, and floor-mounting the sink helps distribute weight. Each bathroom must have a working privacy door. Sole access to a shared bathroom cannot be through a testing bedroom. All restrooms should be minimally furnished with a toilet, sink, hand soap dispenser, paper towel dispenser, wall-mounted mirror, ceiling light, ceiling vent, and an electrical outlet (1).

An ideal sleep center design relative to restroom facilities allows for a private restroom for each patient room. This provides patient privacy, reduces the duration of restroom breaks during the PSG, and allows patients the option of preparing for and departing directly from the sleep center to their daytime job, following the conclusion of the test in the morning. The option of departing directly to work is certainly desirable and convenient for most patients who are tested during weeknights and can be a pivotal marketing point for a sleep center located within a town or city that offers competing sleep center facilities. A fully functional private patient restroom should be designed for access from within the patient room and should include shower facilities.

The presence of shower facilities will introduce patient expectations for personal items such as soap, shampoo, and appropriate towels and linen to be provided, as would commonly be found in a hotel. The presence of shower facilities will also demand increased housekeeping/environmental services involvement, which may increase a facility's operating expenses.

In situations where private restrooms are not possible, a common solution is to incorporate a shared patient restroom design. This can be advantageous from a facility design perspective but may result in patient dissatisfaction. The single shared patient restroom not only limits a patient's morning personal hygiene options, but during the night, there may be patients who leave the restroom soiled or in an undesirable condition for the next patient. This scenario may require staff members to clean the restroom, which can result in staff dissatisfaction and interrupt the PSG procedure.

Private patient restrooms can be constructed without shower facilities for cases in which construction cost restraints are an issue. A single shower area can then be shared by patients, which will most likely be better tolerated relative to patient satisfaction.

If the sleep center facility will include a patient reception or waiting area used during the day to process physician office or clinic appointments, consideration should be given to the facility's proximity to the nearest public restroom, as waiting patients or family members will most likely require this. Construction of a public restroom may be required if a nearby access does not exist.

Reasonable accommodations for disabled persons should be made in all patient, public, and staff restrooms. This would include adequate space for patients using wheelchairs and walkers to access and utilize the area, wall-mounted support bars near the toilet and within the shower area, optional sitting stool for use within the shower area, and a mechanism for patients to activate a call for assistance such as a wall-mounted help button or pull chain. The AASM accreditation standards require that at least one testing bedroom and bathroom be handicap accessible as defined either by local building regulations or by sections 6.3 and 6.4 of the Americans with Disabilities Act (1).

Control Room

A control room must be large enough to comfortably house working space for the PSG technologist staff and required equipment. The control room is the hub of activity within the sleep center, and technologists spend most of their work time within this area. Therefore, it is important to design the control area to be as comfortable as possible for the technical staff, with consideration for the amount of general traffic projected for the area, equipment placement, and individual staff member workstations and related furniture. The AASM accreditation standards require that the dimensions of the control room be not less than 40 ft^2 in total or 20 ft^2 per testing bedroom, whichever is larger (1).

Ideally, the control room should be centrally located a relatively short distance away from patient rooms. As patients will commonly call for assistance from technologists during a sleep study, a short distance between the control room and the patient room will reduce the amount of time it takes for the technologist to enter the patient room in response to the call. This is also an important consideration with regard to technologist reaction time in emergencies such as cardiac arrhythmias or seizure events. In addition, some of the monitoring devices used during a PSG that incorporate connected components in both the control area and the patient room specify maximum cabling lengths that are important for proper equipment operation. These specifications may impact the distance requirements between the control room and the patient rooms as well.

Despite the described importance of maintaining a relatively short distance between the patient rooms and the control room, it is important to maintain strict boundaries between employee areas and patient areas. Patient privacy and confidentiality should be considered when designing the control room. Patients should at no time be allowed to physically enter, or visually observe, the control room. Video monitors should be placed in a manner and location where they cannot be visually observed from patient areas. Patients should not see documents containing another patient's information within the control room. Patients should neither hear telephone conversations within the control room relating to other patients nor be able to hear audio sounds that originate from a patient room. Succeeding in maintaining patient privacy and confidentiality within the control room may result in unique construction or facility renovation requirements (Fig. 67-3).

Once the area of the control room that will house the monitoring equipment has been identified, adequate access to electricity will need to be established in that area. Multiple wall outlets will most likely be required in order to furnish sufficient power to all of the varying monitoring instruments. An ideal wiring design allows for multiple instruments assigned to a particular patient room to be powered by outlets, utilizing a separate independent ground. By providing separate grounds for each patient room, the potential for electrical interference originating in one patient room to travel to the next patient room is significantly reduced. In facilities where emergency auxiliary power is available, such as in a hospital, connecting the primary PSG unit or computer processing unit to an outlet with automatic auxiliary power switching can be advantageous during periods of

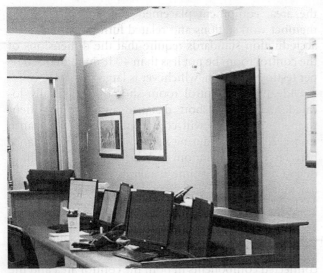

Figure 67-3 Technologist control room for 4-bed acquisition.

power outages in order to minimize the amount of data lost during a power failure. If facility furnished emergency auxiliary power is not available, the use of an uninterrupted battery power supply with surge protection is recommended for the previously mentioned units. If intermittent power outages are common in the facility, then an uninterrupted battery power supply with surge protection is recommended regardless of the presence of emergency auxiliary power.

Cabling is an important consideration in designing the control room area. Many of the monitoring devices housed within the control room are interfaced through cabling to components housed in the patient room. In addition, sleep center entrance security video signals and audio intercom signals may also require a cabled connection to related devices in the control room. The control room design should allow for a designated space, chute, or conduit intended to introduce these multiple cables from above the ceiling, inside the wall, and into the control room near the floor. This design allows for quick access to all incoming and outgoing cables; can improve troubleshooting efficiency; and makes it easier for outside contractors to locate, add, or remove cables. However, it is important to note that when placing multiple cables next to each other such as described, electrical interference originating from within a cable can transmit to other cables. This can be a problem for some instruments that are prone to receiving extraneous AC electrical interference such as a PSG system. In this scenario, using shielded cables can reduce the transmission of this interference. In the case of PSG systems specifically, the use of network or serial cabling is recommended, because it is much less prone to receiving extraneous interference. Network or serial cabling is commonly used with PSG systems.

Lighting preferences within a control area may vary depending on the time of day or the type of job task being performed. Common fluorescent ceiling units can be used in a control room to illuminate the work area. It can be advantageous to wire segments of the ceiling units within the control area to different on/off switches. This gives staff members the ability to alter the amount of illumination in a particular area of the control room. Higher amounts of work area illumination are usually preferred when staff are performing job tasks such as daytime PSG scoring and analysis, and reading or writing patient chart information. When performing PSG procedures during the night, many technologists prefer a lower or softer degree of illumination within the control area. Conversely, in the interest of reinforcing and maintaining the sleep–wake cycle of nightshift technologists, high-intensity fluorescent lights can be used in a control room during the nighttime hours to simulate sunlight. Some research shows this can be of benefit to the nightshift staff, as it can increase employees' total sleep time as well as the quality of sleep during the daytime hours.

Patient Setup Area

An area specifically used for patient setup procedures can be advantageous for the patients as well as the staff. It allows for all of the required sensors and application chemicals to be stored and easily accessed during the setup procedure, saving time for the technologist performing the procedure. Many of the chemicals used to apply electrodes and sensors to patients have strong odors. Maintaining a specific setup area when these chemicals are in use will keep the odors away from patient rooms, thereby avoiding the potential for patient irritation and disruption of a PSG test. Also, it can be advantageous to remove electrodes and sensors the morning following a test within the patient setup area. The sensors can be more easily cleaned and returned to their respective storage area, ready to be used for the next patient.

The size requirements of the room will vary depending on the amount and size of furnishings used and the number of patients being set up simultaneously. A common list of furnishings for a single-patient setup area consists of a chair, a cart with drawers to store disposable supplies, a standard sink used for cleaning sensors, hooks to hang and store sensors and electrodes, a flammable storage container for collodion and acetone if used, and a waste receptacle. A television for the patient to watch during the setup procedure or a radio in this area can often be useful. A reasonable single-patient setup area would require to be at least 6 × 8 ft. Areas used for multiple simultaneous setup procedures will need to be designed and constructed in a much larger space.

Patient setup areas should be constructed and placed within a sleep center facility with patient privacy in mind. Patients or visitors should not be able to view other patients being set up for a PSG, especially as the procedure will commonly require the patient to remove specific parts of clothing. If more than one patient will be set up simultaneously within the area, care should be taken to partition the individual areas to maintain patient privacy.

An extremely important design consideration is a ventilation system. Strong odors resulting from the use of collodion or acetone are common during procedures. A patient setup area ventilation system that will actively remove odors should be located in the ceiling. Ideally, the air should be entirely removed from the area and transferred to the outside of the building, as opposed to filtered and recycled within the area. A variety of ventilation systems are commercially available. The size of the setup area will dictate how many individual ventilation intakes will be required. Issues such as general noise level, electrical power requirements, filtering options, and cleaning requirements should be reviewed before purchasing a system.

As both the patient setup procedure and the sensor removal procedure result in numerous waste items, it is important to provide adequate waste receptacles. The area should facilitate adherence to conventional policies and procedures relating to proper labeling and disposal of contaminated waste. A "sharps" disposal system should be in place for the disposal of blunt tip needles and other sharp objects. Arrangements should be made for the routine removal of waste from the setup area on a daily basis.

Patients who are studied for a variety of neurologic disorders will occasionally display symptoms or behaviors such as seizures or cataplexy. Unfortunately, these events can occasionally occur before the start of the recording phase of a PSG test, often during the setup procedure. Activating a video camera within the patient setup area can be useful for at least capturing the event on video, despite the lack of PSG data. In addition, it is becoming increasingly common for sleep centers to video-record all tech–patient interactions. Some patients may choose to take legal action against a particular sleep facility or sleep technologist, claiming inappropriate contact or communication. Placing a video camera in the setup area and recording the procedure provides video documentation that could become critical evidence in defending one's actions with a patient if brought to litigation.

Scoring/Record Review Room

There can be advantages to creating a room with the sole purpose of conducting PSG scoring and interpretation activities. Although scoring can usually be performed in most control rooms on the computer where the data were acquired, the level of control room traffic and noise during the day, daytime testing activities, and general clerical activities can be a distraction to those scoring and interpreting the data in the control room.

In order to review digital PSG recordings within a scoring/record review room, computer workstations often referred to as review stations are required. PSG data are transferred from the acquisition computer in the control room to the review station or to a central server for scoring and interpretation. Data are usually transferred through a local area network (LAN). The sleep center LAN allows PSG data files located on any computer within the network to be accessed, viewed, and scored on a review station. Special consideration for a network-cabling pathway should be included in the construction design of the scoring/record review room for LAN connectivity.

A scoring/record review room can serve quite well for a PSG archive storage area as well. PSG files can be managed and moved through a LAN, allowing files to be archived to a variety of digital storage devices and stored within the room. This allows for convenient access to past archived PSG files for review as needed.

Other optional uses for a scoring/record review room include conducting PSG scoring education and training, physician dictation stations, Internet research activities, and patient database management.

Patient Lounge

A patient lounge area can be used for a variety of patient needs during the night, as well as daytime operations. A common recommended method for dealing with patients who experience insomnia during an all-night PSG is to have the patient leave the room for a period. A patient lounge provides a comfortable change of environment for these patients away from their room. The room can contain features such as comfortable chairs and sofas, a central telephone access for patients, a television, and small food/snack items. If a television or telephone access will be used, consideration for telephone wiring and television cabling should be included in the facility design.

Often, parents of younger patients, or personal care attendants of disabled patients who are required to accompany the patient while they are being tested in the sleep center, may utilize this area to nap during the night while the patient is undergoing testing.

Depending on the location of the patient lounge within the sleep center facility, the area can also serve as a reception area during daytime operations. For this functionality, the area should ideally be located at the point of entrance into the sleep center, and clerical/reception staff should be present within or adjacent to the area.

Utility Room

An area designated for equipment repair and maintenance can be beneficial in a sleep center facility. It provides a location for broken sensors and electrodes to be placed for subsequent repair. Diagnostic/repair instruments such as a volt ohm meter and replacement batteries can be utilized and stored within the area as well.

Cleaning and cold sterilization can also take place in this area. Reusable items such as electroencephalogram (EEG) electrodes and humidifier canisters can be soaked in this area during cold sterilization procedures.

Facility construction considerations for this area specifically relating to the building and repair of electrical sensors and sterilization procedures would include a counter with electrical wall outlets, a deep sink for cold sterilization, adequate lighting, and ceiling ventilation.

Office Space

It is useful to have office space designated for management personnel. Confidential employee meetings and interviews can take place in this area, as well as storage of confidential employee files, policy and procedures documents, and equipment purchase records. The construction considerations for this area should be similar to those of most conventional offices, including telephone and LAN access; electrical wall outlets; and sufficient space for a desk, chairs, and file storage. A locked door is required to ensure the security of confidential documents.

Of all the primary components of a sleep center facility mentioned earlier, the absolute minimum functional requirements are a control and patient room. Many sleep programs begin very small until a reliable referral base has been established. The three adjacent standard hospital rooms design mentioned earlier in this chapter is a common first-stage scenario implemented within an existing hospital facility. However, with first-stage freestanding facilities, more facility design options will often be available at reasonably low cost.

An additional method of reducing construction costs when establishing or expanding a sleep center facility is to utilize wireless connections between the control room and the patient room, which is available with some digital PSG systems. Labor costs associated with running conventional cables; the cost of the cables themselves; and later labor costs associated with repairing, removing, or adding cables can be eliminated by using wireless technology.

PSG EQUIPMENT

The task of evaluating and replacing diagnostic equipment in a sleep lab is essential not only to ensure a sleep center's diagnostic capabilities when establishing operations but also to maintain and expand a center's diagnostic capabilities and efficiencies as the patient population varies over time. Certainly, the PSG system is the most significant equipment item to evaluate, because it can dictate a center's diagnostic capabilities, and the cost of the system can significantly impact a center's financial condition. However, limitations and/or unique operational requirements of other instrumentation items commonly used in a sleep center can also impact a center's ability to meet the dynamic diagnostic demands of a full-service sleep center. In general, commercially available PSG systems should incorporate the following features as recommended by the AASM (1):

- A toggle switch permitting visual (on-screen) standard negative 50 μV DC calibration signal for all channels to demonstrate polarity, amplitude, and time constant settings for each recorded parameter
- A separate 50/60 Hz filter control for each channel
- The capability of selecting sampling rates for each channel
- A method of measuring actual individual electrode impedance against a reference (the latter may be the sum of all other applied electrodes)
- The capability of retaining and viewing the data in the exact manner in which it was recorded by the attending technologist (i.e., retain and display all derivation changes, sensitivity adjustments, filter settings, temporal resolution)
- A filter design for data collection, which functionally simulates or replicates conventional (analog-style) frequency response curves rather than removing all activity and harmonics within the specified bandwidth

Understanding the general categories of instrumentation in the sleep lab, as well as the primary options and variables associated with PSG systems and ancillary equipment, will be extremely beneficial when evaluating and replacing PSG-related equipment.

PSG Instrumentation
Data Acquisition Hardware

Until the mid-to-late 1990s, conventional PSG acquisition hardware consisted of racks of analog physiologic amplifiers, paper chart drives, and mechanical ink pen systems. More current digital PSG acquisition systems incorporate computer-based hardware, typically consisting of a desktop configuration computer, miniaturized amplifiers with analog-to-digital conversion circuits, and an electrode/sensor signal input box.

When evaluating the hardware components of a PSG system, the number of channels available for physiologic recording is an important consideration. In order to meet all of the diagnostic needs of a full-service sleep center, the number of channels available should meet the channel capacity requirements of the more simple procedures such as an MSLT, to the more extensive procedures such as those required for diagnosing parasomnias that include an extended EEG montage and multiple extremity electromyographic (EMG) channels. Depending on the usage frequency and amount of ancillary equipment used in the center, the number of analog DC input channels available for interfacing ancillary devices is also an important consideration. As a general rule, a PSG system with a channel capacity that exceeds the number of channels used during routine procedures is not only of potential benefit for the expanded recording requirements mentioned earlier, but also allows for channel redundancy, which can help deal with amplifier failure during a recording.

The distance between the control room and the patient room is an important consideration in an evaluation of PSG hardware. Some PSG systems have maximum cable length specifications between the patient sensors and the amplifiers. This particular portion of the signal path is most prone to receiving extraneous electrical interference. In addition, the increased resistance encountered by a signal traveling through a long cable can degrade the signal. A common way of dealing with long distances is to house the amplifiers within the patient room, thereby allowing a short cable between the patient and the amplifiers. The amplified output signal can then be conducted to the control room, because this particular signal is much more suitable for traveling through longer cable.

PSG systems incorporate a sensor input box with input jacks designed to receive a wide variety of sensors, including EEG electrodes, airflow monitoring devices, and respiratory effort sensors. Many PSG system manufacturers also manufacture sensors that are designed with unique jacks that will only fit into their system's sensor input box. A wide variety of sensors are manufactured by companies specializing exclusively in sensors. Although sensor manufacturers commonly provide sensors with a variety of optional jacks designed to interface with a variety of sensor input boxes, compatibility with every system may not always be possible. In addition, the signal strength produced by some third-party sensors may not be compatible with some PSG system amplifiers. Therefore, if there are specific sensor preferences within a center, or if unique sensors are used in a center such as in a research protocol, consideration of these compatibility issues is important when evaluating amplifier and sensor input box hardware.

When performing a PSG, it is often necessary to interface signals provided by ancillary equipment to the PSG system for simultaneous display with physiologic data and to analyze and report the data. These ancillary devices include oximeters, CPAP units, and CO_2 monitors. The typical output signals provided by these devices are analog in nature and range from 1 to 10 V DC. When evaluating and selecting PSG hardware, consideration should be given to the number of DC inputs available and the range of acceptable voltage allowed to ensure compatibility with a center's specific ancillary equipment.

PSG systems allow sleep centers the ability to store and archive PSG data very efficiently. The PSG data acquisition procedure results in a number of digital computer files ranging in total size from 50 to 150 MB per recording, depending on the number of channels being recorded and the varying sampling rates used for each parameter. The AASM accreditation standards specify minimum sampling rates of 1 to 200 Hz, depending on the type of data being recorded (1, 2).

The ability to share and move data between computers within a sleep center can be very advantageous. Technologists or physicians may wish to review data in an area separate from the control room, or simply on a different computer than what was used during the acquisition. This can be accomplished through a LAN. Almost any computer can be networked, but certain hardware is required. The most significant hardware requirement for networking is an Ethernet port. This port or jack provides the computer with the ability to receive a special cable that interconnects the computers within the network. Digital communication technology also allows the option of wireless (WiFi) networking. This method incorporates a hub that receives and transmits wireless data between computers. If networking of hardware is desired in a sleep center, the computer hardware being evaluated should either include an Ethernet port or have integrated WiFi capabilities.

Data Analysis Software

Once physiologic data have been acquired and digitized, software is required to view and manipulate the data. Most data analysis software programs are proprietary and are included as a component of a PSG system. The analysis program provides users with the ability to view, score, and generate reports that communicate analysis values and results.

Although there are a number of stand-alone PSG data analysis programs available, the majority of PSG systems include a proprietary data analysis program. Data acquired using a particular PSG system's acquisition program are commonly formatted in a manner that allows only that PSG system's analysis program to read and interact with the data. As these analysis programs are proprietary, the functionality may vary. According to the AASM standards (1, 2), when evaluating PSG data analysis programs, the following common functions should be included at a minimum:

- Ability to provide a digital screen resolution of at least 1,600 × 1,200 for display and scoring of raw PSG data
- Ability to display a histogram with stage, respiratory events, leg movement events, O_2 saturation and arousals, with cursor positioning on histogram and ability to jump to the page
- Ability to view a screen on a time scale ranging from the entire night to windows as small as 5 seconds
- Recorded video data synchronized with PSG data with an accuracy of at least one video frame per second.

The ability to set a variety of filter settings, background colors, and other features specific to a particular parameter can be accomplished through the use of user-defined display templates. Once all of the display and filtering options available for each parameter have been set to a user's preference, the user can save the settings as a template. Then as the user accesses different patient data in the future, rather than having to repeatedly adjust the display and filtering options for each individual parameter, the user can simply apply his or her template to the recording. This is clearly a time-saving tool for technologists and physicians and should be considered when evaluating analysis software.

A very significant function that analysis software provides is the generation of the PSG analysis report. Most sleep centers will require the ability to configure this report according to the preferences of either their medical staff or their referring physicians. Configurable features within a report will typically include the following:

- Report layouts and templates
- Analysis values
- Graphic summaries
- Color or B/W graphs
- Ability for consolidated split-night reporting
- MSLT reporting
- Configurable analysis start and end times

The PSG analysis report represents the sleep center's entire PSG product and communicates the test results to the sleep center's customers, whether that is the patient or referring physician. From a marketing perspective, the PSG analysis report is the most visible and effective marketing tool a center has, and is certainly critical to its image and customer satisfaction. Therefore, the configurability of presentation options, and the number and categories of available reporting values calculated, is an important consideration when evaluating PSG analysis software.

Ancillary Equipment

There are a variety of optional instruments sometimes not included in a PSG system that require interfacing with the PSG system. Some of the more commonly used devices include pulse oximeters, end-tidal or transcutaneous CO_2 monitors, and clinical CPAP systems.

When evaluating a patient to rule out sleep apnea, the pulse oximeter is a critical tool used to determine the severity of sleep-disordered breathing. Many PSG systems are manufactured with oximetry technology built into the hardware, thereby eliminating the requirement for a stand-alone oximeter device to be interfaced with the PSG system. In addition, some sleep centers prefer the ability to incorporate pulse rate data provided by an oximeter into the PSG data. If this signal is not available from oximetry circuitry, which is built into a PSG system, then a stand-alone unit will need to be interfaced to the PSG system as described. If it is determined that a stand-alone oximetry unit will be required, the unit should have user-configurable alarm limits, because alarms can disrupt patient sleep.

Monitoring a patient's CO_2 levels is often required during PSG procedures. The most noninvasive method of accomplishing this is through the use of an end-tidal CO_2 monitor or a transcutaneous CO_2 monitor. Many of these devices provide printouts or allow recorded, stored data to be downloaded to a printer to display trend data. As with oximetry or pulse rate data, it is important to incorporate real-time CO_2 information into the PSG tracing. The CO_2 monitoring device should provide a DC analog output that can be interfaced with the PSG system hardware. In addition, alarms should be configurable to adjust limits and avoid awakening patients during testing.

To titrate nasal CPAP during a PSG procedure without disrupting the patient by entering the room to change pressures, a CPAP unit that incorporates a remote pressure control is required. Most CPAP manufacturers provide clinical CPAP units that are designed to be used in a sleep center setting and to provide a variety of unique functions, including a remote pressure control. Remote pressure controls are typically connected to the CPAP flow generator unit via a cable, or the controls are software based and installed on the PSG computer. Consideration should be given to the manufacturer's maximum cable length specification and the distance between the patient room and the control area.

Clinical CPAP units commonly allow for a variety of positive airway pressure modes. These modes often consist of standard CPAP, autoadjust, spontaneous bilevel positive airway pressure, bilevel positive airway pressure with backup rate, and auto-servo ventilation. An evaluation of clinical CPAP systems should include a review of the positive airway pressure modes available and the type of pressure mode requirements the center's patients and physician staff require.

Many clinical CPAP systems also provide a variety of analog output signals intended to be interfaced into the PSG system. These signals are usually DC in nature and commonly include flow, machine pressure, mask leak, estimated tidal volume, and nasal pressure–based airflow. The location of these signal outputs may vary between designs, and the signal outputs are usually incorporated into either the flow generator unit or the remote control unit. These signals are typically interfaced to the PSG system through a cable that plugs into the system's DC input hardware. Consideration should be given to the location of a particular clinical CPAP system's output ports and the location of the PSG system's DC input hardware. If output ports are to be located in the patient room, such as those that are incorporated into a flow generator, then the PSG system's DC input hardware must also be located in the patient room. Conversely, if the output ports are located in the control room, as those that are incorporated into the remote pressure control, then the PSG system's DC input hardware must also be located in the control room.

Most clinical CPAP systems incorporate an internal pressure transducer designed to measure intramask pressure changes, detect mask leaks, and provide pressure data for auto-adjusting algorithms. The manufacturer typically calibrates the pressure transducer component of a clinical CPAP unit during production of the unit. The calibration process will usually incorporate the use of a specific nasal mask, most likely a mask produced by the same manufacturer. Given the wide variety of mask designs available, many aspects of the varying designs, particularly the degree of leak allowed for a CO_2 exhaust port, may conflict with a clinical PSG manufacturer's pressure transducer calibration settings and result in flow generator malfunction. Evaluation of clinical CPAP systems should include the manufacturer's supported nasal mask designs.

The ability to communicate with a patient located in the bedroom from the control room is essential. In particular, the sequence of physiologic calibrations performed before beginning a study and ending it requires verbal commands to be communicated to the patient while the technologist is interacting with the acquisition computer in the control room. This is most easily accomplished through an intercom system. Wireless intercom systems that are commercially available are often subject to signal interference. However, depending on the amount of extraneous electrical noise in a particular sleep center environment, a wireless intercom system may be a very efficient, cost-effective solution. Otherwise, a wired intercom system can be used for this purpose. As with most devices that interconnect with cabling, attention must be given to the device manufacturer's maximum cable length specifications. Some intercom systems incorporate a hub that could be located in a control room, which transmits to and receives audio from a number of patient rooms. This is a common intercom configuration found in hospital nursing stations or building security offices. Some may find this configuration useful in a sleep center setting, but others may find that it is more advantageous to have a separate receiver and transmitter for each room located near each computer workstation in the control room. If the patient room component of the intercom system is placed within reach of the patient's bed, then consideration should be given to the potential benefits of a patient call button feature, which is available in some intercom system designs.

Audio visual recording of patient activities is an essential component of a PSG test. In many ways, audio/video information acquired during a PSG plays as significant a role in diagnosing sleep disorders as the physiologic PSG data recorded. A wide variety of equipment options are available relating to digital versus analog video data, wireless versus closed circuit video, color versus black and white, and digital video formatting and editing. Careful review of the key components of a video/audio system is essential when evaluating devices for a new sleep center or when upgrading existing equipment.

Sensors/Electrodes

Many digital PSG systems come with a sensor pack when the equipment is initially purchased. However, a wide variety of manufacturers provide disposable and reusable electrodes and sensors for use in PSG. These sensors include EEG electrodes, airflow monitoring devices, leg movement sensors, and respiratory effort sensors. Some PSG system manufacturers also use proprietary sensors that are manufactured exclusively for use with their PSG system.

Although many PSG systems may provide a starter kit containing the various sensors and electrodes required to perform a PSG, there are typically a wide variety of different sensors and electrodes to choose from. Scalp electrodes are used to record EEG activity. Many are made from either gold or silver–silver chloride material and formed into a cup. An electroconductive material is placed in the cup, and the outer portion of the cup is either glued or pasted to the patient's head. Scalp electrode evaluation should include the preferred length of the electrode lead wire, compatibility of the lead wire jack with the PSG system hardware, the potential for dissimilar metal artifact occurring from the simultaneous use of different electrodes made with different metals, cost, reusable or disposable options, ease of application, and ease of cleaning.

In addition to scalp electrodes, adhesive electrodes are often used to record electrocardiogram (ECG), electrooculography, and other parameters. When evaluating adhesive electrodes, consideration should be given to the length of time the adhesive bond remains strong, the ease of attaining and maintaining acceptable electrode impedances, length of the lead wires, cost, and the general size of the electrode relative to the placement area on the patient.

When evaluating patients for obstructive sleep apnea, the airflow signal is a critical parameter. This is accomplished through the use of an airflow sensor. The most common types of airflow monitoring methods include thermal sensing devices such as a thermistor or thermocouple, polyvinylidene fluoride (PVDF) film, which is thermal and pressure based, and a nonthermal method of nasal pressure monitoring. The AASM specifies that identification of a hypopnea event or flow limitation pattern must be accomplished using the nasal pressure method, whereas the identification of an apnea episode is accomplished using a thermal method (2). Many PSG systems incorporate amplifiers that are especially designed for specific airflow monitoring devices, often produced by the PSG system manufacturer. However, there are many airflow monitoring devices to choose from.

Nasal pressure monitoring incorporates an air pressure transducer connected to a nasal cannula or oral/nasal cannula. This technology has a faster response time than thermistors and thermocouples. The nasal cannula can easily be modified and connected to a standard supplemental oxygen port found on a conventional CPAP mask, which provides an easy method of in-line airflow monitoring during CPAP titration in the lab, without the patient discomfort and mask leaks sometimes experienced with a thermocouple or thermistor placed under a CPAP mask. Nasal pressure monitors are commonly nonlinear. This results in the device exaggerating both apnea and hypopnea waveform changes. Specific filter settings must be incorporated in order to record or display nasal pressure data accurately.

PVDF is a treated plastic film that is polarized with an electric charge, which is used as an airflow monitoring sensor. The sensor has the fast response time (0.005 seconds) of the nasal pressure monitors, while retaining the linear flow measurement of other thermal sensing methods. It is usually smaller than other thermal devices and can be manufactured in a disposable or reusable option. The AASM does not currently accept the use of PVDF sensors for measuring airflow or identifying apneas and hypopneas during PSG. PVDF airflow sensors are acceptable for home sleep apnea testing (HSAT). PVDFsum derived from PVDF effort sensors is an acceptable alternative for identification of apnea or hypopnea during PSG.

When evaluating airflow monitoring devices, the following issues should be considered:

- Do the devices meet the requirements of the American Association of Sleep Technologists for recommended or acceptable sensors for each event type?

- Are the device connectors compatible with the PSG system input hardware?
- Are there external power source requirements (batteries)?
- Can the device provide a combined oral/nasal signal?
- Is the device affordable, and how often will it require replacement?

Monitoring respiratory effort during a PSG is essential in determining whether or not a patient's sleep-disordered breathing is obstructive or central in nature. A number of methods are available to detect and record respiratory effort. The easiest and most cost-effective way is to monitor intercostal EMG activity. This simply requires a number of electrodes to be placed in the correct locations, with the signal amplified and filtered through a conventional differential AC amplifier. Common drawbacks to this method include excessive ECG artifact and the inability to capture the EMG activity as a result of excessive tissue in obese patients.

A number of respiratory effort devices are available that incorporate the method of impedance pneumography. This also requires a number of electrodes to be placed on the patient's chest and abdomen areas, and is a relatively cost-effective method. Common disadvantages of this technology include poor signal quality resulting from limited respiration-related surface area changes in obese patients, as well as cardiogenic pulse artifact. An external power source is typically required with these devices as well.

Another method available for monitoring respiratory effort utilizes a piezoelectric crystal attached to a belt, which is wrapped around the patient. This technology is also not AASM approved for monitoring respiratory effort during PSG, but is acceptable for HSAT. As the patient breathes and the chest or abdomen surface area changes, the belt stretches, causing the crystal to emit a voltage change. The device is easy to apply to the patient and does not typically require an external power source but is typically more expensive than the methods previously described. Common drawbacks to this method include poor signal caused by limited respiration-related surface area changes in obese patients, and the designated abdominal or thoracic belt sliding on the patient into the other belt's source area, resulting in both belts displaying the same effort source.

The AASM standards specify that the detection of respiratory effort be performed using either esophageal manometry, which is fairly invasive, or calibrated or uncalibrated inductance plethysmography (2). Respiratory inductance plethysmography technology uses two sinusoid wire coils insulated and placed within two 2.5 cm (about 1 in) wide, lightweight elastic and adhesive bands. The transducer bands are placed around the rib cage under the armpits and around the abdomen at the level of the umbilicus (belly button). During inspiration, the cross-sectional area of the rib cage and abdomen increases, altering the self-inductance of the coils and the frequency of their oscillation, with an increase in cross-sectional area proportional to lung volumes. The electronics convert this change in frequency to a digital respiration waveform where the amplitude of the waveform is proportional to the inspired breath volume. Additionally, the AASM allows the use of respiratory effort sensors that use PVDF technology for detection of respiratory effort. These effort monitors are also acceptable for monitoring effort during HSAT. When evaluating respiratory effort devices, the following issues should be considered:

- Is the device able to detect minimal effort signals when used on obese patients?
- Is the device able to adequately reject ECG or pulse artifact?
- Are the device connectors compatible with the PSG system input hardware?
- Are there external power source requirements (batteries)?
- Is the device affordable, and how often will it require replacement?

Recording the movement of a patient's extremities is a very important part of studying a patient to rule out periodic limb movements of sleep or other abnormal sleep-related behaviors categorized as parasomnias. Since the advent of clinical sleep centers, monitoring of limb movements has been accomplished by monitoring the EMG activity of specific muscles located in the patient's legs and arms using surface electrodes. This is a very cost-effective method and is usually very reliable. The AASM recommends that surface electrodes be placed longitudinally and symmetrically around the middle of the muscle so that they are 2 cm apart. Both legs should be monitored for the presence of leg movements. Separate channels for each leg are strongly preferred (2). A number of limb movement sensors are available that incorporate piezoelectric materials to generate an electrical response during limb movements. These devices typically tape onto the patient's limbs, thereby greatly reducing the application time when compared with applying EMG surface electrodes. The limb movement sensors are more expensive than the EMG method and are not acceptable alternatives for monitoring EMG during PSG.

It is advantageous to graphically record snoring sounds generated by a patient during a PSG. A common method used to achieve this is to attach a small audio microphone element to the patient's neck and connect the microphone to a standard PSG differential amplifier. The microphone will detect and display not only snoring, but also subtle breathing sounds. However, this method will also result in the detection and display of audio signals generated from extraneous environmental noise, position adjustments, and CPAP mask exhaust port sounds that can be mistaken for snoring. An alternate method of recording snoring sounds is to utilize a commercially available piezoelectric sensor designed specifically for snoring detection. It produces a signal by detecting the movement and vibrations in the patient's neck tissue that are associated with snoring. The device is relatively inexpensive and eliminates the potential artifact mentioned previously.

Identifying and recording the body position of a patient during a PSG is essential in order to document the existence of positional sleep-disordered breathing. A wide variety of body position sensors are commercially available, and they are all based on similar technology. The sensor is typically attached to the midline, anterior chest area of the patient. As the patient changes to a lateral, supine, or prone position, the device changes its output voltage by a small degree. The device is calibrated to the PSG system before the beginning of the test, identifying each voltage output with a particular position. This is a convenient device, especially for the technologist performing the study, because the change in position is recorded automatically. Drawbacks of this method include the internal battery within the device losing power and ultimately failing, and the inability of the device to move enough to trigger the voltage change when it is used with very obese patients. An alternate method of recording body position is for the technologist to manually enter the position changes. This is obviously a much more cost-effective method but eliminates the automated function of the sensor. Not all PSG systems allow manual entry of body position changes, and this is an important feature to consider when evaluating PSG systems.

Audiovisual Equipment

Since the advent of clinical sleep disorders medicine, simultaneous video and audio monitoring of the patient during a PSG has been a standard data parameter. The interpreting physician or analyzing technologist most often uses these data to correlate questionable physiologic data in the PSG with patient or environmental activity that occurred during the test.

For patients suspected of sleeping disorders categorized as parasomnias, video and audio information can be critical for diagnosis. Many parasomnias involve unusual behaviors that occur during sleep and that can only be confirmed visually through video monitoring. These parasomnias include somnambulism, REM sleep behavior disorder, and abnormal movement disorders. In addition, suspected epileptiform activity seen in the

EEG can be correlated with seizure-related motor activity displayed within the video information to assist in diagnosing nocturnal seizures.

Many patients with sleep disorders, particularly those whose disorders result in very mild daytime sleepiness or fatigue, have difficulty being convinced of their condition. In particular, many patients who demonstrate mild-to-moderate obstructive sleep apnea during a sleep study will not believe the physician's interpretation or report and are unwilling to comply with the prescribed treatment. In these cases, the physician may choose to play back the video/audio information for the patient to convince him or her of the condition.

Many sleep centers maintain a library of video clips taken from routine PSGs comprising patient behaviors indicative of a wide range of sleep disorders. This information can be used for training new employees, as well as for educational presentations, with a signed consent from each patient that allows recordings to be used for teaching purposes.

More recently, the video recording of the patient–technologist interaction in the sleep center has become an essential means of liability protection. Some patients may choose to take legal action against a particular sleep center facility or sleep technologist, claiming inappropriate contact or communication. In light of the fact that sleep studies are lengthy, occur in bedrooms, and are often conducted in isolated situations, it is wise for the sleep technologist to video-record all interactions with patients, including sensor hookup. This video documentation can become critical evidence in defending one's actions with a patient if brought to litigation.

Most commercially available PSG data acquisition systems incorporate digital video/audio functionality. During a PSG, digital PSG systems allow the user to view a small video window on the computer screen simultaneously with scrolling physiologic data. The user can easily identify specific video clips of interest for the reviewer the next day. In addition, the reviewers can very easily and quickly locate video data associated with a point in time on the PSG, as the video and PSG data are linked.

General Equipment Considerations

The most important component of the video/audio system in a sleep center facility is the camera. Selecting a camera for use in a sleep center should include considerations within a number of areas. The AASM accreditation standards require that each testing bedroom in the facility have a mechanism for visual monitoring and video recording of patients during testing. Time-delayed photographs are not considered compliant with this standard (1).

The camera must be able to function in low-light environments. Many cameras designed and intended for use within an outdoor security system meet these low-level lighting requirements. When a camera such as this is operating in a low-light environment, the iris adjustment of the camera is typically set wide open. If light were suddenly to be introduced into the environment being recorded by the camera, this wide open iris setting would "white out" the video display, and the user would not be able to recognize objects within the display until the iris was adjusted to a smaller opening. This scenario occurs frequently within a sleep center when the light within a patient's room is turned on and off during the course of a study. Therefore, only cameras with an auto-adjusting iris function should be considered for use in a sleep center. Otherwise, the iris will need to be adjusted manually to view and record events in both lighted and low-light conditions, which is not practical within a sleep center setting.

Because of the general low-light environment of patient rooms in a sleep center, as well as the high cost of color video cameras, video information acquired during a PSG has historically been black and white. As technology has evolved and costs have decreased, color cameras have found a place in the sleep center. Activities such as patient hookup procedures and monitoring patient activity between daytime MSLT trials can be videotaped in color. Ideally, color cameras used for both low-light PSG recording and normal light activities should be able to automatically switch from black and white mode during low-light recording to color mode during normal light recording.

A wide variety of options are available for mounting a camera within a sleep center patient room. The camera should be mounted in a location that will allow the entire patient bed to be viewed in the video display. A fixed camera mount is the most inexpensive method for mounting a camera. This hardware allows for manipulating the angle of the camera and then tightening a number of screws, thereby obtaining a fixed camera angle. In addition, there are mounting systems available that enclose the camera, usually within a plastic mirrored dome. This enclosed mounting method will typically require that the camera be mounted on the ceiling of the room, as opposed to the wall. This can be advantageous in some circumstances involving patients who are overly conscious of a camera in the room and are unable to sleep.

If cost is not a significant issue, a camera mounting system that incorporates pan and tilt functions is ideal in a sleep center patient room. This allows the technologist to move the camera vertically and laterally to capture specific activity or behaviors of the patient during the sleep study. The camera that is typically used with a pan and tilt mounting system will incorporate a zoom lens. The zoom, pan, and tilt functions are all controlled by the user via a remote console typically placed within the sleep center control room or may be integrated into the user interface of the PSG system computer (Fig. 67-4A).

In order to video-record patient activity in a room that is totally dark, the most common type of lighting system used is infrared illumination. An infrared illuminator manufactured as a stand-alone unit can be mounted on the wall or ceiling of the patient room, ideally near the patient (Fig. 67-4B). There are also cameras designed for low-light conditions that have built-in infrared illuminators. This can be a convenient feature, but in this scenario, placement of the camera relative to the patient is critical to ensure that the infrared illumination reaches the patient.

A less costly way to light a patient room for video recording utilizes an incandescent blacklight bulb. The bulb can be placed in a portable or permanent light fixture within the room. A disadvantage to this method is that the black light creates a degree of light within the room that is noticeable to the patient, as opposed to the infrared illuminator, which produces no visible light within the room. Some sleep centers have incorporated both methods in patient rooms, using a conventional dimmer control with the black light to fine-tune the amount of blacklight illumination, ultimately optimizing the overall illumination within the room without disturbing the patient.

The audio portion of the video data is most often used to detect and assess a patient's breathing sounds such as snoring, as well as facilitate communication between the patient and the technologist during a PSG test. The audio data are acquired through a microphone placed in the room. Some cameras have a microphone built into the camera. Also, a number of intercom systems designed specifically for sleep centers provide an audio output signal that can be introduced into the audio recording device. However, to effectively sample the more subtle breathing sounds from a patient, a microphone mounted close to the patient is ideal. Microphones can be omnidirectional or unidirectional. An omnidirectional microphone will receive audio information from a broad 360° angle. A unidirectional microphone will receive audio data from a more focused angle, usually directed through the top of the microphone. If the primary interest in the audio data is to hear and analyze a patient's breathing sounds, a unidirectional microphone will perform best, as extraneous noise within the patient's room will not be sampled. To focus the microphone on the patient, the microphone

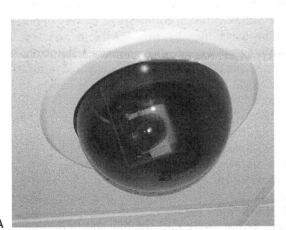

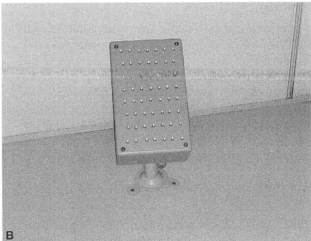

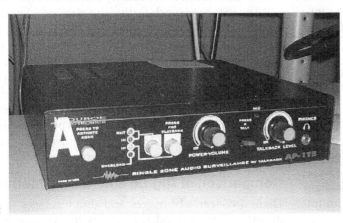

Figure 67-4 The most common analog video components. **A:** Pan-tilt camera. **B:** Wall-mounted infrared light source. **C:** Audio monitoring base station with listen and talkback.

should be mounted on the wall directly above the head of the patient's bed or on the ceiling directly above the patient's bed. An omnidirectional microphone can be placed practically anywhere, as it will be sampling all sounds within the room.

Just as physiologic data recorded during a sleep study can be processed through the use of frequency filters and amplifier gain, so can the audio data. The easiest way to accomplish audio processing is through the use of an audio mixer, which provides processing functions of signal gain or volume, and frequency equalization typically characterized as bass, midrange, and treble controls (Fig. 67-4C). Signal gain or volume controls can be very useful for boosting subtle patient breathing sounds of interest, as well as compensating for low-signal strength caused by long cabling requirements from the patient's room to the control room. Extraneous noise in the patient's room that remains at a constant frequency such as a heating or air-conditioning unit can be filtered out of the audio signal using the equalization controls. Fifty or 60 Hz line interference can be filtered as well. In addition, specific breathing or snoring sounds of particular interest can be focused and boosted using the equalization controls.

Fundamentals of Analog Video/Audio Recording

A conventional analog video system configuration will consist of a camera, microphone, videocassette recorder (VCR), date/time generator, and display monitor. With the exception of the camera and microphone, which are source devices, all other components within the interface chain have signal input and output connections. Analog video/audio systems are rarely used today, as almost all PSG systems currently on the market have built-in digital audiovisual capabilities.

Fundamentals of Digital Video/Audio Recording

Most PSG systems incorporate digital video. Rather than acquiring audio visual data onto a magnetic tape cassette, the video and audio signals are digitized either at the camera source or at the computer, displayed within a window on a PSG system's computer screen simultaneously with scrolling physiologic data, and stored on digital media such as a hard drive or CD-ROM disc. Using a digital camera that converts the images to digital information within the camera eliminates entirely the analog VCR and monitor requirements and interfaces directly into the computer. However, interfacing the video and audio output signals of a VCR to a computer equipped with a video A/D conversion card can easily digitize an analog video system as well.

In order to adequately acquire and play back digital audio/video data during a PSG, there are minimum computer hardware requirements to consider.

1. *Hard disk space:* Minimum of 500 GB. Ideally 1 TB or more. The minimum space will require relatively frequent archiving of video data because these files are large and will use up the disk space.
2. *RAM:* Minimum of 1 GB (2 to 3 GB recommended)
3. *Processor speed:* Minimum of 1 GHz. Although audio visual acquisition has been performed during PSG with slower processors, this minimum recommendation will resolve the "choppy" or fragmented video playback, which is commonly experienced with slower processors.
4. *Monitor resolution:* 15" screen; minimum 1,600 × 1,050 or higher recommended
5. *Analog-to-digital conversion:* This video card will convert incoming video and audio signals from an analog source such as a VCR to digital information to be displayed and stored within the computer.

In general, digitized video in its raw form will utilize a large amount of hard disk space as well as archiving media. For this reason, there are a wide variety of video formats that incorporate degrees of data compression, thereby minimizing disk space requirements. In most cases, digital PSG system manufacturers will determine which format the system will utilize. A specific format will affect not only disk space usage, but also playback quality and editing capabilities. The most common formats are listed in Table 67-1. At the time of this writing, the MPEG-4 format continues to be very popular for its ability to significantly compress the size of raw video files without causing any noticeable effect during playback.

In most cases, digital video acquired during a PSG is viewed in real time on the computer screen, and is unaffected by file compression algorithms. It is only during subsequent playback that the compression scheme may be noticeable.

The use of digital video allows significantly more efficient utilization of PSG time synchronization features. Unlike the analog method, which requires time for the VCR to rewind or fast-forward to a point in time identified within the PSG data, a digital system allows very fast seek and playback functionality within the video data.

The PSG time synch feature can also complement the functions of digital video editing. Once a particular video segment of interest is identified, the segment can be removed from the entire raw video file and saved as a separate file, manipulated for contrast and color, or text can be superimposed into the video display. Not only can this be useful for educational presentations, but the segments of interest can be archived for medicolegal purposes and the rest of the large raw video file can be discarded, significantly reducing the archive media space required.

Comparison of Digital and Analog Methods

There are clear advantages and disadvantages to both digital and analog video methods if only one is used

Table 67-1 Common Digital Video File Formats

Suffix	File Type	Features and Limitations
.mov	QuickTime movie	An industry standard developed as part of an entire multimedia architecture by Apple, the QuickTime movie is an open multimedia format, which has multiplatform, multi-browser support.
.asf	ASF	Developed by Microsoft as a multimedia successor to AVI and other individual media file formats, ASF files can contain up to seven media types, including streaming video. ASF is optimized for network distribution and desktop playback.
.avi	AVI (video for Windows)	The precursor to ASF, AVI files are limited to audio and video only.
.mpg	MPEG	MPEG-4 is the latest standard for video compression and file format developed by an industry group.

ASF, advanced streaming format; AVI, audio–video interleave; MPEG, motion picture experts group.

exclusively. As mentioned previously, it may be to the users' benefit to use both methods (converting analog signals to digital signals through an A/D conversion card) and therefore enjoy the best of both worlds. However, some features are available only through an exclusive commitment to either analog or digital hardware.

Many of the commercially available digital video cameras connect to a computer through a universal serial bus (USB) connection. In light of the fact that the digital camera actually converts and creates digital information as it is being acquired, there is no need for an A/D or video capture card in the computer. Therefore, the camera can be connected directly to the USB port. A USB connection facilitates very fast data communication, which is beneficial for real-time monitoring during a PSG. In addition, some digital cameras can receive power from the computer via the USB cable, thereby eliminating the external power supply requirement for the camera.

Some digital cameras can connect to a computer via an Ethernet connection. An Ethernet connection is typically used within a LAN to connect different computers and peripheral devices to a network. A digital camera that is designed for Ethernet connectivity will transmit its own IP address to other devices. An IP address is a set of numbers that identifies the device to other computers within a network. This can be beneficial in a sleep center setting, because the camera does not need to be interfaced directly to a specific computer, but can be interfaced to any Ethernet entrance into the network (hub, switch, etc.). In addition, any other computer connected to the LAN can view the digital video images.

Clearly, one of the more extraordinary differences between analog and video cameras is size. Digital cameras have progressively diminished in size to where they can very easily be placed in a variety of locations within a sleep center's patient bedroom. This can be advantageous not only in the interest of minimizing construction or facility renovation, but also in "hiding" the camera by mounting it in an inconspicuous location to minimize the patient's awareness of being on camera, which can make sleeping in a center difficult for some patients.

Digital video systems are clearly beneficial with regard to lowering not only the initial hardware purchase expense, but expenses related to archiving the data as well. S-VHS videocassettes and video recorders are becoming obsolete. A recordable DVD will hold from 1.46 to 4.7 GB of data, which will allow a large number of video segments to be archived on a single disc. There is clearly a cost advantage to using digital video as opposed to analog. If the PSG system computers are networked to a LAN server, a larger-capacity storage disk (1 TB or greater) available via the network can be used for data archiving, thereby eliminating the requirement for data storage disks.

In many ways, audio/video information acquired during a PSG plays as significant a role in diagnosing sleep disorders as the physiologic PSG data recorded. Video information can assist clinicians with treatment as well, by convincing patients of their symptoms during sleep. Considering the local patient population, referral patterns, facility issues, and physician preferences, the type of video camera, VCR, digital hardware, and archiving methods used should be tailored to best meet a particular sleep center's requirements. There are clear advantages to digital video acquisition. Lower capital costs, lower archiving media and storage space costs, efficient PSG/video time synchronization functionality, and video editing can all be realized through a digital video system. Current analog equipment can be interfaced to a computer, providing many of the benefits of digital video with minimal replacement of analog hardware. As technology continues to advance, VCR units and video cassettes are likely to become unavailable. Video equipment used in the sleep center can be expected to become smaller, cost less, and continue to play a significant role in the field of sleep disorders medicine.

Data Storage and Archiving Equipment

Once digital PSG files have been accessed and modified during the analysis, and scoring and report generation procedures are completed, the files will continue to reside on the computer's hard drive until they are removed to make space for future recordings. When evaluating computer hardware, consideration should be given to archiving capabilities. Archiving is most commonly accomplished by moving the data to a portable medium such as a recordable CD (CD-R), DVD (DVD-R), optical disc, or external hard drive. To accomplish this task, the computer tower must have access to drives designed to read and write digital information to varying types of portable media or network access to a server and storage space.

Sleep center PSG computers connected via a LAN to a server that contains a drive with the capacity to store large amounts of data are ideal for archiving PSG and video data. PSG files can simply be moved with a click of a computer mouse to a storage location on the LAN. This archive method eliminates the physical storage space required for portable media and allows a more efficient way to retrieve the files when required.

A number of commercially available digital PSG systems incorporate a software function relating to sleep center operational management that includes patient information database features. Archiving digital PSG files through the system's patient database function can facilitate very efficient and quick retrieval of the data when needed.

SUMMARY

Clearly, the process of establishing a new sleep center or upgrading the instrumentation within an existing sleep center requires careful study and consideration of the sleep center's needs and currently available technology before purchasing equipment. Strategies such as upgrading hardware versus purchasing new, as well as combining new and old technology, can often be utilized to reduce costs. Understanding the general components of the sleep center physical plant, categories of instrumentation used within a sleep center, sensor options, and features common to, or expected to be found in, PSG-related software applications is essential. Attention to the requirements outlined in accreditation standards is also essential in order to perform an accurate assessment of the sleep center's physical layout requirements and hardware and software needs, and to adequately evaluate the equipment available.

REFERENCES

1. American Academy of Sleep Medicine. (2018). *Standards for accreditation.* Retrieved from https://j2vjt3dnbra3ps7ll1clb4q2-wpengine.netdna-ssl.com/wp-content/uploads/2018/04/accreditationstandards.pdf
2. Berry, R. B., Albertario, C. L., Harding, S. M., et al.; for the American Academy of Sleep Medicine. (2018). *The AASM manual for the scoring of sleep and associated events: rules, terminology and technical specifications* [Version 2.5]. Darien, IL: American Academy of Sleep Medicine.

chapter 68
The Manager's Role in a Sleep Center

HENRY JOHNS   CONNSTANCE SHIVERS SMITH   ROBERT HENDRICKSON

LEARNING OBJECTIVES

On completion of this chapter, the reader should be able to:

1. Identify the different levels of management and the function of each.
2. Describe the various roles of management and the relationship of management to leadership.
3. Describe the process of recruiting, interviewing, hiring, evaluating, and disciplining employees.
4. Identify the basic steps to establishing a budget.

KEY TERMS

Management structure
Basic management skills
Leadership
Ethics
Job description
Recruiting
Interviewing
Hiring
Team building
Discipline
Budget
Income
Expense

Management and leadership are as important to the function of a sleep diagnostic facility as the electrodes and sensors used to measure sleep. Many in our field will find themselves in a managerial/leadership role by choice or necessity as their careers unfold. This chapter is presented to serve as a guide and building block for a technologist's future in management.

The basic definition of a manager is a person who is responsible for overseeing or administering the day-to-day activities of a business. The most basic job of a manager is to recruit and retain qualified, talented employees, develop and implement budgets, help others meet goals, and get things done. Leadership is the process of enlisting the aid of others to accomplish a common goal. A leader will have basic traits or tendencies that inspire in others the will to achieve.

Management and leadership need to go hand in hand for success. Managers direct activity; leaders inspire the will to achieve. Management can be present without leadership and leadership without management; both concepts will be presented here. Providing motivation, giving direction, removing roadblocks for success, building teams, and providing constructive feedback are the basic tasks of any manager.

MANAGEMENT STRUCTURE

Managers can be categorized into different levels within an organization according to the level of responsibility and the function they serve. Most organizations have three levels of management, which are generally distributed in a pyramid fashion, with upper management at the top, middle managers in the center, and first-line managers at the base. Managers are associated with specific areas, such as finance, marketing, operations, human resources (HR), and administration, as well as specific service lines, such as the sleep center.

Upper or top management is made up of a small group, typically including a president, vice president, chief executive officer (CEO), and so on. Their job is to manage the overall organization. The top managers set the organization's goals, strategies, and operating policies, and they represent the organization to the world outside.

Middle managers are responsible for implementing plans and policies developed by upper management. They make up the largest group of managers in most organizations. Often referred to as operations managers, division heads, or chiefs, they handle such things as inventory control, equipment failures, and routine union issues. Middle managers coordinate the work of supervisors within the organization. Although sometimes creating excess bureaucracy, they serve as a necessary bridge between the front-line managers and the top management. The middle manager translates the organization's mission and goals into action.

First-line managers may be called supervisors, shift managers, coordinators, or office managers. Employees who are entering the ranks of management for the first time hold these positions. First-line managers oversee the day-to-day operations of their respective areas of the organization. They often have authority to hire and evaluate the performance of employees in their section and handle most routine administrative duties. Unlike middle or upper management, first-line managers spend most of their time overseeing the work of subordinates. Many first-line managers are working supervisors, still involved in the hands-on business of patient care.

BASIC MANAGEMENT SKILLS

One of the biggest stumbling blocks a new manager encounters is the realization that he or she is viewed differently by subordinates. Everyone wants to fit into a work group as part of the team, but there are bigger expectations for managers. Successful managers need a number of skills to be at the top of their game. Interpersonal skills and the ability to communicate with both internal and external contacts are necessary to the daily duties of a manager. The ability to convey messages and directions and be clearly understood can often mean the difference between success and failure. Active, empathetic listening assists managers to understand and ensure they are understood. People skills go hand in hand with good communication.

Managers need the ability to think outside the box and envision things in the abstract. This is the conceptual ability to put all the pieces together and grasp how things fit into the organization, which leads to diagnostic skills and the ability to visualize a problem and solution. A good manager is able to examine the organization's symptoms and develop a solution.

Technical skills are also important to a manager at any level and are necessary to understanding how to accomplish a specific kind of work. The ability to do the job is not always as important to a manager as a grasp of how a job is done. Technical skill is most important to the first-line managers because they spent a great deal of time training staff and answering work-related questions. The CEO needs to understand the process; the supervisor needs to be able to turn the knobs and make it happen.

One of the most important skills for a manager is time management. The ability of a manager to prioritize tasks, work efficiently, and appropriately delegate tasks is key to success. However, managerial work does not always follow a logical or systematic progression through the day or week. It is often fraught with change, interruptions, fragmented activities, and uncertainty that can make time very unproductive. Making a habit of keeping a "day book" or notebook, in which a manager can make notes on the events and challenges of the day, is

often very helpful. Some managers include this information on a calendar along with scheduled events. This also helps jog a manager's memory of daily activities in the past.

Leadership

Leadership is an important part of management. In their book *The Leadership Challenge*, Kouzes and Posner indicate that some of the most important traits of leadership are intelligence, competency, honesty, the quality of being forward-looking, and inspiration. The level and skill at which these qualities are displayed directly influence the willingness of staff to follow a manager's lead. It is not sufficient to just possess these qualities; they must be displayed daily. Staff respond positively to seeing them put into practice every day.

Competency in a manager is essential for achieving positive results in the workplace. Managers are often considered to be competent because they are in leadership positions; however, the label of incompetence can be attached to a manager quickly and is difficult to dispel. The ability to make decisions and set the pace for your team is a demonstration of competence. Competent leaders will celebrate the accomplishments and success of the team, thus indirectly pointing out the manager's competence to lead.

Ethical conduct can make or break a manager. Ethics are often referred to as a moral philosophy and encompass the concepts of right and wrong. Every person makes ethical decisions every day on the basis of the individual's own paradigms. In some cultures, it is perfectly acceptable to pay or accept a bribe when doing business. In the United States, we often provide a cash tip for services; however, in Japan, this practice can be seen as offensive. Should a manager accept a resort stay for doing business with a vendor? The answer is an emphatic no; however, this was a standard practice for many years. Managers should always strive to avoid even the appearance of unethical behavior.

In the workplace, ethics can be greatly influenced by the organization's mission, goals, or values and can often influence decisions more strongly than an individual's personal values. Individuals within an organization share a corporate culture that defines goals and values. Organizations develop mission, vision, and value statements to help focus the members of the team to move in a common direction together. Thus, corporate culture creates an ethical climate for the members of the organization.

The quality of being "forward-looking" is essential for any leader. Knowing where you are and where your organization needs to go is of no help unless you are able to communicate your vision to those you lead. When leaders are not seen as forward-looking, it is generally for one of two reasons: the leader has no vision or the leader is unwilling to share the vision with others. Leaders may fear that their vision will not come true or bear fruit. The leader's job is to share a vision of the future with others in the organization, guiding and inspiring them to realize that vision. Ideas and visions may be viewed as a ladder. The leader has an idea, the first rung of the ladder, and a vision of the results, the last rung of the ladder. For success, communication is needed to create all the rungs in between the bottom and top of the ladder. Setting goals for the organization and establishing a timetable to achieve them is leading for success (1).

There are several great myths about management that should be noted.

The Ideal Manager

So what do you need to do to become an ideal manager? Some would argue that there is no such thing, and there may not be. However, we should all strive to become what our staff and our bosses feel is an ideal manager. Success is all about attitude and perception. One of the most popular management styles is that of the "walk around manager." Being out from behind the desk is the best way to know what is going on in your facility. Spend time in each area of the operation for better understanding and communication. It is difficult to lead from behind a desk; it is best to apply the old US Army Infantry motto of "Follow Me." Be a catalyst for positive change and a demonstrator of excellence in business, ethics, and professional practice.

Here are a few keys to successful management and leadership.

Managers should

- keep up with industry changes; be ready to roll with the punches.
- be technically proficient as well as knowledgeable in subject content; you need to be able to provide the answers.
- take an active role in every phase of the operation; earn the respect of employees and other professionals.
- learn to delegate; you can't do it all; if you hire competent staff, they can do the job.
- recruit and hire people who are the cream of the crop and set them to work.
- be there for their staff; support your staff and they will support you.
- give credit where it is due; let your staff shine and give praise—it makes you look good too.
- be fair and consistent; don't show favorites and don't change the rules for different individuals.
- be honest and trustworthy; broken trust may not be repairable.
- communicate; be clear with what you need and expect; remember, information needs to flow both ways.

- share your vision; you can't achieve it alone.
- plan for tomorrow; where do you see your department in 5 years and how will you get there?

Staffing a Sleep Center

A sleep center's ability to grow and stay on top depends largely on the quality of the people working in it. That is because the most important asset of any business is the people. Finding and keeping those quality people is challenging. Turnover costs are high. Getting a reputation for high turnover in a sleep center can have the unwanted result of no one of quality wanting to work there.

HR management is necessary in any business because it is all about people. HR management encompasses federal, state, and local regulatory issues, compensation and benefits, recruiting, interviewing, staffing, retention, job descriptions, policies and procedures, personnel files, team building, training and staff development, creating a safe, healthy, and productive environment, performance evaluation, and discipline.

The type of sleep center determines who is responsible for HR management. A hospital-based sleep center will have an HR department to handle many of these functions for all of its employees. A medium-sized sleep center or a sleep business of multiple centers may have one or two people devoted to HR management. A small freestanding sleep center may have only a manager or supervisor who is responsible for HR management.

Recruiting, Interviewing, and Hiring the People You Need

The hiring process has one purpose, namely, to exchange enough information so that the parties involved can make an informed decision about whether or not to enter into an employment relationship. The usual steps in the hiring process are developing job descriptions, advertising the opening(s), recruiting candidates, reviewing job applications and résumés, interviewing, performing preemployment checks, and extending an offer.

Job Descriptions

Before any recruiting is done, job descriptions must be in place. A job description defines the employment relationship. It includes the following:

1. the position title,
2. the essential duties of the job,
3. the necessary job experience,
4. the educational requirements and/or special skills necessary to perform the job,
5. licensure, registry, or certification requirements,
6. physical requirements such as the demands of the job, the length of the shift, weekend work, rotating shifts, frequent overtime, and exposure to particular conditions (e.g., chemicals and hostile clients),

7. special attendance requirements,
8. a statement that the employee may be asked to perform other duties as needed,
9. satisfactory performance measures,
10. the employee's supervisor, and
11. the date of the most recent update of the job description.

In a sleep center, job descriptions for the technical staff may include trainee, sleep technician, and sleep technologist. The descriptions vary based on the difference in the scopes of practice (2). A trainee is someone who is learning the basic competencies of sleep technology under the direction of a sleep technician or a sleep technologist. A sleep technician is someone who knows the competencies of sleep technology but is not yet credentialed. A sleep technologist is someone credentialed by a board indicating skill mastery. Thus, a sleep technologist should be able to perform all the scope of practice of the sleep technology profession and may provide oversight or training of noncredentialed technical staff. As the role of the sleep technologist expands to include more clinical roles, and technologists seek advanced credentials, higher-level job descriptions may be required to outline the duties of a clinical sleep health educator, patient care coordinator, or shift supervisor.

Administrative assistant job descriptions are developed according to the needs of the individual sleep center, its location, organizational structure, staff size, and amount of business. The administrative staff work closely with the medical director to ensure that sleep center operations comply with federal, state, and local regulations and with other governing bodies such as the American Academy of Sleep Medicine (AASM) and the Joint Commission. In a small sleep center, one person could wear many hats. A manager may have responsibility for day-to-day operations, technical operations, and staffing. As the business grows, with an increasing patient load and increasing staff size, the size of the administrative staff generally increases and the responsibilities diversify. It is the administrative assistant position that usually maintains contact with the technical staff, the medical staff, the insurance industry, and the public. Administrative assistant positions are public relations positions.

Every sleep center must have a medical director who is licensed to practice in the state and is responsible for all the medical personnel in the center. If a sleep center is accredited by the AASM or is seeking such accreditation, then it must have a board-certified or board-eligible sleep physician on staff (3). According to the AASM Standards for Accreditation of Sleep Disorders Centers, the sleep physician must be board-certified by the American Board of Sleep Medicine or board-eligible in sleep medicine by either a member board of the American Board of Medical Specialties or a member board of the American Osteopathic Association.

Job Applications

Once job descriptions are in place, a job application form should be developed for screening purposes and avoidance of possible legal issues. Every applicant must complete an application. This is an opportunity to solicit basic selection criteria and gather the same basic information for all applicants. The application form should contain nothing that the employer is prohibited by law from considering in the hiring process (e.g., age, marital status, religion, gender, number of children, political affiliation, and national origin). All categories of the application must be relevant and job related.

A job application can legally ask the following: name, address, phone number, social security number, employment background with the last three employers (if applicable), educational background, and military service (if applicable to the job). The applicant can be asked questions such as "When can you start?" "Do you have any physical limitations to performing the job?" "Are you legally authorized to work in the United States?" and "Do you have any experience or certifications that are not listed on your application?"

Recruiting

When job descriptions and applications are in place, the recruiting begins. Consider the many ways available to recruit personnel. There are traditional methods: advertisements in newspapers and trade publications, job fairs, open houses, campus recruiting, employee referrals, prerecorded telephone messages, preemployment clinical training, employment agencies, networking, Internet job boards (e.g., American Association of Sleep Technologists and Board of Registered Polysomnographic Technologists), television and radio advertisements, and in-house job postings. More innovative methods include the following: banners and signs, bumper stickers, kiosks, company-sponsored social events, flyers, and competitions. There are pros and cons to all these methods. But using various methods to attract candidates for job positions opens up the candidate pool and encourages workplace diversity.

The Interviewing Process

Before the face-to-face interview, a screening interview is generally performed. This interview is usually performed by the HR department or person. The screening process is used to evaluate candidates to determine if they possess all the qualifications and requirements for the job before a face-to-face interview is scheduled. The job application is reviewed as well as the résumé. However, the HR department or person may not be familiar with the day-to-day duties of the position being applied for, so applications are also screened by the manager or supervisor. The manager or supervisor has knowledge of the position to be filled and the qualities, skills, knowledge, and experience necessary. A review of these items is useful as a tool to identify the best candidates.

The face-to-face interview involves an interviewer or interviewers asking questions and the applicant answering them. A job offer is based on how well the applicant answers the three questions that employers are seeking to answer in the interview process: Does the applicant have the skills and abilities to do the job? Does the applicant have the work ethic that is expected by the employer? Will the applicant be a team player and fit into the sleep center?

The interviewing process should be conducted using a structured format. This kind of format provides interviewers with a checklist to ensure a consistent process and a comprehensive exchange of information. The process generally begins with introductory remarks about what is to take place. Then, questions about prior work experience, qualifications, and education are asked. Next, information is provided about the job, compensation and benefits, and the sleep center. The candidate is given the opportunity to ask questions about the job and the sleep center. In the final step of the process, the candidate is informed about what will occur next and the interview ends on a positive note.

There are different styles of interviewing (4), but the one recognized by HR professionals as being the best interview style is the behavior-based interview. As the name implies, this interview style seeks information on how the applicant behaved in situations at his or her previous job. An example of a behavior-based interview question is "Tell me about a time when you had too many things to do at work and how you prioritized your tasks." Behavior-based interviews avoid asking illegal questions and make it easy to recognize how an applicant behaves and learns from situations both good and bad. There is no such thing as a perfect employee who has never made a mistake or did not learn something from a challenge. All answers are documented on a standard form.

A second type of interview that is useful in a sleep center is the team interview. The team usually comprises three to four people who are the potential coworkers of the applicant. In this type of interview, each team member takes turns asking questions that are in a standardized format, and all answers are documented on a standard form. After the interview, each team member discusses the pros and cons of the applicant. For example, was there a lack of respect shown to any of the team members, or were all the team members treated with respect? The team approach minimizes the likelihood of hiring the wrong person for the job.

The best of both worlds in interviewing is using behavior-based interviewing with a team. Each team member gives input about the applicant and plays a part in determining whether or not the applicant is a good fit to the team.

There are different styles of questioning that can be used during an interview. *Close-ended questions* call for a simple, informational answer, like yes or no. *Open-ended questions* require some thought. These questions require the candidate to reveal attitudes or opinions, for example, "Describe a stressful situation at your previous job and how you handled it," or "How did you improve productivity at your last job?" *Hypothetical questions* allow the candidate to react to a situation or solve an imaginary situation. *Probing questions* let interviewers probe more deeply for additional information. Rational probes request reasons using short questions such as "why?" or "how?" Clarifier probes are used to clarify or expand on previously provided information. Verifier probes check out the honesty of a statement. For example, "You state that you work closely with referral physicians' offices. Tell me what you have done for them." *Leading questions* are asked in such a way that the answer you are looking for is obvious. These are not good questions to ask in an interview. These questions lend themselves to the candidate, giving the interviewer the answers he or she wants to hear.

There are also legal and illegal interview questions (5). Any questions that violate antidiscrimination and consumer protection laws cannot be asked. Avoid questions surrounding age, disability status, national origin, family situation, or legal problems. It is acceptable to ask about availability to work, ability to travel if this is required for the job, and the reason a candidate left a previous position.

Once the interviews are complete, selection and hiring occur. The management team reviews the pool of applicants. A high-impact hiring, based on a systematic review of the applicant's capabilities for performance, recruits high-potential employees, uses various hiring tools (i.e., interviews, personality tests, reference checks, and background checks), and anticipates turnover. Recommendations should be scrutinized by HR and the management team. Once everyone agrees on the applicant to be hired, a written offer of employment should be provided verifying the terms of employment agreed to by both the employer and the soon-to-be employee. An I-9 form for employment must also be filled out by both employer and employee, as required by law. This form attests that the employee is authorized to work and is not an illegal alien. The employer attests that the employee's documents have been reviewed and appear to be in order.

Team Building

On the first day of the job, the new employee should be introduced to all the staff and their job titles and duties; this assists the new employee to understand how he or she fits into the organization. Then orientation begins: outlining the expectations of the employer, including conduct, policies and procedures, diversity, the probationary period, benefits, and dress code.

Policies and procedures manuals work in conjunction with the job description to define the work relationship. The policy manual should contain policies that impact all aspects of employment (i.e., conduct, safety, attendance, paid time off, equal employment opportunity policy, sick leave, compensation, harassment, probationary periods, discipline, leaves of absence, and benefits). The manual should contain a statement indicating to whom the policies apply. Policies must be dated and undergo regular revisions to keep them up-to-date. The procedure manual should include all procedures performed in the operation of the sleep center, namely, emergency procedures (such as code blue, inclement weather, and power outages), starting and ending studies, procedures for performing all studies, hookup equipment, scoring, and how to answer the telephone. Policies and procedures should be reviewed with the employee during the orientation period. The policy and procedure review should be acknowledged by the employee, who should sign documentation acknowledging that he or she has read and understood them. The probationary period is the time (usually 90 days) used by the sleep center and the employee to decide if the employee is a good fit for the center.

In the sleep center, as well as any other business, the people are the most important asset. Therefore, it is in the best interest of the sleep center to create an employee-friendly work environment. This type of environment respects employee well-being as a core value, is sensitive to work–life issues, allows employees autonomy with respect to their jobs, facilitates open communication, rewards initiative, and encourages teamwork.

Focusing on well-being as a core value indicates that your sleep center values its employees. You are concerned about health and safety, so you are compliant with state and federal health and safety standards (e.g., Occupational Health and Safety Administration). A health management program is in place to ensure your employees are physically and mentally able to do their jobs.

You are also concerned about workplace ergonomics. The right tools are provided to avoid workplace injuries. Sleep technologists spend a great majority of their working hours sitting in front of a computer. Adjustable height chairs with good lumbar support and adjustable arms are essential. Adjustable monitors, good lighting, ergonomic keyboard tables, and wrist rests go a long way toward avoiding eyestrain, neck strain, and repetitive wrist injuries.

When businesses are sensitive to work–life issues, employees feel that they are a part of a team. Time off for family special events and family and medical emergencies, flexibility in work shifts, and accessibility to employee assistance programs engender goodwill between employer and employee.

Good communication is necessary for any business to survive and thrive. One definition of communication is the imparting or interchange of thoughts, opinions, or information by speech, writing, or signs (6). In successful businesses, communication flows freely from the top downward, and management encourages communication from the bottom upward. In other words, an interchange of information occurs. The sleep center manager who encourages open communication listens to the concerns and thoughts of the employees and provides the tools necessary for employees to do their job. Management should make it a point to interact with employees in the employees' work area. Praise should always be given publicly, but feedback must be private.

Trust is established between employer and employee when employees have the ability to affect their jobs. Employees with autonomy with respect to their jobs feel empowered to go above and beyond their job descriptions. They are motivated to be creative, resourceful, and responsive to customers' needs without fear of making mistakes. They embrace the team concept because they are unified by a clear sense of mission, and they are rewarded for taking that initiative.

Staff Development

Sleep centers must be committed to training and staff development. The field of sleep technology is constantly changing, and employees must stay current. An investment in staff development is an investment in the current and future success of the sleep center. Training is linked to staff development, but they are not the same thing. Training focuses on learning the necessary skills and acquiring the knowledge to perform a job. For instance, learning to use a new sleep acquisition system is training. It is necessary to perform the job. Development focuses on preparing for a future job. Taking management classes although one is not a manager is an example of staff development. Staff development can be a part of the performance appraisal or independent of it.

Sleep center accreditation and professional registry and certification boards require continuing education. These education credits can be obtained from many sources, including vendor web sites, trade journals, vendors and their representatives, professional associations and registry examination board websites, and through workshops, seminars, courses, and company in-services.

The Multigenerational Staff

Today's workforce is more diverse than ever before. There may be up to five generations working in the same place, with generational characteristics that could prove to be challenging to a manager. Understanding these generational characteristics and developing tactics to help the staff work as a team is a must.

Traditionalists, born before 1945, are those who experienced the Great Depression and both World Wars. There are still a few of them in the workforce. They are hard workers and loyal to the company. They adhere to the rules and respect authority. They are team players. For them work is an obligation. Their satisfaction comes from doing a good job. They need to be respected. They are generally tech-challenged.

Baby Boomers, born between 1946 and 1965, are those who experienced television, the moon landing, the Vietnam War, Watergate, the Civil Rights Act, and other societal changes. They are workaholics, competitive, efficient, and they question authority and want quality. They are loyal to the company and desire job security and upward mobility, and they want money and recognition as the reward for their work. They need to be valued. Some in this group may be tech-challenged. They prefer communication to be face-to-face or by telephone.

Generation X, born between 1966 and 1977, are those who experienced MTV, Nintendo, and personal computers. They find work to be a difficult challenge. They are loyal to the profession but not to the company. They want independence and work–life balance. They want money and a firm financial footing for the future. They are skeptical. They are tech-savvy. They communicate by text and e-mail.

Generation Y, also known as Millennials, born between 1978 and 1995, are those who experienced diversity, natural disasters, and mobile technology. For them, work is a means to an end. They desire freedom, flexibility, and creativity in their work. They want meaningful work and they want to make a difference. They need continuous feedback. They are multitaskers. They are not loyal to the company. They change jobs frequently and are entrepreneurial. They are tech-savvy. They communicate by text, tweet, and instant message (IM) and are always connected.

Generation Z, born after 1995, have experienced global terrorism and economic downturn. They are multitaskers. They change jobs frequently and are entrepreneurial. They are not loyal to the company. They want a fun and flexible workplace, but they also want a clearly defined work structure. They are concerned about their financial and physical well-being. They are tech-savvy. They communicate by text, IM, tweets, and social media.

The manager of a multigenerational staff who understands the characteristics of each generation can improve productivity and the working environment in the sleep center. Some of the biggest challenges the manager faces are communication, team building, and generational stereotyping. These three challenges are interconnected, as it is hard to team-build if stereotyping and poor communication are rife in the sleep center. Encouraging each employee to communicate with his or her coworker in the manner that each employee values goes a long way toward building harmony and toward good teamwork. Having older and younger employees mentor each other in different ways (e.g., technologically vs. organizationally) provides a way for everyone to learn from one another. Giving good reasons for making changes avoids resentment and skepticism. The manager should intervene early when misunderstandings and generational judgments cause problems. The process of team building should involve respect of all staff by all staff, no matter the generation.

Evaluating Performance

Performance evaluations are critical for maintaining appropriate behaviors in the sleep center, providing feedback to employees about their work performance, providing an objective and legally defensible basis for merit raises and promotions, assessing training and staff development needs, guiding and motivating employees to improve job performance, and establishing a set of performance standards that are in line with sleep center values. These written reviews assess the employee's overall job performance on the basis of his or her job responsibilities and include an assessment of achievement, attendance, courteousness, and work ethic.

A good performance review format includes several key elements:

1. clear standards by which performance will be measured,
2. an appropriate rating scale (e.g., surpassed expectations, above expectations, achieved expectations, below expectations, and unacceptable),
3. space for written comments by the immediate supervisor,
4. space for employee self-appraisal,
5. objectives set by both employee and manager at the last evaluation and an accounting of the results,
6. objectives to be met by the next evaluation date, and
7. approvals by all levels of management involved in the process (e.g., supervisor, manager, physician, and HR personnel).

Both formal and informal methods of performance evaluations are used. Informal evaluations are conducted regularly throughout an appraisal year to provide timely feedback and address any performance deficiencies that may need attention long before the annual review. The formal review method is the annual performance evaluation used for compensation purposes.

Discipline

Discipline is an aspect of performance evaluation (7). It is used to shape the behavior of employees and is the road to corrective action. Sleep centers must have in place clear disciplinary standards and evidence that employees were given notice of them. This means that there are written policies and rules that have been communicated to all employees who have acknowledged that they have read and understood the policies and rules.

As much as managers would like for things to go well, there will always be a need for the disciplinary process. The reasons are varied, but employees may have behavioral problems, may not be adequately trained for the job, might not be challenged enough on the job, or may just be insubordinate. Nonetheless, the goal of the disciplinary process is to intervene early when conduct or job performance is not satisfactory. The consequence of managerial inaction is often poor morale among employees. The employee offender may become complacent about not meeting standards. Other employees may then start to emulate the offender, and all employees will eventually lose respect for the manager because of inaction, which can lead to even more problems related to discipline.

The disciplinary process should follow certain rules. These rules include early intervention, focusing on changing behavior, and maintaining privacy. Discipline must be administered fairly and impartially. The employee must be informed of the problem, must be told what to do to fix it, and must be given a reasonable period in which to do so. The employee must understand the consequences of inaction. Discipline must be progressive. It should never be punitive, unfair, or confrontational.

Progressive discipline traditionally follows a process of initial notification, verbal warning, written warning, suspension, and termination. Initial notification is just that—notifying the employee that there is a problem. The focus is on the problem, issue, or behavior, not on the employee. Maintaining the employee's basic self-esteem is a must. If there is no subsequent change in the offense or behavior, discipline progresses to a verbal warning. Verbal warnings are generally documented and placed in the employee file following a discussion with the employee. If the offense continues, the next step is a written warning.

The manager discusses the issue with the employee, outlines the steps necessary to correct it, and sets a timetable for improvement. The consequences of not making the necessary improvements are also spelled out. The employee and the manager should sign and date an acknowledgment of the warning; the employee's signature is not an acknowledgment that he or she agrees with the warning. If the written warning fails to correct the behavior, suspension is the next step. The length of

a suspension is based on the severity of the offense or a continued failure to meet previously indicated expectations. If there are multiple offenses, each suspension should be longer than the previous. Suspension should be unpaid as an incentive to correct behavior. When all else fails and the employee's performance and/or behavior fails to improve, termination may be necessary. However, termination must be defensible in a court of law. Therefore, documentation is very important. A termination interview should be brief, because the time for discussion is over. The employee must still be treated with dignity and respect. Be sensitive as to when the termination interview occurs; try to avoid terminating an employee on holidays, birthdays, Friday afternoons, and before or after a vacation.

As previously indicated, the disciplinary process should be fair and impartial. Policies must be fair and consistently administered among all employees. Two employees who commit the same offense cannot be treated differently. One method for ensuring fairness in the disciplinary process is following a grievance procedure, which includes the right of appeal. This process improves the perception of fairness when it is clearly communicated to all employees.

BUDGETING TIPS FOR THE SLEEP CENTER MANAGER

Good financial planning (budgeting) is essential to developing and maintaining a successful sleep program. The manager must consider budgetary components in a straightforward fashion.

Income is the money available to use to achieve the goals set forth by sleep center ownership. Consider the following when assessing income:

1. *Available beds:* Number of beds in the facility and number of beds available for sleep study scheduling (based on staffing). This will determine the maximum number of procedures possible.
2. *Determine occupancy rates:* Review historical data. Consider anticipated changes related to changes in the number of referring physicians (increasing or decreasing), payer mix, or changes in contracts and staffing availability.
3. *Examine payer data (reimbursement by insurance company):* Review a breakdown of insurance company payment schedules.
4. *Determine estimated income:* Multiply the number of studies predicted for each insurance carrier by the fee schedule. This calculation provides the estimated income for the budgeting year.
5. *Review other sources of income:* Additional income sources may include research projects, equipment validation studies, and so on.

EXPENSES

1. *Building or space rental expenses:* May include rent, mortgage payments, taxes, facility insurance premiums, and so on for the budget year.
2. *Personnel expenses:* Calculate the sum of expenses for all employees for the budget period. Don't forget to add benefit costs (vacation; paid sick time; medical, eye, and dental insurance, etc.). Personnel expenses are invariably one of the largest nonfixed costs related to operating a sleep center.
3. *Capital equipment costs:* Consider replacement costs for computers, software, beds, and audiovisual equipment. Each facility determines the price breakdown for determining what equipment is capital equipment. This point may be as low as $500 or as much as $5,000.
4. *Disposable costs:* Determine disposable costs by evaluating the cost of each piece of disposable equipment per study and how many disposables are used per patient and multiplying by predicted occupancy.
5. *Office equipment costs:* Determine the total costs of all office purchases, including computers not used for polysomnogram collection and scoring, fax machines, copiers, paper and ink/toner, CD/DVDs, even the pencils and paper clips.
6. *Other costs:* Costs for items such as food for multiple sleep latency test/maintenance of wakefulness test patients, breakfast for night patients, positive airway pressure masks dispensed to patients, and so on.

BUILDING NEW BUSINESS

Sleep technology is a fast growing and widely expanding field. Successful sleep centers grow to meet this need for services by adding the following:

- Beds
- Facilities
- Clinics
- Specialty durable medical equipment services
- Service contracts with other facilities/hospitals
- Research/equipment validation services
- Home sleep apnea testing (HSAT)

Start-up costs, maintenance costs, and expected income are evaluated separately. A data review is essential. When a financial history is not available to assess, a reasonable estimation of costs and anticipated revenue becomes critical. Consider that new business ventures may not be immediately profitable. Be prepared to provide predicted time to profit with justification/validation for administration or the finance department.

With rare exceptions, income must exceed costs. No matter how dedicated one may be to the idea that the patient comes first, no facility can stay open for long without generating a profit. If your estimates, after completing a cost/income analysis, indicate costs exceed income, what do you do? Review your data carefully, and develop plans, ideas, and suggestions for changes that may make the proposal profitable before meeting with finance. Provide input that shows your subject matter expertise and skill and commitment as a leader.

Here are some strategies to consider in the financial arena:

Building or sleep center space costs:

- Unless moving the sleep facility is a viable option, building/facility costs are fixed.

Personnel:

- Review and evaluate proposed staffing, scheduling, and workflow processes.
- Eliminate overtime.
- Reduce staff.
- Make patient/staff schedules more efficient.
  - Consider using a setup tech (switching a 12-hour employee for an 8-hour employee). This employee may be able to assist with other duties when not caring for patients, such as scoring, restocking, equipment management, scheduling, and so on.
  - Consider assigning additional duties to night staff, such as scoring.
  - Consider reducing or eliminating employee benefits (use per diem staff).

Patient volumes:

- Assess the reasons for reductions in patient volume.
- Review referral sources.
- Recruit new referring physicians or physician groups.
- Consider insurance company negotiations; a small reduction in cost may increase the number of referrals to your center.
- Insufficient staff.
  - Train additional technical staff.
  - Utilize a temp service.
  - Reevaluate staffing needs and reorganize if possible (i.e., move a day person to nights).
- Review changes in reimbursement.
- Negotiate with major payers.

Equipment (capital and noncapital):

- Postpone purchase of costly equipment; explore less expensive options.
- Assess options for disposable equipment and sensors.
- Consider using nondisposable equipment and sensors (assuming this is less expensive).

- Investigate a more cost-effective way to archive studies.
- Look for opportunities to reduce office equipment expenditures.
- Review all costs (i.e., food for patients and coffee for technologists) and determine if they are essential.
- Consider that small savings add up when volume is taken into account.

New business:

- Is this the best time to start a new venture?
- Can better planning for a new venture reduce start-up costs?
- Will a proposal for new business improve your current financial situation?

All facilities, whether hospitals, medical centers, or independent diagnostic and treatment facilities, vary in the financial information they compile, review, and report. The information provided is intended as a general outline of typical financial procedures.

SUMMARY

A sleep center manager works under the general supervision of the medical director and/or a senior administrator to manage the operations of a sleep program. The manager oversees operations related to in-center and HSAT, diagnostic and therapeutic interventions, comprehensive patient care, and direct patient education.

Ideally, the sleep center manager is credentialed in sleep technology. The manager provides oversight of sleep center staff and is responsible for ensuring that staff adheres to the accepted standards for the evaluation, testing, and treatment of patients in the sleep program.

REFERENCES

1. Cottrell, D., & Adams, A. (2006). *The next level: Leading beyond the status quo.* Dallas, TX: Cornerstone Leadership Institute.
2. Griffin, R. (2005). *Management* (8th ed.). New York, NY: Houghton Mifflin.
3. American Academy of Sleep Medicine. (2018). *Standards for accreditation.* Retrieved from: https://j2v-jt3dnbra3ps7ll1clb4q2-wpengine.netdna-ssl.com/wp-content/uploads/2018/04/accreditationstandards.pdf
4. Arthur, D. (2006). *Recruiting, interviewing, selecting & orienting new employees* (4th ed., pp. 332–336). New York, NY: Amazon.
5. Fry, R. (2006). *Ask the right questions hire the best people* (pp. 52–58). Franklin Lakes, NJ: Career Press.
6. Davila, L., & Kursmark, L. (2005). *How to choose the right person for the right job every time* (pp. 111–120). New York, NY: McGraw-Hill.
7. Buhler, P. (2002). *Streetwise human resources management* (pp. 211–215). Avon, OH: Adams Media Corporation.

chapter 69
Sleep Center Policies and Procedures

ROBIN E. FOSTER

LEARNING OBJECTIVES

On completion of this chapter, the reader should be able to:

1. Recognize the regulatory bodies that require policies and procedures.
2. Define the difference between a policy and a procedure.
3. Describe an alignment continuum.
4. Identify core processes.
5. Determine the number of policy and procedure manuals needed and the relative content material.
6. Utilize guidelines for when a policy needs to be written.
7. Recognize the value of policies and procedures.

KEY TERMS

Accreditation
Accreditation Commission for Health Care
Alignment continuum
American Academy of Sleep Medicine (AASM)
American Association of Sleep Technologists (AAST)
Core processes
Mission statement
Occupational Safety and Health Administration (OSHA)
Strategic plan
Joint Commission (JC)
Vision

Policies and procedures are essential to management and are fundamental to the operation of a sleep center. They are the handbook of operations for managers and employees. They convey the correct work processes for a sleep center that lead to quality services. Everyone needs to know what to do and how to do it. Policies and procedures provide this knowledge for all members of the staff. They include a wide array of applications and vary in degree of specificity. Applications may range from acquisition of supplies to following emergency protocols. Good policies and procedures provide insight into what management believes is important. They define expectations of employees, purpose of these expectations, and consequences of failure to abide by them (1). Consequently, they are used as a measure of employee performance.

Policies and procedures are critical to the evaluation of regulatory compliance because regulatory standards and subsequent levels of compliance are often measured against policies and procedures. The American Academy of Sleep Medicine (AASM) requires specific policies and procedures to be in place for accreditation as do other accrediting organizations such as the Joint Commission (JC) and the Accreditation Commission for Health Care. These organizations set standards for operations and assess compliance for accreditation. When a sleep center is accredited by one of these health care agencies, it is because they have met or exceeded standards of quality imposed upon them by these organizations. Reimbursement for services rendered by sleep centers also depends upon accreditation, especially Medicare.

There is a difference between policies and procedures, but they go hand in hand. Policies define the standards employed for the strategic direction of operations in order to reach goals. They state management's position on a situation, action, or behavior. They are a set of guidelines and rules. Procedures are the specific processes employed to express policies in action for day-to-day operations and to achieve the standards of an organization, resulting in the highest quality of patient care (2). For the most part, a procedure will serve as an adjunct to policy; however, not every policy will require a written procedure. These documents provide direction, guidance, and accountability and are a reflection of the organization's culture. By utilizing policies and procedures, the sleep center will operate with greater efficiency and staff members will have a defined sense of purpose.

ALIGNMENT CONTINUUM

Every organization has a reason for its existence, a sense of purpose. When such a purpose is put on paper, it is iterated as a mission statement. Because goals and objectives progress naturally from the knowledge of why an organization exists, a mission statement provides a sense of direction. In the absence of this direction, decisions and their consequences can drive an organization down the road to failure.

A *mission statement* is the beginning of a policy and procedure manual and serves as a reference to determine the core processes within the written policy. It is the essence of an organization's vision, values, and strategic goals. Writing effective policies and procedures can be challenging if these elements of business have not been defined because the direction of the organization is vague and subsequent management expectations are undefined. The mission of the American Association of Sleep Technologists (AAST), "AAST provides education, resources and advocacy, and leads sleep-care professionals to be the most knowledgeable in the field resulting in the highest quality of care for patients," illustrates this nicely.

Alignment continuum is a term used to describe the relationship between the mission, vision, values, and strategic goals and subsequent core processes. The individual(s) responsible for developing the policy and procedure documents should work to understand the elements of the alignment continuum to ensure continuity with the policies and procedures.

The purpose of the *vision* is to determine whether the direction of the sleep center and its current scope of practice accurately reflect the direction of the organization. The vision captures an organization's purpose and values and embodies the future of the organization. The vision of the AAST, "AAST will play a key role in setting the standard for professional excellence in the evolving practice of sleep healthcare," illustrates this focus on direction.

The *strategic plan* outlines the goals and priorities of the sleep center and assures they are consistent with the direction and focus of the organization. The strategic plan is the road map to accomplish the vision.

Core processes are essential business functions for the organization. There are two types of core processes: operational and clinical. In a sleep center, operational processes establish rules for running the center. Clinical processes regulate patient care. Core processes require a definite course of action or policy. Policies and procedures support these processes and provide a framework for planning, action, and decision making for management and employees. Many core processes for sleep centers have already been identified, so much so that defined supporting policies and procedures are required for accreditation. For instances where there is no precedent, the process of identifying core processes or essential business functions is necessary.

DEVELOPING POLICY AND PROCEDURE MANUALS

Essential business functions can be determined from areas of management that are included in an organizational chart. The manual title represents one of the organization's essential functions (e.g., human resources). If the sleep center is a hospital-based facility, the sleep professional may only need to be concerned with the development of a single manual specific to the operations and core processes of the department. Conversely, a freestanding sleep center typically operates independently and the sleep professional will need to ensure that manuals for all the essential business functions are developed. Careful consideration needs to be given to the number of business functions identified. The fewer manuals that exist, the easier it will be to manage the set of policies and procedures developed to create a desired outcome. The process of development begins the moment a policy topic is selected and is complete only after the document has been distributed and employees have been trained.

References and resources for developing policy and procedure manuals for a sleep center are available online. They include generic templates and downloadable word documents. There are businesses that assist with or develop policies and procedures for sleep centers, as well as online policy and procedures available from established institutions. The JC provides a "standards sampler" pertaining to sleep centers (3). The more specific resources are those available from the AAST and AASM. The AAST offers a manual of policy and procedure templates for sleep centers and a policy and procedure manual for home sleep apnea testing programs (4). The AASM *Accreditation Reference Manual* (5) was created to assist sleep centers in the development of a policy and procedure manual in conjunction with their accreditation.

Another very important regulatory reference and resource for developing policies and procedures is the United States Department of Labor Occupational Health and Safety (OSH) Act (6). Under the Occupational Safety and Health Administration (OSHA) law, employers are responsible for providing a safe and healthful work environment. No manual is complete without established policies and procedures that are in compliance with the employer responsibilities established by the OSHA.

The format for a manual does not have to be printed paper in three-ring binders. Technology has opened the door to online policy and procedure manuals. An electronic format facilitates management of updating and revising content. It also makes it easier for employees to access information by entering key words (7). Whatever format used, it must be kept up-to-date and readily available.

Policies

Policies should be written in plain English, without legal jargon, and in sync with the concepts of the mission statement. When properly aligned with the mission statement, policies will enable the vision and direction of the organization. They are more focused than the mission statement and provide the basis for the code of conduct employed internally within the organization and externally with entities outside the organization.

Policies focus on the rules and regulations of the organization. There are operational and clinical policies. In a sleep center, operational policies regulate the manner of functioning of the sleep center. Consider personnel policies as an example, specifically, a policy pertaining to paid time off (PTO). The policy may indicate the criteria necessary to approve PTO requests. It may also specify how PTO hours are accrued, the maximum PTO hours allowed, and/or whether or not PTO hours could be carried over subsequent years. Other operational policies can include:

- patient acceptance criteria
- method for tracking direct referrals
- verification of insurance
- protecting the privacy and security of patient information
- scheduling of patients
- organization of medical charts
- establishing a quality assurance program and means for monitoring outcomes
- establishing and maintaining a database
- dress code for employees
- recording required employee continuing education
- requirements for attendance at staff meetings
- maintenance of equipment and electrical safety

Clinical policies regulate patient care. Examples of clinical policies are:

- patient education
- practice parameters for all test protocols
- administration of oxygen
- when to contact the physician during a sleep study
- interscorer reliability
- documentation of patient evaluation/management and positive airway pressure assessments.

The policy section of the sample policy and procedure in Figure 69-1 (8–10) provides the general guidelines for performing a split-night study.

Without policy, a recurring situation can take on a life of its own and become "company policy" by virtue of its recurrence; or worse, it may take a life of its own with the refrain, "That's not our policy." Policies are written to clarify the rules of an organization and to ensure a safe, organized, convivial, empowering, and nondiscriminatory workplace for employees and safe, clinically sound environment for patients.

The following guidelines indicate when a policy is needed:

- if the actions of the employees indicate confusion about the most appropriate way to behave (dress codes, e-mail and Internet policies, and cell phone use)
- if guidance is needed about the most suitable way to handle various situations (standards of conduct, travel expenditures, and purchase of sleep center merchandise)
- when needed to protect the sleep center legally (consistent investigation of charges of harassment, nondiscriminatory hiring, and promotion)
- to keep the sleep center in compliance with government policies and laws (e.g., American Disabilities Act, Minimum Wage Act, Affordable Care Act)
- to establish consistent work standards, rules, and regulations (progressive discipline, safety rules, break rules, and smoking rules)
- to provide consistent and fair treatment for employees (benefits eligibility, PTO, bereavement time, and jury duty).

There are additional reasons to develop a policy. Remember, one employee's poor behavior does not require a policy that will affect all employees.

Identifying the appropriate individuals to write and approve policy is crucial. In a hospital setting, the human resources department writes the policies that define appropriate behavior of hospital employees and hospital benefits for employees. The department manager writes operational and clinical policies and procedures specifically for the sleep center. Input from the staff members in this process is invaluable. Their involvement assists management in ensuring that all policies needed exist and increases employee compliance. These policies are approved by hospital administration and the medical director. In a freestanding sleep center, the manager writes the policy and the medical director approves it.

Procedures

A procedure details the implementation of a policy. It is a series of steps with a specific order that are sufficiently detailed to guide the performance of the policy. The procedure section of the sample policy and procedure in Figure 69-1 provides specific guidelines for performing a split-night study.

Policies and procedures provide specific instructions for employees. Well-written procedure documents state explicitly who is supposed to do what and how it is to be done. Consequently, there is less room for misunderstanding and subsequent discord. When misunderstandings occur, and disparity exists between employees or between an employer and employee, policies and procedures provide a reference for clarification and problem solving. Sometimes, legal resolution of a situation is needed. The first course of action to be pursued by legal counsel in a labor dispute is a review of the policies and procedures. Employees are required to

Sleep Facility Policy and Procedure

TITLE: Split-Night Study Guidelines

ORIGINAL DATE:	EFFECTIVE DATE:
REVIEW DATE(s):	REVISION DATE(s):
APPROVAL(s):	
SIGNATURE:	TITLE: Medical Director
SIGNATURE:	TITLE: Sleep Facility Manager
SIGNATURE:	TITLE:

To provide a process to combine the diagnostic and positive airway pressure (PAP) titration portions of the evaluation process. A split-night titration encompasses both continuous PAP and bilevel PAP titration processes.

Split-night studies require that specific requirements are met during the diagnostic portion of the study in order to initiate PAP therapy. Technologists must fit the PAP interface and perform patient teaching prior to lights out, explaining to the patient that PAP therapy may be instituted during the night if the requirements for a split-night study procedure are met.

This policy provides the American Academy of Sleep Medicine (AASM) guidelines for initiating PAP during a diagnostic study and Centers for Medicare and Medicaid Services (CMS) requirement for initiating PAP for home use. The sleep facility medical director may designate adjustments in criteria indicated below.

AASM criteria for initiating PAP during a diagnostic study:
A minimum of 2 hours of diagnostic recording is required.
A minimum of 3 hours of titration time is required.
The titration procedure should be identical to the full night titration protocol.
PAP may be increased at larger increments (2 to 2.5 cm H_2O) during a split-night titration.
Initiate PAP when an apnea–hypopnea index (AHI) >40 per hour is documented during 2 hours of diagnostic recording time OR when an AHI of 20 to 40 per hour is documented and is accompanied by clinical symptoms.

CMS criteria for initiating PAP for home use:
AHI or respiratory disturbance index is >15 events per hour, with a minimum of 2 hours for sleep time OR
AHI is <14 accompanied by clinical symptoms including:

• Excessive daytime sleepiness		
• Impaired cognition	OR	• Hypertension
• Mood disorder		• Ischemic heart disease
• Insomnia		• History of stroke

References
1. Department of Health and Human Services & Centers for Medicare & Medicaid Services. (2016, October). *Positive airway pressure (PAP) devices: Complying with documentation & coverage requirements.*
2. Kapur, V. K., Auckley, D. H., Chowdhuri, S., et al. (2017). Clinical practice guideline for diagnostic testing for adult sleep obstructive apnea: An American Academy of Sleep Medicine clinical practice guideline. *Journal of Clinical Sleep Medicine, 13*(3), 479–504.
3. Medicare Coverage with Evidence Development 1/240.4/ Continuous Positive Airway Pressure (CPAP) Therapy of Obstructive Sleep Apnea (OSA) (March 18, 2015).

Figure 69-1 Sample policy and procedure.

read the entire policy and procedure manual and sign a statement saying they have done so, which will avoid confusion later.

A policy and procedure manual is a reference manual that answers employees' questions. In the sleep center environment, a staff technologist is responsible for data acquisition, patient titrations, and data analysis (scoring). When procedures are communicated to those involved, processes can begin to ensure compliance and accountability for assigned responsibilities.

Policies and procedures define roles and responsibilities and complement the performance expectations outlined in a program's job descriptions. The role of management becomes more efficient when written guidance and direction are established and communicated for operations that occur on an ongoing basis. They give employees defined expectations of their employer.

SUMMARY

Great sleep centers do not just happen, nor do they just stay great. The successful sleep center is made up of individually successful people who do the right things at the right time under the right circumstances. Policies and procedures provide direction for decisions that are made by management and the parameters within which employees can make appropriate judgments. They are a set of documents that establish guidelines for operations, facilitate training of employees, provide a resource for decision making, and promote consistency in delivery of services. Effective policies and procedures are critical to developing competent technical staff, building professionalism, and creating and maintaining a successful sleep center.

REFERENCES

1. Bizfluent. (2018). *What is the difference between a policy & a procedure?* Retrieved from https://bizfluent.com/about-5100532-difference-between-policy-procedure.html. Accessed January 18, 2019.
2. Business Dictionary. (2018). *Policies and procedures.* Retrieved from www.businessdictionary.com/definition/policies-and-procedures.html. Accessed February 2018.
3. The Joint Commission. (2018). *Standards sampler—Sleep centers.* Retrieved from www.joincommission.org
4. American Association of Sleep Technologists. (2018). Retrieved from https://members.aastweb.org/page/online-store. Accessed January 18, 2019.
5. American Academy of Sleep Medicine. (2018). *Accreditation reference manual.* Retrieved from https://learn.aasm.org/Public/Catalog/Details.aspx?id=ZJW6GtHl1fvPCsnGBtnu1Q%3d%3d&returnurl=%2fUsers%2fUserOnlineCourse.aspx%3fLearningActivityID%3dZJW6GtHl1fvPCsnGBtnu1Q%253d%253d. Accessed January 18, 2019.
6. Occupational Safety and Health Administration. (2018). *Employer responsibilities.* Retrieved from https://www.osha.gov/as/opa/worker/employer-responsibility.html. Accessed January 18, 2019.
7. Hamlett, C. (2017). *How to write an office procedures manual.* Retrieved from https://bizfluent.com/how-6241242-write-office-procedures-manual.html. Accessed January 18, 2019.
8. Department of Health and Human Services & Centers for Medicare & Medicaid Services. (October 2016). *Positive airway pressure (PAP) devices: Complying with documentation & coverage requirements.* Retrieved from https://www.cms.gov/Outreach-and-Education/Medicare-Learning-Network-MLN/MLNProducts/downloads/pap_doccvg_factsheet_icn905064.pdf. Accessed January 18, 2019.
9. Kapur, V. K., Auckley, D. H., Chowdhuri, S., et al. (2017). Clinical practice guideline for diagnostic testing for adult sleep obstructive apnea: An American Academy of Sleep Medicine clinical practice guideline. *Journal of Clinical Sleep Medicine, 13*(3), 479–504.
10. Medicare Coverage with Evidence Development 1/240.4/ Continuous Positive Airway Pressure (CPAP) Therapy of Obstructive Sleep Apnea (OSA) (March 18, 2015). Retrieved from https://www.cms.gov/Medicare/Coverage/Coverage-with-Evidence-Development/Continuous-Positive-Airway-Pressure-CPAP-Therapy-For-Obstructive-Sleep-Apnea-OSA-2404.html. Accessed January 18, 2019.

RECOMMENDED READINGS

American Academy of Sleep Medicine. (2017). *Accreditation reference manual (2016) standards.* Westchester, IL: Author.

Occupational Safety and Health Administration. (2017). *OHSA: Compliance guide for medical employers* (14th ed.). Rock Island, IL: Blue Gavel Press.

Page, S. B. (2002). *Establishing a system of policies and procedures.* Westerville, OH: Process Improvement.

Page, S. B. (2016). *Writing effective and successful policies and procedures.* Westerville, OH: Author.

chapter 70

Ethics and Professionalism

ROBYN V. WOIDTKE

LEARNING OBJECTIVES

On completion of this chapter, the reader should be able to:

1. Explain the concepts of professionalism and how the sleep technologist is viewed in the field of allied health.
2. Discuss the contributions of a sleep technologist.
3. Describe the educational aspects of a profession.
4. Assess the implications of social media use for the sleep technologist.

KEY TERMS

Professionalism
Sleep center
Competency
Ethics
Social media

According to the Institute of Medicine (1), sleep disorders and deprivation are considered a public health issue, and as such, sleep technologists not only need to understand professionalism from a personal perspective, but also need to have a sense of how professionalism is encompassed within the field of sleep medicine, as part of a health care organization and the public at large (2).

The field of sleep technology is changing. We now must include in our thinking such aspects of care as wearables (home apnea testing, consumer goods), social media, and incorporating person-centered care. However, our main focus remains unchanged; we watch and monitor individuals while they sleep. In addition, we have a responsibility to shepherd our patients through their therapeutic journey by educating and providing supportive care.

Unlike any other allied health care field, the role and duties of the sleep technologist establish an interesting and unique relationship with patients. The profession is based on an intrusion into a facet of life where few are allowed to enter, with the exception of an occasional health care provider, family, and bed partners. Since patients who are undergoing a sleep study place them in a vulnerable situation, that is, they are sleeping, professional conduct cannot be emphasized enough. Accordingly, patient privacy and welfare must be considered at all times. This fact alone requires additional insight and mindfulness into how we conduct ourselves professionally and ethically. For all health care professionals, conducting themselves with the highest moral and ethical standards and performing their jobs with the utmost care should be paramount (3).

When considering what it means to be a "professional," one might contemplate levels of education, stature within the community, membership in an organization, or employment. These domains are further influenced by culture, personal background, religion, life experiences, and moral and ethical foundations. Being a "health care professional" should optimally include tenets of professionalism. The term *professionalism* takes many forms and can be expressed in many ways. Nevertheless, most of the definitions embrace the foundation of professionalism, which is formed against a backdrop of trust and putting the patient first (4). This term is also encompassed in standards, certification, and licensure (5).

A recent article by Wynia et al. (6) discusses that professionalism is more than just a list of preferred attributes and behaviors to be checked off or measured. They suggest that the goal of professionalism is "ensuring that health professionals are worthy of patient and public trust." They further discuss that the basis of such lists, while they exist, are extensions of the fundamental beliefs that come with the medical profession.

The constructs of professionalism range from simple personal attire to the complex realm of moral and ethical principles. Professionalism can be as uncomplicated as the way by which we greet a patient coming to the sleep disorders center or as multifaceted as our ethical responses to difficult situations; in essence, it is the "social contract" of the conduct of professional interactions, whether a colleague, patient, or family member.

PROFESSIONAL AND HEALTH CARE ORGANIZATIONS

Professional organizations or associations exist for almost every type of group, from craftspeople to the health professional. Nevertheless, the majority of medical professional organizations have no legal jurisdiction, and thus practice under a "self-governing" structure (7). The American Medical Association (AMA) discussed the importance of medical associations as the following: "their conferences, continuing medical education courses, practice guidelines, definitions of ethical norms, and public advocacy positions carry great weight with physicians and the public" (8). It is important to realize that the organization or association is there to protect not only its members but also the public. Moreover, while the AMA does not specifically address the associations in allied health fields, theoretically the same applies.

A professional organization is created by and for people who have a common interest to come together for a common goal, a community. Research indicates that most professional organizations begin with a small core group of committed and enthusiastic individuals in an informal meeting. The ad hoc informal meeting generates a desire to create and carry on a more formal organization. As the organization begins to take form, it begins to define the scope of the profession, standards of practice, and professional guidelines and to create opportunities for education and camaraderie (9).

Hence, the organization provides the foundation from which the profession matures and develops. Although the organization provides an infrastructure that defines the profession, it is up to the individual to remain professionally competent, a component of professionalism. This is accomplished through continuing education, recertification, or ongoing demonstration of competency and daily on-the-job conduct.

Egener et al. (10) state that health care organizations also have a duty to their employees and the public to ensure that professionalism is at the core of its mission. They further state that lack of clarity at the organizational level impacts the ability of the physician to follow the 2002 medical professionalism charter. Organizational professionalism has also been demonstrated to improve the physician moral, improve the trust of the people, and improve the safety and quality of care (11).

WHAT IS PROFESSIONALISM?

The term *professional* connotes knowledge and professional behaviors that are known as professionalism. Brennan and Monson (4) state, "Professionalism is an indispensable element in the compact between the medical profession and society that is based on trust and putting the needs of patients above all other considerations." The sleep technologist must have a fundamental belief that this statement is also true for them and be able to integrate this type of thinking into their professional lives.

The National Board of Medical Examiners (12) has a program directed toward education and evaluation of professional behaviors. To that end, they have developed specific criteria of professional behaviors. Table 70-1 lists the behaviors and gives examples of how those behaviors can be exhibited. As noted earlier, lists are not something just to be checked off but can be used to teach and provide an opportunity to review personal values and conduct.

Although everyone in every profession should exhibit professionalism, it is imperative that the health care professionals practice behavior that is above reproach. They must not only be aware of their own morals and values but have the ability to separate their personal beliefs from their field of practice when cultural and religious values differ from their own, which includes patient autonomy and the right of patients to make their own decisions (13). In some instances, this may create inner conflict, but they must still behave in a professional manner while conducting their jobs.

The fundamental principles of professionalism, as published in 2002 in the *Annals of Internal*

Table 70-1	Categories of Professional Behavior with Examples
Altruism	Contributes to the profession; helps others in the workplace
Honor and integrity	Forthcoming with information; does not withhold information for power; admits errors
Responsibility and accountability	Accountable for deadlines; arrives on time; takes responsibility for their share of the workload
Excellence in scholarship	Masters techniques and technologies in learning; has internal focus and direction; setting own goals
Respect	Respects patients and staff; demonstrates tolerance for a range of behaviors and beliefs
Leadership	Teaches others; perpetuates a culture of professionalism
Caring and compassion	Treats the patient as an individual; supports a balance between work and home with peers and subordinates

Adapted with permission from the National Board of Medical Examiners.

Medicine, are primacy of patient welfare, patient autonomy, and social justice (14). These principles go hand in hand with such responsibilities as commitment to professional competency, honesty with patients, patient confidentiality, appropriateness of relationships, improving quality of care, and improving access to care.

Volunteerism, Social Media, and Leadership

Additional aspects of professionalism occur outside of our conduct within the sleep center. It is important for technologists to be active in their communities. Volunteering not only enhances their professional and personal growth but also provides another avenue to increase their visibility as sleep technologists within their local communities. By networking outside of their "sleep silo," they are demonstrating to others that their profession is important, while creating a new awareness of the impact that sleep deprivation and disorders have on our society.

The proliferation of social media in today's society requires that health care professionals remain professional in their postings. It is beyond the scope of this chapter to adequately address this topic. However, it is important to remember that in addition to patient issues, the sleep technologist should be concerned with ethical behavior, personal–professional boundaries, confidentiality, and professional image (15).

Personal and professional ethics encompass many facets of behavior. Doing good as opposed to harm, showing concern for the well-being of others, preventing harm to your patients, being honest and respectful to patients and others, and respecting the autonomy of others demonstrate personal ethical behavior.

Professional ethics are demonstrated by such traits as impartiality and openness. Being faithful to your duty to your patient, meeting your professional responsibilities, keeping your patient's information confidential, and providing information objectively and with care are important aspects of professionalism. As a health care professional one is expected to always treat patients with impartiality, and faithfully complete all professional duties.

The sleep technologist has a legal and ethical responsibility to maintain patient privacy and confidentiality, fully understand the terms of agreement on social networking sites (i.e., postings can be copied or moved), and follow the same organizational policies required in everyday practice (16). There may also be restrictions on using employer-owned computers (15, 17). A quote from the Mayo Clinic summarizes our obligations to patients and good practices with regard to social media: "Don't Lie, Don't Pry, Don't Cheat, Can't Delete, Don't Steal, Don't Reveal" (18).

Professionalism also requires that we become leaders. Transformational leadership includes such concepts as establishing a vision, raising motivation, instilling pride, confidence building, and empowering others (19). In today's chaotic world of health care reform and changes in which sleep medicine is being transformed, much of this is out of our control; nonetheless, this requires action and a plan for sleep technologists to survive and thrive.

It is important for the leaders of today to provide the vision for tomorrow by actively committing and engaging in this transformation. One such activity would be to ensure that the voice of the sleep technologist is heard in relation to sleep health and technologic advances. Today's leadership can ensure that sleep technologists are a vital part of this change, thereby safeguarding that expertise in this specialized field is not phased out and an ongoing commitment to quality and continuity of care is realized. It is important for the profession to be involved when policy and politics are being considered with regard to our field, such as school start times, commercial safe driving practices, and workplace hours. In this way, these professionals maintain input and the ability to negotiate (19). If the profession is not represented, their voices will not be heard or considered.

MORAL AND ETHICAL BEHAVIOR

Most individuals are taught the difference between right and wrong during their childhood years. The concept of right and wrong provides the foundation of ethical and moral behavior. These are the behaviors that are accepted among society as the correct way to behave and are socially acceptable.

As we mature, we glean the experience to understand that often things are not black and white. As described in Reynolds and Ceranic (20), Rest's four-stage model of moral decision making contributes to responses to situations. These include awareness of the moral issue, making a moral judgment, intention to act morally, and then finally to engage in moral behavior. Our ability to make such decisions and use our life experiences helps us to develop our professional behavior. Health care professionals should be aware of the moral and ethical landscape used within the medical field, and should issues arise, one can confer with others within their profession or consult a standing ethics committee as a sounding board.

As health care professionals, we often struggle with issues that other professions do not have. We deal with individuals who may be in the midst of a health care crisis, who cannot afford treatment, or who do not have adequate transportation to attend to health matters. Because most people are vulnerable during such times, we must show extra consideration to these individuals and in every situation treat all persons with respect and dignity (21).

Certainly, there is a vast array of interpretation of ethical behavior; it is a complex study where many issues, thoughts, feelings, culture, personal beliefs, and the community at large come into play. However, for the majority of people, the golden rule still stands: as we go about our workday, we should question ourselves; are we treating others as we would wish to be treated given the same situation?

In the recent past, our society has been subject to a disturbing lack of ethical behavior in many sectors of business, spanning from banks and the entertainment industry to health care. Inappropriate behaviors by chief executive officers, religious leaders, and other prominent community leaders have increased the spotlight on appropriate ethical and moral behavior (22). Ethical leadership can be defined as "the demonstration of normatively appropriate conduct through personal actions and interpersonal relationships, and the promotion of such conduct to followers through two-way communication, reinforcement, and decision-making" (23). The sleep technologist can use these experiences and information to further define their behavior in the context of the world around them.

Since ethical behavior plays such a large role in professionalism as a condition of employment, places of employment, government, and professional organizations are now requiring ethics training and providing ethics guidelines for employees and/or members. In his article, "A Framework for Universal Principles for Ethics," Larry Colero of the Crossroads Program (24) separates personal, professional, and global ethics. By separating them, one can observe how the different areas build and interact upon each other (Table 70-2).

It is rightly expected that health care professionals maintain the highest rigor of ethical and moral standards. There must be an empathetic approach and a high regard for the frailties of the human race. Ethical treatment of patients, kindness, and a high degree of responsibility should become a natural part of conducting oneself as a member of the allied health profession.

Ethical behavior is linked to our values and morals. According to Frank Navran (25), our values are the principles by which we decide what is right and wrong and what is good and bad. Values can be divided into three areas: moral, pragmatic, and esthetic. As it relates to a profession, we would more likely be concerned with moral and pragmatic values. These encompass such ideals as fairness, truth, justice, health, and thrift.

As a cornerstone of ethical practice, communication is an essential component of professionalism; this includes communication with other health care team members, patients, and their families. Communication includes respect for person and their autonomy,

	Common Guidelines for the Use of Social Media by Health Care Table 70-2 Professionals	
Context	**Concept**
Content credibility	Share only information from credible sources. Refute any inaccurate information you encounter.
Legal concerns	Remember that the content you author may be discoverable. Comply with federal and state privacy laws. Respect copyright laws.
Licensing concerns	Know professional licensure requirements for your state.
Networking practices	Do not contact patients with requests to join your network. Direct patients who want to join your personal network to a more secure means of communication or to your professional site.
Patient care	Avoid providing specific medical advice to nonpatients. Make appropriate disclosures and disclaimers regarding the accuracy, timeliness, and privacy of electronic communications.
Patient privacy	Avoid writing about specific patients. Make sure you are in compliance with state and federal privacy laws. Obtain patient consent when required. Protect patient information through "deidentification." Use a respectful tone when discussing patients.
Personal privacy	Use the most secure privacy settings available. Keep personal and professional profiles separate.
Professional ethics	Disclose any in-kind or financial compensation received. Do not make false or misleading claims.
Self-identification	Identify yourself on professional sites. Make sure that your credentials are correctly stated. Specify whether or not you are representing an employer.

From Ventola, C. L. (2014). Social media and health care professionals: Benefits, risks, and best practices. *Pharmacy and Therapeutics, 39*(7), 491–499.

appropriate forms of communication that are individually tailored, and assessment of comprehension (26).

CODES OF CONDUCT

Most professional organizations have an ethical code of conduct by which their members abide. Our field has similarly created and adopted such a code. In most instances, codes of ethics or professional behaviors are drafted by committees and agreed upon by members. This is the case for the American Association of Sleep Technologists (AAST) membership. The AAST has created a standard of practice (27) that identifies not only the levels of competence but also the associated professional behaviors. Standards of practice become the root of conduct for the sleep technologist professional, from which individual codes may be adopted.

Unlike other allied health professions, sleep technologists provide a unique aspect of patient care. Accordingly, in view of the fact that we work at night, sometimes by ourselves, and possibly in remote areas, the technologist must not veer from the ethical standards and codes of conduct regardless of the circumstance.

PATIENT AND PUBLIC SAFETY AND LEGAL CONCERNS

We must concern ourselves not only with our personal behavior but also with the health and welfare of our patients and society in general. As an example, we must understand the implications of public safety if a patient's excessive sleepiness may cause harm to others and respond accordingly (5). As an allied sleep health professional within the health care community, we have a duty to aid in the continuum of care for the patient, with physicians, social services, durable medical equipment providers, and others as appropriate. It is vital that we work together as a team to ensure that appropriate initiation of therapy and follow-up is conducted (2). As many sleep disorders are considered chronic, it becomes even more imperative that coordination of care includes principles of chronic care management, use of evidence-based practices, and a commitment to remain current in our knowledge.

SUM OF MANY PARTS

Professionalism is the sum of many parts—personal experience, culture, religion, education, and skills. Professional behaviors extend beyond the job; they must be evident in all we do and how we conduct ourselves. The AAST (27) has provided the technologist community with a "Scope of Practice" position statement. This document can provide the technologist a foundation of behaviors and skills, which form the profession.

Professionalism can also lead to improved patient satisfaction. This is important on many levels. When patients have a good experience, they are more likely to feel confident and have more trust in the people who care for them, thus when a technologist greets a patient, educates them, and treats them with respect and dignity, the patient and facility both reap the rewards (28).

The professional conduct practiced by thousands of sleep technologists is ongoing proof that, as individuals and an organization of allied health care workers, they have endorsed a high level of ethical and responsible conduct and understand what that means to how they practice day to day.

Being a professional also means contributing to your field by leading and engaging in educational and organizational pursuits and scholarship. The contributions that sleep technologists have made to the field of sleep medicine are incalculable, and they should not be discounted. For without the sleep technologist, many of the techniques that are now used would not exist, and our knowledge about sleep and its many disorders would not be as complete. Together with physicians and scientific teams, technologists have made important inroads into the understanding of sleep and its disorders.

Outside of the sleep laboratory, sleep technologists have continued to contribute to the education of legislators, teachers, and those in other health-related fields. Some of these activities include organizing and participating in local, state, and national efforts toward the recognition of sleep disorders as a major health problem. Technologists are ongoing advocates of patient education and awareness. Most technologists are familiar with the A.W.A.K.E. (alert, well, and keeping energetic) Network. The A.W.A.K.E. Network was originally created and established by a sleep technologist, Lucy Seger, in the 1980s (29). The ongoing commitment of technologists to patient advocacy is demonstrated by the numerous activities that occur locally and nationally.

In addition, technologists have been instrumental in working with national, state, and local legislative matters to increase sleep awareness among our political leaders. Sleep technologists have aggressively participated in grassroots efforts, including obtaining funding and initiating legislative activities, to ensure that their right to practice as sleep technologists is preserved.

Our individual activities and those of our professional association demonstrate that the field of sleep technology is indeed a profession and that the members of this profession meet high standards for behavior and competence. We are bound together by our skills and abilities to watch while others sleep, to make appropriate clinical decisions, and to conduct ourselves appropriately. Sleep technologists possess the skills required of professionals, including clinical competence, effective communication skills, and ethical decision making regarding the patients' best interest (27). Their ongoing desire for excellence, ensuring the utmost in quality, and compassionate and knowledgeable care of the patients they serve will enhance the ability of the profession of sleep technology to mature and be sustainable in the future. Professionalism is not stagnant, we must continue to learn from our successes and mistakes and put into action these lessons learned.

Standards of Conduct for Registered Polysomnographic Technologists

The standards of conduct for registered polysomnographic technologists are located on the Board of Registered Polysomnographic Technologists web site and consist of five sections (30). These standards focus on ethics, customs, competency, and the law and include sections that address responsibilities to the patient and responsibilities of the technologist to their profession, including dignity, solicitation, and examination. The code of conduct also addresses the relationship of the technologist to other caregivers to include working collegially and ensuring that care is given in an appropriate and ethical manner. The final section of the standards discusses the technologist's appropriate use of their credential. The standards of conduct, while specifically addressing the registered technologist, certainly apply to any technologist who is active in the field.

REFERENCES

1. Institute of Medicine. (2006). *Sleep disorders and sleep deprivation: An unmet public health problem.* Washington, DC: The National Academies Press.
2. Freire, K., Davis, R., Umble, K., et al. (2008). Creating public health management teams that work. *Journal of Public Health Management Practice, 14*(1), 76–79.
3. American Nurses Association. (2001). *Code of ethics for nurses with interpretive statements.* Silver Springs, MD: Author.
4. Brennan, M. D., & Monson, V. (2014). Professionalism: Good for patients and health care organizations. *Mayo Clinic Proceedings, 89*(5), 644–652.
5. Institute of Medicine. (2000). *To err is human: Building a safer health care system.* Washington, DC: The National Academies Press, Institute of Medicine.
6. Wynia, M. K., Papadakis, M. A., Sullivan, W. M., et al. (2014). More than a list of values and desired behaviors: A foundational understanding of medical professionalism. *Academic Medicine, 89*(5), 712–714.
7. Bauchner, H., Fontanarosa, P. B., & Thompson, A. E. (2015). Professionalism, governance, and self-regulation of medicine. *Journal of the American Medical Association, 313*(18), 1831–1836.
8. Rothman, D. J., McDonald, W. J., Berkowitz, C. D., et al. (2009). Professional medical associations and their relationships with industry. *Journal of the American Medical Association, 301*(13), 1367–1372.
9. Brown, S. P. (2000). Professionalization of exercise physiology: A critical essay. *Professionalization of Exercise Physiology (Online), 13*(6). Retrieved from https://www.asep.org/asep/asep/ProfessionalismCriticalEssay.html
10. Egener, B. E., Mason, D. J., McDonald, W. J., et al. (2017). The charter on professionalism for Health Care Organizations. *Academic Medicine, 92*(8), 1091–1099.
11. Brennan, M. D. (2016). The role of professionalism in clinical practice, medical education, biomedical research and health care administration. *Journal of Translational Internal Medicine, 4*(2), 64–65.
12. National Board of Medical Examiners. (2002). *Embedding professionalism in medical education.* Retrieved from http://fliphtml5.com/hzci/dzcr/basic
13. Maurer, F. A., & Smith, C. M. (2009). *Community and public health nursing practice: Health for families and populations.* St. Louis, MO: Saunders Elsevier.
14. ABIM Foundation. (2002). Medical professionalism in the new millennium: A physician charter. *Annals of Internal Medicine, 136,* 243–246.
15. Ventola, C. L. (2014). Social media and health care professionals: Benefits, risks, and best practices. *Pharmacy and Therapeutics, 39*(7), 491–499.
16. National Council of State Boards of Nursing. (2011). *White paper: A nurse's guide to the use of social media.* Retrieved March 3, 2018, from https://www.ncsbn.org/Social_Media.pdf
17. Gagnon, K., & Sabus, C. (2015). Professionalism in a digital age: Opportunities and considerations for using social media in health care. *Physical Therapy, 95*(3), 406–414.
18. Leibtag, A. (2012). *A 12-word social media policy.* Retrieved March 3, 2018, from https://socialmedia.mayoclinic.org/2012/04/05/a-twelve-word-social-media-policy/. Accessed April 5, 2012.
19. Grossman, S. C., & Valiga, T. M. (2009). *The new leadership challenge: Creating the future of nursing* (3rd ed.). Philadelphia, PA: F.A. Davis Company.
20. Reynolds, S. J., & Ceranic, T. (2007). The effects of moral judgment and moral identity on moral behavior: An empirical examination of the moral individual. *Journal of Applied Physiology, 92*(6), 1610–1624.
21. Davies, H. T., Washington, A. E., & Bindman, A. B. (2002). Health care report cards: Implications for vulnerable patient groups and the organizations providing them care. *Journal of Health Politics Policy Law, 27*(3), 379–399.

22. Premeaux, S. (n.d.). The link between management behavior and ethical philosophy in the wake of the Enron convictions. *Journal of Business Ethics, 85*(1), 13–25. doi:10.1007/s10551-008-9745

23. Brown, M., Treviño, L. K., & Harrison, D. A. (2005). Ethical leadership: A social learning perspective for construct development and testing. *Organizational Behavior and Human Decision Processes, 97*(2), 117–134.

24. Colero, L. (n.d.). *A framework for universal principles of ethics*. Retrieved February 24, 2018, from http://www.ethics.ubc.ca/papers/invited/colero.html

25. Prilleltensky, I. (1997). Values, assumptions, and practices: Assessing the moral implications of psychological discourse and action. *American Psychologist, 52*(5), 517–535. Retrieved from http://psycnet.apa.org/doi/10.1037/0003-066X.52.5.517. Accessed January 18, 2019.

26. Donnelly, L. F., & Strife, J. L. (2006). Establishing a program to promote professionalism and effective communication in radiology. *Radiology, 238*(3), 773–779.

27. American Association of Sleep Technologists. (2011). *American Association of Sleep Technologists scope of practice of the sleep technology profession.* Retrieved from http://www.aastweb.org/Resources/Position/ScopeofPractice.pdf

28. Locke, G. R., III, Berndt, M., Woychick, N., et al. (n.d.). *Clinical and health affairs: Professionalism among allied health staff.* Retrieved from http://www.minnesotamedicine.com/PastIssues/PastIssues2007/August2007/ClinicalLockeAugust2007/tabid/2242/Default.aspx

29. A.W.A.K.E. Network. American Sleep Apnea Association (2017). Retrieved from https://www.sleepapnea.org/community/all-about-awake/.

30. Board of Registered Polysomnographic Technologists. (2019). *Standards of conduct.* Retrieved from https://www.brpt.org/ethics/standards-of-conduct/. Accessed January 18, 2019.

chapter 71

Coding, Billing, and Regulatory Compliance

KATHRYN HANSEN

LEARNING OBJECTIVES

On completion of this chapter, the reader should be able to:

1. Define regulatory compliance as it applies to billing and coding of procedures performed in the sleep center.
2. Review coding guidelines used for billing sleep diagnostic procedures.
3. Describe preauthorization requirements that impact sleep center approval processes.
4. Discuss case studies to demonstrate the implementation of regulatory compliance, and coding and billing constructs that impact revenue integrity.

KEY TERMS

Common procedural technology (CPT)
Conditions of Participation (CoP)
Diagnostic related grouping (DRG)
Financial responsibility
Health plan billing rules
Healthcare Common Procedure Coding System (HCPCS)
Informed consent
Insurance contracts
International Classification of Diseases 10th Revision Clinical Modifications (ICD-10 CM)
International Classification of Sleep Disorders, third edition (ICSD-3)
Modifiers

INTRODUCTION

Medical insurance plays an important role in the financial well-being of every health care business. The regulatory environment of medical insurance is evolving faster than ever because of the introduction of Benefits Management Programs, which are mandated to keep control over escalating health care costs through the preauthorization and preapproval processes that have become a normal operational requirement in recent years. These changes have introduced more challenges to maintaining our volume and revenue. As a result, health care professionals must be familiar with the rules and guidelines of each health plan in order to submit proper documentation to assure payment. This familiarity begins with the knowledge of insurance basics.

WHAT IS MEDICAL CODING?

Medical coding is a system of number and letter labels that are unique for each diagnosis, symptom, or symptom set, which is used to track prevalence of diseases and associated diagnoses. Additionally, codes are used for standard communication of procedures used in the treatment of diseases with subsequent treatments. Therefore, accurate medical coding is important for submission of billing claims and in tracking statistics for disease and medical treatment.

Correct coding of the medical claim is essential to obtain insurance reimbursement as well as maintain patient records. Coding claims accurately convey to the insurance payer and other health care entities a standardized reporting of the patient illness or injury and the method of diagnosis and/or treatment.

Medical coding involves using one or more of the following types of codes:

1. International Classification of Diseases (ICD) codes are used to standardize the reporting of diagnoses, symptoms, and causes of health condition in humans into specific categories with approved code sets using numbers and letters to characterize the diseases. Currently, the manual is the 10th revision for clinical modification.
   The World Health Organization (WHO) creates, copyrights, and oversees these classifications, which are recognized by every medical facility and practitioner worldwide. In the United States, the National Center for Health Statistics, which is a part of the Centers for Medicare and Medicaid Services (CMS), manages any amendments to the ICD codes alongside the WHO (1).

2. *International Classification of Sleep Disorders*, third edition (*ICSD-3*) codes provide specific information on sleep disorders, including diagnostic criteria, essential features, and objective findings.
   The American Academy of Sleep Medicine (AASM) creates, copyrights, and maintains these classifications, which are used primarily by sleep specialists. The *ICSD-3* references appropriate *ICD-10* codes for the sleep disorders identified in this manual (2).

3. Common Procedural Technology (CPT) codes are a five-digit number or a four-digit number with one alpha character assigned to every procedure and service, which medical practitioners include in documentation to designate a medical, surgical, or diagnostic service. These codes are used by third-party payers to determine the amount of reimbursement that a practitioner will receive from the payer for the service. They are standardized to define the specific elements of the procedure to describe the same procedure across all providers for the intent of creating uniformity in billing (3).

4. CPT codes are developed, maintained, and copyrighted by the American Medical Association (AMA). They are Level I codes, which means they are used for procedures and services usually provided by physicians or other approved licensed clinical providers, such as Nurse Practitioners, Physician Assistants, and Doctors of Osteopathy. As the practice of health care changes, new codes are developed for new services; current codes may be revised; and old, unused codes are retired. Thousands of codes are in use and they are updated annually (3).
   To search for a CPT code and its description, these options are available:
   a. Purchase the CPT manual from the AMA, which is a comprehensive listing of all CPT and Level I codes.
   b. Perform a CPT code search on the AMA web site by registering (for free) for five searches per day. This allows a limited search for a CPT code or the use of a keyword to identify the associated CPT code description.
   c. Contact the referring doctor's office to request the CPT codes and services requested for the patient.
   d. Contact the payer's billing manual or benefits specialists to obtain clarification of the code and description associated with the procedure.

5. Healthcare Common Procedure Coding System (HCPCS) is a set of codes used and maintained by the CMS and used for billing Medicare, Medicaid, and many other third-party payers. If you are billing a Medicare claim, a HCPCS code will be reported in your paperwork. These are considered Level II codes, which cover health care services and procedures that are not provided by physicians. Examples of items billed with Level II codes are medical equipment, supplies, and home sleep apnea testing (HSAT) for Medicare beneficiaries such as G0399. HCPCS Level

II codes start with a letter and have four numbers. A modifier attached to the code, consisting of either two letters or a letter and a number, may be required for coding integrity. The coding guidelines will reflect the need for an additional modifier, which is generally cross-referenced in the description of the code, or in a paragraph preceding the specific coding chapter or section in the manual (4).
To search for a HCPCS Level II code and its description, these options are available:
a. Purchase the current HCPCS manual
b. Search the CMS web site: https://www.cms.gov/Medicare/Coding/HCPCSReleaseCodeSets/Alpha-Numeric-HCPCS.html
c. Complete a web search online.

6. Diagnostic Related Grouping (DRG) codes are used by Medicare and some other third-party payers to categorize hospitalization costs and determine how much to pay for a patient's hospital stay. Rather than paying the hospital for what it spent caring for a hospitalized patient, Medicare pays the hospital a fixed amount on the basis of the patient's DRG or diagnosis. Essentially, the DRG-based payment means that if a patient admitted to the hospital is treated for less money than the DRG payment, a profit is associated with that admission. Likewise, the opposite is true: if the patient care expenses for the same admission are more than the DRG payment, the facility loses money.
Therefore, instead of paying for each day the patient is hospitalized and each procedure completed, Medicare pays a single amount based on the DRG, which is based on the diagnosis(es), age, and gender of the patient. Each DRG is grouped into a category of clinically similar diagnoses, which require similar resources and care to treat.

7. Modifiers are additional two-digit numbers, two-letter numbers, or alphanumeric characters used with the CPT and HCPCS codes to convey additional information about the procedure being billed. They may be used to identify a change in the procedure or multiple procedures completed in the same patient encounter. For instance, if a procedure is discontinued before the completion of the required monitoring time, a modifier is appended to the CPT code to describe reduced services.

KEY MODIFIER FACTS

a. Inappropriate use of modifiers can cause a delay or reduction in payment in the same manner as not using an appropriate CPT code.
b. For a complete list of modifiers, turn to Appendix A of the CPT manual.
c. Append modifiers only according to individual insurance payer guidelines.

d. Modifier use is different for services provided by licensed providers as opposed to the technical services.

e. Modifier use may be different for services provided in the physician practice compared with those provided in the hospital. These requirements are included in the insurance agreement, a document called the Conditions of Participation (CoP).

Knowledge of these coding tools is important for communication and billing purposes. The use of coding in all types of medical practice is not only important but also imperative because commercial insurance payers, Medicare, Tricare, and Medicaid, will not pay a claim if it is not properly submitted with acceptable diagnosis(es) and procedure codes.

CODES FOR BILLING PROCEDURES PERFORMED

It is time to define the details associated with coding for procedures performed in all monitoring settings.

CPT procedure codes 95800 through 95811 are utilized for diagnostic sleep testing services, which include coding for both sleep studies and polysomnography (PSG).

The respective definitions of these two levels of service are provided in the introduction to the Medicine Chapter of the CPT manual.

They are defined as continuous and simultaneous monitoring and recording of multiple physiologic and pathophysiologic parameters for a minimum of 6 hours of monitoring, which includes the physician's review, interpretation, and reporting of the findings. The monitoring time starts with "lights out" and ends with "lights on." It does not include the time spent completing questionnaires, nor the time to apply and remove all of the monitoring sensors (3).

In 2013, two monitoring codes were added to expand coding and differentiate coding for adult and pediatric sleep monitoring:

1. 95782—younger than 6 years; diagnostic study that requires a documentation of greater than or equal to 7 hours' monitoring time
2. 95783—younger than 6 years; positive airway pressure study that requires a documentation of greater than or equal to 7 hours' monitoring time (3)

Table 71-1 provides a summary of the CPT codes and their respective descriptions for polysomnograms

Table 71-1 **CPT Codes for Sleep Studies**

Codes Associated with Type of Monitoring	Description of CMS Classification for Type of Monitoring
95810 95811	Type I PSG is an adult-attended study performed in a sleep center using sleep staging in addition to EEG, EOG, ECG/heart rate, chin EMG, limb EMG, respiratory effort at thorax and abdomen, nasal and oral airflow and positive airway pressure as indicated, which requires at least 6 h of monitoring.
95782 95783	Type I PSG is an attended study performed in a sleep center using sleep staging in addition to EEG, EOG, ECG/heart rate, chin EMG, limb EMG, respiratory effort at thorax and abdomen, nasal and oral airflow in a patient younger than 6 y, which requires at least 7 h of monitoring.
95805	Multiple sleep latency or maintenance of wakefulness testing, recording, analyzing, and interpreting physiologic measurements of sleep during multiple trials to assess a degree of sleepiness when compared with the ability to remain alert.
G0398	HSAT with type II portable monitor, unattended; minimum of seven channels: EEG, EOG, EMG, ECG/heart rate, airflow, respiratory effort, and oxygen saturation.
G0399 95806	HSAT with type III portable monitor, unattended; minimum of four channels: two respiratory movements/airflow, one ECG/heart rate, and one oxygen saturation.
95800	HSAT with type III portable monitor, unattended; minimum of four channels: respiratory analysis, one ECG/heart rate, and one oxygen saturation with measurement of sleep time.
95801	HSAT with type III portable monitor, unattended; minimum of four channels: respiratory movement/airflow, one ECG/heart rate, and one oxygen saturation.
G0400	HSAT with type IV portable monitor, unattended; minimum of three channels.

CMS, Centers for Medicare and Medicaid Services; ECG, electrocardiogram; EEG, electroencephalogram; EMG, electromyogram; EOG, electrooculogram; HSAT, home sleep apnea test; PSG, polysomnography.

and sleep studies completed in the sleep center as well as those used for HSAT (5). A more detailed discussion on HSAT is available in Chapter 44.

For appropriate billing, these codes must include documentation of the required hours of monitoring time. If less time is reported on the scoring summary sheet, a modifier 52 should be appended to the procedure code to indicate that a reduced service was provided and that the reason for the shortened study is unrelated to the patient's clinical condition or a physician's decision to terminate the study. Appending a 52 modifier will result in the study being paid at a reduced reimbursement. Typically, the reimbursement in this case is one-half of the customary payment. Documentation on the technologist's notes as to the reason for the reduced services is important, because this is to be correlated in the interpretation of the study.

On occasion, during a study, the patient develops a clinical change such as shortness of breath, cardiac arrhythmia, severe headache, or unilateral numbness or weakness. These signs and symptoms may represent an emergency condition, which requires transfer to another level of care and hence a termination of the study before the required monitoring time. Confirmation with a provider supports the need for transfer to another service such as the emergency room. These clinical changes may require initiation of cardiopulmonary resuscitation. In this situation, a modifier 53 is appended to the procedure code, indicating that the study was terminated early because of the patient's condition as ordered by a licensed clinical provider. Again, documentation in the technologist's notes is critical for inclusion in the interpretation.

In 2008, CMS created HCPCS codes or G-codes (G0398, G0399, and G0400) to describe HSAT services. These codes can be found in the HCPCS Level II codebook and on the CMS web site.

Some Medicare contractors and third-party payers will require the use of G-codes and will not accept CPT codes when reporting HSAT. The criteria for use of the appropriate codes for non-Medicare claims may be found in the insurance company's Internet Only Manual or in the CoP associated with the insurance contract for the respective insurance companies.

Be certain to understand the carrier's requirement when submitting the claim. Typically, the code that best describes the procedure is reported. However, in the absence of definitive requirements stipulated by the insurance company, and when services are similar, reporting the CPT code is preferentially accepted rather than using the G-code (3).

Additional definitions of the respective studies completed in the sleep center may be referenced in the CPT coding manuals or online at www.cms.gov.

COMPLIANT BILLING

Having an understanding of the difference between the technical, professional, and global codes is necessary for accurate billing and, in return, getting paid for your work.

If the facility performs the testing and a separate credentialed provider is interpreting the procedure, two modifiers are used on the billing claim: the facility providing the technical services attaches a TC modifier to the CPT code, and the interpreting medical director (MD) attaches a 26 modifier to the same code. If the procedure is recorded in a facility where the doctor owns the equipment to record the procedure *and* interprets the recording, then the claim is submitted as a global charge, meaning it does not use any modifiers. If the procedure is recorded in a facility and the interpreting doctor is employed by the facility, it is necessary to confirm with the Revenue Integrity Team or Coding Department how to submit a charge because it may still use a modifier, depending on the financial relationship of the employed provider.

The following example demonstrates the use of two of the most common modifiers used by the sleep center: "TC" to designate the technical component of a procedure and "26" to designate the professional component of a study:

- 95810-TC—PSG—Code for the diagnostic PSG to bill the technical component, which includes the equipment, space supplies, and personnel.
- 95810-26—PSG—Used to code for the diagnostic PSG for the interpreting physician.
- 95810—PSG—A "global" code to bill both the professional and technical services together in one code. Used for billing a PSG with sleep staging and four or *more* additional parameters of sleep, attended by a technologist, and the review of the study and the interpretation.

To be compliant with coding for a split-night study, use code 95811 for either a continuous positive airway pressure (CPAP) or bilevel titration. If a split-night study is performed, the interpretation should include both the diagnostic and the treatment information in one report. This is how to document it on the billing claim:

- 95811-TC—PSG (CPAP/Bilevel Titration Study) or split-night studies—Code for the PSG to bill the technical component, which includes the equipment, space supplies, and personnel.
- 95811-26—PSG (CPAP/Bilevel Titration Study) or split-night studies—Used to code for the interpreting physician.

- 95811—PSG (CPAP/Bilevel Titration Study) or split-night studies being billed for both the technical and the professional components using a global billing code to include the interpretation.

Coding and billing for the multiple sleep latency test (MSLT) and the maintenance of wakefulness test (MWT) is completed using CPT 95805:

- 95805-TC—MSLT or MWT to bill for the technical component.
- 95805-26—MSLT or MWT to bill for the professional component, which is the interpretation of the study.
- 95805—MSLT or MWT to bill globally for both the technical and professional services.

Alert: If a full study is not recorded and is less than the required hours as stated in the CPT code, then a modifier of 52 (reduced services) on that specific claim for the respective date of service is added to the CPT code. For example, note how to bill only the technical services of a titration study that was monitored for 4 hours: to append the modifier for reduced services and to bill for only the technical services, the documentation on the billing claim will be entered as 95811-TC-52. The insurance company will process this claim for only the titration technical services for less than 6 hours of monitoring.

DISCOVERING THE DIAGNOSIS

It is important to use the correct *ICD-10-CM* code for billing any diagnosis associated with the diagnostic testing, because this describes the reason for completing the procedure. In addition, the correct diagnosis code must be reported to describe the patient's condition. To obtain the most appropriate diagnosis code, take the following steps:

a. Review the medical record to determine what medical conditions or symptoms are described by the documentation to support the medical necessity for performing the procedure.
b. Cross-reference the disease, signs, symptoms, or condition in the front of the *ICD-10-CM* manual, volume II, and locate the corresponding code.
c. To verify the specificity of the code, locate the corresponding code in the volume I tabular list within the *ICD-10-CM* manual and further analyze the most appropriate code that correlates with the documentation.
d. Routinely, refer to the tabular list to locate the most specific code.
e. Coding conventions will reference other diagnoses, which describe in greater detail the information

needed to convey to the third-party payer additional information to justify the medical reason for the procedure.

It is important to review the approved diagnoses codes for associated CPT codes, which are defined by individual insurance payers. Examples of the approved codes accepted by CMS for PSG are listed in the region's Local Coverage Determination (LCD) for PSG. An example of an LCD (6) and these approved codes in one region may be reviewed online.

Compliance with coding and billing requires systematic review of all diagnoses codes commonly used for submitting claims in the sleep center. Ideally, this review is completed semiannually to remain informed of changes to the covered diagnostic codes and to prevent denial of claims.

BILLING AND CODING GUIDELINES

Most insurance payers require that the polysomnogram be performed to include the titration with PAP, that is, CPT code 95811, when clinical criteria support the need for a split-night study. The CPT code 95810 is allowable only when the sleep study does not demonstrate events consistent with sleep apnea and when the PAP titration cannot be completed for unforeseen reasons as documented in the physician's interpretation. Examples include, but are not limited to, the following:

- Insufficient total sleep time;
- Criteria for obstructive sleep apnea (OSA) met late in study with insufficient sleep time left for PAP titration;
- PAP trial attempted but not tolerated by patient.

At this time, many third-party payers will approve only one polysomnogram for a defined number of years, unless there is a significant change in patient status. A repeat polysomnogram will be reviewed for medical necessity with documentation of the following clinical findings:

- Weight gain or loss of a prescribed percentage, with required documentation of body weight;
- After surgical or oral appliance treatment of patients with moderate-to-severe OSA;
- When clinical response is insufficient or when symptoms return despite a good initial response to treatment with PAP device.

For a complete list of the criteria for repeat testing, consult the respective insurance company's CoP for polysomnograms.

Other measurements performed during a sleep study (e.g., vital signs, muscular activity, oximetry, airflow, blood gases, electrocardiogram analyses, gastroesophageal reflux) are also included in the coding for the respective polysomnogram and will not be paid separately. It is important to note that billing for extended electroencephalogram monitoring in addition to the PSG base code is not acceptable practice. The CPT manual does not provide guidelines at this time to support the additional code.

Actigraphy as a stand-alone test (CPT code 95803) is not medically necessary as a routine diagnostic procedure done in the sleep center and requires the insurance company MD's review before completion of the testing.

When seeking preauthorization for a PSG, most commercial insurance companies expect to review clinical information to differentiate between the need for a facility-based test versus HSAT. The following are general contraindications for HSAT:

- Moderate or severe chronic obstructive pulmonary disease—forced expiratory volume in 1 second (FEV1)/forced vital capacity less than or equal to 0.7 and FEV1 less than 80% of predicted
- Moderate or severe congestive heart failure—New York Heart Association Class III or IV
- Cognitive impairment (inability to follow simple instructions)
- Neuromuscular impairment
- Suspicion of a sleep disorder other than OSA (such as central sleep apnea, narcolepsy, restless legs syndrome, circadian rhythm disorder, parasomnias, periodic limb movement disorder)
- Previous technically suboptimal HSAT (two nights of study attempted)
- Previous two-night HSAT that did not diagnose OSA in a patient with ongoing clinical suspicion of OSA
- Patient has demonstrated oxygen desaturation for a defined period of time for any reason
- History of cerebrovascular accident within the preceding 30 days
- History of ventricular fibrillation or sustained ventricular tachycardia
- Pediatric patient under age 18

Documentation of these clinical findings must be included in the history and physical examination from the referring provider and available for the individual completing the preauthorization for the study, if required by the insurance company. The history and physical examination are also required for review by the billing entity because it provides the medical necessity required for payment for the procedure.

REGULATIONS AND COMPLIANCE

All personnel representing your sleep center and respective health care providers are required to adhere to a high level of personal and professional conduct.

Inherent in this conduct is the need to maintain clinical competence and core knowledge of the regulatory standards that govern this changing health care industry. It includes the intent to maintain and protect the confidentiality of patient and organizational information, as well as to ensure the practice of legal and ethical standards in all dealings and transactions. The intent is to observe all laws and regulations that govern the sleep industry.

Therefore, to stay abreast of the changes, continuing education is a must. What exactly does this mean? Knowing the regulations for your respective insurance providers and the state insurance statutes is the first place to start.

FINANCIAL REGULATORY REQUIREMENTS

Clinical personnel are being asked to perform more of the comprehensive tasks that are associated with medical testing, such as documenting the procedure billing code (CPT code) on the practice's encounter or billing form. As a result, it is important to have an understanding of regulatory requirements concerning financial practices.

Follow these steps to embark on getting paid for your work.

a. The process starts with preauthorization or a predetermination for completing the procedure, which is the third-party payers' preliminary commitment to pay for the procedure.
Precertification, preauthorization, or predetermination should be obtained quickly so that the patient's procedure may be carried out without delay. To do this, you need to have the medical history and physical examination from the referring physician, or one that has been completed by the clinic's board-certified sleep specialist. This document must include a chief complaint, which states in the patient's words why he or she is seeking medical care. The chief complaint links to the medical necessity for the procedure and for treatment to be approved for payment. Staff may be asked to assist and instruct the patient to complete a patient information form, as a way of documenting accurate and complete demographic data and a clinical history.
Information that is needed to complete a preauthorization for a procedure includes the sleep history and symptoms including, but not limited to, snoring, daytime sleepiness, observed apneas, choking or gasping during sleep, morning headaches; the Epworth Sleepiness Scale; the physical examination that documents body mass index, neck

circumference, and a focused cardiopulmonary and upper airway system evaluation. Additional detail to have available before calling for preauthorization is listed in the section Billing and Coding Guidelines. Currently, for Medicare patients to qualify for PAP therapy, they must meet either of the following criteria: the apnea–hypopnea index (AHI) is greater than or equal to 15 events per hour with a minimum of 30 events; or the AHI is greater than or equal to 5 and less than or equal to 14 events per hour with a minimum of 10 events and documentation of excessive daytime sleepiness, impaired cognition, mood disorders, or insomnia; or hypertension, ischemic heart disease, or history of stroke.

b. Take time to explain to the patient the sleep center's Notice of Privacy Practices and the Patient Rights and Responsibilities, making sure you are familiar with both notices and are competent in explaining the form accurately. A third form, the Notice of Financial Responsibility, conveys to the patient his or her consent to submit a claim for payment on his or her behalf. It also confers the patient's responsibility for payment of his or her portion of the bill. The facility has the responsibility to inform the patient of the charge, the expected reimbursement for the procedure, and his or her financial responsibility before receipt of the services. To attest to all three of these regulations, written documentation that the patient was informed of the discussion must be in the patient's permanent chart as evidence of adherence to the federal regulations.

c. Informed consent

This is a process in which the patient authorizes medical treatment after a discussion with a physician or a licensed clinical provider that includes the plan of care. During this interview, the assessment, risks, and recommendations are discussed with the patient and documented in the patient's record. The informed consent is required in advance of any testing. It is witnessed by the clinical provider and signed and dated at the time of discussion.

The Consent for Testing and Treatment, generally a requirement for all procedures, is completed in accordance with state and federal requirements. Consent forms also include the permission for release of patient information as required by the Health Insurance Portability and Accountability Act of 1996 (HIPAA).

Under the HIPAA Privacy Rule, providers do not need specific authorization to release patients' personal health information if used for treatment, payment, and health care operations (TPO). Examples of TPO are as follows:

a. Treatment: discussion of the patient's clinical information with other providers,

b. Payment: submission of the billing claim on behalf of the patient, and

c. Operations: activities related to staff training and quality improvement.

SUBMISSION OF THE BILLING CLAIM

Promptly transmit an accurate insurance claim data to the third-party payer so that reimbursement is received in a timely manner. This is usually completed through an electronic data interface. Several areas of complexity with submission of billing claims for sleep studies include the following:

1. An order with diagnosis code(s) is required from the referring physician. Neither the sleep center nor its supervising physicians can prescribe a sleep test for patients they do not treat. If the physician serving as the supervising physician or the MD of the sleep center orders the procedure, the supervising physician/MD must be the patient's treating physician. Therefore, this same provider must have had a relationship with the patient before the performance of the testing and is now managing the care of the patient for his or her specific medical problem.

2. The PSG/sleep study must be performed by the appropriately credentialed technologists. Each insurance plan defines required credentialing. Traditionally, CMS qualifies the required credentials at a minimum as Registered Respiratory Therapist (RRT), Registered Respiratory Therapist–Sleep Disorders Specialist (RRT-SDS), Certified Respiratory Therapist (CRT), Certified Respiratory Therapist–Sleep Disorders Specialist (CRT-SDS), Registered Polysomnographic Technologist (RPSGT). Technologists working in states with state licensure requirements governed by a state practice act are required to demonstrate evidence of meeting all credentialing and licensure requirements by possessing both credentials before working as a direct care provider.

3. Another important credentialing requirement that requires attention concerns direct care providers who work in one state and provide services to a patient living in another state. That provider is required to have a license to work in both the state where the patient resides and the state where the patient is receiving the care and services. Insurance contracts routinely reinforce this expectation as a condition of participation with their plans.

4. The sleep study is completed in accordance with the criteria defined by the respective CPT code. Focus on the parameters required to support the appropriate CPT code and document the duration of the study. This is discussed in additional detail in other sections of this chapter.

5. The sleep study is interpreted by an appropriately credentialed physician. This is defined in each insurance plan and typically requires a board-certified sleep medicine specialist. Evidence of a face-to-face medical interview is required to process the claim. Notes or proof of the physical examination must be placed in the patient's chart. The treating physician is the one who furnishes a consultation or treats a patient for a specific medical problem and uses the results of the test to treat and manage the patient's medical problem.

6. The names of the ordering physician with credentials, interpreting physician with credentials, supervising technologist with credentials, when applicable, and the actual technologist with credentials performing the study must be documented in the patient file and on the interpretation of the procedure to demonstrate compliance with the credentialing regulations.

7. The need for accreditation of the facility must be addressed before submission of billing claims. All CMS regions are rapidly moving toward mandating accreditation through one of the following accrediting entities: Accreditation Commission for Health Care (ACHC) (7), AASM (8), or The Joint Commission (9). All of these entities have established standards that must be in place before the sleep center is awarded an accreditation required by the CMS. This has led the charge for other commercial insurances, who are also changing their CoP to require accreditation of the sleep center. A point of note: if sleep services, including HSAT, are contracted out to another company, both the billing facility and the contracted service must fulfill the standards as written in the accreditation guidelines.

8. Clinicians who complete the insurance claim need to be able to explain complex billing requirements and answer insurance questions to patients. Take time to explain billing parameters to all business and clinical team members associated with your program, so that they have a general understanding of the insurance and billing process and are able to address patient questions correctly.

Tests ordered by physicians who are not treating the patient are rendered medically unnecessary and are not reimbursable in the eyes of the insurance company. When receiving a referral from the attending physician, the sleep center must maintain a record of the attending physician's orders and any test results that may impact the interpretation of the procedure. The interpreting physician must indicate a final diagnosis from the sleep study on the interpretation that correlates with the diagnosis for billing. The diagnosis code for the symptoms or the reason for testing the patient is not to be used on the billing claim.

When billing for a diagnostic test, the ordering physician's National Provider Identifier number must be indicated on the claim form, and the order must be kept on record. If more than two nights of testing are performed, documentation justifying the medical necessity for the additional test(s) must be provided to the insurance company on request.

Ideally, to remain competent, billing and coding staff will need to obtain training in CPT, *ICD-10-CM*, and HCPCS coding and have access to the annually updated coding resources. The billing encounter forms, billing software, and any cheat sheets used need to be updated every year with any changes as defined in the standard coding resources. It is beneficial to subscribe to newsletters or other web site resources to keep abreast of coding changes. Use an official source such as CMS or the AMA to verify any changes or updates received. Ask for information from other third-party payers in writing or verify changes on the payer's online resources page to keep abreast of contracted coding changes. Each quarter, check the CMS National Coverage Determination and LCD requirements to be aware of any changes made by the designated regional Medicare Administrative Contractor who administers the LCD. The responsibilities for knowing what changes are integrated that may affect your practice rests with the sleep center billing and coding experts.

INSURANCE CONTRACTS

Many health insurance companies provide different types of individual and group plans, which many employers offer to their employees. These plans have different coverage, referral restrictions, and payment schedules. They have clinical exclusions, which may be implemented midway in the contract period, in addition to the annual edits. As a result, health insurance plans are always changing, and the patient often has a difficult time understanding what his or her health plans cover.

To obtain a better understanding of the insurance contracts, investigate the following issues when evaluating coverage to ensure correct billing and coding:

a. Medical conditions establish the medical necessity for services

    Documenting the clinical symptoms or reasons for the procedure justifies the medical necessity, which is required to be noted in the medical record, a legal document. Complete and comprehensive documentation is important to show that clinicians have appropriately assessed medical need indicated by medical standards of care.

    Services are medically necessary when they are reasonable and essential for the diagnosis or treatment of illness or injury, or to improve the functioning of an individual's health status. Such services must also be consistent with generally accepted standards of care. Normally, these standards of care are published practice parameters by national professional organizations, such as the AASM, and other professional organizations such as The American College of Physicians. Practice parameters are peer-reviewed, clinically based protocols that have been tested and validated to elicit effective outcomes in care.

b. Evidence of certification requirements by approved accreditation agency
All CMS claims and many other commercial insurances now have certification requirements to obtain payment for diagnostic and therapeutic testing performed in a hospital-based lab, a freestanding facility (includes sleep clinics that are a part of a physician's office), independent diagnostic testing facilities, and all other non–hospital-based facilities where sleep studies are performed. This includes the requirement for the facility to have on file, and available on request, evidence that they are credentialed by one of the approved accreditation agencies.

c. Requirements for patient encounter are documented
Documentation is expected to be generated during a face-to-face encounter with the patient. Insurance contracts have defined criteria for how the encounter occurs: face-to-face is the norm today, and reimbursement is linked to the direct discussion with the patient. If information is not available at the time of this direct discussion, there are requirements for amending the patient encounter.
Delayed entries, documented within a time frame, generally not to exceed 48 hours, are acceptable for purposes of clarification, error correction, addition of information not initially available, and when certain unusual circumstances prevented the generation of the documentation at the time of service. The medical record cannot be altered or redacted, and amendments must be legibly added so the clinician can draw an inference to confirm, clarify, or support the initial entry. Corrections or additions must be dated, timed, and legibly signed or initialed. Delayed written explanations will be considered for clarification only. This explanation is not used for the purpose of increasing the services billed, because of a lack of documentation at the time of service, or retrospectively substantiating medical necessity. All entries must be legible to another person reading the chart signed by the original author. If the signature is not legible and does not identify the clinician, a printed example of the name should be included under the signature with the appropriate credentials to support the required scope of practice.

d. Claim is audited for excluded services prior to submission
Billing federal insurance providers for a noncovered service constitutes fraud. Under Medicare, if a patient elects to have a procedure, and it is not covered under the Medicare health plan, an Advanced Beneficiary Notice is required *before* providing services. This form is obtained from the Medicare web site. Knowledge of the patient's insurance plan is a must to reduce the potential for billing fraud.

e. Health plan billing requirements are met
This may include completion of certain activities before testing, such as preauthorization, completion of a medical questionnaire before approval for the procedure, or a face-to-face interview with the treating physician. Payment for certain treatment devices, such as an oral appliance, may require a failure of PAP therapy before submission of the claim for the device, depending on the insurance plan.

f. Patient financial responsibility education
Discussing the practice's financial policy with the patient and/or his or her guardian is critical to receiving payment for services. To have a constructive proactive discussion, it is necessary to be educated about the sleep center's financial policies. It means one also needs to be in tune with the patient's way of thinking, conveying information in a compassionate positive manner, in an effort to share with the patient that payment of his or her bill is the patient's responsibility. Medical providers are expected to devote time to verifying and understanding each patient's particular insurance coverage to increase collections and cash flow. The first step toward gaining an understanding of the claim management and reimbursement processes is to review the insurance plan contract and clarify the definitions and terminology listed in each insurance plan. This makes a discussion with the patient about the sleep center's payment options more beneficial. Ideally, the copayment is collected at the time of service and, if not paid then, subsequent evidence of the attempt to collect the copayment is documented in the patient's medical chart.

SUMMARY

Understanding how to accurately code and bill for clinical encounters is critical to getting paid for services rendered, reducing risk for fraud and abuse, and making a profit. Regulatory standards expect the integration of financial requirements and statutes that are the basis for compliance with coding and billing requirements. Competency with these financial practices establishes credibility with peers, third-party payers, and the community, because providing services is based on integrity and honesty. When we add the expectation for appropriate documentation, it becomes necessary to have a core structure to coordinate the many facets of sleep center billing. Therefore, completing an annual review of all billing contract requirements will contribute to the financial success of the sleep center. Taking time every year to attend a presentation on the recent coding and billing updates will help to maximize the potential for increased revenue. Completing this education is worth the time and energy required to be successful and sustain a profitable venture.

REFERENCES

1. American Academy of Professional Coders. (2018). *ICD-10-CM expert for providers and facilities*. Salt Lake City, UT: Author.
2. American Academy of Sleep Medicine. (2014). *International classification of sleep disorders* (3rd ed.). Darien, IL: Author.
3. American Medical Association. (2018). *CPT® 2018 professional edition*. Chicago, IL: Author.
4. Optum360. (2018). *HCPCS level II expert codebook*. Salt Lake City, UT: Author.
5. Aronsky, A. J. (2015, April 19). *4 steps to correct coding for home sleep apnea testing*. Retrieved August 6, 2018, from http://www.sleepreviewmag.com/2015/04/4-steps-correct-coding-home-sleep-apnea-testing/
6. Local Coverage Determination (LCD). *Polysomnography and other sleep studies (L34040)*. Retrieved August 6, 2018, from https://med.noridianmedicare.com/documents/10546/6990981/Polysomnography+and+Other+Sleep+Studies+LCD/a30fc4d4-ba1c-4aea-acef-bbb44cf3984e
7. Accreditation Commission for Health Care. *ACHC sleep accreditation standards*. Retrieved August 6, 2018, from https://www.achc.org/sleep.html
8. American Academy of Sleep Medicine. (2018). *AASM standards for accreditation*. Retrieved August 6, 2018, from https://j2vjt3dnbra3ps7ll1clb4q2-wpengine.netdna-ssl.com/wp-content/uploads/2018/05/accreditationstandards-1.pdf
9. The Joint Commission. *Seeking sleep center accreditation*. Retrieved August 6, 2018, from https://www.jointcommission.org/accreditation/ahc_seeking_sleep_centers.aspx

chapter 72

Quality Assurance and Quality Improvement

RICHARD S. ROSENBERG

LEARNING OBJECTIVES

On completion of this chapter, the reader should be able to:

1. Describe the basis for quality assurance and quality improvement.
2. Define structural, process, and outcome measures.
3. Discuss the process for measuring data, what, how, and when.
4. Describe the process for analyzing data and reporting outcomes.

KEY TERMS

Data
Quality assurance
Quality improvement
Continuous quality improvement
Reliability
Validity
Sentinel event
Epworth Sleepiness Scale
Multiple Sleep Latency Test

"I think we can do better". This quote from an Australian comedian is, in six words, the basis for quality assurance and, its close cousin, continuous quality improvement. There are a variety of different elements in the process, beginning with measurement and manipulation. The process requires reliability and validity. Constructs are examined and operationalized. Data are collected and analyzed. Hypotheses are tested. Theories are developed and supported, modified, or abandoned. Does this sound like scientific method? You betcha.

A variety of businesses have benefited from a quality assurance process. This relies on standards of performance, whether in manufacturing screws to exacting specifications or inserting those screws into luxury automobiles with precise torque. An acceptable range of performance is defined. When the range is not met for a certain predetermined percentage of products, an attempt is made to define the problem and propose a solution. Quality assurance is critical when the product has safety implications. If the screw holds the brakes in place, failing to meet the acceptable range of performance can have disastrous consequences. Therefore, the percentage of products meeting specifications must be extremely high, if not 100%. On the contrary, a burnt potato chip may irritate some consumers, but is unlikely to have serious consequences.

Quality improvement does not have an end goal and works in a more continuous fashion. When used in customer service, surveys may be used to obtain satisfaction scores. No matter what the score, an intervention is proposed to try and improve it. When the score is at the top of the range, a new measure of satisfaction is developed that leaves room for improvement.

Quality assurance and improvement processes are both important in medicine, specifically in sleep medicine. There are some areas where the goal should be a total absence of events. For example, patient deaths in the sleep center should not be merely infrequent, they should never happen. These "sentinel events" should result in an immediate change in policies to ensure that they do not happen again. Improving care in sleep medicine is an imperative that benefits sleep centers and patients. The goals are to improve the quality of care, improve the health of populations, and reduce the costs of health care (1).

Measures can be divided into structural, process, and outcomes (1). For example, if you want to know if the number of patients visiting your sleep center is higher today than it was a year ago, you can review billing data or procedure logs. This is considered a structural measure. If you want to know if visiting the sleep center results in reduced blood pressure on the next clinic visit, you can review vital signs from the patient's chart. This would be a process measure. It is nice to have blood pressure in the normal range, but in itself this conveys no specific benefit. The benefit to the patient would be a reduction in the risk of stroke or heart attack, and the number of these events is considered an outcome measure. Outcome measures often require an extended period of time to collect, and as a result may suffer from lower reliability.

> *"Measure that which can be measured and make measurable what cannot be measured."*
>
> Galileo Galilei

The first step in quality assurance or improvement is to measure. The first question is, "What am I interested in?" and the second question is, "How can I measure it?" The first question asks for a construct, and the second asks for an operational definition. This can range from a simple question with obvious measures to more complex constructs that require more complicated measurement tools.

Here's an example from home sleep apnea testing (HSAT) that starts with a simple question and ends with a more complex question. The simple question is, "How many studies do I need to repeat?" The simple measure is to count the number of studies that were considered inadequate and required retesting and divide by the total number of studies run per month. Setting a goal for a small percentage of inadequate studies has implications for patient satisfaction and profit margin. Patients do not want to be told that they need to repeat a study. This delays determination of the results of the study and requires additional work, causing discomfort to the patient. In addition, current reimbursement rates provide a small margin between the cost of the HSAT and the revenue produced. A few inadequate studies per week might make HSAT unprofitable, leading to discontinuation of the service and an increase in patients who are not diagnosed. A high percentage of inadequate tests tells you there is a problem but gives no insight into how to correct the problem. In our fictional sleep center, the Galileo Sleep Measurement Center, more than 20% of our HSATs are rejected by the physicians. Something must be done. But what?

The more complex question is, "Why were the studies considered inadequate?" The idea of an inadequate study is a construct that needs to be defined operationally. That is, we need to make it measurable. This typically starts with observation. We could put a box on the interpretation form that asks the physician, "Why was this study inadequate?" These open-ended questions are difficult to quantify because similar responses can be provided with slightly different language, making it difficult to decide if the causes are actually the same. One physician writes, "oxygen problem" and another physician writes "saturation measurement lost." Can we offer the physicians some options with check boxes? The American Academy of Sleep Medicine (AASM) Scoring Manual (2) provides a starting point. The features of an acceptable HSAT device must be met in order to provide an adequate study. These features include oxygen saturation and heart rate, as well as a measure that allows for

the calculation of a surrogate of the apnea–hypopnea index (typically airflow for the numerator and recording time for the denominator). Of the 20% of recordings rejected by the physicians in our fictional center, 75% are identified as oxygen saturation problems.

Now we are back to a simple measure: How often were HSATs inadequate because of an oxygen saturation problem? During the monthly conference at the Galileo Sleep Measurement Center, we find that Dr. Copernicus rejects studies if the oximeter fails for more than 10% of the study, but Dr. Kepler is willing to accept studies with up to 50% oximeter data lost. In order to be a reliable indicator, the criteria for inadequate must be the same for all of our physicians. After a vigorous discussion, a compromise is reached, and inadequate oximetry is defined as more than 30% of the recording without adequate oximetry data. It is important to document this criterion in the center's Policy and Procedures Manual. This way everyone can create data that can be used for comparisons in later stages of the quality improvement process.

All aspects of the sleep center's activity can be assessed using quality improvement measures. The AASM helpfully provides starting points in a series of articles in the *Journal of Clinical Sleep Medicine*. A range of sleep disorders are covered, but for most centers, the majority of patients have sleep apnea. In a paper devoted to obstructive sleep apnea quality measures (3), the AASM recommends 10 process measures and 3 outcome measures that can be incorporated into a center's quality improvement process. These measures were developed through literature review, evaluation of physician burden, and a consensus meeting.

Process measure #5, for example, assesses sleepiness in patients. The center is required to determine the "Proportion of patients aged 18 years and older diagnosed and treated for obstructive sleep apnea that had sleepiness assessed annually" (3, p. 360). Sleepiness is a construct, and it needs to be operationalized. Some centers use the Epworth Sleepiness Scale, whereas others prefer the Multiple Sleep Latency Test. The AASM does not specify what measure is used, only that a measure is obtained. The outcome measure that is associated with this process measure is to improve quality of life. Again, the AASM does not specify a measure, and a wide variety of instruments can be debated by the center staff.

"Sleepiness" and "quality of life" are constructs, and some may say they are "squishy." But valid and reliable methods for operationalizing these constructs are available. It is important that the measures provide construct validity—that is, they measure the range and breadth of the construct. It would be inadequate to ask, "Do you fall asleep watching television?" as the only measure of sleepiness. Sleepiness involves falling asleep driving, during conversations, after a heavy lunch, and even feelings of sleepiness that do not involve actual loss of consciousness.

"I'm an angel compared to some of my friends."
Lindsay Lohan

The next step in our quality improvement process is to compare our measures with those of other similar entities. As the quote from Lindsay Lohan emphasizes, everything is relative. We will need to set minimum criterion for triggering of an intervention. From a purely business standpoint, this could be based on practical measures such as profit. But patient satisfaction will also be relevant as patients will fail to return to the center or recommend the center to family and friends if they are not satisfied with the treatment they receive. Establishing criteria that are, as much as possible, objective and consistent among staff will improve the validity of measures as they are compared over time.

Equally important, using measures that are the same as the measures that other centers are using will allow comparisons with "industry standards." Unfortunately, there is little consensus among sleep centers in how to measure quality indicators. For example, the AASM deems acceptable measures of quality of life to include the SF-36, SF-12, Nottingham Health Profile, EuroQoL, EQ-5D, FOSQ, and SAQLI (3).

In the Galileo Sleep Measurement Center, 20% of HSATs were inadequate. A study comparing laboratory testing and HSAT (4) found that 147 of 180 patients had acceptable home studies the first time, resulting in 18.3% of studies scored as inadequate. This means your center is in the same ballpark as the centers participating in the research study. But a failure rate of one in five is high and improving this would result in higher patient satisfaction and profit margins. In a competitive market, a 2% difference might be significant, and patients may gravitate away from your center to the competition.

However, the problem remains that your measurement is based on the standard criteria you have established for your center. The research study did not define "inadequate study" and therefore your comparison may be flawed. Fortunately, this does not invalidate the quality improvement process.

"There are no big problems, there are just a lot of little problems."

Henry Ford

When analyzing the data that have been collected, it's often necessary to examine the component parts of the construct. A center may record low scores on a patient satisfaction survey. That's a big problem. What are the little problems that could contribute to the low satisfaction score? Patients may report long wait times, grumpy staff, uncomfortable beds, and a lack of privacy or have a variety of other complaints. As we work through the quality improvement process, we will try to identify areas of concern and seek to investigate changes that can influence our measures.

In the Galileo Sleep Measurement Center, 20% of HSATs were inadequate. Of these, 75% were due to oximeter failure. This means we can reduce our percentage of inadequate studies to only 5% if we can eliminate the oxygen saturation problems. Can we break this problem down into something we can work on?

A review of the technologist notes finds that for 10% of the studies that were inadequate the patient reported being unable to plug in the oximeter. For another 20% of studies the signal was inadequate from the start with evidence that the probe was not attached properly. And for 70% of the studies the patient reported waking up with the probe not attached to the finger. You measure the duration of valid oximetry readings for your patients and find that the average is only 4.5 hours. From these data, it is clear that we can achieve the largest effect on our measure by improving the way the oximeter probe is attached to the patient's finger. What could be done to keep the probe in place?

A brainstorming session at the center leads to a list of possible interventions: buy a different probe, use stronger tape, educate patients to use a pressure relief loop in the probe cable, or have the technologist attach the probe to the patient when he or she comes to pick up the home-testing device. Some of these methods can be eliminated because of cost or logistics. Settling on a method to try can be the result of a consensus.

Because quality improvement is an experiment, it is important to manipulate only one independent variable at a time. This provides experimental control and supports a cause and effect conclusion. In other words, keep the conditions as similar as possible and change only one thing at a time. If you buy a new probe, change to a stickier tape and modify your patient education strategy, you may reduce the number of inadequate home sleep apnea tests. But what caused the reduction? It would be impossible to know. A more effective strategy may be to stop buying tape at Bob's Discount Tape Emporium and instead go to Marty's Medical Tape Shoppe. If this change causes a significant reduction in inadequate tests, you have determined an effective intervention. If not, you can change something else and see if it works.

"You must take your place in the Circle of Life."
Mufasa, the Lion King

Quality improvement is a circular process. First, you measure. Compare your measure with others. Then you analyze. Finally, make a change. But to close the circle you must measure again and follow the circle of life for another cycle. First, you measure. It is important to use the same measures and the same criteria the second time around. This allows for a valid comparison.

Compare your measure with others. Now that you have completed a cycle, you can compare the new results with the results you measured the first time. There are three possible outcomes: things got better, things got worse, or things didn't change. The outcome will determine what you do next.

If things got better, did they exceed what would be expected by chance? You will need to compare your measure before and after the change. Trigger warning—statistics ahead. Slight variations in your measures are to be expected. The best way to know if you have exceeded those slight variations is to run a statistical test, such as an independent samples t-test. It's not hard and it will let you know if moving forward is worth the effort. If possible, do more of what you did to cause the improvement.

If things got worse, stop the change and start over. Again, make sure the difference between before and after is statistically significant before you give up on the change.

The tricky outcome is that things didn't change. This can happen for several reasons. One reason is that there really is an improvement, but your statistical comparison lacks power. The best way to get more power is to keep going and add more patients to your comparison. If your statistical test is close to showing an improvement, this is the best option. A second option is that your manipulation wasn't powerful enough. You can use a stronger manipulation and see if that makes a difference. The third option is that your change really didn't work. If your measure did not change, you will need to analyze your problem again.

At the Galileo Sleep Measurement Center, the staff agreed to buy a higher-priced tape for patients in an attempt to better secure the oximeter probe. Data were collected for 3 months. This improved the number of hours of valid oximetry to 4.8 hours, but this was not statistically different from the 4.5 hours recorded before the

change. In addition, the number of inadequate studies did not change. One staff person related that the Hubble Sleep Scope Center across town uses tape from Tammy's Tape Emporium, and it works fine for them. Another suggested that two rolls of tape should be provided to each patient instead of one. Dr. Kepler recommended trying forehead reflective oximetry. Dr. Kepler won the debate, and they all agreed to continue the quality improvement process with new technology.

It is important to remember that quality improvement is a circular process, and therefore has no end. Even when one change results in a significant improvement, other aspects of job performance, equipment efficacy, and patient satisfaction will present themselves. And in the end, we can all do better.

REFERENCES

1. Morgenthaler, T. I., Aronsky, A. J., Carden, K. A., et al. (2015). Measurement of quality to improve care in sleep medicine. *Journal of Clinical Sleep Medicine, 11*(3), 279–291.

2. Berry, R. B., Albertario, C. L., Harding, S. M., et al. (2018). *The manual for the scoring of sleep and associated events: Rules, terminology and technical specifications* [Version 2.5]. Darien, IL: American Academy of Sleep Medicine.

3. Aurora, R. N., Collop, N. A., Jacobowitz, O., et al. (2015). Quality measures for the care of adult patients with obstructive sleep apnea. *Journal of Clinical Sleep Medicine, 11*(3), 357–383.

4. Rosen, C. L., Auckley, D., Benca, R., et al. (2012). A multisite randomized trial of portable sleep studies and positive airway pressure autotitration versus laboratory-based polysomnography for the diagnosis and treatment of obstructive sleep apnea: The HomePAP study. *Sleep, 35*(6), 757–767.

chapter 73
Research in the Sleep Center

ALLEN BOONE

LEARNING OBJECTIVES

On completion of this chapter, the reader should be able to:

1. Describe the purpose of clinical research conducted in the sleep center.
2. Define the types of clinical research.
3. Describe the regulatory governance of clinical research involving human subjects.
4. Define the methods of data collection.
5. Define the pretrial and posttrial activities.

KEY TERMS

Adverse event
Serious adverse event
Investigational product (IP)
Contract research organization (CRO)
Subjects
Outcomes
Experimental treatments
Treatment research
Prevention research
Screening research
Diagnostic research
Genetic studies
Epidemiologic studies
Human factors engineering
Failure mode and effects analysis
Discovery and development phase
Investigator's brochure
Preclinical research
In vitro
In vivo
Study plan
Investigational new drug (IND) process
Comparator
Placebo
Double-blind randomized crossover trial
Primary efficacy studies
Site qualification visits
New drug application

Institutional Review Board (IRB)
Clinical research associate (CRA)
Clinical research coordinator (CRC)
Principal investigator (PI)
Delegation of Authority log
Protected health information
Informed consent (IC)
Voluntarism
Information disclosure
Decision-making capacity
European Data Format (EDF)

Research is the reconnaissance party of industry, roving the unknown territories ahead independently, yet not without purpose, seeing for the first time what all the following world will see a few years hence.

S. M. Kinter

In the world of medicine, there is an always evolving desire for discovery in the efforts to prolong wellness and prevent or decrease pain and suffering while effectively and safely treating those in need. Since its beginnings, the practice of medicine has evolved hand-in-hand with research, and there remains a close-knit relationship to this day.

Research of sleep and wake has taken several iterations, from investigatory exploration and experimentation in the efforts to better understand just exactly what occurs during this quasi-hibratory physical state. Of greatest significance was the discovery and quantification of the stages and cycles occurring during sleep. From these discoveries and detailed research came the foundations from which impaired or disrupted sleep and wake functions were appropriately evaluated.

As the developing field of sleep medicine progressed, research began shifting from scientific inquiries needed to define the physiologic functions of sleep toward the pathologies and disorders associated with disrupted, excessive, or insufficient sleep. As eloquently described in the 2005 publication of the *History of the Development of Sleep Medicine in the United States* (1), the science-based foundation paved the way for detailed quantifications of disorders such as narcolepsy, restless legs syndrome, and rapid eye movement behavior disorder.

Today's medical research environment involving sleep and wake is considerably different from that of earlier years. There are more medical sites available to conduct research, and rather than being scientifically focused, these sites are clinically based. These sites are involved in the observation and treatment of patients, and many of the participants involved in clinical trial activities are recruited from their practice databases.

Another significant change in today's sleep/wake-related clinical research is the diversity of investigation. Although there will always be the need for basic science, the majority of clinical trials involve pharmaceuticals or device manufacturers who seek to prove their products' clinical effectiveness. But like the electroencephalogram (EEG), polysomnography (PSG) is also playing a role as a safety measure. Just as the EEG has been, and continues to be, used to measure brainwave activity that could be an indication of an adverse event or serious adverse event, the PSG has come into its own as a means to help investigators identify these safety occurrences. As sleep professionals will attest, there are many events that occur primarily during sleep. Thus, if an investigational product (IP) (drug being investigated) predisposes the study participant to an untoward medical condition during sleep, then the PSG removes ambiguity and provides high-quality, robust data for documentation and quite possibly intervention purposes.

DEFINITION OF RESEARCH

Research is defined as the systematic investigation into and study of materials and sources in order to establish facts and reach new conclusions (2). The National Institutes of Health's (NIH's) definition of clinical research indicates the "aim to advance medical knowledge by studying people, either through direct interaction or through the collection and analysis of blood, tissues, or other samples" (3).

Clinical trials involve research participants, referred to as "subjects." Trials follow a predefined and preapproved plan in the form of a protocol to observe, document, and analyze the effects ("outcomes") of an IP, device, or behavioral intervention. Participation in clinical trials not only increases participants' role in their health care but also plays a critical role of increasing the generalizable knowledge gained during the investigation. Participants have the potential opportunity to access experimental treatments, to which their outcomes can directly contribute to medical research. There are numerous terminology and government agencies specific to clinical research protocols and documents. Please refer to Appendix Q—Research Terminology, Acronyms, and Government Agencies.

The Federal Drug Administration (FDA) specifically recognizes the following trial types (4):

- Treatment research typically involves interventions, such as medication/drug, psychotherapy, devices, or new surgery techniques or radiation intervention.
- Prevention research investigates ways or methods to prevent disorders or diseases from developing or recurring. Prevention research may study medicines/drugs, vitamins, vaccines, minerals, lifestyle changes, or combination therapies.
- Diagnostic research investigates new or improved methods to identify a particular disorder, disease, or condition.
- Screening research investigates new or improved methods to identify certain disorders or health conditions.
- Quality of life research investigates new or improved methods to increase comfort and possibly the quality of life for those with chronic illness.
- Genetic studies investigate new or improved methods to improve prediction of disorders by identifying and understanding how genes and illnesses may be related. Research in this area explores the ways in which genes make an individual more or less likely to develop a disorder.
- Epidemiologic studies investigate new or improved methods to identify patterns, causes, and control of disorders in groups of people.

There are other clinical research involving the validation and verification of medical devices. According to the FDA, the goal of human factors engineering is to reduce or eliminate errors that occur during use of a device that could cause harm or degrade medical treatment to the greatest extent possible (5). This involves assessments at one or more stages during the device development process to identify strengths, weaknesses, or deficiencies that could possibly harm the user. The assessment process utilizes market research, competitor research, failure mode and effects analysis (6), formative and summative in small groups, and well-designed protocols for clinical trials. Device manufacturers developing new or improved positive airway pressure (PAP) machines, hoses, and interfaces are reliant upon this process, and they frequently utilize sleep centers, personnel, and patients as trial participants during the usability segments of development. The results of these trials are then used to make improvements on current designs or validate user acceptance criteria.

For the purposes of discussing an area of greatest relevance to the sleep diagnostic and treatment community, this chapter will focus primarily on pharmacologically related clinical trials. Device trials, such as those investigated for premarket release trials (nasal PAP and other sleep-related equipment), are governed by 21 CFR 812 (7).

DRUG DEVELOPMENT PROCESS

The first step in the process of bringing a new compound to market is the discovery and development phase. Researchers discover new drugs using several methods that include:

- Newly revealed knowledge or insights within a disease that allows researchers to formulate a product

that will at the minimum stop the disease progress or possibly reverse the effects of the disease.
- Testing multiple molecular compounds with the intent of identifying beneficial effects when applied to any of a large number of diseases.
- Investigating already existing compounds or treatments that have effects that were not anticipated in the original design.
- Technologic developments that provide new methods or pathways that were not previously available as a means to assist treatment. Examples of this include new surgical devices that allow access within specific areas of the body or genetic coding.

STAGES OF DRUG DEVELOPMENT

The stages of drug development follow a standard process and timeline, as depicted in Table 73-1. The identification of a promising compound leads to further experiments in order to gather information on items like absorption, distribution, metabolization, and excretion. Other information collected includes dosage, delivery route, side effects or adverse reactions, and intractability with other drugs. All of these results are gathered to serve as the basis for what will become the investigator's brochure. This document summarizes the body of knowledge gained through testing and experimentation throughout the development of the IP or study drug.

The second step is preclinical research. Researchers must find out if the newly discovered compound has the potential to cause serious harm before testing is conducted in humans. Specifically, the effort is to identify its toxicity, conducted through two types of preclinical research areas: in vitro and in vivo. An in vitro test is conducted with glass or plastic laboratory vessels ("petri dishes"), whereas in vivo testing is conducted within the body of a living organism.

The FDA requires researchers to use good laboratory practices (GLPs) for preclinical laboratory studies. This requirement is defined in medical product development regulations. GLP regulations are found in 21 CFR Part 58.1: Good Laboratory Practice for Nonclinical Laboratory Studies.

Table **73-1** Stages of Drug Development

Drug discovery preclinical	3–6 y
Clinical trials; Phases I–III	6–7 y
FDA application and review drug production post FDA approval	6 mo–2 y
Postmarketing safety surveillance clinical trials (Phase IV)	Approximately first half of patent life

FDA, Federal Drug Administration.

Following the successful conclusion of preclinical testing, the IP is ready for human application. Preclinical research, as thorough as it is at answering basic safety questions, is no substitute for actual IP applications in the human. Clinical trials reveal a wealth of information when the IP interacts with the human body in ways bench testing cannot. However, before ever making the first human application, the developers carefully design the overall clinical study (or study plan). They consider what is to be accomplished at each phase. This begins the investigational new drug (IND) process, in which an IND application is submitted to the FDA before clinical research begins. This application includes data from animal studies, toxicity, and any prior human research. Additionally, information about the investigator, manufacturing information, and the clinical protocols (study plan) are included in the submission. Only after FDA approval can the development move to clinical trials.

In clinical drug research, there are four phases of trials (8, 9).

Phase 1 Trials

This is when the IP makes its first contact with humans. This is a highly controlled trial that typically includes between 20 and 100 volunteer participants. The primary focus of this phase is to test the IP for safety, tolerance (usually to dose escalation regimens), and pharmacokinetics (or what the body does to the IP). Healthy volunteers are most commonly used during this phase; however, certain drug designs carry a higher toxicity level in order to be effective to a targeted disease. This higher toxicity would be unethical to administer to a healthy person because it carries a high risk of harm. To this end, the Phase 1 trials for these more toxic compounds will include only participants with the targeted disease. An example of this would be anticancer agents or compounds. According to the FDA, approximately 70% of IND moves on to the next phase. Likewise, it is very rare for Phase 1 trials to occur within a sleep testing facility.

Phase 2 Trials

Phase 2 trials are rigid and well controlled and include a small homogeneous patient population, usually no more than 200 participants. These participants have the targeted disease, but no other confounding illnesses. The primary purpose of this phase is to determine whether or not the IP demonstrates efficacy for its intended indication, and within the safe dose range established during the Phase 1 trial. This trial will typically involve use of "double blinding" where neither the investigator nor the participant is aware of which compound is the "active" (IP) or the "comparator" (a similar already-marketed drug for the same indication), or a placebo. In order to be able to measure the effects of these compounds, participants are randomized in different drug sequences (a means to reduce bias) that involve a period of time per drug and then a "crossover" to the next drug. Hence, the terminology of "Double-Blind Randomized Crossover Trial." This trial phase is more commonly seen in sleep facilities and may only include 5 to 10 investigating sites.

At or near the conclusion of the Phase 2 trial, the sponsor (investigating agent) will meet with the FDA to review all the data collected to this point, and the determination to advance to a Phase 3 trial is made. Of the number of INDs that have made it to this point, the FDA estimates only 33% will move forward to Phase 3 trials.

Phase 3 Trials

This trial phase is an expanded clinical trial intended to gather additional evidence of effectiveness for specific indications and to better understand safety and drug-related adverse effects. This is also referred to as "primary efficacy studies" (10). Phase 3 trials typically have large numbers of participants, ranging from 350 to 1,000 patients. Trials involving large numbers of participants require the developer to seek participants from a wide variety of geographic areas. Factors such as culture, race, and ethnicity can impact participant behavior, whereas reduced or limited diversity can place limits on the generalizability of the findings (11). Therefore, the developer will seek to spread the recruitment efforts across a wide area and, in some cases, take their efforts to other countries in order to satisfy statistical diversification needs.

In the world of clinical trials involving a sleep component, sponsors work with their contract research organization (CRO) to identify multiple facilities capable of handling the protocol requirements as well as the participant volumes. It is very common to see study plans written where the participants are required to have multiple sleep studies in order to complete their trial requirements. To put this into perspective, it is typical practice to have a protocol that, among other requirements, is written to include five or more overnight sleep studies. The plan may or may not include a daytime multiple sleep latency test or maintenance of wakefulness test. If, for example, a hypothetical trial is "powered" (statistically required number of participants needed in order to increase the probability of significant results) by 980 participants and if each of these participants completes the protocol requirements of 5 nocturnal polysomnography (NPSG) studies, a total of 4,900 PSG recordings will be produced for this phase of the study plan. If the sponsor awards the trial to 50 sites, on average each site would generate 98 PSGs for roughly 20 participants. This kind of volume can be burdensome for some sites, whereas others can absorb the volume without issue. Site qualification visits are the sponsors' means for performing

due diligence in determining whether or not sites are adequately equipped to handle their specific trial.

Phase 3 trials can be active for long durations in order to meet the enrollment criteria. For sleep-related trials, duration can be from 18 to 36 months in order to meet the threshold. At the conclusion of the Phase 3 trial, the sponsor makes a formal appeal to the FDA in the form of a new drug application. This request to allow for marketing of the new drug essentially tells the FDA that the sponsor has completed the necessary safety and efficacy requirements in order to gain official approval (12). With formal approval from the FDA, the sponsor can then begin actively promoting and selling their new compound.

Phase 4 Trials

Phase 4 trials begin after the marketing application to the FDA has been approved. The primary purpose of Phase 4 trials is to gather long-term safety data as a condition of the FDA approval. These trials are frequently conducted to compare new compounds with other already-marketed products. Because of the length of time it takes to bring a new compound to market, there can be changes in standards of care for the targeted disease or condition. The FDA will often require the sponsor to continue gathering data as a means of postmarketing surveillance.

KEY PERSONNEL IN CLINICAL RESEARCH

There are a variety of people involved in clinical research, and sometimes it's almost necessary to carry a roster of "Who's Who" in different trials.

First, there is the sponsor. According to regulation 21 CFR 312.3(b), the sponsor is defined as "a person who takes responsibility for and initiates a clinical investigation. The sponsor may be an individual or pharmaceutical company, governmental agency, academic institution, private organization, or other organization." This is the individual or group that initiates the development of the IP or device.

Regulatory requirements are detailed in 21 CFR 312, subpart D, Responsibilities of Sponsors and Investigators. Among the sponsor's responsibilities are:

- Selecting qualified investigators,
- Providing them with the information they need to conduct an investigation properly,
- Ensuring proper monitoring of the investigation(s),
- Ensuring that the investigation(s) is conducted in accordance with the general investigational plan and protocols contained in the IND,

- Maintaining an effective IND with respect to the investigations,
- Ensuring that FDA and all participating investigators are promptly informed of significant new adverse effects or risks with respect to the drug.

For the developers (or sponsors) of the new compound, the FDA includes a robust list of additional requirements:

- Control of drug.
- Obtaining information from the investigator, including a signed investigator statement (Form FDA-1572), an Institutional Review Board (IRB) compliance statement, and a list of all subinvestigators (sub-Is). Before the investigation begins, a sponsor shall give each participating clinical investigator an investigator brochure containing the information described in 312.23(a)(5).
- The promissory of all communicating new observations concerning the IP, in accordance with 312.32.
- Monitoring investigator compliance, in accordance with the requirements of 312.59 and shall notify FDA.
- Review and evaluate the evidence relating to the safety and effectiveness of the drug as it is obtained from the investigator.
- Determine if its investigational drug presents an unreasonable and significant risk to subjects and discontinue its use.
- Maintain IP accountability.
- Maintain complete and accurate records showing any financial interest.
- Retain the records and reports for 2 years after a marketing application is approved for the drug.
- Retain reserve samples of any test article.
- Permit FDA inspection of trial-related materials and records.
- Controlled substances accountability.
- Assure the return of all unused supplies of the IP from each individual investigator, or assure appropriate disposition of unused supplies.

THE CONTRACT RESEARCH ORGANIZATION

According to the International Conference on Harmonization Guideline for Good Clinical Practice E6 (R2), a CRO is "A person or an organization (commercial, academic, or other) contracted by the sponsor to perform one or more of a sponsor's trial-related duties and functions" (13).

The term CRO is broad by definition, and it can be extended to those individuals or organizations that are assigned the responsibility of performing even the smallest of tasks by the sponsor. More commonly, CROs are contracted to provide project oversight of clinical trials. They are often the intermediary for contract and budget negotiations, but more commonly the CRO oversees the trial-related performance of the clinical sites.

The CRO can be assigned a spectrum of responsibilities by the sponsor. However, a participating site must be aware of the scope of the CRO's responsibilities in order to properly address various trial functions and communications to the most appropriate party. This is particularly true in the event the sponsor has transferred a limited number of responsibilities to the CRO. The site will not want to communicate information inappropriately to the wrong party. According to 21 CFR 312, if the sponsor assigns all responsibilities to the CRO, a brief statement stating such is to be provided. The same can be applied in the event of a narrowed scope of responsibilities that are assigned to the CRO.

THE CRA VERSUS THE CRC

A CRA is a clinical research associate, whereas a CRC is a clinical research coordinator. A CRA is the representative of either the sponsor or the CRO, and is assigned the task of assuring the clinical site is performing to the expected standards of the protocol. This is a partial list of the many tasks they perform:

- Assess the site initially for ability to perform as needed for an upcoming trial
- Train the site to the protocol and its associated procedures
- Activate the site as a trial becomes open to accepting new subjects
- Routinely monitor activity and document for completeness and accuracy
- Assist the site in developing or improving recruitment plans
- Perform the close-out visits

Although the majority of CRAs have a clinical background, there are very rare circumstances in which they interact with subjects during a trial.

A CRC, on the other hand, represents the principal investigator (PI) at the clinical site. They are directly responsible for direct subject interaction under the direction of the PI. However, the CRC can perform only the tasks they have been assigned and trained to do. The Delegation of Authority log for the site outlines the specific tasks each of the site's personnel has been assigned to perform, and it is the PI's responsibility to assure all personnel remain within their own scope of performance.

It is possible for a sleep technologist to be a clinical coordinator and vice versa. In many clinical sleep research sites, it is necessary for the coordinator to have a strong understanding of sleep medicine and related technology. However, the requirements for sitting for the sleep technologist registry examinations are insufficient to adequately prepare one for clinical research work. Additional research-specific training, trainee–mentorship guidance, and work experience are minimum requirements for a sleep technologist to either augment or transition to a career in clinical research. A list of resources is provided at the end of this section.

THE INVESTIGATOR

In clinical research, the investigator is defined as the person who actually conducts a clinical investigation and is responsible for the participants. This is the person who specifically agrees to all of the requirements in Section 9, Commitments of the FDA Form 1572. In this section, the investigator agrees to protect the rights, safety, and welfare of participants; follow the rules of the protocol; control the IP and obtain informed consent (IC) from all participants. Additionally, it is the investigator's responsibility to ensure trained, licensed, or certified personnel are appropriately selected for inclusion on the Delegation of Authority form for each specific trial. Moreover, the investigator is responsible to ensure all trial-related staff are familiar with the purpose of the trial and the protocol (14).

> The investigator should ensure that any individual to whom a task is delegated is qualified by education, training, and experience (and state licensure where relevant) to perform the delegated task. Appropriate delegation is primarily an issue for tasks considered to be clinical or medical in nature, such as evaluating study subjects to assess clinical response to an investigational therapy (e.g., global assessment scales, vital signs) or providing medical care to subjects during the course of the study. Most clinical/medical tasks require formal medical training and may also have licensing or certification requirements. Licensing requirements may vary by jurisdiction (e.g., states, countries). Investigators should take such qualifications/ licensing requirements into account when considering delegation of specific tasks. (14)

In the event there is more than one investigator on the research project, one person is designated as the principal or primary investigator (PI). All others are recognized as subinvestigators or "sub-I's" (Section 6, Names of Subinvestigators). Sub-Is do not sign the form's attestation; this is signed by the PI only.

The PI role is most commonly filled by a physician, but it is not uncommon to see a PharmD or PhD as the PI. In the case where IP is being investigated, a physician should be included as a sub-I on the trial. As this pertains to sleep/wake-related clinical trial activity, the PIs have extensive clinical training and experience not only in their own subspecialties (i.e., neurology, pulmonology, and otolaryngology) but also in clinical research. Although many subjects are recruited from within active medical practices, the practice of medicine is not always the same as clinical trial oversight.

GOVERNANCE OF CLINICAL RESEARCH

Research involving human subjects is highly regulated by both national and international bodies. It is the responsibility of all clinical research professionals to know and abide by all applicable regulations, policies, guidelines, and standards to protect the health and welfare of human subjects involved in clinical research. Failure to maintain strict adherence can put trial participants in risky conditions that could potentially have catastrophic consequences as well as legal and civil consequences for the professionals conducting the trial.

ACTION AND REACTION

From September through October 1937, over 100 people died in 15 states. The commonality among all the deaths was found to be a sulfanilamide elixir. Sulfanilamide was a highly effective treatment for streptococcal infections and had been safely used in both tablet and powder forms for many years prior. When the S.E. Massengill Company received requests for a liquid formulation, they developed a solution where the active ingredient was dissolved into the liquid carrying agent. In this case, the carrying agent of choice was diethylene glycol. The company tested the product for flavor, appearance, and fragrance, all of which were found to be satisfactory. With this, S.E. Massengill Company compounded the product and shipped 633 cases across the United States.

Although the company had performed observational testing of the product, they failed to conduct scientific pharmacologic tests with the new compound. At that time, food and drug regulations did not require safety studies on new drugs. This meant that although selling toxic drugs was unethical and immoral, it was not illegal. This tragedy prompted the U.S. federal government to pass the 1938 Federal Food, Drug, and Cosmetic Act. The New Drug section of this act enacted a new system for drug control, which was meant to ensure greater

Table 73-2 Regulatory Developments in Clinical Research

1940–1945: Nazi experiments on humans	Nuremberg Code
1950–1970s: Vulnerable groups entered into clinical trials; that is, prisoners, elderly, and handicapped	Declaration of Helsinki
1932–1972: Tuskegee study of untreated syphilis in the Negro male	National Commission for the Protection of Human Subjects of Biomedical and Behavioral Research 1974 Belmont Report 1978 Common Rule 1991 (45 CFR 46)
1962: Thalidomide used to treat morning sickness, resulting in birth defects	1962 Amendment to the 1938 Federal Food, Drug, and Cosmetic Act; Drug Effectiveness Requirement
1980s: Björk–Shiley prosthetic mechanical heart valve failure	1990 Amendment of the 1938 Federal Food, Drug, and Cosmetic Act; Safe Medical Devices Act (SMDA) of 1990

public protection while increasing medical research and development.

Other events that prompted tightened regulations are included in Table 73-2.

BELMONT REPORT

The Belmont Report (15) is considered to be one of the most important works on ethics and health care research. Like its predecessors that addressed ethics, the Belmont Report's primary purpose is to protect subjects who participate in clinical trials or research studies. The report focused on three specific areas: first was defining the differences between practice and research. This was followed by a section on Basic Ethical Principles; Respect for Persons, Beneficence, and Justice. Finally, the committee concluded with a third section on Application, Informed Consent, Assessment of Risks and Benefits, and then Selection of Subjects.

DECLARATION OF HELSINKI

The World Health Organization (16) in 1964 released a document containing a set of ethical principles regarding human experimentation. Its purpose was to outline defining ethical principles for the protection of participants of experimentation. The document contains 37 statements relating to the following principles:

- General principles
- Risks, burdens, and benefits
- Vulnerable groups and individuals
- Scientific requirements and research protocols
- Research ethics committees
- Privacy and confidentiality

- Informed consent
- Use of placebo
- Posttrial provisions
- Research registration and publication and dissemination of results
- Unproven interventions in clinical practice

The Declaration of Helsinki is considered to be the cornerstone statement of research in medical investigations. Nevertheless, the NIH released its own statement of Ethical Guidelines (17) which include:

- Social and clinical value
- Scientific validity
- Fair subject selection
- Favorable risk–benefit ratio
- Independent review
- Informed consent
- Respect for potential and enrolled subjects

NUREMBERG CODE

From 1946 to 1947, three judges and one alternate of the International Military Tribunal heard the case presented against 23 defendants (20 of whom were physicians) who were accused of murder and torture in the conduct of medical experiments on concentration camp inmates. At the conclusion of "The Doctors' Trial," the judges compiled a set of 10 research principles for the protection of human subjects. Where the Hippocratic Oath focused on the physician, The Nuremberg Code focused on the subjects who were participating in research (18).

Widely recognized for its influence on global human rights law and medical ethics, the basic requirement of IC has been accepted as the first step in protecting research subjects. Along with the other nine principles, the Nuremberg Code indicates:

1. The voluntary consent of the human subject is absolutely essential.
2. The experiment should be such as to yield fruitful results for the good of society, unprocurable by other methods or means of study, and not random and unnecessary in nature.
3. The experiment should be so designed and based on the results of animal experimentation and a knowledge of the natural history of the disease or other problem under study that the anticipated results will justify the performance of the experiment.
4. The experiment should be so conducted as to avoid all unnecessary physical and mental suffering and injury.
5. No experiment should be conducted, where there is an a priori reason to believe that death or disabling injury will occur, except, perhaps, in those experiments where the experimental physicians also serve as subjects.
6. The degree of risk to be taken should never exceed that determined by the humanitarian importance of the problem to be solved by the experiment.
7. Proper preparations should be made and adequate facilities provided to protect the experimental subject against even remote possibilities of injury, disability, or death.
8. The experiment should be conducted only by scientifically qualified persons. The highest degree of skill and care should be required through all stages of the experiment of those who conduct or engage in the experiment.
9. During the course of the experiment, the human subject should be at liberty to bring the experiment to an end, if he or she has reached the physical or mental state where continuation of the experiment seemed to be impossible to him or her.
10. During the course of the experiment, the scientist in charge must be prepared to terminate the experiment at any stage, if he or she has probable cause to believe, in the exercise of the good faith, superior skill, and careful judgment required of him or her, that a continuation of the experiment is likely to result in injury, disability, or death to the experimental subject.

INTERNATIONAL COUNCIL FOR HARMONIZATION

The International Council for Harmonization (ICH) Technical Requirements for Pharmaceuticals for Human Use (19) was formed in 1990 as a global entity to address and create the Guidelines on Safety, Quality, and Efficacy. It later added the subcategory of Multidisciplinary Guidelines. As the organization reports,

> The resulting ICH association establishes an Assembly as the overarching governing body with the aim of focusing global pharmaceutical regulatory harmonization work in one venue that allows pharmaceutical regulatory authorities and notably concerned industry organizations to be more actively involved in ICH's harmonization work.

Specific areas of ICH that cover clinical research can be found in the Efficacy Guidelines section. For those working in a clinical research site, the following have the greatest influence in the conduct of a trial:

E6(R2): Guideline for Good Clinical Practice

E2A: Definitions and Standards for Expedited Reporting

E8: General Considerations for Clinical Trials

E9: Statistical Principles for Clinical Trials

E11: Clinical Investigation of Medicinal Products in the Pediatric Population

Clinical trials with origins in non-U.S. countries focus more on ICH guidelines as their regulatory guidance.

U.S. FOOD AND DRUG ADMINISTRATION

An agency within the U.S. Department of Health and Human Services, it is the FDA's responsibility to protect public health by making sure that human and veterinary drugs, vaccines and other biologic products, medical devices, the nation's food supply, cosmetics, dietary supplements, and products that give off radiation are safe, effective, and secure.

Specific sections of the Code of Federal Regulations (20) that apply to clinical research are:

45 CFR 46: Protection of Human Subjects

Subpart A: Basic HHS Policy for Protection of Human Research Subjects ("Common Rule")

Subpart B: Additional Protections for Pregnant Women, Human Fetuses and Neonates Involved in Research

Subpart C: Additional Protections Pertaining to Biomedical and Behavioral Research Involving Prisoners as Subjects

Subpart D: Additional Protections for Children Involved as Subjects in Research

Subpart E: Registration of Institutional Review Boards

21 CFR Part 11 Electronic Records, Electronic Signature

21 CFR Part 50 Protection of Human Subjects

21 CFR Part 54 Financial Disclosure by Clinical Investigators

21 CFR Part 56 Institutional Review Boards

21 CFR Part 312 Investigational New Drug Application

21 CFR Part 812 Investigational Device Exemptions

The FDA recognizes the ICH guidelines and has adopted various sections within the agency (i.e., Good Clinical Practices). But in specific areas of overlap, the FDA sets U.S. CFR as precedent. As an example, if a U.S. sponsor initiates a trial requiring FDA approval, any country outside the United States that participates in clinical trials must do so using the CFR as the regulatory requirement.

HEALTH INSURANCE PORTABILITY AND ACCOUNTABILITY ACT

The *Health Insurance Portability and Accountability Act*, known as HIPAA, originated in the Office of Civil Rights. Although it is not specific to research, it impacts research with the section called the "privacy rule." The "privacy rule" protects the use and disclosure of patient information, also known as protected health information.

PROTOCOL

According to *Merriam-Webster*, one of the four definitions of "protocol" is "a detailed plan of a scientific or medical experiment, treatment, or procedure." In clinical research, the protocol is road map to which the trial is to be conducted. A very detailed document provides the reader with an IP's background, the intention of the trial and its anticipated outcomes, the intended subject population, and the analysis process.

For the site, the protocol can be viewed as the "Rules of Engagement." The protocol will have been signed off by the PI and approved by the IRB, and must be followed as closely as possible. Failure to follow the rules is classified as a divergence, and depending upon what occurred, it can be further defined as either a deviation or violation.

A deviation is a lesser situation that may occur without significant consequences. For example, a subject missed an appointment within the prescribed time frame (or window) because they were traveling, this is a deviation. On the other hand, a violation is a much more serious event. These can range from events that have an

impact on data collection completeness to making IC inaccurate or impacting the subject's health, safety, and welfare. Examples of a violation include mishandling of samples, incomplete or inaccurate record keeping, or intentional deviation from protocol requirements.

Protocol deviations are sometimes unavoidable, but all attempts should be made to minimize these occurrences. On the other hand, violations (especially those that affect safety, health, and welfare) can have dire consequences. Willfully putting the subject in a compromising position can result in legal actions for the individual who perpetrated the action. This can include removal from the trial, loss of clinical licensure, and criminal prosecution if the infraction warrants. To this end, compliance to the protocol is paramount only to the subjects' welfare.

INFORMED CONSENT

IC is a process, not just a form. Albeit, the IC is recorded in a printed document and signed by the PI and the subject. Moreover, it must occur before any subject participation can occur. There are three critical areas and essential elements of an IC: voluntarism, information disclosure, and decision-making capacity.

The subject retains the right to withdraw consent without repercussion at any time during a clinical trial. The PI is obliged to give the subject any and all relevant new information concerning the trial as it occurs during the subject's time of participation. And lastly, it is the subject who retains the final say in the decision to participate or not. No means no, they have the right to refuse.

CLINICAL RESEARCH IN SLEEP

There are many avenues of clinical investigations in today's sleep medical community. Newer trials are diversifying from strictly pharmaceutical IP investigations, to newer technology involving a variety of devices, techniques, and treatments. Of recent development is the proliferation of "wearable technology." Whereas it was once a matter of giving an IP treatment, recording the sleeping subject, and then analyzing the data to measure the effects (or not), today's trials may include indirect or inferred measures of sleep quality.

Early clinical research trials involving the measurement of sleep on analog polygraphs involved two different methods for analysis. The first method was to produce the recording and then ship it to a site where it was scored by either one person or a select small number of scorers. Reducing the number of scorers meant there would be a potential reduction in interscorer differences, thus quality control was easier to maintain. However, this method of centralizing analysis was expensive and slow. In addition, bulky boxes of irreplaceable participant data were subject to shipping losses. Another popular method of the time was to have each site score their own records. This reduced the analysis time as well as shipping costs. Rather than shipping the records, the "scoresheets" could be faxed to the sponsor. This too had its shortfalls when sponsors pressed the CROs to provide proof of scorer competency from the sites. In order to provide proof, CROs produced an oversight process by which select personnel at site would become "certified scorers" for that specific protocol.

As technology evolved and the industry shifted to digital PSG, the problem of assembling data from multiple sites that may have produced the records from many manufacturers prompted additional regulatory requirements placed by the European Union (EU). Consequently, EU regulators made a condition of sale of polysomnographic and electroencephalographic digital recording systems, that is, the condition of providing a data output whereby a third-party independent software reader could import the recording and correctly display the attributes. First published in 1992, European Data Format (EDF) became the de facto standard for the manufacturers to incorporate as a means of record sharing (21). Using EDF, the records could be imported into an EDF reader software, and the manufacturers' native software remained proprietary, including their algorithms for exporting from native to EDF. Nevertheless, this advance allowed for the electronic transmittal of records from the site to a central reader. As with previous methods of certifying scorers, sponsors required the central readers to provide proof of site competency by producing a recording capable of being imported to an EDF reader. Many central readers required sites to produce sample recordings made to the protocol requirements, and if successfully and accurately produced, the central readers would certify the sites as ready to begin enrolling participants. Now, rather than taking days for shipping and analysis, time frames could be drastically reduced to, in some cases, mere hours for reporting results.

Taking their lead from the EU requirements, many of today's PSG, EEG, and electrocardiogram manufacturers have incorporated EDF as their standard data output. Instead of creating a proprietary digital output that no other system could decipher, emphasis was placed on developing their analysis packages and creating robust reporting analytics in order to gain a market advantage. Some of the systems will allow importing of recordings produced by other systems; however, there has been no literature to date where one manufacturer has validated recordings made using another's proprietary software. They can, however, validate their analysis programs to

EDF standards, thus paving the way for large, multisite trials to transmit their records to a centralized site for scoring and analysis.

Not all clinical trials involving sleep parameters require a participant to have an in-lab PSG. Depending on the focus of the trial, it can be more advantageous to use an ambulatory "home sleep test" to collect the participant data. But this is strictly dependent on the data needs of the trial and compliance to the protocol requirements.

To a certain degree, actigraphy can be cited as the first wearable technology. At its core, actigraphy uses a series of accelerometers to measure the velocity of limb movements. In basic, the more frequent, faster movements are associated with purposeful movement associated with wakefulness. Conversely, slower, less frequent movements are associated with sleep. Despite the inability to decipher wake versus sleep via EEG, actigraphy offers the ability to gather days and/or weeks of data, which upon analysis can reveal a glimpse into the subject's circadian rhythm. It's also a common tool in a wide variety of clinical investigations to confirm participant-reported sleep/wake activities during their enrollment phase. The National Aeronautical and Space Administration (NASA) has integrated actigraphy into many experiments from the space shuttles through the current-day International Space Station missions (22). NASA has used the technology as a means for monitoring astronaut sleep/wake cycles during investigative research experiments and as a safety indicator for disrupted patterns while in flight.

Newer trends in research include implantable devices to improve sleep. Recent developments include:

- Implants in the soft palate to increase the diameter of the airway
- Implantable pulse generators to deliver a stimulus to the hypoglossal muscle during an obstructive apnea event (23)

Other devices include vented patches that cover the nares as a means to increase oral airflow for mild to moderate OSA, nasal vents to hold the sinus cavities open during sleep, and oral devices to move the mandible forward to prevent the tongue from falling back onto the soft palate during sleep.

In the course of clinical trials, there are many measures of sleep and wake that can indicate the effects of treatment (Table 73-3). These are referred to as "end points," and they can be the primary focus of the trial or secondary measures of trial outcomes.

Pharmacologic developments and investigations will continue as long as the need remains, and there are many opportunities for sleep technologists to expand their careers in the clinical research arena.

Table 73-3 Sleep and Wake Measurement End Points

Sleep efficiency	How well or how poorly a participant sleeps during the PSG recording can be correlated as an effect of the treatment, whether it's better, worse, or the same. This can apply to both IP and device trials.
LPS	By definition, LPS occurs at the beginning of the first 10 min of sleep after lights out. This measure can be used to gauge treatment effect in relation to sleep-onset arousals that prevent consolidated sleep early in the recording.
WASO	"WASO" is frequently used as a treatment efficacy measure in IP and device trials. As an end point, it reveals how well treatment has impacted the participants' ability to sleep all the way through the recording after initially falling asleep. It is frequently used in insomnia treatment trials.
Arousals	In large part, arousals during sleep occur secondarily to other disrupting factors, such as apnea or periodic limb movements. However, arousals in narcolepsy appear to occur spontaneously and without provocation. Hence, the frequency of arousals is an important treatment indication for these related trials.
REM latency	REM latency during the PSG and/or MSLT can reveal the effects of untreated or undertreated sleep pathologies, whether a circadian rhythm disorder or narcolepsy. Hence, its measurement indicates treatment efficacy.
Sleep stages	Increases in percentages of certain sleep stages with decreases in others when measured in baseline and treatment nights can indicate the effectiveness of the intended treatment. To reduce the chances of bias, IP trials use a randomized double-blind, crossover pattern of IP and placebo. As such, the sleep stage percentages (or time duration) from baseline (no treatment), Night 1 (treatment or placebo), and Night 2 (switch from Night 1) are compared for differences. The most ideal result is when treatment is at least as or more effective than placebo, or $p > 0.05$ for treatment significance.
LM	Reduction of limb movement during sleep in one IP trial may be the intended result, whereas an increase in another IP trial may be indicative of an unanticipated adverse event. Therefore, although the first trial may use the reduction as a primary end point, the second trial might use LM as a secondary end point because this would be an unintended result of treatment.
Respiratory events	Results of respiratory measures can be end point data for both device and IP trials. Clearly, the goal in breathing-related sleep disorders device trials is to reduce the occurrence of events, which is a primary end point of investigation. It may be the same during an IP trial, but it also may be the unintended effect of the IP treatment. In this case, the outcome of respiratory event changes can become a secondary end point with an emphasis on safety.
PROMs	PROMs are used as a means of corroboration of the participants' perspective in relation to trial activities. They are often evaluated immediately after a diagnostic (i.e., PSG, MWT) or treatment evaluation or during the period between measures. Common PROMs include: • Epworth Sleepiness Scale (ESS) • SF-36 Health Survey; Short Form 36 (captures participants' perceptions of their health-related quality of life).

IP, investigational product; LM, limb movements; LPS, latency to persistent sleep; MSLT, multiple sleep latency test; MWT, maintenance of wakefulness test; PROMs, patient-reported outcomes measures; PSG, polysomnography; REM, rapid eye movement; WASO, wake after sleep onset.

REFERENCES

1. Quan, S. F. (2014). The *Journal of Clinical Sleep Medicine*—A decade of progress: Looking backward and forward. *Journal of Clinical Sleep Medicine, 10*(1), 5–6. doi:10.5664/jcsm.3344

2. *Oxford Dictionaries*. Retrieved from https://en.oxforddictionaries.com/definition/research. Accessed June 1, 2018.

3. National Institutes of Health; Eunice Kennedy Shriver National Institute of Child Health and Human Development. *Clinical research*. Retrieved December 30, 2017, from https://www.nichd.nih.gov/health/clinical-research. Accessed May 1, 2018.

4. U.S. Food and Drug Administration. *What are the different types of clinical research?* Retrieved from https://www.fda.gov/forpatients/clinicaltrials/types/default.htm. Updated January 4, 2018. Accessed June 1, 2018.

5. U.S. Department of Health and Human Services, Food and Drug Administration, Center for Devices and Radiological Health, & Office of Device Evaluation. (2016). *Applying human factors and usability engineering to medical devices. Guidance for industry and food and drug administration staff.* Retrieved from https://www.fda.gov/downloads/medicaldevices/.../ucm259760.pdf. The draft of this document was issued on June 21, 2011. Accessed November 23, 2018.

6. American Society for Quality. *Failure mode effects analysis (FEMA).* Retrieved from http://asq.org/learn-about-quality/process-analysis-tools/overview/fmea.html. Accessed July 1, 2018.

7. U.S. Department of Health and Human Services. Medical Device Tracking Requirements, 21 CFR §821. https://www.ecfr.gov/cgi-bin/text-idx?SID=37de800fb45e161d2a4a4c96c98d3e5b&mc=true&node=pt21.8.821&r gn=div5. Accessed December 14, 2018.

8. U.S. Department of Health and Human Services. Investigational New Drug Application, 21 CFR §312.21 Phases of an Investigation. https://www.ecfr.gov/cgi-bin/text-idx?SID=37de800fb45e161d2a4a4c96c98d3e5b&mc=true&node=se21.5.312_121&rgn=div8. Accessed December 14, 2018.

9. U.S. Department of Health and Human Services. Investigational New Drug Application, 21 CFR §312.85 Phase 4 Studies. https://www.ecfr.gov/cgi-bin/text-idx?SID=37de800fb45e161d2a4a4c96c98d3e5b&mc=true&node=se21.5.312_185&rgn=div8. Accessed December 14, 2018.

10. Weeks-Rowe, E., Woodin, K., & Schneider, J. (Eds.). (2016). *The CRA's guide to monitoring clinical research* (4th ed., pp. 41–54). Boston, MA: CenterWatch.

11. Sugden, N., & Moulson, M. (2015). Recruitment strategies should not be randomly selected: Empirically improving recruitment success and diversity in developmental psychology research. *Frontiers in Psychology, 6,* 523.

12. U.S. Department of Health and Human Services. Applications for FDA Approval to Market a New Drug, 21 CFR §314. https://www.ecfr.gov/cgi-bin/text-idx?SID=37de800fb45e161d2a4a4c96c98d3e5b&mc=true&node=pt21.5.314&rgn=div5. Accessed December 14, 2018.

13. International Council for Harmonisation of Technical Requirements for Pharmaceuticals for Human Use. (2016, November). *ICH harmonised guideline. Integrated addendum to ICH E6(R1): Guideline for good clinical practice E6(R2).* Retrieved from https://www.ich.org/fileadmin/Public_Web_Site/ICH_Products/Guidelines/Efficacy/E6/E6_R2__Step_4_2016_1109.pdf

14. U.S. Department of Health and Human Services Food and Drug Administration. (2009, October). *Guidance for industry investigator responsibilities—Protecting the rights, safety, and welfare of study subjects.* Retrieved from https://www.fda.gov/downloads/Drugs/.../Guidances/UCM187772.pdf

15. Department of Health, Education and Welfare. (1974). *The Belmont Report.* Retrieved from https://www.hhs.gov/ohrp/sites/default/files/the-belmont-report-508c_FINAL.pdf

16. World Medical Association. (2018, July 9). *WMA Declaration of Helsinki—Ethical principles for medical research involving human subjects.* Retrieved from www.wma.net/policies-post/wma-declaration-of-helsinki-ethical-principles-for-medical-research-involving-human-subjects/. Accessed November 23, 2018.

17. National Institutes of Health. *Patient recruitment. Ethics in clinical research. Ethical guidelines.* Retrieved from https://www.cc.nih.gov/recruit/ethics.html. Updated March 2018. Accessed June 2018.

18. Shuster, E. (1997). Fifty years later: The significance of the Nuremberg code. *New England Journal of Medicine, 337,* 1436–1440.

19. International Council for Harmonisation. *The International Council for Harmonisation of technical requirements for pharmaceuticals for human use.* Retrieved from https://www.ich.org/home.html. Accessed July 2018.

20. U.S. Department of Health and Human Services, Office for Human Research Protections. *About OHRP.* Retrieved from https://www.hhs.gov/ohrp/about-ohrp/index.html. Accessed May 2018.

21. European Data Format. Retrieved from https://www.edfplus.info/. Accessed August 2018.

22. National Space and Aeronautical Agency. *Sleep-wake actigraphy and light exposure on ISS-12 (Sleep ISS-12).* Retrieved from www.nasa.gov/mission_pages/station/research/experiments/1802.html. Updated April 2018. Accessed August 2018.

23. Hong, S., Chen, Y.-F., Jung, J., et al. (2017). Hypoglossal nerve stimulation for treatment of obstructive sleep apnea (OSA): A primer for oral and maxillofacial surgeons. *Maxillofacial Plastic and Reconstructive Surgery, 39*(1), 27. doi:10.1186/s40902-017-0126-0

chapter 74

The Sleep Technologist in the Medical Office

JULIE DEWITTE

LEARNING OBJECTIVES

On completion of this chapter, the reader should be able to:

1. Define how home sleep apnea testing is influencing sleep centers and practices.
2. Describe the various functions and expanding roles for the sleep technologist.
3. Discuss the comprehensive sleep program models and the use of technology to support patients.
4. Describe how to grow an expanded sleep program.

KEY TERMS

Alternative therapy
Comprehensive sleep program
HSAT
Integration systems
Team based practice
Technology
Utilization management

CHANGES IN SLEEP CENTER FUNCTION

The Effect of Home Sleep Apnea Testing on Sleep Centers

Health care reforms are bringing changes to health insurance plans and pushing providers to improve the continuity and coordination of care, in an effort to improve patient outcomes and provide cost-effective and efficient care. A significant impact of these measures in sleep medicine is the shift toward home sleep apnea testing (HSAT) for diagnosing obstructive sleep apnea (OSA) and increasing attention to developing practices for improving positive airway pressure (PAP) therapy delivery and compliance. The sleep center is moving from a fee-for-service reimbursement model to an outcomes-based model. The purpose is to reduce costs and optimize patient care.

Sleep testing is trending more and more toward HSAT, rather than in-laboratory overnight testing, and this is directly related to the payer policies. Sleep centers have seen different degrees of adoption of HSAT; however, the trend is shifting away from overnight in-laboratory testing because of changes in reimbursement. This trend is affecting the growth of sleep centers and altering the necessary skill level and knowledge base of technologists (1).

Historically, the majority of patients referred for overnight testing were being evaluated for suspected OSA. With the huge impact of HSAT as the primary diagnostic tool for diagnosing these patients, the dynamics of in-laboratory overnight testing needs to focus on evaluating complex patients with multiple comorbidities (2). These patients include those with hypoventilation, chronic respiratory failure, and premature infants with complex breathing problems.

Technologist Involvement

To manage overnight testing for complex patients, sleep technologists require proper education and strong critical thinking skills. Technologists need to perform patient assessments and be familiar with looking at patient test results (e.g., pulmonary function tests, routine blood work, echocardiograms). It is critical that technologists have a good understanding of the underlying pathophysiology of particular disease processes. Complex patients require close monitoring of ventilatory patterns while they are sleeping. Technologists also require the knowledge to manage complex ventilatory devices like volume-assured pressure support and adaptive servo-ventilation.

The changes occurring are providing technologists an opportunity to utilize their skills in an ambulatory sleep center or office-based sleep program. This necessitates that sleep laboratories become comprehensive sleep centers, and that physicians educate and work with technologists to integrate their skills into the patient care process. Services that can benefit from technologist knowledge and skills and reduce physician workload may include a PAP follow-up program, a PAP walk-in clinic, an alternative therapy program, or an insomnia program. Expansion of sleep center services could also include neonatal and pediatric inpatient testing, and a perioperative screening program. The technologist/clinician's role includes utilizing clinical judgment by making clinical assessments, providing patient education, communicating test results to the patient, and communicating with nonsleep department medical staff.

Insurance Authorization

Another function that can benefit from technologist knowledge and experience is management of the testing and treatment authorization processes. With the introduction of HSAT, the majority of basic OSA patients are being referred for a daytime educational instruction and sent home with a cardiorespiratory device for overnight testing. HSAT is much less expensive than in-laboratory testing and can accurately assess the patient suspected to have moderate-to-severe obstructive apnea (3). Patients requiring differential diagnoses, those with complex comorbidities, and pediatric patients will still require overnight polysomnography (PSG).

The insurance type (e.g., Preferred Provider Organization, Health Maintenance Organization, Medicare, Medicaid) will determine how an authorization is obtained. Multiple private insurers not only require preauthorization but regularly make use of utilization management companies to review preauthorization documents. Utilization management incorporates devices and methods for determining if the testing is medically necessary and if the patient can be tested using HSAT versus in-laboratory overnight testing. The utilization management companies' purpose is to assist the insurer to form authorization processes. The downside of utilization management is clinical decision limitations to the physician. In many cases the need for an in-laboratory assessment requires additional effort by the provider to obtain preauthorization.

Some sleep facilities require the physician's office to obtain the insurance authorization before sending the referral to the sleep center; however, sleep center personnel may have the responsibility for obtaining preauthorization. When a referral is received, it should specify the type of study ordered or if a sleep physician consult is necessary before testing. Some facilities consider the referral as the prescription; otherwise, a prescription stating the type of study needs to be provided. A history and physical that includes a sleep history, along with patient demographics and insurance billing information, will need to accompany the referral. The sleep history should include documentation of body mass index, height, weight, and neck size.

Depending on the insurance company and type of insurance plan it may take several days to a couple of weeks to obtain authorization. To obtain insurance authorization, the appropriate *International Classification of Diseases (ICD)-10* diagnosis codes will need to be listed to identify the patient's symptoms. An appropriate procedure code like the Current Procedural Terminology

(CPT) is also required for authorization of the type of study to be conducted. It is important to know which procedure codes a particular insurer accepts. For example, for HSAT testing, some insurers accept a G-code procedure code, whereas others accept the corresponding CPT procedure code. There are also specific procedure codes for pediatric patients less than 6 years of age. It is the provider's responsibility to contact the insurance company to identify which codes are accepted for testing. It is recommended to have a list of procedural codes available for reference. Be mindful to contact the insurance company if the study conducted fell under a different CPT code than what was authorized (e.g., code 95811—PSG with PAP was authorized but 95810—PSG was completed). Sleep center personnel are often also required to verify the patient's insurance benefits and determine any deductible or copayment that may be required. This information should be available to review with the patient at the time of scheduling, so that he or she is informed of payment due before the sleep study date.

These functions often are most easily accomplished by a sleep technologist with a knowledge of sleep disorders and their symptoms as well as comorbidities that might influence the decision to approve in-laboratory testing as against HSAT.

A COMPREHENSIVE SLEEP PROGRAM MODEL

A comprehensive sleep center expands patient services to make the center prosper and provides a wide spectrum of clinical patient care activities. An expanded ambulatory program in a comprehensive program may include services such as PAP trials, a PAP follow-up program, management of non-PAP therapies for OSA, a weekly PAP walk-in clinic, and an insomnia program. Other methods of extending services include working with in-hospital partners. A perioperative screening program can be developed by partnering with anesthesia and surgeons. Inpatient testing or screening programs can be developed by partnering with pulmonologists and neonatologists to identify patients in need of diagnosis, treatment, and continued follow-up after discharge. All of these services include the need for experienced sleep personnel—a natural fit for the sleep technologist.

A comprehensive care model requires a close-knit multidisciplinary team to manage program growth and the use of protocols to drive patient care. Telemedicine and technologies such as video and telephone visits, remote monitoring, and automated care mechanisms will improve efficiency and effectiveness of patient care and workflow. In this care model, the medical director leads a team of case managers comprising respiratory therapists with formal sleep training and sleep technologists.

This type of a sleep care program will not only alter a physician's role but also enhance the role of the sleep technologist and ensure the future of sleep centers.

Technology to Support Patients and Treatment

Technology today can be useful to assist the sleep technologist in efforts to assure patient compliance with therapy. Technology can provide data that patients can see and this is one means of enhancing therapy use in PAP patients. The increasing utilization of HSAT technology has had a huge impact. There are multiple wearable devices that many motivated patients may use to track their caloric intake, exercise, and weight management, as well as an estimation of their sleep.

PAP devices have wireless modems either built-in or attached to the device. This permits patient adherence checks and adjustment of PAPs remotely. Utilizing wireless modems enables the sleep center staff to track patient adherence while decreasing the number of patient office visits required, which, in turn, increases patient satisfaction. Sleep technologists typically manage this type of a therapy monitoring program in either an office-based or comprehensive sleep program.

Much of the work of monitoring patient PAP adherence can benefit from technology. A PAP modem attached to an automated platform can send feedback to the clinician and a message to the patient for any issues detected or be used to motivate the patient who is doing well with treatment. This type of patient feedback has been shown to improve PAP adherence by 66% (4). The automated platform assists clinicians to focus on patients who are struggling and make more efficient use of their time in daily operations.

The integration of automated mechanisms and the creation of a closed-loop system in the sleep program can reduce primary care physician (PCP) visits, improve PAP therapy adherence, and reduce the need for PCPs to manage sleep disorders. A closed-loop system enhances and streamlines the end-to-end patient care continuum. In a closed-loop system, the sleep team works together to provide optimal patient care and continuous long-term management. A closed-loop system means the sleep specialist is responsible not just for diagnosis and study interpretation, but for long-term follow-up care as well, and can also provide inpatient program support.

There are Internet-based patient education programs available that can ease the anxiety of patients and increase their understanding of how to prepare for a sleep study, what to expect when they go to a sleep center, educate them on OSA and PAP therapy, and explain the difference between an HSAT study and a polysomnogram. These programs have soothing voices, animated graphics, and easy-to-read text, and patients are able to watch the program as many times as they wish. They are a helpful adjunct to technologist-provided education and support.

EXTERNAL INTEGRATION SYSTEMS

Traditionally, sleep centers have focused on diagnostic testing, providing PAP therapy, and patient follow-up. Comprehensive care under an end-to-end workflow model begins with population management using risk identification screening, patient preassessment using web-based education, sleep history intake questionnaires, and wearable sensors. However, managing all of these components can be very problematic because of each being independent of the other. The results are not attached to the electronic health record (EHR) and a provider has to "hunt and peck" to find and compile all the information. An external integration system incorporates mechanisms that connect the entire health care team and improve workflow. The system is the core, connecting all aspects of patient care, including self-directed care platforms, automated care processes, and other remote technologies. This results in the patient and provider team being seamlessly connected from one end to the other with the EHR as the hub to facilitate team-based care.

INTERNAL INTEGRATION SYSTEMS

Integrated care involves creating a team-based practice, protocols to drive patient care, and utilizing individual and group patient appointments and technology to enable patient engagement and improve efficiencies.

The physicians create clinical care pathways and protocols for the staff to follow. They provide training material and case studies for staff education, check and assure quality, and conduct chart reviews. The physicians not only read and interpret sleep studies but also provide patient consults and conduct research projects. They function as the leaders within the sleep medicine program and partner with other specialists to create care pathways and improve the management of patients.

In this model, the technologists/clinicians are using clinical judgment and collaborating with the physicians in the diagnosis and treatment of patients by reviewing the preliminary sleep testing results and initiating treatment. They make appropriate referrals from HSAT testing to in-laboratory testing or to other specialties as indicated by protocols or the physician. Integration and automated mechanisms with the sleep technologist at the forefront facilitate efficiency and provide the patient with effective care.

TEAM-BASED CARE

Team-based care structures sleep center programs and services to utilize specific levels of care for a patient's situation. Although all team members should be informed and kept updated with all aspects of the sleep services available, a multidisciplinary team approach allows a sleep program to provide specific levels of care on the basis of patient needs.

There are many potential areas of growth for sleep technologists/clinicians in a focused team-based care approach. There are also additional opportunities for technologists to support programs such as a commercial driver program, a durable medical equipment (DME) program for dispensing PAP devices, or an insomnia program linked with Internet-based cognitive behavior therapy. Technologists with sufficient training can also manage complex sleep patients (e.g., respiratory failure and muscular dystrophy) under the direction of a physician.

Creating an alternative therapy program is another avenue for sleep centers to offer options for nonadherent PAP patients. Technologists/clinicians trained in this specialty area can evaluate the patient for the appropriate pathway to alternative therapy, such as oral appliance therapy (OAT), positional therapy, or, when appropriate, implantable devices.

Workflows need to be developed for each specialty area and team to care for these patients. Complex sleep-disordered patients are fragile and require very close, timely, and consistent follow-up and encouragement. In this model, the technologist/clinician is at the hub of coordinating the patient's care; thorough close management will steer the direction of care that the patient requires.

With the appropriate training and education, the technologist/clinician can review and monitor diagnostic tests, which may include pulmonary function studies, arterial blood gas results, echocardiograms, and chest X-rays. It is important to know and understand such physiologic information as the patient's vital capacity, oxygen and carbon dioxide levels, and cardiac function including ejection fraction percentage. The technologist/clinician may also monitor the patient's adherence to noninvasive ventilation and make adjustments to PAP as needed for comfort and acclimation. Utilization of transcutaneous carbon dioxide monitoring can indicate how well the patient is ventilating. Overnight oximetry is often useful to determine the need for supplemental oxygen during sleep.

PATIENT ENGAGEMENT

All patient care providers need certain skills in order to build rapport with patients. The ability to demonstrate compassion, confidence, patience, and understanding are skill sets that will assist the technologist to gain the patient's trust and assist him or her to successfully implement his or her treatment plan. As providers we perform a routine of day-to-day procedures and we don't necessarily think from a patient's perspective. We need to remember that this is a new experience for patients

and sometimes not a pleasant one. It's important to realize that every patient is unique and each needs to be treated as an individual.

Routine procedures can be very intimidating. Before doing anything medical during a patient visit, take the time to associate on a personal level. During the office visit, it is important to introduce yourself, be at eye level, ask open-ended questions, and actively listen to the patient. The technologist should always be aware of not only the patient's body language but his or her own as well. The investment of a little bit of extra time will establish a connection with the patient and he or she will trust you and the plan of care. By listening not only with your ears, but also with your eyes and heart, you will connect with the patient on a much deeper level, which will build trust.

Explain to patients how sleep apnea will affect them personally, not in generalized terms. It will empower them to make this personal to them, so that they can explore the options and benefits that treatment will have on their life (e.g., ask patients what it would mean to them if they woke up feeling more refreshed and energized). Think about what might motivate them to be adherent to therapy. Will patients have the perception that they are going to stop breathing and die in their sleep, or might they think that they are having some pauses in their breathing and this machine will help them sleep better? Their perception is based upon the technologist's approach to explaining the disorder and treatment options to the patient. When terms like heart attack, stroke, and diabetes are used, it instills fear in the mind of a patient and can sometimes result in resistance. Inform the patient but keep it simple so he or she can understand the information and be less fearful. Communicating using language at a third-grade level improves patient understanding. The use of visual cues and graphics, avoiding the use of technical jargon, and speaking in layman's terms increase the patient's acceptance of information. As a technologist, it is imperative to connect with patients at their level to ensure that they understand the information. Utilize open-ended questions when reviewing information with patients to further strengthen their knowledge and gauge their level of understanding. Keeping patients motivated increases the probability of starting, continuing, and adhering to therapy. Inform patients you are there for them, provide contact information, and educate them regarding additional resources available for support.

CHALLENGES

Growth and a shift to a comprehensive sleep center or program from a testing-based sleep laboratory present many challenges. There must be a change in culture and focus to a new global perspective. People may be very resistant and fearful of change. However, the change will create growth and with utilization of new technology the sleep technologist can have a significant role in the medical office or expanded sleep program. Sleep medicine has become extremely specialized and, therefore, innovation helps improve efficiency by utilizing new technologies.

Employee engagement and performance excellence require continuous education. Learning new methods and understanding current technology are critical to successfully working with patients. The field of sleep medicine is rapidly changing and evolving into a complex specialty. Weekly staff education time should be scheduled for physicians and staff to present patient case studies and participate in learning new technology and programs. This will keep the technologist involved and using critical thinking skills.

The expansion of sleep center services requires a quality improvement tracking system to analyze the many different types of encounters. Quality improvement is not just a regulatory exercise or a program that is required to perform services but is a living dynamic process that drives the procedures in the sleep program. When data show poor outcomes, the workflow will need to change, providing another challenge that sleep programs face.

ALTERNATIVE THERAPY

The sleep technologist in the medical office or expanded sleep program is likely to interact with and educate patients undergoing PAP and other alternative therapies. This requires an expanded view of patient therapies. Alternative therapy is multifaceted and includes many different forms of therapy. Even positional therapy, that is, assisting a patient with positional OSA to avoid the supine position during sleep, is considered an alternative therapy.

ORAL APPLIANCE THERAPY

An oral appliance is a device that may be utilized for the treatment of OSA and snoring. The technologist should be familiar with oral appliances, which primarily comprise tongue retaining and mandibular advancement devices (MADs). These devices are small, easy to use, portable, and designed to pull the tongue forward or hold the jaw in a forward position to keep the airway open during sleep. The most common device is the MAD.

Indications for an oral appliance include OSA of all severities, although efficacy may be limited in those with severe OSA. Contraindications include central sleep apnea, dentures, loose teeth, or a significant number of missing teeth and extensive gum disease. A specialized

dentist trained in sleep dentistry and oral appliances works with the sleep team to customize oral appliance therapy (OAT) for patients with OSA.

A temporary MAD device is a short-term type of therapy to identify responders before prescribing a custom oral appliance. This device is a boil-and-bite apparatus that provides horizontal and vertical adjustments to the mandible. A temporary oral appliance has been shown to predict success of a custom oral appliance (5). The technologist instructs the patient how to use the device and also makes necessary adjustments. The patient should have follow-up sleep testing to check efficacy of the oral appliance (6). If the patient is successful with the temporary oral appliance, the sleep specialist will refer the patient for a custom device consultation. The dentist recommends the style and type of device best suited to the patient. The technologist educates and works with the patient to assure proper follow-up with the dentist and the sleep physician.

EXPIRATORY POSITIVE AIRWAY PRESSURE

This therapy may be prescribed for patients with OSA. The technologist must be familiar with the therapy and contraindications, which include severe breathing disorders such as hypercapnic respiratory failure, respiratory muscle weakness, severe heart disease, and acute upper respiratory infections.

The device provides positive expiratory pressure when a patient breathes out, as a means to keep the airway open. It consists of a pair of oval-shaped devices that fit over the nares. The patient will use one set per night as they are disposable. The technologist should instruct the patient on the use of the device and discuss possible complications before the patient starts therapy.

Explain to the patient that discomfort during wake time is possible because it is difficult to breathe out through the nose while using this device. It is important for the technologist/clinician to instruct the patient to breathe through the mouth while he or she is awake and adjusting to the device. Coach the patient to breathe normally and not force the air out through the nose because this can damage the ear drum. Upon falling asleep, there will be a natural shift to nasal breathing and the patient will not be aware of the expiratory pressure created.

The patient should have a follow-up HSAT study approximately 2 weeks after the start of therapy to validate effectiveness of this therapy.

SURGICAL OPTIONS

Patients who are nonadherent to other forms of sleep apnea therapy may have surgical options; however, this is dependent on whether surgery will be beneficial for them. There are multiple different sites within the upper airway that may be the contributor to OSA and the severity of the apnea. The technologist's role in patients undergoing surgical therapies for sleep-disordered breathing is providing education and support postprocedure if needed. All complications or continuing symptoms must be brought to the attention of the surgeon and/or sleep physician. Surgical patients should be retested once healing from surgery is complete to assure that their sleep-disordered breathing has resolved.

TONSILLECTOMY/ADENOIDECTOMY

In nonobese children, surgery is usually the first line of treatment in the form of tonsillectomy/adenoidectomy. Craniofacial surgeries are helpful for correcting deformities but are not usually considered in otherwise normal children whose facial structure is still growing. If surgery is performed because of OSA, follow-up PSG is highly recommended, particularly in obese children.

UPPER AIRWAY SURGERY

Traditionally, uvulopalatopharyngoplasty (UPPP) was at one time one of the most common surgical procedures performed for OSA. New emerging therapies such as hypoglossal nerve stimulation are promising, although additional evidence regarding long-term impact is needed (7).

Nasal obstruction and nighttime nasal congestion are known risk factors for sleep-related breathing disorders. Common areas of the nasal passage that may contribute to sleep apnea prevalence are deviated septum, enlarged turbinates, and nasal valve collapse. The medical specialist will evaluate the patient to determine the type of procedure that will be most effective for that patient (e.g., septoplasty, turbinate reduction, cartilage graft). Patients with a deviated nasal septum might be corrected simultaneously with UPPP for moderate-to-severe OSA; however, UPPP is not considered to be a primary therapy in itself.

MAXILLOMANDIBULAR ADVANCEMENT AND GENIOGLOSSUS ADVANCEMENT

This surgical procedure moves the jaw forward to enlarge the upper airway. It is normally performed after other forms of surgical treatment have failed. A genioglossus advancement may be done concurrently to pull the tongue forward and prevent it from blocking the airway. Patients with high residual apnea–hypopnea index and respiratory disturbance index after other types of unsuccessful surgical procedures may benefit from maxillomandibular advancement as a subsequent step after UPPP (8).

POSITIVE AIRWAY PRESSURE (PAP) THERAPY

PAP Trial

A continuous positive airway pressure (CPAP) therapy trial program allows patients to try PAP therapy for approximately 7 days. The patient returns to the sleep center for a follow-up adherence check at the end of the trial to assess the efficacy of therapy. If the patient's OSA is well controlled with PAP therapy, home equipment can then be ordered through a DME company. This is an excellent way to assess the likelihood of adherence to therapy in patients who are hesitant to use PAP.

New PAP User Class (or Peer-to-Peer Support)

Another service that sleep programs can provide is a new PAP user class. This is a group setting in which a sleep technologist instructs the patients on the use of PAP therapy and care of their equipment and provides information on an approximate timeline for replacement of supplies. In many cases, the group setting is appropriate as a peer-to-peer support mechanism, but keep in mind some patients may not be comfortable in a group setting.

Troubleshooting Appointments and Follow-Up

Patients often experience anxiety and difficulty with initiation of PAP therapy. Offering support programs assures the patient that there are options and other modalities to help them become and remain adherent with therapy.

PAP therapy troubleshooting and desensitization appointments are a valuable service for patients. The technologist is an integral component—assessing the patient, working out issues with equipment or therapy, and assisting the patient to achieve long-term success with PAP therapy. Technologists must assess the patient's anatomy, sleeping position, air pressure leaks, any disabilities that may hinder application of the mask, and check PAP adherence. Desensitization appointments are useful as a means to assist patients who are struggling with PAP therapy. They may need a different form of treatment for their OSA (e.g., CPAP vs. auto-PAP, or a different type of equipment).

Another useful tool to assist the patient having difficulty using PAP is breathing exercises. The technologist can teach the patients breathing exercises to help them relax and adapt to PAP therapy.

To monitor and evaluate treatment effectiveness, schedule a 90-day follow-up appointment. This is reassuring to patients and indicates you will continue to support the patient to succeed with therapy.

Growing an Extended Sleep Program

The sleep technologist/clinician is well positioned to be a major part of sleep center and program growth. There are many opportunities for the technologist to develop and utilize his or her clinical skills. With the multiple changes occurring in the health care industry and the direct impact to sleep centers, it is critical for the technologist in any setting to be open to change and utilize the many tools that are already available to grow and enhance sleep program services. HSAT offers additional avenues for innovation and to support a successful sleep program. Technology is a key factor that can be used to provide support to patients and to the sleep program. Utilizing all of these tools changes how we deliver care and manage patients with sleep disorders. A program that utilizes all of these modalities together will successfully provide the patient with long-term continuous care and assure sustainability as a comprehensive sleep center or program.

REFERENCES

1. Brooks, R., & Trimble, M. (2014). The future of sleep technology: Report from an American Association of Sleep Technologists summit meeting. *Journal of Clinical Sleep Medicine, 10*(5), 589–593.
2. Parish, J. M., Freedman, N. S., & Manaker, S. (2015). Evolution in reimbursement for sleep studies and sleep centers. *Chest, 147*(3), 600–606.
3. Collop, N. A., Anderson, W. M., Boehlecke, B., et al. (2007). Clinical guidelines for the use of unattended portable monitors in the diagnosis of obstructive sleep apnea in adult patients. *Journal of Clinical Sleep Medicine, 3*(7), 737–747.
4. Hwang, D., Chang, J. W., Benjafield, A. V., et al. (2018). Effect of telemedicine education and telemonitoring on CPAP adherence: The tele-OSA randomized trial. *American Journal of Respiratory and Critical Care Medicine, 197*(1), 117–126.
5. Hwang, D. (2018, June). *Evaluating the use of a titratable pre-fabricated mandibular advancement device to predict response to a custom device.* Abstract Presentation. Associated Professional Sleep Societies, Baltimore, MD.
6. Ramar, K., Dort, L. C., Katz, S. G., et al. (2015). Clinical practice guideline for the treatment of obstructive sleep apnea and snoring with oral appliance therapy: An update for 2015. *Journal of Clinical Sleep Medicine, 11*(7), 773–827.
7. Strollo, P. J., Jr., Soose, R. J., Maurer, J. T., et al; STAR Trial Group. (2014). Upper-airway stimulation for obstructive sleep apnea. *New England Journal of Medicine, 370*(2), 139–149.
8. Zaghi, S., Holty, J. E., Certal, V., et al. (2016). Maxillomandibular advancement for treatment of obstructive sleep apnea: A meta-analysis. *JAMA Otolaryngology— Head & Neck Surgery, 142*(1), 58–66. doi: 10.1001/jamaoto.2015.2678

chapter 75

The Sleep Technologist in the Durable Medical Equipment World

SUSAN HARPHAM   SONIA GARCIA   NICOLE BRECHT   MICHAEL R. WATSON

LEARNING OBJECTIVES

On completion of this chapter, the reader should be able to:

1. Understand testing requirements for coverage of various positive airway pressure devices.
2. Identify when it is appropriate to transfer from continuous positive airway pressure therapy to bilevel therapy.
3. List tips to improving patient adherence to therapy.

KEY TERMS

Durable medical equipment (DME)
Continuous positive airway pressure (CPAP)
Bilevel positive airway pressure (BPAP)
Expiratory positive airway pressure (EPAP)
Inspiratory positive airway pressure (IPAP)
Autotitrating positive airway pressure (APAP)
Adaptive servo ventilation (ASV)
Average volume assured pressure support (AVAPS)
Apnea–hypopnea index (AHI)
Respiratory disturbance index (RDI)
PAP adherence

In the ever-changing world of durable medical equipment (DME), we are faced with many challenges. These challenges include how to balance quality patient care with a decreasing rate of reimbursement and a growing need for documentation. As a DME company, selecting appropriate devices, ensuring that documentation meets reimbursement requirements, managing patient adherence, and utilizing various resources effectively are essential to a successful outcome for the patient.

SELECTING APPROPRIATE DEVICES

A variety of equipment is available for treatment of sleep-disordered breathing (SDB). Selection of the device will depend on diagnosis and the appropriate setting(s) required to treat the condition and requires a physician order. A diagnosis is needed before the insurer will allow dispensing of positive airway pressure (PAP) equipment. Acceptable testing includes an in-laboratory polysomnography (PSG) or a home sleep apnea test (HSAT) that meets the criteria of the Centers for Medicare and Medicaid for type II, III, or IV testing. Many health insurers are leaning toward the more cost-effective use of HSAT when the patient meets criteria for high pretest probability of obstructive sleep apnea (OSA) (1). Table 75-1 provides PSG and HSAT device specifications for diagnosis of OSA.

CONTINUOUS POSITIVE AIRWAY PRESSURE

OSA is typically treated with a continuous positive airway pressure (CPAP) device. The preferred method for determining the appropriate treatment pressure for patients with OSA is an in-laboratory PAP titration. Some patients who undergo in-laboratory PSG for diagnosis meet criteria for severe OSA (an apnea–hypopnea index [AHI] of >40) on the diagnostic night and undergo a split-night study, with PAP titration occurring on the same night. Patients with a high pretest probability of OSA who undergo HSAT for diagnosis sometimes are placed on an autotitrating device at home following diagnosis.

Once OSA has been confirmed via sleep testing, a CPAP device will generally be ordered for home use. Following a standard in-laboratory titration, the physician determines the appropriate PAP pressure and provides an order for home CPAP equipment on the basis of those findings. Standard CPAP pressures range from 4 to 20 cm H_2O. The order may include specific flex settings for patient comfort or a ramp time, and generally will include an order for a specific PAP interface (mask or another interface option).

BILEVEL POSITIVE AIRWAY PRESSURE

In patients with OSA, a bilevel PAP (BPAP) device is often used if a patient is unable to tolerate higher PAP pressures. BPAP may also be used when CPAP is

Table 75-1 Types of Sleep Studies

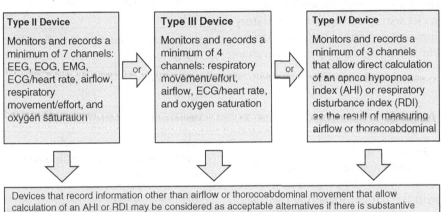

Type I

This polysomnography is performed in a facility-based laboratory to show sleep staging with 1–4 lead electroencephalogram (EEG), electrooculogram (EOG), submental electromyogram (EMG), and electrocardiogram (ECG). It must also include at least the following additional parameters of sleep: airflow; respiratory effort; oxygen saturation by oximetry; and whole night used for diagnosis or split night used for diagnosis and treatment

Type II Device

Monitors and records a minimum of 7 channels: EEG, EOG, EMG, ECG/heart rate, airflow, respiratory movement/effort, and oxygen saturation

or

Type III Device

Monitors and records a minimum of 4 channels: respiratory movement/effort, airflow, ECG/heart rate, and oxygen saturation

or

Type IV Device

Monitors and records a minimum of 3 channels that allow direct calculation of an apnea hypopnea index (AHI) or respiratory disturbance index (RDI) as the result of measuring airflow or thoracoabdominal

Devices that record information other than airflow or thorocoabdominal movement that allow calculation of an AHI or RDI may be considered as acceptable alternatives if there is substantive clinical evidence in the published peer-reviewed medical literature that demonstrates that the results accurately and reliably correspond to an AHI or RDI. This determination will be made on a device-by-device basis. Currently, the only approved type IV device that indirectly measures AHI or RDI is the Watch-PAT device.

ineffective at controlling hypopneas. In some patients, apneas are controlled at lower CPAP pressures, but hypopnea is not controlled until much higher pressures are reached. In this case, BPAP allows the use of a lower expiratory pressure to control apnea and a higher inspiratory pressure to control hypopnea, which is often better tolerated. Standard BPAP pressures range from 4 to 25 cm H_2O, with separate settings for inspiratory positive airway pressure and expiratory positive airway pressure (EPAP) based on the requirements determined to control their SDB determined during an in-laboratory titration study.

AUTOTITRATING POSITIVE AIRWAY PRESSURE

In patients with positional or rapid eye movement (REM)–related SDB, an autotitrating positive airway pressure (APAP) device is also an option. These patients may require relatively high PAP pressures when sleeping supine, but minimal pressure when sleeping in other positions. Similarly, patients with primarily REM-related events may be more comfortable on a lower PAP pressure during other stages of sleep when respiratory events are minimal. Standard APAP pressures range from 4 to 20 cm H_2O. The physician typically orders a setting range for home treatment of patients using APAP on the basis of the pressure needs identified during a titration study.

APAP is also used as a means of titrating and determining PAP pressure requirements at home in patients with uncomplicated OSA, sometimes by requirement of the insurance carrier. The physician ordering APAP to determine treatment needs for OSA patients generally specifies an open APAP pressure range from 4 to 20 cm H_2O and orders APAP for 3 to 7 days at home. A data download can then assist the physician to determine an appropriate CPAP setting for the patient and allows the patient to be switched from APAP to CPAP for long-term treatment or determine the need for further in-laboratory testing.

ADAPTIVE SERVO VENTILATION

Primary central sleep apnea (CSA) is frequently treated with an adaptive servo ventilation (ASV) device. An in-laboratory PSG is required to determine optimal treatment settings for patients who require ASV. The diagnosis of CSA requires an AHI greater than or equal to 5 with the sum of the total central apneas plus central hypopneas greater than 50% of the total apneas and hypopneas; and a central apnea–hypopnea index greater than or equal to 5 per hour; and the presence of either excessive daytime sleepiness, insomnia, frequent awakenings; and no evidence of daytime or nocturnal hypoventilation.

The requirements are stringent, and clinical documentation of symptoms along with a PSG that demonstrates CSA as defined are essential to obtain approval for ASV equipment coverage. Standard ASV pressures range from 4 to 25 cm H_2O and require a determination of the pressure support (PS) minimum and maximum setting; EPAP minimum and maximum setting; and an auto or fixed backup rate setting during an in-laboratory titration. These settings are specified in the physician order for ASV treatment following the physician's evaluation of the titration study.

BILEVEL AND AVAPS

Restrictive thoracic disorders and chronic obstructive pulmonary disease are often treated with a bilevel-S or bilevel ST device. These devices can be used in a spontaneous mode (S) with the patient triggering the inspiratory pressure or a spontaneous timed mode (ST) with a backup rate if needed.

An average volume assured pressure support (AVAPS) device is similar to a bilevel device with auto-titration that occurs on the basis of patient breathing patterns. Home use of bilevel or AVAPS requires documentation of neuromuscular disease or severe thoracic cage abnormality (e.g., kyphosis, scoliosis, or pectus carinatum) in the patients' medical record. Titration must be performed in a sleep laboratory and entails monitoring the patient during the titration to assure that any obstructive events are treated, and that the device is adequately meeting the tidal volume requirements to maintain adequate oxygenation. Standard AVAPS pressures range from 4 to 25 cm H_2O with a PS minimum and maximum setting, EPAP setting, and backup rate setting (2).

DOCUMENTATION AND REIMBURSEMENT REQUIREMENTS

DME coding for sleep therapy falls into two main categories, international classification of diseases (ICD) and healthcare common procedure coding system. The code sets are utilized to report medical diagnoses and procedures for claim reimbursement. All providers, including physicians, use this coding system and it is based on documentation in the patient's medical record. Insurance will use these codes to determine coverage criteria (3). Table 75-2 provides a listing of ICD-10 codes for SDB diagnoses.

Table 75-2 ICD-10 Coding for Common Sleep Disorders

Condition Type	ICD-10 Code
Unspecified sleep apnea	G47.30
Primary central sleep apnea	G47.31
High-altitude periodic breathing	G47.32
Obstructive sleep apnea (adult) (pediatric)	G47.33
Sleep-related nonobstructive alveolar hypoventilation	G47.34
Congenital central alveolar hypoventilation syndrome	G47.35
Sleep-related hypoventilation/ hypoxemia	G47.36
Central sleep apnea in conditions classified elsewhere	G47.37
Other sleep apnea	G47.39
Obesity hypoventilation syndrome	E66.2
Restless legs syndrome	G25.81
Cheyne–Stokes breathing pattern	R06.3

Most insurers have similar requirements for approval of PAP therapy. The patient must have a documented face-to-face clinical evaluation by the treating physician before undergoing a sleep study. The clinical evaluation should include a sleep history, signs and symptoms of OSA, a validated sleep hygiene inventory (i.e., Epworth Sleepiness Scale), and a physical exam. The physical exam should include a measurement of neck circumference, documentation of body mass index, and a focused cardiopulmonary and upper airway evaluation. Some or all of the following elements in the patient's chart notes:

The patient must also have had a covered sleep study that meets criteria for diagnosis of OSA. This is generally defined as an AHI/RDI greater than or equal to 15 with a minimum of 30 events or an AHI/RDI greater than or equal to 5 and less than 15 events per hour with a minimum of 10 events and documentation of excessive daytime sleepiness, impaired cognition, mood disorders, insomnia, hypertension, ischemic heart disease, or a history of stroke (4).

In order to transition a patient to bilevel therapy, they must meet all of the qualifying criteria. This requires documentation that the patient has qualified for PAP, that PAP therapy was tried and proven ineffective during a trial conducted in a facility or home setting, and that the patient met compliance requirements.

Bilevel substitution can occur during several time frames. During the initial PAP therapy from 0 to 60 days, substitution with a bilevel device does not require a new initial face-to-face clinical evaluation or a new sleep study. A patient reevaluation must be completed between the 31st and the 91st day of initiation of the original CPAP therapy. During the 61st and the 91st days following the initial PAP therapy, substitution of a bilevel device still does not require a new initial face-to-face clinical evaluation or a new sleep study. During this time frame, a patient reevaluation must take place before the 120th day after initiation of the original CPAP therapy.

After the 91st day from the initiation of therapy, a new clinical evaluation is required, but a new sleep study is not required. If a bilevel device is substituted at this point, a new 3-month trial begins for the bilevel device therapy and a patient reevaluation must occur between the 31st and the 91st day of initiation of the bilevel therapy (4). Table 75-3 provides a listing of appropriate devices for treatment on the basis of diagnosis and insurance requirements for coverage of the therapeutic device.

MANAGING ADHERENCE

For most insurers, adherence to therapy is defined as the use of PAP greater than or equal to 4 hours per night on 70% of nights during a consecutive 30-day period anytime during the first 3 months of initial therapy. Medicaid adherence guidelines vary from state to state. The patient must also have a face-to-face visit with his or her prescribing physician within the 31st and the 91st day after starting therapy. The physician must document in the patient chart notes that the patient is benefitting from the therapy (4). Adherence must be achieved and documented for payment of the device to be covered as well as for ongoing supply coverage. Adherence can be difficult to achieve for numerous reasons. The most common reasons for nonadherence include poor patient participation, improper mask fitting, poor tolerance of PAP pressures, and side effects of treatment.

The first hurdle to adherence is getting the patient to participate in the therapy. Education is essential because often times the patient interaction with his or her physician after the sleep study is limited. During an initial CPAP setup, some patients only know that a device was ordered, but do not know why. Therefore, it is essential to begin the encounter by educating the patient on the condition that the physician has diagnosed as a result of his or her sleep study. The most effective approach is to review the symptoms that sent the patient for evaluation and testing and the results of his or her sleep study, such as the AHI and what that indicates in layman's terms. At this point, education on PAP therapy and the benefits of use will give the patient the knowledge needed to decide if he or she is going to take an active role in the therapy (5).

Table 75-3 Therapeutic Devices Appropriate for Treatment of SDB by Diagnosis

Condition:	Requirements:				Device:	HCPCS:
Obstructive sleep apnea (OSA)	Attended/home-based polysomnogram with a minimum of 2 h of recorded sleep without device &	Apnea–Hypopnea Index (AHI) ≥ 15/h or	AHI ≥ 5 and ≤14/h and must include at least one of the following: &	EDS Insomnia Mood disorders Impaired cognition Hx of stroke hypertension ischemic heart disease	CPAP APAP Bilevel-S	E0601 E0601 E0470
Central sleep apnea (CSA)	Attended/home-based polysomnogram with a minimum of 2 h of recorded sleep without device &	The Diagnosis of CSA OR Complex sleep apnea (CompSA) &	The ruling out of CPAP as an effective therapy if either OSA or CSA is a component of the initially-observed sleep-associated hypoventilation. &	Significant improvement of the sleep-associated hypoventilation with the use of the bilevel device while breathing the usual FiO_2	Bilevel-S Bilevel S/T Bilevel AVAPS Bilevel ASV	E0470 E0471 E0471 E0471
Restrictive thoracic disorders	Sleep oximetry ≤88% (for at least 5 continuous minutes on usual FiO_2) or	$PaCO_2$ ≥ 45 mmHg OR While awake and breathing normal FiO_2 or	MIP < 60 cm H_2O OR FVC < 50% predicted (progressive neuromuscular diseases only) &	COPD does not contribute significantly to the patient's pulmonary function. Requires documentation in the patient's medical record of a neuromuscular disease or a severe thoracic cage abnormality	Bilevel-S Bilevel S/T Bilevel AVAPS	E0470 E0471 E0471
Chronic obstructive pulmonary disease (COPD)	Sleep oximetry must be ≤88% for at least 5 continuous minutes. &	Liter flow must be on 2 L/min, or the Patient's normal FiO_2, whichever is higher. &	$PaCO_2$ ≥ 45 mm Hg While awake and breathing usual FiO_2 &	Before initiating therapy, OSA and treatment with CPAP have been considered and ruled out.	Bilevel-S	E0470
COPD conversion from S to S/T	Sleep oximetry ≤88% for at least 5 continuous minutes, repeated no sooner than 61 d after initiation of bilevel-S &	Must be breathing on Oxygen at 2 L/min or the patient's normal FiO_2, whichever is greater &	This must be accomplished while the patient is breathing on a bilevel-S device. &	$PaCO_2$ ≥52mmHg, repeated no sooner than 61 d after initiation of compliant use of a bilevel-S system, and while awake and breathing the patient's usual FiO_2.	Bilevel S/T Bilevel AVAPS	E0471 E0471

Proper mask fitting is crucial to patient adherence. A common complaint is the comfort and/or fit of the mask, and an uncomfortable mask may lead a patient to discontinuing therapy. There are three main types of masks; full face, nasal, and nasal pillow. During the initial PAP setup, identifying the correct type of mask that fits the patient's physical features and personal lifestyle is important. Full face masks are generally used for claustrophobic patients, mouth breathers, and patients on higher PAP pressures. Nasal masks and nasal pillows are generally used with lower PAP pressures for patients who can sleep breathing through their nose. Improper fitting can cause leaking, eye irritation, skin breakdown, and restless night of sleep. In most cases, the initial interface fitting would have been performed in the sleep center during the titration study, and often the physician will order a specific mask for the patient. Because of limited time during the titration study, the patient may not have the ability to trial various types of interfaces. Therefore, the patient should be informed that there are other interface options if he or she is having difficulty with the initial mask or interface provided.

Therapeutic settings for PAP are determined by the ordering physician and must be adhered to by the DME provider. The patient should be informed that it will take time for him or her to get used to the pressure and the mask. This desensitization period is different for each individual. If the patient awakens during the night and feels that the pressure is too high, it is important to assure that he or she understands the ramp function and is instructed to use it if necessary. If the patient cannot tolerate the PAP pressure after the desensitization period, evaluating the efficacy data can provide the physician some insight into what pressure settings are appropriate and if the proper device has been prescribed.

Appropriate replacement of PAP supplies is also vital to compliance. Most insurers have guidelines on the frequency of supply replacement and requirements for supply coverage. For instance, some insurers may require current device downloads to document usage in order to approve supply replenishment. Medicaid requirements for resupply will also vary from state to state. The most common resupply coverage frequencies are listed in Table 75-4.

New device technologies such as modem downloads and smartphone applications have provided patients, clinicians, and physicians with new ways to support adherence to therapy and optimize treatment. Modems are able to upload readings daily that show hours of usage, interface leak, and efficacy data. DME companies have varied timelines and frequency for reviewing the information. Some sleep centers and physician staff also monitor these downloads frequently, particularly during the early period of therapy initiation, to assist with patient adherence.

For PAP patients, intervention early and often to address issues could mean the difference between an

Table 75-4 CMS PAP Supply Reimbursement Schedule

Device	Healthcare Common Procedure Coding System	Frequency
Full-face mask	A7030	1/3 mo
Full-face cushion replacement	A7031	1/mo
Nasal cushion replacement	A7032	2/mo
Nasal pillow cushion replacement	A0733	2/mo
Nasal/pillow mask	A7034	1/mo
Headgear	A7035	1/6 mo
Chinstrap	A7036	1/6 mo
Tubing used with PAP device	A7037	1/3 mo
Filter, disposable, used with PAP device	A7038	2/mo
Filter, nondisposable, used with PAP device	A7039	1/6 mo
Water chamber for humidifier, used with PAP device, replacement	A7046	1/6 mo

PAP, positive airway pressure.

adherent user and a nonadherent one. PAP equipment downloads also provide a wealth of information in determining optimal pressure settings for the APAP user, including knowledge of emergent central apneas and AHI reporting to assist with a determination that the best device has been prescribed for treatment. CSA occurs when the effort to breathe is diminished or absent and is usually associated with a reduction in blood oxygen saturation on the download. Downloads also assist to ensure that the interface is working well for the patient. The smart phone application gives patients the ability to be engaged in their treatment and positively reinforces continued use, which assists them to feel they are in control of their treatment.

PEDIATRIC PATIENTS

Pediatric sleep patients are different on every level for a DME company. The qualifications for reimbursement as well as adherence requirements are different for each insurer, and there are many limitations. CPAP, bilevel, and ASV machines cannot be used on any person less than 66 lb. Bilevel S/T and AVAPS cannot be used on a pediatric patient who is less than 7 years old and at least 40 lb. In addition, there are limited pediatric interfaces available.

Some DME companies create their own release form and will set up equipment for pediatric patients outside of the parameters provided by the manufacturers. A noninvasive ventilator is approved for use in the pediatric patient, and it has the capability to treat SDB in this patient without a physician requiring to sign a release form. Adherence to therapy is difficult with this population; in many cases, the patient is too young to understand why the device is ordered or the purpose of its application. With these patients, the caregiver plays a huge role in the success of therapy and the patient's ability to tolerate treatment.

PROFESSIONAL OPPORTUNITIES

With a decreasing rate of reimbursement in the DME industry, providers have had to be creative with how to provide quality education and treatment support for sleep patients. Some companies have opted to drop-ship devices with instructional videos, whereas others utilize nonlicensed, well-trained, and supervised technicians. These individuals can provide education for patients prescribed APAP and CPAP devices but not for bilevel or ventilation devices. Nonlicensed individuals receive in-depth training on symptomology, interfaces, and device treatments. Licensed clinicians complete ongoing monthly competency checks for the nonlicensed individuals. This has opened up opportunities for other health care professionals including sleep technologists, medical assistants, and nursing assistants in the DME industry. In some states, personnel require licensing, so referencing individual state requirements through your regulatory agency for licensure clarification is recommended.

Patients can have admirable sleep therapy outcomes if proper testing, documentation, device consideration, and educational support is provided. Continued monitoring will help ensure that patient treatment needs are addressed as his or her condition changes. So, when referring to DME companies, research their patient care, training, adherence track record, and device knowledge to assure that patients are receiving quality care and are likely to succeed with therapy.

REFERENCES

1. Koninklijke Philips Electronics. (2011). *Helpful hints for filing polysomnography and home sleep test (HST) for diagnosing obstructive sleep apnea (OSA)* [Brochure]. Geyer SB. Retrieved from https://philipsproductcontent.blob .core.windows.net/assets/20170523/e992fd3d72be4f 618b73a77c015724ba.pdf
2. ResMed. (2014). *Respiratory assist device (RAD) qualifying guidelines* [Brochure]. San Diego, CA: Author.
3. Department of Health and Human Services, Centers for Medicare and Medicaid Services. Medicare Learning Network. (2018, May). *ICD-10-CM, ICD-10-PCS, CPT, and HCPCS code sets* (Publication ICN 900943). Retrieved from https://www.cms.gov/Outreach-and-Education/Medicare-Learning-Network-MLN/MLN-Products/Downloads/ICD9-10CM-ICD10PCS-CPT-HCPCS-Code-Sets-Educational-Tool-ICN900943.pdf
4. CGS Administrators, LLC. (2017). *Local coverage article: Positive airway pressure (PAP) devices for the treatment of obstructive sleep apnea* (Article A52467). Retrieved from https://www.cms.gov/medicare-coverage-database/details/article-details.aspx?articleId=52467&ContrID=140#0
5. Good Night Medical. (2016). *What is CPAP?* Retrieved from http://goodnightmedical.com/learn-how-we-can-help-treat-your-sleep-disorder

chapter 76

The Sleep Technologist Working in Industry

JOSEPH W. ANDERSON

LEARNING OBJECTIVES

On completion of this chapter, the reader should be able to:

1. Define the opportunities in industry for the sleep technologist.
2. Describe the role of continuing education for technologists seeking work in the sleep industry.

KEY TERMS

Analog
Continuing education
Digital
Electronic medical record (EMR)
HTML
Computer networking
Positive airway pressure
Registered Polysomnographic Technologist
Telecommute

INTRODUCTION

Opportunities available to the sleep technologist today are not the same as it was several decades ago. It was much easier to gain entrance into a field that was growing extremely fast, and entry-level opportunities could be found almost anywhere. Even if you were not already working in an allied health field, there were sleep laboratories that were willing to train you through their own entry-level "in-house" training or orientation programs.

Education resources in those days were limited, costly, and usually required traveling hundreds or thousands of miles from home for weeks at a time to learn the basics needed to obtain a position in a sleep laboratory that did not have its own training program. After training and considerable time working in a local sleep laboratory, you would need to travel to sit for the board examination in the hopes of obtaining the

Registered Polysomnographic Technologist credential. These boards were given in certain cities and on certain dates. If you did not pass the required testing, it could be months before you would have another opportunity to take the examination.

Although entry into the field was based more on personal initiative and the willingness to learn, career pathways were somewhat limited. Most sleep laboratories were managed under pulmonary or neurology services, often by the supervisors from those departments. Most sleep laboratories were hospital based, and even with the rapid growth of the service, hospitals were often not clear on just how to manage these sleep laboratories, even though they saw the medical need for the service.

The rapid growth of sleep laboratories created a shortage of trained and qualified staff that could safely and accurately perform sleep studies. Most of the studies at the time were done using paper polygraphs; however, the transition to digital technology began on a large scale in the 1990s. This transition created new opportunities for those who wanted to work in sleep, teach sleep technology, or travel. There were growing opportunities beyond clinical practice in both industry and education. We will explore several industry opportunities and look ahead to the future.

EDUCATION

As the need for sleep technologists grew because of the expansion of the industry, the ability of individual sleep laboratories to employ those with little to no experience reduced. Laboratories found themselves needing staff that at minimum were knowledgeable in basic medical terminology, physiology, cardiology, neurology, pulmonary function, and the ability to work with computers because of the transition from paper (analog) to computer (digital) polysomnography.

Sleep training companies, colleges, and schools with accredited sleep technology programs grew and provided trained and educated personnel to meet the expansion in sleep diagnostics and therapy. This matrix of education programs created opportunities for those trained and educated in sleep technology to train those who desired to enter the field.

Even though the number of sleep education programs and institutions has seen a recent decline, the role of the educator continues to be a solid path to advancement in the sleep field. The American Academy of Sleep Medicine–Accredited Sleep Technology Education Program, the Sleep Technology–Approved Resource programs supported by the Board of Registered Polysomnographic Technologists, and other collegiate and sleep education programs ensure that there is a continuing role in the industry for the educator.

PRODUCT DEVELOPMENT AND MANAGEMENT

During the rapid expansion of the industry in the 1980s and the 1990s, an additional career path opened surrounding the need to develop and manage new diagnostic and therapeutic products: recorders, positive airway pressure devices and masks, and the hardware and software to support the conversion to digital media. New vendors developed advanced, improved equipment, and they needed staff who were not only skilled in specific industry needs but also familiar with sleep diagnostics and therapy. The combination of these skill sets presented opportunities for technologists to leave the clinical or education setting and join the engineering, manufacturing, and sales sectors.

As advances in technology continue, the need for experienced sleep technologists in product development and management roles will increase in the coming years.

SOFTWARE DEVELOPMENT AND INFORMATION TECHNOLOGY

With the move to digital equipment during the late 1990s and early 2000s came the need for more information technology (IT) professionals. The next 10 years brought tremendous development in the digital world of acquisition and therapy equipment and software, including various forms of in-lab and global networking. Today, sleep diagnostic systems are networked together in the sleep laboratory or through the facility network and electronic medical record (EMR) software for review and storage of data.

For the sleep technologist to work with IT and software developers, however, it is essential to have a basic knowledge of software, software development, HTML, and computer networking. The sleep technologist with IT knowledge can effectively collaborate with developers and engineers to assist with mapping out the field's needs-based direction for software and product development.

Social media, mobile phone and tablet apps, web sites, and many forms of media provide additional industry opportunities for sleep technologists. The tools needed to create and maintain these platforms are beginning to make it easier for those with moderate software development skills to merge those skills with sleep medicine and technology knowledge to create a medium that can market or support a sleep industry product.

SALES

The equipment and software business is highly competitive, and vendors are always looking to hire sleep technologists who may enjoy and excel in sales. These positions may be either inside or outside sales positions. Inside sales normally involve calling on accounts within a given territory. These accounts can be specialized accounts such as government entities, hospitals, or private sleep laboratories. One benefit of an inside sales position is that you usually stay close to home because the majority of the sales are conducted by phone or via the Internet.

Outside sales generally require face-to-face visits to accounts several times a year. These visits are usually within an assigned territory domestically or globally. Sales trips require travel ranging from 1 day to a week or more. This is a rewarding position for someone who enjoys sales, likes to travel, and has the support on the home front to allow travel. Both inside and outside sales also include travel to and participation in trade shows and conferences, within the United States and sometimes internationally.

Working in sales is not for everyone, because there are downsides. Often, your income is based upon your sales commissions and the business of sales is highly competitive. The software and equipment you are marketing is similar to that of the competition, and the successful sale is often personality driven as much as in the price or equipment performance. For those possessing an outgoing personality and the temperament for sales, the financial rewards afford great potential, as does the opportunity to travel.

MARKETING

For those with a creative side and meticulous attention to detail, marketing may be an interesting career path. Marketing is the connection between product development and sales (*development + marketing = sales*). It's where the tactics and tools for the sales team are developed to assist them in generating interest in the products being sold. These products can be a brand-new platform or design or an upgrade or revamp to an existing system already in use.

Marketing is the arena where new equipment documentation is developed to be filed for national and international compliance and regulatory approvals to sell the product. This includes development of the inserts and labels on the product or in the product packaging. Arrangements are made for product testing and evaluations "outside" of the company for documentation of the safety and other compliance requirements needed to obtain government approvals for domestic or international sales.

The marketing department is where the sales resources are designed and developed. These resources include photographs, videos, brochures, press releases, social media, sales sheets, specification sheets, technical manuals, product manuals, promotional events, and the incentives for sales, promotional items, and campaigns to promote and highlight the product for the intended customer base. Many times, the marketing team is responsible for identifying the appropriate trade shows and conferences for product marketing and they are also often in attendance at these venues.

The price point at which the product will be sold is identified within the marketing department. Price encompasses the development and production costs, licensing and government approval costs and fees, sales commissions, delivery and setup costs, training costs, support costs, and finally the desired margin of profit. Understandably, the sales team wants the product sold at the lowest price point possible to make it most financially competitive, whereas the company prefers a higher profit margin. In marketing, there is a balance between many components that lead to a product's success.

Social media has provided a place to market a product or concept instantly. Marketing information such as release news or marketing materials can be made available through a variety of digital avenues with the information traveling globally within seconds. This is another industry opportunity for the sleep technologist who wishes to showcase their marketing and social media skills.

EQUIPMENT INSTALLATION

Another very important industry role open to the sleep technologist is installing the purchased product or product upgrade. This role requires expertise with the product and the technical skills to use the product and act as the trainer or educator for the product being installed. This usually entails an extended on-site visit to the customer's facility to install the product and teach equipment operations, usually to both the day and night shift staff, including the physicians.

Ideally, the sleep laboratory is closed during the process of installation and training, but this may not always be the case. When the sleep laboratory is closed during installation, a set schedule for installation and training will maximize on-site time. However, when the sleep laboratory remains open, a new installation can cause a lot of confusion and disrupt the day-to-day operations of the sleep laboratory.

Because of the complexity of interfacing with a specific EMR or facility firewall, there is usually participation with the biomed and IT departments during the installation process. The actual physical installation (i.e., running the cables, installing audio and video equipment) is usually contracted out and may or may not be completed before the installation of the equipment. The majority of time during an installation is usually spent positioning the product and creating the interface and internal network setup for the system as well as training the staff on the new or upgraded product.

The preferred method of training is to train the trainer. The facility identifies a few selected individuals, providers, and/or technologists to receive product training and education. In turn, they will disseminate the knowledge to the rest of the staff. This method is efficient in reducing confusion and distractions, especially when the laboratory remains open and operational during installation and training.

TECHNICAL SUPPORT

Once any product is installed and put into actual use, there is a need for product support. Product support ranges from providing a simple refresher on the correct use of the product for maximum efficiency, to supporting product upgrades and making repairs. In the case of a failure of some product component or process, a technical support call is made to the vendor or manufacturer of the product for assistance. Technical support is an area where an experienced technologist can showcase his or her knowledge base not only in the clinical arena but also in the hardware, software, and education realm.

Technical support can be provided from corporate headquarters and a designated support location or may be delivered remotely from the support technologist's own home. Technologic advances and the desire to reduce operating costs make the latter increasingly more popular. Increased Internet speeds have made it possible to provide seamless, complete full-service technical support from just about anywhere. Recent reports show that about one in five workers across the world telecommutes. In some parts of the world such as the Middle East, Latin America, and Asia, nearly 10% of workers work from home. Traditionally, telework is not as common in the United States, but in an attempt to increase profit margins by reducing operation and overhead costs, it is gaining popularity with employers, and it is expected to surge in the future.

SUMMARY

During the past few decades, the skill sets of those who work in all aspects of sleep medicine and technology have increased to meet the technologic advances that have occurred. Entry-level opportunities now mean an educational commitment. Fewer opportunities exist that do not require some level of advanced training or education before beginning a career as a sleep technologist. Changes have taken place both in the clinical setting and within the industries that supply products required to meet the clinical needs of patients. The sleep technologist of today and tomorrow needs to have skill sets that include a wide range of knowledge in areas of electroneurodiagnostics, respiratory therapy, pulmonary function, cardiology, computer technology, customer service, and education. It also means that industry opportunities are limitless among those who are willing to continue their education, stay abreast of current medical and industry trends, and obtain the skill sets needed to meet these demands.

Tomorrow's industry opportunities are varied and vast; they can take you far in the sleep medicine and technology industry. Continuing to grow and expand skill sets and knowledge will certainly prepare the sleep technologist looking for a change for whatever industry opportunity presents itself.

SECTION X
Appendix

Appendix A

Artifact Recognition

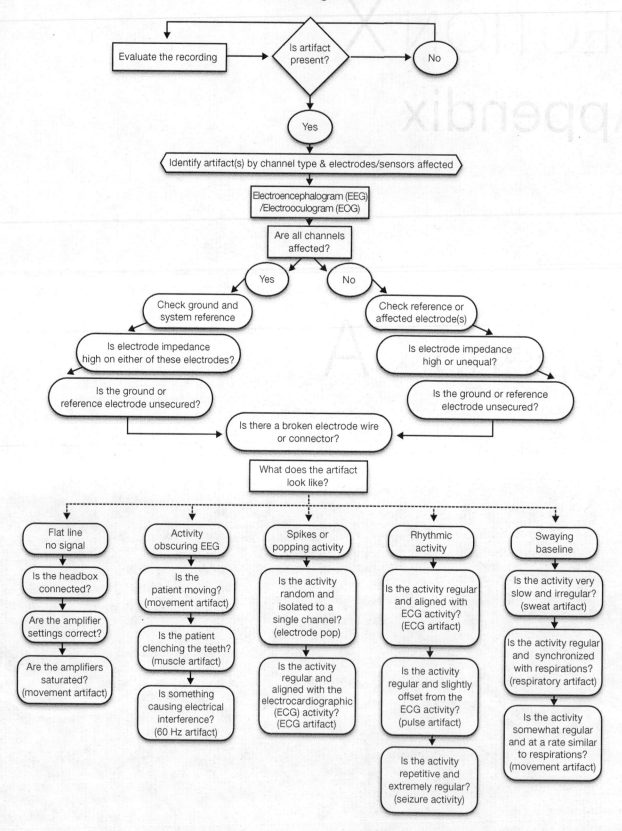

Appendix B
Trouble-shooting EEG

Trouble-Shooting EEG—Part I

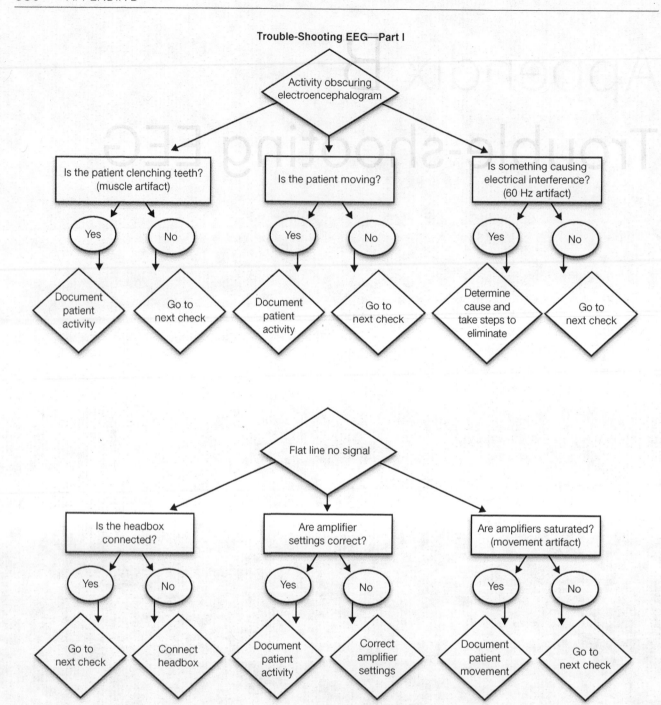

Trouble-Shooting EEG—Part II

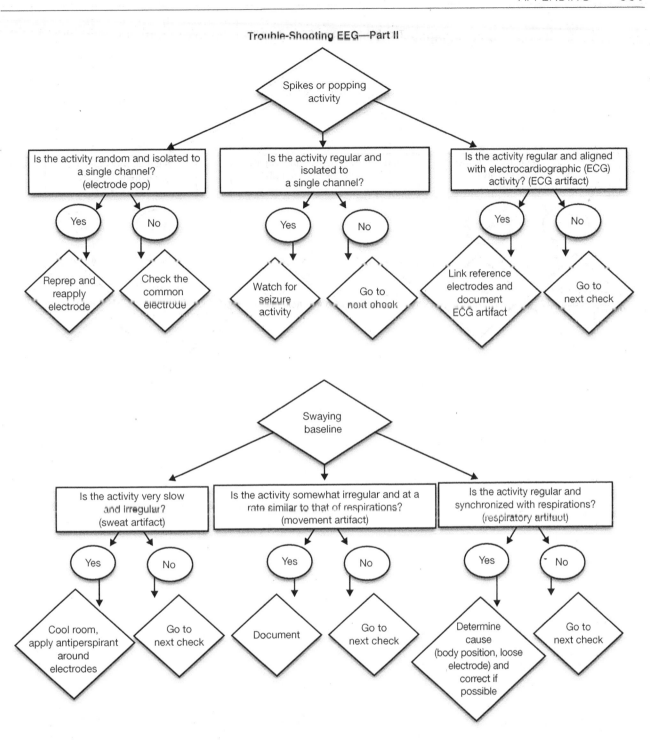

Trouble-Shooting EEG—Part III

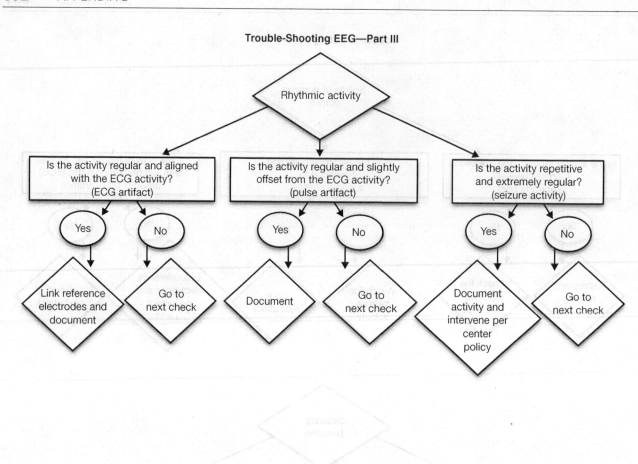

Appendix C

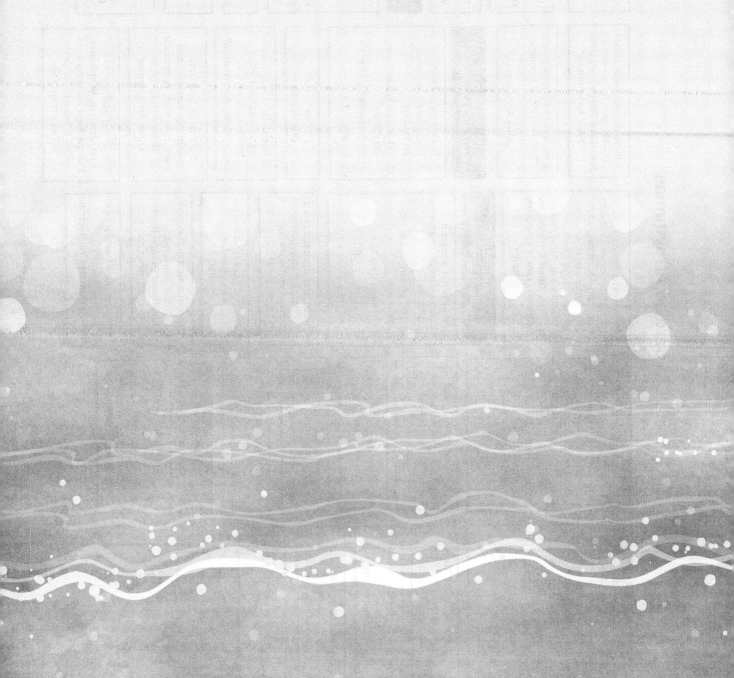

Cardiac Arrhythmias

Group A: Sinus Rhythms

(1) P wave present and all look the same
(2) QRS present and all look the same
(3) PR interval between 0.12 and 0.20 s
(4) QRS interval <0.12 s
(5) P:QRS = 1:1

If "yes" to all, Sinus Rhythm, proceed below. If "no" to (1) proceed to Group B

Rate <40 bpm, asleep for >30 s, **Bradycardia**

Rate >90 bpm, asleep for >30 s, **Sinus Tachycardia**

If R–R interval >3 s, **Asystole**

Group B: Atrial Arrhythmias

(1) P wave present, but all **DO NOT** look the same
(2) QRS present and all look the same
(3) PR interval between 0.12 and 0.20 s
(4) QRS interval <0.12 s

If "yes" to all, proceed below. If "no" to (1) that is, no P wave or inverted P wave and (3) <0.12, proceed to Group C

If abnormal beat occurs earlier than expected, **PAC**

If abnormal beat occurs later than expected, atrial escape beat following sinus pause

If three or more beats at rate > 100/min, **Narrow Complex Tachycardia**

Other Atrial Arrhythmias

If P wave replaced by rapid oscillations of variable size, shape, and timing, and ventricular rate is irregularly irregular, **Atrial Fibrillation**

If P wave replaced by rapid oscillations of well-formed saw tooth—appearing wave, QRS complexes occur every second, third, fourth, etc. sawtooth wave. **Atrial Flutter**, list under **"Other Arrhythmias"** Ventricular rate is irregularly irregular

Group C: Junctional Arrhythmias

(1) P wave not present or inverted before or after QRS
(2) QRS present and all look the same
(3) PR interval <0.12 s
(4) QRS interval <0.12 s
(5) P:QRS = 1:1 or < 1:1

If "yes" to all, proceed below
If "no" to (1) that is, no P wave or inverted P wave and (3) <0.12, proceed to Group D

If abnormal beat occurs earlier than expected, **PJC**

If abnormal beat occurs later than expected, **Junctional Escape Beat** following sinus pause

If three or more beats at rate >100/min, **Narrow Complex Tachycardia**

If three or more beats at rate 60–100/min, **Accelerated Junctional Rhythm**, list under **"Other Arrhythmias"**

If three or more beats at rate 40–60/min, **(Idio) Junctional Rhythm**, list under **"Other Arrhythmias"**

Group D: Ventricular Arrhythmias

(1) P wave not present
(2) QRS present, widened and bizarre
(3) PR interval indeterminate (no P wave)
(4) QRS interval >0.12 s
(5) P:QRS < 1:1

If "yes" to all, proceed below

If abnormal beat occurs earlier than expected, **PVC**, if frequent (>6/min), list under **"Other Arrhythmias"**

If abnormal beat occurs earlier than expected and every other beat, **Ventricular Bigeminy**, list under **"Other Arrhythmias"**

If abnormal beat occurs later than expected, **Ventricular Escape Beat** following sinus pause if frequent, list under **"Other Arrhythmias"**

If three or more beats at rate <40 bpm, **(Idio) Ventricular Rhythm**, list under **"Other Arrhythmias"**

If three or more beats at rate 40–100 bpm, **Accelerated Ventricular Rhythm**, list under **"Other Arrhythmias"**

If three or more beats at rate ≥100 bpm, **Wide Complex Tachycardia**

Group E: Atrioventricular (AV) Blocks

(1) P wave present all look the same
(2) QRS present and all look the same
(3) PR interval >0.20 s
(4) QRS interval <0.12 s
(5) P:QRS 1:1

If "yes" to all, **1st Degree AV block**

If "P:QRS > 1:1" (more P waves than QRS complexes), proceed below

If PR interval progressively increases before non conducted P wave, second **Degree AV Block, Mobitz I (Wenckebach)**

Appendix D

Continuous Positive Airway Pressure (CPAP) Titration for OSA Patient

Before starting the sleep study, all patients should be educated on positive airway pressure (PAP) and have a PAP trial.

1. Establish study type/setting as ordered by the physician.
2. Educate and instruct patient on PAP and assure proper mask fit.
3. Have the patient lie down before Lights Out for a trial on PAP at a basic pressure setting of 4–5 cm H_2O or at a pressure setting that the patient can tolerate. A higher setting may be needed for some patients.
4. Make adjustments to the mask and the PAP pressure setting to insure patient comfort. Allow the patient to ask questions about PAP process before Lights Out.

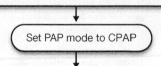

Set PAP mode to CPAP

After Lights Out, start the patient at 5 cm H_2O PAP or a setting the patient can tolerate. Then observe the patient for the following:*

Adults		For <12 y olds	For 12 y olds
≥2	Obstructive apnea or	≥1	≥2
≥3	Hypopnea or	≥1	≥3
≥5	RERAs or	≥3	≥5
≥3	Minute of loud or unambiguous snoring	≥1	≥3

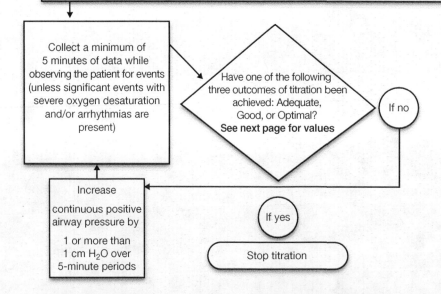

Collect a minimum of 5 minutes of data while observing the patient for events (unless significant events with severe oxygen desaturation and/or arrhythmias are present)

Have one of the following three outcomes of titration been achieved: Adequate, Good, or Optimal?
See next page for values

If no

Increase continuous positive airway pressure by 1 or more than 1 cm H_2O over 5-minute periods

If yes

Stop titration

Recommendations:

1. A higher starting PAP pressure may be needed with an elevated body mass index and for retitration studies.
2. If the patient awakens and complains that the pressure is too high, a lower pressure that the patient reports is comfortable may be used to allow the patient to return to sleep; then titration can be resumed.
3. Bilevel should be tried during the titration study if the patient is uncomfortable, intolerant of a high PAP pressure or if there are continued obstructive respiratory events at 15 cm H_2O of PAP during the titration study.

*By Positive Airway Pressure Titration Task Force of the American Academy of Sleep Medicine. Clinical guidelines for the manual titration of positive airway pressure in patients with obstructive sleep apnea. *J Clin Sleep Med 2008*;4(2):157-171.

Values for Acceptable Titration

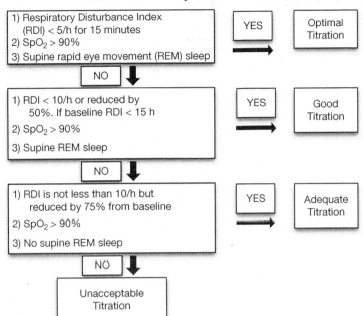

Appendix E

Bilevel Positive Airway Pressure Titration for OSA Patient

Before starting the sleep study, all patients should be educated and have a positive airway pressure (PAP) trial.

1. Establish a study type/setting as ordered by the physician.
2. Educate and instruct the patient on PAP/bilevel protocol and assure proper mask fit.
3. Have the patient lie down before Lights Out for a trial on bilevel at a basic pressure setting of inspiratory positive airway pressure (IPAP) 8 cm H_2O-expiratory positive airway pressure (EPAP) 4 cm H_2O or at a pressure setting the patient can tolerate. A higher setting may be needed for some patients. For those who reach a predetermined pressure threshold on PAP, create a starting pressure support create a starting pressure support level (IPAP/EPAP pressure difference) of at least 4 cm H_2O.
4. Make adjustments to ensure patient comfort.
5. Allow the patient to ask questions about the process before Lights Out.

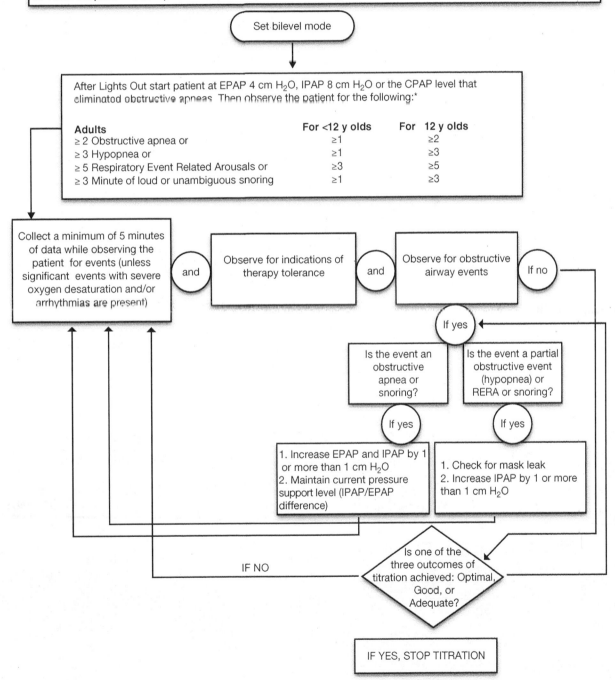

Set bilevel mode

After Lights Out start patient at EPAP 4 cm H_2O, IPAP 8 cm H_2O or the CPAP level that eliminated obstructive apneas. Then observe the patient for the following:*

Adults	For <12 y olds	For 12 y olds
≥ 2 Obstructive apnea or	≥1	≥2
≥ 3 Hypopnea or	≥1	≥3
≥ 5 Respiratory Event Related Arousals or	≥3	≥5
≥ 3 Minute of loud or unambiguous snoring	≥1	≥3

Collect a minimum of 5 minutes of data while observing the patient for events (unless significant events with severe oxygen desaturation and/or arrhythmias are present)

and — Observe for indications of therapy tolerance — **and** — Observe for obstructive airway events — If no

If yes

Is the event an obstructive apnea or snoring?

Is the event a partial obstructive event (hypopnea) or RERA or snoring?

If yes

If yes

1. Increase EPAP and IPAP by 1 or more than 1 cm H_2O
2. Maintain current pressure support level (IPAP/EPAP difference)

1. Check for mask leak
2. Increase IPAP by 1 or more than 1 cm H_2O

IF NO

Is one of the three outcomes of titration achieved: Optimal, Good, or Adequate?

IF YES, STOP TITRATION

Data from Positive Airway Pressure Titration Task Force of the American Academy of Sleep Medicine. Clinical guidelines for the manual titration of positive airway pressure in patients with obstructive sleep apnea. J Clin Sleep Med; 2008;4(2):157-171.

Appendix F

Administration of O₂ during PAP Titration for OSA Patient

```
┌─────────────────────────────────────────────┐
│ SpO₂% < 88% during PAP titration for 5 minutes │
│            or longer cumulative               │
└─────────────────────────────────────────────┘
                      │
                      ▼
      ┌──────────────────────────────────────┐
      │ Check patient (SpO₂% signal quality + ECG) │
      └──────────────────────────────────────┘
```

- Acceptable
- Faulty → Correct problem
- Patient asleep
- Patient awake → Call MD or follow protocol
- Obvious obstructive qualities present → YES → Adjust PAP
  - SpO₂% ≤ 88%
  - SpO₂% > 88% Continue to monitor
  - NO

Add oxygen to PAP mask or circuit follow protocol or 1 LPM wait 15 minutes

- SpO₂% > 88%
- SpO₂% ≤ 88%

Check patient (SpO₂% signal quality + ECG)

- Correct problem ← Faulty
- Acceptable → SpO₂% > 88% Continue to monitor
- SpO₂% ≤ 88%

Add oxygen to PAP mask follow protocol 1 LPM

pressure setting with AHI/RDI < 10/h or if initial AHI/RDI < 10/h, the titration results in further reduction in AHI/RDI.

pressure setting with AHI/RDI >10/h or if initial AHI/RDI < 10/h, the titration does not result in further reduction in AHI/RDI.

- Continue to monitor ← SpO₂% > 88%
- SpO₂% < 88%

ASSUMED: no preexisting cardiopulmonary pathology
REQUIRED: MD prescription/direction/lab protocol
CAVEATS: stated threshold values, wait times, and oxygen flows are guidelines only and should be set by individual laboratory protocol.

Continue to add 1 LPM with 15 minutes wait between increases until SpO₂% is >88% or 5 LPM O₂ has been shown ineffective (call MD ≥ 5 LPM)

Appendix G

Evaluating Movement Disorders

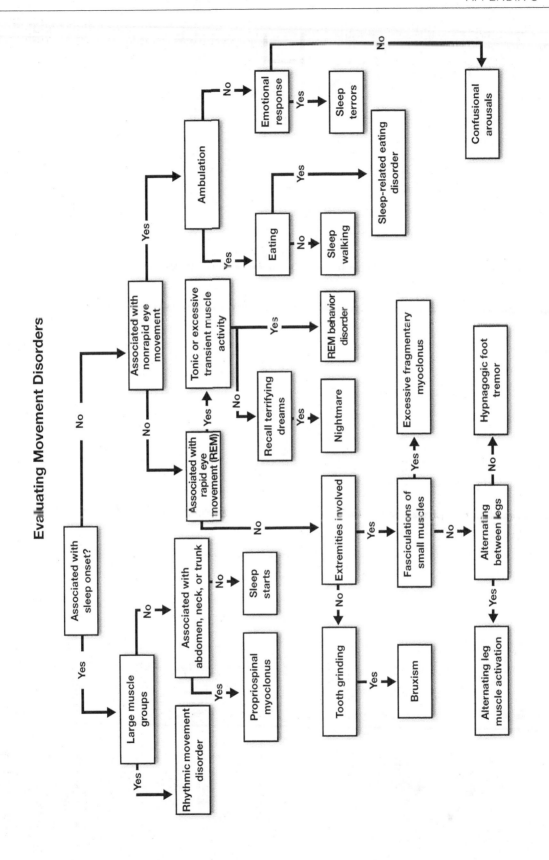

Appendix H

Excessive Daytime Sleepiness (EDS)

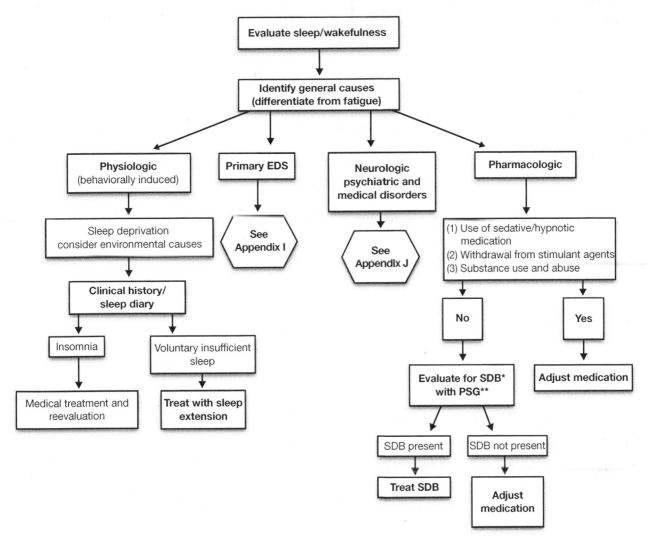

*SDB, sleep disordered breathing.
**PSG, polysomnogram.

Appendix I

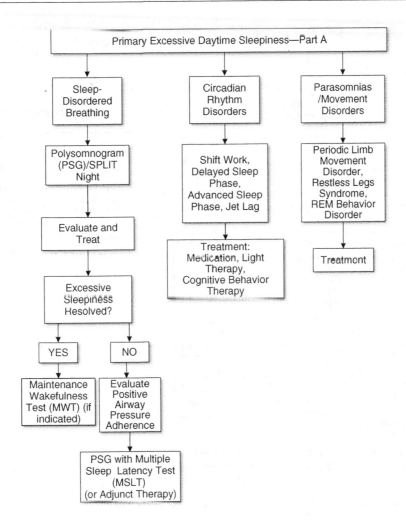

Primary Excessive Daytime Sleepiness—Part A

Sleep-Disordered Breathing

Polysomnogram (PSG)/SPLIT Night

Evaluate and Treat

Excessive Sleepiness Resolved?

YES → Maintenance Wakefulness Test (MWT) (if indicated)

NO → Evaluate Positive Airway Pressure Adherence → PSG with Multiple Sleep Latency Test (MSLT) (or Adjunct Therapy)

Circadian Rhythm Disorders

Shift Work, Delayed Sleep Phase, Advanced Sleep Phase, Jet Lag

Treatment: Medication, Light Therapy, Cognitive Behavior Therapy

Parasomnias /Movement Disorders

Periodic Limb Movement Disorder, Restless Legs Syndrome, REM Behavior Disorder

Treatment

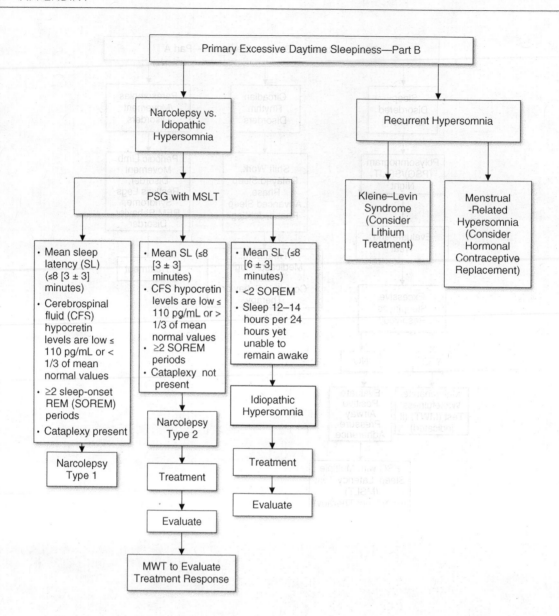

Primary Excessive Daytime Sleepiness—Part B

Narcolepsy vs. Idiopathic Hypersomnia

Recurrent Hypersomnia

PSG with MSLT

Kleine–Levin Syndrome (Consider Lithium Treatment)

Menstrual -Related Hypersomnia (Consider Hormonal Contraceptive Replacement)

- Mean sleep latency (SL) (≤8 [3 ± 3] minutes)
- Cerebrospinal fluid (CFS) hypocretin levels are low ≤ 110 pg/mL or < 1/3 of mean normal values
- ≥2 sleep-onset REM (SOREM) periods
- Cataplexy present

- Mean SL (≤8 [3 ± 3] minutes)
- CFS hypocretin levels are low ≤ 110 pg/mL or > 1/3 of mean normal values
- ≥2 SOREM periods
- Cataplexy not present

- Mean SL (≤8 [6 ± 3] minutes)
- <2 SOREM
- Sleep 12–14 hours per 24 hours yet unable to remain awake

Narcolepsy Type 1

Narcolepsy Type 2

Idiopathic Hypersomnia

Treatment

Treatment

Evaluate

Evaluate

MWT to Evaluate Treatment Response

Appendix J

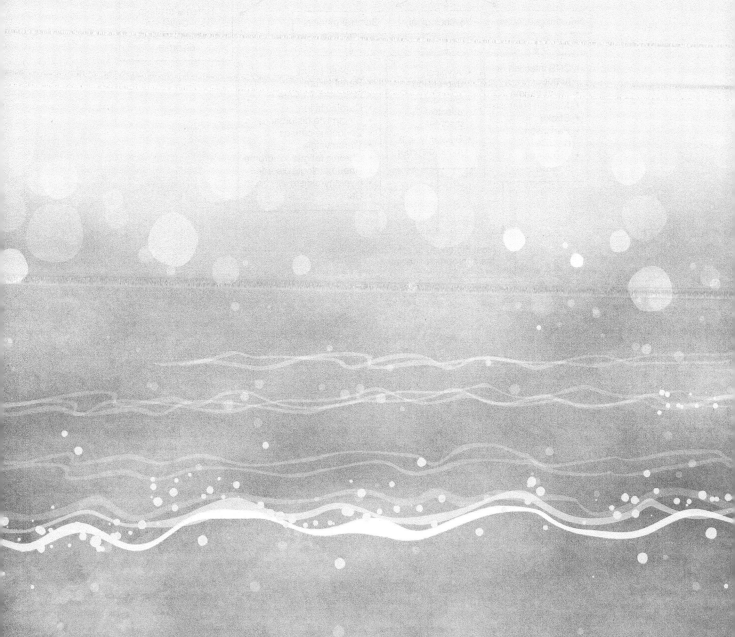

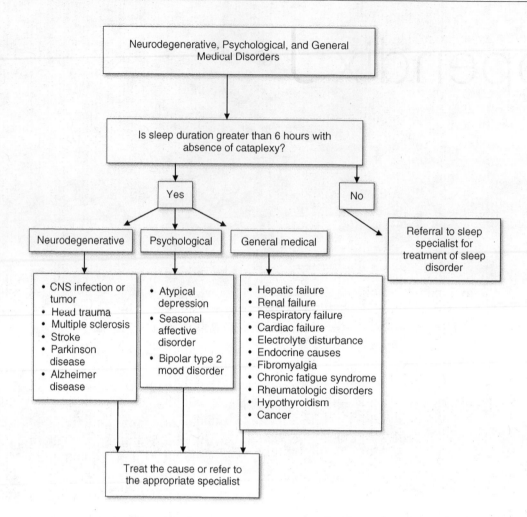

Neurodegenerative, Psychological, and General Medical Disorders

Is sleep duration greater than 6 hours with absence of cataplexy?

Yes

No

Neurodegenerative

Psychological

General medical

Referral to sleep specialist for treatment of sleep disorder

- CNS infection or tumor
- Head trauma
- Multiple sclerosis
- Stroke
- Parkinson disease
- Alzheimer disease

- Atypical depression
- Seasonal affective disorder
- Bipolar type 2 mood disorder

- Hepatic failure
- Renal failure
- Respiratory failure
- Cardiac failure
- Electrolyte disturbance
- Endocrine causes
- Fibromyalgia
- Chronic fatigue syndrome
- Rheumatologic disorders
- Hypothyroidism
- Cancer

Treat the cause or refer to the appropriate specialist

Appendix K

Evaluation and Treatment of Insomnia

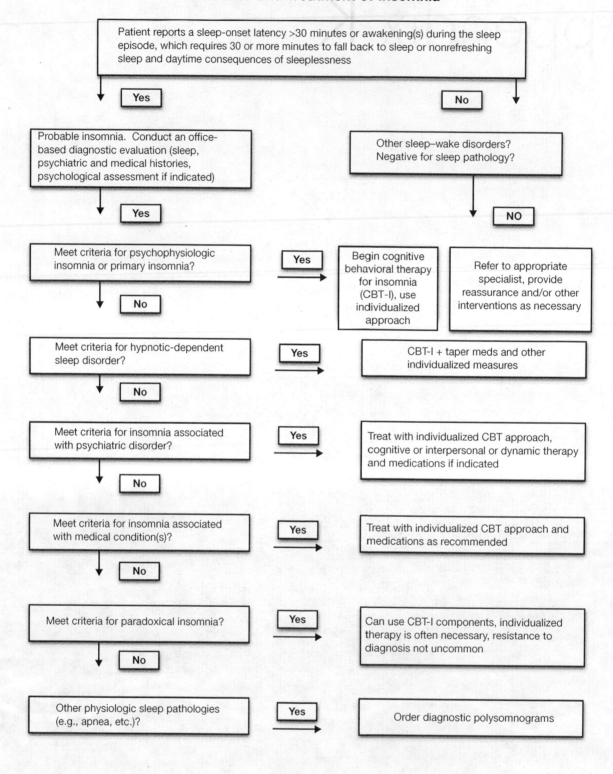

Appendix L

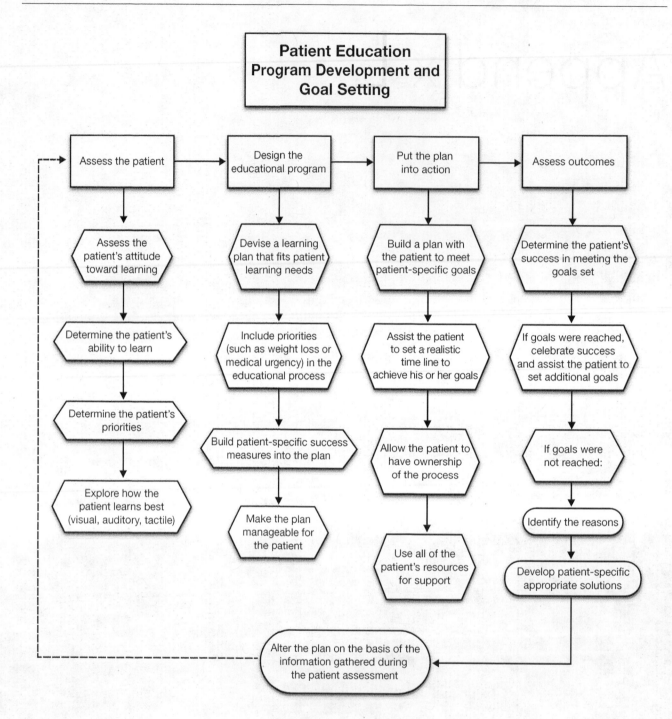

Patient Education Program Development and Goal Setting

Assess the patient → Design the educational program → Put the plan into action → Assess outcomes

Assess the patient's attitude toward learning

Devise a learning plan that fits patient learning needs

Build a plan with the patient to meet patient-specific goals

Determine the patient's success in meeting the goals set

Determine the patient's ability to learn

Include priorities (such as weight loss or medical urgency) in the educational process

Assist the patient to set a realistic time line to achieve his or her goals

If goals were reached, celebrate success and assist the patient to set additional goals

Determine the patient's priorities

Build patient-specific success measures into the plan

Allow the patient to have ownership of the process

If goals were not reached:

Explore how the patient learns best (visual, auditory, tactile)

Make the plan manageable for the patient

Use all of the patient's resources for support

Identify the reasons

Develop patient-specific appropriate solutions

Alter the plan on the basis of the information gathered during the patient assessment

Appendix M

Essential Elements of the Patient Education Plan

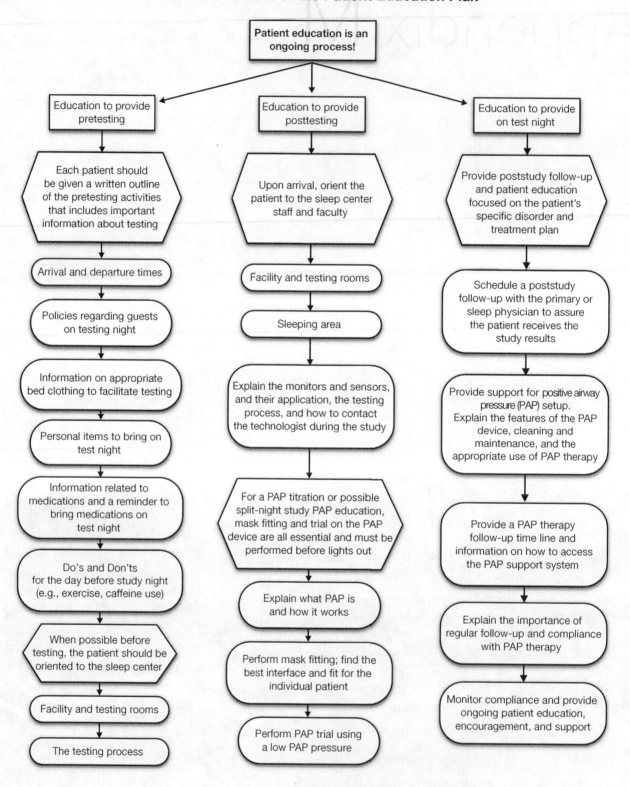

Patient education is an ongoing process!

Education to provide pretesting

Each patient should be given a written outline of the pretesting activities that includes important information about testing

Arrival and departure times

Policies regarding guests on testing night

Information on appropriate bed clothing to facilitate testing

Personal items to bring on test night

Information related to medications and a reminder to bring medications on test night

Do's and Don'ts for the day before study night (e.g., exercise, caffeine use)

When possible before testing, the patient should be oriented to the sleep center

Facility and testing rooms

The testing process

Education to provide posttesting

Upon arrival, orient the patient to the sleep center staff and faculty

Facility and testing rooms

Sleeping area

Explain the monitors and sensors, and their application, the testing process, and how to contact the technologist during the study

For a PAP titration or possible split-night study PAP education, mask fitting and trial on the PAP device are all essential and must be performed before lights out

Explain what PAP is and how it works

Perform mask fitting; find the best interface and fit for the individual patient

Perform PAP trial using a low PAP pressure

Education to provide on test night

Provide poststudy follow-up and patient education focused on the patient's specific disorder and treatment plan

Schedule a poststudy follow-up with the primary or sleep physician to assure the patient receives the study results

Provide support for positive airway pressure (PAP) setup. Explain the features of the PAP device, cleaning and maintenance, and the appropriate use of PAP therapy

Provide a PAP therapy follow-up time line and information on how to access the PAP support system

Explain the importance of regular follow-up and compliance with PAP therapy

Monitor compliance and provide ongoing patient education, encouragement, and support

Appendix N
ResMed AirView™ Diagnostic Report

Diagnostic Report (Signed)

Recording details				07/25/2013
Device		**ApneaLink Air**	Type:	**III**
Recording	Start: **10:27pm**	End: **6:10am**	Duration - hr:	**7:42**
Monitoring time (flow)	Start: **10:37pm**	End: **6:08am**	Duration - hr:	**6:44**
Oxygen saturation evaluation	Start: **10:37pm**	End: **6:10am**	Duration - hr:	**7:32**

Statistics

NORMAL	MILD	MODERATE	34.5 SEVERE	
0	5	15	30	

Events index	REI (AHI): **34.5**	AI: **16.9**	HI: **17.6**
Supine		Time - hr **6:44**	Percentage: **100.**
	REI (AHI): **34.5**	AI: **16.9**	HI: **17.6**
Non-supine		Time - hr **0:00**	Percentage: **0.0**
	REI (AHI): **0.0**	AI: **0.0**	HI: **0.0**
Upright		Time - hr **0:00**	Percentage: **0.0**
	REI (AHI): **0.0**	AI: **0.0**	HI: **0.0**
Events totals		Apneas: **114**	Hypopneas: **119**
Apnea Index Obstructive: **5.8**	Central: **10.2**	Mixed: **0.9**	Unclassified: **0.0**
Cheyne-Stokes respiration		Time - hr: **0:00**	Percentage: **0**
Oxygen desaturation		ODI: **31.5**	Total: **238**
Oxygen saturation %	Baseline: **95**	Avg: **94**	Lowest: **87**
Oxygen saturation - eval time %	<=90%sat: **2**	<=85%sat: **0**	<=80%sat: **0**
		<=88%sat: **0**	<=88%Time - hr: **0:00**
Breaths	Total: **4209**	Avg/min: **10.4**	Snores: **1263**
Pulse - bpm	Min: **49**	Avg: **61**	Max: **93**

Analysis guidelines: **AASM 2012, Automatic scoring**

Apnea[10%; 10s; 80s; 1.0s; 20%; 60%; 8%]; Hypopnea[70%; 10s; 100s; 1.0s]; Snoring[6.0%; 0.3s, 3.5s; 0.5s]; Desaturation[3.0%]; CSR[0.5]. Airflow sensor and respiratory effort sensor: Pressure transducer. Hypopneas were scored only if there was valid oximetry data.

Interpretation

This patient needs ongoing therapy.

Electronically signed by Dr James User, NPI ecodoc@resmed.com123

12/17/2018 7:55pm (-08:00)

Appendix O
Respironics Compliance Report

COMPLIANCE INFORMATION 7/3/2018 TO 7/9/2018

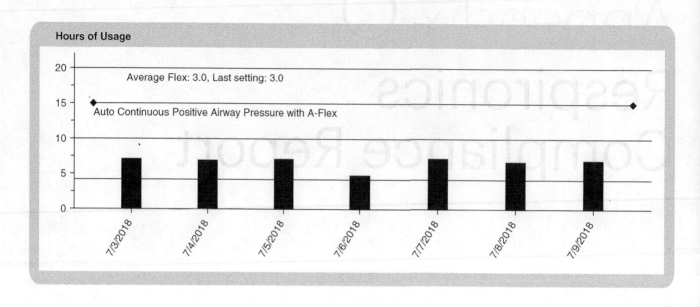

Hours of Usage

Average Flex: 3.0, Last setting: 3.0

Auto Continuous Positive Airway Pressure with A-Flex

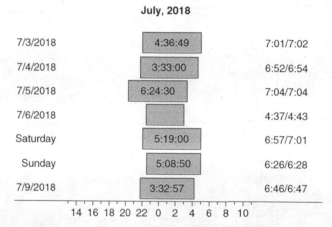

July, 2018

7/3/2018	4:36:49	7:01/7:02
7/4/2018	3:33:00	6:52/6:54
7/5/2018	6:24:30	7:04/7:04
7/6/2018		4:37/4:43
Saturday	5:19:00	6:57/7:01
Sunday	5:08:50	6:26/6:28
7/9/2018	3:32:57	6:46/6:47

14 16 18 20 22 0 2 4 6 8 10

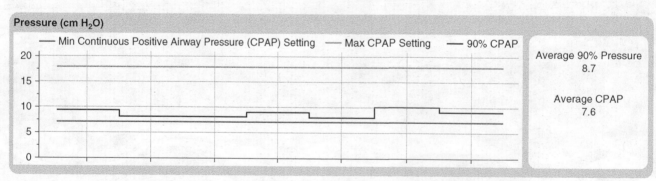

Pressure (cm H$_2$O)

— Min Continuous Positive Airway Pressure (CPAP) Setting   — Max CPAP Setting   — 90% CPAP

Average 90% Pressure
8.7

Average CPAP
7.6

Percent of Night in Periodic Breathing

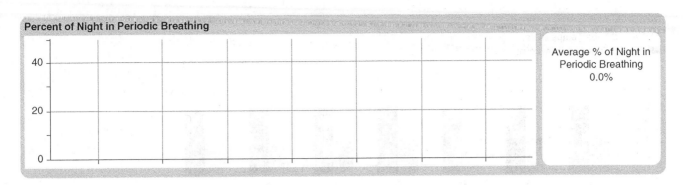

Average % of Night in
Periodic Breathing
0.0%

Clear Airway and Obstructed Airway Apnea Indices

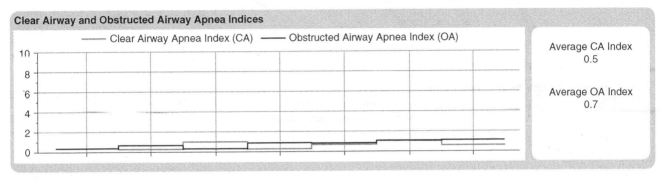

Average CA Index
0.5

Average OA Index
0.7

Hypopnea and Respiratory Disturbance Index Indices

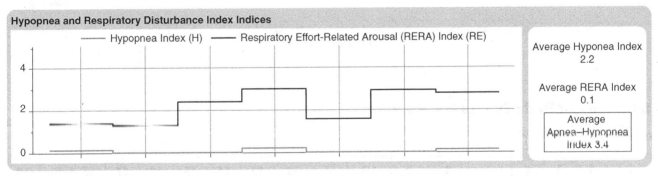

Average Hyponea Index
2.2

Average RERA Index
0.1

Average
Apnea–Hypopnea
Index 3.4

Flow Limitation and Vibratory Snore Indices

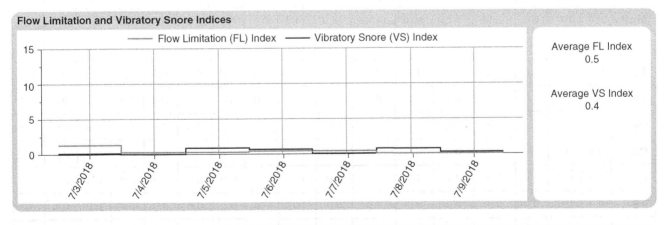

Average FL Index
0.5

Average VS Index
0.4

Percent of Night in Large Leak

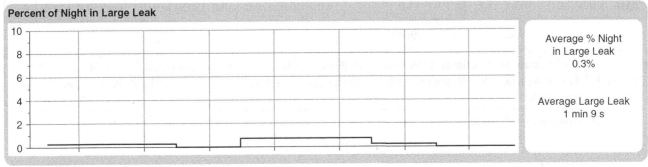

Average % Night
in Large Leak
0.3%

Average Large Leak
1 min 9 s

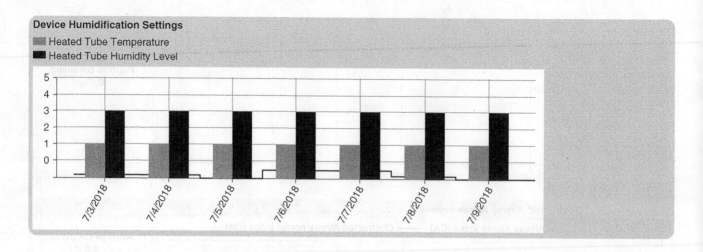

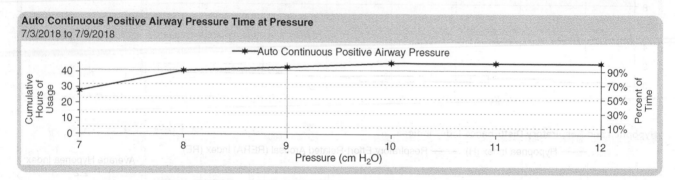

Summary of Daily Events Per Hour

7/3/2018 - 7/9/2018

P	4	5	6	7	8	9	10	11	12	13	14	15	16	17	18	19	20
MaP	0.0	0.0	0.0	1,694	752.7	96.6	173.6	18.0	13.3	0.0	0.0	0.0	0.0	0.0	0.0	0.0	0.0
%	0.0	0.0	0.0	61.6	27.4	3.5	6.3	0.7	0.5	0.0	0.0	0.0	0.0	0.0	0.0	0.0	0.0
FL	0.0	0.0	0.0	0.4	0.4	1.2	0.7	0.0	0.0	0.0	0.0	0.0	0.0	0.0	0.0	0.0	0.0
VS	0.0	0.0	0.0	0.4	0.4	0.6	0.3	0.0	0.0	0.0	0.0	0.0	0.0	0.0	0.0	0.0	0.0
OA	0.0	0.0	0.0	0.6	0.8	0.6	1.0	0.0	0.0	0.0	0.0	0.0	0.0	0.0	0.0	0.0	0.0
CA	0.0	0.0	0.0	0.6	0.5	0.0	0.3	0.0	0.0	0.0	0.0	0.0	0.0	0.0	0.0	0.0	0.0
H	0.0	0.0	0.0	1.9	2.4	4.3	2.8	0.0	0.0	0.0	0.0	0.0	0.0	0.0	0.0	0.0	0.0
RE	0.0	0.0	0.0	0.0	0.2	0.0	0.0	0.0	0.0	0.0	0.0	0.0	0.0	0.0	0.0	0.0	0.0
AHI	0.0	0.0	0.0	3.1	3.7	4.9	4.1	0.0	0.0	0.0	0.0	0.0	0.0	0.0	0.0	0.0	0.0

90%

Legend	P - Pressure, MaP - Minutes at Pressure, % - Percent of Night, FL - Flow Limitation, VS - Vibratory Snore, H - Hypopnea, OA - Obstructed Airway Apnea, CA - Clear Airway Apnea, RE - RERA, AHI - Apnea/Hypopnea Index

Used with permission from Philips Respironics.

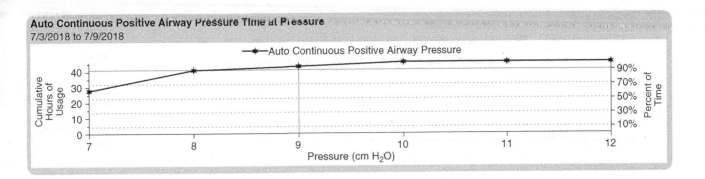

Auto Continuous Positive Airway Pressure Time at Pressure
7/3/2018 to 7/9/2018

DAILY DETAILS

7/3/2018 9:50 PM to 7/4/2018 4:57 AM

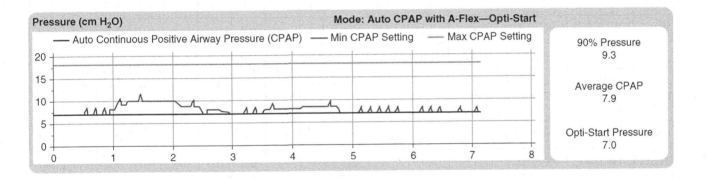

Pressure (cm H₂O)   **Mode: Auto CPAP with A-Flex—Opti-Start**

90% Pressure
9.3

Average CPAP
7.9

Opti-Start Pressure
7.0

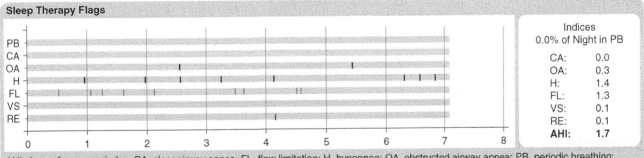

Sleep Therapy Flags

Indices
0.0% of Night in PB

CA:	0.0
OA:	0.3
H:	1.4
FL:	1.3
VS:	0.1
RE:	0.1
AHI:	**1.7**

AHI, Apnea/hypopnea index; CA, clear airway apnea; FL, flow limitation; H, hypopnea; OA, obstructed airway apnea; PB, periodic breathing; RE, RERA; VS, vibratory snore.

Unintentional Leak

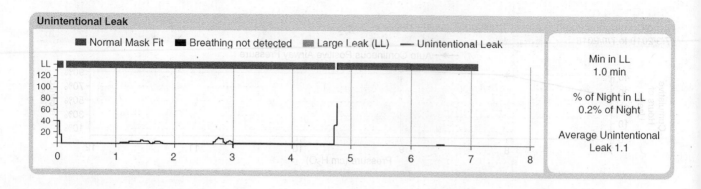

■ Normal Mask Fit   ■ Breathing not detected   ■ Large Leak (LL)   — Unintentional Leak

Min in LL
1.0 min

% of Night in LL
0.2% of Night

Average Unintentional
Leak 1.1

Daily Events Per Hour

7/3/2018

Total AHI: 1.7

P	4	5	6	7	8	9	10	11	12	13	14	15	16	17	18	19	20
MaP	0.0	0.0	0.0	183.3	148.6	30.2	56.8	1.7	0.4	0.0	0.0	0.0	0.0	0.0	0.0	0.0	0.0
%	0.0	0.0	0.0	43.5	35.3	7.2	13.5	0.4	0.1	0.0	0.0	0.0	0.0	0.0	0.0	0.0	0.0
FL	0.0	0.0	0.0	0.7	1.2	4.0	2.1	0.0	0.0	0.0	0.0	0.0	0.0	0.0	0.0	0.0	0.0
VS	0.0	0.0	0.0	0.3	0.0	0.0	0.0	0.0	0.0	0.0	0.0	0.0	0.0	0.0	0.0	0.0	0.0
OA	0.0	0.0	0.0	0.3	0.4	0.0	0.0	0.0	0.0	0.0	0.0	0.0	0.0	0.0	0.0	0.0	0.0
CA	0.0	0.0	0.0	0.0	0.0	0.0	0.0	0.0	0.0	0.0	0.0	0.0	0.0	0.0	0.0	0.0	0.0
H	0.0	0.0	0.0	1.6	1.6	0.0	'1.1	0.0	0.0	0.0	0.0	0.0	0.0	0.0	0.0	0.0	0.0
RE	0.0	0.0	0.0	0.0	0.4	0.0	0.0	0.0	0.0	0.0	0.0	0.0	0.0	0.0	0.0	0.0	0.0
AHI	0.0	0.0	0.0	1.9	2.0	0.0	1.1	0.0	0.0	0.0	0.0	0.0	0.0	0.0	0.0	0.0	0.0

90%

Legend	P - Pressure, MaP - Minutes at Pressure, % - Percent of Night, FL - Flow Limitation, VS - Vibratory Snore, H - Hypopnea, OA - Obstructed Airway Apnea, CA - Clear Airway Apnea, RE - RERA, AHI - Apnea/Hypopnea Index

DAILY DETAILS

7/4/2018 9:42 PM to 7/5/2018 4:37 AM

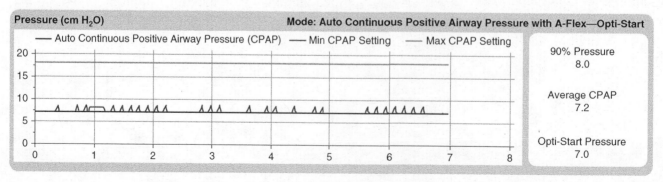

Pressure (cm H₂O)   Mode: Auto Continuous Positive Airway Pressure with A-Flex—Opti-Start

— Auto Continuous Positive Airway Pressure (CPAP)   — Min CPAP Setting   — Max CPAP Setting

90% Pressure
8.0

Average CPAP
7.2

Opti-Start Pressure
7.0

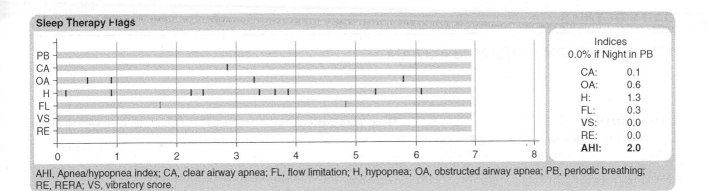

Sleep Therapy Flags

Indices
0.0% if Night in PB

CA:	0.1
OA:	0.6
H:	1.3
FL:	0.3
VS:	0.0
RE:	0.0
AHI:	**2.0**

AHI, Apnea/hypopnea index; CA, clear airway apnea; FL, flow limitation; H, hypopnea; OA, obstructed airway apnea; PB, periodic breathing; RE, RERA; VS, vibratory snore.

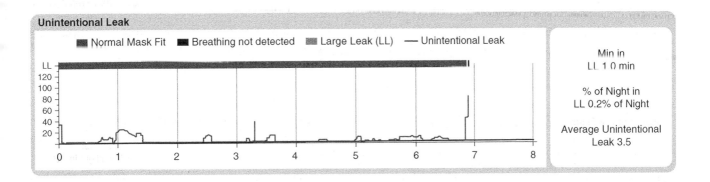

Unintentional Leak

■ Normal Mask Fit   ■ Breathing not detected   ■ Large Leak (LL)   — Unintentional Leak

Min in
LL 1 0 min

% of Night in
LL 0.2% of Night

Average Unintentional
Leak 3.5

Daily Events Per Hour

7/4/2018

Total AHI: 2.0

P	4	5	6	7	8	9	10	11	12	13	14	15	16	17	18	19	20
MaP	0.0	0.0	0.0	317.1	95.8	0.0	0.0	0.0	0.0	0.0	0.0	0.0	0.0	0.0	0.0	0.0	0.0
%	0.0	0.0	0.0	76.8	23.2	0.0	0.0	0.0	0.0	0.0	0.0	0.0	0.0	0.0	0.0	0.0	0.0
FL	0.0	0.0	0.0	0.4	0.0	0.0	0.0	0.0	0.0	0.0	0.0	0.0	0.0	0.0	0.0	0.0	0.0
VS	0.0	0.0	0.0	0.0	0.0	0.0	0.0	0.0	0.0	0.0	0.0	0.0	0.0	0.0	0.0	0.0	0.0
OA	0.0	0.0	0.0	0.6	0.6	0.0	0.0	0.0	0.0	0.0	0.0	0.0	0.0	0.0	0.0	0.0	0.0
CA	0.0	0.0	0.0	0.0	0.6	0.0	0.0	0.0	0.0	0.0	0.0	0.0	0.0	0.0	0.0	0.0	0.0
H	0.0	0.0	0.0	1.3	1.3	0.0	0.0	0.0	0.0	0.0	0.0	0.0	0.0	0.0	0.0	0.0	0.0
RE	0.0	0.0	0.0	0.0	0.0	0.0	0.0	0.0	0.0	0.0	0.0	0.0	0.0	0.0	0.0	0.0	0.0
AHI	0.0	0.0	0.0	1.9	2.5	0.0	0.0	0.0	0.0	0.0	0.0	0.0	0.0	0.0	0.0	0.0	0.0

90%

Legend	P - Pressure, MaP - Minutes at Pressure, % - Percent of Night, FL - Flow Limitation, VS - Vibratory Snore, H - Hypopnea, OA - Obstructed Airway Apnea, CA - Clear Airway Apnea, RE - RERA, AHI - Apnea/Hypopnea Index

DAILY DETAILS

7/4/2018 9:42 PM to 7/5/2018 4:37 AM

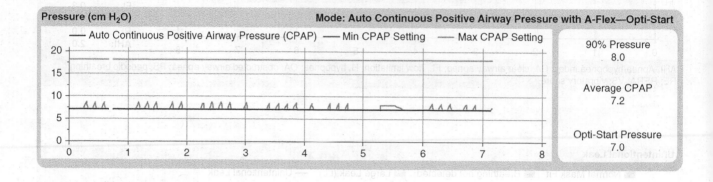

Pressure (cm H$_2$O) — Mode: Auto Continuous Positive Airway Pressure with A-Flex—Opti-Start

— Auto Continuous Positive Airway Pressure (CPAP) — Min CPAP Setting — Max CPAP Setting

90% Pressure
8.0

Average CPAP
7.2

Opti-Start Pressure
7.0

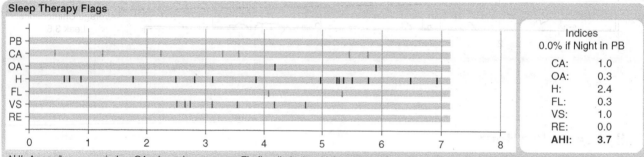

Sleep Therapy Flags

Indices
0.0% if Night in PB

CA:	1.0
OA:	0.3
H:	2.4
FL:	0.3
VS:	1.0
RE:	0.0
AHI:	**3.7**

AHI, Apnea/hypopnea index; CA, clear airway apnea; FL, flow limitation; H, hypopnea; OA, obstructed airway apnea; PB, periodic breathing; RE, RERA; VS, vibratory snore.

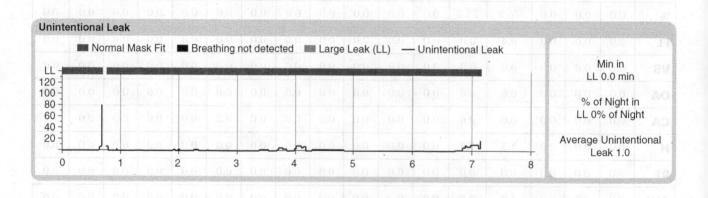

Unintentional Leak

■ Normal Mask Fit　■ Breathing not detected　■ Large Leak (LL)　— Unintentional Leak

Min in
LL 0.0 min

% of Night in
LL 0% of Night

Average Unintentional
Leak 1.0

Daily Events Per Hour

7/5/2018   Total AHI: 3.7

P	4	5	6	7	8	9	10	11	12	13	14	15	16	17	18	19	20
MaP	0.0	0.0	0.0	321.1	103.7	0.0	0.0	0.0	0.0	0.0	0.0	0.0	0.0	0.0	0.0	0.0	0.0
%	0.0	0.0	0.0	75.6	24.4	0.0	0.0	0.0	0.0	0.0	0.0	0.0	0.0	0.0	0.0	0.0	0.0
FL	0.0	0.0	0.0	0.2	0.6	0.0	0.0	0.0	0.0	0.0	0.0	0.0	0.0	0.0	0.0	0.0	0.0
VS	0.0	0.0	0.0	0.9	0.6	0.0	0.0	0.0	0.0	0.0	0.0	0.0	0.0	0.0	0.0	0.0	0.0
OA	0.0	0.0	0.0	0.4	0.0	0.0	0.0	0.0	0.0	0.0	0.0	0.0	0.0	0.0	0.0	0.0	0.0
CA	0.0	0.0	0.0	0.7	1 7	0.0	0.0	0.0	0.0	0.0	0.0	0.0	0.0	0.0	0.0	0.0	0.0
H	0.0	0.0	0.0	2.2	2.9	0.0	0.0	0.0	0.0	0.0	0.0	0.0	0.0	0.0	0.0	0.0	0.0
RE	0.0	0.0	0.0	0.0	0.0	0.0	0.0	0.0	0.0	0.0	0.0	0.0	0.0	0.0	0.0	0.0	0.0
AHI	0.0	0.0	0.0	3.3	4.6	0.0	0.0	0.0	0.0	0.0	0.0	0.0	0.0	0.0	0.0	0.0	0.0

90%

Legend	P - Pressure, MaP - Minutes at Pressure, % - Percent of Night, FL - Flow Limitation, VS - Vibratory Snore, H - Hypopnea, OA - Obstructed Airway Apnea, CA - Clear Airway Apnea, RE - RERA, AHI - Apnea/Hypopnea Index

DAILY DETAILS

7/6/2018 10:16 PM to 7/7/2018 3:00 AM

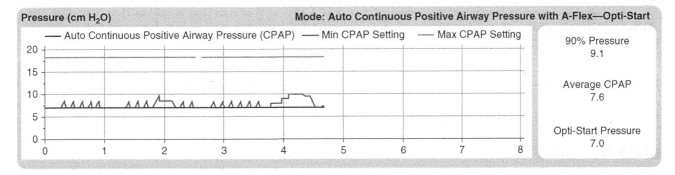

Pressure (cm H₂O)   Mode: Auto Continuous Positive Airway Pressure with A-Flex—Opti-Start

— Auto Continuous Positive Airway Pressure (CPAP) — Min CPAP Setting — Max CPAP Setting

90% Pressure
9.1

Average CPAP
7.6

Opti-Start Pressure
7.0

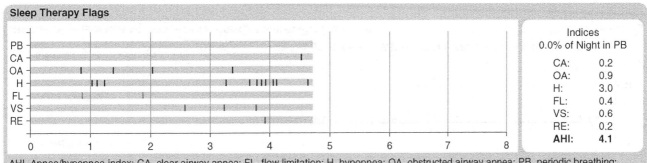

Sleep Therapy Flags

Indices
0.0% of Night in PB

CA:	0.2
OA:	0.9
H:	3.0
FL:	0.4
VS:	0.6
RE:	0.2
AHI:	**4.1**

AHI, Apnea/hypopnea index; CA, clear airway apnea; FL, flow limitation; H, hypopnea; OA, obstructed airway apnea; PB, periodic breathing; RE, RERA; VS, vibratory snore.

Unintentional Leak

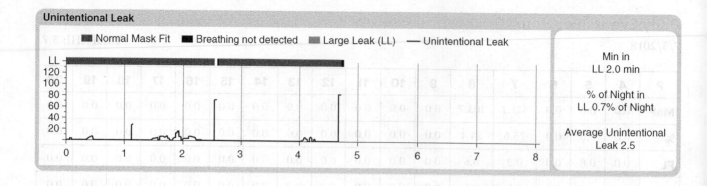

■ Normal Mask Fit   ■ Breathing not detected   ■ Large Leak (LL)   — Unintentional Leak

Min in
LL 2.0 min

% of Night in
LL 0.7% of Night

Average Unintentional
Leak 2.5

Daily Events Per Hour

7/6/2018

Total AHI: 4.1

P	4	5	6	7	8	9	10	11	12	13	14	15	16	17	18	19	20
MaP	0.0	0.0	0.0	165.0	79.0	10.1	23.9	0.0	0.0	0.0	0.0	0.0	0.0	0.0	0.0	0.0	0.0
%	0.0	0.0	0.0	59.4	28.4	3.6	8.6	0.0	0.0	0.0	0.0	0.0	0.0	0.0	0.0	0.0	0.0
FL	0.0	0.0	0.0	0.4	0.8	0.0	0.0	0.0	0.0	0.0	0.0	0.0	0.0	0.0	0.0	0.0	0.0
VS	0.0	0.0	0.0	0.7	0.8	0.0	0.0	0.0	0.0	0.0	0.0	0.0	0.0	0.0	0.0	0.0	0.0
OA	0.0	0.0	0.0	0.7	1.5	0.0	0.0	0.0	0.0	0.0	0.0	0.0	0.0	0.0	0.0	0.0	0.0
CA	0.0	0.0	0.0	0.4	0.0	0.0	0.0	0.0	0.0	0.0	0.0	0.0	0.0	0.0	0.0	0.0	0.0
H	0.0	0.0	0.0	2.5	3.0	11.9	2.5	0.0	0.0	0.0	0.0	0.0	0.0	0.0	0.0	0.0	0.0
RE	0.0	0.0	0.0	0.0	0.8	0.0	0.0	0.0	0.0	0.0	0.0	0.0	0.0	0.0	0.0	0.0	0.0
AHI	0.0	0.0	0.0	3.6	4.5	11.9	2.5	0.0	0.0	0.0	0.0	0.0	0.0	0.0	0.0	0.0	0.0

Legend	P - Pressure, MaP - Minutes at Pressure, % - Percent of Night, FL - Flow Limitation, VS - Vibratory Snore, H - Hypopnea, OA - Obstructed Airway Apnea, CA - Clear Airway Apnea, RE - RERA, AHI - Apnea/Hypopnea Index

DAILY DETAILS

7/7/2018 9:52 PM to 7/8/2018 4:52 AM

Pressure (cm H₂O)   **Mode: Auto Continuous Positive Airway Pressure with A-Flex—Opti-Start**

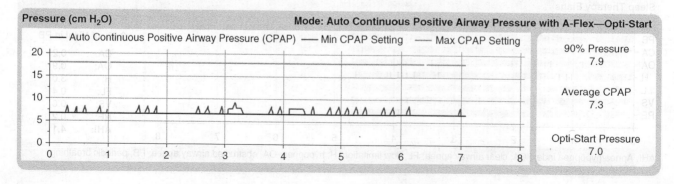

— Auto Continuous Positive Airway Pressure (CPAP)   — Min CPAP Setting   — Max CPAP Setting

90% Pressure
7.9

Average CPAP
7.3

Opti-Start Pressure
7.0

Sleep Therapy Flags

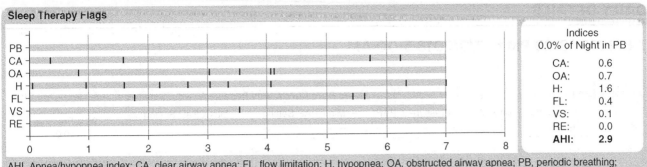

Indices	
0.0% of Night in PB	
CA:	0.6
OA:	0.7
H:	1.6
FL:	0.4
VS:	0.1
RE:	0.0
AHI:	**2.9**

AHI, Apnea/hypopnea index; CA, clear airway apnea; FL, flow limitation; H, hypopnea; OA, obstructed airway apnea; PB, periodic breathing; RE, RERA; VS, vibratory snore.

Unintentional Leak

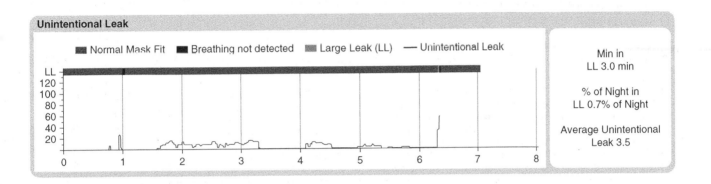

Min in
LL 3.0 min

% of Night in
LL 0.7% of Night

Average Unintentional
Leak 3.5

Daily Events Per Hour

7/7/2018   Total AHI: 2.9

P	4	5	6	7	8	9	10	11	12	13	14	15	16	17	18	19	20
MaP	0.0	0.0	0.0	318.1	98.2	1.3	0.3	0.0	0.0	0.0	0.0	0.0	0.0	0.0	0.0	0.0	0.0
%	0.0	0.0	0.0	76.1	23.5	0.3	0.1	0.0	0.0	0.0	0.0	0.0	0.0	0.0	0.0	0.0	0.0
FL	0.0	0.0	0.0	0.6	0.0	0.0	0.0	0.0	0.0	0.0	0.0	0.0	0.0	0.0	0.0	0.0	0.0
VS	0.0	0.0	0.0	0.2	0.0	0.0	0.0	0.0	0.0	0.0	0.0	0.0	0.0	0.0	0.0	0.0	0.0
OA	0.0	0.0	0.0	0.6	1.2	0.0	0.0	0.0	0.0	0.0	0.0	0.0	0.0	0.0	0.0	0.0	0.0
CA	0.0	0.0	0.0	0.8	0.0	0.0	0.0	0.0	0.0	0.0	0.0	0.0	0.0	0.0	0.0	0.0	0.0
H	0.0	0.0	0.0	1.9	0.6	0.0	0.0	0.0	0.0	0.0	0.0	0.0	0.0	0.0	0.0	0.0	0.0
RE	0.0	0.0	0.0	0.0	0.0	0.0	0.0	0.0	0.0	0.0	0.0	0.0	0.0	0.0	0.0	0.0	0.0
AHI	0.0	0.0	0.0	3.3	1.8	0.0	0.0	0.0	0.0	0.0	0.0	0.0	0.0	0.0	0.0	0.0	0.0

90%

Legend	P - Pressure, MaP - Minutes at Pressure, % - Percent of Night, FL - Flow Limitation, VS - Vibratory Snore, H - Hypopnea, OA - Obstructed Airway Apnea, CA - Clear Airway Apnea, RE - RERA, AHI - Apnea/Hypopnea Index

DAILY DETAILS

7/8/2018 10:29 PM to 7/9/2018 5:00 AM

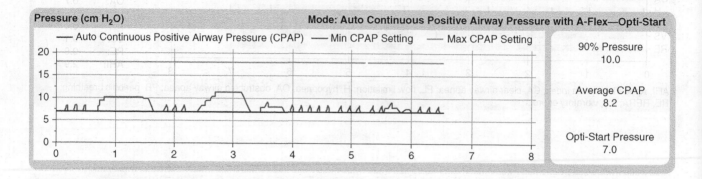

Pressure (cm H₂O) — Mode: Auto Continuous Positive Airway Pressure with A-Flex—Opti-Start

— Auto Continuous Positive Airway Pressure (CPAP) — Min CPAP Setting — Max CPAP Setting

90% Pressure
10.0

Average CPAP
8.2

Opti-Start Pressure
7.0

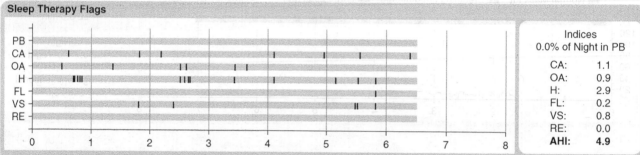

Sleep Therapy Flags

Indices
0.0% of Night in PB

CA:	1.1
OA:	0.9
H:	2.9
FL:	0.2
VS:	0.8
RE:	0.0
AHI:	**4.9**

AHI, Apnea/hypopnea index; CA, clear airway apnea; FL, flow limitation; H, hypopnea; OA, obstructed airway apnea; PB, periodic breathing; RE, RERA; VS, vibratory snore.

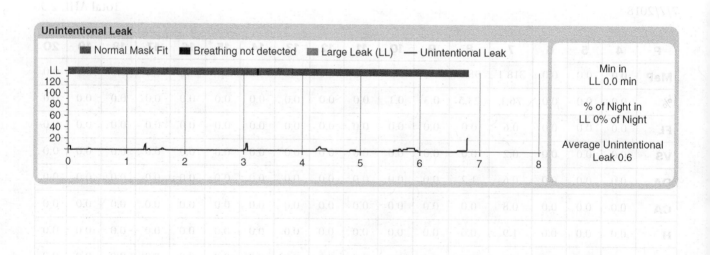

Unintentional Leak

■ Normal Mask Fit ■ Breathing not detected ■ Large Leak (LL) — Unintentional Leak

Min in
LL 0.0 min

% of Night in
LL 0% of Night

Average Unintentional
Leak 0.6

Daily Events Per Hour

7/8/2018   Total AHI: 4.9

P	4	5	6	7	8	9	10	11	12	13	14	15	16	17	18	19	20
MaP	0.0	0.0	0.0	171.9	116.4	9.5	59.7	16.3	12.9	0.0	0.0	0.0	0.0	0.0	0.0	0.0	0.0
%	0.0	0.0	0.0	44.4	30.1	2.5	15.4	4.2	3.3	0.0	0.0	0.0	0.0	0.0	0.0	0.0	0.0
FL	0.0	0.0	0.0	0.3	0.0	0.0	0.0	0.0	0.0	0.0	0.0	0.0	0.0	0.0	0.0	0.0	0.0
VS	0.0	0.0	0.0	1.0	1.0	0.0	0.0	0.0	0.0	0.0	0.0	0.0	0.0	0.0	0.0	0.0	0.0
OA	0.0	0.0	0.0	0.3	1.5	0.0	2.0	0.0	0.0	0.0	0.0	0.0	0.0	0.0	0.0	0.0	0.0
CA	0.0	0.0	0.0	1.7	1.0	0.0	0.0	0.0	0.0	0.0	0.0	0.0	0.0	0.0	0.0	0.0	0.0
H	0.0	0.0	0.0	2.4	2.6	12.6	5.0	0.0	0.0	0.0	0.0	0.0	0.0	0.0	0.0	0.0	0.0
RE	0.0	0.0	0.0	0.0	0.0	0.0	0.0	0.0	0.0	0.0	0.0	0.0	0.0	0.0	0.0	0.0	0.0
AHI	0.0	0.0	0.0	4.4	5.1	12.6	7.0	0.0	0.0	0.0	0.0	0.0	0.0	0.0	0.0	0.0	0.0

90%

Legend	P - Pressure, MaP - Minutes at Pressure, % - Percent of Night, FL - Flow Limitation, VS - Vibratory Snore, H - Hypopnea, OA - Obstructed Airway Apnea, CA - Clear Airway Apnea, RE - RERA, AHI - Apnea/Hypopnea Index

DAILY DETAILS

7/9/2018 9:42 PM to 7/10/2018 4:30 AM

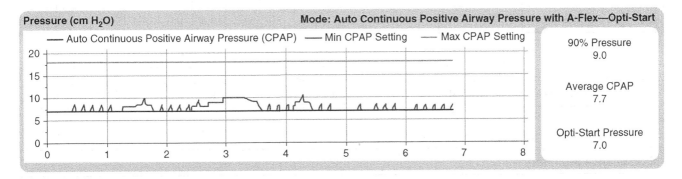

Pressure (cm H₂O)   Mode: Auto Continuous Positive Airway Pressure with A-Flex—Opti-Start

90% Pressure 9.0

Average CPAP 7.7

Opti-Start Pressure 7.0

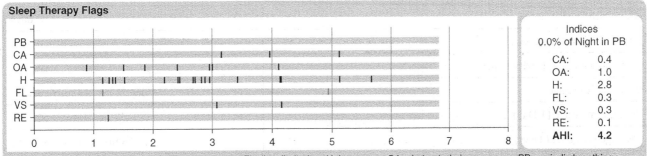

Sleep Therapy Flags

Indices
0.0% of Night in PB

CA: 0.4
OA: 1.0
H: 2.8
FL: 0.3
VS: 0.3
RE: 0.1
AHI: 4.2

AHI, Apnea/hypopnea index; CA, clear airway apnea; FL, flow limitation; H, hypopnea; OA, obstructed airway apnea; PB, periodic breathing; RE, RERA; VS, vibratory snore.

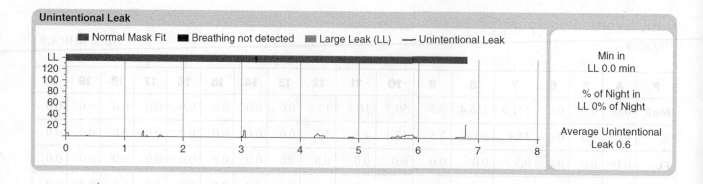

Unintentional Leak

■ Normal Mask Fit   ■ Breathing not detected   ■ Large Leak (LL)   — Unintentional Leak

Min in
LL 0.0 min

% of Night in
LL 0% of Night

Average Unintentional
Leak 0.6

Daily Events Per Hour

7/9/2018

Total AHI: 4.2

P	4	5	6	7	8	9	10	11	12	13	14	15	16	17	18	19	20
MaP	0.0	0.0	0.0	217.6	111.0	45.4	32.9	0.0	0.0	0.0	0.0	0.0	0.0	0.0	0.0	0.0	0.0
%	0.0	0.0	0.0	53.5	27.3	11.2	8.1	0.0	0.0	0.0	0.0	0.0	0.0	0.0	0.0	0.0	0.0
FL	0.0	0.0	0.0	0.6	0.0	0.0	0.0	0.0	0.0	0.0	0.0	0.0	0.0	0.0	0.0	0.0	0.0
VS	0.0	0.0	0.0	0.0	0.5	0.0	1.8	0.0	0.0	0.0	0.0	0.0	0.0	0.0	0.0	0.0	0.0
OA	0.0	0.0	0.0	1.1	0.5	1.3	1.8	0.0	0.0	0.0	0.0	0.0	0.0	0.0	0.0	0.0	0.0
CA	0.0	0.0	0.0	0.6	0.0	0.0	1.8	0.0	0.0	0.0	0.0	0.0	0.0	0.0	0.0	0.0	0.0
H	0.0	0.0	0.0	1.7	4.9	4.0	1.8	0.0	0.0	0.0	0.0	0.0	0.0	0.0	0.0	0.0	0.0
RE	0.0	0.0	0.0	0.3	0.0	0.0	0.0	0.0	0.0	0.0	0.0	0.0	0.0	0.0	0.0	0.0	0.0
AHI	0.0	0.0	0.0	3.4	5.4	5.3	5.4	0.0	0.0	0.0	0.0	0.0	0.0	0.0	0.0	0.0	0.0

90%

Legend	P - Pressure, MaP - Minutes at Pressure, % - Percent of Night, FL - Flow Limitation, VS - Vibratory Snore, H - Hypopnea, OA - Obstructed Airway Apnea, CA - Clear Airway Apnea, RE - RERA, AHI - Apnea/Hypopnea Index

Compliance Summary

Date Range	7/3/2018 - 7/9/2018 (7 days)
Days with Device Usage	7 days
Days without Device Usage	0 days
Percent Days with Device Usage	100.0%
Cumulative Usage	1 day 21 hrs. 48 mins. 8 secs.
Maximum Usage (1 Day)	7 hrs. 4 mins. 51 secs.
Average Usage (All Days)	6 hrs. 32 mins. 35 secs.
Average Usage (Days Used)	6 hrs. 32 mins. 35 secs.

Minimum Usage (1 Day)	4 hrs. 37 mins. 54 secs.
Percent of Days with Usage >= 4 Hours	100.0%
Percent of Days with Usage < 4 Hours	0.0%
Total Blower Time	1 day 22 hrs. 3 mins. 36 secs.
Auto-CPAP Summary	
Auto-CPAP Mean Pressure	7.6 cmH2O
Auto-CPAP Peak Average Pressure	8.2 cmH2O
Average Device Pressure <= 90% of Time	8.7 cmH2O
Average Time in Large Leak Per Day	1 mins. 9 secs.
Average AHI	3.4
Device Settings as of	7/9/2018
Device Mode	AutoCPAP-A-Flex
Device Settings	

Parameter	Value
Min pressure	7 cmH2O
Max Pressure	18 cmH2O
A-Flex Setting	3
Auto Off	Off
Auto On	On
View Optional Screens	On
Ramp Type	SmartRamp
Ramp Time	20 minutes
Ramp Start Pressure	5.0 cmH2O
Mask Resistance	Off
Mask Resistance Lock	Off
Tubing Type	15 HT
Tubing Type Lock	Off
Optl-Start	On
EZ-Start	Disabled
Tube Temperature	1
Humidifier	3
Humidification Mode on Heated Tube Disconnect	Adaptive

Compliance Summary

Date Range	7/3/2018 - 7/9/2018 (7 days)
Days with Device Usage	7 days
Days without Device Usage	0 days
Percent Days with Device Usage	100.0%
Cumulative Usage	1 day 21 hrs. 48 mins. 8 secs.
Maximum Usage (1 Day)	7 hrs. 4 mins. 51 secs.
Average Usage (All Days)	6 hrs. 32 mins. 35 secs.
Average Usage (Days Used)	6 hrs. 32 mins. 35 secs.
Minimum Usage (1 Day)	4 hrs. 37 mins. 54 secs.
Percent of Days with Usage >= 4 Hours	100.0%
Percent of Days with Usage < 4 Hours	0.0%
Total Blower Time	1 day 22 hrs. 3 mins. 36 secs.

Auto-CPAP Summary

Auto-CPAP Mean Pressure	7.6 cmH2O
Auto-CPAP Peak Average Pressure	8.2 cmH2O
Average Device Pressure <= 90% of Time	8.7 cmH2O
Average Time in Large Leak Per Day	1 mins. 9 secs.
Average AHI	3.4

Device Settings as of	7/9/2018

Device Mode	AutoCPAP-A-Flex
Device Settings	

Device Settings

Parameter	**Value**
Min pressure	7 cmH2O
Max Pressure	18 cmH2O
A-Flex Setting	3
Auto Off	Off
Auto On	On
View Optional Screens	On
Ramp Type	SmartRamp
Ramp Time	20 minutes
Ramp Start Pressure	5.0 cmH2O
Mask Resistance	Off
Mask Resistance Lock	Off
Tubing Type	15 HT

Tubing Type Lock	Off
Opti-Start	On
EZ-Start	Disabled
Tube Temperature	1
Humidifier	3
Humidification Mode on Heated Tube Disconnect	Adaptive

Hours of Usage

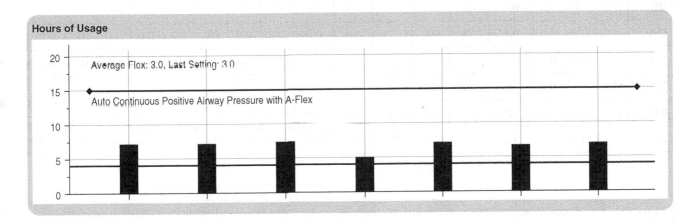

Device Humidification Settings

■ Heated Tube Temperature
■ Heated Tube Humidity Level

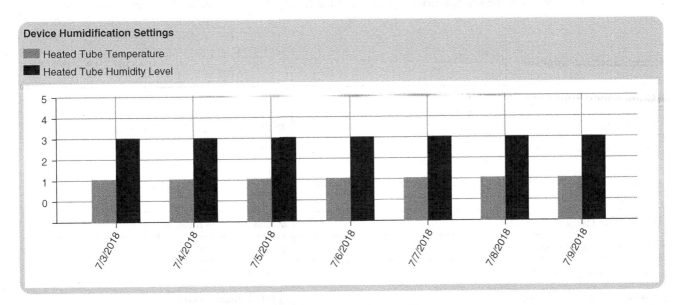

Auto Continuous Positive Airway Pressure Time at Pressure
7/3/2018 to 7/9/2018

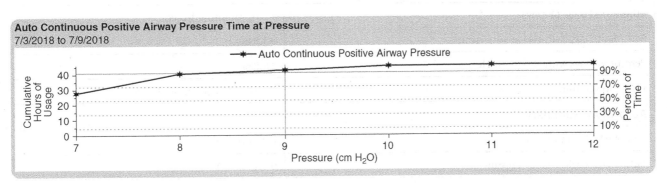

Summary of Daily Events Per Hour

7/3/2018 - 7/9/2018

P	4	5	6	7	8	9	10	11	12	13	14	15	16	17	18	19	20
MaP	0.0	0.0	0.0	1,694	752.7	96.6	173.6	18.0	13.3	0.0	0.0	0.0	0.0	0.0	0.0	0.0	0.0
%	0.0	0.0	0.0	61.6	27.4	3.5	6.3	0.7	0.5	0.0	0.0	0.0	0.0	0.0	0.0	0.0	0.0
FL	0.0	0.0	0.0	0.4	0.4	1.2	0.7	0.0	0.0	0.0	0.0	0.0	0.0	0.0	0.0	0.0	0.0
VS	0.0	0.0	0.0	0.4	0.4	0.6	0.3	0.0	0.0	0.0	0.0	0.0	0.0	0.0	0.0	0.0	0.0
OA	0.0	0.0	0.0	0.6	0.8	0.6	1.0	0.0	0.0	0.0	0.0	0.0	0.0	0.0	0.0	0.0	0.0
CA	0.0	0.0	0.0	0.6	0.5	0.0	0.3	0.0	0.0	0.0	0.0	0.0	0.0	0.0	0.0	0.0	0.0
H	0.0	0.0	0.0	1.9	2.4	4.3	2.8	0.0	0.0	0.0	0.0	0.0	0.0	0.0	0.0	0.0	0.0
RE	0.0	0.0	0.0	0.0	0.2	0.0	0.0	0.0	0.0	0.0	0.0	0.0	0.0	0.0	0.0	0.0	0.0
AHI	0.0	0.0	0.0	3.1	3.7	4.9	4.1	0.0	0.0	0.0	0.0	0.0	0.0	0.0	0.0	0.0	0.0

90%

Legend	P - Pressure, MaP - Minutes at Pressure, % - Percent of Night, FL - Flow Limitation, VS - Vibratory Snore, H - Hypopnea, OA - Obstructed Airway Apnea, CA - Clear Airway Apnea, RE - RERA, AHI - Apnea/Hypopnea Index

Compliance Information

6/10/2018 – 7/9/2018

Compliance Summary	
Date Range	6/10/2018 - 7/9/2018 (30 days)
Days with Device Usage	28 days
Days without Device Usage	2 days
Percent Days with Device Usage	93.3%
Cumulative Usage	7 days 4 hrs. 26 mins. 9 secs.
Maximum Usage (1 Day)	8 hrs. 12 mins. 9 secs.
Average Usage (All Days)	5 hrs. 44 mins. 52 secs.
Average Usage (Days Used)	6 hrs. 9 mins. 30 secs.
Minimum Usage (1 Day)	2 hrs. 16 mins. 38 secs.
Percent of Days with Usage >= 4 Hours	83.3%
Percent of Days with Usage < 4 Hours	16.7%
Total Blower Time	7 days 8 hrs. 37 mins. 35 secs.
Auto-CPAP Summary	
Auto-CPAP Mean Pressure	8.1 cmH2O
Auto-CPAP Peak Average Pressure	9.2 cmH2O

Average Device Pressure <= 90% of Time	9.7 cmH2O
Average Time in Large Leak Per Day	1 mins. 2 secs.
Average AHI	3.6
Device Settings as of	7/9/2018
Device Mode	**AutoCPAP - A-Flex**
Device Settings	

Parameter	Value
Min Pressure	7 cmH2O
Max Pressure	18 cmH2O
A-Flex Setting	3
Auto Off	Off
Auto On	On
View Optional Screens	On
Ramp Type	SmartRamp
Ramp Time	20 minutes
Ramp Start Pressure	5.0 cmH2O
Mask Resistance	Off
Mask Resistance Lock	Off
Tubing Type	15 HT
Tubing Type Lock	Off
Opti-Start	On
EZ-Start	Disabled
Tube Temperature	1
Humidifier	3
Humidification Mode on Heated Tube Disconnect	Adaptive

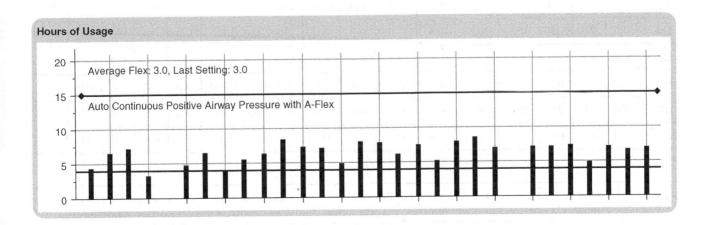

Hours of Usage

Average Flex: 3.0, Last Setting: 3.0

Auto Continuous Positive Airway Pressure with A-Flex

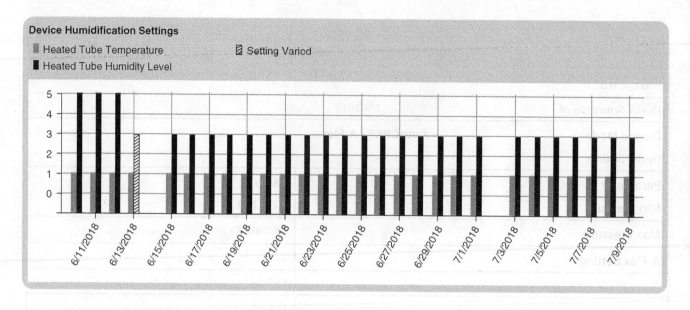

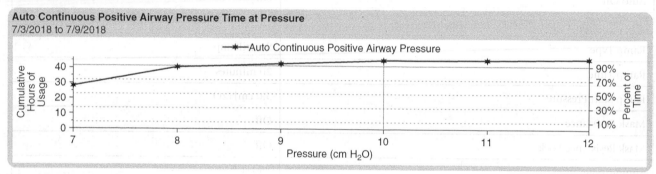

Summary of Daily Events Per Hour

7/3/2018 - 7/9/2018

P	4	5	6	7	8	9	10	11	12	13	14	15	16	17	18	19	20
MaP	0.0	0.0	0.0	1,694	752.7	96.6	173.6	18.0	13.3	0.0	0.0	0.0	0.0	0.0	0.0	0.0	0.0
%	0.0	0.0	0.0	61.6	27.4	3.5	6.3	0.7	0.5	0.0	0.0	0.0	0.0	0.0	0.0	0.0	0.0
FL	0.0	0.0	0.0	0.4	0.4	1.2	0.7	0.0	0.0	0.0	0.0	0.0	0.0	0.0	0.0	0.0	0.0
VS	0.0	0.0	0.0	0.4	0.4	0.6	0.3	0.0	0.0	0.0	0.0	0.0	0.0	0.0	0.0	0.0	0.0
OA	0.0	0.0	0.0	0.6	0.8	0.6	1.0	0.0	0.0	0.0	0.0	0.0	0.0	0.0	0.0	0.0	0.0
CA	0.0	0.0	0.0	0.6	0.5	0.0	0.3	0.0	0.0	0.0	0.0	0.0	0.0	0.0	0.0	0.0	0.0
H	0.0	0.0	0.0	1.9	"2.4	4.3	2.8	0.0	0.0	0.0	0.0	0.0	0.0	0.0	0.0	0.0	0.0
RE	0.0	0.0	0.0	0.0	0.2	0.0	0.0	0.0	0.0	0.0	0.0	0.0	0.0	0.0	0.0	0.0	0.0
AHI	0.0	0.0	0.0	3.1	3.7	4.9	4.1	0.0	0.0	0.0	0.0	0.0	0.0	0.0	0.0	0.0	0.0

90%

Legend.	P - Pressure, MaP - Minutes at Pressure, % - Percent of Night, FL - Flow Limitation, VS - Vibratory Snore, H - Hypopnea, QA - obstructed Airway Apnea, CA - Clear Airway Apnea, RE - RERA, AHI - Apnea/Hypopnea Index

Appendix P

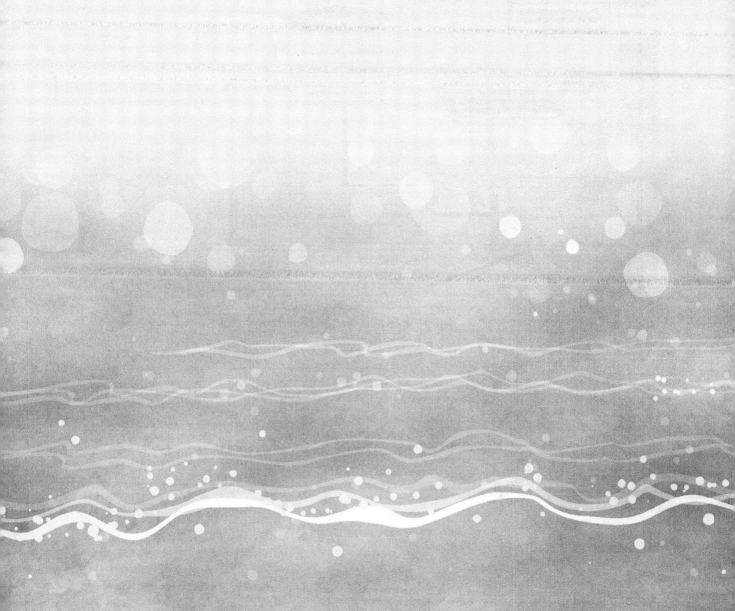

PERIOPERATIVE SCREENING PILOT PROGRAM

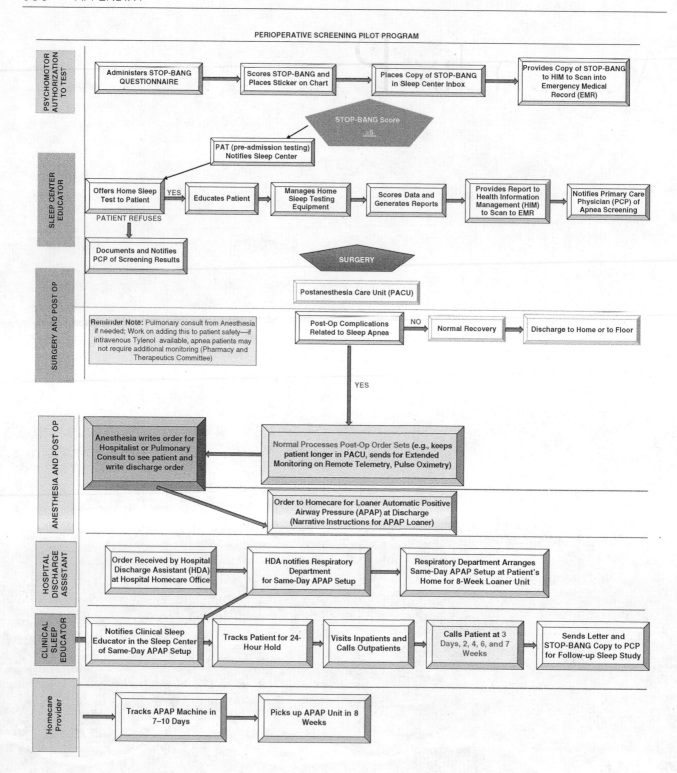

Appendix Q
Research Terminology, Acronyms, and Agencies

Adverse drug reaction Any noxious, unintended, or undesired effect of a drug that occurs at doses used in humans for prophylaxis, diagnosis, or therapy. This World Health Organization definition excludes therapeutic failures, intentional and accidental poisoning (i.e., overdose), and drug abuse. Additionally, this also does not include adverse events due to errors in administration or noncompliance (taking a drug at more or less than the prescribed dosage).

Analysis Comparison of the outcomes for the study and control groups.

Audits, Food and Drug Administration Process by which the U.S. Food and Drug Administration (FDA) reviews the clinical data as part of clinical drug trials.

Benchmark standard A criterion of evaluation or measurement used as a reference point in observation.

Bioresearch Monitoring Program A comprehensive program of on-site inspections and data audits designed to monitor all aspects of the conduct and reporting of FDA-regulated research. This program monitors and sponsors institutional review boards, clinical investigators, and nonclinical laboratories involved in the testing of investigational devices.

Blinding A study design feature that helps ensure that bias does not distort the conduct of a study or the integration of its results. In a single-blind study, only the clinical investigators are aware of which intervention (e.g., investigational drug or control) each patient is receiving. In a double-blind study, neither the patients nor the clinical investigators know the identity of the intervention. In a triple-blind study, neither the patients, the clinical investigators, nor the committee monitoring the response variables is revealed about the identity of the groups.

Carcinogenicity Producing or tending to produce cancer.

Case report form A standardized data entry form used in a clinical trial. Generally, all information collected in trials appears on case report forms (CRFs), or is referred to and explained by CRFs.

Center for Biologics Evaluation and Research (CBER) A center of the FDA whose mission is to protect and enhance public health through regulation of biologic and related products including blood, vaccines, and biologic therapeutics according to statutory authorities (www.fda.gov/cber).

Center for Devices and Radiological Health (CDRH) The center of the FDA whose responsibility is to ensure that medical devices are safe and effective, including ensuring the minimization of exposure from radiation-emitting electronic products (https://www.fda.gov/AboutFDA/CentersOffices/OfficeofMedicalProductsandTobacco/CDRH/default.htm).

Center for Drug Evaluation and Research (CDER) A center of the FDA whose mission is to ensure that safe and effective drugs are available to the American people (www.fda.gov/cder).

Clinical reviewer A person with responsibility for critically evaluating a medical perspective information contained in a marketing application.

Clinical studies The class of all scientific approaches used to evaluate medical means of disease prevention, medical diagnostic techniques, and medical treatments. Investigational and marketed prescription drug evaluations plus over-the-counter drugs are included.

Clinical trial protocol Document describing a clinical study and how it is to be conducted. A protocol includes the objectives of the study, the study design, a description of the drug and the dosage, the experimental procedure, handling of adverse reactions, how the results will be analyzed, and patient consent and clearance provisions.

Clinical trials Medical research studies conducted with volunteers. Each study is designed to answer scientific questions and to find better ways to prevent, detect, or treat human medical conditions.

Comparative studies Studies conducted to determine statistically whether one procedure is better than the other.

Compliance A quantitative indicator of whether a set of procedures or practices was carried out in accordance with established guidelines or standards stated in the protocol of a study.

Concomitant medication An additional therapy or regimen that is either self-administered or prescribed concurrently with a study therapy.

Contract Research Organizations (CROs) Organizations that are hired by companies to perform specific studies on a given topic.

Cooperative Clinical Trials Group (CCTG) A community-based organization that conducts research involving human volunteers under agreement with the National Institutes of Health.

Data All collected and recorded information on patients considered for enrollment or actually enrolled in a trial.

Database A collection of data files that are organized in a specified manner and that are accessed by designated personnel for designated purposes.

Defibrillator An electronic apparatus used to counteract atrial or ventricular fibrillation by the application of brief electroshock to the heart, either directly or through electrodes placed on the chest wall.

Discovery The early phases of the overall drug development process dealing with the synthesis of or search for compounds and the screening process developed to identify lead compounds.

Disease The condition in which the functioning of the body or a part of the body is interfered with or damaged. In a person with an infectious disease, the infectious agent that has entered the body causes it to function abnormally in some way(s). The type of abnormal functioning that occurs is the disease. Usually, the body will show signs and symptoms of the problems that it is having with functioning. Disease should not be confused with infection.

Double blinding In a clinical trial, a procedure for issuing and administering treatment assignments by code number to keep study patients and all members of the clinical staff, especially those responsible for patient treatment and data collection, from knowing the assigned treatments, so that the information does not influence some measurement, observation, or process.

Drug (from the FDA Food, Drug, & Cosmetic Act) (1) a substance recognized by an official pharmacopoeia or formulary; (2) a substance intended for use in the diagnosis, cure, mitigation, treatment, or prevention of disease; (3) a substance other than food intended to affect the structure or function of the body; (4) a substance intended for use as a component of a medicine but not a device or a component, part, or accessory of a device. Biologic products are included within this definition and are generally covered by the same laws and regulations, but differences exist regarding their manufacturing processes (chemical process vs. biologic process).

Drug development process The entirety of the activities and decision making that must be completed from the identification of a lead compound to regulatory agency approval for marketing of a compound as a new drug product.

Effectiveness The desired measure of a drug's influence on a disease condition. Effectiveness must be proven by substantial evidence consisting of adequate and well-controlled investigations, including human studies by qualified experts, which prove that the drug will have the effect claimed in its labeling.

Efficacy A relative concept referring to the ability of a drug to elicit a beneficial clinical effect. This may be measured or evaluated by using objective or subjective parameters and in terms ranging from global impressions to highly precise measurements.

Equivalence trials A trial typically conducted to demonstrate that there is no clinically significant difference between a standard and an experimental treatment. The study is designed with the desired outcome being equivalence in efficacy, whereas immediate toxicity, long-term adverse effects, or costs may be demonstrated to be advantageous for the experimental treatment.

Federal Food, Drug, and Cosmetic Acts of 1938 and 1962 Law that requires a manufacturer to prove the safety and effectiveness of a drug before it can be marketed.

Food and Drug Administration (FDA) A public health agency charged with protecting American consumers by enforcing the Federal Food, Drug, and Cosmetic Act and several related health laws (www.fda.gov).

Food and Drug Administration Modernization Act of 1997 (FDAMA) Major legislation focused on reforming the regulation of food, medical products, and cosmetics. Some of the provisions of the act include prescription drug user fees, FDA initiatives and programs, information on off-label use and drug economics, risk-based regulation of medical devices, and standards for medical products.

Form FDA 483 An official FDA form on which any objectionable conditions and/or practices noted during an inspection are listed. An FDA investigator issues Form FDA 483 to an establishment (e.g., investigator, sponsor, monitor, contract research organization, or Institutional Review Board) at the conclusion of an inspection.

Gene therapy The process of introducing new genes into the DNA of a person's cells to correct a genetic disease or flaw.

Generic Drug Enforcement Act of 1992 A law authorizing the Secretary of Health and Human Services to impose debarments and to take other action to ensure the integrity of abbreviated drug applications under the Federal Food, Drug, and Cosmetic Act.

Genomics The study of genomes, which includes genome mapping, gene sequencing, and gene function.

Good Clinical Practices (GCP) FDA-promulgated guidelines governing the conduct of clinical studies from which data will be used to support applications for marketing permits (New Drug Applications).

Good Clinical Practices (GCP) document An international ethical and scientific quality standard for the design, conduct, recording, and reporting of trials that involve the participation of human subjects.

Good Review Practices An FDA initiative designed to promote standardization of the quality and consistency of reviews of New Drug Applications and Investigational New Drugs.

Institutional Review Board (IRB) Any board, committee, or other group of experts and laypeople formally designated by an institution to review, to approve the initiation of, and to conduct a periodic review of, biomedical research involving human subjects. The primary purpose of such review is to ensure the protection of the rights and welfare of the human subjects.

International Conference on Harmonization (ICH) An organization with representation from the regulatory parties of the European Union, Japan, and the United States, established to create common standards for safety, efficacy, and quality of medical products (www.ich.org).

Investigational agents A medical product (e.g., drug, biologic, or medical device) used for research purposes to diagnose, prevent, or treat disease.

Investigational New Drug (IND) Status given to an experimental drug after the FDA approves an application for it to be tested with humans.

Investigational New Drug (IND) application Application that a drug sponsor must submit to the FDA before beginning tests of a new drug on humans. The IND application contains the plan for the study and is supposed to give a complete picture of the drug, including structural formula, animal test results, and manufacturing information.

Managed care Arrangements for integrated health care delivery and financing that are designed to provide appropriate, effective, and efficient health care through organized relationships with providers. Includes formal programs for ongoing quality assurance and utilization review, financial incentives for covered members to use the plan's providers, and financial incentives for providers to contain costs. Managed care plans vary greatly in the degree to which benefit coverage is offered, monitored, and conditioned upon certain criteria being met by the subscriber and the subscriber's primary care physician.

Medical device A diagnostic or therapeutic contrivance that does not interact chemically with a person's body.

Monitor A person who oversees the ongoing evaluation of a continuing process to determine when and if changes in that process are necessary for reasons of efficiency, data quality, safety, and so forth.

National Cancer Institute (NCI) The federal government's principal agency for cancer research and training. The NCI is a component of the National Institutes of Health (www.nci.nih.gov).

National Institutes of Health (NIH) A group of institutes and related support structures responsible for funding basic and applied research in the health field. The National Institutes of Health also initiates and carries out medical research on an intramural and extramural basis (www.nih.gov).

New Drug Application (NDA) An application requesting FDA approval to market a new drug for human use in interstate commerce. The application must contain, among other things, data from specific technical viewpoints for FDA review, including chemistry, pharmacology, medicine, biopharmaceutics, and statistics, as well as for anti-infectives and microbiology.

Oncology The study of diseases that cause cancer.

Orphan drugs Drugs (and other products) for the treatment of a rare disease that affects fewer than 200,000 people or a drug that may offer little or no profit to the manufacturer but that may benefit people with rare diseases.

Outliers In statistics, an observation so distant from the central mass of data that it is considered an obvious mistake or anomaly that should be removed from the data whether or not a cause of the deviation can be found.

Outsourcing Hiring of contract employees to perform support services rather than use of a company's own employees.

Patient In the clinical trial setting, patient refers to any subject involved in the trial.

Pharmaceutical A medicinal drug.

Pharmacokinetics The action of drugs in the body over a period of time, including the processes of absorption, distribution, localization in tissues, biotransformation, metabolism, and excretion.

Pharmacology The science that deals with the origin, nature, chemistry, and effects of drugs and the uses of drugs for living organisms.

Phase 1 trials The first trials in humans that test a compound for safety, tolerance, and pharmacokinetics. The Phase 1 trials usually use healthy volunteers. For known toxic compounds, such as anticancer agents, only patients with the targeted illness are used.

Phase 2 trials The pilot studies that define efficacy and further test safety with selected populations of patients with the disease or condition to be treated, diagnosed, or prevented. Dose and dosing regimens are assessed for magnitude and duration of effect during this phase.

Phase 3 trials Expanded clinical trials intended to gather additional evidence of effectiveness for specific indications and to better understand safety and drug-related adverse effects. Phase 3 trials are usually large multicenter trials that achieve substantial safety experience and may also include specialized studies needed for labeling.

Pivotal trial A clinical trial for a marketing application that is considered an essential component to supporting the safe and effective use of a medical product.

Placebo A pharmacologically inactive agent given to a patient as a substitute for an active agent. When trials with placebos are conducted, the patient is not informed whether he or she is receiving the active or the inactive agent (the placebo).

Postmarketing surveillance Requirement that drug firms report to the FDA the adverse experiences from the use of all marketed drugs of which they are aware. If the adverse experiences result in death, prolonged hospitalization, or permanent disability, the firm must report the incident within 15 days of its notification of the adverse experience. All other adverse experiences can be reported on an annual basis.

Premarket Approval Application (PMA) An application requesting FDA approval to market a new medical device for human use in interstate commerce. The application must contain, among other things, data from specific technical viewpoints for FDA review.

Prescription Drug User Fee Act of 1992 (PDUFA) Requires manufacturers to pay fees for certain new drug applications and supplements, an annual establishment fee, and annual product fees.

Quality assurance (QA) Any procedure, method, or philosophy for collecting, processing, or analyzing data that is aimed at maintaining or improving the reliability or validity of the data and the associated procedures used to generate them.

Remote data capture A process by which information is entered directly into a computer or a centralized database without being recorded on paper.

Safety A relative concept referring to the freedom from harm or damage resulting from adverse reactions or physical, psychological, or behavioral abnormalities that occur as a result of drug or nondrug use. No drug is completely safe or without the potential for side effects. Before a drug may be approved for marketing, the law requires the submission of the results of tests adequate to show that the drug is safe under the conditions of use in the proposed labeling. "Safety" is thus determined on a case-by-case basis and reflects the drug's risk-versus-benefit relationship.

Site monitoring The act of overseeing the progress of a clinical trial and of ensuring that it is conducted, recorded, and reported in accordance with the protocol, standard operating procedures, Good Clinical Practices, and the applicable regulatory requirements.

Special populations A subset of the population that may be more sensitive than the general public to the effects of a medical product (e.g., pediatric and geriatric populations and patients with compromised liver or kidney function).

Standard operating procedure (SOP) Established or prescribed methods to be followed routinely for the performance of designated operations or in designated situations.

Superiority trial A trial typically conducted to demonstrate that there is a clinically significant difference between a standard and an experimental treatment. The study is designed with the desired outcome being superiority in efficacy in favor of the experimental treatment.

Therapeutic agent A drug, biologic, or medical device used for research purposes in the treatment of disease.

Toxicology The scientific study of poisons, their actions, their detection, and the treatment of the conditions produced by them.

Trial Any tentative or experimental action conducted to obtain data used to make some judgment or conclusion.

Institute of Medicine (US) Roundtable on Research and Development of Drugs, Biologics, and Medical Devices; Davis, J. R., Nolan, V. P., Woodcock, J., et al., (Eds.). (1999). *Assuring data quality and validity in clinical trials for regulatory decision making: Workshop report.* Washington, DC: National Academies Press (US).

Appendix D, Glossary and Acronyms. Association of Clinical Research Professionals. Retrieved from https://www.ncbi.nlm.nih .gov/books/NBK224575

Reprinted with permission from Association of Clinical Research Professionals. (June 2018). *Certification exam abbreviation list.* Retrieved from www.acrpnet.org/download/ certification-exam-abbreviations-list

ADR Adverse Drug Reaction

AE Adverse Event

ALCOAC Accurate, Legible, Contemporaneous, Original, Attributable, and Complete

ALT Alanine Transaminase (liver enzyme)

AST Aspartate Transaminase (liver enzyme)

BID Twice a day

BMI Body Mass Index

BP Blood Pressure

BUN Blood Urea Nitrogen (kidney function test)

C Celsius

CAPA Corrective and Preventive Action

CIOMS Council for International Organizations of Medical Sciences

CK Creatinine Kinase (muscle enzyme)

CRA Clinical Research Associate

CRC Clinical Research Coordinator

CRF Case Report Form

CRO Contract Research Organization

CSR Clinical Study Report

CTMS Clinical Trial Management System

CV Curriculum Vitae

DCF Data Clarification Form

DSMB Data and Safety Monitoring Board

ECG Electrocardiogram

eCRF Electronic Case Report Form

EDC Electronic Data Capture

EHR Electronic Health Record

EKG Electrocardiogram

EMR Electronic Medical Record

ePRO Electronic Patient-Reported Outcomes

eTMF Electronic Trial Master File

F Fahrenheit

FEV1 Forced Expiratory Volume in 1 second

GCP Good Clinical Practices

GI Gastrointestinal

GLP Good Laboratory Practices

GMP Good Manufacturing Practices

hCG Human Chorionic Gonadotropin

HMO Health Maintenance Organization

IB Investigator's Brochure

ICF Informed Consent Form

ICH International Conference on Harmonization

IDMC Independent Data Monitoring Committee

IEC Independent Ethics Committee

IP Investigational Product

IRB Institutional Review Board

IVRS Interactive Voice Response System

IWRS Interactive Web Response System

LAR Legally Acceptable Representative

MAOI Monoamine Oxidase Inhibitor

μg Microgram

mm Hg Millimeters of mercury

NSAID(s) Nonsteroidal Anti-Inflammatory Drug(s)

PI Principal Investigator

PK Pharmacokinetics

p.r.n. as needed

PRO Patient-Reported Outcomes

QA Quality Assurance

QC Quality Control

QD or OD Once a day

QID Four times a day

QTc ECG/EKG QT interval corrected for heart rate

RBCs Red Blood Cells

RBM Risk-Based Monitoring

SAE Serious Adverse Event

SDV Source Document Verification

SMO Site Management Organization

SOP Standard Operating Procedure

SUSAR Suspected Unexpected Serious Adverse Reaction

TID Three times a day

TMF Trial Master File

WBCs White Blood Cells, or leukocytes

Glossary

Accelerometer A device that measures the vibration or acceleration of motion.

Accelerometry The quantitative measurement of acceleration and deceleration in the entire human body or a part of the body in the performance of a task.

Acclimatization A process used to assist a patient to adapt and become accustomed to a new climate or environment such as positive airway pressure (PAP) treatment.

Acetylcholine A chemical that when released, results in wakefulness or rapid eye movement (REM) sleep and when inhibited leads to slow-wave sleep.

Acromegaly A chronic metabolic disorder in which there is excessive growth hormone production after the skeleton and other organs have finished growing.

ACTH A protein hormone of the pituitary gland that stimulates the adrenal cortex.

Actigraphy Durable lightweight device that is worn on the nondominant wrist like a watch and records gross motor movements for a period of time.

Action potential A momentary reversal in the potential difference across a plasma membrane (as of a nerve cell or muscle fiber) that occurs when a cell has been activated by a stimulus.

Activation Understanding one's role in the care process and having the knowledge, skill, and confidence to manage one's health and health care.

Active sleep A sleep state in infants that is distinguished by eye movements, fairly rapid irregular breathing, occasional body movements, vocalizations and facial movements in the way of smiles, frowns, and sucking. Analogous to REM sleep in older children and adults.

Adaptive servoventilation An automatic, minute ventilation-targeted device that performs breath-to-breath analysis and adjusts pressure settings accordingly to maintain a regular breathing pattern.

Addison disease A rare, chronic disorder caused by adrenal gland failure resulting in insufficient production of adrenal hormones including cortisol, aldosterone, androgens (male), and estrogen (female).

Adenotonsillectomy Surgical removal of the tonsils and adenoids.

Adherence Conscious and consistent persistence to remain focused on something (like using PAP).

Advance directives Written instructions, such as a living will or durable power of attorney, for health care, as recognized by the state where the patient resides.

Advanced sleep phase disorder Referred to as "morning larks," individuals with this disorder go to sleep before the normal bedtime and then awaken earlier than what is considered normal.

Airway patency An airway that is open or unblocked.

Alcoholism Generally refers to compulsive and uncontrolled consumption of alcoholic beverages, usually to the detriment of the drinker's health, personal relationships, and social standing. It is medically considered a disease, specifically a neurologic disorder. Acute alcohol use decreases sleep onset latency, suppresses REM sleep in a dose-dependent manner during the first half of the night, and may increase stage N3 sleep.

Algorithm A basic technique that takes in one or more inputs and gives back one or more outputs. It can be called a "list of steps," or a list of operations to solve a problem. Algorithms are mostly written in pseudocode, flow charts, or programming languages.

Alpha intrusion A brief occurrence of alpha activity during a stage of sleep.

Alveolar minute ventilation The amount of minute ventilation that takes part in gas exchange. Alveolar ventilation is calculated by multiplying the tidal volume minus physiologic dead space by respiratory rate (RR).

Alveoli Small hollow sacs at the end of the respiratory tree that are involved in gas-exchange in the lungs.

Alzheimer disease An irreversible, progressive brain disease that slowly destroys memory and thinking skills and eventually even the ability to carry out the simplest tasks.

American Academy of Dental Sleep Medicine The organization for practitioner dentists that promotes research on the use of oral appliances and dental surgery for the treatment of sleep disordered breathing (SDB) and provides training and resources for those who work directly with patients.

American Academy of Sleep Medicine (AASM) The United States-based professional medical society that sets the clinical and technical standards for sleep medicine, including the accreditation of sleep facilities and A-STEP education programs.

American Board of Sleep Medicine (ABSM) The ABSM provides certification examinations, which set the highest standard in clinical sleep medicine, behavioral sleep medicine, and sleep technology.

American Society for Metabolic and Bariatric Surgery (ASMBS) The largest medical organization in the world dedicated to obesity-related diseases and conditions and metabolic and bariatric surgery.

Aminergic Relating to neurons and neural pathways.

Amnesia Partial or total loss of memory, usually resulting from shock, psychological disturbance, brain injury, or illness.

Ampere A measure of electric current.

Amplitude The vertical height of a wave, representing the electrical voltage of the wave.

Amyotrophic lateral sclerosis (ALS) A progressive neuromuscular disease characterized by a gradual destruction of motor neurons in the brain and spinal cord, resulting in progressive weakness and paralysis.

Analog A continuous measurement or transmission of a signal.

Analog to digital converter Converts an analog (continuous) signal into numeric form by assigning a numeric value, at predetermined intervals, to the amplitude of the analog waveform.

Anatomic dead space The volume of the conducting airways of the nose, mouth, and trachea down to the level of the alveoli, representing that portion of inspired gas unavailable for exchange of gases with pulmonary capillary blood.

Anemic hypoxia Occurs when there are insufficient RBCs in the blood to accept oxygen and deliver oxygen to the tissues.

Angiotensin converting enzyme (ACE) inhibitors ACE inhibitors are drugs used to treat heart failure and high blood pressure.

Anhydrous Without water.

Anticonvulsants Medications used in the treatment of epileptic seizures.

Antidepressant medication Psychiatric medication used to alleviate mood disorders. These medications influence REM sleep by lengthening REM latency, decreasing REM density, and decreasing REM percentage, particularly during the first third of the night.

Antihistamines A class of medications used to treat allergies and their symptoms.

Anti-kickback statute The federal Anti-Kickback Statute prohibits anyone from soliciting, receiving, offering, or paying any remuneration, directly or indirectly, overtly or covertly, in cash or in kind, in return for a referral (or to induce a referral) for any item or service that is paid by any federal or state health care program.

Anxiety disorder A disorder characterized by anxiety that is excessive and long standing but is not focused on any particular object or situation.

Aortic bodies A group of chemosensitive cells in the wall of the aortic arch. Along with the carotid bodies, these cells are the main sensors for oxygenation (PO_2) but also respond to PCO_2 and pH.

Apnea Cessation of breathing lasting 10 seconds or longer in adults or the equivalent of two breaths in children.

Apnea index The number of apneas per hour of sleep.

Apnea/hypopnea index The number of apneas and hypopneas per hour of sleep.

Armodafinil A wakefulness promoting agent used in the treatment of narcolepsy, SWSD, and residual daytime sleepiness complaints in obstructive sleep apnea patients treated with continuous positive airway pressure (CPAP).

Arousal Waking during sleep for a very brief period; a sudden shift in EEG frequency lasting for at least 3 seconds with at least 10 seconds of stable sleep preceding the change in N1, N2, N3, or REM sleep. Scoring an arousal during REM sleep requires a concurrent increase in submental EMG.

Arrhythmia Any variation from the normal rhythm in the heartbeat.

Arterial blood gas (ABG) A sampling of arterial blood that directly measures the blood pH and the dissolved amount of carbon dioxide and oxygen in the blood plasma. An ABG also generally reports calculated values for both bicarb and arterial oxygen saturation.

Ascending reticular activating system Composed of several neuronal circuits that travel through the thalamus, connecting the brain stem (reticular formation) to the cerebral cortex.

Assessment The evaluation of the quality of an intervention.

ASTEP Accredited Sleep Technology Education Program developed by the AASM to promote the standardization of sleep technologist education and training.

Asthma An inflammatory disease of the airway characterized by episodic dyspnea and wheezing, reversible episodes of bronchoconstriction, and airway hyperreactivity to a variety of specific and nonspecific stimuli.

ASV Auto or adaptive servoventilation devices, which monitor breathing based on specific technology designed by Philips/Respironics (Auto Servo Ventilation) and ResMed (Adaptive Servo Ventilation) to continuously modify pressure in response to specific breathing pattern changes (central apnea and Cheyne–Stokes respiration) during sleep.

Asystole An interruption of cardiac rhythm lasting more than 3 seconds.

Atelectasis Collapse of a lobe or segment of the lung or the entire lung that prevents the exchange of oxygen and carbon dioxide.

Atrial fibrillation An irregularly irregular ventricular rhythm associated with replacement of consistent P waves by rapid electrical oscillations.

Atrial flutter A cardiac arrhythmia characterized by more atrial contractions than ventricular beats with atrial rates of between 240 and 400 minutes.

Atrioventricular (AV) block Occurs when atrial depolarizations fail to reach the ventricles or when atrial depolarization is conducted with a delay.

Augmentation Stimulation of an increased rate of biologic activity, such as a faster heartbeat.

Automatic behavior Behavior that occurs without conscious awareness.

Automatic bilevel positive airway pressure (ABPAP) A noninvasive treatment for sleep apnea that auto-adjusts the inspiratory and expiratory air pressure levels to keep the airway free of obstructions. The machine has a low expiratory pressure and a higher inspiratory pressure and uses an algorithm to sense changes in breathing and increases and decreases both pressures at the same time to deliver the appropriate pressure setting.

Automatic positive airway pressure (APAP) A noninvasive treatment for sleep apnea that auto-adjusts the pressurized air to keep the airway free of obstructions. The machine has a low-range setting and a high-range setting and uses an algorithm to sense changes in breathing and increases or decreases positive air pressure to deliver the appropriate pressure setting. Auto positive airway pressure adjusts PAP to the minimum needed to maintain an open airway in variable conditions.

Automatisms Unconscious movements that may resemble simple repetitive tics or that may be complex sequences of natural-looking movements. Automatisms involve doing something "automatically" and not remembering afterward how one did it or even that one did it.

Average volume-assured pressure support (AVAPS) A non-invasive treatment for sleep apnea that allows a preset target tidal volume. The patient's tidal volume from each breath is estimated and compared with the preset target tidal volume and inspiratory pressure is adjusted to ensure that the preset tidal volume is maintained.

A.W.A.K.E. A patient support group, Alert, Well, and Keeping Energetic, sponsored by a nonprofit organization, the American Sleep Apnea Association. The organization promotes education and awareness through dedication to reducing injury, disability, and death from sleep apnea and enhancing the well-being of those affected by sleep apnea.

Barbiturates Medications that act on the CNS by depressing or inhibiting nerve signals in the brain.

Bariatric surgery A variety of surgical procedures for selective obese patients that reduce the amount of food the stomach can hold, causing malabsorption of nutrients.

Basal forebrain Activation of the basal forebrain leads to acetylcholine release, resulting in wakefulness or REM sleep.

Benzodiazepines Medications used to treat anxiety disorders. These medications suppress stage N3 sleep and can slightly worsen the AHI in patients with OSAS. They can also decrease the arousal index related to leg movements, but may not actually decrease the number of leg movements.

Beta blockers Medications that treat high blood pressure, which work by blocking the action of epinephrine (adrenaline) and norepinephrine (noradrenaline), two chemicals produced by the body that increase heart rate and raise the blood pressure.

Bicarbonate (H_2CO_3) Normally existing as ions H^+ and HCO_3^-, the main buffer of the body for acidity and a major storage form for CO_2.

Bigeminy A heart arrhythmia in which an abnormal heartbeat occurs every other concurrent beat.

Bilevel positive airway pressure (BPAP) Maintains the patency of the airway using a lower pressure during exhalation than inhalation.

Biocalibrations A series of exercises performed prior to initiating a study, to verify correct input derivations and signal quality.

Bioelectric potentials Voltages generated by the body.

Biofeedback A technique for teaching self-control of autonomic functions, such as the rate of the heartbeat or breathing.

Biopotential An electrical potential generated by electrical activity in living organisms that results from chemical processes.

Bipolar disorder A disorder characterized by the alternating pattern of two emotional extremes: depression and euphoria.

Board of Registered Polysomnographic Technologists (BRPT) An independent, nonprofit certification board that administers the RPSGT credential. The BRPT develops, maintains, and administers the RPSGT exam and establishes the BRPT Standards of Conduct for credentialed technologists.

Body mechanics The way we use our body to accomplish a task.

Body rocking A childhood parasomnia that is classified as a rhythmic movement disorder. Body rocking typically involves rocking the entire body while on the hands and knees. Movements may persist into NREM sleep and may occur following arousals or during waking from sleep.

BPAP (bilevel PAP) A PAP device that delivers two set pressures, one inspiratory positive airway pressure (IPAP) and a lower expiratory positive airway pressure (EPAP).

Bradycardia An EKG rhythm of less than 60 bpm during wake and less than 40 bpm during sleep for ages 6 years through adult.

Brainstem Portion of the brain where most respiratory and cardiovascular control networks reside. Located just anterior to the spinal cord and composed of the medulla and pons.

Breach notification The Health Insurance Portability and Accountability Act of 1996 (HIPAA) Breach Notification Rule requires covered entities to notify affected individuals, health and human services, and in some cases, the media of a breach of unsecured protected health information. . . . The Breach Notification Rule also requires business associates of covered entities to notify the covered entity of breaches at or by the business associate.

Bruxism Grinding the teeth and clenching the jaw during wakefulness and sleep; often associated with arousals during sleep.

Business associate A business associate is an organization that performs functions on behalf of a covered entity that involve use or disclosure of protected health information. Business associates are indirectly regulated by the HIPAA through contractual obligations.

CAAHEP Commission on Accreditation of Allied Health Education Programs is the largest programmatic accrediting body in the health sciences fields. CAAHEP is comprised of committees on accreditation in 23 healthcare professions.

Caffeine An alerting natural component that is found in coffee, tea, and chocolate. It is added to energy drinks, colas, and various over-the-counter medications. Often used for a boost of energy and to improve alertness. Potential side effects are diuresis (dehydration), anxiety, irritability, tremulousness, and insomnia.

Capnography Noninvasive method for assessing alveolar hypoventilation by monitoring of the concentration of CO_2 in the exhaled breath.

Cardiac cycle The rhythmic pattern that is initiated when an electrical impulse is conducted through the heart muscle. One cardiac cycle is one beat of the heart and lasts approximately 0.8 seconds in duration during a normal resting heart rate.

Care coordination The deliberate organization of patient care activities between two or more participants (including the patient) involved in a patient's care to facilitate the appropriate delivery of health care services.

Carotid bodies A bilateral structure located at the bifurcation of the common carotid artery that is comprised of chemosensitive neurons that regulate respiratory control. Along with the aortic bodies of the aortic arch, these are the main sensors for oxygenation (PO_2) but also react to PCO_2 and pH.

Case management The coordination of health care services to assure appropriate medical care is provided. A comprehensive approach to primary services offered to patients, families, and the community for all aspects of care that assesses, monitors, plans, and advocates on behalf of the patient to promote quality, cost-effective outcomes.

Cataplexy Sudden and transient episodes of loss of muscle tone triggered by emotion.

Central apnea A cessation of ventilation greater than 10 seconds without any muscular effort to breathe.

Central chemoreceptors Sensory cell groups in the brain that increase activity to increasing PCO_2 and acidity, producing a compensatory increase in ventilation.

Central nervous system (CNS) The central nervous system is comprised of the brain and spinal cord. It gathers information from all over the body and coordinates activity.

Central sleep apnea Cessation of breathing, characterized by an absence of airflow and effort, due to a transient reduction or withdrawal of central neural output to the respiratory muscles (the diaphragm and intercostal muscles).

Certification in Clinical Sleep Health (CCSH) An advanced certification offered by the BRPT that assesses the professional competence of healthcare providers and educators who work directly with sleep medicine patients, families and practitioners to coordinate and manage patient care while improving outcomes.

Certified Polysomnographic Technologist (CPSGT) An entry-level certification offered by the BRPT for technicians new to the sleep technology profession. It is time limited, and within 3 years, the CPSGT must earn the RPSGT credential.

C-Flex This is a flow-based technology and patient comfort feature designed by Respironics to reduce pressure at the moment of exhalation, giving patients more control over their therapy.

Cheyne–Stokes respiration A breathing pattern of rhythmic waxing and waning of depth of breaths and regularly recurring apneic periods. Abbreviated CSR.

Child life specialist A trained healthcare professional with expertise in assisting children and their families to deal with issues in a healthcare setting such as a sleep center.

Cholinergic A substance associated with the neurotransmitter acetylcholine.

Chronic obstructive pulmonary disease A disease state characterized by airflow limitation that is relatively irreversible.

Chronobiology The study of circadian rhythms on physiologic and pathologic events.

Chronological age (CA) Age since birth.

Chronotherapy Technique used to progressively delay the sleep period by 1 or 2 hours per day.

Circadian rhythm An innate, 24-hour cycle of fluctuation in physiologic and behavioral functions.

Circadian rhythm sleep disorders Those sleep disorders in which the circadian rhythm is disrupted.

Circulatory hypoxia Occurs in patients with normal lung function and arterial oxygen content but there is vascular damage or under perfusion of the vascular tissue and oxygen rich blood cannot reach the site where gas exchange occurs.

Claustrophobia Irrational fear of being in a confined or enclosed space, which can make one feel like they are unable to breathe. A PAP interface may cause this same sensation in some patients.

CoA PSG Committee on Accreditation for Polysomnographic Technologist Education is the CAAHEP committee on accreditation for the sleep technology profession.

Cognitive behavioral therapy (CBT) Goal-oriented therapy focusing on changing attitudes and behaviors to improve health outcomes.

Commercial weight loss program Proprietary products and/or programs marketed to promote weight loss.

Common mode rejection The cancellation of unwanted voltages that are common to both input electrodes.

Common procedural technology (CPT) American Medical Association codes consisting of a 5-digit number or a 4-digit number with one alpha character assigned to every medical procedure and service.

Competency Fundamental knowledge, ability, or expertise in a specific subject area or skill set.

Complex sleep apnea A newly described respiratory pathology in which the application of CPAP for the treatment of obstructive sleep apnea elicits central apneas in the patient. This pathology is often seen in heart failure patients.

Compliance The degree to which patients follow recommended therapeutic intervention. Defined as the use of PAP) for an average of 4 hours a night for a minimum of 70% of nights.

Computer network A computer or data network is a digital network that allows computing devices to exchange data with each other using connections (data links) between nodes.

Conceptional age The weeks from the day of conception to the day of delivery.

Conductivity A measure of a material's ability to conduct an electric current.

Confusional arousals Recurrent episodes of mental confusion or confusional behavior during an arousal or awakening from sleep; characterized by diminished vigilance, excessive sleep inertia, unclear thoughts, and slowed speech.

Congestive heart failure Occurs when cardiac dysfunction requires the body to make compensatory changes to maintain adequate cardiac output. The failure of the heart to pump effectively results in venous congestion, which produces many of the symptoms of CHF.

Conjugate eye movement The two eyes move in a parallel fashion and the eyes move with respect to each other.

Consensus Being in agreement.

Contact-free sleep tracking device A sleep tracking option a patient does not need to wear while sleeping. A recording device that is positioned near the user and that uses accelerometers to sense and record movements.

Continuous positive airway pressure (CPAP) CPAP is a therapeutic treatment for sleep apnea that maintains the airway using continuous air pressure.

Continuous quality assurance A management process that encourages all health care workers to continuously ask questions on how to improve health care. It is a philosophy within an organization used to reduce waste, increase efficiency, and increase employee and client satisfaction.

Corrected age GA + CA —Corrected age "corrects" for prematurity; it is calculated by adding the gestational age and the CA or by subtracting the number of weeks of prematurity from the CA.

Cortisol A hormone released by the cortex of the adrenal gland when an individual experiences stress.

Covered entity A covered entity is defined in the HIPAA rules as (1) health plans, (2) health care clearinghouses, and (3) health care providers who electronically transmit any health information. Covered entities can be institutions, organizations, or persons.

CPAP circuit The machine, air hose, and patient interface that delivers continuous air pressure during inspiration and exhalation to keep the upper airway open.

Craniofacial structure The structure of the cranium and face.

Crescendo–decrescendo breathing An abnormal pattern of breathing where a progressive increase in breathing rate is followed by a decreased breathing rate and ultimately in an apnea. The apnea leads to an increased carbon dioxide (CO_2) level that causes excessive compensatory hyperventilation, creating a spindle-like pattern in the depth of breathing.

Cryptogenic A condition distinguished by an unknown cause.

Cystic fibrosis A multisystem genetic disorder that primarily affects Caucasian infants, children, and young adults characterized by abnormal transport of sodium and chloride across the epithelium in all exocrine tissues, leading to an increase in sweat sodium and chloride concentration.

Data Information that is collected, measured, analyzed, and reported and then examined and used for decision-making.

Data review The analysis of available information, often used to assess and improve outcomes.

Dead space Compartments within the respiratory system that are not actively involved in gas exchange.

Delayed sleep phase disorder Referred to as "night owls," individuals go to bed later and awaken later than what is considered normal.

Dementia with Lewy bodies The second most common cause of degenerative dementia, representing approximately 15% to 20% of cases. The onset of symptoms typically begins between 50 and 80 years of age. The pathologic feature in brain tissue is Lewy bodies, which are inclusions seen within neurons. The clinical features of dementia with Lewy bodies include dementia, psychosis, and mild extrapyramidal symptoms such as spasticity.

Dental device A method of treating snoring and mild to moderate obstructive sleep apnea. Also referred to as an oral appliance.

Depression A mental illness that can affect all aspects of an individual's life and may cause an inability to concentrate, insomnia, loss of appetite, feelings of extreme sadness, guilt, helplessness and hopelessness, and thoughts of death.

Desensitization A process used to decrease an overwhelming fear of artificial circumstances such as claustrophobia caused by PAP by repeated and controlled exposure to the feared situation or object.

Diabetes mellitus A chronic condition associated with abnormally high levels of sugar (glucose) in the blood that results from defects in the body's ability to produce and/or use insulin.

Diagnostic-related groupings (DRG) A patient classification system adopted on the basis of diagnosis within distinct groupings.

Diaphragm The primary respiratory muscle: a dome-shaped sheet of skeletal muscle that segregates the thoracic cavity from the abdominal cavity. During contraction, the dome is pulled down toward the stomach increasing thoracic volume. It is innervated by the phrenic nerve.

Diastole The time when the heart is in a state of relaxation.

Digital Signals or data expressed as a series of the digits 0 and 1, typically represented by the values of a physical quantity such as voltage.

Discharge planning Part of an overall care plan and approach to continuity of care between the hospital and the community. Includes assessment, planning, coordination, and evaluation to ensure patients are receiving the best care and services as they recuperate, reducing hospital length of stay and unplanned readmissions.

Discomfort State of physical unease that makes one feel physically or mentally uncomfortable.

Diurnal Relating to or occurring in a 24-hour period; daily.

Dominant posterior rhythm An EEG pattern, slower than the alpha rhythm in adults, that changes as the child develops from a 3.5- to 4.5-Hz rhythmic activity at 3 to 4 months post-term, to a 5- to 6-Hz activity by 6 months of age. Analogous to alpha activity in older children and adults.

Durable medical equipment (DME) Equipment that benefits or supports a patient in need because of a specific medical condition or illness.

Dyskinesias Equipment that benefits or supports a patient in need because of a specific medical condition or illness.

Dysrhythmias Conditions where the heart rhythm is irregular either too fast (tachycardia) or too slow (bradycardia). Also referred to as arrhythmia and irregular heart rate.

Effusions The escape of fluid from the blood vessels or lymphatics into the tissues or a cavity.

Elastic recoil A force that opposes stretch. Elastic recoil is due to the stretched muscles used to increase thoracic cavity size during an inspiration, as well as some muscles that are incidentally stretched, and the contribution from the stretched lungs.

Electroencephalogram (EEG) A recording of the electrical activity of the brain measured by the application of surface electrodes to determine sleep stages and wakefulness.

Electromyogram (EMG) A recording of the electrical activity of the muscles measured by the application of surface electrodes to monitor specific muscle groups during sleep.

Electronic health record (EHR) A longitudinal electronic record of patient health information generated by one or more encounters in any care delivery setting.

Electrooculogram (EOG) A recording of the electrical activity of the eyes measured by the application of surface electrodes to the outer canthi of the eyes to monitor various eye movements related to wakefulness and sleep stages.

Endocardium The innermost layer of the heart that extends outward to include the valves of the heart; a sheet of endothelium resting on a thin layer of connective tissue.

Endocrine disorders Disorders that involve the overproduction or underproduction of hormone substances from an endocrine gland.

End-tidal CO_2 A CO_2 measurement from a side-stream nasal cannula or a direct measurement of exhaled CO_2 from a tracheostomy or an endotracheal tube. End-tidal CO_2 measurements are subject to breath-to-breath fluctuations and may be affected by varying respiratory patterns such as tachypnea, sighs, or mouth breathing.

Entrain To modify the phase or period of an intrinsic circadian rhythm, or biologic clock, in order to align with external environmental cues, such as light.

Entrainment process A process for resetting the circadian rhythm.

Enuresis Recurrent, involuntary bedwetting occurring during sleep in a child older than 5 years.

Epicardium The outer layer of the heart that contains an outer fibrous connective tissue and an inner serous pericardium that functions as a protective layer.

Epiglottis A flap made of elastic cartilage covered with a mucous membrane attached at the entrance of the larynx. It closes during swallowing to prevent liquids or food from entering the windpipe and lungs and remains open during breathing to allow air into the larynx.

Epileptic seizure A clinical event associated with a transient, hypersynchronous neuronal discharge representing a potential underlying brain pathology.

Epileptiform discharges A pattern on the EEG associated with an increased risk of seizures.

Episodic nocturnal wandering Episodes of wandering with a 1- to 3-minute duration consisting of stereotyped paroxysmal ambulation, accompanied by screaming and bizarre, dystonic movements.

Epworth Sleepiness Scale (ESS) A self-administered questionnaire used to assess a patient's own perception of their sleepiness, which assists sleep professionals to recognize and measure excessive daytime sleepiness (EDS).

Equipment Devices used in the diagnosis or treatment of a patient.

Equipment grounding Refers to a connecting circuit from the equipment to the earth, a low-resistance path to the earth ground intentionally created.

Escape beat A delayed heartbeat originating from an ectopic focus somewhere in the AV junction instead of the atrium.

Ethics A system of moral principles or values. The rules of conduct recognized in respect to an individual's actions or behavior in a group or organization.

Exacerbation An increase in severity of a disease or any of its symptoms.

Excessive daytime sleepiness The experience of persistent sleepiness that is not resolved with adequate sleep. EDS is the often presenting complaint in the sleep clinic.

Excessive fragmentary myoclonus Characterized by small movements of the fingers, toes, or corners of the mouth, or small muscle twitches resembling fasciculations that do not cause gross movement.

Expiration The act of expelling air from the lungs. The portion of the total breathing cycle not devoted to inspiration.

Expiratory positive airway pressure PAP that is applied during the exhalation phase of respiration to prevent the collapse of a patient's airway during sleep.

Expiratory pressure relief (EPR) A patient comfort feature used on Res Med airflow generators to detect the beginning of exhalation and reduce motor speed to decrease exhalation pressure, making PAP therapy more comfortable.

Expiratory reserve volume (ERV) The maximum amount of gas that can be exhaled from the resting end-expiratory level.

External respiration The exchange of gas in the lungs.

Extrinsic sleep disorder Disorders that either originate or develop from causes outside the body.

False Claims Act The federal False Claims Act makes it illegal to knowingly submit or present a false, fictitious, or fraudulent claim to the federal government.

Fasciculation "Muscle twitch"; a small, local, involuntary muscle contraction and relaxation visible under the skin arising from the spontaneous discharge of a bundle of skeletal muscle fibers (muscle fascicles).

Fibromyalgia A common syndrome in which an individual has long-term, body-wide pain and tenderness in the joints, muscles, tendons, and other soft tissues at 11 or more of 18 specific tender point sites. Linked to fatigue, sleep problems, headaches, depression, and anxiety.

Financial responsibility The unpaid balance after insurance payments following a health care encounter that is the patient's responsibility.

Flex-PAP A PAP comfort feature providing a brief decrease in pressure when expiration is detected.

Frequency The period or width of the wave expressed as cycles per second (CPS).

Fugue A pathologic amnesiac condition during which one is apparently conscious of one's actions but has no recollection of them after returning to a normal state. This condition, usually resulting from severe mental stress, may persist for as long as several months.

Functional outcomes of sleep questionnaire A self-reported measurement designed to assess improvement of excessive sleepiness, based on multiple activities of daily living.

Functional residual capacity (FRC) The volume of air left in the lungs at the end of normal expiration.

Galanin An inhibitory neurotransmitter believed to promote non-REM sleep, in particular slow-wave sleep.

Gamma aminobutyric acid (GABA) A major inhibitory brain chemical that blocks the transmission of a signal from one brain cell to another.

Gas exchange The process of carbon dioxide (CO_2) removal and replenishment of oxygen (O_2) in the body. Occurs by diffusion down concentration gradients from tissue to blood, then blood to the alveolar gas in the lungs, which are ventilated with atmospheric air.

Gastroesophageal reflux A backflow of gastric acid and other gastric contents into the esophagus due to incompetent barriers at the gastroesophageal junction.

Gestational age Calculated as age since the end of the last menstrual cycle; the length of time that a fetus grows inside the mother's uterus. Gestational age is related to the fetus's stage of growth as well as its cognitive and physical development.

Hard palate A thin bony plate of skull spanning the arch formed by the upper teeth that is positioned anteriorly. It is immobile and divides the nasal and oral cavities forming the roof of the mouth and floor of the nasal cavity.

Head banging A childhood parasomnia that is classified as a rhythmic movement disorder. Children may bang their head into a pillow, mattress, side of a crib, or even the floor, as they fall asleep or when they wake up in the middle of the night. This is considered to be a self-soothing habit; movements may persist into NREM sleep and may also occur following arousals or during waking from sleep.

Headgear A system of straps, usually material, that keeps the mask interface in place while a patient sleeps.

Health literacy The degree to which individuals have the capacity to obtain, process, and understand basic health information and services needed to make appropriate health decisions.

Healthcare common procedure coding system (HCPCS) Codes used and maintained by the Centers for Medicare & Medicaid Services to bill Medicare, Medicaid, and many other third-party payers.

Hemoglobin (Hb) A complex molecule within red blood cells that binds with four oxygen molecules. Hemoglobin is the oxygen transport facility of the circulatory system.

High frequency filter A filter used to attenuate signals above the cutoff frequency. Usually described in Hz or CPS. At a particular setting, frequencies at or above the cutoff frequency will be attenuated with increasing degree dependent on the frequency response curve.

High-voltage slow activity A moderately rhythmic pattern consisting of medium to high amplitude (50 to 150 μV) activity in the range of 0.5 to 4 Hz.

HIPAA The Health Insurance Portability and Accountability Act of 1996 (HIPAA) is U.S. legislation that provides data privacy and security provisions for safeguarding medical information.

HIPAA Omnibus Rule A composite of four closely connected final rules related to the implementation of the Health Information Technology for Economic and Clinical Health Act mandates for the adoption of the electronic health records (EHR) and meaningful use incentives.

Histamine The chemical (neurotransmitter) that the body produces in response to an allergen.

Histotoxic hypoxia Inability of cells to use oxygen normally when oxygen delivery is normal, usually as a result of a toxic agent.

HITECH Act The Health Information Technology for Economic and Clinical Health Act (HITECH Act) is part of the American Recovery and Reinvestment Act of 2009. The HITECH Act was created to motivate the implementation of EHR and supporting technology in the United States.

Home cardiorespiratory monitor Also known as an apnea monitor; a machine used to monitor breathing and heart rate to detect and inform caregivers of potential life-threatening events.

Home sleep apnea test (HSAT) A sleep study used to aid in the diagnosis of obstructive sleep apnea. HSAT often employs small, portable, unattended equipment for use in the home.

Homeostasis The maintenance of a stable physiologic state through different conditions, for example, mild exercise versus rest, temperature, blood flow, and oxygenation.

Homeostatic drive The sleep drive that balances sleep and wakefulness.

HPA axis The hypothalamic-pituitary-adrenal axis regulates things such as body temperature, digestion, immune system, mood, sexuality, and energy usage. It is also a major part of the system that controls reactions to stress, trauma, and injury.

HTML Hyper Text Markup Language is the standard markup language for creating Web pages. HTML defines the structure and layout of a Web document by using a variety of tags and attributes.

Human immunodeficiency virus (HIV) The virus that causes AIDS. This virus is passed from one person to another through blood-to-blood and sexual contact. Sleep disturbances include complaints of insomnia, recurrent nighttime arousals, and EDS.

Hyperarousal A state of increased psychological and physiologic tension manifested by such things as reduced pain tolerance, anxiety, exaggeration of startle responses, insomnia, fatigue, and accentuation of personality traits. Often referred to as the "fight or flight" response designed to protect us from danger.

Hypercapnia CO_2 level above the normal range.

Hypersomnia Excessive sleepiness; increased tendency or need to fall asleep.

Hypertension High blood pressure.

Hyperthyroidism Results from an overactive thyroid that results in excessive thyroid hormone production. Symptoms include fatigue but difficulty sleeping, mood impairment, difficulty concentrating, muscle weakness, tachycardia, and heat intolerance.

Hyperventilation Ventilation that is in excess of metabolic needs, resulting in decreased CO_2 levels. Breathing is either too fast or too deep, or both, relative to CO_2 production.

Hypnagogic foot tremor (HFT) A rhythmic movement of the feet and toes that occurs at the transition of wake and sleep or during light sleep. The clinical impact is unknown because most patients are unaware of the movements and no treatment has been found to be effective.

Hypnagogic hallucinations Vivid dreamlike images or sounds that occur at sleep onset during the progression from wakefulness to sleep

Hypnopompic hallucinations Vivid dreamlike images or sounds that occur at awakening during the progression from sleep to wakefulness.

Hypnotic A sleep-inducing agent.

Hypocapnia CO_2 level below the normal range.

Hypocretin A hypothalamic neurotransmitter found in the cerebrospinal fluid that is responsible for producing and sustaining wakefulness. Regulates wakefulness and REM sleep as well as appetite and energy expenditure. A lack of hypocretin can account for the EDS and cataplectic attacks seen with narcolepsy; also referred to as orexin.

Hypoglossal stimulation Used in treating obstructive sleep apnea to open the airway; an implantable device that produces an electrical stimulation to the hypoglossal nerve in the tongue.

Hypopnea A specified reduction in airflow lasting at least 10 seconds in adults or the equivalent of two breaths in children with associated O_2 desaturation or arousal.

Hypopnea index The number of hypopneas per hour of sleep.

Hypothalamus Located in the forebrain below the thalamus; controls sleep cycles, body temperature, and growth.

Hypothyroidism Results from an underactive thyroid, which produces insufficient levels of thyroid hormone. The effect is metabolic slowing, which leads to symptoms of weight gain and fatigue.

Hypoventilation Ventilation that does not meet metabolic needs, resulting in increased CO_2 levels. Breathing is either too shallow or too slow, or both, relative to CO_2 production.

Hypoxemia An abnormally low amount of oxygen in the blood; usually refers to arterial blood.

Hypoxia A deficiency of oxygen reaching the tissues of the body.

Hypoxic drive A form of respiratory drive, which regulates the respiratory cycle.

Iatrogenic nasal resistance Nasal resistance induced inadvertently by a treatment or diagnostic procedure.

ICE Institute for Credentialing Excellence; formerly the National Organization for Competency Assurance (NOCA) the membership association for credentialing bodies.

Idiopathic hypersomnia A dyssomnia of unknown cause characterized by constant and severe excessive sleepiness.

Impedance In an electrical circuit opposition to the flow of alternating current by the combination of resistance and capacitance.

Impede To obstruct the progress of.

Implant To insert or embed an object into a person's body, or the object that is inserted or embedded. A medical device surgically embedded in the body.

Indeterminate sleep A transitional sleep state seen in infants at sleep onset, during arousals, or when the infant is transitioning between active and quiet sleep.

Infectious diseases Any disease caused by a pathogen, which causes the development of an infection. These diseases are considered contagious or communicable from person to person.

Information technology (IT) infrastructure Consists of the hardware, software, networks, data centers, facilities, and related equipment used to manage and operate IT services.

Informed consent A process in which the patient authorizes medical treatment that includes the plan of care after a discussion with a physician or a licensed clinical provider.

Infradian Cycles that occur at recurrent intervals of longer than 24 hours.

Insomnia An individual's report of sleeping difficulties. There are three main subtypes of insomnia: difficulty initiating sleep (sleep onset insomnia), awakening frequently during the night (sleep maintenance insomnia), and awakening long before the desired time to get up (early morning awakening or terminal insomnia).

Inspiration The movement of atmospheric air into the airways and lungs. Inspiration is usually due to a more negative intrapleural pressure created by the activation of the diaphragm and external intercostals.

Inspiratory positive airway pressure PAP that is applied during the inspiration phase of respiration to prevent the collapse of a patient's airway during sleep.

Inspiratory reserve volume The maximum amount of gas that can be inhaled from the end-inspiratory position.

Inspire medical upper airway stimulation therapy An implantable device to treat selective PAP-intolerant moderate-to-severe obstructive sleep apnea patients. The device monitors inspiratory effort and provides electrical stimulation to a branch of the hypoglossal nerve, providing coordinated tongue protrusion.

Insufflation Performed using a thin nasopharyngeal tube to administer warm humidified air at 2 to 10 L per minute to treat upper airway obstruction in children.

Interface A group of masks or other nasal or oronasal sealed connections used for the administration of PAP therapy. The type of interface has a significant impact on the acceptance and compliance with PAP. Most patients prefer nasal or pillow mask interfaces for their fit and comfort.

Interictal The period between seizure and convulsion in epilepsy. For most people with epilepsy, it corresponds to more than 99% of their life.

Internal respiration The exchange of gas in the tissues inside the body.

International Classification of Diseases 10th Revision Clinical Modifications (ICD10 CM) A medical classification system used for procedural coding.

International Classification of Sleep Disorders, 3rd Edition (ICSD-3) A medical classification system provided by the AASM used for procedural coding and a reference for sleep clinicians.

Intervene To come, appear, or lie between two things.

Intraoperative The period describing the duration of a patient's surgical procedure.

Intrinsic sleep disorder Disorders that either originate or develop from causes inside the body.

Irregular sleep–wake rhythm A rare disorder in which total sleep time within each 24-hour day remains roughly equal to the amount that would be obtained if sleep was obtained in a single sleep period, but the sleep is distributed throughout the day and night in multiple short episodes.

Isolated sleep paralysis Characterized by a period of inability to voluntarily move skeletal muscles at the beginning of a sleep period (hypnagogic) or immediately after awakening (hypnopompic). Consciousness is maintained but the individual feels paralyzed, and is unable to open the eyes or speak, typically due to persistent active inhibition of alpha motor neurons that persists after cortical waking.

Jet lag disorder Desynchronization and its clinical effect after rapidly crossing several time zones.

The Joint Commission Accredits and certifies healthcare organizations and programs in the United States.

Junctional arrhythmias Junctional arrhythmias can occur if the AV nodal tissue fires prematurely or if the atrial mechanism for initiating the cardiac cycle fails. Junctional arrhythmias feature normal-appearing QRS complexes. When P waves are seen, they will be inverted and can occur before or after the QRS complex. This category of arrhythmias includes premature junctional contraction, junctional and accelerated junctional rhythm, and junctional tachycardia.

Larynx The area of the upper airway between the trachea and the pharynx. It plays a large role in obstructive sleep apnea, especially during sleep.

Latency to persistent sleep Time from "lights out" to the first epoch of continuous sleep.

Licensure Granting a license to practice a profession at the state level.

Light therapy A treatment for circadian rhythm sleep disorders that consists of controlling exposure to either artificial or natural light.

Limit setting This childhood disorder is characterized by difficulty initiating sleep. The child stalls or refuses to go to sleep at the set bedtime.

Locus ceruleus Located in the brainstem; inhibits the ventrolateral preoptic nucleus, leading to wakefulness.

Low-frequency filter A filter used to attenuate signals below the cutoff frequency. Usually described in Hz or CPS. At a particular setting, frequencies at or below the cutoff frequency will be attenuated with increasing degree dependent on the frequency response curve.

Low-voltage irregular activity A pattern of 14 to 35 μV amplitude activity that is characterized by predominantly theta activity in the 5 to 8 Hz range with intermixed 1 to 5 Hz slow activity.

Lyme disease A tick-borne spirochetal illness with clinical symptoms of fatigue, headache, chills, torticollis, nausea, and vomiting. Sleep-related complaints include sleep-onset insomnia, frequent awakenings, EDS, and restless legs/nocturnal leg jerking.

Malingering The intentional creation of false or exaggerated physical or psychological symptoms, motivated by external reasons such as to avoid work.

Mallampati airway classification A rough estimate of tongue size relative to the oral cavity used to assess the risk of upper airway obstruction.

MAO inhibitors A class of drugs effective in treating atypical depression and Parkinson disease. Because of potentially lethal dietary and drug interaction, these drugs are usually used as a last line of treatment, only when other classes of antidepressant drugs have failed.

Mask Any of the several types of noninvasive PAP interfaces, such as nasal pillows, nasal masks, and full-face masks.

Mask fitting A critical process that requires time, patience, and skill to select an interface that will best fit an individual's facial features, needs, and preferences.

Material safety data sheet (MSDS) A summary of the health hazards and associated recommended safe work practices for the use of chemicals in the workplace. OSHA requires that chemical manufacturers provide an MSDS sheet to the purchasers of their chemicals.

Maxillomandibular advancement A surgical procedure that moves the upper and lower jaws forward and enlarges the airway so that soft tissues in the soft palate and tongue are pulled forward.

Medulla a.k.a. medulla oblongata. The lower most anatomical region of the brain, just anterior to the spinal cord. It is the location of the main respiratory and cardiovascular control systems.

Melatonin A secretory product of the pineal gland used to maintain the circadian rhythm and to regulate other hormones.

Metabolic syndrome A constellation of metabolic abnormalities associated with an increased risk of vascular diseases. Symptoms include central obesity with fat deposits centered around the abdomen, glucose intolerance/insulin resistance, hypertension, hypercholesterolemia, and blood-clotting abnormalities.

Minute ventilation (MV) The amount of air a person breathes in 1 minute. Determined by measuring the amount of air either inhaled or exhaled for a full minute. Can also be estimated by multiplying the RR by the patient's average tidal volume .

Mission statement The essence of an organization's vision, values, and strategic goals; serves as a reference in determining the core processes for which policy is written.

Mixed sleep apnea An apnea that is associated with absent inspiratory effort in the initial portion of the event, followed by resumption of inspiratory effort in the second portion of the event.

mm Hg Millimeters of mercury.

Modafinil A wake-promoting agent that improves physiologic sleepiness and neurobehavioral deficits related to sleep disorders such as obstructive sleep apnea, shift work, narcolepsy. Has a half-life of 9 to 14 hours.

Mode Refers to the setting type of the respiratory ventilation system used for the treatment of sleep apnea. Basic PAP machines deliver a continuous air pressure to maintain airway patency. Advanced machines can also deliver pressure support to maintain a consistent tidal volume.

Modifiers A process to expand CPT codes to further describe a service or procedure using 2-digit modifiers.

Motivation Providing reason or incentive for a patient to commit to using PAP on a nightly basis with a positive outlook.

Motivational enhancement (ME) A client-centered, directive method for enhancing intrinsic motivation to change by exploring and resolving ambivalence.

Multimodal analgesia The use of different classes of analgesics and different sites of analgesic administration to provide superior dynamic pain relief with reduced analgesic-related side effects.

Muscular dystrophy (MD) A group of genetically inherited muscle diseases characterized by a loss of muscle protein, causing progressive muscular weakness.

Myocardial infarction Commonly known as a heart attack.

Myoclonus Involuntary twitching of a muscle or a group of muscles.

Narcolepsy A chronic neurologic disorder characterized by EDS and sudden and uncontrollable attacks of sleep that are sometimes accompanied by hallucinations and paralysis (atonia).

Nares The exterior portion of the nose that contains branched bones or cartilages called "turbinates" that open the nasal cavity to allow the inhalation and exhalation of air. Their main function is to warm air on inhalation and remove moisture on exhalation.

Narrow complex tachycardia A rhythm lasting for greater than three consecutive beats at a rate greater than 100 per minute with a QRS duration of ≥120 ms.

Nasal cavity The interior, large air-filled space of the nose lined with a mucous membrane and divided by a vertical fin known as the "nasal septum." It warms, moisturizes, and filters air before it enters the larynx and lungs. There are also little hairs within the nasal cavity that prevent dirt and dust from entering the lungs.

Nasal expiratory positive airway pressure (nEPAP) Expiratory PAP delivered by the patient's own breathing via a valve inserted into each nostril.

NCCA National Commission for Certifying Agencies; the accrediting body for the Institute for Credentialing Excellence.

Neuroimaging The use of X-ray studies and MRI to detect abnormalities or trace pathways of nerve activity in the CNS.

Neuromuscular disease Encompasses many diseases that impair muscle function, either directly, involving pathologies of the voluntary muscle, or indirectly, from pathologies of nerves or neuromuscular junctions.

Neuromuscular disorder A disorder that affects the peripheral nervous system, which includes muscles, the nerve-muscle (neuromuscular) junction, peripheral nerves in the limbs, and the motor-nerve cells in the spinal cord. The disorders most commonly associated with SDB are muscular dystrophy, myotonic dystrophy, ALS, poliomyelitis, and myasthenia gravis.

Neuron Nerve cell that transmits information throughout the body.

Neurotransmitters Chemicals that transmit signals from one neuron to the next across synapses.

Nightmares Nightmares are characterized by a sudden arousal from REM sleep to a fully awake state following a frightening dream. Considered "anxiety dreams" they are clinically quite different from sleep terrors in etiology and presentation. There is generally clear recall of the dream, which may be accompanied by anxiety.

Nocturnal frontal lobe epilepsy Epileptic foci located in the frontal lobe (in particular in the mesial and orbital cortex) that results in seizures emerging almost exclusively from sleep.

Nocturnal paroxysmal dystonia Episodes of intermediate duration (20 seconds–2 minutes) beginning as a paroxysmal arousal but subsequently associated with complex movements including rhythmic movements of the trunk and pelvis, dystonic posturing and vocalization.

Nocturnal stridor A high-pitched inspiratory sound that is frequently unrecognized by the patient but commonly reported by the patient's bed partner.

Noninvasive ventilation (NIV) The administration of ventilatory support in the absence of an artificial airway.

Normal sinus rhythm The characteristic rhythm of the healthy human heart. The heart rate is in the normal range, the P waves are normal on the ECG, and the rate does not vary significantly.

Nosology A classification of diseases.

Notch filter A specialized cutoff filter that attenuates or eliminates a designated frequency. Usually 50 or 60 Hz.

Notice of privacy practices (NPP) The HIPAA Privacy Rule requires health plans and covered health care providers to develop and distribute a notice that provides a clear, user-friendly explanation of individuals' rights with respect to their personal health information and the privacy practices of health plans and health care providers.

Nyquist sampling theory Theory that states that the minimum sampling rate must be twice the rate of the highest frequency sampled in order to adequately resolve the signal and prevent aliasing.

Obesity hypoventilation syndrome (OHS) A disorder including the conditions of obesity, sleep-disordered breathing, and chronic hypoventilation while awake not caused by chronic obstructive lung disease. Decreased chest wall compliance, impaired respiratory drive, and severe obstructive sleep apnea (OSA) are mechanisms that contribute to hypoventilation.

Obsessive-compulsive disorder An anxiety disorder characterized by persistent, upsetting, and unwanted thoughts (obsessions) and repetitive behaviors (compulsions) that the person believes will prevent the events associated with the obsession.

Obstructive sleep apnea Absence of airflow lasting at least 10 seconds in adults or the equivalent of two breaths in children that is associated with continued or increased inspiratory effort throughout the entire period.

Office for Civil Rights (OCR) The OCR is the administrative office that is tasked with enforcing HIPAA.

Office of the Inspector General (OIG) An office under the U.S. Department of Health and Human Services that oversees federal regulations. The OIG is responsible for (1) conducting audits and investigations; (2) reviewing legislation; (3) recommending policies to promote efficiency and effectiveness; and (4) preventing and detecting fraud, waste, and abuse in the operations of the agency.

Ohm A measure of the resistance to the flow of electricity.

Ohm's law A law of electricity, which states that the strength or intensity of an unvarying electric current is directly proportional to the electromotive force and inversely proportional to the resistance of the circuit.

Oneiric Of or relating to dreams.

Opioids Also known as narcotics; they are any synthetic narcotic that has opiate-like activities but is not derived from opium. Opioids are a class of drugs used for pain management. Opioids have a very strong analgesic effect.

Oral appliance A method of treating snoring and mild to moderate obstructive sleep apnea. Also referred to as a dental device.

Orexin A hypothalamic neurotransmitter found in the cerebrospinal fluid that is responsible for producing and sustaining wakefulness. Regulates wakefulness and REM sleep as well as appetite and energy expenditure. A lack of orexin can account for the EDS and cataplectic attacks seen with narcolepsy. Also referred to as hypocretin.

Orofacial Relating to the mouth and face.

Outcomes measures Measurable changes in health as a result of medical intervention.

Overlap syndrome (COPD and OSA) Coexisting obstructive sleep-disordered breathing and obstructive airways disease.

Oxygen conserving device An oxygen delivery device that extends the use time from a supply of oxygen by releasing the prescribed liter flow of oxygen only when the patient inhales. It automatically turns the oxygen supply on/off with every breath.

Oxygen extraction The difference between arterial and venous concentrations of oxygen.

P wave The ECG waveform that represents depolarization.

PaCO$_2$ The partial pressure of CO$_2$ in arterial blood obtained by ABG analysis.

Panic disorder A disorder that consists of recurrent extremely intense terrifying panic attacks that may come without warning or without an obvious cause. Symptoms may include heart palpitations, pressure in the chest, dizziness, nausea, sweating, and faintness.

PAP Above atmospheric pressure administered to the airway, as treatment for sleep apnea.

PAP titration The process of determining therapeutic level(s) of PAP in carefully measured increments of cm H$_2$O until SDB is alleviated.

Paradoxical intention therapy A medical therapy used for such diagnoses as obsessive compulsive disorder, psychophysiologic insomnia, and psychosis.

Parasomnia An undesirable physical phenomena that occurs predominantly or exclusively during the sleep period. Parasomnias have been classified into three groups by the *International Classification of Sleep Disorders (ICSD), 2nd edition*: Arousal disorders, parasomnias associated with REM sleep, and other parasomnias.

Paresthesia Any subjective sensation experienced as numbness, tingling, or a "pins and needles" feeling.

Parkinson disease A progressive degenerative movement disorder with features that include resting tremor, bradykinesia (slowness of movement), rigidity, and gait disturbance.

Paroxysmal arousal A brief (<20 seconds) abrupt arousal from sleep with vocalization and motor activity consisting of head movements, sudden eye opening, head raising or sitting up in bed, often with a frightened expression.

Partial pressure The proportion of a specific gas in a mixture of gases. Usually in mm Hg.

Patient engagement Actions that individuals must take to obtain the greatest benefit from the health care services available.

Patient grounding Prevents line-frequency interference (50 or 60 Hz) by providing a conductive pathway from the patient to ground via the recording system.

PCO$_2$ The partial pressure of carbon dioxide (in blood plasma). The main controlled variable (along with pH) of the respiratory control system. Normal values for arterial blood are near 41 mm Hg; venous blood is approximately 46 mm Hg.

Periodic leg movements in sleep Rhythmic movements of the lower extremities that are measured during sleep that may or may not have clinical relevance.

Perioperative The period extending from when the patient goes into the hospital for surgery until the time the patient is discharged home.

Peripheral chemoreceptors A group of specialized sensory cells residing in the carotid bodies and aortic bodies that respond to decreased oxygenation, increased PCO$_2$ or plasma acidity. These are the primary O$_2$ sensors for the respiratory and cardiovascular systems.

Personal protective equipment Safety equipment employees use to protect themselves from the hazards of their work environment, includes gloves, goggles, masks.

pH A measure of acidity (H$^+$: hydrogen ion concentration) where 7 is neutral and low values [7–0] are most acidic. A critical component of respiratory control and homeostasis. Normal values are near 7.4.

Pharmacology The branch of medicine and biology concerned with the study of drug action.

Pharynx A section of the upper airway behind the nasal turbinates and the tongue. It is a common site of airway collapse, especially in sleep.

Phase response curve (PRC) The magnitude and direction of a phase shift caused by a zeitgeber; expressed in a PRC.

Phase shift The change in circadian timing brought about by a zeitgeber.

Phobia An intense, irrational fear of an object or situation that is not likely to be dangerous.

Phrenic nerve The bilateral motor nerves driving the diaphragm. The phrenic nerve emanates from the phrenic nucleus in the cervical spinal cord.

Phrenic nerve stimulation An implantable device that produces rhythmic stimulation of the diaphragm with electrical impulses to stimulate breathing.

Physiologic Normal healthful functioning, not due to anything pathologic nor significant in terms of causing illness.

Physiologic dead space The total dead space in the entire respiratory system including the alveoli; the sum of anatomical and alveolar dead space.

Pick disease Dementia that is associated with loss of neurons in the frontotemporal region of the brain, occurring most frequently in women around age 60.

Pineal gland Produces melatonin from the amino acid tryptophan.

Pittsburgh Sleep Quality Index A brief clinically useful self-report inventory that evaluates subjective sleep quality and disturbance over the previous month.

Plethysmograph A device for measuring lung volumes and capacities more precisely than conventional spirometry. The patient is recorded while in a sealed box but breathing atmospheric air through a tube to the outside of the box.

Plethysmography The process of measuring the various lung volumes and capacities. The patient sits in an airtight enclosure and breathes through a tube extending out of the box. Plethysmography is more accurate than conventional spirometry.

Pneumothorax An opening between the intrapleural space and either the atmosphere or the lungs.

PO$_2$ The partial pressure of oxygen (in blood plasma). Normal values are 95 to 100 mm Hg in arterial blood and 40 mm Hg in venous blood. Tissue levels can be very low (<5 mm Hg).

Polypharmacy The use of multiple medications by a patient, especially when too many forms of a medication are used by a patient; when more drugs are prescribed than is clinically warranted; or even when all prescribed medications are clinically indicated but there are too many pills to take (pill burden).

Polysomnograph A multiple channel recording instrument comprised of a hardware device (often called an amplifier) that interfaces with software to produce a digital record of biophysical changes to identify sleep stages and related events.

Pons Located in the brainstem, it links the medulla oblongata and the thalamus.

Portable monitoring Nonfacility-based sleep study monitoring of limited channels of data.

Positional sleep apnea Sleep apnea where the patient has an apnea–hypopnea index at least twice as high supine versus a nonsupine position.

Positional therapy Implementation of a strategy to keep the patient in a nonsupine position while sleeping.

Posttraumatic stress disorder A stress reaction to a severe trauma; characterized by anxiety, irritability, inability to concentrate, jumpiness, intense startle reactions, and hypervigilance.

P–R interval The time from the onset of the P wave to the beginning of the QRS complex; the duration is usually 120 to 200 ms.

Precipitating Cause an event or occurrence.

Preclinical Of or relating to the period of a disease before the appearance of symptoms.

Premature atrial contraction A common arrhythmia that produces premature P waves, with normal QRS morphology and normal T waves.

Premature ventricular contraction A common arrhythmia that is produced when a contraction signal originates in the ventricle of the heart. This arrhythmia has an absent P wave and an early and wide and/or aberrant QRS with a compensatory pause.

Professional organization or association A group created by and for people with a common interest and a common goal. A professional organization provides the foundation from which the profession evolves and develops.

Progressive supranuclear palsy A Parkinsonian syndrome with typically less tremor and poor response to Parkinson's medication. It is commonly misdiagnosed as Parkinson's disease.

Propriospinal Distinctively or exclusively spinal.

Propriospinal myoclonus Consists of sudden muscular jerks occurring at sleep onset; mainly involving the abdomen, neck, and trunk.

Protected health information (PHI) Protected information refers to health data created, received, stored, or transmitted by HIPAA-covered entities and their business associates in relation to the provision of health care, health care operations, and payment for health care services.

Psi(g) Pounds per square inch (to the gauge).

Psychogenic Originating in the mind or in mental or emotional processes; having a psychological rather than a physiologic origin.

Psychosocial The relationship between individual thoughts, emotions, behaviors, and social factors.

Pulmonary function test (PFT) A test that measures how well the lungs are expanding and contracting during breathing. It reflects the efficiency of gas exchange between the blood and the air within the lungs.

Pulmonary hypertension A disease defined as a higher-than-normal blood pressure in the arteries of the lungs, primarily affecting the right side of the heart.

Pyrexia Abnormal elevation of body temperature.

QRS The ECG waveform that represents ventricular depolarization.

Quality assurance An implemented plan and systematic activities used to demonstrate services and solutions delivered to meet quality standards.

Quiet sleep A sleep state in infants that is distinguished by slower, more rhythmic breathing, little body movement, and no eye movements. During quiet sleep, infants are usually not as easily aroused or awakened by noise and other disturbances—including a sudden reduction in the oxygen supply. Analogous to slow-wave sleep in older children and adults.

Ramp feature A PAP feature that allows the PAP pressure to be lowered and gradually increased to the set pressure so the patient can fall asleep and/or return to sleep after awakening during the night.

Raphe nuclei Located in the reticular formation of the brainstem. Cells are most active and variable during waking. The serotonin-containing neurons of the raphe nuclei promote the emergence of slow-wave cortical activity.

Regional perfusion A measurement of oxygen levels at the site of transcutaneous O_2 sensors on the skin used to eliminate cardiorespiratory influence; can be used to quantify tissue perfusion in patients with peripheral vascular disease.

Registered Polysomnographic Technologist (RPSGT) An internationally recognized credential offered by the BRPT that represents certification in the sleep technology field for the healthcare professionals who clinically assess patients with sleep disorders.

Registered Sleep Technologist (RST) The ABSM credential for sleep technologists that represents certification in the sleep technology field for the healthcare professionals who clinically assess patients with sleep disorders.

Regulations Regulations are issued by federal government departments and agencies to carry out the intent of legislation enacted by Congress and carried out by administrative agencies. The rules issued by these agencies are called "regulations" and are designed to guide the activity of those regulated by an agency and also the activity of the agency's employees. Regulations also function to ensure uniform application of the law.

Reliability A consistent measurement of data. It is a state where the measurement, test, or experience produces the same results on repeated trials.

REM latency The time from sleep onset to the first epoch of REM sleep.

REM sleep behavior disorder Characterized by a paradoxical increase in muscle tone and frequent limb movements during REM sleep, elaborate, purposeful movements, vocalizations, and occasionally violent behaviors such as punching, kicking, and/or leaping out of bed. This motor activity is associated with dream recall as patients seem to be acting out their dreams.

Renal disease A condition in which the kidneys fail to adequately filter toxins and waste products from the blood. Also referred to as kidney disease. Sleep disturbances reported by those on dialysis for end-stage renal disease include sleep apnea, restless legs syndrome, and periodic limb movement disorder.

Residual AHI (apnea–hypopnea index) Apneas and hypopneas that persist despite treatment.

Residual volume The total gas still in the lung at the end of a maximal exhalation.

Respicardia remedē system An implantable device to treat selective patients with adaptive servo ventilation–intolerant or ineligible central sleep apnea. The device stimulates a phrenic nerve to produce diaphragmatic contractions, causing inspiration. Phrenic nerve stimulation is also referred to as "diaphragmatic pacing."

Respiration In the human body, it refers to the process of gas exchange between oxygen and carbon dioxide at the cellular level.

Respiratory artifact An unwanted physiologic signal in the electrocardiogram or electroencephalogram recording of a polysomnogram. Begins during the inspiratory phase of respiration and correlates precisely with the RR of the patient.

Respiratory disturbance index The number of apneas, hypopneas, and RERAs (respiratory efforts related arousals) per hour of sleep.

Respiratory rate The number of times a person breathes each minute.

Restless legs syndrome Neurosensorimotor disorder that significantly impacts sleep in the first half of the night as patients often must stretch, move, or walk to provide relief of unpleasant sensations in the legs, resulting in significant disruption to sleep quality.

Restrictive lung disease A disorder characterized by reduced lung volumes, either because of an alteration in the lung parenchyma or due to diseases of the chest wall, pleura, or neuromuscular apparatus.

Restrictive thoracic disorder Restrictive thoracic disorder is defined as any of the group of neuromuscular or thoracic cage disorders that impair pulmonary mechanics, restricting the ability of air movement in and out of the lungs.

Reticular formation The part of the brain that regulates essential functions of the body such as the sleep–wake cycle. Consists of diffuse groups of nerve cells that are embedded within a wealth of nerve fibers, giving it a mesh-like appearance, which runs throughout the inner core of the midbrain, pons, and medulla, and fills the spaces between major nuclei and nerve tracts in the brainstem.

Rheumatologic disorders Chronic debilitating diseases of the muscles, tendons, connective tissue, bones and joints causing stiffness, pain, and limited mobility.

Rhythmic anterior theta activity EEG waveforms ranging 5 to 7 Hz.

Rhythmic movement disorder (RMD) A neurologic disorder involving the large muscle groups, where a patient involuntary rocks or moves the body in a repetitive manner immediately before and during sleep. The movements most often include the upper torso, neck, arms, and head and typically are seen in children. Rhythmic humming or other sounds sometimes accompany the body motions.

Rostral Situated toward the oral or nasal region.

Safe harbor Certain categories of activities that are deemed *not* to violate the Anti-Kickback Statute, provided all required elements of the safe harbor are met.

Schizophrenia A psychotic disorder characterized by the occurrence of delusions, hallucinations, incoherence, catatonic behavior, or inappropriate affect that causes impaired social or work functioning.

Seasonal affective disorder Either bipolar or recurrent major depressive disorder where symptoms usually present during winter and remit during the spring. Symptoms improve when the patient is exposed to daylight or bright light therapy.

Sedative Having a soothing, calming, or tranquilizing effect; reducing or relieving anxiety, stress, irritability, or excitement.

Seizure A sudden abnormal discharge of electrical activity of the brain usually affecting how a person acts or feels for a short time.

Selective serotonin reuptake inhibitor Antidepressants that affect serotonin levels in the brain.

Self-management Patients' active participation in their own treatments and decisions, often with the education and assistance of members of the health care team.

Sensitivity The ratio of input voltage (μV) and output amplitude (mm). $S = V/A$.

Sensorimotor Of, relating to, or involving both sensory and motor activity.

Sentinel event An unanticipated event in a health care setting where serious physical or psychological injury or death occurs unrelated to a patient illness.

Sequelae A pathologic condition resulting from a disease, treatment, or injury.

Serotonin A hormone that transmits signals between nerve cells that contribute to feelings of well-being, good mood, and happiness.

Shared decision making (SDM) A process where health care workers and patients work together to select treatments and make other health-related decisions.

Shift work Work schedules outside the hours of the normal work day during a 24-hour period that may follow a different pattern in consecutive periods of days or weeks.

Shift work sleep disorder (SWSD) Can occur when work schedules conflict with the timing and duration of an individual's normal sleep period.

Side effect An effect, often undesirable, of a medication or treatment other than the intended effect.

Sinus A system that consists of a hollow cavity that extends through the cheek bones, the forehead, behind the nose, and between the eyes. It is lined with soft tissue, and as air passes through on the way to the lungs, the mucus helps humidify and filter the air.

Sinus pause A missed pacing stimulus from the SA node producing a pause, during which the heart is electrically silent.

Sinus tachycardia An ECG rhythm during sleep that reflects a sustained sinus heart rate of greater than 90 bpm for adults.

Sleep State of perceptual disengagement from and unresponsiveness to the environment; period of rest and inactivity; the states of sleep are NREM and REM.

Sleep deprivation An insufficient duration of sleep (quantitative), a fragmented or interrupted sleep period (qualitative), or a combination of both factors.

Sleep diary A self-reported log of wake–sleep pattern over a period, allowing the physician the ability to view the patient's sleep schedule over a period. Also referred to as a sleep log.

Sleep disordered breathing Patterns of abnormal breathing including snoring, RERAs, hypopneas, and apneas.

Sleep disruption Disturbed and fragmented sleep patterns that may result in daytime sleepiness.

Sleep efficiency The portion of the total recording time spent asleep. Usually expressed as a percentage.

Sleep fragmentation The interruption of sleep with frequent, brief arousals characterized by increases in EEG frequency or bursts of alpha activity and occasionally, transient increases in skeletal muscle tone.

Sleep history A detailed history of a patient's sleep disruptions, problems, and other related issues taken by a sleep specialist to evaluate clinical signs and symptoms, determine health consequences, and make appropriate recommendations.

Sleep hygiene The behavioral patterns that are consistent with sleeping well.

Sleep latency The time from lights out to sleep onset (first of any epoch of sleep).

Sleep onset The first epoch of sleep.

Sleep-onset REM period A REM period that occurs during the first 15 minutes of an MSLT nap; two or more SOREMPs on MSLT are highly indicative of narcolepsy.

Sleep paralysis Inability to move or speak, sometimes accompanied by the sensation of inability to breathe for a few seconds or a few minutes that occurs during the transition from wakefulness to sleep or from sleep to wakefulness

Sleep-related breathing disorder (SRBD) A group of chronic conditions where partial or complete cessation of breathing occurs several times during the night. These disorders are characterized by abnormal respiratory patterns or insufficient ventilation, resulting in EDS that interferes with a person's ability to function during the daytime.

Sleep restriction therapy A treatment for insomnia that uses a paradoxical approach where less time is spent in bed in an effort to improve sleep.

Sleep terrors A sudden, abrupt, striking, and frightening arousal from slow-wave sleep associated with profound autonomic activity and behavioral manifestations of intense fear. Episodes usually begin suddenly with the individual sitting upright in bed and emitting a powerful, piercing scream.

During the sleep terror, the individual is unresponsive, and efforts to restrain or console the individual tend to exacerbate autonomic and motor activity.

Sleep walking A NREM parasomnia that follows an abrupt arousal from SWS during the first third to first half of the sleep period. May vary in presentation from simple sitting up in bed to agitated running during sleep.

Snoring To breathe during sleep with a rough hoarse noise at various decibel levels due to vibration of the soft palate.

Soft palate The muscular extension of the hard palate positioned posteriorly that consists of muscle fiber and connected tissue giving it support and mobility. It separates the nasal cavity and nasal portion of the pharynx from the mouth and closes the nasal passages during swallowing.

Somnambulism Ambulation that occurs during sleep; also referred to as sleep walking.

Somniloquy Sleep talking; not generally associated with pathology. Sleep talking can be associated with REM sleep behavior disorder and other sleep disorders such as sleep terrors, confusional arousals, or sleepwalking.

Spirometry A technique for measuring or quantifying one or more pulmonary compartments. This usually involves the patient performing various respiratory maneuvers to assess specific compartments.

Split-night sleep study A sleep study consisting of an initial diagnostic assessment followed by a treatment portion. To determine when to initiate CPAP during an overnight sleep study, the AASM standards recommend initiating CPAP during an overnight sleep study when the AHI is greater than 40 during 2 hours of a diagnostic study or AHI is 20 to 40 per hour based on clinical judgment.

Sporadic Occurring occasionally or in irregular or random instances.

Standard precautions (universal precautions) Practices that are performed to prevent the spread of infection and reduce the risk of transmission of blood borne pathogens; includes hand washing and the use of personal protective equipment (e.g., gloves, mask, goggles).

Stanford Sleepiness Scale A subjective measure of sleepiness rating that uses a 7-point Likert rating scale to assess immediate changes in the patient's level of sleepiness. The rating is from "Not sleepy at all" to "Extremely sleepy." This can be used to assess the patient's readiness to fall asleep before their scheduled bedtime in the sleep laboratory or before an MSLT testing situation.

Stark Law A U.S. federal law that prohibits physician self-referral, specifically a physician referral of a Medicare or Medicaid patient to an entity providing designated health services if the physician (or an immediate family member) has a financial relationship with that entity.

Stimulus control therapy A behavioral treatment that is based upon the premise that time spent in bed worrying about sleep is counterproductive to initiating sleep and creates secondary conditioning of sleeplessness.

Subclinical Not manifesting characteristic clinical symptoms of a disease or condition.

Sundowning Confusional behavior, which is often perceived by care-givers to be worse at night, which interferes with sleep. Sundowning is commonly seen in patients with dementing illnesses.

Suprachiasmatic nucleus Controls the circadian rhythm. These nuclei are located in the anterior hypothalamus.

Supraglottoplasty Surgical division or reconstruction of shortened aryepiglottic folds at the entrance to the larynx; generally performed in children with severe stridor or respiratory obstruction due to laryngomalacia.

Surfactant A lipid-based substance that covers the inner walls of the alveoli. This substance reduces surface tension of the aqueous film coating the inner surface of the alveolus, which stabilizes airway and alveolar size.

Susceptible Easily influenced or affected.

Synchronized Occurring simultaneously or in unison.

Systole The active contracting phase of the heartbeat. Systole is the complement of diastole (the relaxation phase)

T wave The ECG waveform that represents ventricular repolarization.

Tachypnea Increased RR.

Telecommunication Transmission of information using two or more stations equipped with transmitter and receiver devices allowing patient–physician interaction.

Telecommuting A work arrangement in which the employee works outside the office, often working from home or a location close to home such as a coffee shop, library, or other locations.

Telemedicine A bidirectional interaction between patients and health care providers, allowing delivery of remote health care services using telecommunications technologies.

Telemonitoring Remotely monitoring patients who are not in the same location as that of the health care provider.

Thalamus Located just above the brainstem; relays signals between the cerebral cortex and the reticular formation.

Thermistor A sensor that indirectly measures nasal and/or oral airflow by detecting changes in temperature. Thermistors are thermally sensitive variable resistors that produce voltage alterations when connected in a low-current (but constant-current) circuit.

Thermocouple A sensor composed of dissimilar metals that detects nasal and/or oral airflow by measuring differences in temperature.

Tidal volume (Vt or V_T) The volume of a single normal breath. Normal values in an adult are 400 to 600 mL.

Time constant The duration of signal responses set by the low- and high-frequency filters. Rise-time constant is the length of time it takes for a signal to rise to 63% of its maximum amplitude (pertinent to the HFF). Fall-time constant is the length of time it takes a signal (i.e., calibration wave) to decay or return to 37% of its original amplitude (pertinent to the LFF).

Titration Implementation of incremental changes in therapeutic pressure levels to determine optimal patient response.

Examples in polysomnography are technologist-monitored PAP and oxygen titration.

Total lung capacity The amount of gas contained in the lung at the end of a maximal inhalation.

Total recording time The total amount of time recorded between lights out and lights on.

Tracé alternant The tracé alternant pattern is seen at approximately 37- to 38-week conceptional age. This quiet sleep pattern consists of short periods of discontinuous background activity in the theta range between bursts of delta activity. Wake–sleep cycles become even easier to differentiate at this age.

Tracé discontinue The tracé discontinue pattern is a quiet non-REM of discontinuous background activity and periods of very low amplitude activity with infrequent bursts of delta and delta brushes. Eye and body movements disappear, respirations are regular, and the EMG is tonic.

Tracheotomy A surgical procedure to make a permanent or semipermanent opening from the neck into the trachea to produce an airway.

Transcutaneous Through the skin.

Transcutaneous CO_2 CO_2 measurement obtained through the skin.

Transtracheal oxygen catheter A flexible, small tube that passes from the lower neck into the trachea and delivers oxygen directly to the lungs.

Tricyclic antidepressant Medications that work by preventing the reabsorption of noradrenaline and serotonin back into the nerve cells. This prolongs the mood-lightening effect of any released noradrenaline and serotonin and in this way helps to relieve depression.

Ultradian rhythm Cycles that occur at recurrent intervals of less than 24 hours.

Upper airway resistance syndrome A pattern of respiratory events that demonstrate flattening or cupping of the nasal transducer signal followed by an arousal that do not meet criteria for scoring hypopneas, resulting in a low AHI.

Uvulopalatopharyngoplasty Surgical procedure that involves removal of the uvula, tonsils, and tonsillar pillars along with the lower part of soft palate.

V_A/Q Ventilation to perfusion ratio.

Validity A well-founded measurement that corresponds with real-world probability. It helps determine the types of tests to use and maintains that the tests are ethical and cost-effective.

Values The principles by which we decide what is right and wrong and what is good and bad.

Vascular dementia Occurs in patients with a history of stroke and cerebrovascular disease.

Ventilation The process of moving air in and out of the lungs.

Ventricular bigeminy A heart arrhythmia in which an abnormal ventricular heart beat occurs every other concurrent beat.

Ventricular fibrillation A condition in which there is uncoordinated contraction of the cardiac muscle of the ventricles in the heart, making them tremble rather than contract properly.

Ventricular tachycardia A faster than normal rhythm that is associated with the generation of electrical impulses within the ventricles and is characterized by an electrocardiogram having a broad QRS complex.

Ventrolateral preoptic area Located in the anterior hypothalamus; contains sleep-active neurons, inhibits arousal, and plays a role in initiating and maintaining sleep.

Videopolysomnography A digital video recording synchronized with the PSG signals, which time-locks the sleep-related events to the PSG signals.

Vital capacity The volume of gas that can be expelled from the lungs from a position of full inspiration.

Volt A measure of the "pressure" under which electricity flows.

Volume-assured pressure support (VAPS) A noninvasive treatment for sleep apnea that provides a constant tidal volume, the volume of air inspired or expired in a single breath during regular breathing. The machine automatically adjusts the pressure support delivered to maintain an optimal and consistent tidal volume.

Wake State of being watchful or vigilant. Stage W is scored when more than 50% of an epoch has alpha rhythm over the occipital region.

Wake after sleep onset The time that the patient was awake following the first epoch of sleep until the end of the study.

Watt A measure of the amount of work done by a certain amount of current at a certain pressure or voltage.

Wearable sleep tracking device A wearable device that tracks a patient's movement while asleep, typically utilizing an actigraph. Software within the device translates the movement into periods of wake and sleep, to improve sleep habits and sleep quality through sleep training.

Wide complex tachycardia A rhythm lasting for greater than three consecutive beats at a rate greater than 100 per minute with a QRS duration of ≥ 120 ms.

Wireless The ability to transmit and/or receive data without a physical connection to a device.

Z-drugs A group of nonbenzodiazepine drugs with effects similar to benzodiazepines, which are used in the treatment of insomnia.

Zeitgebers Zeitgebers or "time givers" entrain or align the internal clock, which cycles with a period slightly longer than 24 hours; about 24.2 hours in adults and 24.3 hours in adolescents.

Index